Cystic Fibrosis

Cystic Fibrosis

Second edition

Edited by

Margaret E. Hodson MD MSc FRCP Dmed Ed
Professor of Respiratory Medicine, Honorary
Consultant Physician, Royal Brompton Hospital and
Harefield NHS Trust, London, UK

Duncan M. Geddes MA MBBS MD FRCP
Professor of Respiratory Medicine, Consultant
Physician, Royal Brompton Hospital and Harefield NHS
Trust, London, UK

A member of the Hodder Headline Group
LONDON
Co-published in the United States of America by
Oxford University Press Inc., New York

First published in Great Britain in 1995
Second edition published in 2000 by
Arnold, a member of the Hodder Headline Group,
338 Euston Road, London NW1 3BH

http://www.arnoldpublishers.com

Co-published in the United States of America by
Oxford University Press Inc.,
198 Madison Avenue, New York, NY 10016
Oxford is a registered trademark of Oxford University Press

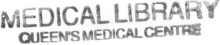

British Library Cataloguing in Publication Data
A catalogue record for this book is available from the British Library

Library of Congress Cataloguing-in-Publication Data
A catalog record for this book is available from the Library of Congress

ISBN 0 340 74208 9

1 2 3 4 5 6 7 8 9 10

Commissioning Editor: Joanna Koster
Project Editor: Catherine Barnes
Production Editor: James Rabson
Production Controller: Iain McWilliams
Project Manager: Alison Nick

Typeset in 10/12 Minion by Phoenix Photosetting, Chatham, Kent
Printed and bound in the United Kingdom by
The Bath Press, Bath

What do you think about this book? Or any other Arnold title?
Please send your comments to feedback.arnold@hodder.co.uk

Contents

Contributors   vii

1   Epidemiology   1
a   Clinical epidemiology of cystic fibrosis   2
S. Walters

b   The epidemiology of cystic fibrosis   13
P. A. Lewis

2   Basic molecular genetics   27
G. Santis

3   Phenotype–genotype relationships   49
G. R. Cutting

4   Applied cell biology   61
E. W. F. W. Alton and S. N. Smith

5   Microbiology of cystic fibrosis   83
N. Høiby and B. Frederiksen

6   Immunology of cystic fibrosis   109
G. Döring, G. Bellon and R. Knight

7   The pathology of cystic fibrosis   141
M. N. Sheppard and A. G. Nicholson

8   Cardiopulmonary physiology   157
A. Bush

9   Diagnostic methods   177
a   Diagnosis   178
B. J. Rosenstein

b   Screening   189
D. J. H. Brock

10   Respiratory system   203
a   Pediatrics   204
S. G. Marshall, M. Rosenfeld and B. W. Ramsey

b   Adults   218
M. E. Hodson

11   Growth, development and nutrition   243
J. M. Littlewood and S. P. Wolfe

12   **Gastrointestinal and pancreatic disease in cystic fibrosis**   **261**
     A. G. F. Davidson

13   **Liver and biliary disease in cystic fibrosis**   **289**
     D. Westaby

14   **Reproductive and sexual health**   **301**
     S. M. Sawyer

15   **Other organ systems**   **313**
     a Other organ systems   314
     C. Koch and S. Lanng

     b Osteoporosis   329
     S. L. Elkin

16   **Psychological aspects of cystic fibrosis**   **339**
     B. Lask

17   **Nontransplant Surgery**   **349**
     D. M. Griffiths

18   **Lung transplantation**   **361**
     B. P. Madden

19   **Paramedical issues**   **375**
     a Physiotherapy   376
     J. A. Pryor and B. A. Webber

     b Dietary treatment of cystic fibrosis   384
     S. Poole, A. McAlweenie and F. Ashworth

     c Nursing   396
     F. Duncan-Skingle and F. Foster

     d Cystic fibrosis home care   406
     F. Duncan-Skingle and E. Bramwell

     e Social work   413
     N. Cloutman

     f Occupational therapy   419
     V. Otley Groom

20   **Exercise and training for adults with cystic fibrosis**   **433**
     A. K. Webb and M. E. Dodd

21   **Future prospects**   **449**
     M. Stern and D. M. Geddes

     Index   **461**

Contributors

E. W. F. W. Alton MA MD FRCP
Professor of Gene Therapy and Respiratory Medicine,
Department of Gene Therapy, National Heart and Lung
Institute, Emmanuel Kaye Building, Manresa Road, London
SW3 6LR, UK

F. Ashworth BSc(Hons) SRD
Chief Dietitian, Department of Nutrition and Dietetics, Royal
Brompton Hospital and Harefield NHS Trust, Sydney Street,
London SW3 6NP, UK

G. Bellon MD
Professor, Centre Hospitalier Lyon Sud, Service de Pédiatrie,
F-69310 Pierre Benite, France

E. C. Bramwell RGN
Department of Cystic Fibrosis, Royal Brompton Hospital and
Harefield NHS Trust, Sydney Street, London SW3 6NP, UK

D. J. H. Brock PhD FRCPE FRCPath FRSE
Formerly Professor of Human Genetics, Human Genetics
Unit, Molecular Medicine Centre, University of Edinburgh,
Western General Hospital, Edinburgh EG4 2XU, UK

A. Bush MD FRCP FRCPCH
Reader in Paediatric Respirology, Royal Brompton Hospital
and Harefield NHS Trust, Sydney Street, London
SW3 6NP, UK

N. Cloutman CQSW
Social Worker, Department of Social Work, Royal Brompton
Hospital and Harefield NHS Trust, Sydney Street, London
SW3 6NP, UK

G. R. Cutting MD
Center for Medical Genetics, CMSC 9-123, Johns Hopkins
University School of Medicine, 600 North Wolfe Street,
Baltimore, Maryland 21287-3914, USA

A. G. F. Davidson BSc MD FRCPC
Professor, Department of Pediatrics, Division of Biochemical
Diseases, University of British Columbia and British
Columbia's Children's Hospital, 4480 Oak Street, Room 2066,
Vancouver BC V6H 3V4, Canada

M. Dodd MCSP
Specialist Physiotherapy Clinician, Bradbury Cystic Fibrosis
Unit, North West Lung Centre, Wythenshawe Hospital,
Southmoor Road, South Manchester M23 9LT, UK

G. Döring PhD Dr rer nat.
Professor, Department of General and Environmental
Hygiene, Hygiene-Institute, University of Tübingen,
Wilhelmstraße 31, D-72074 Tübingen, Germany

F. Duncan-Skingle RGN NDNCert HVCert
Cystic Fibrosis Unit, Royal Brompton Hospital and Harefield
NHS Trust, Sydney Street, London SW3 6NP, UK

S. L. Elkin MCSP MBBS MRCP
Research Fellow, Department of Cystic Fibrosis, Royal
Brompton Hospital and Harefield NHS Trust, Sydney Street,
London SW3 6NP, UK

F. Foster RGN RSCN
Formerly Royal Brompton Hospital and Harefield NHS Trust,
Sydney Street, London SW3 6NP, UK

B. Frederiksen MD PhD
Danish Cystic Fibrosis Center, Pediatric Department G 5003,
Rigshospitalet, Copenhagen, Denmark

D. M. Geddes MA MBBS MD FRCP
Professor of Respiratory Medicine, Consultant Physician,
Royal Brompton Hospital and Harefield NHS Trust, Sydney
Street, London SW3 6NP, UK

D. M. Griffiths MCh FRCS
Consultant Neonatal and Paediatric Surgeon, Wessex
Regional Centre for Paediatric Surgery, Southampton General
Hospital, East Wing, Tremona Road, Southampton SO16 6YD,
UK

V. Otley Groom Dip COT SROT
Head of Occupational Therapy, Department of Occupational
Therapy, Royal Brompton Hospital and Harefield NHS Trust,
Sydney Street, London SW3 6NP, UK

M. E. Hodson MD MSc FRCP Dmed Ed
Professor of Respiratory Medicine, Royal Brompton Hospital and Harefield NHS Trust, Sydney Street, London SW3 6NP, UK

N. Høiby MD Dr Med Sci
Professor and Chairman, Department of Clinical Microbiology, Rigshospitalet, University of Copenhagen, Juliane Maries Vej 22 DK-2100, Copenhagen, Denmark

R. Knight PhD MBBS
Imperial College, National Heart and Lung Institute, Emmanuel Kaye Building, Manresa Road, London SW3 6LR, UK

C. Koch MD Dr Med Sci
Professor, Department of Pediatrics and Danish CF Center, Rigshospitalet, 5003, GGK, Blegdamsvej 9, DK-2100 Copenhagen Ø, Denmark

S. Lanng Dr Med Sci
Department of Pediatrics and Danish CF Center, Rigshospitalet, 5003, GGK, Blegdamsvej 9, DK-2100 Copenhagen Ø, Denmark

B. Lask FRCPsych FRCPCH MPhil MBBS
Consultant Psychiatrist, Department of Psychiatry, St. George's Hospital Medical School, London SW17 0RE, UK

P. A. Lewis PhD Ceng
Senior Lecturer, Public Health Group, School of Postgraduate Medicine, University of Bath, Bath BA2 7AY, UK

J. M. Littlewood OBE MD FRCP FRCPE FRCPCH OCH
Regional Paediatric Cystic Fibrosis Unit, St. James University Hospital, Leeds LS9 7TF, UK

A. McAlweenie BSc SRD
Formerly Dietetics Department, Royal Brompton Hospital and Harefield NHS Trust, Sydney Street, London SW3 6NP, UK

B. P. Madden MD MSc FRCPI FRCP
Consultant Cardiothoracic and Transplant Physician, Cardiothoracic Unit, St. George's Hospital, Blackshaw Road, London SW17 0QT, UK

S. G. Marshall MD
Associate Professor, Department of Pediatrics, Children's Hospital and Regional Medical Center 4800 Sand Point Way N.E., P.O. Box 5371, Seattle WA 98105-0371, USA

A. G. Nicholson MD MRCPath
Consultant in Histopathology, Department of Pathology, Royal Brompton Hospital and Harefield NHS Trust, Sydney Street, London SW3 6NP, UK

S. Poole BSc SRD
Formerly Dietetics Department, Royal Brompton Hospital and Harefield NHS Trust, Sydney Street, London SW3 6NP, UK

J. A. Pryor MSc MBA FNZSP MCSP
Research Fellow Physiotherapy, Department of Cystic Fibrosis, Royal Brompton Hospital and Harefield NHS Trust, Sydney Street, London SW3 6NP, UK

B. W. Ramsey MD
Professor, Department of Pediatrics, Director, Therapeutic Development Network, Children's Hospital and Regional Medical Center, 4800 Sand Point Way N.E., P.O. Box 5371, Seattle WA 98105-0371, USA

M. Rosenfeld MD MPH
Assistant Professor, Department of Pediatrics, Children's Hospital and Regional Medical Center, 4800 Sand Point Way N.E., Seattle WA 98105-0371, USA

B. J. Rosenstein MD
Professor of Pediatrics, Johns Hopkins University, Director, Cystic Fibrosis Center, Johns Hopkins Hospital, 315 Park, Baltimore, Maryland 21287-2533, USA

G. Santis MD FRCP
Senior Lecturer in Respiratory Medicine, Department of Respiratory Medicine and Allergy, Thomas Guy House, Guy's Hospital, St. Thomas' Street, London SE1 9RT, UK

S. M. Sawyer MBBS MD FRACP
Associate Professor, Department of Respiratory Medicine and Center for Adolescent Health, Royal Children's Hospital, Parkville 3052, Victoria, Australia

M. N. Sheppard MD FRCPath
Consultant Histopathologist and Senior Lecturer, Department of Pathology, Royal Brompton Hospital and Harefield NHS Trust, Sydney Street, London SW3 6NP, UK

S. N. Smith CEd BA PhD
Department of Gene Therapy, National Heart and Lung Institute, Emmanuel Kaye Building, Manresa Road, London SW3 6LR, UK

M. Stern MBChB PhD MRCP
Senior Lecturer, Department of Gene Therapy, National Heart and Lung Institute, Emmanuel Kaye Building, Manresa Road, London SW3 6LR, UK

S. Walters BSc MB FRCP FFPHM
Senior Lecturer, Department of Public Health and Epidemiology, University of Birmingham Medical School, Edgbaston, Birmingham B15 2TT, UK

A. K. Webb FRCP
Consultant Physician, Clinical Director of Bradbury Cystic Fibrosis Unit, North West Lung Centre, Wythenshawe Hospital, Southmoor Road, South Manchester M23 9LT, UK

B. A. Webber FCSP DSc(Hons)
Formerly Physiotherapy Department, Royal Brompton Hospital, Sydney Street, London SW3 6NP, UK

D. Westaby MA FRCP
Consultant Physician and Gastroenterologist, Chelsea and
Westminster Hospital, 369 Fulham Road, London SW10 9NH,
UK

S. P. Wolfe BSc SRD
Regional Paediatric Cystic Fibrosis Unit, St. James University
Hospital, Leeds LS9 7TF, UK

Epidemiology

1a Clinical epidemiology of cystic fibrosis

    S. Walters   2

Introduction   2

Diagnosis   2

Clinical features   4

Social and demographic features in adults   7

Prognosis   9

Provision of medical care   11

Treatment of cystic fibrosis   12

1b The epidemiology of cystic fibrosis

    P. A. Lewis   13

Introduction   13

Incidence of the cystic fibrosis phenotype (CFP)   15

Life-span analyses for populations with
CF phenotypes   17

Assessing the effectiveness of healthcare using
international differences in life span   20

The epidemiology of the *CFTR* gene   21

Conclusion   22

References   22

Clinical epidemiology of cystic fibrosis

S. WALTERS

INTRODUCTION

Epidemiology may be defined as the study of the distribution and determinants of disease frequency in human populations[1]. Clinical epidemiology applies epidemiological principles to a clinical population, i.e. to a population already known to have a particular disease. An analogous definition might therefore be that clinical epidemiology is the study of the distribution of disease manifestations and determinants of disease outcome in a clinical population.

Clinical epidemiology is the basic science underpinning the practice of evidence-based medicine. Therefore a knowledge of the clinical epidemiology of cystic fibrosis, and in particular a knowledge of risk factors for development of certain disease manifestations, and factors influencing overall prognosis, will be of value to all clinicians involved in the care of cystic fibrosis patients.

This chapter examines and describes the clinical epidemiology of cystic fibrosis. It includes a description of clinical features and prognostic indicators, social and demographic features of the population, and finally some information about the application of clinical epidemiology to evidence-based practice in cystic fibrosis care. This chapter could not have been written without the high-quality information that has been collected over the years by both the United States and Canadian patient data registries.

DIAGNOSIS

Although genotype analysis is readily available, rare mutations are so many and the phenotype so variable that diagnosis is usually made either on clinical grounds or on the basis of a screening program. In 1996, 6.2 per cent of newly diagnosed patients in the USA were diagnosed by neonatal screening[2]. Regardless of whether the case presents clinically or through screening, diagnosis is confirmed by the sweat test; 98 per cent of patients in the USA had sweat sodium or chloride greater than 61 mEq/L, with a mean sweat chloride of 101.7 mEq/L (standard deviation 18.91 mEq/L). Of the 2 per cent who were sweat-test negative, 75 per cent were diagnosed on the basis of two known mutations, 1 per cent on transepithelial potential difference, and 24 per cent on clinical manifestation[2].

Age at diagnosis

In the USA, 70 per cent of all cystic fibrosis (CF) patients were diagnosed before their first birthday[2], and 90 per cent before their eighth birthday. The proportion diagnosed before 1 year was similar, although slightly lower, in series from New Zealand (61 per cent)[3] and Ireland (55 per cent)[4]. However, late diagnosis continues to be made, with occasional cases being diagnosed as late as the seventh decade of life (Fig. 1.1).

Late diagnosis (after 16 years of age) is associated with a milder clinical syndrome than seen in patients diagnosed as children[5]. This includes better lung function and nutritional status, and a lower prevalence of colonization by *Pseudomonas aeruginosa*. Late-diagnosed patients usually represent the mild end of the clinical spectrum presented by cystic fibrosis. This has very important implications when considering studies looking at the long-term benefits of neonatal screening for cystic fibrosis.

Neonatal screening

Intuitively, it seems reasonable to assume that early diagnosis of patients with cystic fibrosis before the onset of chronic bacterial colonization of the respiratory tract, and before the onset of clinical malnutrition, would lead to an improved clinical outcome. However, there is little good evidence that long-term outcome is improved as a result of neonatal screening.

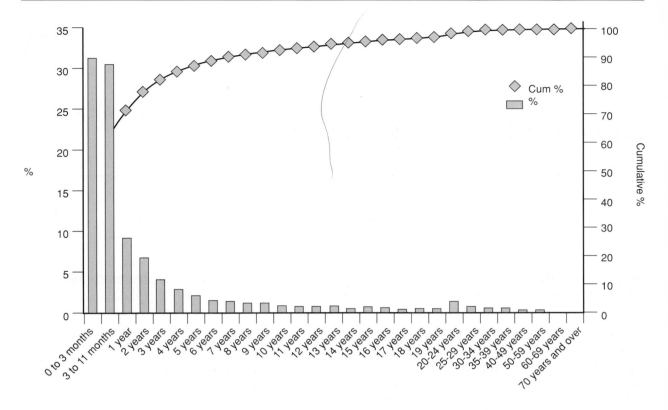

Fig. 1.1 *Age at diagnosis of cystic fibrosis. (Data from US CF Foundation Patient Data Registry, 1996.)*

The reasons for this include the lack of suitable randomized studies, the majority employing either pseudo-randomization, or using historical or geographic controls, or no controls at all. In those studies where randomization has been employed, there is a fundamental difficulty in interpretation of results because of the problem that those diagnosed late in life have milder disease. This means that the screened cohort will include the majority of patients, including those with very mild disease, whereas the control cohort will include, at least initially, only those with more severe disease. Therefore reported differences in clinical outcome might be explained by this bias. Finally, studies with randomized design have been let down by failure to analyze by intention-to-screen (i.e. analyze the groups as originally randomized); this usually means including those missed by screening (false negatives) in the group diagnosed clinically. This would tend to enhance clinical differences between the groups.

In a pseudo-randomized study in the UK, which was not analyzed by intention-to-screen, there were few reported clinical benefits, the main one being reduced time in hospital in the screened cohort in the first year of life. However, this could be explained by the differential rates of inclusion of mild cases in the screened and unscreened cohorts under the age of 1 year[6]. Longer-term results analyzed by intention-to-screen are required. The study with the most robust design and analysis comes from Wisconsin, USA. This study has recently reported results of 10-year follow-up, demonstrating small, but significant differences in favor of the screened cohort for nutritional parameters, especially in those with pancreatic insufficiency and homozygous for ΔF_{508}[7].

It should be remembered that there are other benefits from running a screening program among neonates that have not been considered in published reports. This includes the ability to offer prenatal diagnosis to parents of infants detected by screening, the reduction of stress among parents seeking a diagnosis for their sick child, rapid determination of population prevalence in developing countries or areas where this is unknown, and the ability to research early development of respiratory and nutritional abnormalities in CF patients before clinical symptoms develop.

Clinical presentation

The most common clinical presentation of CF remains acute or persistent respiratory symptoms, appearing in 51 per cent of all cases diagnosed in the USA[2]. Other common clinical features on presentation in this report were failure to thrive or malnutrition (43 per cent),

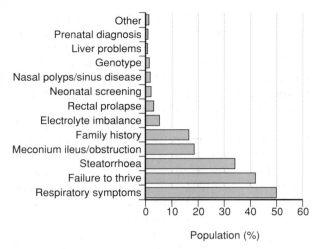

Fig. 1.2 *Clinical features suggesting the diagnosis of CF. These modes of clinical presentation are not mutually exclusive, and therefore the total is greater than 100 per cent. (Data from the CF Foundation US Clinical Patient Database, 1996.)*

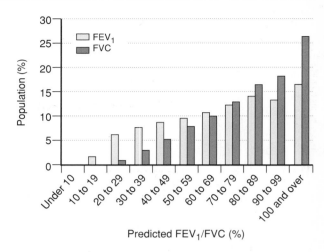

Fig. 1.3 *Lung function (per cent predicted) in the US CF clinical population. (Data from US Patient Data Registry, 1996.)*

steatorrhea or abnormal stools (35 per cent), and meconium ileus or intestinal obstruction (19.1 per cent).

Clinical presentations of US patients are summarized in Fig. 1.2. It is interesting to note that although overall only 3.5 per cent were diagnosed by screening (prenatal or neonatal), in 1996, this method of presentation comprised 9.1 per cent of newly diagnosed patients[2]. Genotype as a means of presentation was 1.5 per cent overall, but 5.8 per cent of newly diagnosed patients in 1996. This suggests that the number of patients with CF diagnosed before the onset of any clinical symptoms is increasing.

Congenital bilateral absence of the vas deferens (CBAVD) is a clinical syndrome recently described in which there is a relatively high prevalence of CFTR (CF transmembrane conductance regulator) mutations, with 14.5 per cent being homozygous for CFTR mutations, 48.1 per cent being heterozygous, and 37.4 per cent having no CFTR abnormalities[8]. A high proportion of patients with CBAVD homozygous for CFTR mutations have abnormal sweat chloride[9], and a few have some clinical symptoms suggestive of CF. The suggestion has been made that CBAVD patients who are homozygous for CFTR mutations represent the mildest form of CF.

CLINICAL FEATURES

Lung function

The US Patient Data Registry[2] recorded that, in 1996, the mean forced expired volume (FEV_1) was 72.3 per cent predicted (SD 27.5 per cent) and the mean FVC was 84.5

per cent predicted (SD 23.3 per cent)[2]. The distribution of per cent predicted FEV_1 and FVC percentiles in the US CF clinical population is summarized in Fig. 1.3. FEV_1 and FVC by age are shown in Fig. 1.4.

These diagrams are difficult to interpret because of age–cohort effects. They represent all CF patients in the US Patient Data Registry, and therefore consist of several different birth cohorts, not all of which were exposed to current treatment practices throughout their life. In addition, there is a survivor effect, meaning that in each cohort, lung function can only be measured in those remaining alive. As age increases, the proportion of each birth cohort that remains as survivors decreases, until those left become the extreme survivors of that birth cohort, and therefore very atypical of the original group.

Difficulties with cohort and survivor effects mean that it is not possible to predict decline in lung function among a cohort of existing patients from these current lung-function measurements. However, Fig. 1.4 demonstrates the pattern that might be expected in a population of patients which develop a progressive predominantly obstructive respiratory function defect, followed by censoring of patients with a severe defect from the population either by death or transplantation. Increase in mean lung-function parameters due to censoring are offset by decline among the remaining members of the cohort. Various cohort studies of CF patients have demonstrated a lung-function decline in individual adult patients of approximately 3–5 per cent predicted per annum in FEV_1.

Figure 1.3 demonstrates that the majority of patients at any point in time have good lung function, with only a minority at any single point in time suffering from severe respiratory function defects. Table 1.1 shows that the majority of those with moderate to severe lung disease are in the older age groups.

Lung function is related to other aspects of clinical

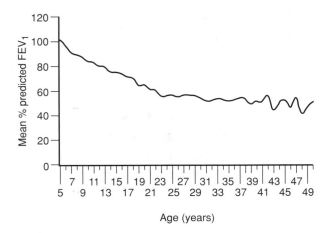

Fig. 1.4 *Mean per cent predicted FEV, by age in the US CF clinical population. (Data from the US Patient Data Registry, 1996.)*

status in CF (Table 1.2). However, it is difficult to determine from cross-sectional data whether these complications of CF arose because of declining lung function or were the cause of it.

Respiratory infection

The organism most frequently reported in sputum culture from cystic fibrosis patients is *Pseudomonas aeruginosa*. This is true in most reported case series. In the US, 60 per cent of patients had *P. aeruginosa* in their sputum or other respiratory cultures[2]. However, the prevalence of

P. aeruginosa infection varies between countries, and between treatment centers within countries. In Canada, for example, the isolation frequency for *P. aeruginosa* was 48 per cent in 1995, but varied between treatment centers from 25 per cent to 52 per cent[11]. The reported prevalence in New Zealand was 44 per cent[3], and in adults in France was 62 per cent[12] and in Ireland, 69 per cent[4].

Likewise, although the overall prevalence of *Burkholderia cepacia* infection was only slightly higher in Canada than in the US (9.2 per cent in Canada, 3.6 per cent in the US), the prevalence varied from 2 per cent to 21 per cent in different treatment centers within Canada. This is likely to represent both differences in the distribution of risk factors for colonization for these organisms, and differences in policies to limit cross-infection operating in the different treatment centers. The frequency of all organisms isolated in US patients in 1996 is shown in Fig. 1.5.

Of the factors that affect infection rates with different microorganisms, one of the most important is age. The prevalence of culture-positivity for *Pseudomonas aeruginosa*, *Burkholderia cepacia*, *Aspergillus* spp. and mycobacteria increase with age. The prevalence of culture-positivity for *Haemophilus influenzae* falls with age. These patterns for the most frequently isolated organisms are shown in Fig. 1.6.

Other suggested risk factors for colonization with *Pseudomonas aeruginosa* include genotype (certain genotypes are associated with lower colonization rates), sex[13] (females may be colonized younger than males), pancreatic insufficient phenotype, and nosocomial

Table 1.1 *Severity of lung function defect by age (data from US Patient Data Registry, 1996[2])*

Severity of FEV, defect	Children		Adults	
	Number	%	Number	%
Normal (> 90% predicted)	3586	41.4	760	12.6
Mild (70–89% predicted)	2762	31.5	1152	19.1
Moderate (40–69% predicted)	1858	21.4	2324	38.5
Severe (<40% predicted)	490	5.7	1805	29.9

Table 1.2 *Association between lung function, microbial colonization, and nutritional status in the US CF clinical population, 1996 (data from US Patient Data Registry, 1996[2])*

FEV, % predicted	Number	%	% cultured *Pseudomonas aeruginosa*	% cultured *Burkholderia cepacia*	% under 5th centile for weight
Normal (90% or more)	4346	32	44.9	1.3	9.5
Mild (70–89%)	3884	24	64.1	3.0	14.4
Moderate (40–69%)	4182	28	80.9	5.6	31.3
Severe (under 40%)	2295	16	87.3	8.4	61.2
Total	14707	100	67.2	4.2	25.1

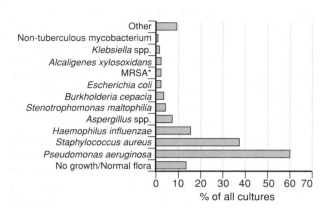

Fig. 1.5 *Organisms cultured from respiratory tract of CF patients in the USA, 1996. Percentage of all cultures. MRSA, methicillin-resistant* Staphylococcus aureus. *(Data from US Patient Data Registry, 1996.)*

transmission within treatment centers where precautions were not taken to prevent cross-colonization[14]. *Pseudomonas aeruginosa* can appear in the respiratory tract of young infants with CF[15] prior to the onset of clinical respiratory disease, suggesting that this may be a primary infection, and prior lung damage by other microorganisms is not necessary for infection to be established.

Growth and nutritional status

The distribution of height and weight percentiles in the US CF clinical population is bimodal[2], with 20 per cent being below the fifth centile for height and 25 per cent below the fifth centile for weight, with the remainder of the patients showing a normal distribution with a mode at centiles 25–49 (Fig. 1.7). In children, there is a close match between distributions for height and weight centiles, but among adults there is a mismatch. Height tends towards normal (mean centile 37.5), but weight tends to be lower than in children (mean centile 23.1).

Again, the explanation of this distribution from cross-sectional data is difficult. Possible explanations include a cohort effect whereby adults did not benefit from current nutritional management when they were children, and hence now suffer from residual effects of malnutrition while young. A survivor effect may also be operating, particularly in respect of the higher height centile, where the smaller and lighter children did not reach adult life, and the selective good prognosis of pancreatic sufficiency. Another cohort effect may be operating, namely the late maturation and growth of children with CF, meaning that full adult height is reached well after the age of 17 years. Finally, low weight among the adult group may be due to deteriorating clinical condition with age.

Complications

In addition to the classical clinical manifestations of CF – respiratory infection and malabsorption – there may be a number of clinical complications affecting individuals with CF that are related to CF, but appear in only a minority of patients.

The most frequent complication recorded in the US CF clinical population is diabetes mellitus requiring treatment with insulin, which appeared in 6 per cent of their patients[2]. Development of complications tends to increase with age (Fig. 1.8), with the exception of DIOS (distal intestinal obstruction syndrome), the annual prevalence of which remains constant with age.

There have been varying reports of annual incidence and overall prevalence of diabetes mellitus in different CF clinical populations. This variation may in part be

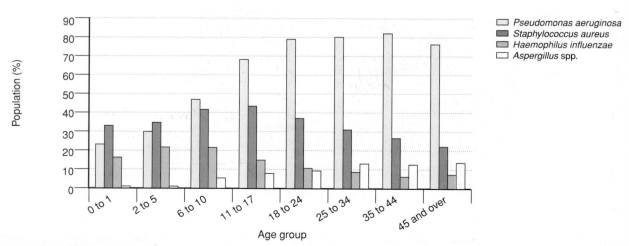

Fig. 1.6 *Microbial colonization rates by age in US CF patients, 1996. (Data from the US Patient Data Registry, 1996.)*

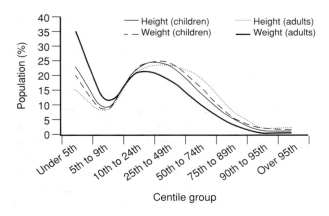

Fig. 1.7 *Distribution of height and weight centiles, US CF clinical population, 1996. (Data from US Patient Data Registry, 1996).*

due to different ages of the clinical populations, in part to differences in the diagnostic tests and criteria applied to define diabetes in the CF population, and in part due to true differences in prevalence. The Danish cohort studies have been the most methodologically precise. In 1994, a prevalence of diabetes mellitus of 14.7 per cent was reported in the Danish CF population[16]. Age was the only reported risk factor for development of diabetes; underlying severity of cystic fibrosis was not a risk factor. This study also reported that CF patients develop

microvascular complications of diabetes at a similar rate to diabetics without CF. In a later report, the same authors recorded a mean age of diagnosis of diabetes at 21 years, and reported that impaired glucose tolerance (IGT) on a previous oral glucose tolerance test conferred a relative risk of 5.6 for development of diabetes, although some patients with IGT on one or more occasion did not go on to develop diabetes[17].

Of recent interest is the question as to whether adults with CF are more susceptible to cancer. A large cohort study from the US concluded that the risk of cancer among patients with CF overall was the same as that for the general population (relative risk (RR) 0.8; 95% confidence interval (CI) 0.6–1.1). However, there was an increased risk of gastrointestinal cancer in both the US and European cohorts enrolled in the study, with a relative risk of 6.5 (3.5–11.1) and 6.4 (2.9–14.0), respectively[18].

SOCIAL AND DEMOGRAPHIC FEATURES IN ADULTS

Reported measurements of clinical outcome in CF have not been very sophisticated in reports of either clinical trials or clinical case series. Measures tend to be confined to either survival, or measurements of lung function, nutritional status, clinical or X-ray

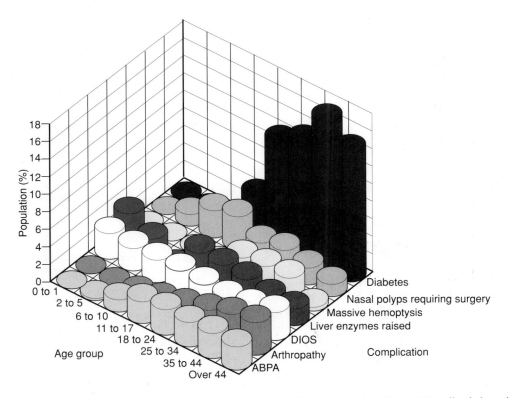

Fig. 1.8 *Prevalence of recorded complications of CF by age in the US CF clinical population, 1996. ABPA, allergic bronchopulmonary aspergillosis. (Data from US Patient Data Registry, 1996.)*

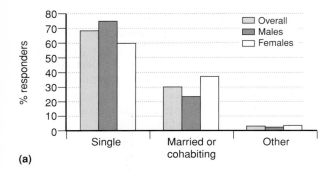

(a)

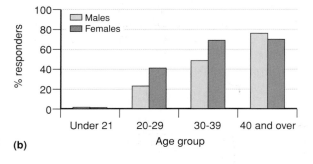

(b)

Fig. 1.9 *Marital status of men and women with CF:* **(a)** *overall marital status;* **(b)** *proportion married or cohabiting by age and sex. (Data from ACFA (UK) Survey, 1994.)*

scores, or biochemical parameters. Although these are important indicators of clinical status, they do not necessarily reflect how the patient feels and, more importantly, whether their lifestyle matches that of their peers without CF.

Demographic features

In the US CF patient population in 1996, 33 per cent of adult patients were married or cohabiting, with a further 5.2 per cent separated, widowed, or divorced[2]. Very similar figures were obtained from the 1994 Association of CF Adults (ACFA) Survey in the UK[19], where 30 per cent were married or cohabiting, and from studies reported elsewhere[20].

The ACFA survey demonstrated, however, that male patients with CF were significantly more likely to remain living with their parents than females, although as age increased, the differences between men and women decreased (Fig. 1.9). This suggested that although it may be harder for young men with CF to achieve independence, this is delayed rather than prevented. A study from The Netherlands suggested that patients with CF were no more likely to be dependent on their parents than other young people[21].

Education

Despite the fact that CF patients from time to time miss periods of education due to episodes of illness, educational attainments of adults with CF are similar to those of the general population. In the US, 30 per cent of adult patients had achieved a college degree or higher. In the ACFA survey, the educational attainments of adults with CF were impressive, and were at least comparable to those of the general population of the same age. Eighty-two per cent achieved GCSE or equivalent qualifications, which are basic school-leaving qualifications taken at age 16 in the UK; 25 per cent achieved A-level or equivalent, a higher school-leaving qualification required for university entrance, taken at age 18 in the UK; and 17 per cent achieved a university or college degree[19].

Any academic qualification is associated with an increased likelihood of employment, even after adjustment for disease severity (Fig. 1.10).

A study in The Netherlands suggested that educational attainments among adults with CF were higher than among the general population, with the CF population concentrating on traditional education, whereas the general population preferred vocational training[21].

Employment

A high proportion of adult patients are able to work, either full- or part-time. In the UK, adults achieved 80 per cent of the employment rate of the general population of the same age and sex[22]. In both the US and the UK, 50 per cent of adults are in paid employment, with a further 24–25 per cent students[2,19]. Half of those not currently employed in the UK were unable to work due to ill health[19] (Fig. 1.11).

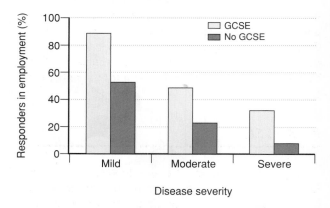

Fig. 1.10 *Association between educational attainments and employment status after adjustment for disease severity in adults with cystic fibrosis. GCSEs (General Certificates of Education) are qualifications taken just prior to leaving school at age 15–16 in the United Kingdom, and signify attainment at a basic level of secondary education, but do not qualify the student for university entrance. (Data from ACFA (UK) Survey, 1994.)*

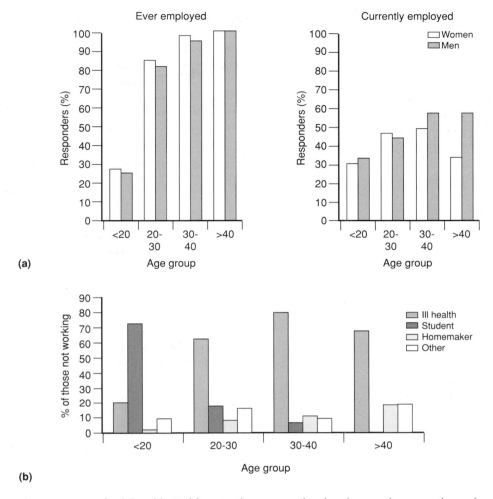

Fig. 1.11 *Employment status of adults with CF:* (**a**) *proportion ever employed and proportion currently employed, by age group;* (**b**) *reasons given for not working, by age. (Data from ACFA(UK) Survey, 1994.)*

Of particular interest is the fact that although survival has been steadily increasing, the proportion of adults able to work has remained similar to those reported a decade ago[20], suggesting that continued survival increases have not been at the expense of quality of life. The majority of patients remain well for the majority of their lives.

PROGNOSIS

There have been many attempts to derive prognostic indicators for CF. This has been made more important by the advent of transplantation as a treatment for end-stage lung disease. It is therefore useful to have an index that will indicate when survival is expected to be poorer for the untreated patient than for a transplanted patient, and hence when referral for transplantation might be considered.

The problem with the studies reported in the literature is that they all start with different baseline popula-

tions: for example, some consider children, others adults, and others all age groups. They also use different survival times as an indicator, ranging from 2 to 10 years and over. They use different analytic methods which may produce different results in the same patient population. They also include slightly different subsets of clinical information in their multivariate models.

Genotype

Initial studies concentrated on the issue as to whether homozygosity for the ΔF_{508} mutation conferred a particularly severe phenotype. However, the majority of these studies took place before a good classification of effects of different mutations on the function of CFTR was produced. The majority of studies employing multivariate modeling that included genotype markers have concluded that homozygosity for ΔF_{508} is not an adverse prognostic indicator. Some genotypes are associated with a mild phenotype, including the ΔF_{508}/R117H compound heterozygote. However, the consensus is that prognosis cannot usually be determined by genotype analysis[23].

Pancreatic-sufficient phenotype

A pancreatic-sufficient phenotype is generally associated with milder clinical manifestations of cystic fibrosis. However, its association with survival is not as clear as for other risk factors, such as pulmonary function. After accounting for major prognostic factors, pancreatic-sufficient phenotype has only been a significant positive prognostic indicator in a few studies[24,25].

Age

As for phenotype, once major prognostic factors are accounted for, age appears not to be a major determinant of survival, appearing as a determinant of survival in only one study[26].

Sex

It is recognized in most countries that the average life expectancy is shorter for females than for males with cystic fibrosis. However, it is not completely clear whether this is a gender-specific phenomenon *per se*, or whether it is related to increased prevalence of other poor prognostic indicators in women, such as poor lung function and nutritional status. In the first year of life, survival is greater for girls, but after that, greater for boys, giving an overall survival advantage for males.

A study in a large US clinical cohort demonstrated that after adjustment for a number of other prognostic factors, such as nutritional status, pulmonary function, pancreatic-sufficient phenotype, age at diagnosis, mode of presentation, race and airway microbiology, female sex conferred an additional risk of death before the age of 20 years (RR 1.6; 95% CI 1.4–1.8), but after the age of 20 years there was no significant difference[24].

In some other studies, female sex emerged as an adverse prognostic indicator[27], but in other careful studies aimed at developing prognostic indices for CF, female sex was not an adverse prognostic indicator after other important markers for survival were accounted for[28].

Possible explanations for the observation of shorter survival in females include poorer nutrition in females, which was felt to account for the reduced survival seen in Canadian females[29], and an earlier age at first colonization with *Pseudomonas aeruginosa*[13].

Pulmonary function

Almost every study employing multivariate modeling

techniques identifies pulmonary function as a major determinant of survival. This includes several of the studies mentioned above[24,26,28,29]. In some studies, FEV_1 was the only lung-function marker associated with survival, in others, FVC[28] or a marker of gas trapping (RV/TLC) were independently associated with survival[30]. In some studies, FEV_1 per cent predicted emerged as the only significant prognostic marker.

Exercise tolerance

A study from the US suggested that exercise tolerance could be a more sensitive prognostic indicator than simple lung-function tests. This study found that peak oxygen uptake (V_{O2peak}) was a better predictor of 8-year survival in patients over 7 years of age than FEV_1[31]. In this study, colonization with *Burkholderia cepacia* was the only other risk factor, age, sex, body mass index, FEV_1 and P_{CO_2} after exercise being unrelated to survival.

However, a more recent UK study in adults found that although univariate analysis identified exercise performance as prognostic markers (including V_{O2peak}, peak work rate, peak minute ventilation (VE) and VE/VO_2 ratio), multivariate analysis revealed only FEV_1 to predict 5-year survival. FEV_1 over 55 per cent predicted gave a 96 per cent 5-year survival, but under 55 per cent predicted, survival was only 46 per cent. In this study, colonization with *Burkholderia cepacia* was not a predictor of survival.

Therefore it remains unclear as to whether exercise testing offers significantly improved prediction of survival when compared to simple pulmonary function tests alone. The populations in the two studies were of different ages, and it may be that exercise testing is more useful in children than in adults.

Bacterial colonization

The majority of studies have considered the role of either *Pseudomonas aeruginosa*, *Burkholderia cepacia* or both in determining survival in cystic fibrosis patients. Most studies employing multivariate modeling techniques have failed to show colonization with either *Pseudomonas aeruginosa* or, more specifically with the mucoid subtype, to be associated with survival, after accounting for other prognostic factors, particularly lung function[25,28,29]. However, mucoid *Pseudomonas aeruginosa* was an adverse prognostic factor in one study, which was also unusual in identifying age as an independent prognostic indicator[26]. In another study confined to infants diagnosed before the age of 2 years, with 10-year follow-up, *Pseudomonas aeruginosa* was associated with poorer survival when *Staphylococcus aureus* had also been isolated before the age of 2 years[32].

The situation with *Burkholderia cepacia* colonization is a little clearer, in that although it appears from some studies to colonize selectively those with poorer lung function and a poorer initial prognosis[33], it is also associated with a poorer prognosis after colonization, even after matching for initial lung function[25,29,31, 34].

Nutritional status

Along with lung function, this appears to be one of the most important prognostic indicators in cystic fibrosis patients. Different studies use different indices of nutrition, but in a majority of studies, poor nutritional status appears to be independently associated with a poor prognosis[24,28,29,30].

Socio-economic indicators

Very few studies have looked at the effect of socio-economic status on survival in cystic fibrosis, despite widespread knowledge that low socio-economic status confers higher mortality rates for a wide variety of other common conditions. In the study by Britton[27], which examined mortality rates by region in the UK, there were only two significant predictors of premature death (death below the median age of survival): female sex (RR 1.47; 1.16–1.87) and manual social class (RR 2.75; 2.16–3.52).

In a recent study from the US, patients who had health insurance, either privately or through Medicaid, had a median survival of 20.5 years, compared with just 6.1 years for those without insurance. Socio-economic status and possession of insurance were both significantly and independently associated with survival in this study[35].

Functional status

There has only been one published study, showing that although functional status appeared to be associated with survival, after adjustment for important clinical prognostic indicators, the association became non-significant[36].

PROVISION OF MEDICAL CARE

Although it seems reasonable to assume that care for patients with cystic fibrosis can best be provided by those specializing in treatment of this condition, it has proved difficult to subject this assumption to formal study and statistical analysis. A randomized controlled trial is not possible, and it is difficult to obtain data about patients who do not attend specialist cystic fibrosis clinics. Patient data registries generally exclude patients who do not attend recognized cystic fibrosis clinics, making construction of cohort survival curves difficult. In addition,

those who attend CF clinics may be a self-selected group with pre-existing good prognosis[27].

Early studies were flawed by using historical controls (i.e. before and after establishment of a CF center)[37], or by relying on comparison of different median survival rates in countries with different methods of organizing healthcare. A study in the UK by the British Paediatric Association demonstrated that those patients attending centers where 40 or more patients were registered had better survival than those attending smaller treatment centers. Although the cut-off point was arbitrary, and it does not address the problem of self-selection of good-prognosis patients, it provided the best evidence at that time that specialist-center care improved outcome in cystic fibrosis[38].

Size of clinic is a crude measure of specialization, as is survival a crude measure of health status. We surveyed over 1000 adults with cystic fibrosis in 1990, and 1800 adults in 1994. One-third of the group surveyed were not attending separate clinics for cystic fibrosis patients at any hospital, and were therefore deemed to be receiving non-specialist care. There were no social-class differences between the groups. Patients attending the specialist clinics were more likely to have had simple clinical investigations recently, more likely to have had access to paramedical personnel (dietitians, physiotherapists, nurse specialists), more likely to have received home intravenous therapy, were taking higher doses of pancreatic enzymes with meals and snacks, had less severe symptom scores, and were more likely to be satisfied with professional aspects of their care[39].

Findings were similar in a follow-up study in 1994, although the proportion not receiving specialist care had fallen to one-quarter. Patients were also asked how they would prefer their care to be organized in this latter survey. This included the option of having care shared between a local hospital and a more distant specialist center. The results are shown in Fig. 1.12. Only 2 per cent of adult patients want care provided by a local general hospital. The rest would be prepared to travel at least 25 miles (40 km) to a local specialist center, and many would be prepared to travel up to 100 miles (160 km) to a major specialist center. These results were similar regardless of the type of care actually being received[19].

There is now wide consensus that specialist-center care is of benefit to patients. The World Health Organization International Cystic Fibrosis (Mucoviscidosis) Association (ICF(M)A) recently recommended the establishment of such care centers as an appropriate model of care in countries where CF is thought to be more widespread than is appreciated by the medical profession[40]. In the UK, the Clinical Standards Advisory Group recommended that health-care purchasers/commissioners ensure that all CF patients resident in their area have access to specialist services[41].

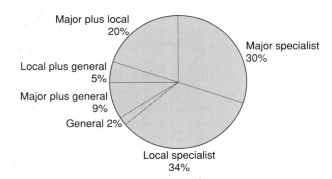

Fig. 1.12 *Preferences for organization of medical care expressed by adults with cystic fibrosis in the United Kingdom, 1994.*

TREATMENT OF CYSTIC FIBROSIS

This chapter on clinical epidemiology would not be complete without mentioning treatment of cystic fibrosis, but cannot possibly hope to cover the whole scope of management of this complex disease, and does not wish to re-visit many areas already addressed in this book. Therefore this section addresses the way in which systematic reviews of the literature can assist the clinician in evidence-based practice in cystic fibrosis, and introduces the Cochrane Collaboration CF Group.

Evidence-based medicine in CF

Evidence-based medicine is the process of applying published evidence regarding the epidemiology, diagnosis, investigation, treatment and prognosis of medical conditions to the individual patient. Although many doctors would contend this is what they do all the time, in practice it is extremely difficult for practitioners to collect together, critically appraise and then put into practice the vast literature on a particular clinical area.

Traditional reviews, such as this chapter, of the medical literature have a number of problems, and are subject to the biased inclusion and exclusion of papers by the author, as well as the author's biased interpretation of the information contained in the selected papers. Therefore, although the primary research may be based on careful methodology and criteria, reviews of the research may be much less rigorous in their criteria for minimization of bias. In addition, traditional reviews may be out of date.

The systematic review of medical literature is an attempt to overcome some of the drawbacks of traditional reviews, while at the same time presenting the clinician with an overview that reduces the need to refer to the extensive primary literature. A systematic review will have a predetermined protocol, with explicit criteria for ensuring a thorough search of the literature, minimization of publication bias, selection of studies for inclusion in the review, predefined outcomes for consideration in the review, protocols for data extraction, and methods for undertaking statistical overviews, including methods for sensitivity analysis to check for bias.

The Cochrane Collaboration is an international collaboration that produces and maintains in perpetuity, systematic reviews of randomized controlled trials of healthcare interventions. This covers the whole of medical practice. Cochrane reviews are produced according to a strict protocol, and updated each time new trials become available. A Cochrane CF group has been established, and both protocols and reviews appear on the Cochrane Library, an electronic publication that is updated several times a year. The advantage of protocols appearing in the library is that criticism and feedback can be received before the review is performed. Input from patients and consumers of healthcare is encouraged to ensure that the outcomes considered in reviews are of relevance to consumers.

More information about the Cochrane Collaboration and the CF Cochrane Group can be obtained from their website:http://web.bham.ac.uk/walterss/Cfcochrane1.htm

The epidemiology of cystic fibrosis

P.A. LEWIS

INTRODUCTION

Epidemiology is the study of disease in well defined populations, often referred to as 'the population perspective'. Thus it is able to document the nature, extent and burden of disease relative to the disease-free population. Such data are essential if informed choices are to be made on the provision of health care and other services. Ideally cohorts, that is, all the people born in a given time period, are studied. An epidemiological study is not truly completed until all the members of a cohort are dead. If a cause of death is available subjects can be retrospectively added to diseased sub-cohorts, thus eventually influencing the cohort's incidence and survival. In addition the method relies on a sophisticated system of birth and death registration as well as routine clinical surveillance. These facilities ensure that comparative data are available for both the base and diseased populations. Thus while epidemiological method can eventually arrive at the best estimate of 'the true state of nature' it cannot produce answers quickly. For this reason clinical populations (survivors who have already been diagnosed) are also studied, this is termed 'clinical epidemiology'. These clinical studies must be interpreted using established epidemiological criteria and provide results which are consistent with the overall population perspective. Often the evidential weight of such studies is low due to a small numbers of subjects (leading to wide confidence intervals), the effects of various forms of bias and, as we shall see, fundamental inconsistencies with other published data.

The etiology of cystic fibrosis

Cystic fibrosis (CF) is a condition caused by genetic defects that lead to a variety of abnormalities in the CF transmembrane conductance regulator (CFTR). The *CFTR* gene is located on the long arm of chromosome 7 and current estimates suggest that there are well over 800 different defects associated with the CF phenotype (CFP).

It is now becoming clear that the CFP is characterized by a very wide phenotypic spectrum, spanning neonates that are not viable, even with the most modern treatment, to those with subclinical disease. The CFP can involve a variety of systems, no one of which is diagnostic. There is a battery of diagnostic procedures available for atypical cases[42] as well as a large literature, which is suggestive of associations between various mutations and genotypes and the CFP.

Attempts at linking the CFP with genotype have only been partially successful because:

- The CF populations studied are biased as they only consist of 'survivors'.
- The effects of the abnormal biochemical pathways have been confounded in these survivors by treatment and environmental effects.
- Some mutations may be phenotypically dominant over other mutations, further confounding individual mutation–phenotype associations.
- There may be other non-CFTR genetic factors influencing the phenotype.
- While some of the abnormal pathologies associated with CF are discrete, e.g. presence or absence of the vas deferens in males, most are characterized by a change in the level of functioning, compared to normal. This change in functioning varies between cases with identical CF mutations to such an extent that there can be overlap both between groups which have different genotypes and between CF cases and non-cases, e.g. measures of lung function.

As two mutant *CFTR* genes are necessary to produce a CFP, over 640 000 CF genotypes may be anticipated. This number of genotypes is likely to be larger than the world population of CF cases, which leads to insurmountable problems in fully documenting the genotype–phenotype associations. Thus while in theory it is only necessary to specify pairs of defective *CFTR* genes which are known to give rise to the CFP to define the disease, the practical problems associated with this may also be insurmountable. A genetic definition of the disease may therefore be impossible.

This absence of a definition of the condition and a categorization of the phenotype–genotype relationship is not a problem to practicing clinicians. They will continue to identify those patients who will benefit from 'treatment for cystic fibrosis', thus considerably improving both patients' life span and quality of life.

However, for the epidemiologist, cystic fibrosis presents a serious challenge. Until the taxonomy of the CFP is more fully understood, comparisons between any groups, where the groups did not arise by random allocation from the same population, will be difficult to interpret due to different phenotypes in each group. This will be particularly true for international comparisons.

Epidemiological method

Clear and unambiguous definitions are a prerequisite for epidemiological studies. The study population needs to be defined in a way that will allow individuals to be allocated exclusively into the study population or not. Populations are best defined by a well-delineated geographical region, while definitions based on clinic attendance are notoriously imprecise as they are subject to important selection biases.

A distinction must be made between the question that the research is trying to answer and the question that is actually answered. For example, the question 'What is the current CF population of England?' cannot be answered directly. A population estimate is a cross-sectional measure and thus is only meaningful on a particular date. Such estimates are usually given for fixed dates, e.g. January 1 or mid-year (July 1). The 'current CF population of England' can be taken to mean a number of things, some possibilities are:

- All people with two CF mutations and alive on (date) and resident in England.
- All people alive on (date) with a clinical diagnosis of CF, even if they were diagnosed after (date), who are British nationals and ordinarily resident in England, which includes those temporarily living abroad, e.g. members of armed forces and their families.
- All people registered as attending specialist CF centers in England as patients on (date).

If (date) is too recent, there can be problems of both underascertainment in the younger ages, due to delays in diagnosis and reporting, and over-reporting in the older ages, due to delays in death notifications.

Careful attention to detail will help in the interpretation of apparently conflicting results and clarify the applicability of one set of results to other populations.

The definition of the cystic fibrosis phenotype

Historically, cases have been diagnosed using accumulated clinical experience to best interpret the symptoms and signs. This experience has been gradually refined with the objective of reducing both the false-positive and false-negative rates, and, more recently, to make the diagnosis as soon as possible to enable therapy to begin before there is long-term lung damage. The combined effect of these factors should be a temporal increase in the likelihood of diagnosis, with some trade-off between decreasing the false-negative rate and increasing the false-positive rate. This effect can be found in incidence studies conducted up to about the mid-1960s[43]. The reported UK CFP incidence from 1968 to 1977 was 1/2414, whereas for 1978–88 it was 1/2416[44], which suggests that changes in diagnostic practice have made little difference to incidence estimates in the UK over this 20-year period.

There has never been a consensus view, agreed and promulgated by a professional body, as to the criteria that should be met to allow a CF diagnosis. Internationally agreed definitions have been of use in the study of other chronic diseases (see, for example, references 45,46). Historically, some clinicians have categorized the diagnostic status of their CFP patients as proven, probable or possible. For example, in one group of 342 patients 249 were categorized as 'proven' (73 per cent), 36 'probable' (11 per cent) and 57 'possible' (16 per cent)[47]; whereas in another group of 234 cases, 177 were classified as 'possible' (76 per cent)[48]. Some studies blandly report 'all patients diagnosed with CF'[38], but in the majority of cases the diagnostic criteria are not specified. This lack of definition of the disease can lead to bias in several ways. For example, the more severe cases are likely to be 'proven' and subject to a greater mortality rate than the others. The proportion of cases in each category therefore depends on the age distribution of the diagnosed population, since a younger population will have more severe cases still surviving compared with an older population. In addition, a physician who favors early aggressive management is more likely to diagnose a condition given the same clinical evidence than is a physician who favors a more conservative treatment policy.

The advent of genetic testing has probably led to shifts in the diagnostic strategies of many clinicians. Patients presenting with apparently very mild CF phenotypes and two CF mutations are categorized as CF. Similar patients but with no detectable CF mutations might not be diagnosed as CF, due to both the social and economic stigmata and the risks of litigation to the clinician.

Defining cystic fibrosis

Ideally, CF cases should be defined as those individuals having two defective *CFTR* genes, where those defects have been previously associated with the CFP. Such a genetic definition has two associated problems. It might lead to completely asymptomatic CF homozygotes, who would be included in a study of the genetics of CF, but not in clinical studies. Also, as has been suggested earlier, it is unlikely that examples of all theoretically possible CF genotypes exist, making a study of the resultant phenotypes problematic. There would seem to be no other option than to continue with the clinical definition of the disease. A genetic investigation in atypical cases might be helpful but cannot be taken to be diagnostically definitive.

INCIDENCE OF THE CYSTIC FIBROSIS PHENOTYPE (CFP)

Racial group differences

As the incidence of the CFP is believed to be rare in non-Caucasian populations[49] these will be dealt with separately.

CAUCASIAN GROUPS

Many authorities give the incidence of the CFP in Caucasian populations in the region of 1/1600 to 1/2000 live births, without citation. An estimate of 1 in 2058 was given in 1965[50], but probably the most influential has been 'A conservative and acceptable figure is an incidence of 1 in 2000 live births for homozygotes for the cystic fibrosis gene in populations of Caucasian descent'[51]. This estimate was based on an appraisal of the evidence available from a number of published studies. It is now clear that this estimate is misleading for a variety of reasons. Too much weight was given to the studies that produced the higher-incidence estimates. One of the studies reviewed[52] gave the incidence for part of the USA as 1 in 3700 live births, which is remarkably close to the latest estimate[53] of 1 in 3400 in 'white' males and females. This latest estimate for the USA attempts to deal with known problems of underascertainment in previous estimates due to the death of cases prior to diagnosis at a participating clinic, using complex statistical modeling techniques. These techniques rely on a number of assumptions, any of which might be invalid. Different populations 'of Caucasian descent' have a different incidence, so it is misleading to quote incidence data for the disease without giving the base population. It has also been suggested that there is a rising trend of ethnic intermarriage[54] which would invalidate historical incidence data based on ethnic groupings.

National variations in reported incidence are very large. In the USA the highest incidence reported is 1/489[55] while the lowest is 1/6667[56]. This wide variation is not uncommon in incidence reports within one country, and although it may be related to a true regional variation in incidence, the possibility that sampling and other methodological biases, as well as publication bias, exist in these studies cannot be discounted. Confidence intervals on incidence estimates are not usually given and there are usually insufficient data in the publication to allow one to be calculated accurately[47]. The extent of the random variation in incidence is not widely appreciated. In a well-defined population of 5.2 million there might be a long term average of 25 CF births per year, i.e. 1 in 2500 live births. Over a 20 year period there should be one year where, soley by chance, there were less than 17 or more than 36 births giving point estimates of incidence of about 1 in 3900 births and 1 in 1700 births respectively. It would take 20 years of data to get an incidence estimate to better than ±10%.

It has been shown that the international variations in published estimates of incidence cannot be explained solely by the method of data collection and analysis[47]. To try to obtain a reliable estimate for the birth incidence, a population-based study, which concentrates on a carefully delineated large population, is highly desirable[47]. In addition, case-finding should be by population screening[47].

Four large population studies have been reported, from The Netherlands[47], Sweden[57], Czechoslovakia[58] and the UK[38,44,59]. All relied on clinical case-finding rather than screening. The Swedish study was for the births between 1950 and 1957, and found 113 cases by the end of 1959 in 0.8 million births, an incidence of 1/7700. The Dutch study covered the birth cohort 1961–65 and found 342 cases in 1.2 million births, giving an incidence of 1/3600. The study of the former Czechoslovakia found 297 cases in 1.5 million births, an incidence of 1/5200 for the period 1960–67. The UK study is following cohorts from 1968 onwards and records over 7000 cases in 17 million births, giving an incidence of 1/2415, although for routine use this may be safely 'rounded' to the more convenient 1/2500. Previous incidence estimates for this time period by the UK study have been slightly lower than this figure, at 1/2475[59], which reflects the effect of cases now being diagnosed in adult life.

Incidence estimates for countries should be based on large, long-term population studies which would negate the random variation seen in year-to-year incidence, even in studies of large populations[44]. An incidence of one case in every 2500 births, giving a CFP carrier frequency of 1 in 25 people and a CF gene frequency of 1 in 50, would seem to be the maximum reasonable estimate for any large Caucasian population.

Table 1.3 *Approximate cystic fibrosis phenotype birth incidence (live births per case) for countries whose populations are European Caucasian*

Country	Incidence	Reference
Ireland	2000	97
UK	2415	44
Australia (Victoria)	2500	98
Former USSR (Moscow)	2500	47
Turkey	3000	99
New Zealand (Auckland)	3000	100
France (parts)	2000–3500	101, 102, 103
USA	3400[a]	53
Spain	3500	64
Greece	3500	64
Netherlands	3500	47
Belgium	3700	64
Former German Democratic Republic	4000	74
Denmark	4500	104
Norway	4500	64
Italy	4700	105
Canada (British Columbia)	5000	47
Ashkenazi Jews in Israel	5000	106
Former Czechoslovakia	5500	57
Poland	6000	64
Sweden	8000	58
Finland	25 000	64

[a]Estimated to have 85 per cent ascertainment.
Modern estimates are only given where they are substantially different to the cited historical data.

Table 1.4 *Approximate cystic fibrosis phenotype birth incidence (live births per case) for countries or populations that are non-Caucasian*

Country	Incidence	Reference
Israeli Jews (Europe–America)	3300	95
Israeli Jews (Asia–Africa)	9400	95
American Blacks	17 000	93
Oriental population of Hawaii	90 000	107
Japan/Japanese	320 000–680 000	65, 66

Many Caucasian populations are reported as having a lower incidence than this. In particular, in Finland the population has been reported as having an incidence as low as 1/40 000[60] and values for Sweden are quoted at 1/8000[52,61,62]. Population subgroups having these antecedents might, therefore, have a substantially lower incidence than the maximum value suggested here.

A summary of estimates of the incidence of CFP in some predominantly Caucasian countries is given in Table 1.3. The disease is found throughout Europe[63,64] but incidence estimates are not reliable for many countries.

NON-CAUCASIAN GROUPS

In this context, 'non-Caucasian' is solely a geographical definition of the original gene pool of the individual. Individuals who are apparently from racial or ethnic groups with a presumed low incidence of the disease should be assessed with caution. When evaluating international data it must be remembered that the relative burden cystic fibrosis places on the populations of different countries varies considerably. Thus in some countries the treatment of cystic fibrosis will be seen as less of a priority because in terms of its contribution to the total infant mortality rate (IMR) there are other more substantial problems, many of which are more easily dealt with than CF. In these countries, incidence reports will be low due to a lack of detection as cases are not being actively sought.

There have been two population-based studies in Japan[65,66]. The first study tried to find all cases reported since 1951 (the first reported case) up to 1993. Each case was reviewed to confirm the diagnosis. In total 104 cases 'of pure Japanese descent' were found in 71 million live births, giving an incidence of 1/680 000. The second study was based solely on death certificates, with no independent confirmation of diagnosis or a check on the ethnic origins of the cases. Deaths between 1968 and 1985 for those born between 1968 and 1980 were used as the numerator in the incidence calculation, which will give an underestimate of the total CF births. In 22 million births (calculated from the data) there were 70 deaths, giving an incidence of 1/320 000. These two studies give a good illustration of how different methods will give different results from the same population.

Table 1.4 gives the approximate CFP birth incidence for some non-Caucasian populations. Good incidence estimates are not available for most non-Caucasian populations, although a small numbers of cases have been reported for most countries where there are pediatricians with an interest in CF. Even if a particular population has been thoroughly screened for CFP cases, this cannot be taken as evidence that there are no CF mutations in that population. CFP cases have been reported for so many parts of the world that it is safest to assume that CF genes, and hence potentially CFPs, are present in every population, even if the incidence is orders of magnitude lower than that of Caucasian populations.

Sex ratio

The sex ratio at birth has been thought to favor males[50], as does the sex ratio among siblings and close relatives[38,67]. Comparisons in the UK suggest that the base population sex ratio varied on an annual basis between 104.8 and 106.1 males per 100 females for the period 1968–88[68,69], while for the same period the overall ratio in CFP cases was 110 to 100. It has not been established whether this difference arises at conception, or because of a differential spontaneous abortion rate or for some other reason. In the USA the sex ratio is reported as 1 for both whites and non-whites[53].

Seasonal effects

Some seasonal effects in the CFP birth rate have been reported[47,70,71], although the effect does not seem to be consistent between reports. Other studies have failed to find an effect[72–74], having made adjustments for the temporal variations in the base population birth rate. In the UK, there is no strong seasonal effect but there do seem

to be noticeable increases in the incidence on an approximate 11-year cycle, one peak being around 1982[59].

LIFE-SPAN ANALYSES FOR POPULATIONS WITH CF PHENOTYPES

Historical improvements

Improvements in general population survival have been reported by many of the nations of the world over the past 50 years. This has been reflected in the reduction in the age- and sex-specific mortality rates over this period and in part by an aging population. These improvements have usually been bettered by the CF populations, although they started from a much lower level.

For the patients of one clinic for the period 1943–64 life-table methods show that meconium ileus usually led to infant death, with about 15 per cent surviving at 1 year. The nonmeconium ileus median survival was about 9 months, with about 20 per cent survival to 4 years[75].

More recent survival data give estimates of median survival in some countries of about 30 years[11,44,76–78].

Mortality-rate comparisons between different populations can be confounded by the different age structures of the populations. Thus while the overall population mortality rate for the UK in 1995 was 10.9 per thousand, for the CFP population it was 21 per thousand, apparently only double the 'normal' rate. A calculation of the standardized mortality ratio (SMR) to adjust for age[78] gives the 1995 SMR for the CFP population of about 3300[44].

Current survival

Up-to-date estimates of survival are impossible, as ascertainment is rarely good until at least 5 years have passed since birth[38]. This is due primarily to delays in diagnosis and reporting. However, when death reporting is prompt, it is appropriate to estimate age-specific mortality rates for older age groups up to the last completed year, and these indicate that improvements continue to be made, e.g. compare UK[38,44], Canada[11,79] and USA[76,80].

A current life table[78] represents the hypothetical survival of the current cohort if the current year's age-specific mortality rates were to apply to them over their life span. As mortality rates are still in a state of flux, estimates of life expectancy are problematical[81].

It is possible that some age-specific mortality rates will start rising in the near future as severe cases who previously died in childhood now die in early adulthood. Recent current survival curves for the USA, Canada, Victoria (Australia) and the UK are given in Fig. 1.13. Age-specific mortality rates for females have usually been higher than those for males, females having a shorter projected life span. If there are accurate annual counts of

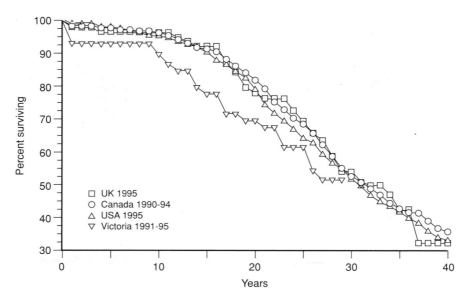

Fig. 1.13 *Current survival, males.*

deaths of CFPs, then a prolonged rise in the number of deaths will indicate that improvements in survival are ending. At the moment, annual UK CFP births are about twice the annual deaths. When annual deaths equal annual births the CFP population will have stopped growing and survival will have stopped improving[44].

Cohort survival

The more reliable method of assessing changes in survival is to compare successive birth cohorts. Although this will give (within the limits of the data collected) an accurate representation of the survival experience of a group, it suffers from the disadvantage of only having complete data once all the group has died. Producing cohort survival[78] is a long process and few researchers have attempted the task.

Cohorts from 1968 are being followed in the UK. The most recent data available[82] suggest that the median survival for males in the 1968–70 cohort is 19.0 years, for the 1971–73 cohort it is 19.9 years and for the 1974–76 cohort the median had not been reached by the end of 1996 but it should be well in excess of 24 years. The equivalent data for the three female cohorts are 14.0 years, 19.1 years and 20.1 years (Figs 1.14 and 1.15). The age-specific mortality rates for females have always been worse than those for males (within the limits of statistical variability), but for those born in more recent years females have achieved equality in survival in the UK. This is illustrated in Table 1.5, which gives the percentage of each 3-year sex cohort surviving to 5 years. Although sexual equality seems to have been achieved in terms of survival, females are still at a disadvantage because in the unaffected population their survival is better than that of males.

Different survival patterns

Most of the attention directed towards life-span analyses has been concerned with single-parameter estimates (the mean and median survival). There are other important features of the curves in Figs 1.13 and 1.14. The graphs of current survival (Fig. 1.13) show that the curves are convex, that is, as age increases they get steeper because, in the current year, the mortality rate increases with age. This has been taken to show that once past a certain age the mortality rate accelerates. This is seen as plausible because this 'crisis' occurs about the time of puberty, a period of profound change. In comparison the UK cohort survival curves are virtually straight lines past the first year of life up to age 28 years (year of birth 1968–70) although each successive cohort is less steep. This indicates that the shoulder-like shape (convexity) of the current survival curve is 'artefactual' and is due to the changing patterns in the cohort survival. The successive age-specific mortality rates in the current survival are taken from cohorts where the mortality rates are greater. Any expectation that the mortality rates in the immediate post-pubertal period are substaintally greater than those found before puberty is misplaced. Comparisons of current survival curves for different years confirm that the 'dip' moves forward each year. These data are consistent with treatment effect which began about 1975.

The observation that the slope of the cohort survival curve decreases with successive cohorts is indicative of a strong 'year of birth' effect on survival. The 'calendar year of treatment' effect seems to be missing, older people have worse survival than younger people in the same year, when it may be presumed that the same

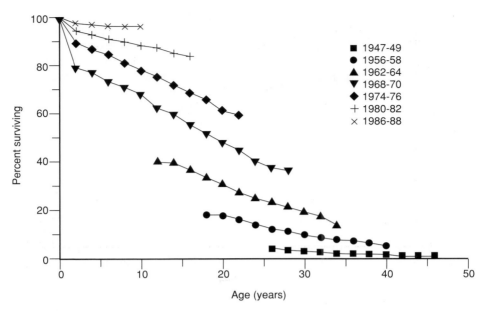

Fig. 1.14 *Selected cohort (males) and interrupted cohort (both sexes) for UK.*

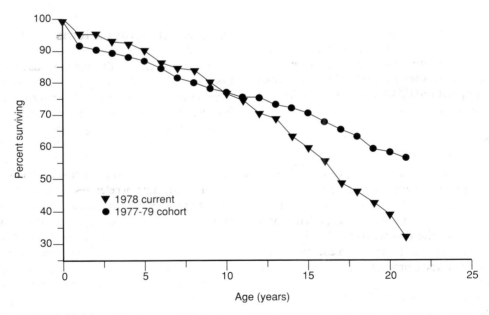

Fig. 1.15 *UK current and cohort survival, females.*

Table 1.5 *Percentage of 3-year cohorts surviving to the fifth year by sex for UK cystic fibrosis cases (adapted from ref. 44)*

Cohort	Males	Females
1968–70	74.7	73.2
1971–73	77.9	76.9
1974–76	85.6	83.6
1977–79	88.2	86.5
1980–82	92.0	90.3
1983–85	92.7	93.6
1986–88	96.5	96.8
1989–91	96.7	97.1

treatments are available. This is possibly the strongest data showing the benefits of early modern treatment, but in the absence of a detailed analysis the observation is only speculative. Such an analysis might provide an insight into the future life span of the CFP. A simple extrapolation of the survival curve for 1986–88 cohort suggest a median survival as high as 60 years. The implications of this possibility are substantial, in terms of fully informing parents taking part in screening programs, in the provision of health care (the adult population would be well over three times larger than the pediatric population), to insurers, to patients and others.

UK and Australian[84] data usually show a relatively high infant mortality rate (IMR). This is not shown in the Canadian or USA data which are clinic based and suggest that referrals are occurring after the period of the high IMR, so that some deaths are missing from these data. The Australian and UK data have no such exclusions as they are population based and are more likely to represent a true picture of the CFP life span.

ASSESSING THE EFFECTIVENESS OF HEALTHCARE USING INTERNATIONAL DIFFERENCES IN LIFE SPAN

The effectiveness of healthcare is the provenance of the clinical epidemiologist. International differences in the life span of CFPs have been used to promote the advantages of different models for the delivery of health care to CFPs. However, any clinical epidemiological data should be consistent with broader epidemiological data if they are to be plausible.

An estimated difference in current survival, for the period 1976–80, to age 20 years, of 18 per cent between Victoria (Australia) and England and Wales has been attributed to the availability of care in a specialist center in Victoria, compared with England and Wales[84]. Easy access to care at specialist centers has also been cited as the reason for improvements in survival in the USA[85].

The specialist center in Victoria managed the care of 90 per cent of the children and adolescents. There are many potential confounding factors in this observational study including possible genetic structures, the different climate and social differences. This large difference in survival led to a campaign to promote specialist centers in England and Wales. These data have been revisited subsequently and placed in an historical context[86]. The England and Wales section of the data are broadly comparable with recently published long-term UK data, some of which are given in this chapter. However, if the Australian data are accurate, then more recent survival data from Australia suggests that in the years subsequent to this study Australian survival actually got worse! This is just not plausible. The most likely explanation is a combination of data from a period of random good survival in Australia and publication bias. Hence some of the strongest data supporting the advantages of specialist centers has been shown to be flawed. It follows, therefore, that historically pediatricians in the UK have delivered to their CF patients a life span as good as any other country.

Canadian CFP patient data registry reported a median survival, as calculated on a current life-table basis, of over 27 years for the decade 1981–90[79], which was superior to UK results[59]. These Canadian data are for patients attending one of 32 specialized clinics. Canadian clinics recruit approximately 120 new CFP cases per cohort. As the births in Canada are approximately 390 000 per year[86], this suggests an incidence of 1/3250. The IMR for the sexes combined for 1986–90 is given as 0.007. This is virtually identical to the Canadian population IMR[87]. Equivalent IMR data for 1980–85 for UK CFP births is 0.050[59]. The apparently superior Canadian survival compared with UK survival can be explained in part by selection bias in the Canadian study population. Neonatal experience suggests that CFP babies have a greater unavoidable mortality rate than non-CFP babies, a feature missing from the Canadian (and USA) data.

Recent estimates of current survival for the Canadian population[11] suggest that after peaking in 1989, median survival has been steadily falling, so that it is now similar to that in other countries (Fig 1.13). Falling survival in the Canadian population is not plausible, given the experience of other similar countries. A more likely explanation is that some of the reported increase in survival during the 1980s was due to both statistical fluctuations in the numbers dying and underreporting of deaths, probably in the very young. Treatment does not prevent death, only delays it, so an eventual rise in deaths should be expected after a sudden fall in deaths. Further, some of the methodological weaknesses in this clinic-based study are perhaps being eliminated gradually with improved reporting. This, too, would lead to an apparent reduction in survival due to the elimination of previous overestimates.

For the first time ever, reported current survival estimates for the USA, Canada, Australia and the UK are similar (Fig. 1.13). This is not surprising, as one would

Table 1.6 *CF case frequency and population incidence of specified CF genotypes*

Genotype	Gene frequency	Case frequency (per 100)	Live births per case (1000s)
$\Delta F_{508}/\Delta F_{508}$	0.67×0.67	45	6
ΔF_{508}/single common	0.67×0.03	2.00	120
ΔF_{508}/all common	0.67×0.18	12	21
ΔF_{508}/single rare	0.67×0.0002	0.013	2×10^4
ΔF_{508}/all rare	0.67×0.15	10	25
Single common/single common	0.03×0.03	0.09	3×10^3
Single rare/single rare	0.0002×0.0002	4.0×10^{-6}	6×10^7
Single common/single rare	0.03×0.0002	6.0×10^{-4}	4×10^5

expect the populations to be broadly comparable, the clinicians and other carers to have similar training and the same therapies to be available. Also, previous international comparisons have drawn attention to methodological weakness in studies which are gradually being eliminated. Should differences reappear, the data currently available are insufficient to determine the cause of the differences.

Seventy-five per cent of CFP patients in Denmark are treated in one center[85] and current survival estimates (i.e. projected not observed) of 80 per cent survival to age 50 years are attributed to 'aggressive treatment'. While the data may be correct and the processing of the data to obtain the survival estimates legitimate, the interpretation of the results is at best naïve. There are no deaths shown past 35 years of age, even though the survival projection is up to 50 years of age. The implication is that in this clinic in Denmark people with a CFP have a better survival than the unaffected population![86] This is difficult to believe especially as the numbers involved are small and a short time period is considered.

The evaluation of different models of medical management of CFPs is far from easy. The publication of flawed data only serves to confuse the issues because they actually contribute nothing to the debate. This confusion leads to delays in starting properly designed studies to answer these important clinical questions.

Heart–lung transplantation

Patients with end-stage lung disease are candidates for heart–lung transplantation. The extent of the transplantation program is limited by the lack of suitable donor organs, and this is particularly true for children[88]. At present transplantation offers the hope of an improved quality of life, but not necessarily of an increased life span, for the recipients.

THE EPIDEMIOLOGY OF THE *CFTR* GENE

Gene and genotype frequency

Many laboratories throughout the world are continuing the quest to discover all the CFTR gene mutations, which give rise to the CFP. The total number of different *CFTR* gene mutations is a matter of speculation; an up-to-date list is available on the Worldwide Web site at http://www.genet.sickkids.on.ca/cftr/ together with other supplementary material. Although the number of mutations that have been identified continues to increase, important conclusions about genotype incidence may be drawn from plausible gene frequency data. In time more precise data will become available, but such are the numerical characteristics of the problem that the conclusions are unlikely to change substantially.

To be able to give a numerical illustration, two plausible assumptions are necessary:

1. The defective *CFTR* gene frequency for populations of Caucasian origin is 1 in 50; that is, the CF heterozygote frequency is 1 in 25.
2. The number of different types of defective *CFTR* genes in Caucasian populations is 800.

There is one common *CFTR* gene mutation (ΔF_{508}), which has an occurrence of about 67 per cent in the UK; six mutations which each have an occurrence of 3 per cent; and therefore the remainder must occur on average 0.5 per cent of the remaining time (approximately 0.08 per cent each). The resultant genotype incidences and frequencies in the base population are given in Table 1.6, which illustrates the rarity of many genotypes. This table provides the basis for calculating the percentage of cases that can be detected readily by genetic screening.

The practical consequences of such data may be illustrated by data for the UK[82]. There have been about 135 different CF mutations found *and* reported in about 11 000 genes tested from 5500 UK cases. There is a single instance of 50 of these genes. There are 198 different genotypes reported, 132 of them having a single instance. About 200 cases have no identified gene and a further 1000 only have one gene identified, although many of these will not have been analyzed exhaustively. For those born since 1990, genetic reports are unavailable for 10 per cent of cases. Thus of the 18 000 (135×135) CF homozygote genotypes which are already known to be theoretically possible in the UK, only a very small number of them have been observed.

In any large population there will be CF mutations, already identified in other populations, that have yet to be detected and there will be others which will only come to light when chance makes them one of a pair of genes in a CFP.

Practical problems in finding rare CF genotypes

The last column of Table 1.6 gives the average number of births that will contain one CF case in a population with a high CFP incidence. The births sample size required to have a 95 per cent chance of containing at least one case is four times as large as the average quoted.

The implications of Table 1.6 are illustrated by the fact that the average number of births per specific 'common/rare' genotype is more than twice the world births in one year[86].

Looking for consistency in the epidemiology of the gene

The defective *CFTR* genes do not exist in isolation. They coexist with all the other genes in the gene pool of a population, and all the genes in the gene pool share similar antecedents. Any patterns found in the distribution of defective *CFTR* genes should be mirrored in the distribution of other genes.

Studies on attendees at individual clinics are suggesting the approximate relative gene frequencies, but only for those genes that can be detected. These will give data on survivors. Only when the genetic characteristics of large cohorts have been established will a full genotypic picture begin to emerge.

The data on the distribution of the most common lesions, by surviving cases and country[63, 64] can only be extrapolated back to estimate relative frequency and population frequency by assuming that there is no survival advantage attached to these alleles. There is already a large body of data published on clines (contours of equal gene frequency) for other genes, e.g. blood groups[89]. There should be an association between these clines and CF clines as the same populations are involved. The relative frequency of ΔF_{508} as a proportion of all CF mutations has been given as clines for Europe[64]. To convert these relative frequency data, obtained by genetic analysis of CFPs, to population gene frequencies requires an accurate estimate of CF incidence, which, as suggested earlier, is problematic. Until there is proper population heterozygote genotyping, all genetic frequency data must be viewed with caution.

Hybridization studies give estimates of the proportion of the genes of a population which come from different racial groups. These allow calculations of the expected frequency of genetic diseases in this population. As an illustration of how these data may be used, assume virtually no CFTR-defective genes in individuals with a pure African pedigree. It has been estimated that African–Americans have about 30 per cent Caucasian genes due to miscegenation[90], but a wide national variation has been reported when data on various genes have been pooled[91,92]. This variation has the range 7–49 per cent. If the Caucasian CF heterozygote rate is 1/25 then the rate for African–Americans should be 1/85, based on 30 per cent hybridization. The expected CF rate in African–Americans can then be calculated as 1/85 × 1/85 × [quarter], which is 1/28 900. The incidence of CF in African–Americans in Washington has been estimated as 1/17 000[93] and in non-whites for all of USA as 1/12 000[53]. Such discrepancies in estimates indicate the lack of precision in the base data used in the calculations.

The matter is further complicated by indications that the American–African cases have much longer life spans than their Caucasian counterparts: a small study shows 95 per cent survival to 18 years[94], suggesting a different pattern of phenotypes. Data exist which will enable similar calculations to be attempted for other countries with hybrid populations. For example, in African populations in Brazil the percentage Caucasian genes has been esti-

mated to be constant between the different states of Brazil at about 50 per cent[92].

Studies of different mutation distributions in different Jewish ethnic groups showed wide variability[95], but the numbers studied were small, so the confidence intervals would be wide.

CONCLUSION

The discovery of the CF gene, with its many mutations, led to the realization that the disease entity, known as CF, was far more complex than had been previously thought. This complexity extends to the epidemiology of the disease, where there are many unresolved issues. The population of the world is not in a Hardy–Weinberg equilibrium[96] so the reported increase in ethnic intermarriage[54] implies a future change in the genetic epidemiology of CF and of the epidemiology of the CFP itself. The challenge to epidemiologists is to report and correctly interpret the epidemiology of CF, allowing for the effects of changes in treatment, population age and sex structure, environment and genetic epidemiology. It is only when people with cystic fibrosis, their families and carers and those responsible for the purchase of healthcare have access to the same accurate data that informed choices can be made and equity ensured.

REFERENCES

Clinical epidemiology of cystic fibrosis

1. McMahon, B. and Pugh, T.F. (1970) *Epidemiology: Principles and Methods*, Boston, Little, Brown.
2. Fitzsimmons, S.C. (1997) *Cystic Fibrosis Foundation Patient Data Registry Annual Data Report 1996*, Bethesda, Maryland.
3. Wesley, A., Dawson, K., Hewitt, C. and Kerr, A. (1993) Clinical features of individuals with cystic fibrosis in New Zealand. *NZ Med. J.*, **106**; 28–30.
4. Mulherin, D., Ward, K., Coffey, M., Keoghan, M. and Fitzgerald, M. (1991) Cystic fibrosis in adolescents and adults. *Irish Med. J.*, **84**, 48–51.
5. Gan, K.H., Geus, W.P., Bakker, W., Lamers, C.B. and Heijerman, H.G. (1995) Genetic and clinical features of patients with cystic fibrosis diagnosed after the age of 16 years. *Thorax*, **50**, 1301–1304.
6. Chatfield, S., Owen, G., Ryley, H.C. *et al.* (1991) Neonatal screening for cystic fibrosis in Wales and the West Midlands: clinical assessment after five years of screening. *Arch. Dis. Child.*, **66**, 29–33.

7. Farrell, P.M., Kosorok, M.R., Laxova, A. *et al*. (1997) Nutritional benefits of neonatal screening for cystic fibrosis. *NEJM*, **337**, 997–999.

8. De Brakeleer, M. and Ferec, C. (1996) Mutations in the cystic fibrosis gene in men with congenital bilateral absence of the vas deferens. *Mol. Human Repro.*, **2**, 669–677.

9. Colin, A.A., Sawyer, S.M., Mickle, J.E., Oates, R.D., Milunsky, A. and Amos, J.A. (1996) Pulmonary function and clinical observations in men with congenital bilateral absence of the vas deferens. *Chest*, **110**, 440–445.

10. Rosenberg, S.M., Howatt, W.F. and Grum, C.M. (1992) Spirometry and chest rontgenographic appearance in adults with cystic fibrosis. *Chest*, **101**, 961–964.

11. Canadian Patient Data Registry National Report (1995), Canadian Cystic Fibrosis Foundation.

12. Dureieu, I., Bellon, G., Vital Durand, D., Calemard, L., Morely, Y. and Gilly R. (1995) Cystic fibrosis in adults (review). *Presse Medicale* **24**, 1882–1887 (in French).

13. Demko, C.A., Byard, R.J. and Davis, P.B. (1995) Gender differences in cystic fibrosis: *Pseudomonas aeruginosa* infection. *J. Clin. Epidemiol.*, **48**, 1041–1049.

14. Tummler, B., Bosshammer, I., Breitenstein, S. *et al*. (1997) Infections with *Pseudomonas aeruginosa* in patients with cystic fibrosis. *Behring Institute Mitteilungen,* 249–255 (in German).

15. Abman, S.H., Ogle, J.W., Harbeck, R.J., Butler-Simon, N., Hammond, K.B. and Accurso, F.I. (1991) Early bacteriologic, immunologic and clinical courses of young infants with cystic fibrosis identified by neonatal screening. *J. Paediatr.*, **119**, 211–217.

16. Lang, S., Thorsteinsson, B., Lund-Anderson, C., Nerup, I., Schiotz, P.O. and Koch, C. (1994) Diabetes mellitus in Danish cystic fibrosis patients: prevalence and late diabetic complications. *Acta Paediatr.*, **83**, 72–77.

17. Lang, S., Hansen, A., Thorsteinsson, B., Nerup, J. and Kock, C. (1995) Glucose tolerance in patients with CF: five year prospective study. *BMJ*, **311**, 655–659.

18. Neglia, J.P., Fitzsimmons, S.C., Maisonneuve, P. *et al*. (1995) The risk of cancer among patients with cystic fibrosis. Cystic fibrosis and cancer study group. *NEJM*, **332**, 494–499.

19. Walters, S. (1995) *Association of CF Adults (UK) Survey: Analysis and Report*, Cystic Fibrosis Trust, Bromley, UK.

20. Penketh, A.R., Wise, A., Mearns, M.B., Hodson, M.E. and Batten, J.C. (1987) Cystic fibrosis in adolescents and adults. *Thorax*, **42**, 526–532.

21. Sinnema, G., Bonarius, J.C., Stoop, J.W. and van der Laag, J. (1983) Adolescents with cystic fibrosis in the Netherlands. *Acta Paediatr. Scand.*, **72**, 427–432.

22. Walters, S., Britton, J. and Hodson, M.E. (1993) Social and demographic characteristics of adults with cystic fibrosis in the United Kingdom. *BMJ*, **306**, 549–552.

23. Anon. (1993) Correlation between genotype and pheno-type in cystic fibrosis. The cystic fibrosis genotype–pheno-type consortium. *NEJM*, **329**, 1308–1313.

24. Rosenfeld, M., Davis, R., Fitzsimmons, S., Pepe, M., and Ramsey, B. (1997) Gender gap in cystic fibrosis mortality. *Am. J. Epidemiol.*, **145**, 794–803.

25. Huang, N.N., Schidlow, D.V., Szatrowski, T.H. *et al*. (1987) Clinical features, survival rate and prognostic factors in young adults with cystic fibrosis. *Am. J. Med.*, **82**, 871–879.

26. Henry, R.L., Mellis, C.M. and Petrovic, K. (1992) Mucoid *Pseudomonas aeruginosa* is a marker of poor survival in cystic fibrosis. *Pediatr. Pulmonol.*, **12**, 158–161.

27. Britton, J.R. (1989) Effect of social class, sex, region of residence on age at death from cystic fibrosis. *BMJ*, **298**, 483–487.

28. Hallyar, K.M., Williams, S.G., Wise, A.E. *et al*. (1997) A prognostic model for the prediction of survival in cystic fibrosis. *Thorax*, **52**, 313–317.

29. Corey, M. and Farewell, V. (1995) Determinants of mortality from cystic fibrosis in Canada 1970–1989. *Am. J. Epidemiol.*, **143**, 1007–1017.

30. Grasemann, H., Wiesemann, H.G., and Ratjen, F. (1995) The importance of lung function as a predictor of two year mortality in mucoviscidosis. *Pneumologie*, **49**, 466–469 (in German).

31. Nixon, P.A., Orenstein, S.M., Kelsey, S.F. and Doershuk, C.F. (1992) The prognostic value of exercise testing in patients with cystic fibrosis. *NEJM*, **327**, 1785–1788.

32. Hudson, V.L., Wielinski, C.L. and Regelmann, W.E. (1993) Prognostic implications of initial oropharyngeal bacterial flora in patients with cystic fibrosis diagnosed before the age of two. *J. Pediatr.*, **122**, 854–860.

33. Lewin, L.O., Byard, P.J. and Davis, P.B. (1990) Effect of *Pseudomonas cepacia* colonisation on survival and lung function in cystic fibrosis patients. *J. Clin. Epidemiol.*, **43**, 125–131.

34. Muhdi, K., Edenborough, R.B., Gumery, L. *et al*. (1996) Outcome for patients colonised with *Burkholderia cepacia* in a Birmingham adult cystic fibrosis clinic and the end of an epidemic. *Thorax*, **51**, 374–377.

35. Curtis, J.R., Burke, W., Kassner, A.W. and Aitken, M.L. (1997) Absence of health insurance is associated with decreased life expectancy in cystic fibrosis. *Am. J. Resp. Crit. Care Med.*, **155**, 1921–1924.

36. Shepherd, S.L., Hovell, M.F., Slymen, D.J. *et al*. (1992) Functional status as an overall measure of health in adults with cystic fibrosis: further validation of a generic health measure. *J. Clin. Epidemiol.*, **45**, 117–125.

37. Hill, D.J., Martin, A.J., Davidson, G.P. and Smith, G.S. (1985) Survival of cystic fibrosis patients in South Australia: Evidence that cystic fibrosis centre care leads to better survival. *Med. J. Australia.*, **143,** 230–232.

38. Dodge, J.A., Goodall, J., Geddes, D.M. *et al*. (1988) Cystic fibrosis in the United Kingdom 1977–85: an improving picture. British Paediatric Association Working Party on Cystic Fibrosis. *BMJ*, **297**, 1599–1602.

39. Walters, S., Britton, J. and Hodson, M.E. (1994) Hospital care for adults with cystic fibrosis: an overview and comparison between special cystic fibrosis clinics and general clinics using a patient questionnaire. *Thorax*, **49**, 300–306.

40. Anonymous (1997) Implementation of cystic fibrosis services in developing countries: memorandum from a Joint WHO/ICF(M)A meeting. *Bull. World Health Org.*, **75**, 1–10.

41. Clinical Standards Advisory Group (1993) *Access and Availability to Specialist Services: Cystic Fibrosis*, HMSO, London.

The epidemiology of cystic fibrosis

42. Wallis, C. (1997) Diagnosing cystic fibrosis: blood, sweat and tears. *Arch. Dis. Child.*, **76**, 85–91.

43. Hall, B.D. and Simpkiss, M.J. (1968) Incidence of fibrocystic disease in Wessex. *J. Med. Genet.*, **5**, 262–265.

44. Dodge, J.A., Morison, S., Lewis, P.A. *et al.* (1997) Incidence, population, and survival of cystic fibrosis in the UK, 1968–95. *Arch. Dis. Child.*, **77**, 493–496.

45. Popes, M.W., Bennett, G.A., Cobb, S. *et al.* (1958) 1958 revision of diagnostic criteria for rheumatoid arthritis. *Bull. Rheum. Dis.*, **9**, 175–176.

46. World Health Organization (1966) *Cardiovascular disease and hypertension*. WHO report series, WHO, Geneva.

47. Ten Kate, L.P. (1977) Cystic fibrosis in the Netherlands. *Int. J. Epidemiol.*, **6**, 23–34.

48. Goodman, H.O. and Reed, S.C. (1952) Heredity of fibrosis of the pancreas. Possible mutation rate of the gene. *Am. J. Hum. Genet.*, **4**, 59.

49. Tsui, L.-C. (1990) Editorial, in *Population Analysis of the Major Mutation in Cystic Fibrosis* (eds C. Romeo and M. Devoto). *Hum. Genet.*, **85**, 391–445.

50. Danks, D.M., Allan, J. and Anderson, C.M. (1965) A genetic study of fibrocystic disease of the pancreas. *Ann. Hum. Genet.*, **28**, 323–356.

51. di Sant'Agnese, P.A. and Talamo, R.C. (1967) Pathogenesis and physiopathology of CF of the pancreas. *NEJM*, **277**, 1287–1294.

52. Steinberg, A.G. and Brown, D.C. (1960) On the incidence of cystic fibrosis of the pancreas. *Am. J. Hum. Genet.*, **12**, 416–424.

53. Kosorok, M.R., Wei, W.-H. and Farrell, P.M. (1994) The incidence of cystic fibrosis. *Stat. Med.*, **15**, 449–462.

54. Gilbert, F., Schoelkopf, J., Li, Z., Arzimanoglou, I., Shaham, M. and Udey, J. (1995) Ethnic intermarriage and its consequences for cystic fibrosis carrier screening. *Am. J. Prev. Med.*, **11**, 251–255.

55. Honeyman, M.S. and Siker, E. (1965) Cystic fibrosis of the pancreas: an estimate of the incidence. *Am. J. Hum. Genet.*, **17**, 461–465.

56. Hanna, B.L. (1965) Genetic studies of family units, in *Genetics and the Epidemiology of Chronic Diseases*, (eds J.V. Neel, M.W. Shaw and J.Schull), United States Public Health Service, Publication number 1163.

57. Brunechy, Z. (1972) The incidence and genetics of cystic fibrosis. *J. Med. Genet.*, **9**, 33–37.

58. Selander, P. (1962) The frequency of cystic fibrosis of the pancreas in Sweden. *Acta Paediatr.*, **51**, 65–67.

59. Dodge, J.A., Morison, S., Lewis, P.A. *et al.* (1993) Cystic fibrosis in the United Kingdom, 1968–1988: incidence, population and survival. *Pediatr. Perinat. Epidemiol.*, **7**, 157–166.

60. Nevanlinna, H.R. (1972) The Finnish population structure, a genetic and genealogical study. *Hereditas*, **71**, 195.

61. Kollnberg, H. (1970) Cystic fibrosis in Sweden. First Annual Meeting of the European Working Group for Cystic Fibrosis, Stockholm.

62. Isolair, J., Witti, J. and Visakorpi, J.K. (1979) Screening of cystic fibrosis in newborn. *Duodecium*, **95**, 1619 (in Finnish).

63. The Cystic Fibrosis Genetic Analysis Consortium (1994) Population variation of common cystic fibrosis mutations. *Hum. Mutat.*, **4**, 167–177.

64. Lucotte, G., Hazout, S. and de Braekeleer, M. (1995) Complete map of cystic fibrosis mutation ΔF_{508} frequencies in Western Europe and correlation between mutation frequencies and incidence of disease. *Hum. Biol.*, **67**, 797–803.

65. Yamashiro, Y., Shimizu, T., Oguchi, S. *et al.* (1993) The estimated incidence of cystic fibrosis in Japan. *J. Pediatr. Gastroenterol. Nutr.*, **24**, 544–547.

66. Imaizumi, Y. (1995) Incidence and mortality rates of cystic fibrosis in Japan, 1969–1992. *Am. J. Med. Genet.*, **58**, 161–168.

67. Pritchard, D.J., Hickman, G.R. and Nelson, R. (1983) Sex ratio and heterozygote advantage in cystic fibrosis families. *Arch. Dis. Child.*, **58**, 290–293.

68. Office of Populations, Censuses and Surveys (1981) *Review of the Registrar General on births and patterns of family building in England and Wales 1980*. Series FM1 No. 7, HMSO, London.

69. Office of Population Censuses and Surveys (1982) *Review of the Registrar General on births and patterns of family building in England and Wales 1990*. Series FMI No.19, HMSO, London.

70. Brackenridge, C.J. (1978) The seasonal variation of births of offspring from couples heterozygous for cystic fibrosis. *Am. J. Hum. Genet.*, **42**, 197–201.

71. Brackenridge, C.J. (1980) Bimodal month of birth distribution in cystic fibrosis. *Am. J. Med. Genet.*, **5**, 295–301.

72. Daigneault, J., Aubin, G., Simard, F. and Braekeler, M.D. (1991) Birth distribution in cystic fibrosis in Saguenay-Lac-St-Jean, Quebec, Canada. *J. Med. Genet.*, **28**, 613–614.

73. David, T.J., Elstow, G.A., Baumer, J.H. and Evans, C.M. (1981) Cystic fibrosis and the month of birth. *J. Med. Genet.*, **18**, 299–300.

74. Machill, G., Gedschold, J. and Kropf, S. (1990) Birth distribution in cystic fibrosis and phenylketonuria. *Eur. J. Pediatr.*, **149**, 406–407.

75. Mantle, D.J. and Norman, A.P. (1966) Life-table for cystic fibrosis. *BMJ*, **2**, 1238–1241.

76. Cystic Fibrosis Foundation Patient Registry (1996) *1995 Annual Data Report*, Bethesda, MD, USA.

77. The Australian Cystic Fibrosis Associations Federation National Data Registry (1996) *Annual Data Report 1995/6*, North Ryde, NSW, Australia.

78. Hill, A.B. (1980) *A short textbook of medical statistics*. Hodder and Stoughton, London.

79. Canadian Cystic Fibrosis Foundation (1990) *Report of the Canadian Patient Data Registry*, Canadian Cystic Fibrosis Foundation.

80. Cystic Fibrosis Foundation Patient Registry (1992) *1990 Annual Data Report*, Bethesda, MD, USA.

81. Corey, M. (1996) Survival estimates in cystic fibrosis: snapshot of a moving target. *Pediatr. Pulmonol.*, **21**, 149–150.

82. UK Cystic Fibrosis Survey (1997) UK CF data, 1996 update (draft). Private communication.

83 Lewis, P.A., Morison, S., Dodge, J.A. *et al*. (1999) Survival estimates for adults with cystic fibrosis born in the United Kingdom between 1947 and 1967. *Thorax*, **54**, 420–422.

84. Phelan, P. and Hey, F. (1984) Cystic fibrosis in England and Wales and in Victoria, Australia 1976–1980. *Arch. Dis. Child.*, **59**, 71–83.

85. Frederiksen, B., Lanng S., Koch C. and Høiby, N. (1996) Improved survival in the Danish Center-treated cystic fibrosis patients: results of aggressive treatment. *Pediatr. Pulmonol.*, **21**, 153–158.

86. Lewis, P.A. (1998) Inferences for health provision from survival data in cystic fibrosis. *Arch. Dis. Child.*, **79**, 297–299.

87. United Nations (1997) Department for Economic and Social Information and Policy Analysis, Statistics Division. Demographic Yearbook: Issue 47, 1995. New York.

88. Balfour-Lynn, I.M., Martin, I., Whitehead, P.G. *et al*. (1997) Heart–lung transplantation for patients under 10 with cystic fibrosis. *Arch. Dis. Child.*, **76**, 38–40.

89. Mourant, A.E., Kopec, A.C. and Domaniewska-Sobczak, K. (1958) *The ABO Blood Groups*, Blackwell, Oxford.

90. McKusick, V.A. (1969) *Human Genetics*, Prentice-Hall, New Jersey.

91. Glass, H.B. and Li, C.C. (1953) Dynamics of racial intermixture – analysis based on American Negro. *Am. J. Hum. Genet.*, **5**, 1–20.

92. Saldanha, P.H. (1962) Taste sensitivity to phenylthiourea among Brazilian Negroes and its bearing on the problem of White–Negro intermixture in Brazil. *Hum. Biol.*, **34**, 179–186.

93. Kulczycki, L.L. and Schauf, V. (1974) Cystic fibrosis in blacks in Washington DC. *Am. J. Dis. Child.*, **127**, 64–67.

94. Stern, R.C., Doerschuk, C.F., Boat, T.F. *et al*. (1976) Course of cystic fibrosis in black patients. *J. Pediatr.*, **89**, 412–417.

95. Kerem, E., Kalman, Y.M., Yahav, Y. *et al*. (1995) Highly variable incidence of cystic fibrosis and different mutation distribution among different Jewish ethnic groups in Isreal. *Hum. Genet.*, **96**, 193–197.

96. Wier, B.S. (1990) *Genetic data analysis*, Sinauer, Mass.

97. O'Reilly, D., Murphy, J., McLaughlin, J. *et al*. (1974) The prevalence of coeliac disease and cystic fibrosis in Ireland, Scotland and Wales. *Int. J. Epidemiol.*, **3**, 247.

98. Allan, J.L., Robbie, M., Phelan, P.D. and Danks, D.M. (1980) The incidence and presentation of cystic fibrosis in Victoria 1955–1978. *Aust. Paediatr. J.*, **16**, 270–273.

99. Gurson, C.T., Sertel, H., Gurkan, M. and Pala, S. (1973) Newborn screening for cystic fibrosis with chloride electrode and neutron activation analysis. *Helv. Paediatr. Acta*, **28**, 165–174.

100. Becroft, D.M.O. (1968) Fibrocystic disease of the pancreas in New Zealand. *NZ Med. J.*, **68**, 113–119.

101. Feingold, J., Hennequet, A., Jehanne, M. *et al*. (1974) Fréquence de la fibrose kystique de pancreas en France. *Ann. Genet.*, **17**, 257–259.

102. Bernheim, M., Monnet, P., Jeune, M. *et al*. (1961) La maladie fibro-kystique des parenchymes glandulaires. Etude génétique de 41 familles. *Pediatrie*, **16**, 17.

103. Gilly, R., Hermier, M., Robert, J.M. *et al*. (1971) Etude génétique de la mucoviscidose. *Arch. Fr. Pediatr.*, **28**, 49–63.

104. Nielsen, E.L. (1972) Cystic fibrosis: incidence in Denmark. *Acta Paediatr. Scand.*, **61**, 377.

105. Bossi, A., Battistini, F., Magno, E.C. *et al*. (1999) Registro Italiano Fibrosi Cistica: 10 anni do attivita. *Epid. Prev.*, **23**, 5–16. (Translated by C. Tilley).

106. Levin, S. (1963) Fibrocystic disease of the pancreas, in *The Genetics of Migrant and Isolate Populations*, (ed. F. Goldschmidt), Williams and Wilkins, Baltimore.

107. Wright, S.W. and Morton, N.E. (1968) Genetic studies on CF in Hawaii. *Am. J. Hum. Genet.*, **20**, 157–169.

2

Basic molecular genetics

G. SANTIS

Introduction	27	Origin of *CFTR* gene mutations and heterozygote		
Positional genetics and the identification of the cystic		advantage		37
fibrosis gene	27	Molecular pathology of cystic fibrosis		37
The structure of the CF gene (*CFTR*) and its promoter	30	Prenatal diagnosis and screening for heterozygote		
CFTR: structure, function and regulation	32	detection		39
Cellular localization of the CFTR mRNA and protein	33	Animal models		41
CF (*CFTR*) gene mutations	35	References		42

INTRODUCTION

Cystic fibrosis (CF) is one of the most common lethal genetic disorders affecting Caucasian populations, particularly those of northern European origin. A large number of population studies, some dating back almost 50 years, have shown that CF is an autosomal recessive disorder[1]. However, the identification of the CF gene had to await the development of an entirely new approach in the study of genetic diseases. This approach, known as reverse or positional genetics, makes no prior assumptions about the pathogenesis of the disease. It involves the use of restriction fragment length polymorphisms (RFLPs) to screen DNA obtained from families with two or more affected individuals in order to establish the chromosomal localization of the disease locus or loci. This approach has been greatly facilitated by the identification of polymorphic markers that span the whole of the genome and the use of automated systems that allow for rapid DNA analysis. Chromosomal localization allows the characterization of the physical and genetic map of the region and the step-by-step search for sequences that are candidates for the gene in question. Identification of candidate genes is followed by analysis of their nucleotide sequence in order to characterize disease-specific mutations. This has proved highly successful in identifying the gene responsible for CF, partly because of the clear-cut definition of the disease pheno-type and the availability of large, multigenerational families with more than one affected individual. CF was one of the first diseases to be characterized at the molecular level by this approach. The search for the CF gene is therefore described in some detail.

POSITIONAL GENETICS AND THE IDENTIFICATION OF THE CYSTIC FIBROSIS GENE

The isolation of the genes responsible for genetic diseases such as the hemoglobinopathies, α_1-antitrypsin deficiency, phenylketonuria and other inborn errors of metabolism was facilitated by knowledge of the amino-acid sequence of the protein that is defective in these disorders. Because the basic biochemical defect in CF was unknown, research was directed initially towards the identification of the protein that, when abnormal, causes CF. Candidate proteins included the ciliary dyskinesia factor found in the serum; the sodium inhibitory factor, which was isolated from the saliva of CF patients[2]; and the CF antigen, a protein encoded by a gene localized on chromosome 1[3]. None of these proteins proved to be the primary products of the CF gene. Other approaches to the identification of the CF gene included cytogenetic studies to look for chromosomal abnormalities, and linkage studies looking for nonrandom association between CF and different blood groups, HLA-antigens and conventional protein markers[4,5]. None of these studies provided clues for the chromosomal localization of the CF gene.

Rapid advances in molecular biology provided powerful new approaches to the analysis of genetic diseases, including CF, where the basic biochemical defect is unknown. By 1986, these new strategies were employed successfully in the identification of the defective genes for Duchenne muscular dystrophy[6], chronic granulomatous disease[7] and retinoblastoma[8]. However, the search for the primary defect in CF posed an additional degree of complexity. Unlike Duchenne muscular dystrophy, chronic granulomatous disease and retinoblastoma, where deletions and/or translocations focused the search to specific chromosomal regions, in CF no such clues were available. Despite these enormous difficulties, the CF gene was localized to the long arm of chromosome 7 in 1985[9-13] and was finally cloned and sequenced in 1989[14,15].

The first step in the attempt to identify the primary defect in CF was to establish the chromosomal localization of the disease locus. This approach, known as reverse or positional genetics, requires the use of DNA markers defined by RFLPs[16,17] and sequence polymorphisms defined by variable numbers of tandem and dinucleotide repeats[18,19]. The search for the CF locus involved the use of RFLPs to screen DNA obtained from families with two or more affected CF individuals. This was facilitated by the relatively clear-cut diagnostic definition of CF and the availability of a large number of CF families. Although RFLP markers covering a significant portion of the human genome were screened, the initial results were negative. In 1985, linkage was demonstrated between CF and the polymorphic markers D7S15[9,10], MET[11], D7S8[12] and COL1 A2[13], all known to be on chromosome 7. These results established unequivocally that the CF locus was on the long arm of chromosome 7, between bands 22 and 31. By looking at recombination events between CF and these linked markers in a panel of 100 CF families with two or more affected children, the order between these markers and the CF locus was established[20].

Following the localization of the CF gene to chromosome 7, and the isolation of the flanking markers MET and pJ3.11, a number of strategies were employed to identify the CF gene. One approach was to attempt to isolate the CF gene directly, by looking for sequences that are preferentially expressed in cultured epithelial cells. cDNA copies of these transcripts could then be used as radioactively labeled probes to look for hybridization with DNA fragments from flow-sorted chromosome 7 libraries[21].

A second broad strategy was to define the physical map of the region between flanking markers MET and pJ3.11, and to look for sequences that were candidates for the CF gene. The task of moving from the genetic map of the region to the precise molecular definition of the disease was a very formidable one because of the physical distance involved. For example, the region between MET and pJ3.11 was thought to represent 5000 kb of DNA sequence. A region of this size could contain as many as 100–200 genes. The development of novel techniques for cloning and resolving large DNA fragments facilitated the search for the CF locus. Chromosome walking, which utilizes the end of one clone to re-screen a recombinant library (constructed by partial digestion of DNA) in order to identify an overlapping clone, was used to clone and analyze DNA fragments as large as 100 kb. However, regions of DNA can be encountered which are difficult to cross, either because that part of the genome cannot be cloned into a vector, or because it contains many repetitive sequences. Because of these problems, and because chromosome walking can be time consuming, chromosome jumping was developed. In this approach, total DNA is partially digested and then circularized so that fragments that are distant from each other when the DNA is linear are brought close together. By this approach, jumps as great as 400–500 kb can be achieved successfully. The ability to link DNA molecules at great distances from each other was also facilitated by the development of pulse-field gel electrophoresis and the discovery of restriction enzymes that cut human DNA at rare sites. By digesting total DNA with these enzymes, it is possible to obtain large DNA fragments. These can be separated by subjecting them to an electric field whose orientation is changed periodically during electrophoresis. By altering the orientation of the current, differently sized DNA fragments alter their direction of movement according to their size, making it possible to resolve DNA fragments of 100–1000 kb in size. These fragments can then be analyzed by conventional hybridization techniques. These new molecular cloning techniques were successfully applied in the search for the CF gene.

The successful strategy involved the saturation cloning of large numbers of DNA markers from the 7q31 region of chromosome 7[14,21,22]. New probes were tested for associated RFLPs useful in genetic linkage analysis. By looking for recombination events between the CF locus and the new probes, it was possible to construct a restriction map of the region, and to localize the CF locus with respect to a number of closely linked markers[21,22] (Fig. 2.1). In order to clone and sequence the large DNA region separating the CF locus from its closely linked markers, each one of these was used as the starting point for a series of chromosome walking and jumping experiments. The orientation of markers cloned from the various jumps and walks was defined by restriction mapping and pulse-field gel electrophoresis. By this approach, a large contiguous stretch of DNA was cloned and searched for the CF gene. The first step was to analyze the cloned DNA for candidate coding sequences by looking for cross-species hybridization. This involved

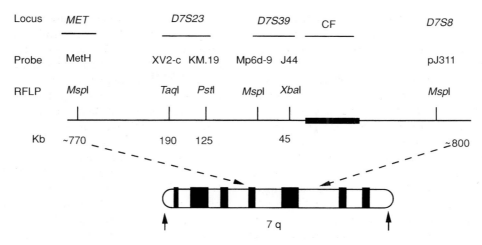

Fig. 2.1 *RFLPs linked to the cystic fibrosis gene on chromosome 7q.*

the use of cloned genomic DNA as hybridization probes to screen rodent, bovine, mouse and chicken genomic DNA. A positive signal indicates that the DNA fragment used as a probe is conserved among different species, and that it is therefore a potential coding sequence. Another feature of human genes is that they may be preceded by a region of DNA that is rich in the nonmethylated dinucleotide CpG[23]. The methylation status of CpG-rich regions of DNA is examined by digesting it with the restriction enzymes *Hpa*II and *Msp*I. Unmethylated regions are digested by both enzymes, in contrast to methylated regions, which are only digested by *Msp*I.

By screening cloned DNA fragments for conserved sequences, and by determining, when appropriate, the methylation status of these sequences, a number of candidate genes were identified[14]. Two of these putative coding sequences were excluded from further analysis on the basis of genetic data showing that they mapped to a different region of chromosome 7 from the CF gene[14].

The DNA segments that revealed sequence conservation were then tested for RNA hybridization. In these experiments, the conserved fragments were used as hybridization probes to screen cDNA libraries of various tissues[14,15]. After screening multiple cDNA libraries with a DNA segment that was shown to be conserved, and whose nucleotide sequence included an unmethylated CpG-rich region, a single clone was isolated from a cDNA library constructed from cultured sweat gland cells of a non-CF individual. By using this cDNA clone as a probe, a 6.5 kb transcript was then obtained from the T84 colon cancer cell line (this cell is known to express the chloride conductance that is associated with CF)[15]. Transcripts of identical size were also obtained from pancreas, lung, cultured epithelial cells from sweat glands, nasal polyps, liver, parotid and placenta. No hybridization signal was detected in the brain, the adrenal gland, skin fibroblast or lymphoblast cell lines[15]. This pattern of expression of the candidate CF gene was

in full accordance with the concept of CF as a disease affecting predominantly epithelial cells.

By screening a variety of cDNA libraries with the original cDNA clone, a total of 18 additional clones were isolated, and their nucleotide sequence determined[15]. The nucleotide sequences of the 5′ and 3′ ends of the transcript, which were not isolated by the hybridization experiments, were determined by using anchored polymerase chain reaction (PCR)[15]. The complete cDNA sequence spanned 6129 base pairs and contained an open reading frame capable of coding a polypeptide of 1480 amino acids. The universal start site, AUG, was present at the beginning of the transcript and it corresponded to the first methionine residue of the candidate polypeptide. The deduced amino-acid sequence of the candidate CF gene cDNA indicated that the gene product was part of a family of transmembrane proteins that are involved in the transport of substances across the cell membrane. This putative protein was named as the CF transmembrane conductance regulator, or CFTR[15].

In order to provide additional support that this was indeed the CF gene, Riordan and colleagues compared the cDNA sequences derived from normal and CF individuals[15]. A 3 base pair deletion was identified which would result in the loss of a phenylalanine residue at position 508 (ΔF_{508}) in CF but not in normal individuals[15,24]. By screening DNA obtained from CF patients and from normal individuals, it was found that the mutation accounted for 68 per cent of CF chromosomes analyzed[24]. None of the normal chromosomes studied carried the ΔF_{508} mutation, suggesting that this alteration in the *CFTR* coding sequence was disease causing, and not a sequence polymorphism. Final proof that the correct gene had been identified was provided almost 1 year later, when it was shown that the expression of the normal *CFTR* cDNA in CF epithelial cells resulted in the correction of the chloride transport defect that is characteristic of CF epithelial cells[25,26].

THE STRUCTURE OF THE CF GENE (*CFTR*) AND ITS PROMOTER

The whole genomic sequence of the *CFTR* gene was identified by using overlapping cDNA clones as hybridization probes, to screen recombinant phage and cosmid libraries[14]. The orientation of DNA fragments isolated by this approach, and their relationship to the physical map of the region, revealed that the *CFTR* gene spans approximately 250 kb of nucleotide sequences, a much larger region of DNA than was previously anticipated[14].

Following the isolation of the genomic DNA segments corresponding to the cDNA clones, the nucleotide sequence of the exons, and of the exon–intron boundaries was then determined. Initial analysis identified a minimum of 24 exons, spanning 6.5 kb of nucleotide sequence[14]. However, after more detailed restriction mapping of the genomic DNA segments, the number of exons has been revised to a total of 27[27]. Moreover, exons 6, 14 and 17 are interrupted by previously unknown noncoding sequences. Because of these intronic sequences within the above three exons, exons 6, 14 and 17 are now referred to as exons 6a/b, 14a/b and 17a/b. Exon 13 was the largest of the 27 exons, encompassing a total of 724 base pairs, whereas exon 14b is the smallest (38 base pairs)[27]. Despite these new findings, the size of the open reading frame, and of the total number of amino-acid residues it encodes, are as reported in reference[14].

The sequence of the *CFTR* coding region predicted a polypeptide of a molecular mass of 168 138 Da[15]. The most striking feature of the predicted protein was that it contained two repeated motifs, each containing a membrane-spanning domain and a hydrophilic region which showed sequence similarities to the nucleotide-binding domains (NBD) of membrane-bound transport proteins[15] (Fig. 2.2). Each of the membrane-spanning domains consisted of six hydrophobic regions capable of spanning a lipid bilayer, and composed of 234 amino acids[15] (Fig. 2.2). Ten of the 12 transmembrane regions contained one or more amino acids with charged side chains, a feature of at least two known channels[15]. The two hydrophilic domains consisted of approximately 150 amino acids each[15]. The phenylalanine residue deleted in the most common mutation is in a region of the first NBD which shares significant homology with other nucleotide-binding proteins[15]. The two symmetrical motifs of the putative protein are separated by a highly charged cytoplasmic domain, named the regulatory, or R domain[15] (Fig. 2.2). This domain, which is encoded by exon 13, contains 9 of the 10 consensus sequences for phosphorylation by protein kinase A (PKA), and seven of the binding sites for protein kinase C[15]. Most of the sequence of the protein is predicted to be either intracytoplasmic, or tightly bound to the membrane[15]. A small

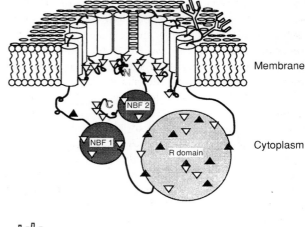

N-linked CHO

▲ Potential site for phosphorylation by protein kinase A

▽ Potential site for phosphorylation by protein kinase C

Fig. 2.2 *Structure of the CFTR protein and its relationship to the plasma membrane.*

region of the protein, between transmembrane domains 7 and 8, contains two potential glycosylation sites, and is predicted to be exposed to the exterior surface[15]. Although the two halves of the protein are similar in structure, the sequence identity between them is only modest. This observation indicates that the two halves of *CFTR* did not arise from duplication of a single gene. The organization of the 27 exons, and their relationship to the proposed domains of the protein is shown in Fig. 2.2.

The nucleotide sequence of the coding region of the *CFTR* gene shared sequence homology with a group of membrane-bound proteins which are involved in the transport of molecules across membranes[15]. The transmembrane domains and the nucleotide-binding folds are shared by all members of this superfamily of proteins, whereas the R domain is unique to *CFTR*. The presence of ATP- binding sites suggests that hydrolysis is involved in the transport function of *CFTR*, whereas the large number of possible phosphorylation sites suggest that *CFTR* might be regulated by covalent modulation. Since most of the protein is orientated towards the cytoplasm, it was thought likely that regulation was by means of cytosolic factors.

Cross-species analysis of the DNA sequence encoding *CFTR* shows significant conservation in structure between the human CFTR cDNA and its bovine, mouse, rat and dogshark homologs[29-32]. There is 90 per cent sequence homology between the bovine and human CFTR cDNA[28] and 76 per cent sequence homology between the mouse and human molecules[29]. There is striking conservation in the sequences encoding the first, second, fifth, sixth, eleventh and twelfth transmembrane domains (95–100 per cent), and to a lesser extent in the sequences encoding the two nucleotide-binding folds. Both potential glycosylation sites are preserved in the mouse, rat, bovine and dogshark CFTR cDNAs[28-31]. Although the sequences encoding the R domain in human, cow, mice and dogshark show significant differences, there is preservation of almost all the serine residues that are putative PKA-binding sites[28]. These cross-species studies support the hypothesis that the transmembrane domains, the nucleotide-binding folds and the R domain are functionally important, and that the function of CFTR may be similar in evolutionarily very diverse organisms. The sequence conservation between human and shark CFTR is remarkable considering that sharks predate in evolutionary terms the earliest reptiles and mammals by approximately 50 and 300 million years, respectively.

CFTR messenger RNA (mRNA) and protein show a pattern of expression *in vivo* that is highly regulated both spatially and temporally, and which varies depending on the species. Spatial expression of CFTR is mainly restricted to epithelial cells in the lung, intestine, pancreas, gallbladder, kidney, salivary and sweat glands, testis and uterus. In these tissues, only a subpopulation of cells may express CFTR. In the lung, the predominant site of expression is in a subpopulation of cells in the submucosal glands. In the rat intestine, a decreasing gradient of expression on the crypt–villus and proximal–distal axis was noted. The expression of the CFTR mRNA is also highly regulated in the rat male and female genital tract. The levels of CFTR mRNA in the endometrial lining of the rat uterus change during the estrus cycle[32]. In the testis, the abundance of the CFTR transcript varies according to the cycle of the seminiferous epithelium[33]. The regulation of expression of CFTR in the uterus was investigated further by inducing ovulation in immature female rats[34]. The administration of gonadotropin hormones to these animals was associated with an increase in the levels of CFTR mRNA and protein, which suggests that CFTR expression in the female reproductive tract is regulated by estrogens[34]. The effect of estrogens on CFTR expression is probably tissue specific, since expression of CFTR in the respiratory tract and intestine remained unchanged during the estrus cycle in female rats[35]. The complexity of the mechanisms regulating expression of CFTR was demonstrated from a study of CFTR expression during differentiation of intestinal cell lines[36]. A tenfold increase in the level of CFTR mRNA was found during differentiation of Caco-2 and HT-29 intestinal cell lines, which was independent of enhanced CFTR gene transcription. This indicates that CFTR mRNA stabilizing factor(s) were responsible for the increased CFTR mRNA levels. Despite higher CFTR mRNA levels, the amount of CFTR protein in differentiated cells was lower than in undifferentiated cells,

indicating that CFTR expression is also under post-translational control[36].

The basal CFTR promoter has been identified as a 250 bp fragment upstream of the ATG translation start codon. Its structure suggests regulatory characteristics that are consistent with the CFTR gene belonging to a group of genes that have characteristics of 'housekeeping genes', but in addition have tissue-specific functions[37-40]. The suggestion that the CFTR gene may be a housekeeping gene is based on five observations:

1. there was no TATA or CAAT box element within the first 500 base pairs upstream of the major transcription start site;
2. the GC content of the promoter region was high, averaging 65 per cent of the first 500 base pairs;
3. in addition to the major transcription start site, multiple minor transcription start sites were also identified;
4. a number of potential SP1 binding sites were identified;
5. the level of expression of the CFTR gene within bronchial epithelium was found to be low.

Determination of the nucleotide sequence of the CFTR promoter of eight mammalian species, representing four different orders, indicates great divergence in sequence conservation in *cis*-transcriptional regulatory elements between two groups:

- one that includes human, nonhuman primates, cow and rabbit (nonrodent); and
- the second group that includes rodents[41].

The promoter region of the CFTR gene also contains sequences that suggest that CFTR could be under transcriptional regulation. Deletion and mutation analysis of the proximal promoter of the human CFTR gene suggest that basal expression and cAMP-mediated transcription depend on an inverted CCAAT sequence, located between 132 and 119 nucleotides upstream of the translational start site[42]. Members of the C/EBP and activating transcription factor/cyclic AMP response-element-binding protein families bind to this element and may contribute to the transcriptional regulation of the CFTR gene. Potential AP-1 and AP-2 binding sites have been identified, as well as candidate sequences for cAMP and glucocorticoid response elements[43]. Regulation of CFTR mRNA expression by the AP-1 nuclear transcription factor was demonstrated when phorbol myrisate acetate (PMA), which is known to induce AP-1, was added to the colon carcinoma cell line T84, and caused a reduction in the rate of transcription of the CF gene[39]. Moreover, reduction of CFTR mRNA in the T84 cell line was associated with the development of a defect in chloride secretion consistent with defective CFTR function[43].

Regulatory sequences that confer tissue-specific and regulated levels of CFTR expression have yet to be characterized. Multiple DNase-I hypersensitive sites, which in general correlate with open chromatin structure *in vivo*, have been identified 5′ to *CFTR* or within the first intron. A putative regulatory element, at 181 + 10 kb within the first intron, was identified as a DNase-I hypersensitive site that is present in cells that express *CFTR* but is absent in cells that do not[44]. This element is thought to be functional because it binds to DNA-binding proteins, as determined by gel mobility assays and DNase-I footprinting, and because it enhances *CFTR* expression when used in transient expression systems[44]. The functionality of this element in transgenic mice was not determined. Using DNase-I hypersensitive site mapping in tissues, combined with phylogenetic mapping, four conserved DNase-I hypersensitive sites were defined[45]. Two of these, at −1.3 and −0.1 kb relative to the initiation codon, correspond to a PMA-response element (TRE) and a nonconsensus cAMP-responsive element (CRE), respectively[45]. Additional DNase-I hypersensitive sites that are nonconserved and appear to regulate *CFTR* expression in rodents were also defined. Some of these correspond to regions of purine–pyrimidine strand asymmetry that may be of physiological significance in the regulation of *CFTR* expression[45]. When a large (310 kb) yeast artificial chromosome (YAC) that contains the intact human *CFTR* gene (270 kb) and approximately 50 kb of 5′ DNA was transfected in Caco-2 cells that constitutively express *CFTR*, a copy-number-dependent expression was observed. This indicates that the YAC clone contains all the regulatory elements that confer full levels of expression[46]. It is unclear, however, whether all high-order regulatory elements are present in this clone, as spatial and temporal expression in mice was not assessed[46].

CFTR gene transcription initiation start sites, including a major one, were described in human cells in culture[37-39]. However, their precise location was not consistent in all studies. Transcription initiation start sites were also determined in primary human and mouse tissues, which could be a more accurate assessment of the *in vivo* regulation of transcription than experiments performed in long-term cell culture systems[47]. These experiments demonstrated a distinct, tissue-specific pattern of transcription start-site usage. In humans, different tissue-specific start sites, leading to the production of *CFTR* transcripts that differ in the length of the 5′ untranslated region were observed, predominantly in the adult and fetal lung[47]. In the mouse, there was variation in the length of the murine CFTR mRNA along the length of the intestine, with different start sites being utilized in the ileum and duodenum[47]. In the mouse, a novel 5′-untranslated exon of murine *CFTR* was identified[47]. This is confined to the testis, it represents more than 95 per cent of *CFTR* transcripts in this tissue and may have an important role in the function of *CFTR* in the testis, or in the regulation of its expression.

CFTR: STRUCTURE, FUNCTION AND REGULATION

CFTR is an ATP-dependent Cl^- channel that mediates cAMP-mediated Cl^- secretion by epithelia, predominantly those in the pancreas, airway and intestine. Although its primary function is to mediate cAMP-mediated Cl^- secretion, it may have additional functions. Its role as a Cl^- channel was established after a series of important experiments: transfection of the normal CFTR cDNA into cultured CF airway and pancreatic epithelial cell lines[25,48] corrected their chloride permeability defect, which confirmed CFTR as the protein that is defective in CF. Transfection of nonepithelial cell lines with the normal CFTR cDNA resulted in a plasma-membrane chloride conductance that was stimulated by cAMP[49,50]. Since chloride conductance was conferred to cells that do not normally have such membrane function, and as these cells do not normally express *CFTR*, it was argued that CFTR is a chloride channel and not a regulator of chloride channels[49,50]. This was demonstrated conclusively by Bear and colleagues who showed that purified CFTR reconstituted in a lipid bilayer functioned as a 9–10 pS chloride channel[51].

Protein kinase A (PKA) is the primary activator of CFTR Cl^- channels in humans[52,53]. Protein kinase C (PKC) also stimulates CFTR Cl^- channels, although it is much less potent than PKA[54,55]. Other, non-PKA kinases may also regulate CFTR[56]. Tissue-specific expression of alternative kinases may contribute to the variability of the steady-state open probability of CFTR when it is expressed in various cell types[56]. Phosphorylation alone is insufficient to open CFTR channels. Nucleotides are also required, probably in order to allow hydrolysis at one of the two nucleotide-binding folds. Membrane-associated phosphatases probably dephosphorylate CFTR once cAMP stimulation is removed, resulting in falls in chloride secretion[56].

The function of the various domains of the CFTR protein, and the regulation of its chloride-channel activity have been investigated in detail. The two membrane-spanning domains are thought to represent the pore of the channel. This is based on *in vitro* mutagenesis experiments in which the mutation of specific charged amino acids in the transmembrane domain resulted in changes in the ion permeability of CFTR to iodide, chloride, fluoride and bromide[57]. The CFTR chloride channel is regulated by phosphorylation of the R domain and activated by the direct action of nucleoside triphosphates on phosphorylated CFTR chloride channels[52]. The R domain contains 9 of 10 serine residues which are putative sites for cAMP-dependent PKA-mediated phosphorylation[15]. By mutating four of these serines to alanines, the activation of the channel by PKA was abolished[52], whereas the partial deletion of the R domain resulted in a channel that was active without requiring PKA[58].

Prestimulation with PKC potentiates the subsequent response to PKA by enhancing its rate of activation and by increasing the fraction of time that the channel remains open (steady-state open probability)[56,59]. This effect is still observed when all strong and several weak PKA consensus sites were removed, indicating that the potentiation site is yet to be characterized. It is possible that phosphorylation by PKC alters the structural conformation of CFTR to expose neighboring sites to PKA[56,59]. This was assessed by circular dischroism spectroscopy which showed no effect of PKC on the structure of recombinant CFTR R domain[56,59]. Phosphorylation alone does not activate the CFTR chloride channel, since chloride movement requires the addition of ATP. The activation of CFTR is mediated through the direct interaction between ATP and the two NBDs, since mutagenesis of highly conserved amino acids in both NBDs altered the potency with which ATP stimulates the channel.

CFTR may have functions other than those of a small-conductance chloride channel in the apical membrane of epithelial cells:

- There is good evidence that CFTR regulates amiloride-sensitive epithelial sodium channels. Basal sodium absorption is higher in CF airway epithelial cells and, also, sodium absorption is further increased by cAMP in CF airway cells but not in normal cells[60]. This indicates that there is altered regulation of epithelial sodium channels in CF. Transfection of the three sodium-channel subunits in canine kidney cells resulted in a 30 per cent increase in amiloride-sensitive sodium transport after forskolin administration[61]. Transfection of CFTR cDNA in these cells altered their response to forskolin from stimulation to inhibition, and decreased basal sodium transport by 30 per cent[61]. The mechanism by which CFTR regulates amiloride-sensitive sodium channels remains to be elucidated.
- It has also been proposed that the CFTR channel conducts ATP, and that extracellular ATP serves as an autocrine activator of CFTR itself[62], of the outwardly rectifying Cl⁻ channels[63,64] and possibly of other transporters in the apical membrane[65]. However, the ability of CFTR to conduct ATP was questioned.
- Bradbury et al.[66] showed that endocytosis and exocytosis are defective in a CF pancreatic cell line (CFPAC), and that this defect is corrected by the expression of wild-type *CFTR*. Membrane recycling regulates the secretion and localization of proteins through and on the cell membrane. A defect in this process may have diverse effects and could explain the multiple biochemical abnormalities found in CF.
- The CFTR protein may also function as a chloride channel in intracellular compartments. For example, it has been argued that in CF there is a defect in the acidification of cells of the *trans*-Golgi network, of prelysosomes and of endosomes because of

diminished chloride conductance in the membrane of these intracellular organelles[67]. However, it has not been shown that this chloride conductance is directly mediated by CFTR.

In many epithelial cells there is heterogeneity of CFTR transcripts, which may lead to CFTR protein isoforms with potentially diverse functions. However, the functional significance of multiple CFTR transcripts is unknown, and there is no evidence that transcripts other than the full CFTR mRNA are translated into protein. Heterogeneity of CFTR transcripts occurs probably because of alternative splicing. For example, alternative splicing removes exon 9 from the full-length CFTR mRNA in nasal epithelial cells of normal individuals, in some of whom transcripts without exon 9 account for almost 88 per cent of the total mRNA[68,69]. Splicing of exon 9 from CFTR transcripts segregates with a sequence variation at the intron 8/exon 9 splice acceptor site[68,69]. Individuals with more than 50 per cent of their CFTR transcripts lacking exon 9 have five consecutive thymidines at that site, in contrast to others who have polythymidine tracts of 7 and 9[69]. Alternative splicing of exons 4 and 12 of the CFTR mRNA from non-CF individuals has also been reported, but the proportion of these alternatively spliced transcripts was not determined[70]. Removal of exon 9 from mRNA may have a regulatory function during differentiation of an intestinal epithelial cell line, but its role in other epithelial cells of normal individuals and of patients with CF is unknown[71]. These findings suggest either that the exons removed are not important for the function of the CFTR protein, or that only small amounts of normal CFTR protein are necessary to obtain a normal clinical phenotype. The latter is the most likely explanation, since all exons removed by alternative splicing encode regions of the protein that are functionally important, and are also the sites of missense mutations that cause CF. Moreover, expression of CFTR cDNA lacking exon 9 or exon 5 in HeLa cells, CFPAC cells or *Xenopus* oocytes was associated with immature, incompletely glycosylated CFTR and with lack of chloride conductance in response to cAMP[72,73]. These findings argue strongly that even abundant splice variants do not retain normal function and are unlikely to have any physiological role.

CELLULAR LOCALIZATION OF THE CFTR mRNA AND PROTEIN

The pattern of expression of the CFTR mRNA and protein in different organs has been investigated by the techniques of *in situ* hybridization and immunohistochemistry. In the human pancreas, the CFTR protein was localized predominantly to the apical surface of epithelial cells lining the intercalated ducts of the exocrine pancreas[74-76]. There was no staining of the apical membranes of acinar cells, and large ducts stained weakly at high antibody titers[74]. In the human intestine, the CFTR mRNA and protein were detected in cells lining the crypts throughout the small and large intestine, and in particular in cells at the base of the crypts. No staining was seen of cells on the luminal surface of the colon[32,74–76]. The CFTR protein was localized to the apical membrane of these cells[74–76]. In the human sweat gland, staining with monoclonal antibodies was most pronounced on the apical membrane of the reabsorptive duct, with very little staining on the secretory coil[74]. CFTR was also localized in the basolateral membrane of the inner cell layer of the duct[77]. In the human liver, high levels of expression of the CFTR mRNA were detected exclusively in epithelial cells lining the bile duct[77]. In the salivary gland, CFTR protein was localized to the apical membrane of a subpopulation of epithelial cells lining the intralobular ducts, which is thought to be the site of active salt reabsorption[74]. In the human airway, CFTR mRNA was detected in the surface epithelium, the ciliated and collecting ducts and the serous ducts of the submucosal glands[78]. The highest levels of expression of the CFTR mRNA were detected in the serous tubules, in a minority of cells in the ciliated and collecting ducts, but not in the surface epithelium[78]. Immunolocalization studies confirm expression of the CFTR protein predominantly in the serous tubules of the submucosal glands and in a small proportion of cells of the surface epithelium, as well as the ciliated and collecting ducts[78]. In the bovine trachea, CFTR immunoreactivity is localized at the apical membrane of the surface epithelium[79]. However, in the bovine submucosal glands, CFTR shows intracytoplasmic localization, probably in the membrane of secretory vesicles[79].

The pattern of expression of CFTR mRNA in rat tissue was similar to the pattern of expression observed in human tissues. For example, CFTR mRNA is expressed in ductal cells in the pancreas and submandibular glands, in the crypts of the small and large intestine, in the epithelium lining the uterus and in the seminiferous tubules[33]. Expression in the seminiferous tubules is stage specific, which led to the suggestion that CFTR plays an important role in spermatogenesis[33]. Expression of the CFTR mRNA in the mucosa and submucosa of the bronchi and bronchioles was at low levels, and in agreement with the levels of expression reported in human airway tissues[33]. In contrast, the level of expression of the CFTR mRNA in rodent pancreas and submandibular gland was much lower than in human tissues[74].

Expression of the *CFTR* gene and protein in human fetal tissues was detected by reverse transcription PCR, by *in situ* hybridization and by immunohistochemistry. CFTR mRNA was detected in hepatocytes and myocardial cells by week 8 of gestation[80,81], in the surface epithelium of the trachea and bronchi from week 11 of gestation, and in pancreatic ducts from week 12 of gestation[80–83]. In the pancreas, CFTR mRNA was present in precursor duct cells early in gestation, and in centroacinar and ductal cells at later stages, resembling CFTR expression in the adult pancreas[83,84]. In the intestine, CFTR expression was seen in progenitor cells of the intestinal crypt, with decreasing gradient of expression along the crypt–villous axis, again as seen in the corresponding adult tissues[83,84]. In the developing liver, CFTR expression was confined to epithelial cells lining the bile duct and ductules and the gallbladder[83]. No expression was detected in hepatocytes[83]. By week 30 of gestation, CFTR was also localized to the apical domain of ciliated cells in the developing glands in the airway[80]. There was a decreasing gradient of expression of CFTR mRNA from the proximal to the distal pulmonary epithelium[82,83,84], whereas alveolar type II cells from second-trimester human lung tissue expressed the CFTR transcript in culture. This suggested that alveolar type II cells secrete chloride and therefore lung fluid, which was consistent with the secretory properties of the human fetal lung[82]. Expression of CFTR mRNA in trachea and large bronchi was diffuse in the first trimester but became more restricted at later stages[83]. The relatively high levels of CFTR expression in fetal lung were in marked contrast to the low levels of CFTR expression in adult lung. The age at which downregulation of CFTR mRNA occurs is unknown, as is the relationship between this event and the change of the airway epithelium from a chloride-secreting into a sodium-absorbing tissue. Expression of CFTR was detected in the fetal epididymis at week 18 of gestation, but at lower levels than in the intestine[81,83,84]. No expression was detected in the first- and second-trimester female reproductive tissues[83]. Amounts of CFTR mRNA in pancreatic epithelial cells, lung and intestine were similar to those detected in respective tissues from non-CF fetuses[81].

Studies on the cellular localization of CFTR in different species, combined with knowledge of the electrophysiology of cells expressing CFTR and with knowledge of CF pathology, have provided important insight into the function of CFTR in different tissues. The detection of CFTR mRNA in ductal cells in the pancreas and submandibular glands, which are the main sites for chloride and fluid reabsorption, along with the localization of CFTR in the crypts of the intestine, supports the notion that in these cells, CFTR functions as a bidirectional chloride channel. The very low levels of expression of CFTR mRNA in the villi of the intestine, coupled with evidence that the characteristics of chloride channel in guinea-pig villi are not those of CFTR[85], indicate that fluid absorption in the intestine, in contrast to secretion, is not mediated by CFTR. In the absorptive duct of the sweat gland, CFTR was localized not only to the apical but also to the basolateral membrane of the epithelial cells, which is in agreement with electrophysiological data[86]. The low levels of expression in human and rodent airway surface epithelium, and the much higher expression in the submucosal glands, questions the current notion that the airway epithelium is primarily responsible for the development of lung disease in CF. Expression of CFTR not only in the male genital duct but also in the seminiferous tubules suggests an explanation for the abnormal spermatozoa reported in CF patients[33]. Although the expression of CFTR mRNA in the rat uterus is highly regulated[32,33], the precise function of CFTR in this tissue remains unknown. Finally, the localization of CFTR in the membrane of secretory vesicles in bovine submucosal glands in the airway is currently the only immunohistochemical evidence that CFTR may have an intracellular function[79].

CF (*CFTR*) GENE MUTATIONS

Prior to the identification of the *CFTR* gene, extensive haplotype associations between closely linked DNA markers and the CF locus indicated that CF was caused by a small number of mutations[22,24]. For example, a single mutation was thought to account for the disease in the majority of CF patients of northern European origin, whereas a separate mutation was thought to be prevalent in the southern European populations. Additional haplotype data, from different ethnic groups such as the African–American CF population, indicated that there may be several other mutations specific to these ethnic groups[87].

Following the cloning of the CF gene, the sequence of overlapping cDNA clones derived from normal and CF individuals was compared. Sequence analysis revealed a 3 bp deletion which would result in the loss of a phenylalanine residue at position 508 of the putative protein[15]. This mutation was identified on 68 per cent of French Canadian CF chromosomes, but none of the normal chromosomes tested[24]. Following the identification of this mutation, extensive screening of various CF populations worldwide has confirmed that it is the most common disease-causing mutation[88]. However, the frequency of the ΔF_{508} differs significantly among various ethnic groups[88]. The highest frequency was reported from Denmark, where the ΔF_{508} mutation accounts for 82 per cent of CF chromosomes, whereas the lowest frequency was found in Algeria, where it accounts for only 26.3 per cent of the CF chromosomes analyzed. In northern Europe, the overall frequency is approximately 71 per cent, whereas in southern Europe it varies from 45 to 55 per cent[88].

Extensive, worldwide efforts have since identified an unexpectedly large number of mutations, in both northern and southern European CF chromosomes[89]. By convention, mutations are named by using the single-letter code for the normal and mutant amino acids. For example, N1303K is a substitution of a lysine (N) by an asparagine (K) residue at codon 1303 of the CFTR cDNA. Mutations producing a termination codon are indicated by an X. Frame-shift and splice-junction mutations are indicated by their location relative to the numbered nucleotide sequence of the *CFTR* gene. A number of large, or complex deletions, such as the deletion of exons 4–7 and 9–13 have been identified. Mutations are distributed throughout the gene (Fig. 2.3).

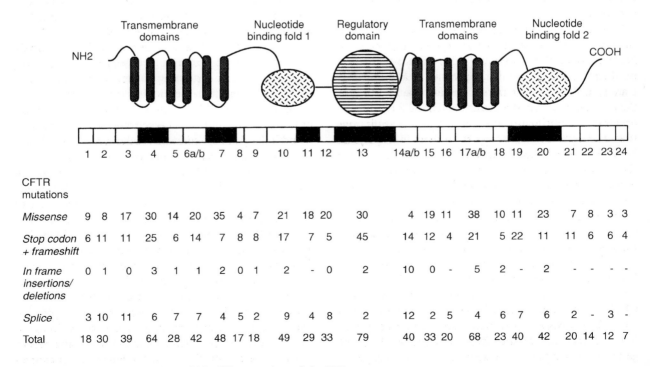

CFTR mutations	1	2	3	4	5	6a/b	7	8	9	10	11	12	13	14a/b	15	16	17a/b	18	19	20	21	22	23	24
Missense	9	8	17	30	14	20	35	4	7	21	18	20	30	4	19	11	38	10	11	23	7	8	3	3
Stop codon + frameshift	6	11	11	25	6	14	7	8	8	17	7	5	45	14	12	4	21	5	22	11	11	6	6	4
In frame insertions/ deletions	0	1	0	3	1	1	2	0	1	2	-	0	2	10	0	-	5	2	-	2	-	-	-	-
Splice	3	10	11	6	7	7	4	5	2	9	4	8	2	12	2	5	4	6	7	6	2	-	3	-
Total	18	30	39	64	28	42	48	17	18	49	29	33	79	40	33	20	68	23	40	42	20	14	12	7

Fig. 2.3 *Distribution of mutations within different regions of the CFTR gene.*

Although the overall frequency worldwide of mutations other than the ΔF_{508} mutation is extremely low, some of the rare alleles appear to segregate with specific ethnic groups[90]. The distribution of 272 CF mutations were studied by assessing the origin of 27 177 CF chromosomes from 29 European countries and three countries from North Africa[90]. The most common mutations were: ΔF_{508} (66.8 per cent), G542X (2.6 per cent), N1303K (1.6 per cent), G551D (1.5 per cent) and W1282X (1.0 per cent). There is wide distribution of mutations, suggesting an ancient origin. Some mutations are extremely common in selected ethnic populations. The most striking example is the W1282X mutation that accounts for 36.2 per cent of CF chromosomes in the Ashkenazi Jewish population in Israel[90,91] and is also relatively common in Mediterranean countries and northern Africa (mean frequency 6.1 per cent). The N1303K mutation is found in most of the Western and Mediterranean countries and is particularly common in Tunisia, where it accounts for 17.2 per cent of the CF alleles[90]. The G542X mutation is also common in Mediterranean countries[90] and the 621 + 1 G→T mutation which accounts for 23 per cent of French Canadian CF chromosomes[92]. In African–American and Asian populations, the frequency of non-ΔF_{508} mutations occurring in 11 exons of the *CFTR* gene is the same as in Caucasian CF patients, which indicates that the high incidence of CF in populations of European origin is due to the high frequency of the ΔF_{508} mutation[93]. Some mutations are relatively common in specific geographic regions[90].

The majority of missense mutations affect highly conserved residues of the gene, predominantly those coding for the putative nucleotide-binding folds of the CFTR protein. Missense mutations are probably more informative than other mutations in terms of defining important functional domains of CFTR. For example, there is a cluster of 11 missense mutations in one region of exon 11 that spans only five codons. This region is in the first NBF, termed motif C, which appears to be a unique feature of the ATP transporters[94]. The fact that this represents a mutation 'hot spot' suggests that ATP binding or hydrolysis is probably critical for CFTR function. Missense mutations occur less commonly in the second NBF, including the region corresponding to the putative motif C of the first NBF[89]. This indicates that the functional importance of the first and second NBFs may be different. There is also a missense mutation 'hot spot' in exons spanning the first transmembrane domain, in particular exons 4, 7 and 17b. Mutations in this region, which is thought to correspond to the pore of the CFTR Cl⁻ channel, would be expected to cause changes in ion conductivity. A large number of mutations also occur in exon 13 which encodes the putative R domain of the protein. The R domain contains multiple potential phosphorylation sites for cAMP-dependent protein kinase A (PKA). So far, there is absence of CF-causing mutations affecting these phosphorylation sites.

By altering single amino acids, missense mutations are associated with a protein that is of normal size but functions abnormally. In contrast, nonsense and frame-shift mutations are expected to result in either absent or truncated, nonfunctioning protein. Evidence for this was provided by reverse transcription PCR of mRNA obtained from airway epithelial cells from a CF patient homozygous for two nonsense mutations in the *CFTR* gene. CFTR mRNA was undetectable by this method, which suggests absence, or severe reduction of CFTR protein in the airway epithelium[95]. Splice mutations, which will be expected to result in abnormal splicing of the pre-mRNA, represent the minority of the mutations identified so far. The majority of these splice mutations are predicted to cause disease because they alter either the acceptor or donor splice sites at the intron–exon boundaries. Direct evidence for aberrant splicing was shown for two putative mutations, the Q1291H mutation, which results in the substitution of histidine for a glutamine residue in exon 20[96], and for the 717 + 1 G→T mutation, which results in a threonine residue instead of a glycine residue at position + 1 of the splice donor site of intron 5[97].

All but one of the known *CFTR* mutations occur either within one of the exons or at one of the intron–exon boundaries of the *CFTR* gene. The exception is a mutation found deep within intron 20 of the *CFTR* gene, which creates a new splice acceptor site and results in aberrant splicing of exon 21[89].

Despite extensive molecular studies, a number of CF chromosomes in various populations remain uncharacterized. Ferec *et al.*[98] and Fanen *et al.*[99] used denaturing gradient gel electrophoresis (DGGE) to screen all 27 exons and the intron–exon boundaries of the *CFTR* gene of 191 and 105 French CF patients, respectively. Ferec *et al.*[98] characterized 98 per cent of CF chromosomes studied, and Fanen *et al.*[99] defined the molecular defect in 88 per cent of the CF chromosomes analyzed. Fanen *et al.*[99] also screened a region spanning 225 nucleotides upstream of the first methionine codon of the *CFTR* gene, without identifying mutations or polymorphisms in that region. Similar results were also reported by Gasparini and colleagues[100], who determined the nucleotide sequence of 90 per cent of the *CFTR* gene, and of the corresponding intron–exon boundaries, in eight southern European CF patients who lacked the ΔF_{508} mutation on both of their CF chromosomes. These findings suggest that CF may be caused by mutations in the promoter region of the *CFTR* gene, in distant regulatory sequences or in one of the introns. Linkage disequilibrium data in the southern European populations suggest that promoter mutations may be common, since the highest association with CF was shown with polymorphic markers located to the 5′ region of the *CFTR* gene[101].

The extensive sequence analysis of the *CFTR* gene has revealed a number of polymorphisms. A total of 69 sequence variations have been reported, 40 of which are within the coding region, two are in the 5′ untranslated region, and the remainder within introns of the *CFTR* gene (CF Genetic Analysis Consortium). Of the 40 sequence variations affecting sequences in the coding region of the gene, 19 do not alter the encoded amino acid, whereas the remainder result in a conservative amino-acid substitution. In addition to these polymorphisms, a number of repetitive DNA elements, and a number of simple sequence repeats, have also been identified[101,102].

ORIGIN OF *CFTR* GENE MUTATIONS AND HETEROZYGOTE ADVANTAGE

The stark difference in the relative frequency of ΔF_{508} in the different populations was addressed by a number of studies. Kerem and colleagues[24] found a strict association of the ΔF_{508} mutation with a single extended linked marker haplotype, which suggested that the mutation occurred only once. Analysis of ΔF_{508} carrying CF chromosomes in Europe showed significant association between the ΔF_{508} mutation and the B haplotype, as defined by the polymorphic markers XV-2c and KM.19, which supports the theory of a single origin for this mutation[103]. Additional support for this hypothesis was provided by the finding of an association between the ΔF_{508} mutation and a single haplotype for three intragenic polymorphic markers[104], and the finding that a dimorphic 4-base pair tandem repeat (GATT) at the 3′ end of intron 6 was in absolute linkage disequilibrium with the ΔF_{508} mutation[102]. The most comprehensive analysis of the evolution and age of the mutation was based on analysis of chromosomes from 15 European countries, using three intragenic CFTR microsatellites (IVS8CA, IVS17BTA and IVS17BCA)[105]. These microsatellites, or short tandem repetitive polymorphic sequences, are due to additions or deletions of nucleotides. The evolution of such microsatellites from the ancestral haplotype in which a mutation occurred provides a valuable tool for the study of the origin and evolution of a given mutation. Analysis of the intragenic and extragenic markers flanking the ΔF_{508} mutation suggest that it had a single origin[105]. By constructing a parsimony tree and by calculating the number of mutations necessary to generate the number of different haplotypes, it has been proposed that the ΔF_{508} mutation occurred a minimum of 52 000 years ago, and probably before 173 000 years ago. This is in contrast to previous estimates based on recombination frequencies of extragenic markers, which estimated the age as 2940–5200 years[106]. These are based on whole CF population and not on ΔF_{508} chromosomes as the microsatellite study, which may account for the different estimates. The ancestral population is thought to be genetically distinct from present European populations[105]. It was also proposed that the mutation was introduced to Europe at different periods, the first during the Paleolithic period[105]. Two other CFTR mutations, G542X and N1303K, may also have occurred on the same microsatellite haplotype as the ΔF_{508} mutation, presumably in the same geographic region[107].

It has been estimated that in the absence of ΔF_{508}, CF would have been observed at a frequency of 1 in 30 000 children. The high frequency of the ΔF_{508}, and the single origin of this mutation, suggest that the high prevalence of CF in the Caucasian population may be due to heterozygote advantage. Alternative explanations such as a strong founder effect, high mutation rate, meiotic drive and genetic drift have not received significant support and have been discarded or excluded[108].

Selective advantage might be conferred at the individual, gamete or gene level. At the gene level it may be conferred by the mutations themselves, or by a separate gene in close linkage to the CF gene and its mutations. The proposed age of the ΔF_{508} mutation suggests that a selective advantage must exist at least for chromosomes bearing the ΔF_{508} mutation[105]. This is because the time required to lower the frequency of a recessive lethal allele from any high value in the absence of a selective advantage to its present frequency of 1.4 per cent is much less than the estimated minimum age of the ΔF_{508} mutation[105]. Several hypotheses have been proposed to account for the CF heterozygote selective advantage. These include resistance to pulmonary tuberculosis[109], resistance to influenza[110] and resistance to cholera[108,111]. Resistance to cholera represents the only hypothesis that links the heterozygote selective advantage to the known physiological function of the CFTR protein (CFTR functions as a small-conductance chloride channel in epithelia, in particular those in the lung, pancreas and intestine)[56]. This hypothesis was tested in the CF exon 10 replacement mouse models ('null' mutant mouse) which express no functional CFTR. These studies provided conflicting results[112,113]. In one study, a direct correlation was found between fluid and Cl⁻ secretion in response to cholera toxin and the number of each CFTR allele in each mouse[112]. In contrast, the Cl⁻ secretory responses of colonic and ileal epithelia in normal and CF heterozygote mice to multiple secretagogues, including cholera toxin, were similar[113]. It is possible that most advantage is conferred by ΔF_{508} CFTR. Alternatively, the association of ΔF_{508} and at least three other relatively common mutations with the same intragenic haplotype may indicate that selective advantage might be conferred by the genetic background on which the mutations arose[104]. Recently resistance to typhoid has been suggested as a heterozygote advantage. One study of reproductive advantage gave equivocal results.

MOLECULAR PATHOLOGY OF CYSTIC FIBROSIS

The molecular mechanisms by which mutations in the *CFTR* gene disrupt the function of CFTR as a membrane-bound cAMP-regulated chloride channel are now being unraveled. It is now established that CFTR is glycosylated first in the endoplasmic reticulum and then in the Golgi, from which it is ultimately transported to the plasma membrane[26,114]. In the endoplasmic reticulum, the glycosylated form of wild-type CFTR undergoes an ATP-dependent conformational change in order to become stable before it exits the endoplasmic reticulum and becomes further glycosylated in the Golgi[115]. This process is inefficient, with only 20–25 per cent of immature CFTR achieving the stable form and being transported to the plasma membrane. In contrast, ΔF_{508} mutation was shown to be processed abnormally and retained in the endoplasmic reticulum[116]. ΔF_{508} was shown to remain associated with at least two chaperones, Hsp70 and calnexin, which prevent proteins from folding inappropriately during processing[117,118]. ΔF_{508} rarely matures into a stable form and is degraded by the ubiquitin–proteosome system in the endoplasmic reticulum[119,120]. This observation was demonstrated in heterologous cells overexpressing the protein and in native epithelia. An investigation of the cellular localization of CFTR in tissues obtained from CF patients with various CFTR genotypes found no CFTR at the apical membrane of the absorptive part of the sweat duct of CF patients who are homozygous for the ΔF_{508} mutation, or compound heterozygotes for the ΔF_{508}, 621 + 1 G→T and 171 + 1 G→A mutations[74]. In tissues obtained from normal individuals and from CF patients with the ΔF_{508}/G551D genotype, CFTR was correctly localized to the apical membrane of the reabsorptive part of the sweat duct[74]. Similar observations were made when the localization of normal and mutant CFTR in the airway of CF patients was investigated[78]. These findings are in complete agreement with other *in vitro* studies and are thought to represent the molecular basis for the ΔF_{508} defect. The findings have important implications. If no CFTR is correctly localized in the epithelial cells of most CF patients, therapeutic measures aimed at stimulating or correcting the function of the protein will not succeed. In such patients, therapy will therefore need to be directed towards the replacement or bypassing of the protein. The hypothesis that cells from most CF patients lack mature CFTR at its correct cellular location also raises the possibility of novel approaches to CF therapy, such as the development of drugs that can promote intracellular transport of CFTR. Recent studies showed that blocking the ubiquitin-directed degradation pathway failed to overcome the ΔF_{508} processing defect[119,120], while treatment with the chemical chaperone, glycerol, was shown to overcome it[121].

The success of such an approach assumes that mutant CFTR such as ΔF_{508}-CFTR, retains functional activity. Some *in vitro* studies suggest that ΔF_{508}-CFTR is able to function as a chloride channel, but less efficiently than wild-type CFTR. It has been shown that ΔF_{508}-CFTR overexpressed in Vero cells reaches the plasma membrane, but at markedly lower amounts than wild-type CFTR[122] and that in ΔF_{508}-CFTR transfected Vero cells there was a cAMP-activated chloride channel which remained closed a greater proportion of the time than the wild-type CFTR channel[122]. When ΔF_{508} and wild-type CFTR mRNA was introduced into *Xenopus* oocytes, comparable chloride currents were generated[123]. However, the doses of forskolin and isobutylmethylxanthine (IBMX) required to induce these currents were much higher for the mutant than for the wild-type CFTR[123]. This would suggest that ΔF_{508}-CFTR would not function normally in CF epithelial cells, even if the processing defect described above is rectified. However, others have shown that the ΔF_{508}-CFTR chloride-channel activity is indistinguishable from that of wild-type CFTR and that, in the endoplasmic reticulum, wild-type CFTR and ΔF_{508}-CFTR form functional chloride channels[124,125]. Based on these findings, it now appears that the structural alterations that cause ΔF_{508}-CFTR to be retained in the endoplasmic reticulum do not drastically alter channel function.

Although abnormal processing represents the most common mechanism by which *CFTR* gene mutations disrupt CFTR function, some mutations cause CF by alternative mechanisms. Frame-shift and stop-codon mutations result in truncated or absent CFTR protein. Some missense mutations in the first transmembrane region generate the mature, fully glycosylated form of CFTR and are presumably transported to the plasma membrane like wild-type CFTR[123]. Expression of these mutations in Fischer rat thyroid epithelial cells resulted in regulated, cAMP-stimulated chloride-channel activity[123]. However, chloride current generated by these channels was lower than that generated by wild-type CFTR[123]. These mutant CFTR channels, like wild-type CFTR channels, were regulated by phosphorylation and intracellular nucleotides. However, they displayed reduced pore properties that impaired chloride efflux through the channel, but retained their chloride selectivity[123]. Another transmembrane mutant, R347H, functioned as a single-ion pore, unlike wild-type CFTR which functions as a multi-ion pore, containing many chloride ions at once[126].

The bioelectric properties of two NBF1 mutant CFTR proteins, A455E and P547H, which are associated with pancreatic sufficiency and mild lung disease, provide additional insight into the molecular pathology of CF[127,128]. These mutants formed regulated chloride channels in epithelia, generated reduced amounts of apical chloride current, but did not disrupt the function of individual chloride channels. The A455E and P547H are, however, incorrectly processed; mature protein constitutes only 10–15 per cent of the total[128]. However, the amount of mature protein produced by these mutants is greater than that of ΔF_{508}[128]. Using immunohistochemistry and confocal microscopy, P574H protein was present on the apical surface of Vero cells at levels that were between that of wild-type CFTR and ΔF_{508}[127].

Proline residues located in membrane-spanning domains of transport proteins, like CFTR, are thought to play a structural role. The transmembrane regions of CFTR contain four prolines which are conserved among different species. Mutations of two of these prolines, P99L and P205S, are associated with CF. By mutating these residues, it was shown that proline 205 is critical for CFTR folding and that proline 99 contributes to the Cl⁻ channel pore[129].

These molecular mechanisms explain how various CFTR mutations alter normal CFTR function and processing and provide a partial explanation of the variable clinical phenotype associated with CF. However, lung disease, the major determinant of morbidity and mortality in CF, does not correlate with CF genotype or chloride function. Some studies suggest a correlation between another chloride channel, a calcium-activated channel and disease activity in CF mice[130]. CF mutations may have effects on CFTR functions other than its role as a small-conductance chloride channel, in particular its role as a regulator of other chloride channels[61]. It has been shown so far that the A455E mutation, which is associated with pancreatic sufficiency and less-severe lung disease, is able to regulate outwardly rectifying chloride channels (ORCCs)[131]. In contrast, the G551D mutation, which is associated with pancreatic insufficiency, failed to regulate ORCCs, raising the possibility that the severity of lung disease may depend more upon the regulatory function of CFTR than its chloride function[131].

PRENATAL DIAGNOSIS AND SCREENING FOR HETEROZYGOTE DETECTION

Prenatal diagnosis

Prior to the cloning of the *CFTR* gene, genetic counseling of couples with an affected child with CF used indirect DNA diagnosis with RFLP markers in linkage disequilibrium with the CF gene[132]. For these studies, parents must be heterozygous for an RFLP, and DNA from an affected individual must be available. By identifying polymorphic markers which were very tightly linked to the CF gene, prenatal diagnosis in informative families was at least 98 per cent accurate[133]. Diagnostic error was due to recombination between the polymorphic marker and the CF locus. After the identification of a large number of *CFTR* gene mutations, it is now possible to provide direct and accurate detection of CF fetuses. DNA from at-risk fetuses is obtained from chorionic villus samples (commonly between the eleventh and twelfth weeks of gestation) or amniotic fluid cells (usually at 16 weeks of gestation). In a limited number of studies to date, most couples with no positive family his-

tory of CF choose to terminate a pregnancy if a fetus with CF is identified.

For some couples, therapeutic abortion of a CF fetus is not an option. Under these circumstances, it is possible to use *in vitro* fertilization techniques to establish the CF status of eight-cell embryos *in vitro* by single-cell aspiration and PCR amplification of DNA, and then fertilize only those embryos that lack one or two copies of the parental *CFTR* mutations[134].

Heterozygote detection (see also Chapter 9)

The development of tests that identify the major mutation associated with CF raised the possibility of using this technology for large-scale population based screening for CF. This led to considerable debate on the merits of screening the population for CF heterozygotes, on the most appropriate way to implement such a program, and on the optimal time to institute it.

Initial policy documents by the National Institutes of Health[135] suggested that carrier screening should only be instituted if 90–95 per cent of mutations can be detected. Combining detection of the ΔF_{508} with other mutations common to specific ethnic groups, it appears that there are several populations for which 95 per cent sensitivity can now be achieved with existing technology. These include Ashkenazi Israeli populations[91], Celtic Britons[98], French Canadians from Quebec and some native Americans. In Denmark, where the ΔF_{508}-CFTR mutation accounts for 82 per cent of CF chromosomes, analysis of selected exons of the *CFTR* gene by single-strand conformation polymorphism (SSCP) identified 90.5 per cent of mutations[136], whereas in north-west England, a similar detection rate was achieved by screening for known CFTR mutations in exons 4, 10, 11, 20 and 21[137]. In unselected populations in northern Europe and North America, lower detection rates (82–90 per cent) have been reported. By detecting 85 per cent of CFTR mutations, it will be possible to identify 72 per cent of couples at risk. For couples in whom only one of the two partners tests positive, the risk for CF in their first offspring would be approximately 1 in 600.

In certain populations, detection rates have proved significantly lower. In Hispanics, the detectable alleles account for only 57 per cent of all CFTR mutations in this population, while in African–Americans the detection rate is approximately 75 per cent. In Asian–Americans, in whom the carrier rate is very low (1 in 90), only 30 per cent of alleles can be identified. In southern European populations, systematic examination of some, or all exons of the *CFTR* gene identified only 60 per cent of CFTR mutations[90]. It is unlikely that the sensitivity of mutation analysis would substantially improve by screening for an expanded number of mutations, because these are rare and unlikely to account for a significant proportion of uncharacterized CF alleles.

Genetic testing, as part of research programs, has so far been offered to the general public as well as in the prenatal and antenatal context. Screening programs aimed at identifying CF heterozygotes in the general population separate the test from any immediate decisions concerning reproduction, allowing for unpressured informed reproductive decisions in the future. This could also be a disadvantage, since the information provided to those screened might not be retained, and therefore not utilized when reproductive decisions are taken. Concern has also been expressed that such an approach will not reach a broad range of the population and might be biased towards uptake by the educationally and socially advantaged[138]. Testing during pregnancy might be associated with higher uptake, and provides information when it is of immediate relevance, thus minimizing the risk of misinformation. The major disadvantage of this approach is that it offers very limited time for reflection at what is already a time of stress.

Studies so far suggest that uptake of genetic screening by the general population is variable[139–141]. Rates of acceptance are higher when young adults near reproductive age are targeted and when offers are made by personal invitation[139–141]. Offers made by mail or leaflet were associated with the lowest uptake[139–141]. The most satisfactory results were obtained when offers of participation in genetic education and testing were offered to pregnant women and those with positive family history of CF[141,142]. Even under these circumstances, uptake was variable, with acceptance of offers for testing varying from 50 per cent to up to 78 per cent. There are multiple reasons offered for refusal to take up genetic testing. These include personal views on the moral basis of abortion, the sensitivity of the test, convenience, and when relevant, the cost of the test and its potential impact on health insurability. In addition, psychological reasons such as reluctance to know the outcome in individuals with a positive family history also influence decision making. Positive reasons for accepting participation include autonomy and informed decision-making in the event of the fetus being shown to be affected by CF.

In the prenatal testing context, two models were assessed. In sequential screening, women are screened first and their partners are tested only if the women are found positive for a CF allele. In couple screening both partners are tested at the same time and are reported to be 'high risk' only if both results are positive. A number of studies, including a randomized trial of stepwise versus couple screening, addressed the merits of these approaches[138, 140–146]. There were modest differences in anxiety levels experienced by the participants[144]. With sequential screening, there was anxiety during the period when women who had tested positive awaited their partner's results[144]. Couple screening allowed carriers to avoid transient levels of anxiety, but was associated with more anxiety and false reassurance among most screeners who tested negative[144]. Women screened by the sequential method were found to be significantly better informed on the implications of the test and the significance of being a single gene carrier than the counterparts tested by the couples method. Overall, sequential screening and couple screening proved efficient, relatively trouble free and 'consumer friendly'[140].

In an early pilot study, based at the Simpson Memorial Maternity Pavilion, Edinburgh, 3165 of 4384 pregnant women attending antenatal clinics for the first time were screened[138]. Six mutations were screened (for ΔF_{508}, R117H, R553X, G542X, G551D, 621 + 1 G→T), accounting for 85 per cent of CFTR mutations in Scottish CF chromosomes. A total of 111 CF heterozygotes were identified among the 3165 pregnant women analyzed. Partners were only screened if the woman tested positive. When both partners were found to be heterozygotes for a CFTR mutation, prenatal diagnosis was offered. Of the 110 male partners screened, four were found to be positive. All four couples opted for prenatal diagnosis, which identified one ΔF_{508} homozygote fetus and three unaffected fetuses. The woman carrying the CF fetus opted for termination. Preliminary cost–benefit analysis suggested that this model for prenatal screening for CF is cost effective. After 5 years, 25 000 couples were tested in the setting, initially as part of a research program and then routinely[142]. Uptake of the sequential and couple models was similar, at 70 per cent. There was no change in the rates of acceptance once screening moved from research to a routine basis[142]. Twenty-two high-risk couples (both parents were found to be CF heterozygotes) were identified through screening, of which 20 (91 per cent) opted for prenatal diagnosis[142]. Eight affected fetuses were identified; in all, pregnancy was terminated. Similar outcomes, over shorter periods, were reported by others, demonstrating that screening programs achieve their intended result[142].

The short- and long-term psychological impact of population-based carrier testing for CF is being systematically assessed[147]. No difference was found in the degree of general anxiety, reproductive intentions, behavior between carriers and screen-negative individuals at 3 years. Carriers had a poorer perception of their health than non-carriers, despite being told that that the carriers status did not adversely affect their health. In the long term, retention of the meaning of the test results from CF screening was poor. Understanding the limitations of the test because of its failure to identify all CF mutations was shown to be poor, irrespective of the method used.

National Institutes of Health consensus development statement on genetic testing for cystic fibrosis

An independent consensus development panel of medical and health policy experts was convened by the National Institutes of Health to provide healthcare professionals, patients and the general public with a responsible assessment of optimal practice for genetic testing for cystic fibrosis[141]. Its key conclusions and recommendations were:

1. The goal of genetic testing is to provide individuals with information that will permit them to make informed decisions.
2. CF genetic testing should be offered to adults with a positive family history of CF, to partners of people with CF, to couples currently planning a pregnancy and to couples seeking prenatal care.
3. Offering CF genetic testing to the general population or to newborn infants is not recommended.
4. Access to genetic testing in the prenatal setting enhances the ability of couples to make reproductive choices. The cost is reasonable in relation to the benefits obtained.
5. Comprehensive educational programs for healthcare professionals and the public were recommended. Accurate counseling services should be provided.

ANIMAL MODELS (see also Chapter 4)

The cloning and characterization of the mouse gene equivalent to human CFTR gene[29] has allowed the development of mouse models of CF. The coding region of the mouse CFTR gene shows significant sequence homology to the human CFTR cDNA, and in particular to the regions encoding the two nucleotide-binding folds, to the R domain and to many of the potential protein kinase A and protein kinase C phosphorylation sites[29].

Initially, three independent groups produced, almost simultaneously, mouse models which mimic many important features of CF[148–150]. The murine models of CF were generated from an embryonic stem cell line in which the mouse CFTR gene was disrupted at exon 10. The targeted cell lines were injected into blastocysts and transferred into pseudopregnant female mice in order to obtain chimeric animals. Mice homozygous for the disrupted exon 10 were generated by mating chimeric animals capable of germ-line transmission of the defective CFTR gene. Although these animal models share important features with the human disease, there are also clear differences between them. The murine model generated by Snouwaert et al. (replacement or 'null' mutant mouse) is characterized by failure to thrive, bowel obstruction resembling meconium ileus, alteration of mucous and serous glands in the bowel, nasal mucosa and submaxillary glands, and gallbladder disease[149]. There was no evidence of pancreatic or pulmonary involvement, and male mice had normal vas deferens and were fertile[149]. The lethal phenotype of these mice was corrected by expression of human CFTR under the control of the rat intestinal fatty acid binding protein promoter[151]. These mice survived and showed functional correction of ileal goblet cell and crypt cell hyperplasia[151]. Nasal, tracheal and intestinal epithelial cells from the homozygous mutant mice had no cAMP-mediated chloride response, in contrast to chloride responses to triphosphate nucleotides and calcium, which were preserved[152]. CF murine and intestinal epithelia exhibited Na$^+$ hyperabsorption, providing evidence of a strong link between CFTR and Na$^+$ channel activity in airway and intestinal epithelia[153–155]. These investigators also observed upregulation of Ca^{2+}-mediated chloride secretion and argued that this may buffer the severity of airway disease in CF mice[130]. The CF mouse oviduct epithelium exhibited defective cAMP but not Ca^{2+}-mediated Cl$^-$ secretion[156]. Similar findings were observed in CF mice epididymides and seminal vesicles, which led to the speculation that the fertility of male CF mice and normal oviduct function may be due to functioning Ca^{2+}-mediated Cl$^-$ secretion[157]. The severe intestinal obstruction that was characteristic of the exon 10 'null' mice was also observed in two other CF mouse models; one that was generated by the introduction of a termination codon mutation in exon 2 of the CF gene[158] and another that was constructed by duplication of exon 3[159].

The murine model described by Dorin et al. differs from that of Snouwaert et al. in several respects. The bioelectric properties of the exon 10 insertional mutant mouse demonstrate reduced cAMP-related Cl$^-$ secretion throughout the respiratory and intestinal tracts both in vivo and in vitro; calcium-related Cl$^-$ secretion that is preserved in the airways but is reduced in the intestine; and increased amiloride response and a more negative nasal potential difference compared to wild-type animals. These findings suggest that the exon 10 insertional mutant mouse displays most of the bioelectric properties of humans with CF, apart from sodium absorption, which, in contrast to humans, it is not increased in the small intestine and is reduced in the trachea of these mice[160]. Post-mortem histological analysis of homozygous mutant mice showed colonic dilatation with abnormal mucus accumulation, dilatation of the salivary glands, mucin accumulation in the vas deferens, focal pulmonary atelectasis, but no pancreatic or pulmonary disease in all or most of the animals analyzed[148]. Although there was no overt pulmonary disease, the mucociliary transport velocity in the trachea was significantly lower in these mutant mice than in normal animals. In addition, there was an increase in the number of inflammatory cells in the lamina propria of mutant mice, implying that these may represent early alterations in the lung that precede infection[161]. In contrast to the mouse model described by Snouwaert et al.[149], the mice generated by Dorin et al. had no overt clinical disease and thrived normally up to 30 days postpartum. This variation in phenotype probably reflects the different strategies employed by the two groups. Snouwaert et al.

disrupted the mouse *CFTR* gene by using a replacement vector to insert a neomycin gene and to create an in-frame stop-codon mutation in exon 10[149]. In contrast, Dorin *et al.* used an insertional vector to introduce a duplication of DNA sequence spanning intron 9 and exon 10[148]. The normal exon 10 was retained, thus allowing for the production of wild-type CFTR mRNA by alternative splicing. In fact, trace levels of normal message were detected by multiplex RNA polymerase chain reaction in mice homozygous for the disrupted exon 10, which is compatible with the expression of very low levels of residual wild-type protein[119]. These observations are of relevance to future treatment strategies in humans, because they suggest that small amounts of wild-type CFTR might have major clinical benefit.

Mice carrying the most common CF mutation, ΔF_{508}, were also generated[150,162,163]. Mutant animals showed pathological and electrophysiological changes compatible with CF. The animals died of peritonitis and showed deficient cAMP-activated Cl$^-$ secretion. These mice showed normal ΔF_{508} mRNA levels in all tissues studied and demonstrated the temperature-sensitive transport defect first described for the human ΔF_{508}. The biophysical characteristics of the mutant channel were not significantly different from normal.

Mice carrying another common CF mutation, G551D, were also generated[164]. These mice displayed a phenotype that resembled the human disease. In contrast to null mice, the G551D mice had reduced risk of intestinal obstruction. Electrophysiological studies showed a level of CFTR-related chloride conductance that was intermediate between that of 'null' and the insertional exon 10 mutant mice[164].

Although murine models of CF demonstrate many of the important features of the human disease, they differ in two important respects. Pancreatic disease is absent in all mutant mice, in contrast to CF patients who are homozygous for stop-codon or frame-shift mutations and in whom pancreatic insufficiency is a universal finding[165]. CFTR mRNA and protein are found at low levels in the murine pancreas, in contrast to humans, where *CFTR* is expressed in the pancreas at high levels[74]. These observations suggest that CFTR is functionally less important in the murine than in the human pancreas. Male CF patients are infertile because of bilateral vasal aplasia, in contrast to the great majority of male mice homozygous for the 'null' mutation which have normal vas deferens and are fertile[148–150]. The basis for this difference is unclear, but may be accounted for by normal Ca^{2+}-mediated Cl$^-$ secretion in the 'null' CF mice epididymides and seminal vesicles[157].

The development of murine models of CF will be of enormous value in the evaluation of novel therapies aimed at curing or arresting the progression of CF, and will facilitate our understanding of the pathogenesis of the disease. For example, the observation that mutant mice develop a meconium ileus-like illness in the absence of pancreatic disease has led to re-evaluation of the etiology of meconium ileus in humans. The relative contribution of the airway surface epithelium and of the submucosal glands to the development of lung disease in CF patients is a subject of controversy. The nature of lung pathology found in the murine models of CF will address this question, since the mouse lower respiratory tract is devoid of submucosal glands.

REFERENCES

1. Danks, D.M., Allan, J. and Anderson, C.M. (1965) Genetic study of fibrocystic disease of the pancreas. *Am. J. Hum. Genet.*, **28**, 323–356.
2. Mangos, J.A., McSherry, N.R. and Benke, P.J. (1967) A sodium inhibitory factor in the saliva of patients with cystic fibrosis of the pancreas. *Pediatr. Res.*, **1**, 436–442.
3. Dorm, J.R., Novak, M. and Hill, R.F. *et al.* (1987) A clue to the basis defect in cystic fibrosis from cloning the CF antigen gene. *Nature*, **326**, 614–617.
4. Goodchild, M.C., Edwards, J.H. and Glenn, K.P. (1976) A search for linkage in CF. *J. Med. Genet.* **13**, 417–419.
5. Polypenidis, A., Ludwig, H. and Gotz, M. (1973) CF and HLA antigens. *Lancet*, **ii**, 1452.
6. Monaco, A.P., Neve, R.L., Colletti-Feener, C., *et al.* (1986) Isolation of candidate cDNAs for portions of the Duchenne muscular dystrophy gene. *Nature*, **323**, 646–650.
7. Royer-Pokora, B., Kunkel, L.M., Monaco, A.P. *et al.* (1986) Cloning the gene for an inherited human disorder – chronic granulomatous disease – on the basis of its chromosomal localisation. *Nature* **322**, 32–37.
8. Friend, S.H., Bernards, R., Rogelj, S. *et al.* (1986) A human DNA segment with properties of the gene that predisposes to retinoblastoma and osteosarcoma. *Nature*, **323**, 64–46.
9. Tsui, L.-C., Buchwald, M., Barker, D. *et al.* (1985) Cystic fibrosis locus defined by a genetically linked polymorphic DNA marker. *Science*, **230**, 1054–1057.
10. Knowlton, R.G., Cohen-Haguenauer, O., Nguyen, V.C. *et al.* (1985) A polymorphic DNA marker linked to cystic fibrosis is located on chromosome 7. *Nature* **318**, 380–382.
11. White, R., Woodward, S., Leppert, M. *et al.* (1985) A closely linked genetic marker for cystic fibrosis. *Nature*, **318**, 382–384.
12. Wainwright, B., Scrambler, P., Schmidtke, J. *et al.* (1985) Localisation of the cystic fibrosis locus to human chromosome 7 cen-q22. *Nature*, **318**, 384–385.
13. Scambler, P.J., Wainwright, B., Farrall, M. *et al.* (1985) Linkage of COLIA 2 collagen gene to cystic fibrosis and its clinical implications. *Lancet*, **ii**, 1241–1242.
14. Rommens, J.M., Iannuzzi, M.C., Kerem, B.-S. *et al.* (1989) Identification of the cystic fibrosis gene: chromosome walking and jumping. *Science*, **245**, 1059–1065.

15. Riordan, J.R., Rommens, J.M., Kerem, B.-S. *et al*. (1989) Identification of the cystic fibrosis gene: cloning and characterisation of complementary DNA. *Science*, **245**, 1066–1073.

16. Kan, Y.W. and Dozy, A.M. (1978) Polymorphism of DNA sequence adjacent to the human β-globin structural gene: relation to sickle mutation. *Proc. Natl Acad. Sci., USA*, **75**, 5631.

17. Botstein, D., White, R., Scolnick, M. and Davis, R.W. (1980) Construction of a genetic linkage in man using restriction fragment length polymorphisms. *Am. J. Hum. Genet.*, **32**, 314.

18. Nakamura, Y., Leppert, M., O'Connell, P. *et al*. (1987) Variable number of tandem repeat (VNTR) markers for human gene mapping. *Science*, **235**, 1616–1622.

19. Weber, J.L. (1990) Informativeness of human dinucleotide (dC–dA)n. (dC–dT)n polymorphisms. *Genomics*, **7**, 524–526.

20. Beaudet, A., Bowcock, A., Buchwald, M. *et al*. (1986) Linkage of cystic fibrosis to two tightly linked DNA markers: joint report from a collaborative study. *Am. J. Hum. Genet.*, **39**, 681–693.

21. Tsui, L.-C., Rommens, J.M., Burns, J. *et al*. (1988) Progress towards cloning the cystic fibrosis gene. *Phil. Trans. R. Soc. Lond.*, **319**, 263–273.

22. Rommens, J.M., Zengerlin, S., Burns, J. *et al*. (1988) Identification and regional localisation of DNA markers on chromosome 7 for the cloning of the cystic fibrosis gene. *Am. J. Hum.Genet.*, **43**, 645–663.

23. Bird, A. (1986) CpG-rich islands and the function of DNA replication. *Nature*, **321**, 209–213.

24. Kerem, B.-S., Rommens, J.M., Buchanan, J.A. *et al*. (1989) Identification of the cystic fibrosis gene: genetic analysis. *Science*, **245**, 1073–1080.

25. Drumm, M.L., Pope, H.A., Cliff, W.H. *et al*. (1990) Correction of the cystic fibrosis defect *in vitro* by retrovirus mediated gene transfer. *Cell*, **62**, 1227–1233.

26. Gregory, R.A., Cheng, S.H., Rich, D.P. *et al*. (1990) Expression and characterisation of the cystic fibrosis transmembrane conductance regulator. *Nature*, **347**, 382–386.

27. Zielinski, J., Rozmahel, R., Bozon, D. *et al*. (1991) Genomic DNA sequence of the cystic fibrosis transmembrane conductance regulator. *Genomics*, **10**, 214–218.

28. Diamond, G., Scanlin, T.F., Zasloff, M.A. and Bevins, C.L. (1991) A cross-species analysis of the cystic fibrosis transmembrane conductance regulator. *J. Biol. Chem.*, **266**, 22761–22769.

29. Tata, F., Stanier, P., Wicking, C. *et al*. (1991) The mouse homologue of the cystic fibrosis gene. *Genomics*, **10**, 298–299.

30. Fiedler, M.A., Nemecz, Z.N. and Shull, G.E. (1992) Cloning and sequence analysis of the rat cystic fibrosis transmembrane conductance regulator. *Am. J. Physiol.*, **262**, L779–L784.

31. Grzelczak, A., Dubel, S., Alon, N. *et al*. (1990) A highly conserved cystic fibrosis gene homologue is expressed in the salt-secreting shark rectal gland. *J. Cell. Biol.*, **111**, 310(A).

32. Trezise, A.E.O., Linder, C.C., Grieger, D. *et al*. (1993) *CFTR* expression is regulated during both the cycle of the seminiferous epithelium and the oestrous cycle of rodents. *Nature Genet.*, **3**, 157–164.

33. Trezise, A.E.O. and Buchwald, M. (1991) *In vivo* cell-specific expression of the cystic fibrosis transmembrane conductance regulator. *Nature*, **353**, 434–437.

34. Rochwerger, L. and Buchwald, M. (1992) Stimulation of *CFTR* expression by oestrogens *in vitro*. *Pediatr. Pulmonol. Suppl.*, 25A.

35. Tizzano, E.F., Trezise, A.E.O., Rochwerger, L. *et al*. (1992) Characterisation of *CFTR* expression in rat tissues during embryogenesis and estrous cycle. *Pediatr. Pulmonol.*, **8**, 247A.

36. Sood, R., Bear, C., Auerbach, W. *et al*. (1992) Regulation of CFTR expression and function during differentiation of intestinal epithelial cells. *EMBO J.* **11**, 2487–2494.

37. Chou, J.L., Rozmahel, R. and Tsui, L.-C. (1993) Characterization of the promoter region of the cystic fibrosis transmembrane conductance regulator gene. *J. Biol. Chem.*, **266**, 24271–24476.

38. Koh, J., Sferra, T.J. and Collins, F.S. (1993) Characterization of the cystic fibrosis transmembrane conductance regulator propmoter region. Chromatin context and tissue-specificity. *J. Biol. Chem.*, **268**, 15912–15921.

39. Yoshimura, K., Nakamura, I., Trapnell, B.C. *et al*. (1991) The cystic fibrosis gene has a 'housekeeping' promoter and is expressed at low levels in cells of epithelial origin. *J. Biol. Chem.*, **266**, 9140–9144.

40. Denamur, E. and Chehab, F.F. (1995) Methylation status of CpG sites in the mouse and human CFTR promoters. *DNA Cell Biol.*, **14**, 811–815.

41. Vuillaumier, S., Kaltenbock, B., Lecointre, G., Lehn, P., Denamur, E. (1997) Phylogenetic analysis of cystic fibrosis transmembrane conductance regulator gene in mammalian species argues for the development of a rabbit model for cystic fibrosis. *Mol. Biol. Evol.*, **14**, 372–380.

42. Mathews, R.P. and McKnight, G.S. (1996) Characterization of the cAMP response element of the cystic fibrosis transmembrane conductance regulator gene promoter. *J. Biol. Chem.*, **271**, 31869–31877.

43. Trapnell, B.C., Zeitlin, P.L., Chu, C.-S. *et al*. (1991) Down-regulation of the cystic fibrosis gene mRNA transcript levels and induction of the cystic fibrosis secretory phenotype in epithelial cells by phorbol esters. *J. Biol. Chem.*, **266**, 10319–10323.

44. Smith, A.N., Barth, M.L., McDowell, T.L. *et al*. (1996) A regulatory element in intron 1 of the cystic fibrosis transmebrane conductance regulator. *J. Biol. Chem.*, **271**, 9947–9954.

45. Vuillaumier, S., Dixmeras, I., Messai, H. *et al*. (1997) Cross-species characterization of the promoter region of the cystic fibrosis transmebrane conductance regulator gene reveals multiple levels of regulation. *Biochem. J.* **327**, 618–623.

46. Vassoux, G., Manson, A.L. and Huxley, C. (1997) Copy number-dependent expression of a YAC-cloned human CFTR gene in human epithelial cell line. *Gene Ther.*, **4**, 618–623.

47. White, N.L., Higgins, C.F. and Trezise, A.E.O. (1998) Tissue-specific *in vivo* transcription start sites of the human and murine cystic fibrosis genes. *Hum. Mol. Genet.*, **7**, 363–369

48. Rich, D.P., Anderson, M.P., Gregory, R.I. *et al*. (1990) Expression of the cystic fibrosis transmembrane conductance regulator corrects defective chloride channel regulation in cystic fibrosis airway epithelial cells. *Nature*, **347**, 358–363.

49. Anderson, M.P., Rich, D.P., Gregory, R.J. *et al*. (1992) Generation of cAMP-activated chloride currents by expression of CFTR. *Science*, **251**, 679–682.

50. Kartner, N., Hanrahan, J.W., Jensen, T.J. *et al*. (1991) Expression of the cystic fibrosis gene in non-epithelial invertebrate cells produces a regulated anion conductance. *Cell*, **64**, 681–689.

51. Bear, C.E., Li, C., Kartner, N. *et al*. (1992) Purification and functional reconstitution of the cystic fibrosis transmembrane conductance regulator (CFTR). *Cell*, **68**, 809–818.

52. Cheng, S.H., Rich, D.P., Marshall, J. *et al*. (1991) Phosphorylation of the R-domain by cAMP-dependent protein kinase regulates the CFTR chloride channel. *Cell*, **66**, 1027–1036.

53. Chang, X.-B., Tabcharini, J.A., Hou, Y.-X. *et al*. (1993) Protein kinase A still activates CFTR chloride channel after mutagenesis of all ten PKA consensus phosphorylation sites. *J. Biol. Chem.*, **268**, 11304–11311.

54. Tabcharini, J.A., Chang, X.-B., Riordan, J.R. and Hanrahan, J.W. (1991) Phosphorylation-regulated Cl− channel in CHO cells stably expressing the cystic fibrosis gene. *Nature*, **352**, 628–631.

55. Berger, H.A., Travis, S.M. and Welsh, M.J. (1993) Regulation of the cystic fibrosis transmembrane conductance regulator Cl− channel by specific protein kinases and phosphotases. *J. Biol. Chem.*, **268**, 2037–2047.

56. Hanrahan, J., Mathews, C., Grygorczyk, R. *et al*. (1996) Regulation of the CFTR chloride channel from humans and sharks. *J. Exp. Zool.*, **275**, 283–291.

57. Anderson, M.P., Gregory, R.J., Thompson, S. *et al*. (1991) Demonstration that CFTR is a chloride channel by alteration of its anion selectivity. *Science*, **253**, 202–205.

58. Rich, D.P., Gregory, R.J., Anderson, M.P. *et al*. (1991) Effect of deleting the R domain on CFTR-generated chloride channels. *Science*, **253**, 205–207.

59. Dulhanty, A. and Riordan, J.R. (1994) Phosphorylation by cAMP-dependent protein kinase causes a conformational change in the R domain of the cystic fibrosis transmembrane conductance regulator. *Biochemistry*, **33**, 4872–4879.

60. Boucher, R.C., Stutts, M.J., Knowles, M.R., Cantley, L. and Gatzy, J.T. (1986) Na+ transport in cystic fibrosis respiratory epithelia. *J. Clin. Invest.*, **78**, 1245–1252.

61. Stutts, M.J., Canessa, C.M. and Olsen, J.C. (1995) CFTR as a cAMP-dependent regulator of sodium channels. *Science*, **269**, 847–850.

62. Cantiello, H.F., Prat, A.G., Reisin, L.B. *et al*. (1994) External ATP and its analogs activate the cystic fibrosis transmembrane conductance regulator by a cyclic AMP-independent mechanism. *J. Biol. Chem.* **269**, 11224–11232.

63. Reisin, I.L., Prat, E.H., Abraham, J.F. *et al*. (1994) The cystic fibrosis transmembrane conductance regulator is a dual ATP and chloride channel. *J. Biol. Chem.*, **269**, 20584–20591.

64. Schwiebert, E.M., Egan, M.E., Hwang, T.-H. *et al*. (1995) CFTR regulates outwardly rectifying chloride channels through an autocrine mechanism involving ATP. *Cell*, **81**, 1063–1073.

65. Al-Aqwati, Q. (1995) Regulation of ion channels by ABC transporters that secrete ATP. *Science*, **269**, 805–806.

66. Bradbury, N.A., Jiling, T., Berta, G. *et al*. (1992) Regulation of plasma membrane re-cycling by CFTR. *Science*, **256**, 530–532.

67. Barasch, J., Kiss, B., Prince, A. *et al*. (1991) Defective acidification of intracellular organelles in cystic fibrosis. *Nature*, **352**, 70–73.

68. Chu, C.S., Trapnell, B.C., Murtagh, J.J. *et al*. (1991) Variable deletion of exon 9 coding sequences in cystic fibrosis transmembrane conductance regulator gene mRNA transcripts in normal bronchial epithelium. *EMBO J.*, **10**, 1355–1363.

69. Chu, C.-S., Trapnell, B.C., Curristin, S.M. *et al*. (1992) Extensive posttranscriptional deletion of the coding sequence for part of nucleotide-binding fold 1 in respiratory epithelial mRNA transcripts of the cystic fibrosis transmembrane conductance regulator gene is not associated with the clinical manifestations of cystic fibrosis. *J. Clin. Invest.*, **90**, 785–790.

70. Bremer, S., Hoof, T., Wilke, M. *et al*. (1992) Quantitative expression patterns of multi-drug-resistance P-glycoprotein (MDR1) and differentially spliced cystic fibrosis transmembrane. *Eur. J. Biochem.*, **206**, 137–149.

71. Montrose-Rafizadeh, C., Blackmon, D.L., Hamosh, A. *et al*. (1992) Regulation of cystic fibrosis transmembrane conductance regulator (*CFTR*) gene transcription and alternative RNA splicing in a model of developing intestinal epithelium. *J. Biol. Chem.*, **267**, 19299–19305.

72. Delaney, S.J., Rich, D.P., Thompson, S.A. *et al*. (1993) Cystic fibrosis transmembrane conductance regulator splice variants are not conserved and fail to produce chloride channels. *Nature Genet.*, **4**, 426–431.

73. Strong, T.V., Wilkinson, D.J., Mansoura, M.K. *et al*. Expression of an abundant alternatively spliced form of the *CFTR* gene is not associated with a cAMP activated chloride conductance. *Hum. Mol. Genet.*, **2**, 225–230.

74. Kartner, N., Augustinas, O., Jensen, T.L. *et al*. (1992) Mislocalisation of ΔF508 *CFTR* in cystic fibrosis sweat gland. *Nature Genet.*, **1**, 321–327.

75. Crawford, I., Maloney, P.C., Zeitlin, P. *et al*. (1991) Immunocytochemical localisation of the cystic fibrosis gene product, CFTR. *Proc. Natl Acad. Sci. USA*, **88**, 9262–9266.

76. Marino, C.R., Matovsic, L.M., Gorelick, F.S. and Cohn, J.A. (1991) Immunolocalisation of CFTR using a polyclonal. *J. Clin. Invest.*, **88**, 712–716.

77. Strong, T.V., Boehm, K., Watson, S.J. and Collins, F.S. (1992) Characterisation of *CFTR* expression in human tissues by in situ hybridisation. *Pediatr. Pulmonol. Suppl.*, **8**, 248A.

78. Engelhart, J.F., Yankaskas, J.R., Ernst, S.A. *et al*. (1992) Submucosal glands are the predominant site of *CFTR* expression in the human bronchus. *Nature Genet.*, **2**, 240–248.

79. Lacquot, J., Hinnrasky, J., Spilmont, C. *et al*. (1992) Immunocytochemical localisation of the cystic fibrosis gene product CFTR in tracheal submucosal secretory cells. *Eur. Resp. J.*, **5**, (Suppl. 15), 298.

80. Gailard, D., Lallemand, A., Ruocco, S. *et al*. (1992) Immunohistochemical localisation of the CFTR during human foetal development. *Eur. Resp. J.*, **5**, Suppl. 15, 298.

81. Harris, A., Chalkley, G., Goodman, S. and Coleman, L. (1991) Expression of the cystic fibrosis gene in human development. *Development*, **113**, 305–310.

82. McCray, P.B., Wohlford-Leanne, W. and Snyder, J.M. (1992) Localisation of cystic fibrosis transmembrane conductance regulator mRNA in human fetal lung tissue by *in situ* hybridisation. *J. Clin. Invest.*, **90**, 619–625.

83. Trezise, A.E.O., Chambers, J.A., Wardle, C.J., *et al*. (1993) Expression of the cystic fibrosis gene in human foetal tissues. *Hum. Mol. Genet.*, **2**, 213–218.

84. Tizzano, E.F., Chitayat, D. and Buchwald, M. (1993) Cell-specific expression of the CFTR mRNA shows developmentally regulated expression in human fetal tissues. *Hum. Mol. Genet.*, **2**, 219–224.

85. Sepulveda, F.V., Fargon, F. and McNaughton, P.A. (1991) K$^+$ and Cl$^-$ currents in enterocytes isolated from guinea pig small intestine. *J. Physiol.*, **434**, 351–367.

86. Reddy, M.M. and Quinton, P.M. (1989) Localisation of Cl conductance in normal and Cl impermeability in cystic fibrosis sweat duct epithelium. *Am. J. Physiol.*, **257**, C727–C735.

87. Cutting, G.R., Antonarakis, S.E., Buetow, K.H. *et al*. (1989) Analysis of DNA polymorphisms haplotypes linked to the cystic fibrosis locus in North American Black and Caucasian families supports the existence of multiple mutations of the cystic fibrosis gene. *Am. J. Hum. Genet.*, **44**, 307–318.

88. Cystic Fibrosis Genetic Analysis Consortium (1990) Worldwide survey of the ΔF508 mutation: report from the Cystic Fibrosis Genetic Analysis Consortium. *Am. J. Hum. Genet.*, **47**, 354–359.

89. Tsui, L.-C. (1992) Mutations and sequence variations in the cystic fibrosis (*CFTR*) gene. *Hum. Mutat.*, **1**, 392–398.

90. Estivill, X., Baucells, C. and Ramos, C. (1997) Geographic distribution and regional origin of 272 cystic fibrosis mutations in European populations. The Biomed CF Mutation Analysis Consortium. *Human Mutat.*, **10**, (2), 135–154.

91. Shoshani, T., Augarten, A., Gazit, E. *et al*. (1992) Association of a nonsense mutation (W1282X), the most common mutation in the Ashkenazi Jewish cystic fibrosis patients in Israel, with presentation of severe disease. *Am. J. Hum. Genet.*, **50**, 222–228.

92. Rozen, R., De Braekeleer, M., Daingneault, J. *et al*. (1992) Cystic fibrosis mutations in French Canadians: three CFTR mutations are relatively frequent in a Quebec population with an elevated incidence of cystic fibrosis. *Am. J. Med. Genet.*, **42**, 361–364.

93. Cutting, G.R., Curristin, S.M., Nash, F. *et al*. (1992) Analysis of four diverse populations indicates that a subset of cystic fibrosis mutations occur in common among caucasians. *Am. J. Hum. Genet.*, **50**, 1185–1194.

94. Cutting, G.R., Kasch, L.M., Rosenstein, B.J. *et al*. (1990) A cluster of cystic fibrosis mutations in the first nucleotide binding fold of the cystic fibrosis transmembrane conductance regulator protein. *Nature*, **346**, 366–369.

95. Amosh, A., Trapnell, B.C., Zeitlin, P.L. *et al*. (1991) Severe deficiency of cystic fibrosis transmembrane conductance regulator mRNA carrying nonsense mutations R553X and W1316X in respiratory epithelial cells of patients with cystic fibrosis. *J. Clin. Invest.*, **88**, 1880–1885.

96. Jones, C.T., Mcintosh, I., Keston, M. *et al*. (1992) Three novel mutations in the cystic fibrosis gene detected by chemical cleavage: analysis of variant splicing and a nonsense mutation. *Hum. Mol. Genet.*, **1**, 11–18.

97. Fonknechten, N., Chomel, J.-C., Kitzis, A. *et al*. (1992) Skipping of exon 5 as a consequence of the 711 + 1G→T mutation in the *CFTR* gene. *Hum. Mol. Genet.*, **1**, 281–282.

98. Ferec, C., Audrezet, M.P., Mercier, B. *et al*. (1992) Systematic screening for mutations in the cystic fibrosis gene: new implications for carrier detection. *Nature Genet.*, **1**, 188–191.

99. Fanen, P., Ghanem, N., Vidaud, M. *et al*. (1992) Molecular characterisation of cystic fibrosis: 16 novel mutations identified analysis of the whole cystic fibrosis transmembrane conductance regulator (CFTR) coding regions and splice site junctions. *Genomics*, **13**, 770–776.

100. Gasparini, P., Nunes, V., Savoia, A. *et al*. The search for Southern European cystic fibrosis mutations: identification of two new mutations, four variants, and intronic sequences. *Genomics*, **10**, 193–200.

101. Farrall, M., Law, H.-Y., Rodeck, C.H. *et al*. (1986) First-trimester prenatal diagnosis of cystic fibrosis with linked DNA probes. *Lancet*, **i**, 1402–1404.

102. Chehab, F.F., Johnson, J., Louie, E. *et al*. (1991) A dimorphic 4-bp repeat in the cystic fibrosis gene is in absolute linkage disequilibrium with the ΔF508 mutation: implications for prenatal diagnosis and mutation origin. *Am. J. Hum. Genet.*, **48**, 223–226.

103. Tsui, L.-C. (1990) Population analysis of the major mutation in cystic fibrosis. *Hum. Genet.*, **85**, 391–392.

104. Sereth, H., Shoshani, T., Bashan, N. and Kerem, H.-S. (1992) The selective advantage hypothesis for CF

mutations and variable intragenic haplotype. *Pediatr. Pulmonol. Suppl.*, **8**, 245A.

105. Morral, N., Bertranpetit, J., Estivill, X. *et al.* (1994) The origin of the major cystic fibrosis mutation (delta F508) in European populations. *Nature Genet.*, **7**, (2), 169–175.

106. Serre, J.L., Serre, J., Simon-Bouy, B. *et al.* (1990) Studies of RFLPs closely linked to the cystoc fibrosis locus throughout Europe lead to new considerations in population genetics. *Hum. Genet.*, **84**, 449–454.

107. Morral, N. (1993) Microsattelite haplotypes for cystic fibrosis: mutation frameworks and evolutionary tracers. *Hum. Molec. Genet.*, **2**, 1015–1022.

108. Romeo, G., Devoto, M. and Galietta, L.J. (1989) Why is the cystic fibrosis gene so frequent? *Hum. Genet.*, **84**, 1–5.

109. Meindl, R.S. (1987) Hypothesis: a selective advantage for cystic fibrosis heterozygotes. *Am. J. Phys. Anthropol.*, **74**, 39.

110. Shier, W.T. (1979) Increased resistance to influenza as a possible source of heterozygote advantage in cystic fibrosis. *Med. Hypoth.*, **5**, 661.

111. Rodman, D.M. and Zamudio, S. (1991) The cystic fibrosis heterozygote advantage in surviving cholera? *Med. Hypoth.*, **36**, 253.

112. Gabriel, S.E., Brigman, K.N., Koller, B.H. *et al.* (1994) Cystic fibrosis heterozygote resistance to cholera toxin in the cystic fibrosis mouse model. *Science*, **266**, 107–109.

113. Cuthbert, A.W., Halstead, J., Ratcliff, R. *et al.* (1995) The genetic advantage hypothesis in cystic fibrosis heterozygotes: a murine study. *J. Physiol.*, **482**, (Pt 2), 449–454.

114. Gregory, R.J., Rich, D.P., Cheng, S.H. *et al.* (1991) Maturation and function of cystic fibrosis transmembrane conductance regulator variants bearing mutations in putative nucleotide domains 1 and 2. *Mol. Cell. Biol.*, **11**, 3886–3893.

115. Ward, C.L. and Kopito, R.R. (1994) Intracellular turnover of cystic fibrosis transmembrane conductance regulator . Inefficient processing and rapid degradation of wild-type and mutant proteins. *J. Biol. Chem.*, **269**, 25710–25718.

116. Cheng, S.H., Gregory, R.J., Marshall, J. *et al.* (1990) Defective intracellular traffick and processing of CFTR is the molecular basis of most cystic fibrosis. *Cell*, **63**, 827–834.

117. Yang, Y., Junich, S., Cohn, J.A. and Wilson, J.M. (1993) The common variant of the cystic fibrosis transmembrane conductance regulator is recognised by hsp70 and degraded in a pre-Golgi nonlysosomal compartment. *Proc. Natl Acad. Sci. USA*, **90**, 9480–9484.

118. Pind, S., Riordan, J.R. and Williams, D.B. (1994) Participation of the endoplasmic reticulum chaperone calnexin (p88, IP90) in the biogenesis of the cystic fibrosis transmembrane conductance regulator. *J. Biol. Chem.*, **269**, 12784–12788.

119. Ward, C.L., Omura, S. and Kopito, R.R. (1995) Degradation of CFTR by the ubiquitin–proteasome pathway. *Cell*, **83**, 121–127.

120. Jensen, T.J. (1995) Multiple proteolytic systems, including the proteasome, contribute to CFTR processing. *Cell*, **83**, 129–135.

121. Sato, S. (1996) Glycerol reverses the misfolding phenotype of the most common cystic fibrosis mutation. *J. Biol. Chem.*, **271**, 635–638.

122. Dalemans,W., Barbry, P., Champigny, G. *et al.* (1991) Altered chloride ion channel kinetics associated with the ΔF_{508} cystic fibrosis mutation. *Nature*, **354**, 526–528.

123. Drumm, M.L., Wilkinson, D.J., Mansoura, M. *et al.* (1992) Function of NBF1-mutant CFTRs correlates with clinical phenotype. *Pediatr. Pulmonol. Suppl.*, **8**, 260A.

124. Li, C. (1993) The cystic fibrosis mutation does not influence the chloride channel activity of CFTR. *Nature Genet.*, **3**, 311–316.

125. Pasyk, E.A. and Foskett, J.K. (1995) Mutant (Delta F508) cystic fibrosis transmembrane conductance regulator chloride channel is functional when retained in the endoplasmic reticulum of mammalian cells. *J. Biol. Chem.*, **270**, 12347–12350.

126. Tabcharani, J.A. (1993) Multi-ion pore behaviour in the CFTR chloride channel. *Nature*, **366**, 79–82.

127. Champigny, G. (1995) A change in gating mode leading to intrinsic Cl-channel activity compensates for defective processing in a cystic fibrosis mutant corresponding to a mild form of the disease. *EMBO J.*, **14**, 2417–2423.

128. Sheppard, D.N., Ostedgaard, L.S., Winter, M.S. and Welsh, M.J. (1995) Mechanism of dysfunction of two nucleotide binding domain mutations in cystic fibrosis transmembrane conductance regulator that are associated with pancreatic sufficiency. *EMBO J.*, **14**, 876–833.

129. Sheppard, D.N., Travis, S.M., Ishihara, H. and Welsh, M.J. (1996) Contribution of proline residues in the membrane spanning domains of the cystic fibrosis transmembrane conductance regulator to chloride channel function. *J. Biol. Chem.*, **271**, 14995–15001.

130. Clarke, L.L., Grubb, B.R., Yankaskas, J.R. *et al.* Relationship of a non-cystic fibrosis transmembrane conductance regulator-mediated chloride conductance to organ-level disease in CFTR (–/–) mice. *Proc. Natl Acad. Sci. USA*, **91**, (2), 479–483.

131. Fulmer, C.F. (1995) Two cystic fibrosis transmembrane conductance regulator mutations have different effects on both pulmonary phenotype and regulation of outwardly rectified chloride currents. *Proc. Natl Acad. Sci. USA*, **92**, 6832–6836.

132. Estivill, X., Gasparini, P., Novelli, G. *et al.* (1989) Linkage disequilibrium for DNA haplotypes near the cystic fibrosis locus in two Southern European populations. *Hum. Genet.*, **83**, 175–178.

133. Beaudet, A.L., Feldman, G.L., Ferbach, S.D. *et al.* (1989) Linkage disequilibrium, cystic fibrosis, and genetic counselling. *Am. J. Hum. Genet.*, **44**, 319–326.

134. Handyside, A.H., Lesko, J.G., Taren, J.J. *et al.* (1992) Birth of normal girl after IVF and pre-implantation diagnosis for CF. *NEJM*, **327**, 905–909.

135. Workshop on Population Screening for the Cystic Fibrosis Gene (1990) Statement from the National Institutes of

Health Workshop on Population Screening for the Cystic Fibrosis Gene. *NEJM*, **323**, 70–71.

136. Schwartz, M. and Brand, N.J. (1991) Carrier screening for cystic fibrosis among pregnant women in Denmark. *Am. J. Hum. Genet*, **49**, (Suppl.), 330A.

137. Super, M. and Schwarz, M.J. (1992) Mutations of the cystic fibrosis gene locus within the population of north-west England. *Eur. J. Pediatr.*, **151**, 108–111.

138. Mennie, M.E., Gilfillan, A., Liston, W.A. *et al*. (1992) Prenatal screening for cystic fibrosis. *Lancet*, **340**, 214–217.

139. Clayton, E.W., Hannig, V.L., Pfotenhauer, J.P. *et al*. (1996) Lack of interest by nonpregnant couples in population-based cystic fibrosis carrier screening. *Am. J. Hum. Genet.*, **58**, (3), 617–627.

140. Brock, D.J. (1996) Population screening for cystic fibrosis. *Curr. Opin. Pediatr.*, **8**, (6), 635–638.

141. National Institutes of Health (1997) *Genetic Testing for Cystic Fibrosis*, NIH Consensus Statement, NIH, USA.

142. Brock, D.J. (1995) Prenatal screening for cystic fibrosis: 5 years' experience reviewed. *Lancet*, **347**, 148–150.

143. Mennie, M.E., Axworthy, D., Liston, W.A. and Brock, D.J. (1997) Prenatal screening for cystic fibrosis carriers: does the method of testing affect the longer-term understanding and reproductive behaviour of women? *Prenat. Diagn.*, **17**, (9), 853–860.

144. Miedzybrodka, Z.H., Hall, M.H., Mollison, J. *et al*. (1995) Antenatal screening for carriers of cystic fibrosis: randomised trail of stepwise v. couple screening. *BMJ*, **310**, (6976), 353–357.

145. Levenkron, J.C., Loader, S. and Rowley, P.T. (1997) Carrier screening for cystic fibrosis: test acceptance and one year follow-up. *Am. J. Med. Genet.*, **73**, (4), 378–386.

146. Harris, H., Scotcher, D., Hartley, N. *et al*. (1993) Cystic fibrosis carrier testing in early pregnancy by general practitioners. *BMJ*, **306**, (6892), 1580–1583.

147. Axworthy, D., Brock, D.J., Bobrow, M., Marteau, T.M. (1996) Psychological impact of population-based carrier testing for cystic fibrosis: 3-year follow-up. UK Cystic Fibrosis Follow-Up Study Group. *Lancet*, **347**, (9013), 1443–1446.

148. Dorin, J., Dickinson, P., Alton, E.W.F.W. *et al*. (1992) Cystic fibrosis in the mouse by targeted insertional mutagenesis. *Nature*, **359**, 211–215.

149. Snouwaert, J.N., Brigman, K.K., Latour, A.M. *et al*. (1992) An animal model for cystic fibrosis made by gene targetting. *Science*, **257**, 1083–1088.

150. Colledge, W.H., Abella, B.S., Southern, K.W. *et al*. Generation and characterization of a delta F508 cystic fibrosis mouse model. *Nature Genet.*, 10, (4), 445–452.

151. Zhou, L., Dey, C.R., Wert, S.E. *et al*. (1994) Correction of lethal intestinal defect in a mouse model of cystic fibrosis by human CFTR. *Science*, **266**, (5191), 1705–1708.

152. Clarke, L.L., Grubb, B.R., Gabriel, S.F. *et al*. (1992) Defective epithelial chloride transport in a gene-targeted mouse model of cystic fibrosis. *Science*, **257**, 1125–1128.

153. Grubb, B.R., Paradiso, A.M. and Boucher, R.C. (1994) Anomalies in ion transport in CF mouse tracheal epithelium. *Am. J. Physiol.*, **267**, (1, Pt 1), C293–C300.

154. Grubb, B.R. (1995) Ion transport across the jejunum in normal and cystic fibrosis mice. *Am. J. Physiol.*, **268**, (3, Pt 1), G505–G513.

155. Grubb, B.R. and Boucher, R.C. (1997) Enhanced colonic Na$^+$ absorption in cystic fibrosis mice versus normal mice. *Am. J. Physiol.*, **272**, (2 Pt 1), G393–G400.

156. Leung, A.Y., Wong, P.Y., Gabriel, S.E. *et al*. (1995) cAMP- but not Ca(2+)-regulated Cl-conductance in the oviduct is defective in mouse model of cystic fibrosis. *Am. J. Physiol.*, **268**, (3, Pt 1), C708–C712.

157. Leung, A.Y., Wong, P.Y., Yankaskas, J.R. and Boucher, R.C. (1996) cAMP- but not Ca(2+) regulated Cl-conductance is lacking in cystic fibrosis mice epididymides and seminal vesicles. *Am. J. Physiol.*, **271**, (1, Pt 1), C188–C193.

158. Hasty, P., O'Neal, W.K., Liu, K.Q. *et al*. (1995) Severe phenotype in mice with termination mutation in exon 2 of cystic fibrosis gene. *Somatic Cell and Molec. Genet.*, **21**, (3), 177–187.

159. O'Neal, W.K., Hasty, P., McCray, P.B. *et al*. (1993) A severe phenotype in mice with a duplication of exon 3 in the cystic fibrosis locus. *Hum. Molec. Genet.*, **2**, (10), 1561–1569.

160. Smith, S.N., Steel, D.M., Middleton, P.G. *et al*. (1995) Bioelectric characteristics of exon 10 insertional cystic fibrosis mouse: comparison with humans. *Am. J. Physiol.*, **268**, C297–C307.

161. Zahm, J.M., Gaillard, D., Dupuit, F. *et al*. (1997) Early alterations in airway mucociliary clearance and inflammation of the lamina propria in CF mice. *Am. J. Physiol.*, **272**, (3, Pt 1), C853–C859.

162. van Doorninck, J.H., French, P.J., Verbeek, E. *et al*. (1995) A mouse model for the cystic fibrosis delta F508 mutation. *EMBO J.*, **14**, (18), 4403–4411.

163. Zeiher, B.G., Eichwald, E., Zabner, J. *et al*. (1996) A mouse model of the delta F508 allele of cystic fibrosis. *J. Clin. Invest.*, **96**, 2051–2064.

164. Delaney, S.J., Alton, E.W., Smith, S.N. *et al*. (1996) Cystic fibrosis mice carrying the missense mutation G551D replicate human genotype–phenotype correlations. *EMBO J.*, **15**, (5), 955–963.

165. Hamosh, A. (1992) Preliminary results of the Cystic Fibrosis Genotype–Phenotype Consortium Study. *Pediatr. Pulmonol. Suppl.*, **8**, S144–S145.

3

Phenotype–genotype relationships

G. R. CUTTING

Introduction	49	Genes other than *CFTR* that may influence the CF genotype	55
Variability of the cystic fibrosis phenotype	49	Summary	56
Relationship between genotype and organ disease	50	References	57

INTRODUCTION

For inherited disorders, the interplay among three elements determines disease severity. These elements are: the nature of the defect in the responsible gene, the context in which the defective gene operates (i.e. genetic background) and environmental influences. The contribution of the first component can be assessed by study of the relationship between gene defects and disease severity. Cystic fibrosis (CF) is caused by abnormal function of a chloride channel called CFTR. Identification of the gene encoding CFTR and the discovery of numerous mutations in this gene has provided a wealth of material for genotype–phenotype analysis. Insight into this relationship has also been provided by the discovery that patients with other disorders that clinically overlap with CF have mutations in each *CFTR* gene. Furthermore, animal studies have demonstrated the importance of genetic background. Emerging from this mosaic is a theme not uncommon to inherited disorders; certain aspects of the CF phenotype are primarily determined by the type of CFTR mutation, while some features are heavily influenced by other factors. This chapter will review the studies underlying this concept.

VARIABILITY OF THE CYSTIC FIBROSIS PHENOTYPE

Cystic fibrosis is a genetic disease of epithelia and is manifest in the lungs, pancreas, sweat glands and, in the male, vas deferens. The disorder is highly variable; some patients die in early childhood due to respiratory or hepatic complications while others live into their sixth decade before succumbing to the illness. Lung disease is the major life limiter, variable even among affected siblings. Pancreatic disease ranges from complete loss of exocrine and endocrine functions while other patients have some preserved function and some only develop pancreatitis. Sweat gland dysfunction results in increased concentrations of sodium and chloride in sweat. The level of sweat chloride does vary considerably among patients; from near normal range (40–60 mM) to 120 mM, with the average level being about 100 mM. Although useful for diagnostic purposes, abnormal sweat chloride concentrations do not cause illness. Malformation of reproductive structures in males is probably the most consistent feature of CF. Virtually all males with CF are infertile due to abnormalities in structures derived from the wolffian duct, most common of which is bilateral absence of the vas deferens. The diagnostic criteria for CF in the United States has been revised to incorporate our increased understanding of the molecular and electrophysiologic abnormalities in this disorder[1] (Table 3.1).

Although a range of dysfunction in each of these organs is observed, there is some degree of correlation of severity among the different organs. For example, the degree of pancreatic dysfunction and level of chloride concentration in sweat electrolytes appears to be correlated. Patients with some preservation of pancreatic function have less abnormal elevations in sweat chloride concentration. Furthermore, the severity of disease in certain organs is consistent among affected siblings. The degree of pancreatic function and occurrence of neonatal intestinal blockage due to meconium appear to be two manifestations that show a high degree of concor-

Table 3.1 *Criteria for the diagnosis of cystic fibrosis*

One or more clinical features consistent with CF:
- chronic sinopulmonary disease
- gastrointestinal and nutritional abnormalities
- salt loss syndromes
- male urogenital abnormalities resulting in obstructive azoospermia

OR

A history of CF in sibling

OR

A positive newborn screening test

AND

Evidence of CFTR dysfunction:
- elevated sweat chloride concentration (>60 mM)
- presence of CF-producing mutations in each *CFTR* gene
- characteristic abnormalities on nasal potential difference measurement

dance within sibships. Since siblings share the same abnormal *CFTR* genes, it appears that these features of the disease correlate with the nature of mutations in the *CFTR* gene.

RELATIONSHIP BETWEEN GENOTYPE AND ORGAN DISEASE

CFTR genotype and lung disease

Pulmonary disease is the major cause of morbidity and mortality in cystic fibrosis. Over 90 per cent of patients succumb to this complication, making it an area of intense investigation[2]. The degree to which CFTR mutations influence this aspect of CF has been unclear, since the severity of lung disease varies considerably among affected individuals in the same family. However, studies comparing siblings and identical twins have suggested that there is an inherited component to CF lung disease[3,4]. Hodson and colleagues have shown that one measure of lung function (%FEV$_1$) correlated among adult siblings, especially those with milder pancreatic disease[3]. The latter observation is in agreement with other studies indicating that patients with less severe pancreatic disease have less severe lung disease[5–7].

Cloning of the *CFTR* gene and identification of disease-associated mutations enabled comprehensive studies of the relationship between genotype and the lung phenotype. About half of CF patients are homozygous for the mutation, ΔF_{508}. These patients provide an ideal group for comparison with patients with other genotypes[6,8]. The ΔF_{508} homozygotes showed a relatively consistent picture in regards to pancreatic disease, and, to a lesser degree, sweat gland dysfunction[6,8]. The severity of lung disease, however, was highly variable. Lung disease was similarly variable in patients heterozygous for the

ΔF_{508} mutation or those carrying two mutations other than ΔF_{508}. Furthermore, the latter two groups of patients did not manifest more or less severe pulmonary disease than the ΔF_{508} homozygotes[6,8]. Consistent with prior reports, patients with residual pancreatic function (i.e. pancreatic sufficient) had evidence of milder lung disease. Patients carrying nonsense mutations were also studied to evaluate whether absence of CFTR produced a different phenotype from that observed in patients expressing mutant protein. Again, no differences were apparent when patients carrying two nonsense mutations were compared to ΔF_{508} homozygotes[8].

Despite early evidence that genotype was poorly correlated with phenotype, studies of two missense mutations, A455E and R117H, suggested that this relationship may be more subtle than first realized. The mutation A455E occurs at a relatively high frequency in The Netherlands. This mutation had been associated with mild pancreatic disease[9] and preliminary studies suggested that patients carrying A455E and ΔF_{508} had less severe lung disease[10]. A more extensive study involving 33 compound heterozygotes revealed better pulmonary function tests and reduced rates of colonization with *Pseudomonas aeruginosa* than ΔF_{508} homozygotes from the same population[11]. These results suggest that A455E does produce less severe lung disease in the Dutch. A study of nine French-Canadian patients with the genotype A455E/ΔF_{508} revealed better pulmonary function (%FVC and %FEV$_1$) than five ΔF_{508} homozygotes drawn from the same population[12]. These studies indicate that presence of one copy of the A455E mutation confers milder lung disease. Thus, A455E acts in a dominant fashion to the severe alleles such as ΔF_{508}. The same situation is observed for mutations that are associated with pancreatic sufficiency (see below)[9,13].

The R117H mutation has been reported in CF patients with mild pancreatic disease and in otherwise healthy males with a form of infertility identical to that seen in men with CF[14,15]. A major question was how the

Table 3.2 *Association between mutations and specific features of the CF phenotype*

Mutation	% pancreatic sufficient (n)	Sweat chloride concentration in mM (n)	Age at diagnosis in years (n)	Reference
ΔF_{508}	2.5 (396)	106 ± 22 (328)	1.7 ± 3.0 (392)	8
P67L[a]	77 (12)	57 ± 9 (12)	22.5 ± 11.3 (12)	107
R117H[b]	87 (23)***	82 ± 19 (20)***	10.2 ± 10.5 (23)**	8
R334W[b]	40 (15)***	108 ± 16 (15)	7.6 ± 6.6 (15)**	33
A455E[b]	79 (33)***	Not reported	15.0 ± 10.6 (33)***	11
A455E[b]	78 (9)*	80 ± 19 (9)**	5.7 ± 1.6 (9)**	12
3849 + 10 kb C→T[b]	67 (15)	62 ± 17 (14)	12.5 ± 8.8 (15)	42
3849 + 10 kb C→T[a]	77 (13)	39 (13)	Not reported	41

[a]Statistical comparison with Δ_{508} homozygotes was not performed.
[b]*, $P < 0.05$; **, $P < 0.01$; ***, $P < 0.001$ compared to a group of age- and sex-matched ΔF_{508} homozygote controls.

same mutation gave rise to CF lung disease in some individuals while, in other cases, the individuals had normal lung function. A second genetic variation was found to be associated with the R117H mutation in patients with CF. It was proposed that the combination of the two alterations reduces the amount of partially functional protein to a level that is insufficient for normal lung function[16]. Presence of the R117H mutation alone results in enough partially functional protein to escape CF lung disease but not male infertility (see below). Thus, variation within the *CFTR* gene can influence lung phenotype.

CFTR genotype may be predictive of another aspect of CF lung disease; bacterial colonization. A study of 267 children and adolescents with CF indicated that patients with pancreatic sufficiency had lower colonization rates with *Pseudomonas aeruginosa*[17]. Furthermore, there was the suggestion that the risk of colonization correlated with the nature and location of the mutations[17]. Colonization with the latter organism is almost pathognomic for CF, although its role in the rate of progression of lung disease in this disorder is not clear[18–21]. However, more recent studies suggest that the altered salt concentration of CF airway fluid plays an important role in *Pseudomonas* infection due to decreased activity of antimicrobial peptides[22]. These observations indicate that a more complete understanding of CF biology may point to elements of the pulmonary phenotype that are more directly related to CFTR dysfunction. Correlation of these elements to genotype may produce stronger and more meaningful associations.

CFTR genotype and pancreatic disease

The exocrine pancreas is affected in virtually all patients with cystic fibrosis[23]. Most patients (85–95 per cent) have a deficiency of digestive enzymes due to obstruction of pancreatic ducts[23,24]. This process begins *in utero* and continues for the life of the patient, eventually leading to the destruction of the entire organ. The remaining 5–15

per cent of patients retain some degree of pancreatic function and produce sufficient amounts of pancreatic enzymes for adequate absorption of protein, fat and fat-soluble vitamins[23].

Preservation of pancreatic function was found to be highly concordant among affected siblings[25]. Since siblings have identical genotypes at the *CFTR* locus, this observation indicated that the nature of the CF mutation was strongly correlated with pancreatic status. This concept was supported by a study of DNA markers surrounding the *CFTR* gene, which indicated that individuals who were pancreatic sufficient carried different mutations than those who were pancreatic insufficient[26]. Following the cloning of the *CFTR* gene, a subset of mutations were found to be highly associated with preserved pancreatic function[9]. A multicenter collaborative study confirmed this result, but also emphasized that genotype is not completely predictive of the pancreatic phenotype[8]. For example, the vast majority of 396 ΔF_{508} homozygotes were pancreatic insufficient, but 10 of these patients had preserved pancreatic function[8]. Similarly, patients carrying a mutation associated with preserved pancreatic function (R117H) were predominantly, but not exclusively, pancreatic sufficient (Table 3.2). Other mutations associated with mild pancreatic disease show a high but not exclusive association with preservation of pancreatic function (Table 3.2). Thus, CFTR mutations associated with pancreatic sufficiency retain partial function whereas nonfunctional mutations give rise to severe pancreatic disease[27]. However, other factors such as environment or genetic background must play some role in determining the severity of pancreatic disease in CF patients. The high degree of variability in the cystic fibrosis phenotype raises a note of caution in interpreting whether a mutation has mild or severe consequences in small numbers of patients. Evidence that pancreatic status, the feature of CF most closely related to genotype, does not show an absolute correlation with mutation reaffirms this cautionary note.

CFTR genotype and sweat gland disease

Dysfunction of the sweat gland has been recognized as a part of the cystic fibrosis phenotype since the early 1950s. The gland is composted of two structures: a coil that produces an ultrafiltrate of the plasma and a duct which resorbs sodium and chloride from sweat. CFTR is present in both the coil and the duct. Loss of CFTR function results in a reduced absorption of sodium and chloride in the duct, producing sweat with high concentrations of salt[28]. Elevation of the chloride concentration above 60 mM has been a diagnostic standard for cystic fibrosis for over 40 years[29,30]. As with other features of the CF phenotype, sweat chloride concentrations can vary widely. The average sweat chloride concentration in CF patients is about 100 mM and sweat chloride in patients can range from 60 mM to 160 mM[2]. While the vast majority of patients with cystic fibrosis have chloride concentrations of 60 mM, a small fraction, approximately 1–2 per cent, have a sweat chloride value in the normal range (60 mM)[31]. Individuals with sweat chloride concentrations below 60 mM represent a special class known as atypical CF and will be discussed in more detail below. Although there is no clear-cut correlation between the level of sweat chloride abnormality and severity of lung disease, there is evidence to suggest that patients with pancreatic sufficiency have less abnormal sweat chloride concentrations[8,32].

Patients with two, one or no copies of the ΔF_{508} mutation had similar concentrations of chloride in sweat, suggesting no relation between sweat-gland function and genotype[6]. A subsequent study comparing ΔF_{508} homozygotes to patients carrying ΔF_{508} and one of seven mutations found the same result for six of the seven mutations[8]. However, patients carrying ΔF_{508} and the mutation R117H had lower sweat concentrations than age- and sex-matched ΔF_{508} homozygotes[8]. Since this study involved a statistically robust cohort of patients (n = 23), it provided the evidence that genotype could be predictive of sweat-gland phenotype. The R117H mutation was also associated with pancreatic sufficiency, indicating that mutations producing mild pancreatic disease may be associated with less abnormal sweat chloride concentrations. This appears to be the case for some mutations but not others. For example, patients with the mutation R334W were frequently pancreatic sufficient but sweat chloride concentrations were similar to those of ΔF_{508} homozygotes (Table 3.2)[33]. A mutation associated with a highly variable phenotype, G85E, has been associated with mild and severe pancreatic disease. Some patients with G85E had low sweat chloride levels (60 mM) while a majority appear to have levels comparable to those of ΔF_{508} homozygotes[34,35]. Considering the high degree of variability associated with the mutation, it is likely that genetic background plays a significant role in determining outcome in a patient with the G85E mutation.

On the other hand, there are examples where patients with mild pancreatic disease have less significant elevations in sweat chloride concentrations, as was observed with the R117H mutation. Two examples are the missense mutations L206W and A455E (Table 3.2). The latter mutation is of particular interest because it is associated with milder lung, pancreatic and sweat gland status. These genotype–phenotype observations suggest that there may be a subset of mutations associated with pancreatic sufficiency that also allow more normal sweat gland function. This subset probably represents mutations that have the highest levels of residual CFTR function. Indeed, patients carrying mutations that were associated with a partially functional cAMP-activated CFTR channel had significantly less abnormal sweat chloride concentrations[32]. These types of mutations have been termed class I or class IV and are splice mutations that allow synthesis of very reduced amounts of normal protein, or missense mutations that permit residual function of the mutant CFTR.

Genetic studies of patients with the atypical form of cystic fibrosis also support the concept that there is a connection between CFTR mutation and sweat-gland dysfunction. The diagnosis of atypical CF has primarily been made in adult patients who presented with clinical features such as pulmonary disease, and/or pancreatic dysfunction consistent with cystic fibrosis, but with sweat chloride concentrations below the range typical for cystic fibrosis (i.e. 60 mM)[36–38]. In addition, some of the male patients with this phenotype were found to be fertile; a situation highly unusual in patients with classic forms of cystic fibrosis. Two mutations have been shown to be associated with the atypical phenotype. The missense mutation G551S was discovered in homozygosity in two sisters with pulmonary disease consistent with cystic fibrosis but sweat chloride concentrations in the normal range for adults (49–54 mM)[39]. Subsequently, three Mexican CF patients have been found to be heterozygous for the G551S mutation and ΔF_{508}[40]. These individuals were pancreatic sufficient and had moderately elevated sweat chloride concentrations. These observations suggest that one copy of G551S paired with a severe mutation like ΔF_{508} produces mild pancreatic disease and moderately elevated sweat chloride concentrations, while two copies of G551S creates an even milder phenotype manifest by normal sweat chloride concentrations.

An mRNA splicing mutation termed 3849 + 10 kbC→T has also been associated with the atypical CF phenotype. This is an unusual alteration, distant from the coding region of the gene, which alters the splicing of the *CFTR* gene[41]. The consequence is production of very reduced amounts of normal protein. The level of the RNA has been estimated to be about 8 per cent of that found in normal subjects[41]. The 3849 mutation has been consistently associated with normal to borderline abnormal sweat chloride concentrations[41–45]. Most but not all patients carrying this mutation are pancreatic sufficient and the diagnosis of CF was suspected due to mild, but characteristic, lung disease. A high proportion of affected males carrying the 3849 mutation are fertile[41] (see below).

CFTR genotype and male infertility

One of the most consistent features in cystic fibrosis is male infertility. It has been estimated that between 96 and 97 per cent of male CF patients are infertile due to azoospermia[46]. Autopsy and detailed clinical studies reveal that the vast majority of CF males have abnormalities in structures derived from the wolffian duct. This includes the epididymis, vas deferens and seminal vesicles[47–49]. A variety of abnormalities involving the testes has also been observed[50]. Spermatogenesis is also abnormal in CF males[51]. Since virtually all CF males are infertile, it appears that normal development of the male reproductive tract requires functional CFTR. Healthy male carriers of CF mutations (e.g. fathers of CF patients) are fertile, indicating that 50 per cent of the normal level of CFTR function is sufficient for male fertility. Interestingly, a very small number of fertile males carry the 3849 mutation (see above) which is associated with reduced amounts of normally functioning CFTR. However, not all males carrying this mutation are fertile. This observation suggests that the 3849 mutation allows production of CFTR protein at or near the threshold level for development of the male reproductive tract. Individual variation in proteins involved in the splicing process may affect the level of functional CFTR, thereby accounting for the fertile and infertile males with this mutation.

The concept that male reproductive structures require a certain level of functional CFTR suggested that very mild defects in CFTR may be found in males that exhibit only infertility. Indeed, a separate recessive genetic disorder affecting 1 in 125 males, called congenital bilateral absence of the vas deferens (CBAVD), had been reported[52]. Detailed clinical studies revealed that some patients had features observed in cystic fibrosis such as bronchiectasis, chronic sinusitis and elevated concentrations of sweat chloride[15,53]. Thus, some males described with this recessive disorder actually have a mild form of cystic fibrosis. However, other males with CBAVD manifest no evidence of clinical features consistent with CF or evidence of CFTR dysfunction[53]. Nasal potential difference measurements in males with CBAVD can be abnormal but different from readings in CF patients, further substantiating that the CBAVD phenotype is distinct from CF[54]. When the most recent diagnostic criteria for cystic fibrosis are applied (see Table 3.1), males with absent vas deferens and normal sweat chloride concentration, and the absence of any other clinical features, do not meet the criteria for diagnosis of CF.

The appropriateness of distinguishing CBAVD from CF is further substantiated by analysis of the *CFTR* genes in CBAVD males. Between 70 and 75 per cent of these males carry mutations in each *CFTR* gene[15,55,56]. The most common genotype is ΔF_{508}/R117H[56]. This is intriguing since this genotype has been associated with pancreatic-sufficient CF. However, the gene bearing the R117H mutation found in males with CBAVD is different from the gene bearing the R117H found in patients with cystic fibrosis (see above)[16]. The latter contains a variant in intron 8 of the *CFTR* gene, called 5T, which reduces the splicing efficiency of RNA transcripts[57]. The net effect is low levels of RNA transcripts encoding partially functional CFTR protein with the R117H mutation. This produces lung disease observed in R117H/ΔF_{508} patients. Males with CBAVD carry R117H associated with a more efficient variant of splicing, called 7T. This combination is predicted to produce higher levels of partially functional protein, allowing these individuals to escape the pulmonary disease of CF, but not abnormalities in the male reproductive tract. Interestingly, the 5T variant has also been associated with CBAVD when found in males carrying a severe CF mutation such as ΔF_{508}[55,56,58–60]. Thus, a reduction of functional CFTR due to this splice variant also causes reproductive abnormalities in the male.

Two problems are immediately apparent in appreciating the relationship between the 5T variant and CBAVD. First, why does a mutation involved with abnormal splicing of CFTR cause infertility in otherwise healthy males when another splice mutation, 3849 (discussed above), is associated with fertility in CF patients? Second, why is the 5T mutation variably penetrant? In other words, there are fathers of patients with cystic fibrosis who carry the ΔF_{508} mutation in one gene and the 5T variant in the other gene who are fertile. Conversely, screening studies have revealed a convincingly high rate of the same genotype in infertile males due to CBAVD. Explanations have been provided for both questions. It appears that the intron splice variant is handled differently in different tissues. In the vas deferens, the 5T variant results in much higher levels of abnormally spliced CFTR than is observed in respiratory epithelial cells[61–63]. It has been suggested that this situation allows the production of higher levels of normal CFTR in epithelial tissues outside the reproductive tract, thereby accounting for the lack of pulmonary and pancreatic disease in the ΔF_{508}/5T males. The molecular basis of the incomplete penetrance of the 5T polymorphism may also have been solved. A DNA polymorphism preceding the poly(T) tract in intron 8 of the *CFTR* gene varies between 11 and 13 copies[57]. A recent report suggests that splicing efficiency varies depending on whether the 5T variant is accompanied by 11, 12 or 13 copies of the polymorphism[64]. The combinations proposed to have the least efficient splicing, 5T with 12 or 13 copies, is almost exclusively observed in males with CBAVD. Conversely, most fertile males have 5T associated with 11 copies[64]. This situation is somewhat analogous to that observed with the R117H mutation; two genetic variables have to be taken into account to understand the phenotypes produced.

CFTR genotype and other phenotypic features

The wide clinical spectrum of CF has encouraged investigators to search for an association between CF mutations and symptoms of the disease in tissues other than lung, pancreas, sweat gland or male reproductive system. Neonatal intestinal obstruction due to viscous meconium is a condition highly suggestive of a CF diagnosis. This problem, termed meconium ileus, was reported in 17.4 per cent of all CF patients[2]. Family studies have recorded a higher than expected rate of meconium ileus in affected siblings, suggesting a possible genetic basis for this complication[65]. Prior to the cloning of the CFTR gene, DNA polymorphism analysis suggested that a high-risk allele for CF and meconium ileus may exist[66]. The problem with the proposal was that the polymorphism differentiating between high and low rates of meconium ileus was distant from the CFTR gene. Not unexpectedly, later studies failed to find the same association[67]. The meconium ileus (MI) issue was revisited following identification of the CFTR gene. MI appeared to be more frequent than expected in patients ($n = 9$) with the genotype G542X/ΔF_{508}[9]. A subsequent study involving 57 patients with the same genotype did not uncover a statistically significant difference in the frequency of MI from ΔF_{508} homozygotes. However, another CF mutation, G551D, conferred a reduced risk of meconium ileus in a group of 79 patients from Europe and North America[68]. Subsequently, CF mice bearing the G551D mutation were shown to have reduced rates of fatal intestinal blockage, consistent with human studies[69]. Finally, African–Americans with CF were found to have lower rates of MI than Caucasians. This difference disappeared when genotype was taken into account. Patients homozygous for ΔF_{508} had the highest rate of MI (African–Americans 19.2 per cent; Caucasians 21.8 per cent), those without the ΔF_{508} mutation had the lowest rate (9.3 per cent and 11.9 per cent, respectively), while patients with one ΔF_{508} mutation were in between (15.6 per cent and 16.8 per cent, respectively)[70]. These rates were independent of race, indicating that the ΔF_{508} mutation was associated with an increased risk for meconium ileus. The reduced rate of MI in African–Americans was predicted to be a result of the lower frequency of the ΔF_{508} mutation (about 50 per cent of CF alleles in that population)[71].

Sinus disease is a very common feature of CF[72]. Radiographic evidence of nasal sinus abnormalities were found in 185 of 187 patients[73]. Nasal polyps, a complication of sinus disease, occurs in about 25 per cent of patients with cystic fibrosis[74]. Nasal polyposis is relatively uncommon in the general population, and so uncommon in children that it is seen as a reason to evaluate a child for the diagnosis of CF. Isolated nasal polyposis is rarely observed in CF. One study reported two unusual mutations in male twins with nasal polyps and elevated sweat chloride concentrations[75]. These patients had no evidence of pulmonary or pancreatic disease. The authors speculated that one of the mutations (591del18) had a very mild effect on CFTR function, allowing the patient to manifest only the sinus and sweat-gland abnormality. Since nasal polyposis is so common in CF, it has been speculated that CFTR abnormality may predispose to the formation of nasal polyps. Investigators in Germany discovered a higher than expected frequency of a relatively common CF mutation, G551D, in surgical specimens of nasal polyps[76]. Four of 56 samples studied had one copy of the G551D mutation, a highly significant increase from the frequency of the G551D mutation in the general population[76]. The latter study has not been reproduced so the role of CFTR in isolated nasal polyposis is uncertain.

Disease of the liver occurs in about 25 per cent of patients with cystic fibrosis, while overt clinical liver disease affects about 2–3 per cent of children and 5 per cent of adults[77]. According to the Cystic Fibrosis Foundation report of 1996[2], liver disease is responsible for about 1.6 per cent of deaths. Patients with liver disease do not have a different distribution of CF mutations than their counterparts without liver disease[78–80]. Furthermore, three out of four sibships with multiple affected children were discordant for liver disease[79]. Together, these observations indicate that hepatic disease is not defined by the nature of the CF mutation but by other factors.

The resting metabolic rate in cystic fibrosis patients is higher than in normal subjects[81–83]. Since there is a great deal of variability in the age of onset of this increase in metabolic rate and the degree to which the metabolic rate is increased, studies have tried to discern whether there is a relationship between metabolic rate and genotype. The results have been mixed. Two studies have indicated a relationship between CFTR mutations and basal metabolic rate. In particular, ΔF_{508} homozygotes appeared to have higher rates than other genotypes, even after correction for differences in severity of pulmonary disease[84,85]. On the other hand, a study investigating aerobic exercise capacity found no significant differences when they compared 10 ΔF_{508} homozygotes with 20 CF patients heterozygous for ΔF_{508}[86]. Similarly, a study of 32 males aged 7–39 years found a strong correlation between declining pulmonary function and increased resting energy expenditure. However, the energy expenditure did not correlate with presence or absence of the ΔF_{508} mutation[87]. Therefore, it appears that resting energy expenditure increases as lung disease worsens. However, it is unclear whether the nature of the mutation in the CFTR gene has any influence on resting metabolic rate independent of a severity of lung function. Considering that the correlation between genotype and lung function is tenuous, perhaps it is not surprising that resting metabolic rate, which depends on many variables, may be even less dependent upon CFTR genotype.

CFTR genotype and other forms of lung disease

In light of the fact that males with reproductive abnormalities similar to that seen in CF carry CFTR mutations, investigators have studied patients with lung disease similar to that seen in cystic fibrosis for CF mutations. Three diseases have been most heavily studied: chronic bronchitis, disseminated bronchiectasis and allergic bronchopulmonary aspergillosis (ABPA). The first group comprises a rather large and diverse population of patients under the category of chronic obstructive pulmonary disease due to bronchial hypersecretion, and includes patients with the diagnosis of chronic bronchitis. A study in 1990 suggested that the ΔF_{508} mutation frequency was higher than expected in 65 adults with bronchial hypersecretion[88]. One of six individuals carrying the ΔF_{508} mutation had an elevated sweat chloride concentration, and two other patients had borderline elevated sweat chloride concentrations, suggesting the diagnosis of atypical CF. The remaining three patients had normal sweat chloride concentrations. However, several other studies have failed to find increased frequency of CF mutations in patients with chronic bronchitis[89–92].

The second pulmonary disorder, disseminated bronchiectasis, appears to have a higher than expected incidence of CFTR mutations. Bronchiectasis is defined as a chronic infection of the airways that eventually leads to dilatation of the bronchi and bronchioles. A study of 10 adult patients with this phenotype found a higher than expected frequency of the ΔF_{508} mutation; however, several of the patients had features consistent with cystic fibrosis, such as pancreatic insufficiency or elevated sweat chloride concentrations[93]. Clinical studies and mutation analysis of the remaining patients raised some questions as to whether they might have had mild forms of CF. A more extensive mutational analysis of 60 patients with disseminated bronchiectasis revealed a higher than expected frequency of CF mutations and the 5T variant[94,95]. Again, lack of complete clinical information, such as sweat chloride concentrations and nasal potential difference measurements, on each patient leaves open the possibility that some of these patients may have had a mild form of cystic fibrosis. A third study involving 32 patients with disseminated bronchiectasis identified a variety of CFTR mutations, some which have been previously identified as causing CF[96]. None of the patients had CF mutations on both chromosomes, lead-ing the authors to conclude that defects in the *CFTR* gene may be a risk factor for the development of disseminated bronchiectasis.

The third condition, ABPA, is a complication of asthma that has been reported in about 10–12 per cent of patients with cystic fibrosis[97]. Eleven patients meeting stringent diagnostic criteria for ABPA were studied for CFTR mutations, and five were found to carry one CF mutation[98]. This frequency was higher than expected in the general population and in a study of 53 patients with chronic bronchitis. One of the 11 patients was found to have a mild form of cystic fibrosis. Although this study involves a small number of well-characterized patients, it suggests that CFTR mutations may play an etiologic role in other forms of lung disease, as suggested by a recent study of patients with atypical sinopulmonary disease[99]. For these disorders, studies of larger groups of patients will be critical in defining whether a reduction in the level of functioning CFTR is a predisposing factor to other forms of pulmonary disease.

GENES OTHER THAN *CFTR* THAT MAY INFLUENCE THE CF GENOTYPE

The high degree of variability in cystic fibrosis suggests that other factors must be important in the development of disease in the individual patient. The observation of variability within sibships supports this contention. However, assessing the contribution of other genes to the CF phenotype is difficult in human populations, due to our high degree of genetic diversity. These studies are better performed in animal models, where selective breeding can create more homogeneous genetic backgrounds to observe the phenotypic consequences of select CFTR mutations. The creation of numerous CF mouse lines has facilitated study of the contribution of genetic background to CF phenotype in mice[100,101]. As suspected from human studies, the genetic background of mice can influence the severity of the disease, both in the intestine and in the lungs[102,103].

One of the problems with CF mice is that they do not develop a phenotype that is similar to that of humans. Intestinal obstruction leading to early death is a common feature in mice, whereas disease of the pancreas and lungs is minimal[100,101,104]. It has been suggested that CF mice do not develop lung disease due to the fact that they have elevated levels of chloride conductance via a calcium-mediated channel[105]. In support of this hypothesis, inbred congenic mice carrying a CFTR defect appear to develop lung disease due to lack of a non-CFTR chloride channel normally found in outbred mice[103]. Although the physiologic status of airway cells in humans is not precisely the same as in mice, the murine studies clearly point out the importance of other gene products in the development of lung and intestinal disease. These studies suggest that it is likely that humans have genetic modifiers, and the study of the human homologs of modifiers found in mice may be fruitful in the search for the cause of phenotype variation. For example, the locus in humans corresponding to the intestinal modifier gene from mice has been identified and DNA markers from this region appear to show different distributions in CF siblings with concordant and discordant features[106]. This locus involves a large amount of DNA, so identification on the responsible gene may be a difficult task.

Evidence that genetic background may play an important role in the CF phenotype has been inferred by a difference approach. Cystic fibrosis is commonly observed in European Caucasians but also occurs in African–Americans in the United States. Since each group retains a certain degree of genetic difference, due to their origins on different continents, the clinical features of African–American and Caucasian CF patients have been compared. A group of 47 ΔF_{508} homozygotes were matched by age, sex and geographic location with 188 Caucasians with the same genotype. The patient groups were similar in many respects; however, nutritional parameters such as height and weight percentiles differed significantly among the two groups[70]. The latter may be an indication of dietary differences, aggressiveness of nutritional therapy, or possibly differences in the genetic background that influence nutritional status. The latter interpretation is consistent with the finding that a modifier gene affects the severity of intestinal disease in CF mice and suggests that genes may play an important role in determining nutritional status. The identification of specific genes that play a role in the development of the CF phenotype will await cloning of genes in mice and/or identification of genes whose products interact directly with the CFTR protein.

SUMMARY

The genotype–phenotype relationship in cystic fibrosis is complex despite its being a monogenic disorder. The discovery and investigation of factors that contribute to variability among individuals with the same genotype is an area of intense study. At this time, some conclusions can be drawn regarding the importance of CFTR in the development of the CF phenotype. It is clear that defects in each copy of this gene causes the CF phenotype. Homozygosity for the common mutation, ΔF_{508}, or compound heterozygosity for ΔF_{508} and one of the less common, but not rare, mutations, causes the classic phenotype: progressive obstructive lung disease, exocrine pancreatic insufficiency, male infertility and elevated sweat chloride concentrations. Variability can be observed among patients with the classic form of CF, especially in the severity of pulmonary disease, the most common cause death of in CF. Although our under-

standing of the role of other genes and environment in the development of lung disease is incomplete, evidence that other factors are important raises the possibility that therapeutic intervention for CF lung disease may be possible at several levels.

A second conclusion that can be drawn at this time is that genotype correlates more closely with certain features of the CF phenotype than others. Mutations that allow partial function of CFTR consistently ameliorate the severity of pancreatic disease. It appears that a subset of these mutations permit enough CFTR function to modulate the degree of sweat-gland dysfunction, and a select few produce less-severe lung disease. Most of the latter mutations affect the development of the male reproductive tract, suggesting that this process has the highest requirement for CFTR function. One exception is the splice mutation 3840 + 10 kb C→T, but tissue-specific splicing may lead to higher levels of full-length CFTR transcript in reproductive structures than observed in airway cells, such as has been reported for the 5T splicing variant. The emerging theme suggests that each organ affected in CF requires a different level of CFTR function. Mutations that allow minimal residual function of CFTR are associated with mild pancreatic disease, indicating that the pancreas requires only low levels of CFTR function. On the other hand, mutations that cause only moderate reduction in the level of functional CFTR cause male infertility but do not produce disease in other organs. This suggests that the development of the male reproductive structures requires CFTR function at levels higher than those necessary for normal operation of the pancreas, sweat gland and lungs (see Fig. 3.1). With this understanding in hand, future studies can focus on the variation of disease severity in specific organs, after accounting for the contribution by CFTR. For example, comparison of the severity of lung

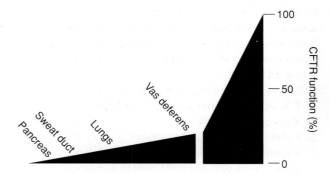

Threshold for normal organ function

Fig. 3.1 *Representation of the level of CFTR function required for normal function of the major organ systems involved in cystic fibrosis. Genotype–phenotype studies indicate that decreasing levels of CFTR function are associated with progressive involvement of more organ systems.*

disease among patients carrying pancreatic-sufficient mutations should uncover subtle differences among partially functional mutants. A greater appreciation for the genotype–phenotype relationship will be crucial for therapeutic interventions aimed both at the basic defect and approaches to circumvent the loss of CFTR function.

REFERENCES

1. Rosenstein, B. and Cutting, G.R. (1998) The diagnosis of cystic fibrosis; A consensus statement. *J. Pediatr.*, **132,** 589–595.

2. Fitzsimmons, S.C. (1997) *Cystic Fibrosis Foundation, Patient Registry 1996 Annual Report*, Bethesda, MD.

3. Santis, G., Osborne, L., Knight, R.A. and Hodson, M.E. (1990) Independent genetic determinants of pancreatic and pulmonary status in cystic fibrosis. *Lancet*, **336,** 1081–1084.

4. Santis, G. (1992) Pulmonary disease and genotypes. *Pediatr. Pulmonol. Suppl.*, **8**, 140–141.

5. Gaskin, K.J., Gurwitz, D., Durie, P., Corey, M., Levison, H. and Forstner, G. (1982) Improved respiratory prognosis in patients with cystic fibrosis with normal fat absorption. *J. Pediatr.*, **100**, 857–862.

6. Kerem E., Corey M., Kerem B. *et al*. (1990) The relation between genotype and phenotype in cystic fibrosis – analysis of the most common mutation (ΔF_{508}). *NEJM*, **323**, 1517–1522.

7. Santis, G., Osbourne, L., Knight, R.A. and Hodson, M.E. (1990) Linked marker haplotypes and the deltaF508 mutation in adults with mild pulmonary disease and cystic fibrosis. *Lancet*, **336**, 1426–1429.

8. Cystic Fibrosis Genotype/Phenotype Consortium (1993) Correlation between genotype and phenotype in cystic fibrosis. *NEJM*, **329**, 1308–1313.

9. Kristidis, P., Bozon, D., Corey, M. *et al*. (1992) Genetic determination of exocrine pancreatic function in cystic fibrosis. *Am. J. Hum. Genet.*, **50**, 1178–1184.

10. Gan, K.H., Heijerman, H.G.M. and Bakker, W. (1994) Correlation between genotype and phenotype in patients with cystic fibrosis. *NEJM*, **330**, 865–866 (letter to the editor).

11. Gan, K., Veeze, H.J., van den Ouweland, A.M.W. *et al*. (1995) A cystic fibrosis mutation associated with mild lung disease. *NEJM*, **333**, 95–99.

12. DeBraekeleer, M., Allard, C., Leblanc, J., Simard, F. and Aubin, G. (1997) Genotype–phenotype correlation in cystic fibrosis patients compound heterozygous for the A455E mutation. *Hum. Genet.*, **101**, 208–211.

13. Kerem, B., Rommens, J.M., Buchanan, J.A. *et al*. (1989) Identification of the cystic fibrosis gene: genetic analysis. *Science*, **245**, 1073–1080.

14. Dean, M., White, M.B., Amos, J. *et al*. (1990) Multiple mutations in highly conserved residues are found in mildly affected cystic fibrosis patients. *Cell*, **61**, 863–870.

15. Anguiano, A., Oates, R.D., Amos, J.A., *et al*. (1992) Congenital bilateral absence of the vas deferens – a primarily genital form of cystic fibrosis. *JAMA*, **267**, 1794–1797.

16. Kiesewetter, S., Macek, M. Jr, Davis, C. *et al*. (1993) A mutation in the cystic fibrosis transmembrane conductance regulator gene produces different phenotypes depending on chromosomal background. *Nature Genet.*, **5**, 274–278.

17. Kubesch, P., Dörk, T., Wulbrand, U. *et al*. (1993) Genetic determinants of airways' colonization with *Pseudomonas aeruginosa* in cystic fibrosis. *Lancet*, **341**, 189–193.

18. Kulczycki, L.L., Murphy, T.M. and Bellanti, J.A. (1978) *Pseudomonas* colonization in cystic fibrosis: a study of 160 patients. *JAMA*, **240,** 30–34.

19. Wilmott, R.W., Tyson, S.L. and Matthew, D.J. (1985) Cystic fibrosis survival rates: The influences of allergy and *Pseudomonas aeruginosa*. *Am. J. Dis. Child.*, **139**, 669–671.

20. Kerem, E., Corey, M., Gold, R. and Levison, H. (1990) Pulmonary function and clinical course in patients with cystic fibrosis after pulmonary colonization with *Pseudomonas aeruginosa*. *J. Pediatr.*, **116,** 714–719.

21. Abman, S.H., Ogle, J.W., Harbeck, R.J., Butler-Simon, N., Hammond, K.B. and Accurso, F.J. (1991) Early bacteriologic, immunologic, and clinical courses of young infants with cystic fibrosis identified by neonatal screening. *J. Pediatr.*, **119**, 211–217.

22. Smith, J.J., Travis, S.M., Greenberg, P. and Welsh, M.J. (1996) Cystic fibrosis airway epithelia fail to kill bacteria because of abnormal airway surface fluid. *Cell*, **85**, 229–236.

23. di Sant 'Agnese, P.A. and Hubbard, V. (1984) The pancreas, in *Cystic Fibrosis*, (ed. L.M. Taussig), Thième Stratton, New York, pp. 230–295.

24. Figarella, C. and Carrère, J. (1994) The evolution of pancreatic disease in cystic fibrosis, in *Cystic Fibrosis – Current Topics*, (eds J.A. Dodge, D.J.H. Brock and J.H. Widdicombe), John Wiley & Sons Ltd, New York, pp. 255–275.

25. Corey, M., Durie, P., Moore, D., Forstner, G. and Levison, H. (1989) Familial concordance of pancreatic function in cystic fibrosis. *J. Pediatr.*, **115**, 274–277.

26. Kerem, B.S., Buchanan, J.A., Durie, P. *et al*. (1989) DNA marker haplotype association with pancreatic sufficiency in cystic fibrosis. *Am. J. Hum. Genet.*, **44**, 827–834.

27. Sheppard, D.N., Rich, D.P., Ostedgaard, L.S., Gregory, R.J., Smith, A.E. and Welsh, M.J. (1993) Mutations in CFTR associated with mild-disease-form Cl⁻ channels with altered pore properties. *Nature*, **362**, 160–164.

28. Quinton, P.M. and Bijman, J. (1983) Higher bioelectric potentials due to decreased chloride absorption in the sweat glands of patients with cystic fibrosis. *NEJM*, **308**, 1185–1189.

29. di Sant 'Agnese, P.A., Darling, R.C., Perera, G.A. and Shea, E. (1953) Abnormal electrolyte composition of sweat in cystic fibrosis of the pancreas. *Pediatrics*, **12**, 549–563.

30. Gibson, L.E. and Cooke, R.E. (1959) A test for

concentration of electrolytes in sweat in cystic fibrosis of the pancreas utilizing pilocarpine by iontophoresis. *Pediatrics*, **23**, 545–549.

31. di Sant 'Agnese, P.A. and Powell, G.F. (1962) The eccrine sweat defect in cystic fibrosis of the pancreas (mucoviscidosis). *Ann. NY Acad. Sci.*, **93**, 555–599.

32. Wilschanski, M., Zielenski, J., Markiewicz, D. *et al.* (1995) Correlation of sweat chloride concentration with classes of the cystic fibrosis transmembrane conductance regulator gene mutations. *J. Pediatr.*, **127**, 705–710.

33. Estivill, X., Ortigosa, L., Peréz-Frias, J. *et al.* (1995) Clinical characteristics of 16 cystic fibrosis patients with the missense mutation R334W, a pancreatic insufficiency mutation with variable age of onset and interfamilial clinical differences. *Hum. Genet.*, **95**, 331–336.

34. Vazquez, C., Antinolo, G., Casals, T. *et al.* (1996) Thirteen cystic fibrosis patients, 12 compound heterozygous and one homozygous for the missense mutation G85E: a pancreatic sufficiency/insufficiency mutation with variable clinical presentation. *J. Med. Genet.*, **33**, 820–822.

35. Kerem, E., Nissim-Rafinia, M., Argaman, Z. *et al.* (1997) A missense cystic fibrosis transmembrane conductance regulator mutation with variable phenotype. *Pediatrics*, **100**, E5

36. Stern, R.C., Boat, T.F., Abramowsky, C.R., Matthews, L.W., Wood, R.E. and Doershuk, C.F. (1978) Intermediate-range sweat chloride concentration and *Pseudomonas* bronchitis. *JAMA*, **239**, 2676–2680.

37. Stern, R.C., Boat, T.F., Doershuk, C.F., Tucker, A.S., Miller, R.B. and Matthews, L.W. (1977) Cystic fibrosis diagnosed after age 13. *Ann. Intern. Med.*, **87**, 188–191.

38. Huff, D.S., Huang, N.N. and Arey, J.B. (1979) Atypical cystic fibrosis of the pancreas with normal levels of sweat chloride and minimal pancreatic lesions. *J. Pediatr.*, **94**, 237–239.

39. Strong, T.V., Smit, L.S., Turpin, S.V. *et al.* (1991) Cystic fibrosis gene mutation in two sisters with mild disease and normal sweat electrolyte levels. *NEJM*, **325**, 1630–1634.

40. Orozco, L., Lezana, J.L., Villarreal, M.T., Chávez, M. and Carnevale, A. (1995) Mild cystic fibrosis disease in three Mexican delta-F508/G551S compound heterozygous siblings. *Clin. Genet.*, **47**, 96–98.

41. Highsmith, W.E. Jr, Burch, L.H., Zhou, Z. *et al.* (1994) A novel mutation in the cystic fibrosis gene in patients with pulmonary disease but normal sweat chloride concentrations. *NEJM*, **331**, 974–980.

42. Augarten, A., Kerem, B., Yahav, Y. *et al.* (1993) Mild cystic fibrosis and normal or borderline sweat test in patients with the 3849 + 10 kb C→T mutation. *Lancet*, **342**, 25–26.

43. Stewart, B., Zabner, J., Shuber, A.P., Welsh, M.J. and McCray, P.B. Jr (1995) Normal sweat chloride values do not exclude the diagnosis of cystic fibrosis. *Am. J. Resp. Crit. Care Med.*, **151**, 899–903.

44. Stern, R.C., Doershuk, C.F. and Drumm, M.L. (1995) 3849 + 10 kb C→T mutation and disease severity in cystic fibrosis. *Lancet*, **346**, 274–276.

45. Dreyfus, D., Bethel, R. and Gelfand, E. (1996) Cystic fibrosis 3849 + 10 kb C→T mutation associated with severe pulmonary disease and male fertility. *Am. J. Resp. Crit. Care Med.*, **153**, 858–860.

46. Brugman, S.M. and Taussig, L.M. (1984) The reproductive system, in *Cystic Fibrosis*, (ed. L.M. Taussig), Thième Stratton, New York, pp. 323–337.

47. Kaplan, E., Shwachman, H., Perlmutter, A.D., Rule, A., Khaw, K.T. and Hosclaw, D.S. (1968) Reproductive failure in males with cystic fibrosis. *NEJM*, **279**, 65–69.

48. Taussig, L.M., Lobeck, C., di Sant 'Agnese, P.A., Ackerman, D. and Kattwinkel, J. (1972) Fertility in males with cystic fibrosis. *NEJM*, **287**, 586–589.

49. Dodge, J.A. (1995) Male fertility in cystic fibrosis. *Lancet*, **346**, 587–588.

50. Wilschanski, M., Corey, M., Durie, P. *et al.* (1996) Diversity of reproductive tract abnormalities in men with cystic fibrosis. *JAMA*, **276**, 607–608.

51. Denning, C.R., Sommers, S.C. and Quigley, H.J. Jr (1968) Infertility in male patients with cystic fibrosis. *Pediatrics*, **41**, 7–17.

52. McKusick, V.A. (1994) *Mendelian Inheritance in Man*, 11th edn, Johns Hopkins University Press, Baltimore, MD, pp.1–3009.

53. Colin, A.A., Sawyer, S.M., Mickle, J., Oates, R.D., Milunsky, A. and Amos, J. (1996) Pulmonary function and clinical observations in men with congenital bilateral absence of the vas deferens. *Chest*, **110**, 440–445.

54. Osborne, L.R., Lynch, M., Middleton, P.G. *et al.* (1993) Nasal epithelial ion transport and genetic analysis of infertile men with congenital bilateral absence of the vas deferens. *Hum. Mol. Genet.*, **2**, (10), 1605–1609.

55. Chillòn, M., Casals, T., Mercier, B. *et al.* (1995) Mutations in the cystic fibrosis gene in patients with congenital absence of the vas deferens. *NEJM*, **332**, 1475–1480.

56. Dörk, T., Dworniczak, B., Aulehia-Scholz, C. *et al.* (1997) Distinct spectrum of CFTR gene mutations in congenital absence of vas deferens. *Hum. Genet.*, **100**, 367–377.

57. Chu, C., Trapnell, B.C., Curristin, S., Cutting, G.R. and Crystal, R.G. (1993) Genetic basis of variable exon 9 skipping in cystic fibrosis transmembrane conductance regulator mRNA. *Nature Genet.*, **3**, 151–156.

58. Zielenski, J., Patrizio, P., Corey, M. *et al.* (1995) CFTR gene variant for patients with congenital absence of vas deferens. *Am. J. Hum. Genet.*, **57**, 958–960.

59. Costes, B., Girodon, E., Ghanem, N. *et al.* (1995) Frequent occurrence of the CFTR intron 8 (TG)$_n$ 5T allele in men with congenital bilateral absence of the vas deferens. *Eur. J. Hum. Genet.*, **3**, 285–293.

60. Dumur, V., Gervais, R., Rigot, J.M. *et al.* (1996) Congenital bilateral absence of the vas deferens (CBAVD) and cystic fibrosis transmembrane regulator (CFTR) – correlation between genotype and phenotype. *Hum. Genet.*, **97**, 7–10.

61. Teng, H., Jorissen, M., Poppel, H., Legius, E., Cassiman, J.J. and Cuppens, H. (1997) Increased proportion of exon 9 alternatively spliced CFTR transcripts in vas deferens

compared with nasal epithelial cells. *Hum. Mol. Genet.*, **6**, 85–90.

62. Mak, V., Jarvi, K., Zielenski, J., Durie, P. and Tsui, L.-C. (1997) Higher proportion of intact exon 9 CFTR mRNA in nasal epithelium compared with vas deferens. *Hum. Mol. Genet.*, **6**, 2099–2107.

63. Rave-Harel, N., Kerem, E., Nissim-Rafinia, M. *et al.* (1997) The molecular basis of partial penetrance of splicing mutations in cystic fibrosis. *Am. J. Hum. Genet.*, **60**, 87–94.

64. Cuppens, H., Lin, W., Jaspers, M. *et al.* (1998) Polyvariant mutant cystic fibrosis transmembrane conductance regulator genes. *J. Clin. Invest.*, **101**, 487–496.

65. Allan, J.R., Robbie, M., Phelan, P.D. and Danks, D.M. (1981) Familial occurence of meconium ileus. *Eur. J. Pediatr.*, **135**, 291–292.

66. Mornet, E., Simon-Bouy, B., Serre, J.L. *et al.* (1988) Genetic differences between cystic fibrosis with and without meconium ileus. *Lancet*, **1**, 376–378.

67. Kerem, E., Corey, M., Kerem, B., Durie, P., Tsui, L. and Levison, H. (1989) Clinical and genetic comparisons of patients with cystic fibrosis, with or without meconium ileus. *J. Pediatr.*, **114**, 767–773.

68. Hamosh, A., King, T.M., Rosenstein, B.J. *et al.* (1992) Cystic fibrosis patients bearing the common missense mutation Gly→Asp at codon 551 and the deltaF508 are indistinguishable from deltaF508 homozygotes except for decreased risk of meconium ileus. *Am. J. Hum. Genet.*, **51**, 245–250.

69. Delaney, S.J., Alton, E., Smith, S. *et al.* (1996) Cystic fibrosis mice carrying the missense mutation G551D replicate human genotype–phenotype correlations. *EMBO J.*, **15**, 955–963.

70. Hamosh, A., Fitzsimmons, S., Macek, M. Jr, Knowles, M., Rosenstein, B. and Cutting, G.R. (1998) Comparison of the clinical manifestations of cystic fibrosis in black and white patients. *J. Pediatr.*, **132**, 255–259.

71. Macek, M. Jr, Macková, A., Hamosh, A. *et al.*(1997) Identification of common CF mutations in African-Americans with cystic fibrosis increases the detection rate to 75%. *Am. J. Hum. Genet.*, **60**, 1122–1127.

72. Ramsey, B. and Richardson, M.A. (1992) Impact of sinusitis in cystic fibrosis. *J. Allergy Clin. Immunol.*, **90**, 547–552.

73. Ledesma-Medina, J., Osman, M.Z. and Girdany, B.R. (1980) Abnormal paranasal sinuses in patients with cystic fibrosis of the pancreas. *Pediat. Radiol.*, **9**, 61–64.

74. Stern, R.C., Boat, T.F., Wood, R.E., Matthews, L.W. and Doershuk, C.F. (1982) Treatment and prognosis of nasal polyps in cystic fibrosis. *Am. J. Dis. Child.*, **136**, 1067–1070.

75. Varon, R., Magdorf, K., Staab, D. *et al.* (1995) Recurrent nasal polyps as a monosymptomatic form of cystic fibrosis associated with a novel in-frame deletion (591del18) in the CFTR gene. *Hum. Mol. Genet.*, **4**, 1463–1464.

76. Burger, J., Macek, M. Jr, Stuhrmann, M., Reis, A.,

Krawczak, M. and Schmidtke, J. (1991) Genetic influences in the formation of nasal polyps. *Lancet*, **337**, 974 (letter).

77. di Sant 'Agnese, P.A. and Hubbard, V.A. (1984) The hepatobiliary system, in *Cystic Fibrosis*, (ed. L.M. Taussig), Thième Stratton, New York, pp. 296–322.

78. Ferrari, M., Colombo, C., Sebastio, G. *et al.* (1991) Cystic fibrosis patients with liver disease are not genetically distinct. *Am. J. Hum. Genet.*, **48**, 815–816 (letter).

79. DeArce, M., O'Brien, S., Hegarty, J. *et al.* (1992) Deletion delta F508 and clinical expression of cystic fibrosis-related liver disease. *Clin. Genet.*, **42**, 271–272.

80. Colombo, C., Apostolo, M.G., Ferrari, M. *et al.* (1994) Analysis of risk factors for the development of liver disease associated with cystic fibrosis. *J. Pediatr.*, **124**, 393–399.

81. Buchdahl, R., Cox, M. and Fulleylove, C. (1988) Increased resting energy expenditure in cystic fibrosis. *J. Appl. Physiol.*, **64**, 1801–1806.

82. Shepherd, R., Holt, T., Vasquez-Velasquex, L., Coward, W., Prentice, A. and Lucas, A. (1988) Increased energy expenditure in children with cystic fibrosis. *Lancet*, **i**, 1300–1303.

83. Vaisman, N., Pencharz, P., Corey, M., Canny, G. and Hahn, E. (1987) Energy expenditure of patients with cystic fibrosis. *J. Pediatr.*, **111**, 496–500.

84. O'rawe A., McIntosh I., Dodge J.A. *et al.* (1992) Increased energy expenditure in cystic fibrosis is associated with specific mutations. *Clin. Sci.*, **82**, 71–76.

85. Tomezski, J.L., Stallings, V., Kawchak, D.A., Goin, J.E., Diamond, G. and Scanlin, T.F. (1994) Energy expenditure and genotype of children with cystic fibrosis. *Pediatr. Res.*, **35**, 451–460.

86. Kaplan, T.A., Moccia-Loos, G., Rabin, M. and McKey, R.M. Jr (1996) Lack of effect of delta F508 mutation in aerobic capacity in patients with cystic fibrosis. *Clin. J. Sport Med.*, **6**, 226–231.

87. Fried, M., Durie, P.R., Tsui, L., Corey, M., Levison, H. and Pencharz, P. (1991) The cystic fibrosis gene and resting energy expenditure. *J. Pediatr.*, **119**, 913–916.

88. Dumur, V., Lafitte, J., Gervais, R. *et al.* (1991) Abnormal distribution of cystic fibrosis deltaF508 allele in adults with chronic bronchial hypersecretion. *Lancet*, **335**, 1340

89. Gasparini, P., Savoia, A., Luisetti, M., Peona, V. and Pignatti, P.F. (1990) The cystic fibrosis gene is not likely to be involved in chronic obstructive pulmonary disease. *Am. J. Resp. Cell Mol. Biol.*, **2**, 297–299.

90. Gervais, R., Lafitte, J., Dumur, V. *et al.* (1993) Sweat chloride and deltaF508 mutation in chronic bronchitis or bronchiectasis. *Lancet*, **342**, 997.

91. Artlich, A., Boysen, A., Bunge, S., Entzian, P., Schlaak, M. and Schwinger, E. (1995) Common CFTR mutations are not likely to predispose to chronic bronchitis in Northern Germany. *Hum. Genet.*, **95**, 226–228.

92. Muller, E., Entzian, P., Boysen, A., Arlich, A., Schwinger, E. and Schlaak, M. (1995) Frequency of common cystic fibrosis gene mutations in chronic bronchitis patients. *Scand. J. Clin. Lab. Invest.*, **55**, 263–266.

93. Poller, W., Faber, J., Scholz, S., Olek, K. and Müller, K.M. (1991) Sequence analysis of the cystic fibrosis gene in patients with disseminated bronchiectatic lung disease. *Klin. Wochenschrift*, **69**, 657–663.

94. Pignatti, P.F., Bombieri, C., Marigo, C., Benetazzo, M. and Luisetti, M. (1995) Increasd incidence of cystic fibrosis gene mutations in adults with disseminated bronchiectasis. *Hum. Mol. Genet.*, **4**, 635–639.

95. Pignatti, P.F., Bombieri, C., Benetazzo, M. *et al.* (1996) CFTR gene variant EVS8-5T in obstructive pulmonary disease. *Am. J. Hum. Genet.*, **58**, 889–892.

96. Girodon, E., Cazeneuve, C., Lebargy, F. *et al.* (1997) CFTR gene mutations in adults with disseminated bronchiectasis. *Eur. J. Hum. Genet.*, **5**, 149–155.

97. Nelson, L.A., Callerame, M.L. and Schwartz, R.H. (1979) Aspergillosis and atopy in cystic fibrosis. *Am. Rev. Respir. Dis.*, **120**, 863–878.

98. Miller, P.W., Hamosh, A., Macek, M. Jr *et al.* (1996) Cystic fibrosis transmembrane conductance regulator (CFTR) gene mutations in allergic bronchopulmonary aspergillosis. *Am. J. Hum. Genet.*, **59**, 45–51.

99. Friedman, K., Heim, R., Knowles, M. and Silverman, L. (1997) Rapid characterization of the variable length polythymidine tract in the cystic fibrosis (CFTR) gene: Association of the 5T allele with selected CFTR mutations and its incidence in atypical sinopulmonary disease. *Hum. Mutat.*, **10**, 108–115.

100. Snouwaert, J.N., Brigman, K.K., Latour, A.M. *et al.* (1992) An animal model for cystic fibrosis made by gene targeting. *Science*, **257**, 1083–1088.

101. Dorin, J.R., Dickinson, P., Alton, E.W.F.W. *et al.* (1992) Cystic fibrosis in the mouse by targeted insertional mutagenesis. *Nature*, **359**, 211–215.

102. Rozmahel, R., Wilschanski, M., Matin, A. *et al.* (1996) Modulation of disease severity in cystic fibrosis transmembrane conductance regulator deficient mice by a secondary genetic factor. *Nature Genet.*, **12**, 280–287.

103. Kent, G., Hes, R., Bear, C. *et al.* (1997) Lung disease in mice with cystic fibrosis. *J. Clin. Invest.*, **100**, 3060–3069.

104. Clarke, L.L., Grubb, B.R., Gabriel, S.E., Smithies, O., Koller, B.H. and Boucher, R.C. (1992) Defective epithelial chloride transport in a gene-targeted mouse model of cystic fibrosis. *Science*, **257**, 1125–1128.

105. Clarke, L.B., Grubb, B.R., Yankaskas, J.R., Cotton, C.U., McKenzie, A. and Boucher, R.C. (1994) Relationship of a non-cystic fibrosis transmembrane conductance regulator-mediated chloride conductance to organ-level disease in CFTR (–/–) mice. *Proc. Natl Acad. Sci. USA*, **91**, 479–483.

106. Zielenski, J., Corey, M., Rozmahel, R. *et al.* (1999) Detection of a cystic fibrosis modifier locus for meconium ileus on human chromosome 19q13. *Nature Genet*, **22,** 128–129.

107. Gilfillan, A., Warner, J.P., Kirk, J.M. *et al.* (1998) P67L: a cystic fibrosis allele with mild effects found at high frequency in the Scottish population. *J. Med. Genet.*, **35**, 122–125.

4

Applied cell biology

E.W.F.W. ALTON AND S.N. SMITH

Introduction	61	Other organs	71
Sweat gland	61	Intracellular defects	72
Respiratory tract	64	CFTR	72
Gastrointestinal tract	68	Heterozygotes	75
Pancreas	69	Relationship of the basic defect to pathology	75
Blood	69	CF model systems	76
Kidney	70	Conclusion	76
Skin	70	References	77
Salivary glands	71		

INTRODUCTION

Over the past decade arguably more has become known about the basic defect in cystic fibrosis (CF) than in the preceding four centuries since the first astute observations recorded in Swiss–German folklore:

> Woe to that child, which when kissed on the forehead tastes salty;
> he is 'bewitched' and soon must die

The transport of sodium (Na^+) and chloride (Cl^-) ions, and particularly the latter, is central to the basic defect in CF. The aim of this chapter is first to describe the ion transport defects present in the various affected organs, preceded in the sweat gland and airways by a brief summary of the normal counterpart of these processes. This is followed by sections on the CF gene product, cystic fibrosis transmembrane conductance regulator (CFTR), and speculation on how abnormalities in this protein might cause disease in patients. Finally, recent studies on cultured cells and animal models as the basis for future studies on the basic defect in this disease are reviewed.

SWEAT GLAND

Normal physiology

Since salt appears on the skin surface through the sweat glands, the above-noted 'salty kiss', as well as the more objective sweat test, indicate that the CF defect must be present in this organ. The primary secretion which is formed in the secretory coil at the base of the sweat gland is isotonic with plasma and its production is under the regulation of both temperature and efferent nerve endings, cholinergic control being markedly more important than adrenergic regulation in humans. As sweat passes up through the sweat duct Na^+ is reabsorbed by an active energy-requiring process, dependent on the activity of the Na^+, K^+-ATPase in the epithelial cells lining the duct. To maintain electrical neutrality, Cl^- is secondarily reabsorbed with the Na^+ and, since the ductal cells are impermeable to water, a hypotonic solution is produced at the skin surface.

All epithelial cells, whether lining the sweat duct, respiratory or gastrointestinal tracts, generate a potential difference (PD) between their luminal and serosal (vascular) surfaces. This voltage is produced by the separation of charge across these surfaces, related to the activity of the Na^+, K^+-ATPase noted above. By actively pumping Na^+ out of the cell, low intracellular Na^+ levels are produced which can be used by the cell to transport ions passively across cell membranes. Thus, for example, Na^+ will enter ductal cells through specific proteins (channels) down such a favorable concentration gradient. The accompanying Cl^- can also move into the cell through anion channels on the luminal membrane and exit through channels at the basolateral surface.

Cystic fibrosis

SECRETORY COIL

The volume and rate of sweat production in CF is normal[1], suggesting that under physiologic conditions the secretory coil is unaffected. However, if sweating is stimulated through the β-adrenergic pathway either *in vivo* or *in vitro*[2], CF tissues fail to produce sweat. Furthermore, isoprenaline also fails either to increase (make more negative) the PD of, or produce Cl^- secretion in, the CF secretory coil, in contrast to normal glands. α-Adrenergic and cholinergic stimulation, however, produce normal rates of sweating[2], as well as normal Cl^- movement in CF glands, likely via calcium-dependent potassium and chloride conductances. A recent study has shown that of the three cell types present in the secretory coil, it is only the β-adrenergic-sensitive cells which are affected in CF. Importantly, the stimulation of the plasma membrane enzyme, adenylate cyclase, by adrenergic agonists, such as isoprenaline, produces an elevation in intracellular cAMP, which is indistinguishable in CF and non-CF glands[2].

These important studies were some of the first to indicate that the basic defect in CF is linked to defective regulation through cAMP-linked pathways, and that this abnormality lies distal to the production of this second messenger. Furthermore, these studies distinguish between a normally functioning calcium-linked intracellular pathway (stimulated through cholinergic inputs) and defective cAMP-linked control, the former allowing for normal sweat production in the CF secretory coil. Protein kinase C (PKC) activity does not appear to regulate Cl^- movement in the secretory coil.

REABSORPTIVE DUCT

Chloride transport

Since there is excessive salt on the skin surface in the face of normal rates of sweating, the basic defect must also be present in the reabsorptive portion of the sweat duct. A series of elegant studies on this part of the gland provided the first indications for the cause of this abnormality[1]. The PD produced by the epithelial cells of the duct *in vivo* was measured and demonstrated that CF epithelium has a markedly more negative PD than normal tissue[1] (Fig. 4.1). Furthermore, although the rates of reabsorption of both Na^+ and Cl^- were reduced, this was markedly more so for Cl^-. To extend these findings, individual ducts were dissected from skin biopsies and the lumen microperfused *in vitro*[3]; these ducts also showed the difference in PD noted *in vivo*. When non-CF glands were perfused with a lower salt solution (50 mM) than was present in the external bath solution (150 mM), the PD became more negative, indicating that the duct cells were readily permeable to Cl^- ions moving down the created concentration gradient into the lumen of the duct. The same experiment repeated in CF ducts caused the PD to become more positive, indicating that these cells were impermeable to Cl^- (Table 4.1). Furthermore, if instead of NaCl, non-CF ducts were perfused with sodium sulfate, their PD became identical to CF glands. Because sulfate ions are too large to pass across the epithelial cells, such conditions mimic those present in CF glands, namely one of Cl^- impermeability. A number of studies have confirmed and elaborated on these findings. The basal conductance (G, a measure of permeability to ions) of normal duct epithelium comprises an approximately 90 per cent contribution from Cl^- and 5 per cent from Na^+. In CF ducts G is approximately sixfold less than in normal glands and this is entirely related to the reduced Cl^- movement. Studies have addressed whether the site of defective Cl^- transport is within or between the ductal cells. If the former predominates in

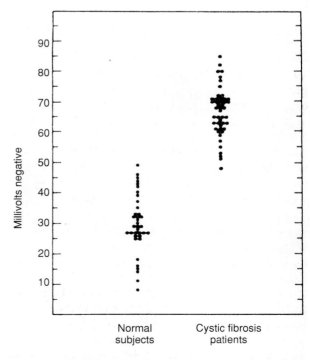

Fig. 4.1 *Sweat duct potential difference. (Reproduced with permission from ref. 136.)*

Table 4.1 *Average luminal potential differences in cystic fibrosis and normal sweat ducts perfused with solutions of varying composition*

	150 mM NaCl	50 mM NaCl	75 mM Na$_2$SO$_4$
Pre-ouabain control ($n = 7$)	-6.8 ± 2.5	-24.2 ± 2.4	-75.5 ± 11.1
CF ($n = 5$)	-76.9 ± 13.2	-47.6 ± 12.3	-33.3 ± 19.5

normal cells then, by analogy with other epithelia, it is likely that this will occur through anion channels. Evidence for this has come from studies using Cl$^-$ channel blockers and the identification of at least four types of anion channels within sweat gland cells. Furthermore, bumetanide, an inhibitor of Na$^+$/2Cl$^-$/K$^+$ cotransport used to allow Cl$^-$ entry into epithelial cells, markedly reduces Cl$^-$ permeability in normal cells. Finally, evidence that the Cl$^-$ impermeability is intrinsic to these cells is shown by the retention of the defect in cultured cells, as well as the lack of effect of CF sweat on the ion transport properties of non-CF ducts.

That the defective Cl$^-$ transport in CF is linked to these cellular pathways has been shown in a number of ways. Thus, microelectrode studies have shown that the inner surface of the luminal membrane of normal ductal cells is negatively charged with reference to the outer surface. In CF cells this charge is significantly less negative (depolarized) than in normal cells, related to reduced Cl$^-$ permeability into the cell. Direct measurement of intracellular Cl$^-$ movement using the fluorescent indicator, SPQ, has confirmed this reduced transcellular transport, which is present at both the mucosal and serosal surfaces of these cells. Furthermore, the anion selectivity of ductal cells is altered from the normal Cl$^-$ > I$^-$, indicating that Cl$^-$ transport occurs through altered pathways in CF. Finally, bromide transport (likely to occur through channels) is also reduced in CF. Elevation of cAMP in ductal cells increases Cl$^-$ reabsorption in normal glands but, in accordance with the secretory coil data, has little or no effect in CF cells. With the discovery of the CF gene and its protein product, CFTR, has come the possibility of introducing antisense DNA to the CF gene into the cell. This will prevent transcription and translation of CFTR and, when introduced into normal ductal cells, will induce Cl$^-$ impermeability[4]. Since CFTR is known to form a cAMP-regulatable Cl$^-$ channel, this study provides an important link with the studies noted above. Antibodies to CFTR localize it to the epithelial cells of the normal reabsorptive duct, particularly at the apical membrane but also near the basolateral surface, in keeping with the demonstration of defective cAMP-related Cl$^-$ transport at both cell surfaces. As in other tissues, ΔF_{508} CFTR appears to be mislocalized[5], being retained in the cytoplasm, little or none appearing at the apical membrane. Thus, there is conclusive evidence that transcellular Cl$^-$ transport through ductal cells involves the CF gene product CFTR acting as a Cl$^-$ channel, a process that can be regulated by cAMP. This process is defective in CF glands and represents the basic defect in this tissue.

Sodium transport

Na$^+$ absorption is, as evidenced by the sweat test, reduced in CF ducts. However, this is likely to represent a secondary abnormality related to the Cl$^-$ impermeability, the more negative intraluminal PD in these ducts retaining Na$^+$ within the lumen. That Na$^+$ absorption is not primarily abnormal in CF has been demonstrated in several studies. The increased affinity constant of the Na$^+$-channel blocker amiloride in CF ductal cells is again likely to relate to the increased charge, causing increased binding to the channel. Such Na$^+$ transport can be regulated through agonists elevating intracellular calcium which activate potassium efflux from the cell through a calcium-activated channel. This hyperpolarizes (makes more negative) the cell interior and increases the driving forces promoting Na$^+$ absorption. Such calcium-related regulation of Na$^+$ is not altered in CF, in keeping with the demonstration of a normally functioning calcium-activated potassium channel.

Other

A variety of measured parameters in sweat show no abnormalities in CF, including cAMP and cGMP levels, lactate, bicarbonate and pH. In normal sweat, Cl$^-$ and sulfate levels are positively correlated, but sulfate levels in CF sweat are reduced, a finding of uncertain significance. In many tissues prostaglandin E$_2$ (PGE$_2$) exerts its effects through elevation of cAMP and, unsurprisingly, this agent has no effect in stimulating Cl$^-$ absorption in CF glands. However, this study has suggested a further effect on Cl$^-$ transport over and above that related to cAMP production, which is also defective in CF tissues. A noteworthy observation is the demonstration that the vasoactive intestinal polypeptide (VIP)-ergic innervation of CF sweat glands is markedly reduced in comparison to normal tissues. The VIP gene in humans maps to chromosome 6 and the significance of this finding is presently unknown. Finally, prolactin has been suggested to have a role in sweat formation and this process may be altered in CF glands, perhaps related to overglycosylation of prolactin in CF.

RESPIRATORY TRACT

Normal physiology

The luminal surface of airway epithelial cells is lined by hair-like cilia which beat in synchrony to sweep inhaled particles and potential pathogens out of the respiratory tract. To function effectively these cilia must be bathed in a layer of fluid. The source of this fluid is presently uncertain, but it is hypothesized that it is produced in the lung periphery and moved cranially by ciliary movement[6]. Since the surface area of the alveolar region of the lung is vast in comparison to that of the trachea, large volumes of fluid are likely to be pushed into such a bottleneck. Airway epithelial cells are able to reabsorb fluid using the processes shown in Fig. 4.2. As in sweat duct cells, Na^+ is absorbed through sodium channels in the apical membrane and extruded through the basolateral membrane by the Na^+, K^+-ATPase. Na^+ enters the cell through channels down the favorable gradient created by the ATPase. Once inside the cell, the Na^+ ions are pumped out onto the basolateral surface of the cell by the ATPase and, since such transport of ions results in the consequent movement of water by osmosis, this cycle of sodium absorption will also result in water absorption. It is likely that these processes operate to limit the volume of the periciliary fluid layer. Ion transport mechanisms also exist to rehydrate the airway surface. The low intracellular concentration of Na^+ created by the Na^+, K^+-ATPase can also be used to allow movement of Na^+ into the cell from the basolateral surface through a $Na^+/2Cl^-/K^+$ cotransporter. Cl^- is thus able to enter the cell down the favorable Na^+ gradient created by the ATPase. Cl^- ions will now exit the cell down the created gradient towards the luminal surface through Cl^- channels. Water will follow the movement of Cl^-, enabling rehydration of the airway surface. In the basal state Na^+ absorption predominates, but it is likely that during periods of activity during which the potential for airway dehydration exists, Cl^- secretion can be activated to maintain periciliary fluid volume.

Cystic fibrosis

CHLORIDE TRANSPORT

At a similar time to the sweat-gland studies noted above, chloride impermeability of airway epithelial cells was also demonstrated, both *in vitro* and *in vivo*. The PD of nasal epithelium can be relatively easily measured and provides a convenient bioelectric window onto the lung. As in the sweat gland, this PD is more negative in CF[7] and can be used as a clinical diagnostic test for this disease (Fig. 4.3). Perfusion of the nasal mucosa with a low Cl^- containing solution creates a favorable gradient for Cl^- exit into the lumen, measured as an increased PD. In CF there is a markedly reduced response to this maneuver[8], even in the presence of amiloride (Fig. 4.4). This sodium-channel blocker, by hyperpolarizing the apical cell membrane, will increase the driving force for Cl^- exit from the cell. Very similar results have been obtained *in vitro* from CF nasal polyps[9] and the Cl^- impermeability of CF nasal and airway epithelia has now been confirmed in many studies. That the abnormality is intrinsic to the epithelium and not due to circulating factors has been shown in several ways. Dissociated cells from CF nasal tissue were seeded onto a trachea denuded of cells and this in turn was transplanted into an immunocompromised mouse, the CF cells continuing to demonstrate Cl^- impermeability[10]. CF airway cells have been grown in primary culture

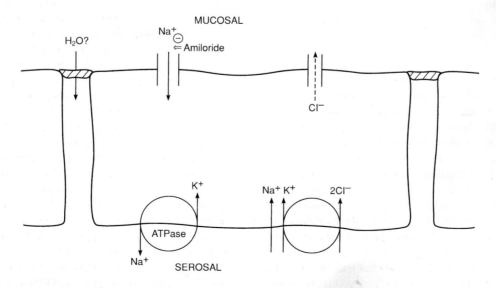

Fig. 4.2 *Normal airway ion transport processes.*

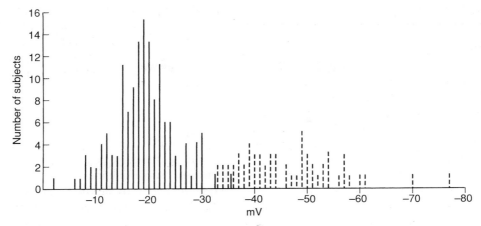

Fig. 4.3 *Frequency distribution of nasal PD in CF (---) and controls (—).*

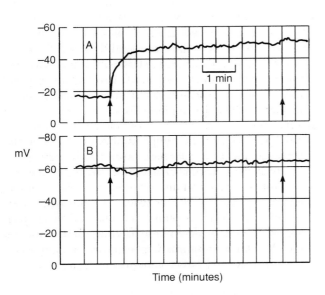

Fig. 4.4 *Effect of perfusion of nasal epithelium with low chloride solution. A, non-CF; B, CF. (Reproduced with permission from ref. 8.)*

in many laboratories and again shown to retain this reduced Cl⁻ conductance. Finally, CF saliva or serum shows no difference in comparison to their normal counterparts in stimulating Cl⁻ secretion in dog trachea.

As in the sweat duct, the abnormal Cl⁻ conductance can be shown to be due to defective transcellular, rather than paracellular, Cl⁻ movement, localized in particular to the luminal membrane. Thus, microelectrode studies show that the apical membrane of CF cells is depolarized relative to its non-CF counterpart and that this is not altered by low Cl⁻ perfusion of the luminal surface of the cell[11,12]. Cl⁻ entry into the cell via the basolateral cotransporter functions normally in CF[12] and intracellular Cl⁻ activity is normal[12]. However, preventing Cl⁻ entry into

the cell by blocking this cotransporter with bumetanide has no effect on Cl⁻ secretion in CF tissues, as expected if there is Cl⁻ impermeability of the apical membrane. Finally, the single-channel studies noted below clearly localize the absent Cl⁻ permeability in CF to the apical membrane. No abnormality of paracellular pathways has been shown in CF airways.

Cl⁻ transport in normal airway epithelium can be stimulated through four second-messenger pathways: cAMP, cGMP, calcium and protein kinase C[13]. Numerous studies have documented the lack of Cl⁻ secretion in response to agents acting through the cAMP pathway in CF airways[10,13,14], as in sweat glands the hallmark of the CF defect. Both cAMP production[15,16] and protein kinase A (PKA) activity[13] have been assayed and are not defective in CF. Single-channel studies of airway epithelium initially identified a Cl⁻ channel[17–19], given the acronym ORDIC because of its biophysical properties of outward rectification of the current–voltage relationship and increased open probability induced by depolarization (DI). This channel has been shown clearly to be different from CFTR. The patch–clamp technique allows such channels to be studied within the normal cell membrane (cell-attached) as well as when removed from this environment (excised). In the cell-attached mode, β-agonists were shown to open this channel in normal airway cells[17,18], but failed to do so in CF cells[16,18]. However, if the CF channel was excised from the cell or subjected to depolarizing voltages, it opened normally[18], suggesting that the regulation of this channel through the cAMP pathway is defective in CF. In the excised mode, PKA failed to activate the channel in CF cells[19–21]. Cl⁻ secretion in response to stimulation through the PKC pathway is also defective in CF nasal polyps[13] and in support of this, PKC activation of the ORDIC channel has also been shown to be defective in CF cells[19,22], despite normal PKC activity[13]. The finding that the ORDIC channel can be activated in both non-CF and CF cells by excision from the cell has led to studies investigating the presence of a possible cytosolic inhibitor. These have identified a heat- and proteolysis-stable substance of between 0.7 and 1.5 kDa, which produces dose-dependent inhibition of the ORDIC channel.

As discussed on p. 72 below, the cloning of the CF gene has led to studies of the function of its product, CFTR. There is now unequivocal evidence that at least one function of this protein is to form a Cl⁻ channel which is regulated by type II PKA[23,24]. Although this corresponds well with the evidence accumulated prior to the identification of the gene, the biophysical properties of the CFTR Cl⁻ channel are indisputably different from those of the ORDIC channel. Thus, the CFTR channel has a linear current–voltage (I–V) relationship, is not activated or inactivated by voltage and has a much smaller conductance[24,25] and resembles a channel previously described in pancreatic duct cells[26]. Thus the ORDIC, or as it has been more recently termed the ORCC channel, is one example of a channel regulated by CFTR (see below).

CFTR has been localized to the apical membrane of airway cells[27]. This occurs principally in submucosal glands (see below) and in the bronchiolar and alveolar regions. Within the bronchioles expression was seen in non-ciliated cells which more proximally accorded with Clara cells, but more distally were in an unspecified non-ciliated population[28]. CFTR has been suggested to be the most common conductance within the respiratory epithelium. Expression of normal CFTR in cultured CF airway cells corrects the cAMP-mediated Cl⁻ defect[29], whereas antisense DNA to CFTR induces the CF phenotype in non-CF cells[30]. In common with the sweat gland, CFTR in CF airway cells may not reach the apical surface but appears to be mislocalized (see below).

Elevation of intracellular calcium is also able to produce Cl⁻ secretion in the airway epithelium, and this process appears to function normally in CF[13,14]. Although the single-channel basis for this Cl⁻ current has not been identified, it has differing biophysical properties to cAMP-induced currents and is likely, therefore, to be linked to proteins other than CFTR[14]. Stimulation requires calmodulin kinase as an intermediate and is not blocked by inhibitors of PKC[31]. One possible candidate for this calcium-activated channel activity is the ClC-2 channel[32].

In the presence of extracellular hypotonicity, cell swelling is quickly followed by the protective response known as regulatory volume decrease (RVD). This response has been well characterized in a number of epithelia and usually involves both chloride and potassium secretion. Although the candidate chloride channel is uncertain, studies have suggested that a channel described as a voltage-sensitive organic osmolyte/anion channel (VSOAC) may be involved, with intracellular ionic strength responsible for channel activation. This process appears to function normally in CF.

NA⁺ TRANSPORT

As noted above, Na⁺ transport predominates in human airways and is largely responsible for the PD across respiratory epithelia[9]. The Na⁺-channel blocker, amiloride, reduces airway PD to approximately the same values in CF and non-CF, suggesting that Na⁺ absorption is increased two- to threefold in this disease[7,8]. This *in vivo* finding has been confirmed *in vitro*, both in Ussing chamber studies[15] and with the demonstration that the ouabain-sensitive oxygen component of CF cells is increased[33], suggesting increased activity of the Na⁺, K⁺-ATPase and, in turn, Na⁺ absorption. The Na⁺ abnormality has been localized to the apical membrane by microelectrode studies[11], but, as for Cl⁻, the basal intracellular Na⁺ activity is normal in CF. Furthermore, Na⁺ is transported normally into the CF cell by the basolateral cotransporter. The abnormality is retained in cell culture[10] and is, therefore, clearly intrinsic to CF epithelium and not related to a circulating factor. Single-channel studies have proved more difficult than for Cl⁻ channels, but reports suggest that when studied in the cell-attached mode, CF cells either demonstrate an increased number of Na⁺ channels or an increased channel open probability in comparison to normal cells[34] and a compensatory increase in Na⁺, K⁺-ATPase activity.

The recent cloning of the amiloride-sensitive sodium channel (ENaC) has helped to elucidate the relationship of this channel to CFTR (see below). CFTR appears to downregulate its activity, operating at the level of channel gating by switching the response to cAMP from an increase to a decrease in channel open probability. This regulatory process is lost in CF, thus producing the increase in sodium absorption. There is no increase in ENaC mRNA expression in CF[35], whereas the expression of both CFTR and ENaC is enhanced by female sex hormones, at least in the rat.

Na⁺ transport is under the regulation of both calcium- and PKC-related pathways in normal airways, cAMP having little effect. In CF these responses have not been well documented, but isoprenaline produces a paradoxical increase in Na⁺ absorption[15]. Aldosterone, a regulator of renal Na⁺ absorption, has been shown not to be elevated in CF, and spironolactone, an aldosterone antagonist, does not reduce the elevated PD in CF. The gene for an amiloride-binding protein flanks the CF gene on chromosome 7, but is not affected by CF mutations. Thus, this Na⁺ defect, which may be of crucial importance in the airways, again appears to be secondary to the Cl⁻ defect, as in sweat glands.

SUBMUCOSAL GLANDS

These tissues are the predominant site of CFTR expression in the airways[36]. CFTR is localized most abundantly in the serous cells of the acinar regions of the glands, particularly in association with their secretory granules. It has also been localized, using immunogold electron microscopy, to both the apical and basolateral plasma membranes of glandular mucous cells. Further functional studies comparing different cell populations indicate that serous cells mediate chloride secretion. Developmental studies in the ferret have shown that differentiation of stem cells to CFTR-expressing gland cells occurs very early within fetal gland development.

Several studies have shown that the cAMP-mediated Cl⁻ defect is also present in the epithelium of these glands. Whether the calcium-linked pathway is intact is more controversial. Thus, two studies have shown normal calcium-regulated chloride transport in airway glands in CF, whereas a further two have indicated that both cAMP- and calcium-linked stimuli appear to be defective with respect to Cl⁻ secretion and mucin output, differing from airway surface epithelium and resembling the gastrointestinal tract (see p. 68). Thus CFTR has been suggested to be the exclusive chloride conductance in submucosal glands. Calcium-linked stimuli would then produce increased basolateral potassium exit through calcium-sensitive potassium channels. This, in turn, leads to intracellular hyperpolarization and thus an increase in the driving force for chloride exit through CFTR. Interestingly, bicarbonate-dependent chloride secretion has been shown to be the major ion movement in serous cells under baseline (unstimulated) conditions, and, in an *in vivo* pig model, clearance of mucin from the ducts of submucosal glands is via liquid generated through both chloride- and bicarbonate-linked transport[37,38].

It is now known that mucus is generated principally from the more proximal cells in the gland, whereas a more fluid secretion with a lower protein content comes from the distally located serous cells. More specifically, of the various mucin genes, *MUC5B* and *MUC7* are expressed only in submucosal glands, with the former confined to mucous tubules and the latter to serous tubules. No differences in the expression of these two genes were detected between CF and non-CF tissues. Thus CFTR may be involved in flushing the secretions from the ducts; these findings may help to explain the low levels of CFTR in airway surface epithelium and may have important implications for CFTR function and pathogenesis of CF. Finally, when incubated with serous cells, CF sputum was a potent inducer of macromolecule secretion. This could be prevented by neutrophil protease inhibitors, suggesting that a positive feedback loop may exist in the airways for excessive mucus production.

OTHER

The role of CF serum in producing airway abnormalities has been much debated. As noted above, a circulating factor is clearly not responsible for the basic defect. However, a number of studies have demonstrated that CF serum increases airway mucin secretion, although not always to a greater extent than normal serum. Furthermore, this (or other) factors in CF serum or saliva can produce ciliary dyskinesia. A sequence of goblet-cell swelling, mucus discharge and disruption of synchronized ciliary activity has been demonstrated to occur with CF but not normal serum. However, other studies have failed to demonstrate such changes and, in particular, when human respiratory tract ciliary beat frequency was studied (as opposed to animal models), CF serum showed no effect on ciliary function.

Calcium has been hypothesized to be important in mediating the CF defect, with reports of increased baseline levels in airways secretions as well as within the cell. Reduced responses of intracellular calcium to histamine and PGE_1 have also been reported. However, other studies have demonstrated normal values, both basally and in response to stimulation, and the relevance of these findings is uncertain. A recent study has shown that the calcium-linked generation of arachidonic acid is increased in CF cells, suggested to be important given the proinflammatory role of this lipid mediator. Further, the analysis of annexin expression in CF and non-CF cell lines showed an overexpression of annexin V – a protein that functions as a calcium channel – in the former

Potassium is predominantly transported into the cell by the Na⁺, K⁺-ATPase and exits across the basolateral membrane through potassium channels whose function is probably not altered in CF[16]. Very little potassium appears to be transported across the mucosal surface in airway epithelium[8]. Bicarbonate can also be secreted across the respiratory epithelium and the regulation of this by cAMP, but not by calcium, is also defective in CF[39], suggesting conduction of this anion through the CFTR channel. This is further underlined by the submucosal gland studies noted above. Basal intracellular pH is normal in CF cells, and a Na⁺/H⁺ exchanger that can be upregulated through PKC also appears to function normally in CF.

Increased sulfation of mucus glycoproteins has been demonstrated in CF cells and has been hypothesized to link with the Cl⁻ defect. Thus, sulfate ions will pass through the apical anion channels and if this passage through CFTR is prevented, intracellular sulfate will increase. This may lead to increased movement of sulfate into the Golgi and, in turn, increased packaging into macromolecules. However, increased sulfation of macromolecules has also been demonstrated in the mucus of patients with other chronic respiratory conditions and may be a nonspecific finding. Finally, altered cell-surface glycosylation present in a CF cell line has been suggested not to relate directly to the absence of CFTR.

Water movement, perhaps one of the most important factors in producing CF lung disease, has been little studied, related at least in part to the difficulties of such measurements. An indirect approach recorded water vapor partial pressure and temperature in the pharynx of non-

CF and CF subjects[40]. At ambient temperatures there was no significant difference in these parameters between the two groups, but once the temperature of the inspired air had been raised to 48°C, both water vapor partial pressure and relative humidity of the inspired air were lower in CF subjects, together with a higher airway surface temperature. Thus, when stressed, such water transport may provide the rate-limiting step in these patients. Interestingly, a recent study has shown that when CFTR mRNA is injected into *Xenopus* oocytes, the resultant protein can function not only as a Cl$^-$ channel but also as a water channel[41]. Using a capacitance probe technique, one group has compared fluid transport across surface epithelial and submucosal gland cultures from CF and non-CF subjects[42]. In the latter, the direction of fluid transport was determined by a balance between sodium absorption and cAMP-mediated chloride secretion through CFTR. In contrast, CF cultures showed only basal absorption and a lack of cAMP- but not calcium-mediated fluid secretion. Similar findings of an increase in basal fluid absorption were also shown using human bronchial xenografts[43]. These findings may help to explain the characteristic airway CF pathophysiology noted above.

GASTROINTESTINAL TRACT

Chloride transport

Chloride transport contributes to the basal PD in the rectal mucosa of normal subjects. Thus, alterations in either the baseline values or the proportion of this voltage which can be inhibited by amiloride would indicate changes in basal Cl$^-$ conductance in CF. Several studies have demonstrated a normal PD in CF rectal mucosa, whereas others show reduced values[44]. Similarly the effect of amiloride has been reported to be not different[44,45], reduced or enhanced in this region of the gut. Although discrepancies exist with regard to basal Cl$^-$ conductance, as expected from preceding sections cAMP-induced Cl$^-$ secretion is abnormal in various regions of the CF gastrointestinal tract, including jejunum[46,47], small intestine, colon and rectum[44,48], demonstrable both *in vitro* and *in vivo*. Production of cAMP or its binding proteins in response to various agonists is not altered[44], and secretion appears to be through the CFTR channel. These findings accord with the intestinal distribution of CFTR, which is low in the stomach, and high in the small and large intestines, expression being principally in the crypts and decreasing towards the villi[49]. Other Cl$^-$ channels have been identified and some shown not to be altered in CF. In CF colonic tissues, agents elevating cAMP tend to reduce PD, through induction of potassium secretion[48], a process which is probably unaffected in CF.

Several studies have addressed whether calcium-mediated responses are abnormal in CF gut. Most studies indicate that, unlike in CF airways, Cl$^-$ secretion cannot be induced through increases in free intracellular calcium in the jejunum, small intestine, colon or rectum[45,48]. Again, K$^+$ secretion may be seen following such stimulation in CF[48]. Basal calcium levels and the induced increases in response to agonists are, however, normal. Some residual Cl$^-$ secretion in response to calcium-mediated agonists was demonstrable in compound heterozygotes in the colon and also in jejunal tissues[46]. PKC-induced stimulation of Cl$^-$ secretion is also abnormal in the jejunum. This reduction in both cAMP- and calcium-stimulated Cl$^-$ secretion suggests that in the gastrointestinal tract both may occur through the CFTR channel, these tissues lacking a calcium-linked channel as in the airways.

However, several recent studies indicate some discrepancies in this hypothesis. Thus, an antibody to CFTR introduced into the T84 Cl$^-$ secreting cell line reduced only the cAMP-stimulated current in whole-cell patch–clamp studies. Calcium-mediated responses were intact, whereas cell-swelling-induced responses were only partially attenuated. Antisense DNA to the CF gene introduced into the same cell line reduced CFTR expression and cAMP-induced Cl$^-$ secretion, but did not alter calcium-stimulated Cl$^-$ transport[30]. Another Cl$^-$ secreting cell line of gut origin (HT29) was studied at different stages of cell polarity. Unpolarized cells demonstrated calcium- but not cAMP-inducible Cl$^-$ secretion, but both were present when cells became polarized. Finally, a cell line derived from CF fetal intestine demonstrates defective cAMP-induced but normal calcium-induced Cl$^-$ transport.

Sodium transport

The variability in amiloride response of the rectum has been noted above and may reflect varying basal Cl$^-$ transport. Esophageal PD is not altered by amiloride superfusion in CF. Na$^+$–glucose cotransport has been studied in CF small intestine and shows an increase in response to a glucose load in most studies. Further, both in rat and human small intestine the Na$^+$–glucose cotransporter is co-localized with CFTR. Na$^+$ absorption was also shown to increase in CF jejunum following stimulation with the phosphodiesterase inhibitor, IBMX. Thus, it is likely that Na$^+$ transport is also increased at least in some regions of the CF gut. The effect of putative circulating factors on Na$^+$ transport has been studied on several occasions, with variable results. Thus CF saliva induces a larger inhibition of Na$^+$ reabsorption in rat colon than normal saliva, whereas no difference was noted in the effects of CF and non-CF serum on Na$^+$–glucose cotransport in one study, but an increased inhibition by CF serum in another.

Other

Baseline esophageal PD is unaltered in CF, whereas analysis of CF gastric juices showed decreased volume, increased viscosity, Na^+ and calcium levels. Indirect evidence for normal potassium-channel function in labial glands has been shown by normal potassium release in response to cholinergic stimulation. In keeping with other organs, CFTR has recently been shown to mediate the HCO_3^- secretion that occurs in all segments of the small intestine, irrespective of whether this occurred through stimulation by cAMP, cGMP or calcium[50].

PANCREAS

Although less information is available on the pancreatic abnormalities in CF, it is clear that the cAMP-mediated Cl^- defect is also present in this organ. Thus, *in vivo*, in response to an infusion of secretin and cholecystokinin, the CF pancreas produces reduced Cl^-, Na^+, K^+ and HCO_3^- levels. Fluid secretion is also reduced but is normal when adjusted for Cl^- and HCO_3^- levels, suggesting that this is secondary to the reduction in these ions. Since the Cl^-/HCO_3^- ratio is not altered in CF, it is likely that the secretion of both these ions is abnormal in CF. The finding that HCO_3^- passes readily through the ORDIC channel (and other Cl^- channels) suggests that the same defect may be responsible for both abnormalities.

Normal pancreatic duct cells provided the first demonstration of the CFTR Cl^- channel[26] and several studies demonstrate the likely involvement of this channel in pancreatic abnormalities in CF. Thus, insertion of a normal copy of the CF gene into CF pancreatic cells complements the cAMP-mediated defect in Cl^- secretion[51] and the single-channel basis for this complementation is likely through the CFTR channel. Furthermore, antibodies to CFTR localize it principally to the proximal ducts of the pancreas, with some seen in the acinar regions. Obstruction of human CF pancreatic ducts has been shown to relate to accumulation of the mucin gene *MUC6*.

In vitro, an immortalized CF pancreatic cell line (CFPAC) having the ΔF_{508} genotype shows no cAMP-mediated Cl^- secretion but normal calcium-mediated transport. As expected, cAMP production and PKA activity are normal in these cells which demonstrate the presence of the ORDIC channel but, as in other organs, there is no correlation between this channel and CFTR mRNA. Inhibition of CFTR function has been shown by both progesterone and estradiol, in contrast to the upregulation of expression seen in the airways. The above noted calcium-linked chloride conductance has been well characterized with a view to possible therapeutic intervention, and angiotensin II, as well as purinergic receptor-linked responses, identified as possible agonists for this calcium-linked pathway. Furthermore, the protein kinase C pathway modulates both the magnitude and stability of CFTR currents in pancreatic cells.

BLOOD

Plasma

One report has identified decreased plasma Na^+ and Cl^- and increased K^+ in CF patients, whereas Zn^{2+} and Mg^{2+} have been shown to be normal. Copper and caeruloplasmin levels are also normal. Ca^{2+} has been suggested to be slightly decreased and Fe^{2+} markedly reduced in these patients. Circulating aldosterone, norepinephrine and dopamine β-hydroxylase levels have been shown to be normal. The renin–angiotensin system of CF subjects compensates so well for volume depletion that salt depletion or dehydration cannot easily be recognized by routine clinical measurements. CF subjects show no change in vitamin C levels compared with non-CF values, but levels correlate with indexes of increased inflammation. Finally, one study has assessed levels of calprotectin as a marker of inflammation, showing it to be significantly elevated in CF.

Red blood cells

Ca^{2+} levels and the transport of Ca^{2+} in CF red blood cells (RBCs) has been the subject of many publications. Free intracellular Ca^{2+} has been shown not to be different from controls nor elevated in CF. Similarly Ca^{2+}-ATPase pump activity has been recorded to be normal or decreased in these patients. One study has differentiated activity as being normal in pancreas-sufficient and reduced in pancreas-insufficient patients, but showed no correlation between pump activity and clinical well-being. Other RBC pumps (Mg^{2+}-ATPase, Na^+, K^+-ATPase) and cotransporters appear to function normally in CF patients, as does their anion and noncarrier-mediated cation permeability. However, one study showed increased sodium–lithium counter transport and Na^+,K^+-ATPase activity in CF subjects. CF RBC Na^+ levels have been shown to be decreased, as have Mg^{2+} and Zn^{2+} levels in one study but not in others. One study has assessed the activity of acrylamine *N*-acetyltransferase in CF red cells, the enzyme involved in the metabolism of the drug sulfamthoxazole, showing no difference to non-CF values. Copper–zinc superoxide dismutase activity has been shown to be significantly reduced, in conjunction with a similar decrease in the levels of cytochrome oxidase in mononuclear cells. The significance of these changes in the activity of copper-dependent enzymes in the face of normal copper serum levels is uncertain. Finally, CF saliva showed no difference from saliva from non-CF subjects in eliciting Na^+ efflux from RBCs.

White blood cells

As in RBCs, there is debate as to calcium levels in CF neutrophils and lymphocytes. Free calcium in both these cells has been shown to be increased or normal, whereas total calcium has been shown to be raised. Calcium release by N-formylmethionyl-leucyl-phenylalanine has been recorded as reduced in CF neutrophils, with consequent alterations in neutrophil secretory activity, as well as not different from controls. However, the responses to the calcium ionophore A23187 and opsonized zymosan were normal, as were basal superoxide production and membrane degranulation. Elevation of cAMP produces inhibition of superoxide production and membrane degranulation in neutrophils and these responses were not altered in CF. Despite an earlier report of normal Cl$^-$ transport in CF lymphocytes, it has been possible to demonstrate the cAMP-related defect in both B and T cells. An initial report showed the presence of the ORDIC channel in these cells and demonstrated altered regulation by PKA[52]. This response is, however, cell-cycle specific, normal lymphocytes showing an increased Cl$^-$ conductance in the G_1 phase which can be further increased by either cAMP[53], Ca^{2+}[53] or cell swelling. CF lymphocytes show no cell-cycle alteration in Cl$^-$ conductance and no increase in this transport in response to elevated cAMP[53]. CFTR mRNA is expressed in lymphocytes and insertion of wild-type CFTR into CF lymphocytes restores both G_1-related Cl$^-$ transport and cAMP-related regulation[54]. An intriguing finding has been the reduced in vitro killing of Pseudomonas aeruginosa by neutrophils in the presence of low levels of sodium[55]. This is related to reduced phagocytosis of the bacteria and may be relevant to airway surface pathology if such low sodium levels can be documented at this site. Finally, one study has shown that both eosinophils and neutrophils from CF subjects degranulate more readily, and that this correlates with clinical variables.

CF antigen

Many studies have described the effect of a factor from CF serum/plasma on cellular function in a variety of organs and these are outlined in the appropriate sections. Initial partial purification of this factor indicated it has a molecular weight of 4.5–11 kDa and was present in very low concentrations in the IgG-rich fraction of plasma. Subsequently the gene coding for the so-called CF antigen was localized to chromosome 1[56] and immunopurification indicated two gene products, named calgranulin A and B. These have been shown to be expressed in circulating neutrophils and monocytes, although not in normal tissue macrophages. They are also expressed in the stratified squamous epithelium of the tongue, esophagus and buccal mucosa, but not in lung, pancreas or skin. CF antigen shows sequence homology with calcium-binding proteins and one of its constituents can be phosphorylated by increasing intracellular calcium. The expression of these proteins is altered during inflammation and they can act as bacteriostatic agents when released from neutrophils.

KIDNEY

The kidney transports Na$^+$ and Cl$^-$ avidly and is also a site where marked expression and function of CFTR has been demonstrated[57]. Evidence for CFTR chloride-channel function has been provided for the distal tubule principal cells in the cortical and inner medullary collecting ducts. There is some debate over the involvement of CFTR in the rodent renal cortex brush border.

Studies have examined whether ion-transport abnormalities are present in CF subjects. An increase in glomerular filtration rate has been demonstrated in some but not other studies, with one identifying an increased creatinine excretion and clearance. Basal Na$^+$ excretion has been shown to be decreased or normal, whereas the response to sodium loading has been shown to be abnormally reduced, indicating increased Na$^+$ reabsorption, probably in the proximal tubules. However, one study has suggested a reduced tubular reabsorptive capacity in CF. Following lithium ingestion, CF subjects showed higher levels than non-CF controls, with a lower fractional excretion. As previously noted, the amiloride-binding protein located on chromosome 7 is unaltered by CF mutations. Basal excretion of K$^+$, phosphate and calcium have been shown to be unaltered in CF.

Two groups have demonstrated the interesting finding that CFTR is involved in the genesis of the renal cysts characteristic of the autosomal dominant adult polycystic kidney disease[58,59]. Immunohistochemistry shows apical labeling of CFTR within the cells lining the cysts, with the Na$^+$, K$^+$-ATPase sited basolaterally. Chloride secretion through CFTR is thought to drive the accumulation of fluid, in conjunction with water, into the cysts.

SKIN

Cultured normal and CF keratinocytes have been examined for cAMP and Ca^{2+}-regulated Cl$^-$ transport. Despite substantial rises in cAMP levels and demonstration of the ORDIC channel in these cells, neither CF nor normal keratinocytes produced Cl$^-$ transport in response to activation of this second-messenger pathway. In contrast, the calcium ionophore A23187 induced Cl$^-$ transport in both CF and non-CF cells. As with red and white cells, fibroblasts have been suggested to have a greater intracellular calcium pool size, as well as reduced Ca^{2+}-ATPase activity. Furthermore, a normal aging phenomenon for fibroblasts in culture is a rise in intracellular calcium.

This appears to occur at a 'younger age' in CF fibroblasts and to a greater magnitude. The culture medium from CF fibroblasts when incubated with non-CF fibroblasts produces an increase in intracellular Ca^{2+} in these cells, although it does not inhibit the Ca^{2+}-ATPase. Culture medium from non-CF cells does not reduce the high intracellular calcium levels in CF fibroblasts.

CF fibroblasts also appear to show abnormalities related to the Na^+, K^+-ATPase inhibitor, ouabain. Thus, they show increased resistance to toxicity caused by this agent when cells are bathed in K^+-free, but not K^+-replete medium. CF fibroblasts also accumulate less sodium in the presence of ouabain than their non-CF counterparts[60]. Culture medium from non-CF fibroblasts increases intracellular Na^+ in CF fibroblasts to normal levels.

As noted above, the significance of these different abnormalities and their link with the basic Cl^- defect is presently uncertain. However, the number of these early reports in a wide variety of cells, if not always reproducible, suggests they are worthy of reinterpretation in the light of present knowledge about CFTR.

Basal Cl^- efflux in CF fibroblasts has been suggested to show a reduced component, although one study demonstrated only a reduced total Cl^- content in CF. As expected, cAMP levels in response to agonists are not different in CF fibroblasts. However, fibroblasts (non-CF or CF) appear to show little or no cAMP-related Cl^- transport, although, as in keratinocytes, the ORDIC channel is present and can be activated through the PKA pathway in normal fibroblasts. Ca^{2+}-mediated Cl^- movement has been shown to be present in non-CF fibroblasts in one study but not in another, both agreeing that CF cells did not differ in their respective findings. However, hypotonicity does appear to induce Cl^- movement in both CF and non-CF cells. A SO_4^{2-}/Cl^- exchanger has been shown to have an increased V_{max} in CF fibroblasts, producing increased SO_4^{2-} uptake, whereas fibroblast membrane vesicles demonstrated several defects of ion transport, suggesting a generalized membrane defect in these cells.

Since fibroblasts do not appear to possess a substantial degree of cAMP-related Cl^- transport, they have been used as a suitable target for introducing CFTR cDNA. This resulted in production of a cAMP-related Cl^- conductance with the previously noted biophysical characteristics typical of the CFTR Cl^- channel. This was not found in mock-transfected fibroblasts or those treated with ΔF_{508} CFTR DNA.

SALIVARY GLANDS

The function of the parotid and submandibular salivary glands has been examined in several studies. CF serum has been shown to stimulate K^+ efflux from rat sub-mandibular glands, an effect that was reduced by a Ca^{2+}-channel blocker. This effect can also be produced by medium from cultured CF fibroblasts, which also induces an increase in calcium and decrease in sodium in these cells. As with many studies on a presumed CF factor, these findings on increased K^+ efflux could not be reproduced in other studies.

CF serum also causes greater stimulation of mucin release from rat submandibular glands, an effect which was shown not to be due to cell lysis and which did not extend to alterations in amylase secretion by the rat pancreas. Both human submandibular and parotid saliva, when stimulated by citric acid show increased Ca^{2+} levels in CF, the former also showing increased PO_4^{2-} and reduced Na^+ and Cl^- levels. CF flow rates were also decreased. Perhaps most importantly, β-agonist-induced mucin and amylase secretion in CF submandibular glands is reduced compared to non-CF glands[61], indicating involvement of this organ in the CF basic defect. A recent study has provided evidence for CFTR expression both in the acinus and ducts of rodent submandibular glands.

OTHER ORGANS

The cAMP-modulated Cl^- channel which is present in the heart and is involved in autonomic responses of this organ has been shown to have identical electrophysiological properties to the CFTR Cl^- channel. Further, the amino-acid sequence of the myocardial product shows 98 per cent homology with CFTR. How this links with the relatively well-preserved myocardial function in CF is unknown. Ocular aqueous humor formation in CF patients shows no differences in the circadian rhythm of flow rates, nor those following application of a β-antagonist, suggesting that CFTR is not involved in this process. The composition of milk from mothers with CF was initially suggested to show an increased Na^+ concentration but this has not been subsequently confirmed. The seminal ejaculate from two CF patients showed an increased Ca^{2+} concentration but normal amounts of Ca^{2+}-ATPase, whereas analysis of other components suggested dysfunction, principally in the seminal vesicles rather than the prostate. CFTR has now been shown to be expressed in the Sertoli cells of the testis, the epididymis and vas deferens. It is also expressed in the human endocervix and fallopian tubes. Endometrial expression is only high after puberty and is downregulated by progesterone and increased by estrogen. The gallbladder, bile ducts, the thyroid and the brain (including thalamus and hypothalamus) add to the long list of organs also showing CFTR expression. Two studies of the nails of CF patients show increased concentrations of Na^+, K^+ and Cl^-. Finally, placental brush-border membranes have been shown to have a Cl^- conductance which is probably not altered in CF, as well to possess CFTR.

INTRACELLULAR DEFECTS

For many years a CF mitochondrial abnormality has been debated. Thus, mitochondrial Ca^{2+} uptake is increased in CF cells and this has been suggested to be linked to altered respiratory system activity in the mitochondrial membrane. With the many studies in a variety of organs describing intracellular calcium abnormalities in CF, the role of calcium-binding proteins such as calmodulin has been examined. The circulating CF antigen[56] has been noted above to show marked homology with calcium-binding proteins. Calmodulin itself shows no structural abnormality in CF and a cDNA probe for this protein did not link to the CF locus. However, calmodulin activity has been shown to be altered in CF and a calmodulin acceptor protein hypothesized to be defective.

Recently, attention has focused on endosomes, the Golgi apparatus and the regulation of endocytosis and exocytosis. The intracellular pH of many of these intracellular organelles is regulated through a pump, moving protons into the organelle interior. To maintain electroneutrality this must be buffered either by inward anion or outward cation movements. There are suggestions that Cl^- conductance may be important in this process and that this may be defective in CF cells[62]. This, in turn, leads to defective acidification of these organelles and hence altered organelle enzyme function, including those involved in glycoprotein processing. This attractive hypothesis is, however, not supported by several studies. The pH of CFPAC lysosomes is lower than in non-CF cells and is not altered in either by elevation of cAMP. Furthermore, ATP-dependent acidification is not altered in CF and is not regulated by cAMP. Also, although transfection of with CFTR does result in a PKA-activated Cl^- conductance in the endosomes of these, but not mock-transfected cells, activation of the PKA-linked pathway produces no alteration in endosomal[63,64,65] or *trans*-Golgi pH[66].

One study has shown that the increase in exocytosis and decrease in endocytosis caused by elevation of cAMP in normal cells is defective in their CF counterparts. This could be restored by transfection with wild-type CFTR cDNA[67]. However, other studies have failed to confirm an effect of CFTR on exocytosis or of mutant CFTR on endocytosis[65,68]. Finally, CFTR has been shown to be involved in endosome–endosome fusion.

CFTR

The cloning of the CF gene in 1989[69] prompted the beginning of studies into the structure and function of its product, CFTR. The protein is symmetrically arranged with two predicted hydrophobic membrane-spanning regions linked by two nucleotide-binding folds (NBFs) and a so-called regulatory, or R, domain, the latter having many potential phosphorylation sites. This predicted structure shows homology with a large superfamily of proteins known as the ABC (ATP-binding cassette) transporters which function as ATP-requiring pumps, exporting macromolecules from the cell interior[70]. One example of this family is the product of the multiple drug resistance (MDR) gene, P-glycoprotein, which is likely to be involved in producing a substantial proportion of resistance to chemotherapeutic agents used in the treatment of solid tumors. Several aspects of CFTR suggested it would not itself be a Cl^- channel, including its lack of resemblance to any known channel, the homology with known transporters and the presence of ATP-binding sites generally not associated with or required by channels. Thus, the most probable function for CFTR was, at one stage, thought to be macromolecule transport, a defect in which led to abnormal regulation of ion transport. In order to study its function, CFTR was expressed in a variety of cells which are believed not to produce this protein endogenously. These have included mammalian (fibroblasts, HeLa cells, Chinese hamster ovary cells) as well as nonmammalian (*Xenopus* oocytes, Cf9, Vero) cells. These studies unanimously demonstrated that CFTR expression produces a Cl^- conductance which can be regulated through the cAMP/PKA pathway. This strongly suggested that CFTR was actually a Cl^- channel, or the more remote possibility that in the presence of CFTR, these cells expressed such a Cl^- channel which had previously lain dormant. To distinguish these two possibilities, site-directed mutagenesis was used to mutate basic lysine to acidic amino acids at sites within the predicted membrane-spanning region of CFTR[23]. If CFTR is a Cl^- channel then these changes should alter its ability to conduct Cl^-. In particular, the anion selectivity of the channel (relative permeability, for example, of Cl^- and I^-) depend both on the hydrated size of the ion as well as the electrostatic forces between the interior of the channel and the ion. These mutations reversed this permeability sequence from $Cl^- > I^-$ for unaltered CFTR, to $I^- > Cl^-$ for the mutated protein, clearly indicating that CFTR itself is a Cl^- channel. Confirmation of this was provided by the purification of the protein and its incorporation into lipid bilayers where it functions as a cAMP/PKA-regulated Cl^- channel[24].

As previously noted, the whole cell current or single-channel characteristics of CFTR[24,25] differ markedly from those of the ORDIC channel. CFTR has a relatively small conductance of approximately 10 pS, shows a linear I–V relationship and no voltage-dependent activation or inactivation. As noted, the halide permeability sequence includes $Cl^- > I^-$ (indeed I^- can be shown to block channel activity) and channel open probability is not altered by the stilbenes DIDS (4, 4′-Diisothiocyanostilbene-2, 2′-disulphonic acid) and SITS (4-Acetamido-4′-isothiocyano-2, 2′-disulphonic acid stibene) and very little reduced by other Cl⁻ channel blockers such as NPPB (5-Nitro-2-(3-phenylpropylamino) benzoic acid) and DPC (Diphenylamine-2-carboxylate). CFTR can be regulated by PKC as well as PKA and the two kinases together appear to produce a synergistic effect[71]. Recently a cGMP-dependent protein kinase has also been shown to be involved in CFTR regulation, and NBD2 has been shown to act as a GTP-binding subunit.

A plethora of studies has assessed the function of different parts of CFTR using site-directed mutagenesis and other techniques. Clearly, it would be of particular interest to introduce mutations which mimic those found in CF patients, of which over 700 have now been identified. Initially it was thought that the nucleotide-binding domains (NBDs) were the principal focus for these alterations, although recently a more even spread of these mutations throughout CFTR has been demonstrated. Site-directed mutagenesis mimicking CF mutations in the NBDs virtually all result in CFTR which lacks functional activity. Interestingly, NBD1 is more sensitive to a given mutation than is NBD2. Since the NBDs bind ATP, the relationship between ATP, the NBDs and CFTR function has been examined.

For channel opening, hydrolysis of ATP at NBD1 is required[72], and direct evidence for intrinsic ATPase activity has now been provided using the purified protein[73], and shown to be present at least within NBF1[74]. The open state can be stabilized by ATP binding at NBD2[75], which produces a raised open probability, and which can be prevented by competition with ADP[76]. This can be terminated by ATP hydrolysis at this domain[72,77] or by dephosphorylation at the R domain. Continuous modulation of CFTR activity is maintained by subtle changes in phosphorylation which affect whether the channel proceeds beyond its initial opening, or how long the subsequent stable state is maintained, and this switching may involve NBD2.

NBF1 has been expressed and reconstituted into planar bilayers, producing Cl⁻ channel activity, suggesting that this region may also act as part of the conduction pathway. Further support for this is direct interaction of this domain with the plasma membrane and the fact that the amino-terminal portion of CFTR alone can form a regulated chloride channel[78]. The role of the transmembrane-spanning regions has also been examined for their contribution to pore formation, and segments 5 and 6 have been shown to contribute to the anion selectivity filter of CFTR[79]. One study has suggested that these regions of the protein mediate association between the two halves of CFTR.

The R domain has been deleted[80] and the consequent CFTR function studied. The channel in this mutant protein now conducts Cl⁻ independently of cAMP, although cAMP still stimulates Cl⁻ transport. This has led to the suggestion that the R domain acts as a 'ball and chain' type regulator of the conduction pathway. Support for this was provided by mutating the four serine residues

found in the R domain, which are the sites of PKA phosphorylation[81]. Three of these serines can be mutated without alteration of function but removal of all four abolishes PKA-related Cl⁻ transport. This led to the suggestion that phosphorylation of these serines induces an electrostatic charge which repels the R domain, producing channel opening. Deletion of the R domain also suppresses the inactivating effect of a NBD2 mutation (but not a NBD1 mutation) suggesting that NBD2 interacts with the channel through the R domain[80]. Further, covalent modification of the R domain stimulates CFTR function, underlining the importance of this region of the protein. The R domain in its unphosphorylated state appears to interact with NBD1 by preventing ATP binding, ATP hydrolysis or the transducing effect of this sequence on the channel pore[82]. Phosphorylation of the R domain then enhances the rate of channel opening by increasing sensitivity to ATP[83], the present weight of evidence likely favoring this rather than the 'ball and chain' model noted above. This is consistent with overexpression of the R domain preventing CFTR chloride-channel function, and exogenously added R domain having a similar effect[84]. In turn, nucleotide binding to NBD1 inhibits R-domain phosphorylation.

CFTR function is also controlled by enzymes which terminate its phosphorylation, namely phosphatases. A number of studies have begun to identify which of the many cellular phosphatases may be involved in this. Evidence has been provided for protein phosphatases 1, 2A[85,86], 2B101, 2C[86] and tyrosine phosphatases. Further, phosphodiesterases which downregulate cAMP levels are also regulators of CFTR function, the type III enzyme being involved in the airways. Control of *CFTR* gene expression has also been studied and shown to be downregulated by phorbol esters and calcium, both acting in a time- and dose-dependent fashion and both probably functioning through protein kinases[85]. Elevation of cAMP for greater than 8 h, however, produces increased transcription of *CFTR*, suggesting the presence of a cAMP-responsive element in the *CFTR* gene promoter. The site of this within the *CFTR* promoter has been mapped, including its interactions with transcription factors. Further, one study has shown that basal expression of *CFTR* also requires protein kinase A activity. Expression is regulated by cell differentiation, at least in certain cell types, and, therefore, may be of importance at various stages in the cellular life cycle. However, in other cells, CFTR mRNA was shown to be expressed throughout cellular development despite alterations in cAMP-mediated Cl⁻ secretion with time.

The normal and CF-related localization of CFTR has been studied extensively. Undoubtedly in normal cells it is present in the apical region of most epithelia studied, as demonstrated by antibody labeling and laser confocal microscopy[27,57,87,88]. Elevation of cAMP did not alter this localization nor induce vehicle fusion[27], suggesting CFTR Cl⁻ channels are already present in the membrane prior to the cAMP stimulus. Studies have presented evidence for membrane insertion following CFTR stimulation, and for the role of heterotrimeric G proteins in mediating exocytosis and thus delivery of CFTR to the cell surface. CFTR is recovered from its surface location at a rate of approximately 5 per cent/minute via endocytosis through a clathrin-linked mechanism. This internalization is reduced by activation of protein kinase A or C[89]. Mutant CFTR has been suggested to have a markedly shorter half-life (<4 hours) than the normal protein (>24 hours)[90]. Further, the glycosylation status of CFTR does not affect its targeting to the cell membrane. Interestingly CFTR can be activated either by disruption of the actin cytosleleton or the addition of actin, factors which may link with the regulation by protein kinase A.

The effect of CFTR mutations can be divided into five classes[91]. Class I includes mutations inducing frameshift, nonsense or other changes in which no protein is produced. Class II, including the most common ΔF_{508} mutation, results in little or no CFTR detectable at the apical membrane[5], corresponding to the demonstrable presence of CFTR within the endoplasmic reticulum (ER). This is due to impaired trafficking through the ER/Golgi compartments. Interestingly, the normal chloride-channel function of the mislocalized mutant ΔF_{508} protein in the endoplasmic reticulum is, however, retained[92] as is the function of the purified mutant protein[93], although other studies have disputed this normal functioning[94,95]. Class III mutations allow for normal trafficking but an altered control of channel open probability at the cell surface. Class IV mutants show normal trafficking and gating but altered single-channel conductance, whereas class V relates to the reduced production of the CFTR protein.

The biochemical basis of the class II mutations has been studied extensively. As noted above, trafficking is temperature dependent[96] and the mutant protein can be rescued by the administration of agents such as glycerol, which may act as chemical 'chaperones'. This has prompted investigations of the normal processes for 'escorting' CFTR to the cell surface. Crucial components of this pathway include the chaperones, including Hsc70, Hsp90 and calnexin[97], and an increasing number of regulatory cofactors, such as Hsp40, Hip, Hop and BAG-1, the overall function of which is to provide the environment necessary for the attainment of the required final structure. Several of these agents have been specifically implicated in CFTR processing, where molecules can be recognized as imperfect by a 'quality control' element. Such imperfect molecules are retained at the level of the ER as type A (unglycosylated) protein and are ultimately degraded[98]. The net result is a final loss of some 65 per cent of normal CFTR[99] and more than 99 per cent of the original mutant molecules[100], by degradation involving proteolytic mechanisms which include the ubiquitin-proteosome system[101,102]. Ubiquitination marks a protein for degradation and is an early process (within 20 min-

utes of protein synthesis) and likely occurring cotranslationally[103]. Indeed the ΔF_{508} mutation affects steps in CFTR folding before the formation of the ATP binding site in NBD1. This mutation reduces the folding yield of CFTR, but does not alter its thermodynamic stability. The ongoing elucidation of the above mechanisms is likely to provide opportunities for pharmacological interventions.

One of the most important developments in CFTR biology over the past few years has been the demonstration that CFTR acts as a regulator of a number of other channels. As noted above, CF airways and intestinal tissues show increased sodium absorption. The molecular basis of this has now been shown in a number of studies in which CFTR and the ENaC sodium channel have been coexpressed in a variety of systems. In the absence of CFTR, expression of ENaC produces large amiloride-sensitive sodium currents which are stimulated by cAMP. When CFTR is coexpressed, much smaller sodium currents are produced which are inhibited by cAMP[104]. Thus, normally CFTR acts as a downregulator of ENaC. Mutant CFTR, irrespective of whether it can conduct chloride or not, does not produce this inhibition[105], thus explaining the increased sodium absorption in CF. Studies have begun to explore the mechanism of this inhibition, showing that the intracellular domains of CFTR are sufficient. At the single-channel level the open probability of ENaC is changed from an increase in the presence of cAMP, to a decrease when CFTR is coexpressed[106]. The inhibition is dose-dependent, with increasing cAMP-stimulated chloride currents mediating greater sodium decreases[107]. Finally, the presence of actin significantly increases the inhibitory effect of CFTR.

Two other chloride channels also appear to be regulated by CFTR. The ORCC channel has been discussed above, including the initial studies suggesting this channel may be the basis of CF. This apparently confusing finding has been clarified by several studies. In knockout CF mice ORCC can still be found in the absence of CFTR[108]. Second, studies have shown that CFTR regulates ORCC, likely through the autocrine transport of ATP and the subsequent stimulation of P2U receptors[109,110,111]. Interestingly, upon cooling of cells to temperatures permissive for CFTR trafficking, the incidence of ORCC channels decreased in CF cells. A further anomaly, which may be resolved by the regulatory functions of CFTR, is the presence of upregulated calcium-activated chloride secretion in CF mice. A recent study has shown that CFTR may act to downregulate the function of this channel, at least in the Xenopus oocyte expression system[112]. Thus, mutant CFTR would allow the increased function of this channel in a manner analogous to that described above for ENaC. Yet another channel, the renal ATP-sensitive potassium channel, ROMK2, also appears to be regulated by CFTR. In this case CFTR confers sensitivity of the channel to the sulfonylurea glibenclamide, itself a blocker of the CFTR channel[113]. Mutation studies showed that this interaction is via the NBF1 site of CFTR. Further, CFTR conferred cAMP sensitivity on a potassium current in a CF pancreatic cell line. Clues as to how these various regulatory functions of CFTR occur are just beginning to emerge. At its C-terminal end CFTR possesses an amino-acid sequence previously recognized to interact with so-called PDZ motifs on a number of proteins. One of these, ezrin-binding protein 50 (EB50) can bind CFTR and EB50 itself binds ezrin[114]. The latter protein then links through the cytoskeleton with many other cellular molecules. The Na^+/H^+ exchanger also has PDZ motifs and, in turn, can also bind to CFTR[115]. Finally, the membrane protein syntaxin also binds to and regulates CFTR[116]. Thus a complex network of interactions may explain the pleiotropic actions of CFTR.

As noted above, it has been proposed that CFTR can transport ATP. The original observation has produced intense debate, with many studies addressing this issue. At present it is still unclear whether the measured extracellular ATP may occur as a result of experimental perturbation (it is well recognized that ATP may be released by very small mechanical stimuli[117]). Thus studies are divided into whether this represents genuine flow through CFTR or an associated channel gated by CFTR[118,119], or whether CFTR does not mediate ATP transport[117,120,121]. Studies have also identified other molecules which may be transported by CFTR, including water, probably at a site separate from that used to transport chloride. Further, CFTR can mediate transport of large organic anions, this requiring ATP hydrolysis.

HETEROZYGOTES

Many studies have examined whether obligate heterozygotes exhibit a 'halfway defect' in comparison to CF patients. Several have identified an intermediate or greater than normal response of airway glycoprotein release in response to serum. Furthermore, the increase in Ca^{2+} entry into these cells produced by serum was also noted to be intermediate in heterozygotes. Fibroblasts from heterozygotes have been reported to show an increased Ca^{2+}-binding capacity in comparison to normal cells, an intracellular Ca^{2+} midway between normal and CF subjects, and to accumulate less ^{22}Na in the presence of ouabain. Similarly, red cells show Na^+ and Mg^{2+} levels in between those for CF and normal cells. Following 3 days of loading with NaBr, multivariate analysis of Na^+, K^+, Cl^- and Br^- in sweat and serum could distinguish between normals and heterozygotes. One study has shown a mild but significant increase in sweat chloride in heterozygote infants under the age of 6 weeks.

In contrast, many studies have been unable to identify heterozygotes in comparison with normal subjects. Thus baseline nasal PD[7], response to amiloride[7] or to Cl^- free perfusion[8] does not differentiate heterozygotes. Furthermore Br^- and Cl^- reabsorption in sweat ducts is not different in these subjects. Thus, at present, no reliable screening test exists for heterozygote detection apart from the genetic analysis described in Chapter 2.

RELATIONSHIP OF THE BASIC DEFECT TO PATHOLOGY

How the above-noted abnormalities link with abnormalities in CFTR structure is unknown, but several possibilities exist:

1. The long-held view that abnormal functioning of a mucosal Cl^- channel will lead to reduced water secretion onto this surface is still an attractive hypothesis. In the airways this could occur both in the surface and/or submucosal gland epithelial cells and result in altered hydration of mucus and reduced periciliary fluid. Both of these would tend to impair mucociliary clearance and hence encourage bacterial adherence. Increased sodium absorption would tend to exacerbate this process.

2. The demonstration that CFTR is likely to be involved in the functioning of intracellular processes, particularly endocytosis and exocytosis, may provide a link with disease causation. Thus, if CFTR acts at an early stage in the processing of proteins, a wide spectrum of abnormalities could be produced. These could include abnormal mucus and aberrant channel protein production, as well as altered synthesis of proteins involved in mucosal surface defense mechanisms and abnormal production of bacterial binding sites (see below).

3. As noted, CFTR shows many similarities to P-glycoprotein, which can demonstrate both Cl^- channel and macromolecule transport function. It is thus possible that CFTR, a related protein, can also do so and the debate relating to ATP transport by CFTR has been highlighted above.

4. A number of studies have shown that CF cells show a two- to threefold increase in the number of binding sites for *Pseudomonas aeruginosa*[122]. *CFTR* gene transfer reduces the increased binding[123], indicating that this is directly related to the mutated protein. This may provide an important mechanism both for the predeliction for this organism for CF airways and the chronic inflammation characteristic of this disease. Thus the binding of this organism stimulates the NFκB transcription factor pathway This in turn could produce the increased levels of proinflammatory cytokines seen in this disease[124,125], as well as the increased mucin production.

5. Airway epithelial cells secrete antimicrobial

substances, including defensins, lysozyme and lactoferrin. The function of these molecules may be in part salt-sensitive, with reduced activity at higher concentrations. Although CF cells secrete normal levels of these proteins, the potentially altered salt composition of the airway surface liquid may provide a link between the basic defect and reduced bacterial clearance[126,127]. However, these findings depend on the demonstration of increased salt concentrations in surface fluid, something that has been hard to document to date[128,129].

6. A provocative recent finding has been the report that epithelial cells may ingest *Pseudomonas* as a host defense mechanism[130], and that this may be defective in CF, the CFTR protein acting as a receptor for these organisms[131].

7. The increased inflammation characteristic of CF has also been suggested to be directly linked to CFTR mistrafficking. Thus it is known that increased retention of proteins within the endoplasmic reticulum can lead to activation of the NFκB transcription pathway. However, severe lung disease develops in CF subjects with the G551D and other mutations which traffic normally to the apical membrane. This may be compounded by reduced levels of the anti-inflammatory cytokine, interleukin-10 (IL-10)[132].

8. One study has shown that CFTR has a role in intracellular acidification, an important event during the initiation of programmed cell death (apoptosis). A failure to undergo such regulated apoptosis may lead to release of intracellular contents and the liberation of potentially toxic enzymes which, in turn, may play a role in disease pathogenesis[133].

The relative contribution of any of these factors is at present only conjecture, and represents an important focus of research.

CF MODEL SYSTEMS

One of the traditional problems with CF research has been the lack of suitable tissue for experimental studies. Prior to the identification of the CF gene a large number of studies were devoted to the production of a suitable animal model, using a variety of long-term pharmacological interventions. Mice, rabbits and, in particular, rats have been chronically treated with isoprenaline, reserpine, pilocarpine, frusemide, amiloride, acetazolamide and combinations of these agents. Interestingly, many facets of disease in CF patients could be reproduced in these animal models. Histological examination demonstrated alterations concomitant with blocked ducts in the submandibular and parotid glands, as well as the pancreas. These may relate to a general decrease in fluid secretion in these organs, also seen in the epididymis of these animals. Intracellular Ca^{2+} is generally increased in these tissues, which is likely related to increases in intracellular mucus, the constituent glycoproteins of which appear to bind more Ca^{2+} than in untreated animals. Abnormalities of Cl^- transport have also been identified in a variety of tissues. However, there is no evidence for an altered PD in the trachea of these animals or of the characteristic cAMP-related defect in the gastrointestinal tract.

Cell culture to amplify the available quantities of CF tissue has also been investigated extensively. Techniques for maintenance of cells from many organs in primary culture have been described, with demonstration of the relevant ion-transport defects. Furthermore, 'immortalized' CF cell lines produced through viral transfection have been produced by many laboratories[134]. Again, these demonstrate various aspects of the CF phenotype and are widely used in studies of the basic defect.

With the cloning of the CF gene came the possibility of producing a genetic CF animal model. To date, 10 CF mice have been generated, including knockout animals which do not produce any CFTR, as well as mice carrying specific human mutations, such as ΔF_{508} and G551D. An excellent review is available[135], and only the key points of these models will be summarized here. Each of the models largely replicates the bioelectrical characteristics seen in humans, with the notable exception that sodium hyperabsorption is not seen in the airways. No model spontaneously develops the lung pathology representative of human CF subjects, although forms of lung disease can be induced depending on exposure to microorganisms and the genetic background of the mice. Intestinal blockage resembling meconium ileus is, however, a characteristic feature of all the animals. The reasons for the lack of lung disease are not clear. A number of possibilities include the presence of an endogenous calcium-mediated chloride channel which subserves the function of CFTR, the lack of sodium hyperabsorption, the relative paucity of submucosal glands and, finally, the short life span of these animals in comparison to humans. As expected, these animals have proved of enormous value in studies of pharmacologic and genetic rescue, and, despite the above limitations, have also contributed importantly to studies of pathogenesis.

CONCLUSION

Clearly, rapid progress in defining the basic defect in CF has been made over the past decade. A unifying hypothesis of altered Cl^- transport in response to elevation of cAMP proposed by electrophysiologists has been linked to the demonstration of the CF gene product acting as such a Cl^- channel. Less clear at present is how this links with the numerous other described cellular abnormalities in this disease and, most importantly, how this defect produces the pathology found in CF patients. The next steps of linking defect to pathology and devising treatment based on these abnormalities are likely to proceed in parallel over the next few years.

REFERENCES

The second edition of this text has necessitated a severe reduction in the number of references. Many outstanding studies, whose findings have been summarized in the text, have accordingly not been quoted directly.

1. Quinton, P.M. and Bijman, J. (1983) Higher bioelectric potentials due to decreased chloride absorption in the sweat glands of patients with cystic fibrosis. *NEJM*, **308**, 1185–1189.
2. Sato, K. and Sato, F. (1984) Defective beta adrenergic response of cystic fibrosis sweat glands in vivo and in vitro. *J. Clin. Invest.*, **73**, 1763–1771.
3. Quinton, P.M. (1983) Chloride impermeability in cystic fibrosis. *Nature*, **301**, 421–422.
4. Sorscher, F.J., Kirk, K.L., Weaver, M.L. *et al.* (1991) Antisense oligodeoxynucleotide to the cystic fibrosis gene inhibits anion transport in normal cultured sweat duct cells. *Proc. Natl Acad. Sci. USA*, **88**, 7759–7762.
5. Kartner, N., Augustinas, O., Jensen, T.J. *et al.* (1992) Mislocalization of ΔF508 CFTR in cystic fibrosis sweat gland. *Nature Genet.*, **1**, 321–327.
6. Kilburn, K.H. (1967) A hypothesis for pulmonary clearance and its implications. *Am. Rev. Resp. Dis.*, **98**, 449–463.
7. Knowles, M., Gatzy, J. and Boucher, R. (1981) Increased bioelectric potential difference across respiratory epithelia in cystic fibrosis. *NEJM*, **305**, 1489–1495.
8. Knowles, M., Gatzy, J. and Boucher, R. (1983) Relative ion permeability of normal and cystic fibrosis nasal epithelium. *J. Clin. Invest.*, **71**, 1410–1417.
9. Knowles, M.R., Stutts, M.J., Spock, A. *et al.* (1983) Abnormal ion permeation through cystic fibrosis respiratory epithelium. *Science*, **221**, 1067–1070.
10. Yankaskas, J.R., Knowles, M.R., Gatzy, J.T. and Boucher, R.C. (1985) Persistence of abnormal chloride ion permeability in cystic fibrosis nasal epithelial cells in heterologous culture. *Lancet*, **i**, 954–956.
11. Cotton, C.U., Stutts, M.J., Knowles, M.R. *et al.* (1987) Abnormal apical cell membrane in cystic fibrosis respiratory epithelium. An *in vitro* electrophysiologic analysis. *J. Clin. Invest.*, **79**, 80–85.
12. Willumsen, N.J., Davis, C.W. and Boucher, R.C. (1989) Cellular Cl⁻ transport in cultured cystic fibrosis airway epithelium. *Am. J. Physiol.*, **256**, C1045–C1053.
13. Boucher, R.C., Cheng, E.H., Paradiso, A.M. *et al.* (1989) Chloride secretory response of cystic fibrosis human airway epithelia. Preservation of calcium but not protein kinase C- and A-dependent mechanisms. *J. Clin. Invest.*, **84**, 1424–1431.
14. Anderson, M.P. and Welsh, M.J. (1991) Calcium and cAMP activate different chloride channels in the apical membrane of normal and cystic fibrosis epithelia. *Proc. Natl Acad. Sci. USA*, **88**, 6003–6007.
15. Boucher, R.C., Stutts, M.J., Knowles, M.R. *et al.* (1986) Na⁺ transport in cystic fibrosis respiratory epithelia. Abnormal basal rate and response to adenylate cyclase activation. *J. Clin. Invest.*, **78**, 1245–1252.
16. Welsh, M.J and Liedtke, C.M. (1986) Chloride and potassium channels in cystic fibrosis airway epithelia. *Nature*, **322**, 467–470.
17. Welsh, M.J. (1986) An apical-membrane chloride channel in human tracheal epithelium. *Science*, **232**, 1648–1650.
18. Frizzell, R.A., Rechkemmer, C. and Shoemaker, R.U. (1986) Altered regulation of airway epithelial cell chloride channels in cystic fibrosis. *Science*, **233**, 558–560.
19. Hwang, T.C., Lu, L., Zeitlin, P.L. *et al.* (1989) Cl⁻ channels in CF: lack of activation by protein kinase C and cAMP-dependent protein kinase. *Science*, **244**, 1351–1353.
20. Schoumacher, R.A., Shoemaker, R.L., Halm, D.R. *et al.* (1987) Phosphorylation fails to activate chloride channels from cystic fibrosis airway cells. *Nature*, **330**, 752–754.
21. Li, M., McCann, J.D., Liedtke, C.M. *et al.* (1988) Cyclic AMP-dependent protein kinase opens chloride channels in normal but not cystic fibrosis airway epithelium. *Nature*, **331**, 358–360.
22. Li, M., McCann, J.D., Anderson, M.P. *et al.* (1989) Regulation of chloride channels by protein kinase C in normal and cystic fibrosis airway epithelia. *Science*, **244**, 1353–1356.
23. Anderson, M.P., Gregory, K.J., Thompson, S. *et al.* (1991) Demonstration that CFTR is a chloride channel by alteration of its anion selectivity. *Science*, **253**, 202–205.
24. Bear, C.E., Li, C.H., Kartner, N. *et al.* (1992) Purification and functional reconstitution of the cystic fibrosis transmembrane conductance regulator (CFTR). *Cell*, **68**, 809–818.
25. Berger, H.A., Anderson, N.H., Gregory, K.J. *et al.* (1991) Identification and regulation of the cystic fibrosis transmembrane conductance regulator-generated chloride channel . *J. Clin. Invest.*, **88**, 1422–1431.
26. Gray, M.A., Harris, A., Coleman, L. *et al.* (1989) Two types of chloride channel on duct cells from human fetal pancreas. *Am. J. Physiol.* **257**, C240–C251.
27. Denning, G.M., Ostedgaard, T.S., Cheng, S.H. *et al.* (1992) Localization of cystic fibrosis transmembrane conductance regulator in chloride secretory epithelia. *J. Clin. Invest.*, **89**, 339–349.
28. Engelhardt, J.F., Zepeda, M., Cohn, J.A. *et al.* (1994) Expression of the cystic fibrosis gene in adult human lung. *J. Clin. Invest.*, **93**, 737–749.
29. Rich, D.P., Anderson, M.P., Gregory, R.J. *et al.* (1990) Expression of cystic fibrosis transmembrane conductance regulator corrects defective chloride channel regulation in cystic fibrosis airway epithelial cells. *Nature*, **347**, 358–363.

30. Wagner, J.A., McDonald, T.V., Nghiem, P.T. *et al.* (1992) Antisense oligodeoxynucleotides to the cystic fibrosis transmembrane conductance regulator inhibit cAMP-activated but not calcium-activated chloride currents. *Proc. Natl Acad. Sci. USA*, **89**, 6785–6789.

31. Wagner, J.A., Cozens, A.L., Schulman, H., *et al.* (1991) Activation of chloride channels in normal and cystic fibrosis airway epithelial cells by multifunctional calcium/calmodulin dependent protein kinase. *Nature*, **349**, 793–796.

32. Schwiebert, E.M., Cid-Soto, L.P., Stafford, D. *et al.* (1998) Analysis of the ClC-2 channels as an alternative pathway for chloride conduction in cystic fibrosis airway cells. *Proc. Natl Acad. Sci. USA*, **95**, 3879–3884.

33. Stutts, M.J., Knowles, M.R. and Gatzy, J.T. (1986) Oxygen consumption and ouabain binding sites in cystic fibrosis nasal epithelium. *Pediatr. Res.*, **20**, 1316–1320.

34. Chinet, T.C., Fullton, J.M., Yankaskas, J.R., Boucher, R.C. and Stutts, M.J. (1994) Mechanism of sodium hyperabsorption in cultured cystic fibrosis nasal epithelium: a patch–clamp study. *Am. J. Physiol.*, **266**, C1061–C1068 .

35. Burch, L.H., Talbot, C.R., Knowles, M.R., Canessa, C.M., Rossier, B.C., and Boucher, R.C. (1995) Relative expression of the human epithelial channel subunits in normal and cystic fibrosis airways. *Am. J. Physiol.*, **269**, C511–C518.

36. Engelhardt, J.F., Yankaskas, J.R., Ernst, S.A. *et al.* (1992) Submucosal glands are the predominant site of CFTR expression in the human bronchus. *Nature Genet.*, **2**, 240–248.

37. Inglis, S.K., Corboz, M.R. and Ballard, S.T. (1998) Effect of anion secretion inhibitors on mucin content of airway submucosal gland ducts. *Am. J. Physiol.*, **274**, L762–L766.

38. Trout, L., King, M., Feng, W., Inglis, S.K. and Ballard, S.T. (1998) Inhibition of airway liquid secretion and its effect on the physical properties of airway mucus. *Am. J. Physiol.*, **274**, L258–L263.

39. Smith, J.J. and Welsh, M.J. (1992) cAMP stimulates bicarbonate secretion across normal, but not cystic fibrosis airway epithelia. *J. Clin. Invest.*, **89**, 1148–1153.

40. Primiano, F.P. Jr, Saidel, G.M., Montague, F.W. Jr *et al.* (1988) Water vapour and temperature dynamics in the upper airways of normal and CF subjects. *Eur. Resp. J.*, **1**, 407–414.

41. Hasegawa, H., Skach, W., Baker, O. *et al.* (1992) A multifunctional aqueous channel formed by CFTR. *Science*, **258**, 1477–1479.

42. Jiang, C., Finkbeiner, W.E., Widdicombe, J.H., McCray, P.B. and Miller, S.S. (1993) Altered fluid transport across airway epithelium in cystic fibrosis. *Science*, **262**, 424–427.

43. Zhang, Y., Yankaskas, J., Wilson, J. and Englehardt, J.F. (1996) In vivo analysis of fluid transport in cystic fibrosis airway epithelia of bronchial xenografts. *Am. J. Physiol.*, **270**, C1326–C1335.

44. Goldstein, J.L., Nash, N.T., al-Bazzaz, F. *et al.* (1988) Rectum has abnormal ion transport but normal cAMP-binding proteins in cystic fibrosis. *Am. J. Physiol.*, **254**, C719–C724.

45. Hardcastle, J., Hardcastle, P.T., Taylor, C.J. and Goldhill, J. (1991) Failure of cholinergic stimulation to induce a secretory response from the rectal mucosa in cystic fibrosis. *Gut*, **32**, 1035–1039.

46. Taylor, C.J., Baxter, P.S., Hardcastle, J. and Hardcastle, P.T. (1988) Failure to induce secretion in jejunal biopsies from children with cystic fibrosis. *Gut*, **29**, 957–962.

47. Teune, T.M., Timmers-Reker, A.J., Bouquet, J., Bijman, J., De Jonge, H.R. and Sinaasappel, M. (1996) In vivo measurement of chloride and water secretion in the jejunum of cystic fibrosis patients. *Paediatr. Res.*, **40**, 522–527.

48. Goldstein, J.L., Shapiro, A.B., Rao, M.C. and Uayden, T.J. (1991) *In vivo* evidence of altered chloride but not potassium secretion in cystic fibrosis rectal mucosa. *Gastroenterol.*, **101**, 1012–1019.

49. Strong, T.V., Boehm, K. and Collins, F.S. (1994) Localization of cystic fibrosis transmembrane conductance regulator mRNA in the human gastrointestinal tract by in situ hybridization. *J. Clin. Invest.*, **93**, 347–354.

50. Seidler, U., Blumenstein, I., Kretz, A. *et al.* (1997) A functional CFTR protein is required for mouse intestinal cAMP-, cGMP- and Ca(2+)-dependent HCO_3^- secretion. *J. Physiol.*, **505**, 411–423.

51. Drumm, M.L., Pope, H.A., Cliff, W.H. *et al.* (1990) Correction of the cystic fibrosis defect in vitro by retrovirus-mediated gene transfer. *Cell*, **62**, 1227–1233.

52. Chen, J.H., Schulman, H. and Gardner, P. (1989) A cAMP-regulated chloride channel in lymphocytes that is affected in cystic fibrosis. *Science*, **243**, 657–660.

53. Bubien, J.K., Kirk, K.L., Rado, T.A. and Frizzell, R.A. (1990) Cell cycle dependence of chloride permeability in normal and cystic fibrosis lymphocytes. *Science*, **248**, 1416–1419.

54. Krauss, R.D., Bubien, J.K., Drumm, M.L. *et al.* (1992) Transfection of wild-type CFTR into cystic fibrosis lymphocytes restores chloride conductance at G1 of the cell cycle. *EMBO J.*, **11**, 875–883

55. Mizgerd, J.P., Kobzik, L., Warner, A.E. and Brain, J.D. (1995) Effects of sodium concentration on human neutrophil bactericidal functions. *Am. J. Physiol.*, **269**, L388–L393.

56. Dorm, J.R., Novak, M., Hill, R.E. *et al.* (1987) A clue to the basic defect in cystic fibrosis from cloning the CF antigen gene. *Nature*, **326**, 614–617.

57. Crawford, I., Maloney, P.C., Zeitlin, P.L. *et al.* (1991) Immunocytochemical localization of the cystic fibrosis gene product CFTR. *Proc. Natl Acad. Sci. USA*, **88**, 9262–9266.

58. Hanaoka, K., Devuyst, O., Schwiebert, E.M., Wilson, P.D. and Guggino, W.B. (1996) A role for CFTR in human autosomal dominant polycystic kidney disease. *Am. J. Physiol.*, **270**, C389–C399.

59. Brill, S.R., Ross, K.E., Davidow, C.J., Ye, M., Grantham, J.J. and Caplan, M.J.(1996) Immunolocalization of ion

transport proteins in human autosomal dominant polycystic kidney epithelial cells. *Proc. Natl Acad. Sci. USA*, **93**, 10206–10211.

60. Breslow, J.L., McPherson, I. and Epstein, J. (1981) Distinguishing homozygous and heterozygous cystic fibrosis fibroblasts from normal cells by differences in sodium transport. *NEJM*, **304**, 1–5.

61. McPherson, M.A., Dormer, R.L., Bradbury, N.A. *et al.* (1986) Defective beta-adrenergic secretory responses in submandibular acinar cells from cystic fibrosis patients. *Lancet*, **ii**, 1007–1008.

62. Barasch, J., Kiss, B., Prince, A. *et al.* (1991) Defective acidification of intracellular organelles in cystic fibrosis. *Nature*, **352**, 70–73.

63. Lukacs, G.L., Chang, X.B., Kartner, N. *et al.* (1992) The cystic fibrosis transmembrane regulator is present and functional in endosomes. Role as a determinant of endosomal pH. *J. Biol. Chem.*, **267**, 14568–14572.

64. Root, K.V., Engelhardt, J.F., Post, M., Wilson, J.W. and Van-Dyke, R.W. (1994) CFTR does not alter acidification of L cell endosomes. *Biochem. Biophys. Res. Comm.*, **205**, 396–401.

65. Dunn, K.W., Park, J., Semrad, C.E., Gelman, D.L., Shevell, T. and McGraw, T.E. (1994) Regulation of endocytic trafficking and acidification are independent of the cystic fibrosis transmembrane regulator. *J. Biol. Chem.* **269**, 5336–5345.

66. Seksek, O., Viwersi, J. and Verkman, A.S. (1996) Evidence against defective trans-Golgi acidification in cystic fibrosis. *J. Biol. Chem.*, **271**, 15542–15548.

67. Bradbury, N.A., Julling, T., Berta, G. *et al.* (1992) Regulation of plasma membrane recycling by CFTR. *Science*, **256**, 530–532.

68. Santos, G.F. and Reenstra, W.W. (1994) Activation of the cystic fibrosis transmembrane regulator by cyclic AMP is not correlated with inhibition of endocytosis. *Biochim. Biophys. Acta*, **1195**, 96–102.

69. Riordan, J.R., Rommens, J.M., Kerem, B.S. *et al.* (1989) Identification of the cystic fibrosis gene: cloning and characterisation of complementary DNA. *Science*, **245**, 1066–1073.

70. Hyde, S.C., Emsley, P., Harshorn, M.J. *et al.* (1990) Structural model of ATP-binding proteins associated with cystic fibrosis, multidrug resistance and bacterial transport. *Nature*, **346**, 362–365.

71. Tabcharani, J.A., Chang, X.B., Riordan, J.R. and Hanrahan, J.W. (1991) Phosphorylation-regulated Cl⁻ channel in CHO cells stably expressing the cystic fibrosis gene. *Nature*, **352**, 628–631.

72. Hwang, T.C., Nagel, G., Naairn, A.C. and Gadsby, D.C. (1994) Regulation of the gating of cystic fibrosis transmembrane conductance regulator Cl channels by phosphorylation and ATP hydrolysis. *Proc. Natl Acad. Sci. USA*, **91**, 4698–4702.

73. Li, C., Ramjessingh, M., Wang, W. *et al.* (1996) ATPase activity of the cystic fibrosis transmembrane conductance regulator. *J. Biol. Chem.*, **271**, 28463–28468.

74. Ko, Y.K. and Pedersen, P.L. (1995) The first nucleotide binding fold of the cystic fibrosis transmembrane conductance regulator can function as an active ATPase. *J. Biol. Chem.*, **270**, 22093–22096.

75. Ko, Y.H., Thomas, P.J. and Pedersen. P.L. (1994) The cystic fibrosis transmembrane conductance regulator. Nucleotide binding to a synthetic peptide segment from the second predicted nucleotide binding fold. *J. Biol. Chem.*, **269**, 14584–14588.

76. Gunderson, K.L. and Kopito, R.R. (1994) Effects of pyrophosphate and nucleotide analogs suggest a role for ATP hydrolysis in cystic fibrosis transmembrane regulator channel gating. *J. Biol. Chem.*, **269**, 19349–19353.

77. Carson, M.R., Travis, S.M. and Welsh, M.J. (1995) The two nucleotide-binding domains of cystic fibrosis transmembrane conductance regulator (CFTR) have distinct functions in controlling channel activity. *J. Biol. Chem.*, **270**, 1711–1717.

78. Sheppard, D.N., Osteddgaard, L.S., Rich, D.P. and Welsh, M.J. (1994) The amino-terminal portion of CFTR forms a regulated Cl⁻ channel. *Cell*, **76**, 1091–1098.

79. Schwiebert, E.M., Morales, M.M., Devidas, S., Egan, M.E. and Guggino, W.B. (1998) Chloride channel and chloride conductance regulator domains of CFTR, the cystic fibrosis transmembrane conductance regulator. *Proc. Natl Acad. Sci. USA*, **95**, 2674–2679.

80. Rich, D.P., Gregory, R.J., Anderson, MP. *et al.* (1991) Effect of deleting the R domain on CFTR-generated chloride channels. *Science*, **253**, 205–207.

81. Cheng, S.H., Rich, D.P., Marshall, J. *et al.* (1991) Phosphorylation of the R domain by cAMP-dependent protein kinase regulates the CFTR chloride channel. *Cell*, **66**, l027–1036.

82. Ma, J., Zhao, J., Drumm, M.L., Xie, J. and Davis, P.B. (1997) Function of the R domain in the cystic fibrosis transmembrane conductance regulator chloride channel. *J. Biol. Chem.*, **272**, 28133–28141.

83. Winter, M.C. and Welsh, M.J. (1997) Stimulation of CFTR activity by its phosphorlyated R domain. *Nature*, **289**, 294–296.

84. Ma, J., Tasch, J.E., Tao, T., Zhao, J., Xie, J., Drumm, M.L. and Davis, P.B. (1996) Phosphorylation-dependent block of cystic fibrosis transmembrane conductance regulator chloride channel by exogenous R domain protein. *J. Biol. Chem.*, **271**, 7351–7356.

85. Berger, H.A., Travis, S.M. and Welch, J. (1993) Regulation of the cystic fibrosis transmembrane conductance regulator Cl⁻ channel by specific protein kinases and protein phosphatases. *J. Biol. Chem.*, **268**, 2037–2047.

86. Luo, J., Pato, M.D., Riordan, J.R. and Hanrahan, J.W. (1998) Differential regulation of single CFTR channels by PP2C, PP2A and other phosphatases. *Am. J. Physiol.*, **274**, C1397–C1410.

87. Zeitlin, P. L., Crawford, I., Lu, L. *et al.* (1992) CFTR protein expression in primary and cultured epithelia. *Proc. Natl Acad. Sci. USA*, **89**, 344–347.

88. Trezise, A. E. and Buchwald, M. (1991) In vivo cell specific

expression of the cystic fibrosis transmembrane conductance regulator. *Nature*, **353**, 434–437.

89. Lukacs, G.L, Segal, G., Kartner, N., Grinstein, S. and Zhang, F. (1997) Constitutive internalization of cystic fibrosis transmembrane conductance regulator occurs via clathrin-dependent endocytosis and is regulated by protein phosphorylation. *Biochem. J.*, **328**, 353–361.

90. Lukacs, G.L., Chang, X.B., Bear, C. *et al.* (1993) The delta F508 mutation decreases the stability of cystic fibrosis transmembrane conductance regulator in the plasma membrane. Determination of functional half-lives on transfected cells. *J. Biol. Chem.*, **268**, 21592–21598.

91. Welsh, M.J. and Smith, A.E. (1993) Molecular mechanisms of CFTR chloride channel dysfunction in cystic fibrosis. *Cell*, **73**, 1251–1254.

92. Pasyk, E.A. and Foskett, J.K. (1995) Mutant (delta F508) cystic fibrosis transmembrane conductance regulator Cl⁻ channel is functional when retained in endoplasmic reticulum of mammalian cells. *J. Biol. Chem.*, **70**, 12347–12350.

93. Li, C., Ramjeesingh, M., Reyes, E. *et al.* (1993) The cystic fibrosis mutation (delta F508) does not influence the chloride channel activity of CFTR. *Nature Genet.*, **3**, 311–316.

94. Drumm, M.L., Wilkinson, D.J., Smit, L.S. *et al.* (1991) Chloride conductance expressed by delta F508 and other mutant CFTRs in Xenopus oocytes. *Science*, **254**, 1797–1799.

95. Dalemans, W., Barbry, P., Champingny, G. *et al.* (1991) Altered chloride ion channel kinetics associated with the delta F508 cystic fibrosis mutation. *Nature*, **354**, 526–528.

96. Penning, G.M., Anderson, M.P., Aniara, J.F. *et al.* (1992) Processing of mutant cystic fibrosis transmembrane conductance regulator is temperature-sensitive. *Nature*, **358**, 761–764.

97. Pind, S., Riordan, JR. and Williams, D.B. (1994) Participation of the endoplasmic reticulum chaperone calnexin (p88, IP90) in the biogenesis of the cystic fibrosis transmembrane conductance regulator. *J. Biol. Chem.*, **269**, 12784–12788.

98. Yang, Y., Janich, S., Cohn, J.A. and Wilson, J.M. (1993) The common variant of cystic fibrosis regulator is recognized by hsp70 and degraded in a pre-Golgi nonlysosomal compartment. *Proc. Natl Acad. Sci. USA*, **90**, 9480–9484.

99. Ward, C.L. and Kopito, R.R. (1994) Intracellular turnover of cystic fibrosis transmembrane conductance regulator. Inefficient processing and rapid degradation of wild-type and mutant proteins. *J. Biochem.*, **269**, 25710–25718.

100. Lukacs, G.L., Mohamed, A., Kartner, N., Chang, Z.B. and Grinstein, S. (1994) Conformational maturation of CFTR but not its mutant counterpart (delta F508) occurs in the endoplasmic reticulum and requires ATP. *EMBO J.*, **13**, 6076–6086.

101. Jensen, T.J., Loo, M.A., Pind, S., Williams, D.B., Goldberg, A.L. and Riordan, J.R. (1995) Multiple proteolytic systems, including the proteasome, contribute to CFTR processing. *Cell*, **83**, 129–135.

102. Ward, C.L., Omura, S. and Kopito, R.R. (1995) Degradation of CFTR by the ubiquitin-proteasome pathway. *Cell*, **83**, 121–127.

103. Sato, S., Ward, C.L., and Kopito, R.R. (1998) Contranslational ubiquitination of cystic fibrosis transmembrane conductance regulator *in vitro*. *J. Biol. Chem.*, **271**, 7189–7192.

104. Stutts, M.J., Canessa, C.M., Olsen, J.C. *et al.* (1995) CFTR as a cAMP-dependent regulator of sodium channels. *Science*, **269**, 847–850.

105. Ismailov, I.I., Awayda, M.S., Jovov, B. *et al.* (1996) Regulation of epithelial sodium channels by the cystic fibrosis transmembrane conductance regulator. *J. Biol. Chem.*, **271**, 4725–4732.

106. Stutts, M.J., Rosier, B.C. and Boucher, R.C. (1997) Cystic fibrosis transmembrane conductance regulator inverts protein kinase A-mediated regulation of epithelial sodium channel single channel kinetics. *J. Biol. Chem.*, **272**, 14037–14040.

107. Briel, M., Greger, R. and Kunzelmann, K. (1998) Cl⁻ transport by cystic fibrosis transmembrane conductance regulator (CFTR) contributes to the inhibition of epithelial Na⁺ channels (ENaCs) in enopus oocytes co-expressing CFTR and ENaC. *J. Physiol.*, **508**, 825–836.

108. Gabriel, S.E., Clarke, L.L., Boucher, R.C. and Stutts, M.J. (1993) CFTR and outward rectifying chloride channel share distinct proteins with a regulator relationship. *Nature*, **363**, 263–268.

109. Schwiebert, E.M., Flotte, T., Cutting, G.R. and Guggino, W.B. (1994) Both CFTR and outwardly rectifying chloride channels contribute to cAMP-stimulated whole cell chloride currents. *Am. J. Physiol.*, **266**, C1464–C1477.

110. Schwiebert, E.M., Egan, M.E., Hwang, T.H. *et al.* (1995) CFTR regulates outwardly rectifying chloride channels through an autocrine mechanism involving ATP. *Cell*, **81**, 1063–1073.

111. Jovov, B., Ismailov, I.I., Berdiev, B.K. *et al.* (1995) Interaction between cystic fibrosis transmembrane conductance regulator and outwardly rectified chloride channels. *J. Biol. Chem.*, **270**, 29194–29200.

112. Kunzelmann, K., Mall, M., Briel, M. *et al.* (1997) The cystic fibrosis transmembrane conductance regulator attenuates the endogenous Ca^{2+} activated Cl⁻ conductance for Xenopus oocytes. *Eur. J. Physiol.*, **435**, 178–181.

113. McNicholas, C.M., Guggino, W.B., Schwiebert, E.M., Hebert, S.C., Giebisch, G. and Egan, M.E. (1996) Sensitivity of a renal K⁺ channel (ROMK2) to the inhibitory sulfonylurea compound glibenclamide is enhanced by coexpression with the ATP-binding cassette transport cystic fibrosis transmembrane regulator. *Proc. Natl Acad. Sci. USA*, **93**, 8083–8088.

114. Short, D.B., Trotter, K.W., Reczek, D. *et al.* (1998) An apical PDZ protein anchors the cystic fibrosis transmembrane conductance regulator to the cytoskeleton. *J. Biol. Chem.*, **273**, 19797–19801.

115. Wang, S., Raab, R.W., Schatz, P.J., Guggino, W.B. and Li, M. (1998) Peptide binding consensus of the NHE-RF-PDZ1

domain matches the C-terminal sequences of cystic fibrosis transmembrane conductance regulator (CFTR). *FEBS Lett.*, **427**, 103–108.

116. Naren, A.P, Nelson, D.J., Xie, W. *et al.* (1997) Regulation of CFTR chloride channels by syntaxin and Munc18 isoforms. *Nature*, **390**, 302–305.

117. Grygorczyk, R. and Hanrahan, J.W. (1997) CFTR-dependent ATP release from epithelial cells triggered by mechanical stimuli. *Am. J. Physiol.*, **272**, C1058–C1066.

118. Reisin, I.L., Prat, A.G., Abraham, E.H. *et al.* (1994) The cystic fibrosis transmembrane conductance regulator is a dual ATP and chloride channel. *J. Biol. Chem.*, **269**, 20584-20591.

119. Sugita, M., Yue, Y. and Foskett, J.K. (1998) CFTR Cl− channel and CFTR associated ATP channel: distinct pores regulated by common gates. *EMBO J.*, **17**, 898–908.

120. Reddy, M.M., Quinton, P.M., Haws, C. *et al.* (1996) Failure of the cystic fibrosis transmembrane conductance regulator to conduct ATP. *Science*, **271**, 1876–1879.

121. Li, C., Ramheesingh, M., and Bear, C.E. (1996) Purified cystic fibrosis transmembrane conductance regulator (CFTR) does not function as an ATP channel. *J. Biol. Chem.*, **271**, 11623–11626.

122. Imundo, L., Barasch, J., Prince, A. and Al-Aqwati, Q. (1995) Cystic fibrosis epithelial cells have a receptor for pathogenic bacteria on their apical surface. *Proc. Natl Acad. Sci. USA*, **92**, 3019–3023.

123. Davies, J.C., Stern, M., Dewar, A. *et al.* (1997) CFTR gene transfer reduces the binding of *Pseudomonas aeruginosa* to cystic fibrosis respiratory epithelium. *Am. J. Resp. Cell Molec. Biol.*, **16**, 1–7.

124. DiMango, E., Zar, H.J., Bryan, R. and Prince, A. (1995) Diverse *Pseudomonas aeruginosa* gene products stimulate respiratory epithelial cells to produce interleukin-8. *J. Clin. Invest.*, **96**, 2204–2210.

125. Di Mango, E., Ratner, A.J., Bryan, R., Tabibi, S. and Prince, A. (1998) Activation of NF-kappaB by adherent *Pseudomonas aeruginosa* in normal and cystic fibrosis respiratory cells. *J. Clin. Invest.*, **101**, 2598–2605.

126. Smith, J.J., Travis, S.M., Greenberg, E.P. and Welsh, M.J. (1996) Cystic fibrosis airway epithelia fail to kill bacteria because of abnormal airway surface fluid. *Cell*, **85**, 229–236.

127. Goldman, M.J., Anderson, G.M., Stolzenberg, E.D., Kari, U.P., Zasloff, M. and Wilson, J.M. (1997) Human beta-defensin-1 is a salt-sensitive antibiotic in lung that is inactivated in cystic fibrosis. *Cell*, **88**, 553–560.

128. Knowles, M.R., Robinson, J.M., Wood, R.E. *et al.* (1997) Ion composition of airway surface liquid of patients with cystic fibrosis as compared with normal and disease-control subjects. *J. Clin. Invest.*, **100**, 2588–2595.

129. Ull, J., Skinner, W., Robertson, C. and Phelan, P. (1998) Elemental content of airway surface liquid from infants with cystic fibrosis. *Am. J. Resp. Crit. Care Med.*, **157**, 10–14.

130. Pier, G.B., Grout, M., Zaidi, T.S. *et al.* (1996) Role of mutant CFTR in hypersusceptibility of cystic fibrosis patients to lung infections. *Science*, **271**, 64–67.

131. Pier, G.B., Grout, M. and Zaidi, T.S. (1997) Cystic fibrosis transmembrane conductance regulator is an epithelial cell receptor for clearance of *Pseudomonas aeruginosa* from the lung. *Proc. Natl Acad. Sci. USA*, **94**, 12088–12093.

132. Bonfield, T.L., Konstan, M.W., Burfeind, P., Panuska, J.R., Hilliard, J.B. and Berger, M. (1995) Normal bronchial epithelial cells constitutively produce the anti-inflammatory cytokine interleukin-10 which is down regulated in cystic fibrosis. *Am. J. Resp. Cell Mol. Biol.*, **13**, 257–261.

133. Gottlieb, R.A. and Dosanjh, A. (1996) Mutant cystic fibrosis transmembrane conductance regulator inhibits acidification and apoptosis in C127 cells: possible relevance to cystic fibrosis. *Proc. Natl Acad. Sci. USA*, **93**, 3587–3591.

134. Jetten, A.M., Yankaskas, J.R., Stutts, M.J. *et al.* (1989) Persistence of abnormal chloride conductance regulation in transformed cystic fibrosis epithelia. *Science*, **244**, 1472–1475.

135. Grubb, B.R. and Boucher, R.C. (1999) Pathophysiology of gene-targeted mouse models for cystic fibrosis. *Physiol. Rev.*, **79** (1 suppl), S193–214.

136. Bijman, J. and Quinton, P.M. (1984) Influence of abnormal Cl− impermeability on sweating in cystic fibrosis. *Am. J. Physiol.*, **247**, C3–C9.

5

Microbiology of cystic fibrosis

N. HØIBY AND B. FREDERIKSEN

Introduction	83	Bacterial infections	85
Microbiology and immunology of CF	83	Conclusion	94
Respiratory virus infections	85	References	95

INTRODUCTION

The cystic fibrosis (CF) gene product, which is the membrane-bound CF transmembrane conductance regulator (CFTR) protein, has been shown to be the chloride-ion channel regulating the transport of chloride ions across fluid-transporting epithelial cells such as exocrine glands[1]. The CF defect of the CFTR protein leads to altered secretions (salty sweat; dehydrated, thick mucus), blocked ducts and reduced noninflammatory defense of the respiratory tract, which leads to recruitment of the inflammatory defense mechanisms and thereby lung tissue damage[2–4]. Scientific progress has been tremendous since discovery of the gene, and trials of gene therapy are now being carried out in several countries[5]. However, in spite of the scientific progress, CF patients continue to suffer from recurrent and chronic respiratory tract infections, and most of their morbidity and mortality is due to such infections throughout their life[6]. When CF was described, most patients died before the age of 5 years due to *Staphylococcus aureus* infection (Table 5.1)[7–11]. The introduction of penicillin improved the prognosis dramatically: the mortality of Andersen's CF cases 1–28 until 1944 was 61 per cent, decreasing to 18 per cent of the cases 29–107 from 1944 to 1948[10]. The prognosis of CF has improved steadily due to a comprehensive therapeutic program and centralized treatment in CF centers. The median survival in the best centers is now more than 40 years, and new prophylatic measures and treatment modalities for critically ill patients, including heart–lung transplantation, will further improve the survival and quality of life of CF patients[6,12]. The most significant CF pathogen during the past three decades has been *Pseudomonas aeruginosa*, which causes most of the morbidity and mortality in these patients (Table 5.2). In spite of that, progress of the treatment implies that CF is no longer a pediatric disease, since more than 20 per cent of CF patients are adults. It is, therefore, essential that the general and specific strategies of prophylaxis and treatment of respiratory tract infections in CF are conveyed to other medical specialties.

MICROBIOLOGY AND IMMUNOLOGY OF CF

CF patients have no detectable immune deficiency and, except for the respiratory tract, they are not more susceptible to infections than normal children of the same age, and bacteremia is rarely recorded in CF patients[3,13,14]. As a consequence of antibiotic treatment, however, *Clostridium difficile* colitis[15] and *Candida* vaginitis may occur. The altered secretions of the respiratory tract leading to dehydrated, thick mucus is thought to be the reason why CF patients suffer from recurrent and chronic respiratory tract infections. Additional explanations are:

1. increased sulfation of mucus glycoproteins due to defective acidification of intracellular organelles[16,17];
2. defective function of human β-defensin-1 in the fluids of the lower respiratory tract due to the high NaCl concentration in CF patients[18]; and
3. defective CFTR-mediated uptake of *P. aeruginosa* from the respiratory tract[19].

The congenital defect of the noninflammatory defense mechanisms of the CF lungs leads to recruitment of the

Table 5.1 *Bacterial flora of the lower respiratory tract recovered shortly before death or at autopsy in CF patients*[13]

Reference	Number of CF patients	Prevalence of different species (%)			
		S. aureus	P. aeruginosa	H. influenzae	Miscellaneous
Andersen[8]	15	80	a		Strep.: 7
di Sant'Agnese and Andersen[11]	13	92	8	8	S. pn.: 15
Zuelzer and Newton [313]	28	79	4		Strep.: 4
Bodian et al.[314]	23	83	9		E. coli: 26
					S.f.: 4
Esterly and Oppenheimer[315]	14 (-1948)	86	14		E.coli: 14
	32 (1948–60)	50	60		E.coli: 9
	9 (1960–66)		89		E.coli: 11
Margaretten et al.[316]	23	a	48		
Iaocca et al.[317]	22	86	96	5	
May et al.[318]	11	36	73 (M)	36	Kleb.: 36
Lloyd-Still et al.[319]	96 (<1 year)		67		E.coli: 33
					Kleb.: 11
					Prot.: 11
					Her.: 11
Harrison and Doggett[320]	51	27	88 (M)		Prot.: 22
			47 (NM)		E.coli: 14
Mitchell-Heggs et al.[321]	7 (>12 years)	14	86	43	
Bedrossian et al.[322]	58	a	57		
Høiby[13]	18	22	94	6	E.coli: 22
			(61 M, 33 ND)		Kleb.: 11
					Prot.: 11
					P.st.: 6

a Figures for other pathogens not given.
Strep., β-hemolytic streptococci; S.f., *Streptococcus faecalis*; Prot., *Proteus* species; Kleb., *Klebsiella* species; Her., *Herellae*; P.st., *Pseudomonas stutzeri*; M, mucoid; NM, nonmucoid; ND, not determined.

Table 5.2 *Lethality of cystic fibrosis patients with and without chronic* P. aeruginosa *lung infection*[257]

	Total number of patients	Number of patients alive	Number of patients dead
Number of patients with chronic P. aeruginosa infection[a]	56	41 (73%)	15 (27%)*
Number of patients with intermittent P. aeruginosa colonization	37	35 } (96%)	2 } (4%)*
Number of patients never colonized with P. aeruginosa	40	39	1
Total number of patients	133	115 (86%)	18 (14%)

a ≥6 months' continuous colonization.*P < 0.0005.

inflammatory defense mechanisms dominated by polymorphonuclear leukocytes (PMNs) and antibodies, and PMN proteases and oxygen radicals gradually destroy the lung tissue. The inflammation is therefore already present in CF infants[4,20] and it is therefore important to treat any bacterial lung colonization and infection aggressively in CF patients. Acute exacerbations of the chronic respiratory disease in CF patients were found to be caused by bacteria (63 per cent), bacteria and virus (13 per cent) and virus (6 per cent), whereas no etiology could be detected in 18 per cent of the exacerbations[21]. In order to prevent such infections, it is necessary to correct the basic defect of the respiratory tract. One such approach is inhalation of the diuretic amiloride, which improves the mucociliary and cough clearance in CF patients. Hopefully such approaches[22,23] or gene therapy[24] will prevent some of the respiratory infections of CF patients. Once the respiratory tract infections persist, most of the viscosity of sputum is due to DNA from the neutrophil granulocytes as a consequence of the persistent recruitment of the inflammatory defense mechanisms, leading to chronic inflammation. An efficient treatment leading to reduced viscosity of CF sputum is therefore inhalation with recombinant DNase[25].

RESPIRATORY VIRUS INFECTIONS

Diagnosis of respiratory virus infections is currently achieved either by detection of virus antigens using the ELISA technique or the direct immunofluorescence microscopy technique, or by raising antibody titers against these viruses. However, the polymerase chain reaction for detection of virus DNA or RNA is also likely to be commercially available in this diagnostic field in the near future. Respiratory viruses (influenza virus A and B, parainfluenza virus 1 and 3, rhinovirus, adenovirus and, especially, respiratory syncytial virus (RSV)) are responsible for some of the acute exacerbations of the pulmonary disease in CF, as mentioned above[21,26–32]. As a consequence, the pulmonary function of CF patients may decrease by 30 per cent for up to 1 month during respiratory viral infections[31]. The patients are susceptible to secondary colonization and infection with bacteria, notably P. aeruginosa, following such viral infections[21,33]. In spite of the significant negative effect of virus infections, vaccination against influenza A is the only generally used prophylactic measure and treatment with amantadine or ribavirin is rarely used, but this is likely to change in the future[27,34].

BACTERIAL INFECTIONS

Bacterial infections of the lower respiratory tract are diagnosed by microscopy and culture of secretions from the lower respiratory tract. Some of the major bacterial pathogens of the lung, e.g. Streptococcus pneumoniae, Haemophilus influenzae, Staphylococcus aureus, are members of the normal flora of the pharynx and the mouth, although in low numbers. Other bacteria, e.g. Enterobacteriaceae, Pseudomonas spp., Alcaligenes spp., are seldom or never found in the normal flora, but E. coli (and also yeast, such as Candida albicans) may colonize the mouth following broad-spectrum antibacterial therapy which eradicates the sensitive normal flora. Because of the insidious nature of some of the lower respiratory tract infections in CF patients, frequent (monthly) bacteriological investigations of sputum or tracheal secretions are necessary. The techniques used to evaluate the lower respiratory tract flora in patients who do not produce large amounts of sputum comprise deep throat culture[35], endolaryngeal suction[36] and bronchoscopy[37,38]. Obviously, bronchoscopy is not suitable for

routine screening purpose. Results obtained by that method and deep-throat culture simultaneously indicate that the predictive values of throat cultures positive for S. aureus or P. aeruginosa were 91 per cent and 83 per cent, respectively, whereas the negative predictive values were 80 per cent and 70 per cent[37]. In children <5 years of age the positive predictive values are poor, whereas the negative predictive values are still high[37b]. In the Danish CF Center, tracheal secretion is obtained by endolaryngeal suction and the bacteriological examination of the secretion comprises microscopy and culture of the secretion. Gram-stained films of the specimens are examined by microscopy, and the bacterial flora associated with areas consisting of respiratory epithelial cells and pus cells but without squamous epithelial cells is described, whereas the flora associated with oral epithelial cells is considered to be predominantly of oral or pharyngeal origin, and is not described[39,40]. Based upon these criteria, 85 per cent of the culture-positive samples (P. aeruginosa, 91 per cent; S. aureus, 81 per cent; H. influenzae, 87 per cent and S. pneumoniae, 85 per cent) were in accordance with the results obtained by microscopy[39]. A presumptive bacteriological diagnosis can frequently be obtained by the microscopic examination (Fig. 5.1) as a guideline for urgent chemotherapy if this is indicated, but in most cases the chemotherapy can be withheld until the result of the culture is obtained. Indication for antimicrobial chemotherapy includes that the bacteria in question have been cultured, as well as found by microscopy according to the principles described above.

The media used for culturing the bacteria from CF sputum includes enriched standard media – chocolate agar and horse-blood agar; selective media for Gram-negative enteric and nonfermentive bacteria (Enterobacteriaceae, Pseudomonas spp., Burkholderia spp., Stenotrophomonas (Xanthomonas) maltophilia, Comamonas acidovorans, Alcaligenes xylosoxidans, etc.; selective media containing colistin and gentamicin for B. cepacia[41]; media containing 7.5 per cent NaCl for S. aureus; in some centers, also selective media for H.

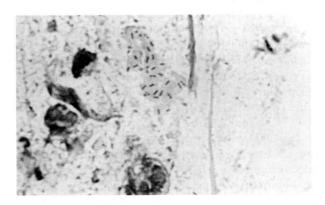

Fig. 5.1 Gram-stained smear of sputum from a cystic fibrosis patient. A small mucoid microcolony of P. aeruginosa and a polymorphonuclear leukocyte are seen. Magnification ×1000.

influenzae[42,43], Sabouraud agar for fungi (*C. albicans, Aspergillus fumigatus*) and Löwenstein–Jensen medium for atypical mycobacteria (but decontamination of the secretion with 0.25 per cent *N*-acetyl-L-cysteine and 1 per cent NAOH followed by 5 per cent oxalic acid is necessary to detect the mycobacteria in the presence of, for example, *P. aeruginosa*[44]. In the Danish CF Center a blood agar plate for primary sensitivity testing with antibiotics (tablets or disks) active to *P. aeruginosa* (colistin, tobramycin, piperacillin, ceftazidime, aztreonam, imipenem, meropenem, ciprofloxacin) is also used. Incubation takes place at 35°C for 48 h (6 weeks for mycobacteria, but frequently atypical mycobacteria isolated from CF patients are rapidly growing species (*M. cheloni, M. fortuitum*) and colonies are detected within 1 week). The chocolate agar medium is incubated in an atmosphere of 5 per cent CO_2. Anaerobic culture is generally not useful, due to heavy growth of the normal anaerobic flora from the throat and the facultative anaerobic pathogens from the lungs. The isolated bacteria are then identified to the species level using standard biochemical tests, and secondary testing of sensitivity to relevant antibiotics is carried out (e.g. *S. aureus*: penicillin, methicillin, fusidic acid, rifampicin, erythromycin, clindamycin and vancomycin; *H. influenzae*: ampicillin, ampicillin + clavulanic acid, cefuroxime, ceftriaxon, ciprofloxacin, sulfonamide, trimethoprin, chloramphenicol, rifampicin, erythromycin, azithromycin and tetracycline; *P. aeruginosa*: see above; *B. cepacia*: as for *P. aeruginosa* but, in addition, tetracycline, chloramphenicol, sulfonamide + trimethoprim and rifampicin. The mucoid colony morphology, which is so characteristic of especially *P. aeruginosa* (but also sometimes found in other species), is described in the report from the laboratory (Fig. 5.2). Typing methods are useful in order to discriminate between reinfection and persisting infection with a given bacterial species. Phage typing is adequate for *S. aureus*[45], biotyping may be used for *H. influenzae*[46,47], whereas the conventional typing methods, such as serotyping, pyocin typing and phage typing, are often inadequate for *P. aeruginosa* because this bacterial species becomes polyagglutinable and nontypeable due to loss of the repeating polysaccharide chain of the O antigen (rough or semi-rough) concurrent with the change to mucoid morphology[48]. Such strains can be typed by the DNA techniques (genomic fingerprinting, toxin A probe, ribotyping, multilocus isoenzyme electrophoresis)[49–52]. These methods have proved that a single individual strain of *P. aeruginosa* predominates for years in most CF patients. For *B. cepacia*, bacteriocin typing and DNA methods such as ribotyping have been used[53–55]. Methods employing DNA technology to detect *P. aeruginosa* have also been developed but are hardly justified in the routine bacteriological surveillance of CF patients[56].

Chronic *P. aeruginosa* colonization in CF is defined as persistence of these bacteria for 6 months or more continuously, and/or development of a significant antibody

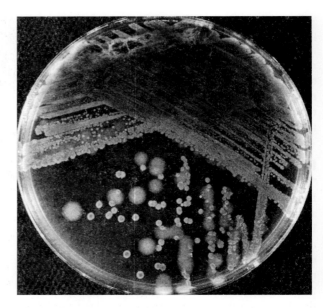

Fig. 5.2 *Mucoid (large) and nonmucoid (small) colonies of* P. aeruginosa *from a cystic fibrosis patient, cultured on solid medium.*

response[13]. The antibody response to *P. aeruginosa* (Fig. 5.3) and other bacteria (*S. aureus, H. influenzae, B. cepacia* and others if isolated repeatedly from sputum) is measured in CF patients at the Danish CF Center routinely at least once a year to rule out undetected chronic infection caused by these bacteria, or more often if clinical deterioration occurs. IgG and IgE antibodies to *Aspergillus fumigatus* are also measured in cases of suspected ABPA[57–65].

Bacteria are still the most important microorganisms responsible for the progression of the lung pathology[6,66–70]. Among the bacteria, *P. aeruginosa* was associated with 51 per cent of the acute exacerbations, *S. aureus* with 19 per cent, *H. influenzae* with 14 per cent, *S. pneumoniae* with 5 per cent and Enterobacteriaceae with

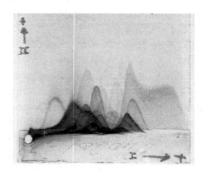

Fig. 5.3 *Crossed immunoelectrophoresis of water-soluble antigens from* P. aeruginosa *against serum from a patient with chronic* P. aeruginosa *pulmonary infection. Many precipitating antibodies are seen (normal: 0–1 precipitating antibody specificity).*

Table 5.3 *Point prevalence rate (%) of the major bacterial pathogens in 192 cystic fibrosis patients treated in the Danish Center (1984) (modified from ref. 71)*

Bacterial species	Prevalence (%) in different age groups			Total
	0–9 years	10–19 years	>20 years	
S. aureus	55	35	30	42
H. influenzae	30	9	8	17
S. pneumoniae	21	1	3	10
E. coli	10	1	8	6
P. aeruginosa	25	81	81	57

10 per cent[21]. However, since the chronic infections are often insidious in onset, many CF centers rely on monthly examinations of all patients in the outpatient clinic, and the microbiology of the lower respiratory tract is routinely checked during these examinations. In small children the bacteria most frequently involved are *S. aureus* and *H. influenzae*, but pneumococci and sometimes Enterobacteriaceae are also isolated during childhood (Table 5.3)[36,71]. In older children and adult patients these bacteria may still play a role, but the major pathogen is *P. aeruginosa* and, in some centers, also *B. cepacia* and other pathogens[36,39,71,72]. Probably reflecting the different efficacy of the chemotherapy, *S. aureus*, *H. influenzae* and *S. pneumoniae* cause mainly recurrent infections, whereas *P. aeruginosa*, *B. cepacia* and mycobacteria mainly cause chronic infections[36,39]. Anaerobic infections seem not to be a major problem[73]. No difference between the two sexes has been found as regards the occurrence of any of the bacterial species[39]. In summary, the bacteriology of CF patients is very complex[74] and detailed studies require epidemiological terms (incidence, prevalence, etc.) in order to facilitate comparison between different centers[73].

Staphylococcus aureus

These Gram-positive cocci are carried in clusters in the nose and on the skin of approximately 10 per cent of normal human beings. They are spread in the air on shed epidermal cells; they can survive in the dust on the floor, etc. They cause a variety of infections, such as abscesses, osteomyelitis, septicemia and postoperative wound sepsis. They are a major cause of nosocomial infections. Ever since the discovery of the disease, *S. aureus* has been considered an important pathogen in CF, although no immune deficiency to these bacteria has been described in CF patients (Tables 5.1 and 5.3)[36,75]. Its peculiar association with CF has been ascribed to the high electrolyte content, the changed composition of lipids in CF sputum, to the presence or absence *in vivo* of a polysaccharide capsule or to the effect of protein A as an IgC scavenger[36,76–78]. No specific phage type of *S. aureus* is characteristic[36,78], but most CF siblings carry the same

strain[45,79]. In CF patients treated with antifolate antibiotics (sulfamethoxazole + trimethoprim) small-colony variants of *S. aureus* are sometimes found, which are associated with persistent infections[80]. These small-variant colonies are nonhemolytic and nonpigmented, and they are auxotrophic, dependent on hemin, thymidine and/or menadione for growth.

Staphylococcus aureus is still the most frequently isolated pathogen in CF children but, due to the efficient antibiotics available today, it is no longer a major problem. In some centers[81], however, it still causes a considerable number of chronic infections, but does not lead to increased mortality as it used to do in virtually all CF patients in the pre-antibiotic era[8,10]. *Staphylococcus aureus* infections may cause some of the early damage of the respiratory tract in CF infants and thereby pave the way for *P. aeruginosa*[36,82–84]. Based on this hypothesis, some CF centers successfully use prophylactic antibiotics

Table 5.4 *Three different approaches to antimicrobial chemotherapy in cystic fibrosis*

(1) Only when clinical signs of lower respiratory infection are present[96]. Mean number of treatment courses/year and the duration of the selective pressure on the microbial flora is lower than in (2) and (3), but there is risk of colonization and low-grade inflammation[4]

(2) Always when microbiological examinations at the monthly visit in the outpatient clinic show the presence of pathogens in the lower respiratory tract[87]. Mean number of treatment courses/year and the duration of the selective pressure on the microbial flora in the CF cohort (1999; 280 patients) in the Danish CF Centre is on average 7.5 months/year, distributed thus:

125 CF patients *without* chronic *P. aeruginosa* infection: 2.7 months/year
131 CF patients *with* chronic *P. aeruginosa* infection: 12 months/year (2 months' intravenous treatment and every day inhalation of colistin)

3. Prophylactic, continuously, from the time of CF diagnosis, orally or by aerosol, to prevent especially *S. aureus* infection. Mean duration of treatment and selective pressure/year on the microbial flora is: 12 months/year[85]

Table 5.5 *Principles of chemotherapy of lung infections in cystic fibrosis patients*[323]

1. Microbial diagnosis based on secretions from the lower respiratory tract is required before chemotherapy is initiated
2. High doses of preferably bactericidal antibiotics for 14 days
3. Preferably use of antibiotics with rare occurrence of resistant variants or use of combination of antibiotics
4. Avoid prophylactic chemotherapy[a]
5. Be aware of cumulative side-effects due to frequent use of antibiotics
6. Be aware of changed pharmacokinetics of some antibiotics in CF patients, especially as regards increased renal excretion
7. Inhalation of antibiotics may be useful as a support of systemic chemotherapy or as replacement of systemic treatment[324–326]

[a]Flucloxacillin against *S. aureus* is an exception[85].

during childhood against *S. aureus*[85]. Other centers, like the Danish, try to eradicate *S. aureus* whenever it is present in the lower respiratory tract (Tables 5.4–5.7)[86–90]. The result of such an aggressive attitude is that chronic *S. aureus* infection has become rare in these centers[36]. Probably due to the efficacy of the treatment in comparison with antipseudomonal treatment, there are very few controlled clinical studies in the literature comparing various antistaphylococcal treatments and prophylaxis regimes, e.g. oral antistaphylococcal prophylaxis in contrast to inhalation showed beneficial prophylactic effect [85,91,92]. The principles and drugs used in the Danish CF Center are given in Tables 5.5–5.7. In nearly all cases, oral treatment is preferred, and the patient does not have to be admitted to hospital during treatment. The bacteriological efficacy (eradication) of each repeated treatment course does not decrease, but remains around 75 per cent, and resistance to the various antibiotics used occurs rarely[87,93]. In case of treatment failure, 4 weeks' treatment with one of the combinations of oral antibiotics (Table 5.7) and, sometimes, inhalation with methicillin is used, and dicloxacillin is given as monotherapy for 2 months more. The efficacy of that regime means that less than 10 per cent of patients are chronically infected (for more than 6 months, continuously) with *S.*

aureus and the antibody response remains low[87]. In case of methicillin-resistant *S. aureus* (MRSA), fusidic acid is combined with rifampicin or clindamycin or, in case of resistance to these drugs, with vancomycin or teicoplanin. Other less aggressive regimes, and the basis for rational selection and dosing of antistaphylococcal antibiotics for CF patients, are described in excellent recent surveys, some of which also deal with methicillin-resistant strains (MRSA), which are frequent in some centers[68,74,75,86,89,94–96].

Haemophilus influenzae

These fastidious, small, Gram-negative rods are found in humans as members of the normal flora in the upper respiratory tract (pharynx, mouth). Most are acapsulate and may cause purulent sputum and fever in patients suffering from chronic bronchitis. Capsulate strains of type *b* cause invasive infections such as meningitis in nonvaccinated infants. Most *H. influenzae* strains isolated from CF patients are noncapsulated and belong to different types, and several different strains may coexist in the respiratory tract[43,97]. No immune deficiency to these bacteria has been described in these patients[36,75,98,99]. Although not recognized by all authors[75], these bacteria are probably responsible for some acute exacerbations of the chronic lung disease in CF[21]. In a few patients, however, chronic *H. influenzae* infection becomes established. Due to the frequent use of ampicillin and other β-lactam antibiotics in CF, β-lactamase-producing strains are often isolated[100]. In the Danish CF Center, 10–20 per cent of the strains are β-lactamase producers. Such strains have been found to emerge during ampicillin or amoxicillin therapy[101]. Combination of ampicillin or amoxicillin with β-lactamase inhibitors, or use of other drugs such as the fluoroquinolones, are efficient in such cases[87,102]. As is the case with *S. aureus*, controlled studies comparing different treatment regimes are rare in the literature. The principles and drugs used in the Danish CF Center are given in Tables 5.5–5.7. The patients are treated in the outpatient clinic with oral antibiotics. The bacteriological efficacy of each treatment course does not decrease but remains around 75 per cent[87]. In case of treatment failure, repeated treat-

Table 5.6 *Specific principles of chemotherapy of lung infections in cystic fibrosis patients*[323]

S. aureus, H. influenzae, P. aeruginosa[a]	Should be eradicated when present in the lower respiratory tract whether there are clinical symptoms or not
P. aeruginosa[b]	Two precipitating antibodies against *P. aeruginosa* means chronic infection; chemotherapy is given regularly at least 4 times/year
Other pathogens	Rather seldom pathogenic in CF; chemotherapy is given when indicated due to clinical or aerological findings. ABPA is treated with steroid hormones even if the patient is colonized with other pathogens

[a] Intermittently colonized.
[b] Chronically colonized.

Table 5.7 *Antibiotics used to treat lung infections in cystic fibrosis patients*[323,326a]

S. aureus	Dicloxacillin (25 mg/kg every 24 hours orally) + fusidic acid (50 mg/kg every 24 hours). Alternative drugs that can replace one of the above-mentioned: rifampicin (15 mg/kg every 24 hours) and clindamycin (20–40 mg/kg/24 hours) or vancomycin (40 mg/kg/24 hours) or teicoplanin (10 mg/kg/24 hours)
H. influenzae	Pivampicillin (35 mg/kg/24 hours orally) or amoxicillin (25–50 mg/kg/24 hours). Alternative drugs: amoxicillin + clavulanate (50 mg + 12.5 mg/kg/24 hours) or rifampicin (15 mg/kg/24 hours) in combination with erythromycin (30–50 mg/kg/24 hours) or azithromycin (10mg/kg/24 hours)
P. aeruginosa[a]	Ciprofloxacin (20–30 mg/kg/24 hours orally) + colistin (2–4 million units/24 hours, aerosolized, for 3 weeks–3 months)
P. aeruginosa[b]	Tobramycin (10 mg/kg/24 hours intravenously) + piperacillin (300 mg/kg/24 hours) or + ceftazidime (150–250 mg/kg/24 hours) or + aztreonam (150–250 mg/kg/24 hours) or + imipenem (50–75 mg/kg/24 hours) or + meropenem (120 mg/kg/24 hours) and + colistin (2–4 million units/24 hours, aerosolized) and/or + ciprofloxacin (20–40 mg/kg/24 hours)

Probenecid is given orally to all patients receiving β-lactam antibiotics eliminated by tubular excretion.
Dosage of other antibiotics for aerosol treatment:
tobramycin, 200–600 mg/24 hours;
ceftazidime, 2–6 g/24 hours

[a] Intermittently colonized.
[b] Chronically colonized.

ment, sometimes over 4 weeks, with one of the combinations given in Table 5.7, ciprofloxacin or ofloxacin orally is used. The efficacy of the regime means that less than 10 per cent of the patients are chronically infected (for more than 6 months, continuously) and the antibody response remains low[87]. Other less aggressive regimes and the basis for rational selection and dosing of anti-haemophilus antibiotics for CF patients are described in recent reviews[68,74,75,94,96].

Burkholderia (Pseudomonas) cepacia

These Gram-negative, motile rods occur in the environment (soil) and are pathogens for vegetables. They are occasionally isolated from samples obtained from homes of CF patients or from food stores, salad bars or greenhouses[103–105]. They are frequently auxotrophic when isolated from CF sputum[106]. Several characteristics of *B. cepacia* isolated from CF patients have been described[107]: production of giant cable-like pili correlated with epidemic spread between CF patients[108]; invasion of respiratory cells and intracellular replication may be characteristic of CF strains[109]; production of a lipopolysaccharide (LPS) that stimulates TNFα production more strongly than LPS from *P. aeruginosa*; and a hemolysin capable of inducing apoptosis and degranulation of phagocytes[110,111]. A major methodological problem is the occurrence of multiple, closely related genomovars within the *B. cepacia* complex, which are nearly impossible to distinguish by the usual phenotypic methods used in microbiological laboratories[112].

Genomovars I, III and IV are named *B. cepacia* and can only be differentiated by DNA techniques and wholeorganism protein electrophoresis. Genomovar II is renamed *B. multivorans*, and the fifth related species is named *B. vietnamiensis*. Another related species found in CF patients is *B. gladioli*[112,113]. *Burkholderia cepacia* is seldom isolated from human infections and it is rarely found as a pathogen in non-CF patients[114]. This species emerged as a pathogen in CF about 20 years ago and has now become endemic in some large centers and has recently been introduced as an epidemic species in other centers where, together with *P. aeruginosa*, it frequently co-colonizes patients[36,72,115–129].

Burkholderia cepacia is frequent in some, but not in other, CF centers[130–132], but the overall prevalence is low (e.g. 3.6 per cent in the USA in 1996 compared to the 59.9 per cent prevalence of *P. aeruginosa*[70]). The prevalence of *B. cepacia* in 0–1-year-old patients was 0.5 per cent, increasing to 3.4–5.7 per cent in adult patients[70]. One reason for the different prevalence of *B. cepacia* in different centers seems to be cross-infection, which was first described in the CF center in Cleveland and subsequently elsewhere, but not in some other centers[133–136]. By cohorting the patients, it was possible to prevent further spreading of the bacteria in the Cleveland center[133]. Recently *B. cepacia* has spread among CF patients in some European centers[125,136,137], and spread outside centers between CF patients during social contact has also been reported from the UK[126]. A large transatlantic epidemic spread of *B. cepacia* between patients attending two CF centers in Manchester and Edinburgh took place in 1990–92. The responsible genomovar III *B. cepacia* was originally acquired by a Manchester patients during a visit to a Canadian CF camp. The further spread took place during social contact at weekly fitness classes held at a local school[138] and several of the patients succumbed due to the infection. Further analysis identified numerous strains of *B. cepacia* in CF patients in the UK and Ireland, but one epidemic strain had spread to at least eight CF centers[139]. Other authors have reported similar results[140]. Cross-infection has also been described between CF patients already harboring *B. cepacia*[141]. Several possible routes of transmission of *B. cepacia* have been identified (e.g. hands of the staff and nebulizers[142,143], and summer camps, which have now been abandoned in North America[144]).

Three distinct clinical patterns of *B. cepacia* infection in CF have been observed[115,117,120,125]:

1. chronic asymptomatic carriage of *B. cepacia*, either alone or in combination with *P. aeruginosa*;
2. progressive deterioration over many months, with recurrent fever, progressive weight loss and repeated hospitalization;
3. rapid, usually fatal deterioration in previously mildly affected patients.

Burkholderia cepacia is more resistant to antibiotics than *P. aeruginosa* and resistance develops very easily[90,145–149]. Eradication of the infection is virtually never obtained by antibiotic treatment with, for example, ceftazidime and tobramycin or co-trimoxazole (trimethoprim (20 mg/kg/24 hours) and sulfamethoxazole (100 mg/kg/24 hours) orally for 2 weeks). Chronic suppression with doxycycline or co-trimoxazole may give rise to some improvement of the clinical symptoms, but since no controlled study has been undertaken, it is very difficult in such cases to ascribe the improvement to causality or covariation. In the Danish CF Center *B. cepacia*-infected patients are kept isolated from other CF patients in and outside the center, and the incidence and prevalence has always been low and no cross-infection detected[150,151]. Similar results have subsequently been reported from other centers employing a segregation policy[152–155]. More detailed hygienic guidelines used in the Danish CF Center are given in the section on *P. aeruginosa* and guidelines for prevention of transmission of *B. cepacia* during social activities are given in reference[156]. According to these authors, the risk of transmission of *B. cepacia* is *low* during social gatherings and casual conversations, *medium* when shaking hands, sharing cups, food, etc., sharing rooms, attending fitness classes and performing social kissing, and *high* for sibling contacts and sexual relationships[156].

Pseudomonas aeruginosa

This Gram-negative, motile rod is an environmental species, which is found especially in fresh water and soil contaminated by animals or humans, poorly chlorinated swimming pools, whirly pools and hydrotherapy pools[53]. *Pseudomonas aeruginosa* is rarely found in the stools of normal humans and then only in small numbers. They are important pathogens in neutropenic patients (septicemia), those with burns, and artificially ventilated patients in intensive care units, where they may cause nosocomial infections. They cause otitis and folliculitis in swimmers. The most prevalent and severe chronic lung infection in CF patients is caused by *P. aeruginosa*[36,68,69], which has become endemic in CF patients in all countries. In addition to the lungs, CF patients are often colonized in the sinuses by these bacteria[157] and they may be present in the stools, probably originating from swallowed sputum[158,159]. They may be auxotrophic when isolated from CF sputum[160].

A seasonal variation of the initial colonization, as well as the onset of the chronic infection, has been observed during a 25-year period: two-thirds of these colonizations and infections were initiated during the winter season (October to March), correlating to the occurrence of respiratory virus infections[33]. It has also been shown that respiratory syncytial virus infection may predispose to chronic *P. aeruginosa* infection[21]. Whether colonization of the upper respiratory tract precedes establishment of bronchial infection with *P. aeruginosa* is unknown. *Pseudomonas aeruginosa* shows chemotaxis towards mucin-rich mucosal surfaces[161]. In animal studies, *P. aeruginosa*[162] adheres to buccal, nasal turbinate and tracheobronchial epithelial cells and to mucus[163,164]. Five types of adhesion factors have been identified on *P. aeruginosa* – pili, alginate, hemagglutinin, exoenzyme 5 and flagella – which bind to corresponding receptors on the host cells: laminin, glycolipids, glycosphingolipids and glycoproteins containing lactosyl and sialosyl residues[164–169]. Injury to epithelial cells of mucus membranes by trypsin or human leukocyte elastase exposed new receptors for *P. aeruginosa* pili, including asialo GM1[170], but increased bacterial adhesion to the CFTR protein has also been shown[19]. These observations are interesting because such damage may follow inflammatory reactions provoked by viruses or by bacteria such as *S. aureus*, which are common in cystic fibrosis.

Infected patients do not spread *P. aeruginosa* to family members not suffering from CF, but siblings with CF often carry the same strain of *P. aeruginosa*, indicating cross-infection or colonization from the same environmental source[171,172]. Environmental sources have been identified in CF centers and in dentistry equipment, a hydrotherapy pool[68,173–179] and hands of the staff on CF wards[142]. Previous studies from holiday camps for CF patients showed that the risk of cross-infection was low[180,181], but during a winter camp in Lanzerote organized by the Danish CF Association, the segregation of infected and noninfected CF patients was violated, and all noninfected patients became infected with *P. aeruginosa*[341]. Large centers seem to have a higher prevalence of

P. aeruginosa infection than smaller centers[182]. The mean prevalence of *P. aeruginosa* in CF patients in the USA was 60.7 per cent, but even in 0–1-year-old patients the prevalence was 20.8 per cent, increasing to 80.1 per cent in 30–35-year-old patients[70]. A number of reports published since 1975 show that cross-infection occurred in the Danish CF Center[173,182–184] and results from some other centers have also indicated the possibility of cross-infection, whereas still other centers could not identify evidence of nosocomial infection[174,176,185–188]. By improving the hygienic measures in the center and by segregating the infected and noninfected patients in different wards in the center and on different days in the outpatient clinic, it was possible to prevent such cross-infection in the Danish CF Center[173,182]. Similar experience has been published from other centers[188,189].

The hygienic principle is to segregate patients in different cohorts according to lower respiratory tract bacteriology:

1. no *P. aeruginosa*;
2. intermittent colonization, and
3. chronic infection with sensitive strains of *P. aeruginosa*;
4. chronic infection with multiply resistant strains of *P. aeruginosa*; and
5. intermittent colonization or chronic infection with *B. cepacia*.

Five separate wards with separate nursing staff are used for hospitalization of these five groups. The first four groups are seen on separate days in the same outpatient clinic, which is thoroughly cleaned using hypochlorite-containing disinfectants every morning, and patients with *B. cepacia* are seen only in a special isolation room. Staff are required to disinfect hands with chlorhexidine–ethanol and change gowns when moving from one ward to another. The lung function recordings use an 'open' electronic spirometer with disposable mouthpieces to avoid contamination of equipment. Other equipment is disinfected by alcohol. Separate holiday camps and social meetings are advised for each group. Inhalation masks are stored in chloramine solution. The yearly incidence of new chronic *P. aeruginosa* infection was thus reduced to the 'natural background' level not associated with treatment at the center, which is assumed to be 1–2 per cent per year (Table 5.8)[182] and similar experience of the efficacy of cohort isolation has been obtained in another CF center[185]. The median age of acquisition of the chronic *P. aeruginosa* infection in the Danish CF Center has consequently increased from 7 years to greater than 12 years during the past decade[190,191]. In order to further study the risk of cross-infection and the efficacy of preventive measures, it is necessary to use classical epidemiological research tools (e.g. cohort studies, case-control studies and intervention studies[192]), which previously have been used in only a few studies[39,182,183,185].

In most patients (82 per cent) a period (median 12 months) of intermittent colonization precedes the persistent colonization, which in the Danish CF Center is defined as continuous presence of *P. aeruginosa* in the lungs for more than 6 months and/or more than two precipitating antibodies against these bacteria[33]. The factors which, in addition to virus infection, determine the

Table 5.8 *Cross-infection between cystic fibrosis patients with and without* P. aeruginosa *pulmonary infection in the Danish CF Center in relation to contact possibility between the patients*[182]

Period	Number of days/patient/year spent in the CF center (outpatient clinic + ward)		Contact density ratio		Mean period incidence of new CF + P	Probability/ day/patient in the center to acquire chronic *P. aeruginosa* infection
1970–75	CF+P	25	2.1		8.4%	
	CF–P	12		2.2		0.73%
1976–80	CF+P	55[a]	4.6		17%	1.54%
	CF–P	12				
				0		
1981–85–87	CF+P	55 ——————[b]	0		6.5–3%	0.56–0.25%
	CF–P	12				

[a]Intensive maintenance treatment program started[327].
[b]Separation of CF+P (CF patients with chronic *P. aeruginosa* infection) and CF–P (CF patients without chronic *P. aeruginosa*) in the outpatient clinic and in the wards, so that contact was avoided[182].

Table 5.9 *Some virulence factors of* P. aeruginosa *and their interaction with the host*

Virulence factor	Function
Pili	Adherence[328]
Alginate	Adherence, microcolony formation[163,210,329]
Phenazin pigments	Interfere with nonspecific and specific lung defense mechanisms[195]
Lipopolysaccharide	Endotoxic activity, major component of immune complexes[250,330,331]
Elastase, alkaline protease	Interfere with the nonspecific and specific humoral and cellular immune response of the lungs, present in immune complexes [194,209]
Leucocidin	Cytotoxic for cells by increasing membrane permeability[332]
Rhamnolipid	Enhances monocyte oxidative burst[194]
Phospholipase C	Degrades lecithin in the lungs[333]
Lipase	Inhibits monocyte chemotaxis and chemiluminescence[194]
Exotoxin A	Inhibits protein synthesis[334]
Exotoxin S	Adhesin, inhibits protein synthesis[166,335]
β-Lactamase	Resistance to β-lactam antibiotics[229]

transition to persistent colonization are probably the toxins produced by *P. aeruginosa*, although this point of view is supported only by circumstantial evidence (Table 5.9). *Pseudomonas aeruginosa* produces many toxins and other virulence factors with potential effect on the lungs of CF patients[107,190,193–195]. Some of these toxins are thought to play a role during establishment of the initial persistent colonization of the CF respiratory tract, notably elastase and alkaline protease, which have been shown to interfere with the nonspecific (phagocytes) and immunologically specific (T cells, NK cells, immunoglobulins) defense mechanisms[196], but also lipopolysaccharide (LPS) and sometimes against alginate, as antibodies can be detected early before the infection becomes chronic against LPS[196–203] and sometimes against alginate [107,190,204–207]. The initial colonization is accompanied by an inflammatory response[208]. Later during the infection, the significance of the action of the toxins becomes doubtful, since specific antibodies are produced by the CF patients (e.g. free elastase and alkaline protease can only be detected in bronchial secretions during the first few months of the infection, before neutralizing antibodies develop[209]).

CHRONIC *P. AERUGINOSA* INFECTION

The most characteristic feature of the persistent *P. aeruginosa* infection is the production of mucoid alginate and the formation of microcolonies in the lungs of the patients[13,68,107,195,210–215]. Alginate is an unbranched, linear heteropolysaccharide, consisting of polymannuronic–polyguluronic acid, and it is the only antigen that is clinically correlated to poor prognosis in CF patients[216]. The biochemistry and genetics of alginate biosynthesis is to a large extent known[107], and we have recently provided experimental evidence supporting the hypothesis that the oxygen radicals produced by the inflammatory response (PMNs) induce the phenotypic change from nonalginate-producing to alginate-producing phenotypes of *P. aeruginosa*[217]. The microcolony form of growth (biofilm) is the survival strategy of environmental bacteria[218,219] and the major component of the matrix of the microcolony is alginate[220] (Figs 5.1 and 5.2). The median concentration of the mucoid exopolysaccharide (alginate) in sputum from CF patients is 35.5 mg/mL[221]. Although mucoid strains are also found in other chronically colonized patients, such strains are characteristic of CF[222]. It has been shown *in vitro* that *P. aeruginosa* growing in alginate biofilms are highly resistant to antibiotics, probably due to slow growth, the penetration barrier and β-lactamase production[223–227], and they are protected against phagocytes and complement[220,228]. Likewise, β-lactamase production has been shown to be the major resistance mechanism of *P. aeruginosa* to β-lactam antibiotics *in vivo* in CF patients[227,229]. A modified system for testing of antimicrobial susceptibility of biofilm bacteria has therefore been suggested[230].

In most patients nonmucoid strains initiate the infection, and the transition to the mucoid variant correlates with the development of a pronounced antibody response against virtually all antigens and toxins of *P. aeruginosa*[216,231], and the occurrence of mucoid variants also correlates to a poor prognosis[211,216,232–235]. Complement deposition on the surface of mucoid microcolonies may be deficient in CF patients[236], favoring the survival of such colonies, although the embedded bacteria are unusual in several other aspects. *Pseudomonas aeruginosa* from CF patients therefore upregulate the production of alginate, leading to biofilm formation, and downregulate other virulence factors, probably by means of quorum sensing[236a]: they become serum sensitive[237,238], polyagglutinable[239,240], lacking the lipopolysaccharide side chain[241], nonmotile, and expressing iron-regulated outer-membrane proteins, indicating that the bacteria grow under iron-restricted conditions in CF lungs[242–244]. The polyagglutinability is due to the semi-rough nature of

Table 5.10 *The pathogenesis of chronic* P. aeruginosa *infection in cystic fibrosis: immune complex mediated tissue damage*[211]

Stage of infection	Mechanisms of pathogenesis	Clinical signs
Acquisition	Cross-infection[173,182]. Concomitant virus infection[182]	None Acute exacerbation
Attachment	Pili, hemagglutinin, exotoxin S, alginate[163,166]	None
Initial persistent colonization	Bacterial toxins: elastase, alkaline protease, exotoxins A and S, phospholipase, lipase, etc.[194]	None or minimal
Chronic infection	Persistence: microcolonies embedded in alginate; PMN–*Pseudomonas* mismatch; tissue damage: immune complexes, PMN elastase, cytokines[242,336]	Chronic suppurative lung inflammation, progressive loss of lung function
Modifying mechanisms	PMN elastase cleaves immune complexes; increase of antibodies to *P. aeruginosa*, especially of IgG_3 subclass; ΔF508 homozygotes versus other mutations; mannose-binding lectin deficiency[340] α_1-antitrypsin deficiency[257,337–339]	Individual clinical course of the infection

the LPS and the presence of a common A band of LPS, and it seems to be related to bacteriophages, which are present in sputum of CF patients[241,245–247]. The semi-rough nature of LPS in strains from CF patients is also in accordance with *in vitro* results from *P. aeruginosa* growing in biofilm[248] and with the change of their hydrophobicity[249].

LPS has been found to be the major component of immune complexes in sputum of CF patients with chronic *P. aeruginosa* infection[250] and such complexes are potent inducers of TNFα production and oxidative burst from phagocytes[251,252]. Actually, increased concentrations of TNFα and the other proinflammatory cytokines, IL-1, IL-6 and IL-8, were found in bronchoalveolar lavage fluids from CF patients, whereas the concentration of the immunomodulatory cytokine, IL-10, was lower than in controls[253,254]. This unique adaptability to the environment in the CF lung is also reflected in the high frequency of development of antibiotic resistance during chemotherapy[254a,254b].

The most remarkable host response to the infection is the pronounced antibody response, which continues to increase over several years, and which is correlated to poor prognosis. As mentioned, these antibodies are eventually directed against most, if not all, antigens of *P. aeruginosa*, including alginate and chromosomal β-lactamase[255], and they belong to all classes and subclasses of immunoglobulins. Some individual differences between the IgG subclass antibody response (high IgG_3 response) is, however, correlated to a more severe course of the lung infection[256]. The correlation between the antibody response and poor prognosis has been shown to be due to immune complex mediated chronic inflammation in the lungs of CF patients[257–262]. This inflammatory reaction is dominated by polymorphonuclear leukocytes, and released leukocyte proteases, myeloperoxidase and oxygen radicals are the main mechanisms of lung tissue damage (Table 5.10)[211,263–270].

The principles and results of early treatment of initial *P. aeruginosa* colonization with oral ciprofloxacin and colistin inhalation[271–273] and the principles and results of maintenance therapy of the chronic *P. aeruginosa* infection with intravenous tobramycin and β-lactam antibiotics every 3 months, combined with colistin inhalation between the courses or by using nebulized tetramycin are described elsewhere[6,274,275,326,326a,326b,326c]. It should, however, be realized that the inflammation continues between courses of chemotherapy[276], so anti-inflammatory therapy is also used[277–279]. The combination of cohort isolation and early intensive treatment of intermittent colonization provides 90 per cent of Danish CF patients with a 2-year protection against the onset of chronic *P. aeruginosa* infection, equal protection to that of an efficient vaccine (Table 5.11). The survival of CF patients treated according to the described principles has increased steadily, so that more than 80 per cent will reach the age of 40 years in the Danish CF Center[6] (Fig. 5.4).

Other pathogens

Many other pathogens may colonize the lower respiratory tract of CF patients. *Streptococcus pneumoniae* was

Table 5.11 *Calculation of 2-year period prevalence (%) of chronic* P. aeruginosa *infection (CF + P) in 100 noninfected CF patients (CF − P) if the yearly incidence is 1%, 5%, 10% and 20%*

| Incidence | 2-year period prevalence | | Protection (%) | |
	CF + P	CF − P	Total	(1 − odds ratio ± protection) × 100
20%	36	64	100	
10%	19	81	100	47% 72%[a] 94%
5%	10	90	100	
1%	2	98	100	

[a](1) 2-year protection by cohorting/isolation in the Danish CF Center: 81 % (calculated from ref. 182).
(2) 2-year protection by early treatment of intermittent colonization in the Danish CF Center: 76% (calculated from ref. 271).
(1) + (2) combined 2-year protection in the Danish CF Center: 90% (calculated from refs. 182 and 271).

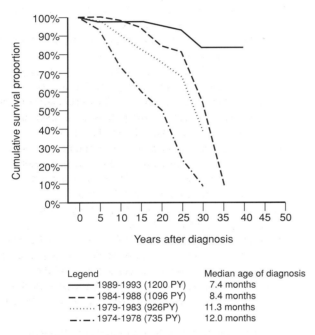

Legend	Median age of diagnosis
——— 1989–1993 (1200 PY)	7.4 months
− − − 1984–1988 (1096 PY)	8.4 months
·········· 1979–1983 (926PY)	11.3 months
−·−· 1974–1978 (735 PY)	12.0 months

Fig. 5.4 *Survival of CF patients treated in the Danish CF Center 1974–93. Modified life tables in 5-year intervals using 5-year age bands. Analysis by years after diagnosis. P < 0.0001 (Poisson regression). PY, person years. (Reproduced from ref. 6 with permission from the editor.)*

found to be associated with 5 per cent, and Enterobacteriaceae with 10 per cent, of acute exacerbations of the respiratory symptoms in CF patients followed in the Danish CF Center[21] but no specific types of these bacteria are connected with CF. *Streptococcus pneumoniae* never cause chronic infections in CF patients, whereas a few patients may suffer from chronic infection caused by mucoid strains of *Klebsiella* species, *E. coli,*

Citrobacter species and even *Proteus* species[36]. In order to discriminate between superficial colonization and chronic infection, the antibody response against the offending pathogen is used in the Danish CF Center (Table 5.6). Occasionally, *Moraxella catarrhalis* and *Lautropia mirabilis* are isolated from CF sputum, but the clinical significance is uncertain[280,281]. *Legionella pneumophila*[26] is also difficult to identify as a pathogen in CF since serological cross-reactions between these bacteria and *P. aeruginosa* invalidate the interpretation of antibody titers[282]. *Pasteurella multocida, Alcaligenes faecalis, Achromobacter (Alcaligines) xylosoxidans* and *Stenotrophomonas (Xanthomonas) maltophilia* colonize the occasional CF patient[36,127,283–286] and atypical mycobacteria have been detected in the respiratory tract of CF patients, but the clinical significance remains uncertain in most cases[286–294], and the result of antibiotic therapy disappointing. *Mycoplasma pneumoniae* and *Chlamydia* species seem not to be of greater importance in CF patients than in other persons[21]. *Aspergillus fumigatus* is frequently isolated from sputum of CF patients and allergic bronchopulmonary aspergillosis develops in a few (5–10 per cent of) patients[57,58,295–311]. This condition is treated with steroid hormones as in other patients, and sometimes with itraconazole[296,308,312]. The significance of *Candida albicans* and related species is uncertain[59].

CONCLUSION

The improved knowledge of the pathology of the recurrent and chronic infections and their intensive treatment has continued to improve the survival and the quality of life of CF patients. Many patients will probably be treated in adult clinics for chest diseases. Hopefully, the described principles can be adapted and improved to further normalize the life of CF patients.

REFERENCES

1. Davidson, D.J. and Porteous, D.J. (1998) The genetics of cystic fibrosis lung disease. *Thorax*, **53**, (5), 389–397.

2. Høiby, N., Giwercman, B., Jensen, E.T. *et al.* (1993) Immune response in cystic fibrosis – helpful or harmful? in *Clinical Ecology of Cystic Fibrosis*, (eds H. Escobar, C.F. Baquero, L. Suarez), Exerpta Medica, Amsterdam, pp. 133–141.

3. Davis, P.B., Drumm, M. and Konstan, M.W. (1996) Cystic fibrosis. *Am. J. Respir. Crit. Care Med.*, **154**, (5), 1229–1256.

4. Armstrong, D.S., Grimwood, K., Carlin, J.B. *et al.*(1997) Lower airway inflammation in infants and young children with cystic fibrosis. *Am. J. Respir. Crit. Care Med.*, **156**, (4), 1197–1204.

5. Alton, E.W.F.W. and Geddes, D.M. (1995) Gene therapy for cystic fibrosis: A clinical perspective. *Gene Therapy*, **2**, (2), 88–95.

6. Frederiksen, B., Lanng, S., Koch, C. and Høiby, N. (1996) Improved survival in the Danish cystic fibrosis center: results of aggressive treatment. *Pediatr. Pulmonol.*, **21**, 153–158.

7. Fanconi, G., Uehlinger, E. and Knauer, C. (1936) Das coeliakiesyndrom bei angeborener zystischer pankreasfibromatose und bronchiektasien. *Wien. Med. Wochenschr.*, **86**, 753–756.

8. Andersen, D.H. (1938) Cystic fibrosis of the pancreas and its relation to celiac disease: a clinical and pathologic study. *Am. J. Dis. Child.*, **56**, 344–399.

9. Blackfan, K.D. and May, C.D. (1938) Inspissation of secretion, dilatation of the ducts and acini, atrophy and fibrosis of the pancreas in infants. *J. Pediatr.*, **13**, 627–634.

10. Andersen, D.H. (1949) Therapy and prognosis of fibrocystic disease of the pancreas. *Pediatrics*, **3**, 406–417.

11. di Sant'Agnese, P.A. and Andersen, D.H. (1946) Celiac syndrome: Chemotherapy in infections of the respiratory tract associated with cystic fibrosis of the pancreas; observations with penicillin and drugs of the sulfonamide group, with special reference to penicillin aerosol. *Am. J. Dis. Child.*, **72**, 17–61.

12. Orenstein, D.M. and Kaplan, R.M. (1991) Measuring the quality of well-being in cystic fibrosis and lung transplantation – the importance of the area under the curve. *Chest*, **100**, (4), 1016–1018.

13. Høiby, N. (1977) *Pseudomonas aeruginosa* infection in cystic fibrosis. Diagnostic and prognostic significance of *Pseudomonas aeruginosa* precipitins determined by means of crossed immunoelectrophoresis. A survey. *Acta Pathol. Microbiol. Scand. Suppl.*, **262**, (C), 3–96.

14. Fahy, I.V., Keoghan, M.T., Crummy, E.J. and Fitzgerald, M.X. (1991) Bacteraemia and fungaemia in adults with cystic fibrosis. *J. Infect.*, **22**, (3), 241–245.

15. Rivlin, J., Lerner, A., Augarten, A., Wilschanski, M.,

16. Kerem, E. and Ephros, M.A. (1998) Severe *Clostridium difficile*-associated colitis in young patients with cystic fibrosis. *J. Pediatr.*, **132**, (l), 177–179.

17. Barasch, J. and Al-Aqwati, Q. (1993) Defective acidification of the biosynthetic pathway in cystic fibrosis. *J. Cell Sci., Suppl.*, **17**, 229–233.

18. Zhang, Y.L., Doranz, B., Yankaskas, J.R. and Engelhardt, J.F. (1995) Genotypic analysis of respiratory mucous sulfation defects in cystic fibrosis. *J. Clin. Invest.*, **96**, (6), 2997–3004.

19. Goldman, M.J., Anderson, G.M., Stolzenberg, E.D., Kari, U.P., Zasloff, M. and Wilson, J.M. (1997) Human beta-defensin-1 is a salt-sensitive antibiotic in lung that is activated in cystic fibrosis. *Cell*, **88**, 553–560.

20. Pier, G.B., Grout, M. and Zaidi, T.S. (1997) Cystic fibrosis transmembrane conductance regulator is an epithelial cell receptor for clearance of *Pseudomonas aeruginosa* from the lung. *Proc. Natl Acad. Sci. USA*, **94**, (22), 12088–12093.

21. Khan, T.Z., Wagener, J.S., Bost, T., Martinez, J., Accurso, F.J. and Riches, D.W.H. (1995) Early pulmonary inflammation in infants with cystic fibrosis. *Am. J. Respir. Crit. Care Med.*, **151**, (4), 1075–1082.

22. Petersen, N.T., Høiby, N., Mordhorst, C.-H., Lind, K., Flensborg, E.W. and Bruun, B. (1981) Respiratory infections in cystic fibrosis cause by virus, chlamydia and mycoplasma – possible synergism with *Pseudomonas aeruginosa*. *Acta Paediatr. Scand.*, **70**, 623–628.

23. Knowles, M.R., Olivier, K., Noone, P. and Boucher, R.C. (1995) Pharmacologic modulation of salt and water in the airway epithelium in cystic fibrosis. *Am. J. Respir. Crit. Care Med.*, **151**, (3 Suppl.), S65–S69.

23. Rosenstein, B.J. and Zeitlin, P.L. (1998) Cystic fibrosis. *Lancet*, **351**, (9098), 277–282 .

24. Knowles, M.R., Noone, P.O., Hohneker, K. *et al.* (1998) A double-blind, placebo controlled, dose ranging study to evaluate the safety and biological efficacy of the lipid–DNA complex GR213487B in the nasal epithelium of adult patients with cystic fibrosis. *Hum. Gene Ther.*, **9**, (2), 249–269.

25. Hodson, M.E. (1995) Clinical studies of rhDNase in moderately and severely affected patients with cystic fibrosis – An overview. *Respiration*, **62**, (Suppl. l), 29–32.

26. Efthimiou, J., Hodson, M.E., Taylor, P. and Batten, J.C. (1984) Importance of viruses and *Legionella pneumophila* in respiratory exacerbations of young adults with cystic fibrosis. *Thorax*, **39**, 150–154.

27. Prober, C.G. (1991) The impact of respiratory viral infections in patients with cystic fibrosis. *Clin. Rev. Allergy*, **9**, (1–2), 87–102.

28. Ramsey, B.W., Gore, E.J., Smith, A.L., Cooney, M.K., Redding, G.J. and Foy, H. (1989) The effect of respiratory viral infections on patients with cystic fibrosis. *Am. J. Dis. Child.*, **143**, 662–668.

29. Abman, S.H., Ogle, J.W., Butler-Simon, N., Rumack, C.M. and Accurso, F.J. (1988) Role of respiratory syncytial virus

in early hospitalizations for respiratory distress of young infants with cystic fibrosis. *J. Pediatr.*, **113**, 827–830.

30. Wang, E.L., Prober, C.G., Manson, B., Corey, M. and Levison, H. (1984) Association of respiratory viral infections with pulminary deterioration in patients with cystic fibrosis. *NEJM*, **311**, 1653–1658.

31. Hordvik, N.L., König, P., Hamory, B. *et al.* (1989) Effects of acute viral respiratory infections in patients with cystic fibrosis. *Pediatr. Pulmonol.*, **7**, 217–222.

32. Conway, S.P., Simmonds, E.J. and Littlewood, J.M. (1992) Acute severe deterioration in cystic fibrosis associated with influenza-A virus infection. *Thorax*, **47**, (2), 112–114.

33. Johansen, H.K. and Høiby, N. (1992) Seasonal onset of initial colonisation and chronic infection with *Pseudomonas aeruginosa* in patients with cystic fibrosis in Denmark. *Thorax*, **47**, (2), 109–111.

34. Shale, D.J. (1992) Viral infections – a role in the lung disease of cystic fibrosis. *Thorax*, **47**, (2), 69.

35. Abman, S.H., Ogle, J.W., Harbeek, R.J., Butler-Simon, N., Hammond, K.B. and Accurso, F.J. (1991) Early bacteriologic, immunologic, and clinical courses of young infants with cystic fibrosis identified by neonatal screening. *J. Pediatr.*, **119**, (2), 211–217.

36. Høiby, N. (1982) Microbiology of lung infections in cystic fibrosis patients. *Acta Paediat. Scand. Suppl.*, **301**, 33–54.

37. Ramsey, B.W., Wentz, K.R., Smith, A.L. *et al.* (1991) Predictive value of oropharyngeal cultures for identifying lower airway bacteria in cystic fibrosis patients. *Am. Rev. Respir. Dis.*, **144**, (2), 331–337.

37a. Rosenfeld, M., Emerson, J., Accurso, F. *et al.* (1999) Diagnostic accuracy of oropharyngeal cultures in infants and young children with cystic fibrosis. *Pediatr. Pulmonol.*, **28**, 321–328.

38. Armstrong, D.S., Grimwood, K., Carlin, J.B., Carzino, R., Olinsky, A. and Phelan, P. (1996) Bronchoalveolar lavage or oropharyngeal cultures to identify lower respiratory pathogens in infants with cystic fibrosis. *Pediatr. Pulmonol.*, **21**, 267–275.

39. Høiby, N. (1974) Epidemiological investigations of the respiratory tract bacteriology in patients with cystic fibrosis. *Acta Pathol. Microbiol. Scand. Sect. B*, **82**, 541–550.

40. Heineman, H.S., Chawla, J.K. and Lofton, W.M. (1977) Misinformation from sputum cultures without microscopic examination. *J. Clin. Microbiol.*, **6**, 518–527.

41. Henry, D.A., Campbell, M.E., LiPuma, J.J. and Speert, D.P. (1997) Identification of *Burkholderia cepacia* isolates from patients with cystic fibrosis and use of a simple new selective medium. *J. Clin. Microbiol.*, **35**, (3), 614–619.

42. Bauernfeind, A., Rotter, K. and Weisslein-Pfister, C. (1987) Selective procedure to isolate haemophilus influenza from sputa with large quantities of *Pseudomonas aeruginosa*. *Infection*, **15**, 64–67.

43. Bilton, D., Pye, A., Johnson, M.M. *et al.* (1995) The isolation and characterization of non-typeable *Haemophilus influenzae* from the sputum of adult cystic fibrosis patients. *Eur. Resp. J.*, **8**, (6), 948–953.

44. Whittier, S., Hopfer, R.L., Knowles, M.R. and Gilligan, P.H. (1993) Improved recovery of mycobacteria from respiratory secretions of patients with cystic fibrosis. *J. Clin. Microbiol.*, **31**, (4), 861–864.

45. Hoff, G.E. and Høiby, N. (1975) *Staphylococcus aureus* in cystic fibrosis: Antibiotic sensitivity and phage types during the latest decade. Investigations on the occurrence of protein A and some other properties of recently isolated strains in relation to the occurrence of precipitating antibodies. *Acta Pathol. Microbiol. Scand. Sect. B.*, **83**, 219–225.

46. Høiby, N. and Kilian, M. (1976) *Haemophilus* from the lower respiratory tract of patients with cystic fibrosis. *Scand. J. Resp. Dis.*, **57**, 103–107.

47. Watson, K.C., Kerr, E.J.C. and Hinks, C.A. (1985) Distribution of biotypes of *Haemophilus influenzae* and *H. parainfluenzae* in patients with cystic fibrosis. *J. Clin. Pathol.*, **38**, 750–753.

48. Speert, D., Campbell, M., Puterman, M.L. *et al.* (1994) A multicenter comparison of methods for typing strains of *Pseudomonas aeruginosa* predominantly from patients with cystic fibrosis. *J. Infect. Dis.*, **169**, (l), 134–142.

49. Grothues, D., Koopmann, U., Hardt Hvd and Tümmler, B. (1988) Genome fingerprinting of *Pseudomonas aeruginosa* indicates colonization of cystic fibrosis siblings with closely related strains. *J. Clin. Microbiol.*, **26**, 1973-1977.

50. Ogle, J.W. and Vasil, M.L. (1991) Genetic heterogeneity in strains of *Pseudomonas aeruginosa* from patients with cystic fibrosis. *J. Clin. Microbiol.*, **29**, (3), 663–664.

51. Bingen, E., Denamur, E., Picard, B. *et al.* (1992) Molecular epidemiological analysis of *Pseudomonas aeruginosa* strains causing failure of antibiotic therapy in cystic fibrosis patients. *Eur. J. Clin. Microbiol.*, **11**, (5), 432–437.

52. Ojeniyi, B. and Høiby, N. (1991) Comparison of different typing methods of *Pseudomonas aeruginosa*. *Pseudomonas aeruginosa in Hum.*, **44**, 13–22.

53. Govan, J.R.W. and Nelson, J.W. (1992) Microbiology of lung infection in cystic fibrosis. *Br. Med. Bull.*, **48**, (4), 912–930.

54. Lipuma, J.J., Fisher, M.C., Dasen, S.E., Mortensen, J.E. and Stull, T.L. (1991) Ribotype stability of serial pulmonary isolates of *Pseudomonas cepacia*. *J. Infect. Dis.*, **164**, (l), 133–136.

55. Kostman, J.R., Edlind, T.D., Lipuma, J.J. and Stull, T.L. (1992) Molecular epidemiology of *Pseudomonas cepacia* determined by polymerase chain reaction ribotyping. *J. Clin. Microbiol.*, **30**, (8), 2084–2087.

56. Mcintosh, I., Govan, J.R.W. and Brock, D.J.H. (1992) Detection of *Pseudomonas aeruginosa* in sputum from cystic fibrosis patients by the polymerase chain reaction. *Mol. Cell Probe*, **6**, (4), 299–304.

57. Schønheyder, H. (1987) Pathogenetic and serological

aspects of pulmonary Aspergillosis. *Scand. J. Infect. Dis. Suppl.*, **51**, 1–62.

58. Forsyth, K.D., Hohmann, A.W., Martin, A.J. and Bradley, J. (1988) IgG antibodies to *Aspergillus fumigatus* in cystic fibrosis: a laboratory correlate of disease activity. *Arch. Dis. Child.*, **63**, 953–957.

59. Przyklenk, B., Bauernfeind, A., Hørl, G. and Emminger, G. (1987) Serologic response to *Candida albicans* and *Aspergillus fumigatus* in cystic fibrosis. *Infection*, **15**, 308–310.

60. Vazquez, C., Aramburu, N., Sojo, A., Vitoria, J.C. and Pascual, C. (1989) IgG antibodies to *Aspergillus fumigatus* in cystic fibrosis. *Arch. Dis. Child.*, **64**, 1094–1095.

61. Drent, M., Vanrens, M.T.M., Wagenaar, S.S., Dejongh, B.M., Vanvelzenblad, H. and Vandenbosch, J.M.M. (1995) Invasive aspergillosis after bilateral lung transplantation in cystic fibrosis. *Resp. Med.*, **89**, (6), 449–451.

62. Arruda, L.K., Muir, A., Vailes, L.D., Selden, R.F., Plattsmills, T.A.E. and Chapman, M.D. (1995) Antibody responses to *Aspergillus fumigatus* allergens in patients with cystic fibrosis. *Int. Arch. Allergy Immunol.*, **107**, (1–3), 410–411.

63. Becker, J.W., Burke, W., Mcdonald, G., Greenberger, P.A., Henderson, W.R. and Aitken, M.L. (1996) Prevalence of allergic bronchopulmonary aspergillosis and atopy in adult patients with cystic fibrosis. *Chest*, **109**, (6), 1536–1540.

64. Murali, P.S., Pathial, K., Saff, R.H. *et al.* (1994) Immune responses to *Aspergillus fumigatus* and *Pseudomonas aeruginosa* antigens in cystic fibrosis and allergic bronchopulmonary aspergillosis. *Chest*, **106**, (2), 513–519.

65. Milla, C.E., Wielinski, C.L. and Regelmann, W.E. (1996) Clinical significance of the recovery of *Aspergillus* species from the respiratory secretions of cystic fibrosis patients. *Pediatr. Pulmonol.*, **21**, 6–10.

66. Mearns, M.B. (1985) Cystic fibrosis. *Arch. Dis. Child.*, **60**, 272–277,

67. Mearns, M.B., Hunt, G.H. and Rushworth, R. (1972) Bacterial flora of respiratory tract in patients with cystic fibrosis, 1950–1971. *Arch. Dis. Child.*, **47**, 902–907.

68. Govan, J.R.W. and Glass, S. (1990) The microbiology and therapy of cystic fibrosis lung infections. *Rev. Med. Microbiol.*, **1**, 19–28.

69. Gilligan, P.H. (1991) Microbiology of airway disease in patients with cystic fibrosis. *Clin. Microbiol. Rev.*, **4**, (l), 35–51.

70. Fitzsimmons, S.C. (1993) The changing epidemiology of cystic fibrosis. *J. Pediatr.*, **122**, (l), 1–9.

71. Petersen, S.S., Jensen, T., Pressler, T., Høiby, N. and Rosendal, K. (1986) Does centralized treatment of cystic fibrosis increase the risk of *Pseudomonas aeruginosa* infection? *Acta Paediatr, Scand.*, **75**, 840–845.

72. Johansen, H.K., Kovesi, T.A., Koch, C., Corey, M., Høiby, N. and Levison, H. (1998) *Pseudomonas aeruginosa* and *Burkholderia cepacia* infection in cystic fibrosis patients treated in Toronto and Copenhagen. *Pediatr. Pulmonol.*, **26**, 89–96.

73. Høiby, N. and Hertz, J.B. (1979) Precipitating antibodies against *Escherichia coli*, *Bacteroides fragilis* ss. *thetaiotaomicron* and *Pseudomonas aeruginosa* in sera from normal persons and cystic fibrosis patients determined by means of crossed immunoelectrophoresis. *Acta Paediatr. Scand.*, **68**, 495–500.

74. Bauernfeind, A., Marks, M.I. and Strandvik, B. (1996) *Cystic Fibrosis Pulmonary Infections: Lessons From Around the World*, Birkhäiuser, Basel, pp. 1–333.

75. Greenberg, D.P. and Stutman, H.R. (1991) Infection and immunity to *Staphylococcus aureus* and *Haemophilus influenzae*. *Clin. Rev. Allergy.*, **9**, (1–2), 75–86.

76. Albus, A., Fournier, J.-M., Wolz, C. *et al.* (1988) *Staphylococcus aureus* capsular types and antibody response to lung infection in patients with cystic fibrosis. *J. Clin. Microbiol.*, **26**, 2505–2509.

77. Herbert, S., Worlitzsch, D., Dassy, B. *et al.* (1997) Regulation of *Staphylococcus aureus* capsular polysaccharide type 5: CO_2 inhibition *in vitro* and *in vivo*. *J. Infect. Dis.*, **176**, (2), 431–438.

78. Goering, R.V., Bauernfeind, A., Lenz, W. and Przyklenk, B. (1990) *Staphylococcus aureus* in patients with cystic fibrosis – an epidemiological analysis using a combination of traditional and molecular methods. *Infection*, **18**, (l), 57–60.

79. Renders, N.H.M., van Belkum, A., Overbeek, S.E., Mouton, J.W. and Verbrugh, H.A. (1997) Molecular epidemiology of *Staphylococcus aureus* strains colonizing the lungs of related and unrelated cystic fibrosis patients. *Clin. Microbiol. Infect.*, **3**, 216–221.

80. Kahl, B., Herrmann, M., Everding, A.S. *et al.* (1998) Persistent infection with small colony variant strains of *Staphylococcus aureus* in patients with cystic fibrosis. *J. Infect. Dis.*, **177**, (4), 1023–1029.

81. Ericsson Hollsing, A. (1987) Serological markers of pulmonary infection in patients with cystic fibrosis [Survey] Stockholm.

82. Burns, M.W. and May, J.R. (1968) Bacterial precipitins in serum of patients with cystic fibrosis. *Lancet*, **1**, 270–272.

83. Lawson, D. (1970) Bacteriology of the respiratory tract in cystic fibrosis – a hypothesis, in *The Control of Chemotherapy*, (ed. P.J. Watte), Livingstone, Edingburgh, pp. 69–77.

84. Couetdic, G., Estavoyer, J.M. Fournier, J.M. and Michelbriand, Y. (1991) Anti-lipoteichoic acid antibodies in 45 cystic fibrosis patients with *Staphylococcus aureus* infection. *Presse Med.*, **20**, (28), 1342.

85. Weaver, L.T., Green, M.R., Nicholson, K. *et al.* (1994) Prognosis in cystic fibrosis treated with continuous flucloxacillin from the neonatal period. *Arch. Dis. Child.*, **70**, (2), 84–89.

86. Bauernfeind, A., Przyklenk, B., Matthias, C., Jungwirth, R., Bertele, R.M. and Harms, K. (1990) Selection of antibiotics for treatment and prophylaxis of staphylococcal infections in cystic fibrosis patients. *Infection*, **18**, (2), 126–130.

87. Høiby, N., Friis, B., Jensen, K. *et al.* (1982) Antimicrobial chemotherapy in cystic fibrosis patients. *Acta Paediat. Scand. Suppl.*, **301**, 75–100.

88. Jensen, T., Pedersen, S.S., Høiby, N., Koch, C. and Flensborg, E.W. (1989) Use of antibiotics in cystic fibrosis: the Danish approach, in *Pseudomonas aeruginosa* infection, (ed. N. Høiby, S.S. Pedersen, G.H. Shand, G. Döring and I.A. Holder), *Antibiotics Chemother.*, **42**, 237–246.

89. Marks, M.I. (1989) Antibiotic therapy for bronchopulmonary infections in cystic fibrosis, in Pseudomonas aeruginosa *infection*, (ed. N. Høiby, S.S. Pedersen, G.H. Shand, G, Döring, A. Holder), *Antibiotics Chemother.*, **42**, 229–236.

90. Geddes, D.M. (1988) Antimicrobial therapy against *Staphylococcus aureus, Pseudomonas aeruginosa*, and *Pseudomonas cepacia*. *Chest*, **94**, (Suppl.), 140S–144S.

91. Loening-Baucke, V.A., Mischler, E. and Myers, M.G. (1979) A placebo-controlled trial of cephalexin therapy in the ambulatory management of patients with cystic fibrosis. *J. Pediatr.*, **95**, 630–637.

92. Nolan, G., McIvor, P., Levison, H., Fleming, P.C., Corey, M. and Gold, R. (1982) Antibiotic prophylaxis in cystic fibrosis: inhaled cephaloridine as an adjunct to oral cloxacillin. *J. Pediatr.*, **101**, 626–630.

93. Jensen, T., Lang, S., Faber, M., Rosdahl, V.T., Høiby, N. and Koch, C. (1990) Clinical experiences with fusidic acid in cystic fibrosis patients. *J. Antimicrob. Chemother.*, **25**, (Suppl. B), 45–52.

94. Spino, M. (1991) Pharmacokinctics of drugs in cystic fibrosis. *Clin. Rev. Allergy*, **9**, (1–2), 169–210.

95. Mouton, J.W. and Kerrebijn, K.F. (1990) Antibacterial therapy in cystic fibrosis. *Med. Clin. North Am.*, **74**, (3), 837–850.

96. Ramsey, B.W. (1996) Drug therapy: management of pulmonary disease in patients with cystic fibrosis. *NEJM*, **335**, (3), 179–188.

97. Moller, L.V.M., Regelink, A.G., Grasselier, H., Dankertroelse, J.E., Dankert, J. and VanAlphen, L. (1995) Multiple *Haemophilus influenzae* strains and strain variants coexist in the respiratory tract of patients with cystic fibrosis. *J. Infect. Dis.*, **172**, (5), 1388–1392.

98. Harper, J.J. and Tilse, M.H. (1991) Biotypes of *Haemophilus influenzae* that are associated with noninvasive infections. *J. Clin. Microbiol.*, **29**, (11), 2539–2542.

99. Watson, K.G., Kerr, E.J.C. and Baillie, M. (1988) Temporal changes in biotypes of *Haemophilus influenzae* isolated from patients with cystic fibrosis. *J. Med. Microbiol.*, **26**, 129–132.

100. Moller, L.V.M., Regelink, A.G., Grasselier, H., VanAlphen, L. and Dankert, J. (1998) Antimicrobial susceptibility of *Haemophilus influenzae* in the respiratory tracts of patients with cystic fibrosis. *Antimicrob. Agents Chemother.*, **42**, (2), 319–324.

101. Pedersen, M., Støvring, S., Mørkassel, E., Koch, C. and Høiby, N. (1986) Persistent *Haemophilus influenzae* infection in the lower respiratory tract of children with chronic lung disease. A comparative study of amoxicillin and pivampicillin. *Scand. J. Infect. Dis.*, **18**, 245–254.

102. Jensen, T., Pedersen, S.S., Stafanger, G., Høiby, N., Koch, C., and Bondesson, G. (1988) Comparison of amoxycillin/clavulannate (Spektramox) with amoxycillin in children and adults with chronic obstructive pulmonary disease and infection with *Haemophilus influenzae*. *Scand. J. Infect. Dis.*, **20**, 517–524.

103. Fisher, M.C., Lipuma, J.J., Dasen, S.E. *et al.* (1993) Source of *Pseudomonas cepacia* – ribotyping of isolates from patients and from the environment. *J. Pediatr.*, **123**, (5), 745–747.

104. Butler, S.L., Doherty, C.J., Hughes, J.E., Nelson, J.W. and Govan, J.R.W. (1995) *Burkholderia cepacia* and cystic fibrosis: Do natural environments present a potential hazard? *J. Clin. Microbiol.*, **33**, (4), 1001–1004.

105. Holmes, A., Govan, J. and Goldstein, R. (1998) Agricultural use of *Burkholderia (Pseudomonas) cepacia*: a threat to human health? *Emerging Infect. Dis.*, **4**, 221–227.

106. Barth, A.L. and Pitt, T.L. (1995) Auxotrophy of *Burkholderia (Pseudomonas) cepacia* from cystic fibrosis patients. *J. Clin. Microbiol.*, **33**, (8), 2192–2194.

107. Govan, J.R.W. and Deretic, V. (1996) Microbial pathogenesis in cystic fibrosis: mucoid *Pseudomonas aeruginosa* and *Burkholderia cepacia*. *Microbiol. Rev.* **60**, (3), 539.

108. Sajjan, U.S., Sun, L., Goldstein, R. and Forstner, J.F. (1995) Cable (Cbi) type 11 pili of cystic fibrosis-associated *Burkholderia (Pseudomonas) cepacia*: Nucleotide sequence of the cblA major subunit pilin gene and novel morphology of the assembled appendage fibers. *J. Bacteriol.*, **177**, (4), 1030–1038.

109. Burns, J.L., Jonas, M., Chi, E.Y., Clark, D.K., Berger, A. and Griffith, A. (1996) Invasion of respiratory epithelial cells by *Burkholderia (Pseudomonas) cepacia*. *Infect. Immun.*, **64**, (10), 4054–4059.

110. Shaw, D., Poxton, I.R. and Govan, J.R.W. (1995) Biological activity of *Burkholderia (Pseudomonas) cepacia* lipopolysaccharide. *FEMS Immunol. Med. Microbiol.*, **11**, (2), 99–106.

111. Hutchison, M.L., Poxton, I.R. and Govan, J.R.W. (1998) *Burkholderia cepacia* produces a hemolysin that is capable of inducing apoptosis and degranulation of mammalian phagocytes. *Infect. Immun.*, **66**, (5), 2033–2039.

112. Vandamme, P., Holmes, B., Vancanneyt, M. *et al.* (1997) Occurrence of multiple genomovars of *Burkholderia cepacia* in cystic fibrosis patients and proposal of *Burkholderia multivorans* sp. nov. *Int. J. Syst. Bact.*, **47**, (4), 1188–1200.

113. Barker, P.M., Wood, R.E. and Gilligan, P.H. (1997) Lung infection with *Burkholderia gladioli* in a child with cystic fibrosis: acute clinical and spirometric deterioration. *Pediatr. Pulmonol.*, **23**, 123–125.

114. Ledson, M.J., Gallagher, M.J. and Walshaw, M.J. (1998)

Chronic *Burkholderia cepacia* bronchiectasis in a non-cystic fibrosis individual. *Thorax*, **53**, (5), 430–432.

115. Isles, A., Maclusky, I., Corey, M. *et al*. (1984) *Pseudomonas cepacia* infection in cystic fibrosis: an emerging problem. *J. Pediatr.*, **104**, 206–210.

116. Baltimore, R.S., Radnay-Baltimore, K., Graevenitz, A.v. and Dolan, T.F. (1982) Occurrence of nonfermentative gram-negative rods other than *Pseudomonas aeruginosa* in the respiratory tract of children with cystic fibrosis. *Helv. Paediatr. Acta*, **37**, 547–554.

117. Lewin, L.O., Byard, P.J. and Davis, P.B. (1990) Effect of *Pseudomonas cepacia* colonization on survival and pulmonary function of cystic fibrosis patients. *J. Clin. Epidemiol.*, **43**, (2), 125–13 1.

118. Laraya-Cuasay, L.R., Lipstein, M. and Huang, N.N. (1977) *Pseudomonas cepacia* in the respiratory flora of patients with cystic fibrosis (CF). *Am. Soc. Ped. Dis.*, 502.

119. Thomassen, M.J. (1985) *Pseudomonas cepacia* colonization among patients with cystic fibrosis. *Am. Rev. Resp. Dis.*, **131**, 791–796.

120. Tomashefski, J.F. Jr, Thomasse, M.J., Bruce, M.C., Goldberg, H.I., Konstan, M.W. and Stern, R.C. (1988) *Pseudomonas cepacia*-associated pneumonia in cystic fibrosis. *Arch. Pathol. Lab. Med.*, **112**, 166–172.

121. Tablan, O.C., Chorba, T.L., Schidlow, D.V. *et al*. *Pseudomonas cepacia* colonization in patients with cystic fibrosis: risk factors and clinical outcome. *J. Pediatr.*, **107**, 382–387.

122. Tablan, O.C., Martone, W.J., Doershuk, C.F. *et al*. (1987) Colonization of the respiratory tract with *Pseudomonas cepacia* in cystic fibrosis. Risk factors and outcomes. *Chest*, **91**, 527–532.

123. Simmonds, E.J., Conway, S.P., Ghoneim, A.T.M., Ross, H. and Littlewood, J.M. (1990) *Pseudomonas cepacia* – a new pathogen in patients with cystic fibrosis referred to a large center in the United Kingdom. *Arch. Dis. Child.*, **65**, (8), 874–877.

124. LiPuma, J.J., Mortensen, J.E., Dasen, S.E. *et al*. (1988) Ribotype analysis of *Pseudomonas cepacia* from cystic fibrosis treatment centers. *J. Pediatr.*, **113**, 859–862.

125. Nelson, S.W., Doherty, C.J., Brown, P.H., Greening, A.P., Kaufmann, M.E. and Govan, J.R.W. (1991) *Pseudomonas cepacia* in inpatients with cystic fibrosis. *Lancet*, **338**, (8781), 1525.

126. Smith, D.L., Smith, E.G., Gumery, L.B. and Stableforth, D.E. (1992) *Pseudomonas cepacia* infection in cystic fibrosis. *Lancet*, **339**, (8787), 252.

127. Gladman, G., Connor, P.J., Williams, R.F. and David, T.J. (1992) Controlled study of *Pseudomonas cepacia* and *Pseudomonas maltophilia* in cystic fibrosis. *Arch. Dis. Child.*, **67**, (2), 192–195.

128. Gessner, A.R. and Mortensen, J.E. (1990) Pathogenic factors of *Pseudomonas cepacia* isolates from patients with cystic fibrosis. *J. Med. Microbiol.*, **33**, (2), 115–120.

129. Mckenney, D., Brown, K.E. and Allison, D.G. (1995) Influence of *Pseudomonas aeruginosa* exoproducts on virulence factor production in *Burkholderia cepacia*:

Evidence of interspecies communication. *J. Bacteriol.*, **177**, (23), 6989–6992.

130. Pedersen, S.S., Jensen, T., Pressler, T., Høiby, N. K. R. (1986) Does centralized treatment of cystic fibrosis increase the risk of *Pseudomonas aeruginosa* infection? *Acta Paediatr. Scand.*, **75**, 840–845.

131. Editorial (1992) *Pseudomonas cepacia* – more than a harmless commensal. *Lancet*, **339**, (8806), 1385–1386.

132. Segonds, C., Chabanon, G., Couetdic, G., Michelbriand,Y. and Bingen, E. (1996) Epidemiology of pulmonary colonization with *Burkholderia cepacia* in cystic fibrosis patients. *Eur. J. Clin. Microbiol. Infect. Dis.*, **15**, (10), 841–842.

133. Thomassen, M.J., Demko, C.A., Doershuk, C.F., Stern, R.C. and Klinger, J.D. (1986) *Pseudomonas cepacia*: decrease in colonization in patients with cystic fibrosis. *Am. Rev. Resp. Dis.*, **134**, 669–671.

134. Hardy, K.A., McGowan, K.L., Fisher, M.C. and Schidlow, D.V. (1986) *Pseudomonas cepacia* in the hospital setting: lack of transmission between cystic fibrosis patients. *J. Pediatr.*, **109**, 51–54.

135. Lipuma, J.J., Dasen, S.E., Nielson, D.W., Stern, R.C. and Stull, T.L. (1990) Person-to-person transmission of *Pseudomonas cepacia* between patients with cystic fibrosis. *Lancet*, **336**, (8723),1094–1096.

136. Millar-Jones, L., Paull, A., Saunders, Z. and Goodchild, M.C. (1992) Transmission of *Pseudomonas cepacia* among cystic fibrosis patients. *Lancet*, **340**, 491.

137. Editorial (1992) *Pseudomonas cepacia* – more than a harmless commensal? *Lancet*, **339**, 1385–1386.

138. Covan, J.R.W., Brown, P.H., Maddison, J. *et al*. (1993) Evidence for transmission of *Pseudomonas cepacia* by social contact in cystic fibrosis. *Lancet*, **342**, (8862), 15–19.

139. Pitt, T.L., Kaufmann, M.E., Patel, P.S., Benge, L.C.A., Gaskin, S. and Livermore, D.M. (1996) Type characterisation and antibiotic susceptibility of *Burkholderia (Pseudomonas) cepacia* isolates from patients with cystic fibrosis in the United Kingdom and the Republic of Ireland. *J. Med. Microbiol.*, **44**, (3), 203–210.

140. Mahenthiralingam, E., Campbell, M.E., Henry, D.A. and Speert, D.P. (1996) Epidemiology of *Burkholderia cepacia* infection in patients with cystic fibrosis: Analysis by randomly amplified polymorphic DNA fingerprinting. *J. Clin. Microbiol.*, **34**, (12), 2914–2920.

141. Ledson, M.J., Gallagher, M.J., Corkill, J.E., Hart, C.A. and Walshaw, M.J. (1998) Cross infection between cystic fibrosis patients colonised with *Burkholderia cepacia*. *Thorax*, **53**, (5), 432–436.

142. Döring, G., Jansen, S., Noll, H. *et al*. (1996) Distribution and transmission of *Pseudomonas aeruginosa* and *Burkholderia cepacia* in a hospital ward. *Pediatr. Pulmonol.*, **21**, 90-100.

143. Hutchinson, G.R., Parker, S., Pryor, J.A. *et al*. (1996) Home-use nebulizers: A potential primary source of *Burkholderia cepacia* and other colistin-resistant, gram-

negative bacteria in patients with cystic fibrosis. *J. Clin. Microbiol.*, **34**, (6), 1601.

144. Pegues, D.A., Carson, L.A., Tablan, O.C. *et al.* (1994) Acquisition of *Pseudomonas cepacia* at summer camps for patients with cystic fibrosis. *J. Pediatr.*, **124**, (5, Part I), 694–702.

145. Aronoff, S.C. (1988) Outer membrane permeability in *Pseudomonas cepacia*: diminished porin content in a B-lactam-resistant mutant and in resistant cystic fibrosis isolates. *Antimicrob. Agents Chemother.*, **32**, 1636–1639.

146. Kumar, A., Wofford-McQueen, R. and Gordon, R.C. (1989) Ciprofloxacin, imipenem and rifampicin; in vitro synergy of two and three drug combinations against *Pseudomonas cepacia. J. Antimicrob. Chemother.*, **23**, 831–835.

147. Klinger, I.D. and Aronoff, S.C. (1985) *In vitro* activity of ciprofloxacin and other antibacterial agents against *Pseudomonas aeruginosa* and *Pseudomonas cepacia* from cystic fibrosis patients. *J. Antimicrob. Chemother.*, **15**, 679–684.

148. Bosso, J.A., Saxon, B.A. and Matsen, J.M. (1987) *In vitro* activity of aztreonam combined with tobramycin and gentamicin against clinical isolates of *Pseudomonas aeruginosa* and *Pseudomonas cepacia* from patients with cystic fibrosis. *Antimicrob. Agents Chemother.*, **31**, 1403–1405.

149. Cohn, R.C. and Rudzienski, L. (1991) Observations on amiloride–tobramycin synergy in *Pseudomonas cepacia. Curr. Ther. Res.*, **50**, (6), 786–793.

150. Nir, M., Johansen, H.K. and Høiby, N. (1992) Low incidence of pulmonary *Pseudomonas cepacia* infection in Danish cystic fibrosis patients. *Acta Paediatr.*, **81**, 1042–1043.

151. Ryley, H.C., Ojeniyi, B., Hoiby, N. and Weeks, J. (1996) Lack of evidence of nosocomial cross-infection by *Burkholderia cepacia* among Danish cystic fibrosis patients. *Eur. J. Clin. Microbiol. Infect. Dis.*, **15**, (9), 755–758.

152. Govan, J.R.W., Brown, P.H., Maddison, J. *et al.* (1993) Evidence for transmission of *Pseudomonas cepacia* by social contact in cystic fibrosis. *Lancet*, **342**, (8862), 15–19.

153. Muhdi, K., Edenborough, F.P., Gumery, L. *et al.* (1996) Outcome for patients colonised with *Burkholderia cepacia* in a Birmingham adult cystic fibrosis clinic and the end of an epidemic. *Thorax*, **51**, (4), 374–377.

154. Paul, M.L., Pegler, M.A.M. and Benn, R.A.V. (1998) Molecular epidemiology of *Burkholderia cepacia* in two Australian cystic fibrosis centers. *J. Hosp. Infect.*, **38**, 19–26.

155. Webb, A.K. and Govan, J.R. (1998) *Burkholderia cepacia*: another twist and a further threat. *Thorax*, **53**, (5), 333–334.

156. Govan, J.R.W. and Nelson, J.W. (1993) Micobiology of cystic fibrosis lung infections – themes and issues. *J. R. Soc. Med.*, **86**, (Suppl. 20), 11–18.

157. Taylor, R.F.H., Morgan, D.W., Nicholson, P.S., Mackay, I.S.,

158. Agnarsson, U., Glass, S. and Govan, J.R.W. (1989) Fecal isolation of *Pseudomonas aeruginosa* from patients with cystic fibrosis. *J. Clin. Microbiol.*, **27**, 96–98.

159. Speert, D.P., Campbell, M.E., Davidson, G.F. and Wong, L.T.K. (1993) *Pseudomonas aeruginosa* colonization of the gastrointestinal tract in patients with cystic fibrosis. *J. Infect. Dis.*, **167**, 226–229.

160. Barth, A.L. and Pitt, T.L. (1995) Auxotrophic variants of *Pseudomonas aeruginosa* are selected from prototrophic wild-type strains in respiratory infections in patients with cystic fibrosis. *J. Clin. Microbiol.*, **33**, (I), 37–40.

161. Nelson, J.W., Tredgett, M.W., Sheehan, J.K., Thornton, D.J., Notman, D. and Govan, J.R.W. (1990) Mucinophilic and chemotactic properties of *Pseudomonas aeruginosa* in relation to pulmonary colonization in cystic fibrosis. *Infect. Immunity*, **58**, 1489–1495.

162. Lamblin, G. and Roussel, P. (1993) Airway mucins and their role in defence against micro-organisms. *Resp. Med.*, **87**, (6), 421–426.

163. Baker, N.R. and Svanborg-Edn, C. (1989) Role of alginate in the adherence of *Pseudomonas aeruginosa*, in Pseudomonas aeruginosa *Infection*, (ed. N. Høiby, S.S. Pedersen, G.H. Shand, G. Döring and I.A. Holder), *Antibiot. Chemother.*, **42**, 72–79.

164. Ramphal, R., Guay, C. and Pier, G.B. (1987) *Pseudomonas aeruginosa* adhesins for tracheobronchial mucin. *Infect. Immun.*, **55**, 600–603.

165. Plotkowski, M.C., Tournier, J.M. and Puchelle, E. (1996) *Pseudomonas aeruginosa* strains possess specific adhesins for laminin. *Infect. Immun.*, **64**, (2), 600–605.

166. Baker, N.R., Minor, V., Deal, C., Shahrabadi, M.S., Simpson, D.A. and Woods, D.E. (1991) *Pseudomonas aeruginosa exoenzyme-S is an adhesin. Infect. Immun.*, **59**, (9), 2859–2863.

167. Hata, J.S. and Fick, R.B. (1991) Airway adherence of *Pseudomonas aeruginosa* – mucoexopolysaccharide binding to human and bovine airway proteins. *J. Lab. Clin. Med.*, **117**, (5), 410–422.

168. Feldman, M., Bryan, R., Rajan, S. *et al.* (1998) Role of flagella in pathogenesis of *Pseudomonas aeruginosa* pulmonary infection. *Infect. Immun.*, **66**, (I), 43–51.

169. Arora, S.K., Ritchings, B.W., Almira, E.C., Lory, S. and Ramphal, R. (1998) The *Pseudomonas aeruginosa* flagellar cap protein, FliD, is responsible for mucin adhesion. *Infect. Immun.*, **66**, (3), 1000–1007.

170. Debentzmann, S., Plotkowski, C. and Puchelle, E. (1996) Receptors in the *Pseudomonas aeruginosa* adherence to injured and repairing airway epithelium. *Am. J. Respir. Crit. Care Med.*, **154**, (Suppl. 4), S155–S162.

171. Kelly, N.M., Tempany, E., Falkner, F.R., Fitzgerald, M.X., O'Boyle, C. and Keane, C.T. (1982) Does pseudomonas cross-infection occur between cystic fibrosis patients? *Lancet*, **11**, 688–689.

172. Renders, N.H.M., Sijmons, M.A.F., van Belkum, A.,

Hodson, M.E. and Pitt, T.L. (1992) Extrapulmonary sites of *Pseudomonas aeruginosa* in adults with cystic fibrosis. *Thorax*, **47**, (6), 426–428.

Overbeek, S.E., Mouton, J.W. and Verbrugh, H.A. (1997) Exchange of *Pseudomonas aeruginosa* strains among cystic fibrosis siblings. *Res. Microbiol.*, **148**, (5), 447–454.

173. Zimakoff, J., Høiby, N., Rosendal, K. and Guilbert, J.P. (1983) Epidemiology of *Pseudomonas aeruginosa* infection and the role of contamination of the environment in a cystic fibrosis clinic. *J. Hosp. Infect.*, **4**, 31–40.

174. Döring, G., Ulrich, M., Muller, W. *et al.* (1991) Generation of *Pseudomonas aeruginosa* aerosols during hand-washing from contaminated sink drains, transmission to hands of hospital personnel, and its prevention by use of a new heating device. *Zbl. Hyg. Umweltmed.*, **191**, (5–6), 494–505.

175. Botzenhardt, K., Wolz, C. and Döring, G. (1991) Cross-colonization and routes of infection assessed with a DNA probe, in Pseudomonas aeruginosa *in Human Disease*, (ed. J.Y. Homma, H. Tanimoto, I.A. Holder, N. Høiby and G.Döring), *Antibiotics Chemother.*, **44**, 8–12.

176. Wolz, C., Kiosz, G., Ogle, J.W. *et al.* (1989) *Pseudomonas aeruginosa* cross-colonization and persistence in patients with cystic fibrosis. Use of a DNA probe. *Epidem. Infec.*, **102**, 205–214.

177. Döring, G, Bareth, H., Gairing, A., Wolz, C. and Botzenhart, K. (1989) Genotyping of *Pseudomonas aeruginosa* sputum and stool isolates ftom cystic fibrosis patients – evidence for intestinal colonization and spreading into toilets. *Epid. Inf.*, **103**, (3), 555–564.

178. Döring, G. (1991) *Pseudomonas aeruginosa* epidemiology: major environmental reservoirs, routes of transmission and strategies for prevention. *Pediatr. Pulmonol. Suppl.*, **6**, 280.

179. Jensen, E.T., Giwercman, B., Ojeniyi, B. *et al.* (1997) Epidemiology of *Pseudomonas aeruginosa* in cystic fibrosis and the possible role of contamination by dental equipment. *J. Hosp. Infect.*, **36**, 117–122.

180. Hoogkamp-Korstanje, J.A.A. and Laag, Jvd. (1980) Incidence and risk of cross-colonization in cystic fibrosis holiday camps. *Anton Leeuwenhock J. Microbiol.*, **46**, 100–101.

181. Speert, D.P., Lawton, D. and Damm, S. (1982) Communicability of *Pseudomonas aeruginosa* in a cystic fibrosis summer camp. *Clin. Lab. Obs.*, **101**, 227–229.

182. Høiby, N. and Pedersen, S.S. (1989) Estimated risk of cross-infection with *Pseudomonas aeruginosa* in Danish cystic fibrosis patients. *Acta Paediatr. Scand.*, **78**, 395–404.

183. Pedersen, S.S., Koch, C., Høiby, N. and Rosendal, K. (1986) An epidemic spread of multiresistant *Pseudomonas aeruginosa* in a cystic fibrosis center. *J. Antimicrob. Chemother.*, **17**, 505–516.

184. Ojeniyi, B. (1994) Polyagglutinable *Pseudomonas aeruginosa* from cystic fibrosis patients – A survey. *APMIS*, **102**, (Suppl. 46), 1–44.

185. Tümmler, B., Koopmann, U., Grothues, D., Weissbrodt, H., Steinkamp, G. and Vonderhardt, H. (1991) Nosocomial acquisition of *Pseudomonas aeruginosa* by cystic fibrosis patients. *J. Clin. Microbiol.*, **29**, (6), 1265–1267.

186. Speert, D.P. and Campbell, M.E. (1987) Hospital epidemiology of *Pseudomonas aeruginosa* from patients with cystic fibrosis. *J. Hosp. Infect.*, **9**, 11–21.

187. Cheng, K., Smyth, R.L., Govan, J.R.W. *et al.* (1996) Spread of beta-lactam-resistant *Pseudomonas aeruginosa* in a cystic fibrosis clinic. *Lancet*, **348**, (9028), 639–642.

188. Farrell, P.M., Shen, G.H., Splaingard, M. *et al.* (1997) Acquisition of *Pseudomonas aeruginosa* in children with cystic fibrosis. *Pediatrics*, **100**, (5), E21–E29.

189. Denton, M., Littlewood, I.M., Brownlee, K.G., Conway, S.P. and Todd, N.J. (1996) Spread of beta-lactam-resistant *Pseudomonas aeruginosa* in a cystic fibrosis unit. *Lancet*, **348**, (9041), 1596–1597.

190. Pedersen, S.S. (1992) Lung infection with alginate-producing, mucoid *Pseudomonas aeruginosa* in cystic fibrosis. *APMIS*, **100**, (Suppl. 28), 5–79.

191. Frederiksen, B., Koch, C. and Høiby, N. (1998) The changing epidemiology of *Pseudomonas aeruginosa* infection in Danish cystic fibrosis patients, 1974–1995. *Pediatr. Pulmonol.*, **28**, 159–166.

192. MacMahorn, B. and Pugh, T.F. (1970) *Epidemiology, principles and methods*, Little, Brown and Company, Boston, pp. 1–376.

193. Liu, P.Y. (1974) Extracellular toxins of *Pseudomonas aeruginosa*. *J. Infect. Dis.*, **130**, S94–S99.

194. Kharazmi, A. (1991) Mechanisms involved in the evasion of the host defence by *Pseudomonas aeruginosa*. *Immunol. Lett.*, **30**, (2), 201–206.

195. Sorensen, R.U., Waller, R.L. and Klinger, J.D. (1991) Infection and immunity to *Pseudomonas*. *Clin. Rev. Allergy*, **9**, (1–2), 47–74.

196. Kharazmi, A. (1989) Interactions of *Pseudomonas aeruginosa* proteases with the cells of the immune system, in Pseudomonas aeruginosa *infection*, (ed. N. Høiby, S.S. Pedersen, G.H. Shand, G. Döring and I.A. Holder), *Antibiot. Chemother.*, **42**, 42–49.

197. Döring, G., Obernesser H.-J., Botzenhart, K., Flehmig, B., Høiby, N. and Hofman, A. (1983) Proteases of *Pseudomonas aeruginosa* in patients with cystic fibrosis. *J. Infect. Dis.*, **147**, 744–750.

198. Döring, G. and Høiby, N. (1983) Longitudinal study of immune response to *Pseudomonas aeruginosa* antigens in cystic fibrosis. *Infect. Immun.*, **42**, 197–201.

199. Döring, G., Buhl, V., Botzenhart, K., Høiby, N. (1983) Immune response to protease of *Pseudomonas aeruginosa* followed by immune complex formation in cystic fibrosis. *Proc. EWGCF, 12th Ann. Meeting*, pp. 74–77.

200. Döring, G., Goldstein, W., Röll, A., Schiotz, P.O., Høiby, N. and Botzenhart, K. (1985) The role of *Pseudomonas aeruginosa* exoenzymes in lung infections of patients with cystic fibrosis. *Infect. Immun.*, **49**, 557–562.

201. Shand, G.H., Pedersen, S.S., Lam, K., Høiby, N. (1989) Iron regulated outer membrane proteins and virulence in *Pseudomonas aeruginosa*, in Pseudomonas

aeruginosa *Infection*, (eds N. Høiby, S.S. Pedersen, G.H. Shand, G. Döring, I.A. Holder), *Antibiot. Chemother.*, **42**, 15–26.

202. De Kievit, T.R. and Lam, J.S. (1994) Monoclonal antibodies that distinguish inner core, outer core, and lipid A regions of *Pseudomonas aeruginosa* lipopolysaccharide. *J. Bacteriol.*, **176**, 7129–7139.

203. Kronborg, G. (1995) Lipopolysaccharide (LPS), LPS-immune complexes and cytokines as inducers of pulmonary inflammation in patients with cystic fibrosis and chronic *Pseudomonas aeruginosa* lung infection. *APMIS*, **103**, (Suppl. 50), 1.

204. Brett, M.M., Simmonds, E.J., Ghoneim, A.T.M. and Littlewood, J.M. (1992) The value of serum IgG titres against *Pseudomonas aeruginosa* in the management of early pseudomonal infection in cystic fibrosis. *Arch. Dis. Child.*, **67**, (9), 1086–1088.

205. Fomsgaard, A. (1990) Antibodies to lipopolysaccharides – some diagnostic and protective aspects. *APMIS*, **98**, (518), 5–38.

206. Fomsgaard, A., Shand, G.H., Freudenberg, M.A. *et al.* (1993) Antibodies from chronically infected cystic fibrosis patients react with lipopolysaccharides extracted by new micromethods from all serotypes of *Pseudomonas aeruginosa*. *APMIS*, **101**, (2), 101–112.

207. Rocchetta, H.L. and Lam, J.S. (1997) Identification and functional characterization of an ABC transport system involved in polysaccharide export of A-band lipopolysaccharide in *Pseudomonas aeruginosa*. *J. Bacteriol.*, **179**, (15), 4713–4724.

208. Elborn, J.S., Cordon, S.M. and Shale, D.J. (1993) Host inflammatory responses to first isolation of *Pseudomonas aeruginosa* from sputum in cystic fibrosis. *Pediatr. Pulmonol.*, **15**, 287–291.

209. Döring, G., Buhl, V., Høiby, N., Schiøtz, P.O. and Botzenhart, K. (1984) Detection of proteases of *Pseudomonas aeruginosa* in immune complexes isolated from sputum of cystic fibrosis patients. *Acta Pathol. Microbiol. Scand. Sect. C*, **92**, 307–312.

210. Baltimore, R.S., Christie, C.D.C. and Smith, G.J.W. (1989) Immunohistopathologic localization of *Pseudomonas aeruginosa* in lungs from patients with cystic fibrosis – Implications for the pathogenesis of progressive lung deterioration. *Am. Rev. Resp. Dis.*, **140**, 1650–1661.

211. Høiby, N., Döring, G. and Schiøtz, P.O. (1986) The role of immune complexes in the pathogenesis of bacterial infections. *Ann. Rev. Microbiol.*, **40**, 29–53.

212. May, T.B., Shinabarger, D., Maharaj, R. *et al.* Alginate synthesis by *Pseudomonas aeruginosa* – a key pathogenic factor in chronic pulmonary infections of cystic fibrosis patients. *Clin. Microbiol. Rev.*, **4**, (2), 191–206.

213. Deretic, V., Mohr, C.D. and Martin, D.W. (1991) Mucoid *Pseudomonas aeruginosa* in cystic fibrosis – signal transduction and histone-like elements in the regulation of bacterial virulence. *Mol. Microbiol.*, **5**, (7), 1577–1583.

214. Roychoudhury, S., Zielinski, N.A., Devault, J.D. *et al.*

(1991) *Pseudomonas aeruginosa* infection in cystic fibrosis – biosynthesis of alginate as a virulence factor, in Pseudomonas aeruginosa *in Human Diseases*, (ed. J.Y. Homma, I.A. Holder, N. Høiby, G. Döring, *Antibiot. Chemother.*, **44**, 63–67.

215. Lam, J., Chan, R., Lam, K. and Costerton, J.W. (1980) Production of mucoid microcolonies by *Pseudomonas aeruginosa* within infected lungs in cystic fibrosis. *Infect. Immun.*, **28**, 546–556.

216. Pedersen, S.S., Høiby, N., Espersen, F. and Koch, C. (1992) Role of alginate in infection with mucoid *Pseudomonas aeruginosa* in cystic fibrosis. *Thorax*, **47**, 6–13.

217. Mathee, K., Ciofu, O. Sternberg, C. *et al.* (1999) Mucoid conversion of *Pseudomonas aeruginosa* by hydrogen peroxide: a mechanism for virulence activation in the cystic fibrosis lung. *Microbiol.*, **145**, 1349–1357.

218. Costerton, J.W., Cheng, K.-J., Geesey, G.G. *et al.* (1987) Bacterial biofilms in nature and disease. *Annu. Rev. Microbiol.*, **41**, 435–464.

219. Costerton, J.W., Lewandowski, Z., Caldwell, D.E., Korber, D.R., Lappinscott, H.M. (1995) Microbial biofilms. *Annu. Rev. Microbiol.*, **49**, 711–745.

220. Jensen, E.T., Kharazmi, A., Lam, K., Costerton, J.W. and Høiby, N. (1990) Human polymorphonuclear leucocyte response to *Pseudomonas aeruginosa* grown in biofilm. *Infect. Immun.*, **58**, 2383–2385.

221. Pedersen, S.S., Kharazmi, A., Espersen, F. and Høiby, N. (1990) *Pseudomonas aeruginosa* alginate in cystic fibrosis sputum and the inflammatory response. *Infect. Immun.*, **58**, (10), 3363–3368.

222. Høiby, N. (1975) Prevalence of mucoid strains of *Pseudomonas aeruginosa* in bacteriological specimens from patients with cystic fibrosis and patients with other diseases. *Acta Pathol. Microbiol. Scand. Sect. B*, **83**, 549–552.

223. Brown, M.R.W., Collier, P.J. and Gilbert, P. (1990) Influence of growth rate on susceptibility to antimicrobial agents – modification of the cell envelope and batch and continuous culture studies. *Antimicrob. Agents Chemother.*, **34**, (9), 1623–1628.

224. Anwar, H., Dasgupta, M., Lam, K. and Costerton, J.W. (1989) Tobramycin resistance of mucoid *Pseudomonas aeruginosa* biofilm grown under iron limitation. *J. Antimicrob. Chemother.*, **24**, (5), 647–655.

225. Anwar, H. and Costerton, J.W. (1990) Enhanced activity of combination of tobramycin and piperacillin for eradication of sessile biofilm cells of *Pseudomonas aeruginosa*. *Antimicrob. Agents Chemother.*, **34**, (9), 1666–1671.

226. Anwar, H., Dasgupta, M.K. and Costerton, J.W. (1990) Testing the susceptibility of bacteria in biofilms to antibacterial agents. *Antimicrob. Agents Chemother.*, **34**, (1l), 2043–2046.

227. Giwercman, B., Jensen, E.T., Hoiby, N., Kharazmi, A. and Costerton, J.W. (1991) Induction of beta-lactamase production in *Pseudomonas aeruginosa* biofilm. *Antimicrob. Agents Chemother.*, **35**, (5), 1008–1010.

228. Anwar, H., Strap, J.L., and Costerton, J.W. (1992) Susceptibility of biofilm cells of *Pseudomonas aeruginosa* to bactericidal actions of whole blood and serum. *FEMS Microbiol. Lett.*, **92**, (3), 235–242.

229. Giwercman, B., Lambert, P.A., Rosdahl, V.T., Shand, G.H. and Høiby, N. (1990) Rapid emergence of resistance in *Pseudomonas aeruginosa* in cystic fibrosis patients due to in vivo selection of stable partially derepressed beta-lactamase producing strains. *J. Antimicrob. Chemother.*, **26**, (2), 247–259.

230. Domingue, G., Ellis, B., Dasgupta, M. and Costerton, J.W. (1994) Testing antimicrobial susceptibilities of adherent bacteria by a method that incorporates guidelines of the National Committee for Clinical Laboratory Standards. *J. Clin. Microbiol.*, **32**, (10), 2564–2568.

231. Pedersen, S.S., Møller, H., Espersen, F., Sørensen, C.H., Jensen, T. and Høiby, N. (192) Mucosal immunity to *Pseudomonas aeruginosa* alginate in cystic fibrosis. *APMIS*, **100**, (4), 326–334.

232. Henry, R.L., Mellis, C.M. and Petrovic, L. (1992) Mucoid *Pseudomonas aeruginosa* is a marker of poor survival in cystic fibrosis. *Pediatr. Pulmonol.*, **12**, (3), 158–161.

233. Høiby, N. (1974) *Pseudomonas aeruginosa* infection in cystic fibrosis. Relationship between mucoid strains of *Pseudomonas aeruginosa* and the humoral immune response. *Acta Pathol. Microbiol. Scand. Sect. B.*, **82**, 551–558.

234. Pedersen, S.S., Høiby, N., Shand, G.H., and Pressler, T. (1989) Antibody response to *Pseudomonas aeruginosa* antigens in cystic fibrosis, in Pseudomonas aeruginosa *infection*, (ed. N. Høiby, S.S. Pedersen, G.H. Shand, G. Döring, I.A. Holder), *Antibiot. Chemother.*, **42**, 130–153.

235. Macdougall, J., Hodson M.E. and Pitt, T.L. (1990) Antibody response of fibrocystic patients to homologous 0-typable and 0-defective isolates of *Pseudomonas aeruginosa*. *J. Clin. Pathol.*, **43**, (7), 567–571.

236. Pier, G.B., Grout, M. and Desjardins, D. (1991) Complement deposition by antibodies to *Pseudomonas aeruginosa* mucoid exopolysaccharide (MEP) and by non-MEP specific opsonins. *J. Immunol.*, **147**, (6), 1869–1876.

236a. Hastings, J.W., Greenberg, E.P. (1999) Quorum sensing: the explanation of a curious phenomenon reveals a common characteristic of bacteria. *J. Bacteriol.*, **181**, 2667–2668.

237. Høiby, N. and Olling, S. (1977) *Pseudomonas aeruginosa* infection in cystic fibrosis. Bactericidal effect of serum from normals and patients with cystic fibrosis on *P. aeruginosa* strains from patients with cystic fibrosis or other diseases. *Acta Pathol. Microbiol. Scand. Sect. C*, **85**, 107–114.

238. Penketh, A.R.L., Pitt, T.L., Hodson, M.E. and Batten, J.C. (1983) Bactericidal activity of serum from cystic fibrosis patients for *Pseudomonas aeruginosa*. *J. Med. Microbiol.*, **16**, 401–408.

239. Pitt, T.L., MacDougall, J., Penketh, A.R.L. and Cooke, E.M. (1986) Polyagglutinating and non-typable strains of *Pseudomonas aeruginosa* in cystic fibrosis. *J. Med. Microbiol.*, **21**, 179–186.

240. Ojeniyi, B., Høiby, N. and Rosdahl, V.T. (1991) Prevalence and persistence of polyagglutinable *Pseudomonas aeruginosa* in isolates from cystic fibrosis patients. *APMIS*, **99**, (2), 187–195.

241. Ojeniyi, B., Baek, L. and Høiby, N. (1985) Polyagglutinability due to loss of 0-antigenic determinants in *Pseudomonas aeruginosa* strains isolated from cystic fibrosis patients. *Acta Pathol. Microbiol. Scand. Sect. B*, **93**, 7–13.

242. Høiby, N. and Koch, C. (1990) *Pseudomonas aeruginosa* infection in cystic fibrosis and its management. *Thorax*, **45**, 881–884.

243. Brown, M.R.W., Anwar, H. and Lambert, P.A. (1984) Evidence that mucoid *Pseudomonas aeruginosa* in the cystic fibrosis lung grows under iron-restricted conditions. *FEMS Microbiol. Lett.*, **21**, 113–117.

244. Shand, G.H., Pedersen, S.S., Brown, M.R.W. and Høiby, N. (1991) Serum antibodies to *Pseudomonas aeruginosa* outer-membrane proteins and iron-regulated membrane proteins at different stages of chronic cystic fibrosis lung infection. *J. Med. Microbiol.*, **34**, 203–212.

245. Lam, M.Y.C., McGroarty, E.J., Kropinski, A.M. *et al*. (1989) The occurrence of a common lipopolysaccharide antigen in standard and clinical strains of *Pseudomonas aeruginosa*. *J. Clin. Microbiol.*, **27**, 962–967.

246. Ojeniyi, B., Rosdal, V.T. and Høiby, N. (1987) Changes in serotype caused by cell to cell contact between different *Pseudomonas aeruginosa* strains from cystic fibrosis patients. *Acta Pathol. Microbiol. Scand. Sect. B*, **95**, 23–27.

247. Ojeniyi, B. (1988) Bacteriophages in sputum of cystic fibrosis patients as a possible cause of *in vivo* changes in serotypes of *Pseudomonas aeruginosa*. *APMIS*, **96**, 294–298.

248. Giwercman, B., Fomsgaard, A., Mansa, B. and Høiby, N. (1992) Polyacrylamide gel electrophoresis analysis of lipopolysaccharide from *Pseudomonas aeruginosa* growing planktonically and as biofilm. *FEMS Microbiol. Immunol.*, **89**, (4), 225–229.

249. Allison, D.G., Brown, M.R.W., Evans, D.E. and Gilbert, P. surface hydrophobicity and dispersal of *Pseudomonas aeruginosa* from biofilms. *FEMS Microbiol. Lett.*, **71**, (1–2), 101–104.

250. Kronborg, G., Shand, G.H., Fomsgaard, A. and Høiby, N. (1992) Lipopolysaccharide is present in immune complexes isolated from sputum in patients with cystic fibrosis and chronic *Pseudomonas aeruginosa* lung infection. *APMIS*, **100**, 175–180.

251. Kronborg, G., Fomsgaard, A. Høiby, N. (1993) Enhancement of lipopolysaccharide-induced tumor necrosis factor secretion by hyperimmune serum from chronic infected patients. *Med. Microbiol. Immunol.*, **182**, (6), 305–316.

252. Kronborg, G., Fomsgaard, A., Jensen, E.T., Kharazmi, A. and Høiby, N. (1993) Induction of oxidative burst

response in human neutrophils by immune complexes made *in vitro* of lipopolysaccharide and hyperimmune serum from chronically infected patients. *APMIS*, **101**, (11), 887–894.

253. Kronborg, G., Hansen, M., Svenson, M., Fomsgaard, A., Høiby, N. and Bendtzen, K. (1993) Cytokines in sputum and serum from patients with cystic fibrosis and chronic *Pseudomonas aeruginosa* infection as markers of destructive inflammation in the lungs. *Pediatr. Pulmonol.*, **15**, 292–297.

254. Bonfield, T.L., Panuska, J.R., Konstan, M.W. *et al.* (1995) Inflammatory cytokines in cystic fibrosis lungs. *Am. J. Resp. Crit. Care Med.*, **152**, (6), 2111–2118.

254a. Ciofu, O., Giwercman, B., Pedersen, S.S. and Høiby, N. (1994) Development of antibiotic resistance in *Pseudomonas aeruginosa* during two decades of antipseudomonal treatment at the Danish CF Center. *APMIS*, **102**, 674–680.

254b. Burns, J.L., Dalfsen, J.M. van, Shawar, R.M. *et al.* (1999) Effect of chronic intermittent administration of inhaled tobramycin on respiratory microbial flora in patients with cystic fibrosis. *J. Infect. Dis.*, **179**, 1190–1196.

255. Ciofu, O., Pressier, T., Pandey, J.P. and Høiby, N. (1997) The influence of allotypes on the IgG subclass response to chromosomal beta-lactamase of *Pseudomonas aeruginosa* in cystic fibrosis patients. *Clin. Exp. Immunol.*, **108**, (1), 88–94.

256. Pressler, T. (1996) IgG subclasses and chronic bacterial infection. Subclass antibodies and the clinical course of chronic *Pseudomonas aeruginosa* lung infection in cystic fibrosis. *APMIS*, **104**, (Suppl. 66), 1–41.

257. Høiby, N., Flensborg, E.W., Beck, B., Friis, B., Jacobsen, L. and Jacobsen, S.V. (1977) *Pseudomonas aeruginosa* infection in cystic fibrosis. Diagnostic and prognostic significance of *Pseudomonas aeruginosa* precipitins determined by means of crossed immunoelectrophoresis. *Scand. J. Resp. Dis.*, **58**, 65–79.

258. Schiøtz, P.O. (1981) Local humoral inununity and immune reactions in the lungs of patients with cystic fibrosis. *Acta Pathol. Microbiol. Scand. Sect. C, Suppl.*, **276**, 3–25.

259. Dasgupta, M.K., Lam, J., Döring, G. *et al.* (1987) Prognostic implications of circulating immune complexes and *Pseudomonas aeruginosa*-specific antibodies in cystic fibrosis. *J. Clin. Lab. Immunol.*, **23**, 25–30.

260. Dasgupta, M.K., Zuberbuhler, P., Abbi, A. *et al.* (1987) Combined evaluation of circulating immune complexes and antibodies to *Pseudomonas aeruginosa* as an immunologic profile in relation to pulmonary function in cystic fibrosis. *J. Clin. Immunol.*, **7**, 51–57.

261. Hodson, M.E., Beldon, I. and Batten, J.C. (1985) Circulating immune complexes in patients with cystic fibrosis in relation to clinical features. *Clin. Allerg.*, **15**, 363–370.

262. Wisnieski, S.J., Todd, E.W., Fuller, R. *et al.* (1985) Immune complexes and complement abnormalities in patients with cystic fibrosis. *Am. Rev. Respir. Dis.*, **132**, 770–776.

263. Suter, S. (1989) The imbalance between granulocyte neutral proteases and antiproteases in bronchial secretions from patients with cystic fibrosis, in Pseudomonas aeruginosa *Infection*, (ed. N. Høiby, S.S. Pedersen, G.H. Shand, G. Döring and I.A. Holder), *Antibiot. Chemother.*, **42**, 158–168.

264. Goldstein, W. and Döring, G. (1986) Lysosomal enzymes ftom polymorphonuelear leukocytes and proteinase inhibitors in patients with cystic fibrosis. *Am. Rev. Respir. Dis.*, **134**, 49–56.

265. Bruce, M.C., Ponez, L., Klinger, J.D., Stern, R.C., Tomashefski, J.F. and Dearborn, D.G. (1985) Biochemical and pathologic evidence for proteolytic destruction of lung connective tissue in cystic fibrosis. *Am. Rev. Respir. Dis.*, **132**, 529–535.

266. Ammitzbøll, T., Pedersen, S.S., Espersen, F. and Schiøler, H. (1988) Excretion of urinary collagen metabolites correlates to severity of pulmonary disease in cystic fibrosis. *Acta Paediatr. Scand.*, **77**, 842–846.

267. Zach, M.S. (1991) Pathogenesis and management of lung disease in cystic fibrosis. *J. R. Soc. Med.*, **84**, (Suppl. 18), 10–17.

268. Brown, R.K. and Kelly, F.J. (1994) Evidence for increased oxidative damage in patients with cystic fibrosis. *Pediatr. Res.*, **36**, (4), 487–493.

269. Döring, G., Frank, F., Boudier, C., Herbert, S., Fleischer, B. and Bellon, G. (1995) Cleavage of lymphocyte surface antigens CD2, CD4, and CD8 by polymorphonuclear leukocyte elastase and cathepsin G in patients with cystic fibrosis. *J. Immunol.*, **154**, (9), 4842–4850.

270. Delacourt, C., Lebourgeois, M., Dortho, M.P. *et al.* (1995) Imbalance between 95 kDa type IV collagenase and tissue inhibitor of metalloproteinases in sputum of patients with cystic fibrosis. *Am. J. Respir. Crit. Care Med.*, **152**, (2), 765–774.

271. Valerius, N.H., Koch, C. and Høiby, N. (1991) Prevention of chronic *Pseudomonas aeruginosa* colonisation in cystic fibrosis by early treatment. *Lancet*, **338**, (8769), 725–726.

272. Frederiksen, B., Koch, C. and Høiby, N. (1997) Antibiotic treatment of initial colonization with *Pseudomonas aeruginosa* postpones chronic infection and prevents deterioration of pulmonary function in cystic fibrosis. *Pediatr. Pulmonol.*, **23**, 330–335.

273. Wiesemann, H.G., Steinkamp, G., Ratjen, F. *et al.* (1998) Placebo-controlled, double-blind, randomized study of aerosolized tobramycin for early treatment of *Pseudomonas aeruginosa* colonization in cystic fibrosis. *Pediatr. Pulmonol.*, **25**, 88–92.

274. Sheldon, C.D., Assoufi, B.K. and Hødson, M.E. (1993)Regular 3 monthly oral ciprofloxacin in adult cystic fibrosis patients infected with *Pseudomonas aeruginosa*. *Resp. Med.*, **87**, (8), 587–593.

275. Regelmann, W.E., Elliott, G.R., Warwick, W.J. and Clawson, C.C. (1990) Reduction of sputum *Pseudomonas aeruginosa* density by antibiotics improves lung function

in cystic fibrosis more than do bronchodilators and chest physiotherapy alone. *Am. Rev. Resp. Dis.*, **141**, 914–92 1.

276. Meyer, K.C., Lewandoski, J.R., Zimmerman, J.J., Nunley, D., Calhoun, W.J. and Dopico, G.A. (1991) Human neutrophil elastase and elastase/alphal-antiprotease complex in cystic fibrosis – comparison with interstitial lung disease and evaluation of the effect of intravenously administered antibiotic therapy. *Am. Rev. Respir. Dis.*, **144**, (3), 580–585.

277. Sordelli, D.O., Macri, C.N., Maillie, A.J. and Cerquetti, M.C. (1994) A preliminary study on the effect of anti-inflammatory treatment in cystic fibrosis patients with *Pseudomonas aeruginosa* lung infection. *Int. J. Immunopathol. Pharmacol.*, **7**, (2), 109–117.

278. Konstan, M.W., Byard, P.J., Hoppel, C.L. and Davis, P.B. (1995) Effect of high-dose ibuprofen in patients with cystic fibrosis. *NEJM*, **332**, (13), 848–854.

279. Bisgaard, H., Pedersen, S.S., Nielsen, K.G. *et al.* (1997) Controlled trial of inhaled budesonide in patients with cystic fibrosis and chronic bronchopulmonary *Pseudomonas aeruginosa* infection. *Am. J. Respir. Crit. Care Med.*, **156**, (4), 1190–1196.

280. Deneuville, E., Dabadie, A., Donnio, P.Y. *et al.*, (1995) Pathogenicity of *Moraxella catarrhalis* in cystic fibrosis. *Acta Paediatr.*, **84**, (10), 1212.

281. Dekhil, S.M.B., Peel, M.M., Lennox, V.A., Stackebrandt, E. and Sly, L.I. (1997) Isolation of *Lautropia mirabilis* from sputa of a cystic fibrosis patient. *J. Clin. Microbiol.*, **35**, 1024–1026.

282. Collins, M.T., McDonald, J., Høiby, N. and Aalund, O. (1984) Agglutinating antibody titers to Legionellaceae in cystic fibrosis patients as a result of cross-reacting antibodies to *Pseudomonas aeruginosa*. *J. Clin. Microbiol.*, **19**, 757–762.

283. Dunne, W.M. and Maisch, S. (1995) Epidemiological investigation of infections due to *Alcaligenes* species in children and patients with cystic fibrosis: Use of repetitive-element-sequence polymerase chain reaction. *Clin. Infect. Dis.*, **20**, (4), 836–841.

284. Burdge, D.R., Noble, M.A., Campbell, M.E., Krell, V.L. and Speert, D.P. (1995) *Xanthomonas maltophilia* misidentified as *Pseudomonas cepacia* in cultures of sputum from patients with cystic fibrosis: A diagnostic pitfall with major clinical implications. *Clin. Infect. Dis.*, **20**, (2), 445–448.

285. Denton, M., Todd, N.J. and Littlewood, J.M. (1996) Role of anti-pseudomonal antibiotics in the emergence of *Stenotrophomonas maltophilia* in cystic fibrosis patients. *Eur. J. Clin. Microbiol. Infect. Dis.*, **15**, (5), 402–405.

286. Demko, C.A., Stern, R.C. and Doershuk, C.F. (1998) *Stenotrophomonas maltophilia* in cystic fibrosis: Incidence and prevalence. *Pediatr. Pulmonol.*, **25**, 304–308.

287. Hjelte, L., Petrini, B., Kallenius, G. and Strandvik, B. (1990) Prospective study of mycobacterial infections in patients with cystic fibrosis. *Thorax*, **45**, (5), 397–400.

288. Boxerbaum, B. (1980) Isolation of rapidly growing mycobacteria in patients with cystic fibrosis. *J. Pediatr.*, **96**, 689–691.

289. Smith, M.J., Efthimiou, J., Hodson, M. and Batten, J.C. (1984) Mycobacterial isolations in young adults with cystic fibrosis. *Thorax*, **39**, 369–375.

290. Mulherin, D., Coffey, M.J., Halloran, D.O., Keogan, M.T. and Fitzgerald, M.X. (1990) Skin reactivity to atypical mycobacteria in cystic fibrosis. *Resp. Med.*, **84**, (4), 273–276.

291. Kilby, J.M., Gilligan, P.H., Yankaskas, J.R., Highsmith, W.E., Edwards, L.J. and Knowles, M.R. (1992) Nontuberculous mycobacteria in adult patients with cystic fibrosis. *Chest*, **102**, (l), 70–75.

292. Efthimiou, J., Smith, M.J., Hodson, M.E. and Batten, J.C. (1984) Fatal pulmonary infection with *Mycobacterium fortuitum* in cystic fibrosis. *Br. J. Dis. Chest*, **78**, 299–302.

293. Hjelt, K., Hojlyng, N., Howitz, P. *et al.* (1994) The role of mycobacteria other than tuberculosis (MOTT) in patients with cystic fibrosis. *Scand. J. Infect. Dis.*, **26**, (5), 569–576.

294. Aitken, M.L., Burke, W., Mcdonald, G., Wallis, C., Ramsey, B. and Nolan, C. (1993) Nontuberculous mycobacterial disease in adult cystic fibrosis patients. *Chest*, **103**, (4), 1096–1099.

295. Mearns, M., Longbottom, J. and Batten, J. (1967) Precipitating antibodies to *Aspergillus fumigatus* in cystic fibrosis. *Lancet*, **1**, 538–539.

296. Knutsen, A.P. and Slavin, R.G. (1991) Allergic bronchopulmonary aspergillosis in patients with cystic fibrosis. *Clin. Rev. Allergy.*, **9**, (1–2), 103–118.

297. Batten, J.C. (1967) Allergic aspergillosis in cystic fibrosis. *Mod. Probl. Pediatr.*, **10**, 227–236.

298. Vazquez, C., Elorz, J., Sojo, A. *et al.* (1993) Immune response to *Pseudomonas aeruginosa* but not to *Aspergillus fumigatus* is independently correlated with pulmonary status in cystic fibrosis, in *Clinical Ecology of Cystic Fibrosis*, (ed. H. Escobar, C.F. Baquero and L. Suarez), Excerpta Medica, Amsterdam, pp. 157–161.

299. Carswell, F. and Hamilton, A. (1990) Pathogenesis and management of aspergillosis in cystic fibrosis. *Arch. Dis. Child.*, **65**, (11), 1288.

300. Edwards, J.H., Alfaham, M., Fifield, R., Philpot, C., Clement, M.J. and Goodchild, M.C. (1990) Sequential serological responses to *Aspergillus fumigatus* in patients with cystic fibrosis – use of antigen stretching to delineate IgG and IgE activity. *Clin. Exp. Immunol.*, **81**, (1), 101–108.

301. Knutsen, A.P., Hutcheson, P.S., Mueller, K.R. and Slavin, R.G. (1990) Serum immunoglobulin-E and immunoglobulin-G anti-*Aspergillus fumigatus* antibody in patients with cystic fibrosis who have allergic bronchopulmonary aspergillosis. *J. Lab. Clin. Med.*, **116**, (5), 724–727.

302. Hutcheson, P.S., Rejent, A.J. and Slavin, R.G. (1991) Variability in parameters of allergic bronchopulmonary aspergillosis in patients with cystic fibrosis. *J. Allerg. Clin. Immunol.*, **88**, (3), 390–394.

303. Hiller, E.J. (1990) Pathogenesis and management of aspergillosis in cystic fibrosis. *Arch. Dis. Child.*, **65**, (4), 397–398.

304. Maguire, S., Moriarty, P., Tempany, E. and FitzGerald, M. (1988) Unusual clustering of allergic bronchopulmonary aspergillosis in children with cystic fibrosis. *J. Pediatr.*, **82**, 835–839.

305. Maguire, C.P., Hayes, J.P., Hayes, M., Masterson, J. and Fitzgerald, M.X. (1995) Three cases of pulmonary aspergilloma in adult patients with cystic fibrosis. *Thorax*, **50**, (7), 805–806.

306. Pinel, C., Grillot, R., Gout, J.P., Lebeau, B., Bost, M. and Ambroisethomas, P. (1991) Cystic fibrosis and allergic bronchopulmonary aspergillosis. *Pathol. Biol.*, **39**, (6), 617–620.

307. Simmonds, E.J., Littlewood, J.M. and Evans, E.G.V. (1990) Cystic fibrosis and allergic bronchopulmonary aspergillosis. *Arch. Dis. Child.*, **65**, (5), 507–511.

308. Knutsen, A.P., Mueller, K.R., Hutcheson, P.S., and Slavin, R.G. (1994) Serum anti-*Aspergillus fumigatus* antibodies by immunoblot and ELISA in cystic fibrosis with allergic bronchopulmonary aspergillosis. *J. Allerg. Clin. Immunol.*, **93**, (5), 926–931.

309. Eldahr, J.M., Fink, R., Selden, R., Arruda, L.K., Plattsmills, T.A.E. and Heymann, P.W. (1994) Development of immune responses to *Aspergillus* at an early age in children with cystic fibrosis. *Am. J. Respir. Crit. Care Med.*, **150**, (6), 1513–1518.

310. Nikolaizik, Y.M., Moser, M., Crameri, R. *et al.* (1995) Identification of allergic bronchopulmonary aspergillosis in cystic fibrosis patients by recombinant *Aspergillus fumigatus* I/a-specific serology. *Am. J. Respir. Crit. Care Med.*, **152**, (2), 634–639.

311. Skov, M., Pressler, T., Jensen, H.E., Høiby, N. and Koch, C. (1999) Specific IgG subclass antibody pattern to *Aspergillus fumigatus* in patients with cystic fibrosis with allergic bronchopulmonary aspergillosis (ABPA). *Thorax*, **54**, 44–50.

312. Denning, D.W., Vanwye, J.E., Lewiston, N.J. and Stevens, D.A. (1991) Adjunctive therapy of allergic bronchopulmonary aspergillosis with itraconazole. *Chest*, **100**, (3), 813–819.

313. Zuelzer, W.W. and Newton, W.A. Jr (1949) The pathogenesis of fibrocystic disease of the pancreas. *Pediatrics*, **4**, 53–69.

314. Bodian, M., Norman, A.P. and Carter, C.O. (1952) A congenital disorder of mucus production – mucosis, in Fibrocystic Disease of the Pancreas, (ed. M. Bodian), Heineman, William, Medical Books Ltd, London, pp. 1–241.

315. Esterly, J.R. and Oppenheimer, E.H. (1968) Observations in cystic fibrosis of the pancreas. III. Pulmonary lesions. *Johns Hopkins Med. J.*, **122**, 94–101.

316. Margaretten, W., Nakai, H. and Landing, B.H. (1961) Significance of selective vasculitis and the 'Bone-marrow' syndrome in *Pseudomonas* septicemia. *NEJM*, **265**, 773–776.

317. Iacocca, V.F., Sibinga, M.S. and Barbero, G.J. (1963) Respiratory tract bacteriology in cystic fibrosis. *Am. J. Dis. Child.*, **106**, 315–324.

318. May, J.R., Herrick, N.C. and Thompson, D. (1972) Bacterial infection in cystic fibrosis. *Arch. Dis. Child.*, **47**, 908–913.

319. Lloyd-Still, J.D., Khaw, K.-T. and Shwachman, H. (1974) Severe respiratory disease in infants with cystic fibrosis. *Pediatrics*, **53**, 678–682.

320. Harrison, G.M. and Doggett, R.G. (1975) Terminal sputum flora in patients with cystic fibrosis. *CF Quart. Ann. Ref.* **XIII**, 30.

321. Mitchell-Heggs, P., Mearns, M. and Batten, J.C. (1976) Cystic fibrosis in adolescents and adults. *Quart. J. Med.*, **45**, 479–504.

322. Bedrossian, C.W.M., Greenberg, S.D., Singer, D.B., Hansen, J.J. and Rosenberg, H.S. (1976) A quantitative study including prevalence of pathologic findings among different age groups. *Hum. Pathol.*, **7**, 195–204.

323. Høiby, N. (1991) Cystic fibrosis: infection. *Schweiz. Med. Wschr.*. **121**, (4), 105–109.

324. Hodson, M.E., Penketh, A.R.L. and Batten, J.C. (1981) Aerosol carbenicillin and gentamicin treatment of *Pseudomonas aeruginosa* infection in patients with cystic fibrosis. *Lancet*, **ii**, 1137–1139.

325. Jensen, T., Pedersen, S.S., Garne, S., Heilmann, C., Høiby, N. and Koch, C. (1987) Colistin inhalation therapy in cystic fibrosis patients with chronic *Pseudomonas aeruginosa* lung infection. *J. Antimicrob. Chemother.*, **19**, 831–838.

326. Ramsey, B.W., Dorkin, H.L., Eisenberg, J.D. *et al.* (1993) Efficacy of aerosolized tobramycin in patients with cystic fibrosis. *NEJM*, **328**, (24), 1740–1746.

326a Ramsey, B., Pepe, M.S., Quan, J.M. *et al.* (1999) Intermittent administration of inhaled tobramycin in patients with cystic fibrosis. *NEJM*, **340**, 23–30.

326b. Vic, P., Ategbo, S., Turck, D. *et al.* (1998) Efficacy, tolerance, and pharmacokinetics of once daily tobramycin for pseudomonas exacerbations in cystic fibrosis. *Arch. Dis. Child.*, **78**, 536–539.

326c. Smith, A.L., Doershuk, C., Goldmann, D. *et al.* (1999) Comparison of a β-lactam alone versus a β-lactam and an aminoglycoside for pulmonary exacerbation in cystic fibrosis. *J. Pediatr.*, **134**, 413–421.

327. Szaff, M., Høiby, N., Flensborg, E.W. (1983) Frequent antibiotic therapy improves survival of cystic fibrosis patients with chronic *Pseudomonas aeruginosa* infection. *Acta Paediat. Scand.*, **72**, 651–657.

328. Woods, D.E., Straus, D.C., Johanson, W.G. Jr, Berry, V.K. and Bass, J.A. (1980) Role of pili in adherence of *Pseudomonas aeruginosa* to mammalian buccal epithelial cells. *Infect. Immun.*, **29**, 1146–1151.

329. Pedersen, S.S., Høiby, N., Espersen, F. and Kharazmi, A. (1991) Alginate and infection, in Pseudomonas aeruginosa *in Human Disease*, (ed. J.Y. Homma, H. Tanimoto, I.A. Holder, N. Høiby and G. Döring), *Antibiot. Chemother.*, **44**, 68–79.

330. Fomsgaard, A., Høiby, N., Shand, G.H., Conrad, R.S. and Galanos, C. (1988) Longitudinal study of antibody response to lipopolysaccharides during chronic *Pseudomonas aeruginosa* lung infection in cystic fibrosis. *Infect. Immun.*, **56**, 2270–2278.

331. Pitt, T.L.(1989) Lipopolysaccharide and virulence of *Pseudomonas aeruginosa*, in Pseudomonas aeruginosa *Infection*, (eds N. Høiby, S.S. Pedersen, G.H. Shand, G. Döring and I.A. Holder), *Antibiot. Chemother.*, **42**, 1–7.

332. Lutz, F., Xiong, G., Jungblut, R., Orlik-Eisel, G., Göbel-Reifert, A. and Leidolf, R. (1991) Pore-forming cytotoxin of *Pseudomonas aeruginosa*: Molecular effects and aspects of pathogenicity, in: Pseudomonas aeruginosa *in Human Disease*, (eds J.Y. Homma, H. Tanimoto, I.A. Holder, N. Høiby and G. Döring), *Antibiot. Chemother.*, **44**, 54–58.

333. Vasil, M., Graham, L.M., Ostroff, R.M., Shortride, V.D. and Vasil, A.I. (1991) Phospholipase C: Molecular biology and contribution to the pathogenesis of *Pseudomonas aeruginosa*, in Pseudomonas aeruginosa *in Human Disease*, (eds J.Y. Homma, H. Tanimoto, I.A. Holder, N. Høiby and G. Döring), *Antibiot. Chemother.*, **44**, 34–47.

334. Saelinger, C.B. and Morris, R.E. (1987) Intracellular trafficking of *Pseudomonas* exotoxin A, in: *Basic Research and Clinical Aspects of* Pseudomonas aeruginosa, (eds G. Döring, I.A. Holder and K.Botzenhart), *Antibiot. Chemother.*, **39**, 149–159.

335. Woods, D.E., To, M. and Sokol, P.A. (1989) *Pseudomonas aeruginosa* exoenzyme S as a pathogenic determinant in respiratory infections, in Pseudomonas aeruginosa *Infection*, (eds N. Høiby, S.S. Pedersen, G.H. Shand, G. Döring and I.A. Holder), *Antibiot. Chemother.*, **42**, 27–35.

336. Tosi, M.F., Zakem, H. and Berger, M. (1990) Neutrophil elastase cleaves C3Bi on opsonized *Pseudomonas* as well as Crl on neutrophils to create a functionally important opsonin receptor mismatch. *J. Clin. Invest.*, **86**, (I), 300–308.

337. Döring, G., Goldstein, W., Schiøtz, P.O., Høiby, N., Dasgupta, M. amd Botzenhart, K. (1986) Elastase from polymorphonuelear leukocytes – a regulatory enzyme in immune complex disease. *Clin. Exp. Immunol.*, **64**, 597–605.

338. Johansen, H.K., Nir, M., Høiby, N., Koch, C. and Schwartz, M. (1991) Severity of cystic fibrosis in patients homozygous and heterozygous for DeltaF508 mutation. *Lancet*, **337**, 631–634.

339. Döring, G., Krogh, Johansen, H., Weidinger, S. and Hø, N. (1994) Allotypes of alpha-l-antitrypsin in patients with cystic fibrosis, homozygous for deltaF508. *Pediatr. Pulmonol.*, **18**, 3–7.

340. Garred, P., Pressler, T., Madsen, H.O. *et al.* (1999) Association of mannose-binding lectin gene heterogeneity with severity of lung disease and survival in cystic fibrosis. *J. Clin. Invest.*, **104**, 431–437.

341. Ojeniyi, B., Frederiksen, B., Høiby, N. (2000) *Pseudomonas aeruginosa* cross-infection among patients with cystic fibrosis during a winter camp. *Pediatr. Pulmonol.* **29**, 177–181.

6

Immunology of cystic fibrosis

G. DÖRING, G. BELLON AND R. KNIGHT

Introduction	109	The lymphocyte response	122
Host factors in bacterial airway colonization	110	Cytokines	123
Bacterial phenotypes in acute and chronic lung infection	113	Nitric oxide	124
The humoral immune response: antibody production and		Immunological strategies for therapy and prevention	124
immune complexes	115	Summary	127
Neutrophil activation	117	References	127
Bronchial hyperreactivity and allergic bronchopulmonary			
aspergillosis (ABPA)	121		

INTRODUCTION

Damage to host defense barriers such as the skin and mucous membranes allows microorganisms access to the internal environment of the host. In response to chemoattractants produced by the host and the invading microorganisms, phagocytic cells such as polymorphonuclear leukocytes (or neutrophils) and macrophages reach the infected site. Antigen presentation by macrophages and dendritic cells leads to activation and proliferation of the helper T cells and eventually antibody production and cell-mediated cytotoxicity.

The complex cellular interactions, which are a feature of the generation of an immune effector response, are mediated by a large number of chemical agents. These include enzymes, interleukins, interferons and peptide hormones. One theme of this chapter is the possibility that some of these mediators, if produced in sufficient amounts for a sufficient time, can have effects outside the immune system itself and may directly damage the lung.

If the injury and infection are trivial, there are no systemic symptoms other than minor discomfort at the site of the injury. When the infection is systemic (for example, influenza) the patient feels subjectively unwell in ways similar to noninfected patients receiving interleukin or interferon therapy. In other words, the subjec-

tive pathology is produced by the immune response and not by the infection *per se*. In both these cases, of course, the immune response is normally successful in eradicating the invading microorganisms and promoting healing.

In a chronic infective disease such as cystic fibrosis (CF), however, the immune system is clearly ineffective in regaining sterility. Since it retains the ability to react to the persisting microorganisms, chronic infective disease is also chronic inflammatory disease. One of the themes of this chapter is that chronic inflammation and its soluble products, as well as having beneficial effects in achieving a host–parasite equilibrium, can also be actively harmful and, in the context of CF, can contribute to lung pathology. We need to consider, therefore, not only antibiotic and other strategies that minimize infection, but also ways by which these pathogenic effects of chronic inflammation may be reduced.

It is interesting how ideas on the role of inflammation in CF have come full circle. The apparent inability of the immune system to keep the airways free of bacterial pathogens led to early speculation that the then unknown genetic abnormality causes an immunological defect and that CF was, in fact, an immunological disorder (reviewed in ref. [1]). With the knowledge that the CF gene codes for an epithelial ion-transport protein (see Chapter 4), and extensive data showing essentially normal systemic immune function in CF, immunology of

CF was regarded no differently from the immunology of any chronic infection. However, recent data suggest again that CF respiratory epithelial cells differ from epithelial cells from normal individuals with regard to inflammation control. The consequences of these findings – if confirmed – imply that before onset of infection, inflammation may be present in CF airways, triggering infection. Thereafter, the chronicity of the infection and the chronic inflammatory response it induces mean that potent inflammatory products are constantly present in the airways. These have the potential for damaging not only airway cells but also cells of the inflammatory infiltrate. This, in turn, contributes to the chronicity of bacterial infection, a situation which indeed deserves the description of 'vicious cycle'[2].

Understanding of the chronic immunological reactions occurring in the CF lung is as important as investigations of other fields of CF research, since anti-inflammatory agents may well have clinical benefit. Moreover, knowledge of which particular inflammatory products are contributing to the disease pathology will allow more selective anti-inflammatory intervention, rather than risking the side-effects associated with potent but unselective anti-inflammatories such as steroids.

The immunology of CF is, therefore, a particular example of the immunology of the host–parasite relationship, and the present chapter will focus on:

1. host and bacterial factors leading to bacterial colonization, and subsequently to acute and chronic infection;
2. the humoral and cellular immune response against the major pathogens, particularly *Staphylococcus aureus* and *Pseudomonas aeruginosa*; and
3. based on this analysis, on new immunological treatment and prevention strategies for infection and inflammation in CF.

HOST FACTORS IN BACTERIAL AIRWAY COLONIZATION

Mucosal surfaces are the major portals of entry for microbes into the human host. To maintain sterile lungs, the mucosal or secretory immune system acts in concert with the constituents of the nonspecific (or innate) immune system, including secretory IgA, lymphocytes, sessile alveolar macrophages, mast cells, mobile neutrophils, antimicrobial peptides and proteins, complement components and the mucociliary clearance system. The secretory immune system generally clears bacterial organisms such as *P. aeruginosa* rapidly, even when large doses are administered to normal lungs[3]. This rapid clearance is mostly due to the influx of neutrophils which, as an immediate response to bacterial infection, reach the involved tissue site in high numbers within hours[4], eliminate the pathogens by phagocytosis and disappear by apoptosis[5]. What are the reasons that this does not happen in CF airways? Although much has been learned, due to the complexity of the immune system and the lack of suitable animal models for CF (CF mice do not show the characteristic signs of chronic lung infection), the answer to this question is still not clear. Several hypotheses have been proposed, as follows.

Inflammation precedes bacterial lung infection

The CF lung is regarded as being essentially normal *in utero* and shortly after birth[6]. Already in the first months of life, however, inflammatory infiltrates in bronchi and mucopurulent plugging of airways can be detected histologically[7]. Both the number of neutrophils and levels of a neutrophil-attracting interleukin (IL), IL-8, were increased in bronchoalveolar lavage (BAL) of CF infants as young as 4 weeks who had negative cultures for common bacterial CF-related pathogens[8,9]. Most probably, the neutrophils detected in BAL fluids are activated, since increased levels of the neutrophil lysosomal enzyme elastase have also been measured in plasma samples of uninfected CF infants[8] (Fig. 6.1). Further support for this hypothesis comes from a study in CF mice raised in a germ-free environment, which showed signs of inflammation[10]. Additionally, CF BAL fluids contain low levels of IL-10, a cytokine which decreases proinflammatory mechanisms[11], probably because CF bronchial epithelial cells do not produce IL-10 in sufficient amounts[12]. These observations strongly suggest (but do not rigorously prove) that airway inflammation is already present before the onset of infection.

However, other groups have not confirmed these findings. For instance, differences between CF and normal individuals concerning IL-10 BAL concentrations have not been detected[13]. Furthermore, since large regional variability of lung infection and inflammation is present in different lung lobes, sampling of BAL fluids in the left lobe may yield inflammatory markers yet no bacterial organisms, whereas both can be found in the upper right lobe[14]. Finally, in a study of 46 newly diagnosed CF infants under the age of 6 months, inflammatory BAL markers correlated with the presence of infection and decreased when pathogens were eradicated or were absent in uninfected patients[15].

How does inflammation relate to infection? Neutrophil activation, characterized by lysosomal enzyme release and enhanced production of reactive oxygen species, may facilitate bacterial infection. There is a large body of evidence that release of host proteinases during acute and chronic infection may damage epithelial cells[16–18] thereby facilitating *P. aeruginosa* adhesion *in vitro* and *in vivo*[16,19–21]. If damaged tissues are remodeled, *P. aeruginosa* may bind to them avidly[22].

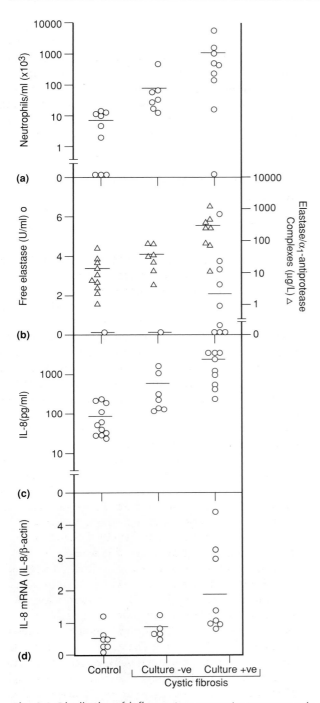

The reason for the increased influx of blood neutrophils into the CF airways without an infectious stimulus is unclear. It may be a result of airway gland obstruction as a consequence of the basic defect (see Chapter 4). However, irrespective of which view is taken, at a very early age most CF patients show signs of lung inflammation[9,15,23–24] which persists even in mildly affected and stable patients[25].

Different membrane composition of CF epithelial airway cells

Several observations argue for an increased binding of bacterial pathogens to CF epithelial cells. Increased or different sulfation of the glycocalix of CF epithelial cells has been demonstrated[26–29] which may facilitate binding of *S. aureus*[30,31]. Furthermore, it has been proposed that the apical membrane of CF bronchial epithelial cells is undersialylated[32]. Both findings have been linked to the hypothesis that CFTR functions in the endosomal compartment as a cAMP-regulated CF channel that regulates endosomal acidification[32]. Since many pathogenic bacteria bind to asialoganglioside 1 (aGM1)[33], this hypothesis would predict increased binding of *S. aureus* or *P. aeruginosa* to CF bronchial epithelial cells, which indeed has been demonstrated [34,35].

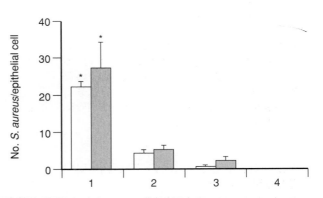

Fig. 6.1 *Distribution of inflammatory parameter measurements in infants with CF, expressed according to their BALF bacterial and viral culture results.* **(a)** *Neutrophils per milliliter in the BALF.* **(b)** *Free elastase and elastase/α₁-antiprotease complexes.* **(c)** *IL-8 protein in the cell-free BALF.* **(d)** *Macrophage IL-8 mRNA levels. The culture-negative group was defined as subjects with no growth (<200 cfu/mL of BALF), while the culture-positive group was defined as subjects with >200 cfu/mL of BALF. The bars represent the means of each measurement. The P values for the negative infants compared to the disease control group were as follows: (1) neutrophil count: P = 0.04; (2) elastase/α₁-antiprotease complexes: P = 0.05; (3) IL-8: P = 0.003. (Reproduced with permission from ref. 8)*

Fig. 6.2 *Adherence of* S. aureus *to primary nasal epithelial cell balls of five patients with cystic fibrosis (CF) (open columns) and five normal healthy individuals (N) (closed columns). Nonwashed (with mucus) (1) and washed (without mucus) (2) cell balls were incubated with* S. aureus *for 2 h, nonadherent bacteria were removed using a cell strainer and centrifugation, and adherent bacteria quantified by scanning electron microscopy. 1: Unwashed cell balls; 2: washed, mucus-depleted cell balls; 3: cell balls, treated with 1 μg/mL neutrophil elastase prior to bacterial incubation; 4: cell balls, treated with 1 μg/mL neutrophil elastase after bacterial incubation. For quantification of adherent bacteria, about 500 cells from 10 cell balls were examined. Values represent means ± SD of five independent experiments for each of the individuals. *, CF 1–2, P < 0.001; N, CF 1–2, P < 0.007; Student's t-test. (Reproduced with permission from ref. 38.)*

However, in other studies this notion has not been confirmed[36], and significant differences in binding of *S. aureus*[37,38] or *P. aeruginosa*[39] to primary epithelial cells from CF patients and healthy individuals were not detected (Fig. 6.2).

Impaired mucociliary clearance

A number of studies demonstrated that *S. aureus*[38,40–43], *P. aeruginosa*[44,45], *Burkholderia cepacia*[46] or *Haemophilus influenzae*[47] bind to respiratory mucins (Fig. 6.3). Significantly less binding is observed when mucus-producing cell balls of primary nasal epithelial cells from CF patients or healthy normal individuals are mucus depleted[38] (Fig. 6.2). Further support for this notion comes from the same study in which *S. aureus* was located in CF airways by immunofluorescence[38]. Only a negligible amount of *S. aureus* cells were adherent to the lung epithelium, whereas nearly all bacteria were found embedded in the mucus, distant from the epithelium. Provided that bacterial pathogens preferentially bind to the mucus layer on top of ciliated cells which cover most of the upper respiratory tract, defects in mucociliary clearance (see Chapter 4) allow rapid bacterial multiplication followed by infection. Defective mucociliary clearance proposed in CF patients has also been demonstrated in CF mice[10]. The nature of the factors that are responsible for impaired mucociliary clearance in CF are still a matter of debate (see Chapter 4).

Mutated CFTR

A direct connection between mutations in CFTR and bacterial lung infections was provided by the findings that normal CFTR functions as an epithelial cell receptor for *P. aeruginosa*[48,49] which also endocytoses bound *P. aeruginosa*, followed by intracellular killing of the pathogen. Since mutant CFTR (ΔF_{508}) does not bind *P. aeruginosa*, the organism would accumulate in the airway lumen, leading to infection[48,49]. In contrast to *P. aeruginosa*, *B. cepacia* may invade airway epithelial cells and resist killing[50]. Interestingly, certain CFTR mutations may predispose CF patients to chronic airways' colonization with *P. aeruginosa*[51].

Abnormal sodium chloride concentrations in CF airway epithelial lining fluids

This attractive hypothesis also links the basic CF defect to the bacterial lung infection. It is based on the observations that cultured airway cells of normal individuals killed bacteria, whereas cells from CF patients did not, and that addition of salt to the bathing fluid on the apical membrane of normal cells prevented killing whereas dilution of this fluid from CF cells became bactericidal[52]. This led to the investigation of the salt-sensitive human antimicrobial peptides such as β-defensin in human airways[53,54]. Although the *in vitro* results showed high significance and the CF defect in bacterial killing was mimicked in a human bronchial xenograft model[54], the

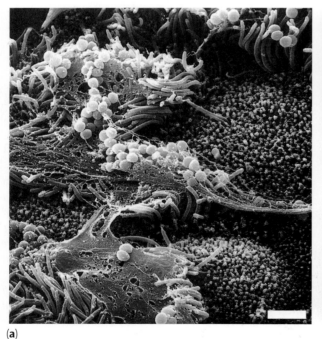

(a)

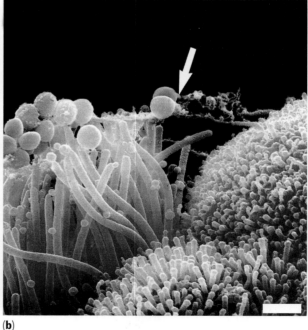

(b)

Fig. 6.3 *Scanning electron micrograph of primary nasal epithelial cells of a cystic fibrosis patient* (**a**) *and a healthy individual* (**b**), *grown as three-dimensional cell balls. Unwashed cell balls were inoculated with* S. aureus *for 2 hours.* S. aureus *can be seen adhering to mucus on cell balls. Note the* S. aureus-*free membranes. Magnifications:* (**a**), ×5000; (**b**), ×8000. *Bars:* (**a**) 1.5μm; (**b**) 1.3μm. *(Reproduced with permission from ref. 38.)*

major problem which prevents the unequivocal acceptance of this hypothesis is a clear demonstration of the abnormally high salt concentrations in CF airways[55]. In contrast to this hypothesis are findings of an increased sodium reabsorption into CF bronchial cells, leading to hypotonic epithelial lining fluids[56].

Impaired neutrophil functions

Neutrophils are the predominant phagocytic cells in CF lung infections. Do neutrophils reach the airways in time? Neutrophils released from the marrow leave the circulation in response to chemoattractants which stimulate the cell via specific cell receptors. They adhere to the endothelial cells lining the blood vessels through integrins and then move through the space between the endothelial cells by a process known as diapedesis. They then move directly to the site of infection along a chemotactic gradient. In human newborns decreased neutrophil chemotaxis until the age of 2 years[57,58] is caused by a reduced number of C3bi receptors (CD11b) on the neutrophil surface. Studies in infant animals show that pulmonary bacterial infections may be due to delayed recruitment of neutrophils into the airways[59,60]. Similarly, a delayed influx of neutrophils soon after birth in CF babies may facilitate bacterial lung infection. Furthermore, based on the hypothesis that CF airway epithelial lining fluids may be hypotonic[56], neutrophils may only function suboptimally[61].

Taken together, several mechanisms, including lung inflammation, altered cell-surface composition, impaired mucociliary clearance, mutated CFTR, inactivated defensins and immature neutrophil function may act together and cause the increased colonization and reduced clearance of microorganisms in the CF lungs.

BACTERIAL PHENOTYPES IN ACUTE AND CHRONIC LUNG INFECTION

During initial colonization and subsequent acute infection with *P. aeruginosa* many of its enzymes and other compounds may act as virulence determinants, and *P.* *aeruginosa* virulence is generally regarded as being multifactorial. It is not within the scope of this chapter to discuss in detail all of these; the interested reader is referred to excellent reviews on their structure, biochemical function and their putative role in infection[62-64]. In general, one can distinguish, first, extracellular or membrane-bound protein toxins which will elicit a specific antibody response shortly after onset of infection and thus will be neutralized or inactivated. Second, there are low molecular weight secondary metabolites which will escape immune recognition and which therefore may be active in the chronic state of the infection. These include rhamnolipids which may act as cell detergents and impair macrophage function[65,66], pyoverdin which scavenges iron[67] and phenacin pigments which may act as T-cell modulators (see section on The lymphocyte response, p. 122) or scavenge oxygen radicals[62-64,68].

Although many pathological effects in the chronic CF lung pathology have been directly attributed to *P. aeruginosa* protein toxins, up to now no one has isolated a free bacterial toxin from *P. aeruginosa*-infected CF sputum or BAL fluids. Most likely, specific antibodies to *P. aeruginosa*, e.g. alkaline protease and elastase, neutralize these enzymatic activities[69] and both antigens have been detected in immune complexes, isolated from CF sputa (Table 6.1)[70].

Thus, cleavage of immunoglobulins, complement components, transferrin, cytokines and cell-surface receptors on immunocompetent cells, etc. by *P. aeruginosa* proteinases, which has been demonstrated *in vitro* or in animal models, may, at most, take place only very early after lung colonization when antibodies are lacking. Indeed, free *P. aeruginosa* alkaline proteinase and elastase have only been detected in bronchial secretions of the minority of CF patients who lack antibodies to them[71]. Similarly, only early in infection and in the absence of antibodies will *P. aeruginosa* lipopolysaccharide (LPS) trigger airway mucus secretion[72], exoenzyme S stimulate lymphocytes[73] and exotoxin A, the most toxic enzyme of *P. aeruginosa*, induce cell necrosis[74]. Moreover, exotoxin A is not only neutralized by specific antibodies, but also readily cleaved by neutrophil elastase and thus may not induce toxicity in the highly proteolytic

Table 6.1 *Immune complexes (IC) containing* Pseudomonas aeruginosa *alkaline protease (AP) or elastase (ELA) in sputum samples of cystic fibrosis patients*

Patients	Sputum IC (mg AHG/mL)	Proteases (ng/mL)		Proteases in IC after cleavage (ng/mL)	
		AP	ELA	AP	ELA
1	16.5	–	–	32	>22
2	3.0	–	–	200	>40
3	3.4	–	–	60	>10
4	6.4	–	–	20	>6

With changes from ref. 70.

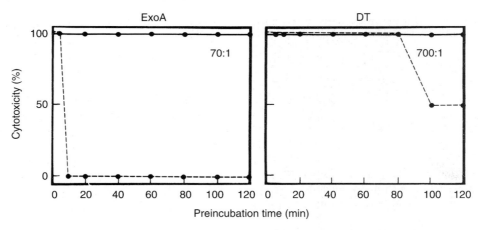

Fig. 6.4 *Influence of PMN enzymes on cytotoxicity of diphtheria toxin (DT) and exotoxin A (Exo A). Exo A (16 ng) or DT (1.6 ng) were incubated with PMN elastase at the indicated ratio (w/w) for various periods and the reaction mixtures then added to 2 ×10⁴ Chinese hamster ovary (CHO) cells. Cytotoxicity was assessed after 3–4 days by medium color change and by cell counting after trypsin treatment in the Neubauer cell chamber. Values represent means of six values in three independent assays. SD was < 20%. The lower limit of the CHO cell assay was about 10 ng for Exo A and about 1 ng for DT. ----, Toxin : PMN elastase incubations; ———, toxin controls. (Reproduced with permission from ref. 154.)*

environment of the CF airways (Fig. 6.4)[75] even when expressed there in considerable quantities[76].

Bacteria sense their environment and may change their phenotype accordingly. The questions of which environmental (or host) factors determine the bacterial phenotype, and how this phenotype is characterized, are of considerable importance in general, and particularly in the CF airways. Transcript analysis of known virulence factors[76,77] and the isolation of genes induced by host factors[78] are potential methods for investigating this problem.

A pathogenically important phenotypic switch of *P. aeruginosa* during the course of chronic infection is the conversion from a nonmucoid to a mucoid strain[79,80]. Several mechanisms have been proposed for this switch, including mutation[81,82] hydrogen peroxide (H_2O_2)[83], nutrient deprivation[84], elevated osmolarity[85], dehydration[86] or energy inhibition[87]. Whereas one study suggested that oxygen selects for mucoid growth of *P. aeruginosa*[88,89], interestingly mucosity is maintained *in vitro* under strict anaerobic growth conditions in the presence of nitrate[90]. High nitrate levels have been detected in CF sputa[90], possibly derived from neutrophils[91], which may be used by *P. aeruginosa* for anaerobic respiration and concomitant alginate production[90].

The production of mucoid exopolysaccharide (alginate) has the effect of enlarging the bacterial surface many times, rendering phagocytosis inefficient[92,93]. Additionally, alginate is a negatively charged polyuronic acid which could enhance electronegative repulsive forces between the bacterium and the phagocyte[93]. Thus, in experimental animal models mucoid strains persist more than nonmucoid variant[94].

The production of alginate is costly for *P. aeruginosa* and various genes are involved[79]. However, besides reducing engulfment by phagocytes, alginate also confers on the pathogen a unique resistance against extracellularly released weapons of phagocytes. Professional phagocytes such as neutrophils are equipped mainly with three different kinds of weapons: reactive oxygen species[95,96], antimicrobial substances with molecular masses of 2–750 kDa[97] and proteolytic enzymes (see below). Alginate is a sink for reactive oxygen species[98] and even restricts diffusion of oxygen[90]. Alginate also protects *P. aeruginosa* against highly positively charged antimicrobial peptides and proteins, possibly due to its negative surface charge. However, although nonmucoid *P. aeruginosa* is readily killed by activated neutrophils[99], nonmucoid *B. cepacia* is resistant to oxidative killing by neutrophils[99]. Alginate also protects *P. aeruginosa* against highly positively charged antimicrobial peptides and proteins, possibly due to its negative surface charge.

Finally, mucoid *P. aeruginosa* profits directly from host serine proteinases, since these enzymes may provide the split products of proteins for bacterial growth. A comparison of substrate specificities of proteases of *P. aeruginosa* and neutrophil origin supports this hypothesis[100], which may also explain why persisting auxotrophic mutants of *P. aeruginosa* (i.e. mutants requiring amino acids for growth) are often found in CF lung infection[101]. Furthermore, other neutrophil and lymphocyte functions[102] may be suppressed by alginate.

Until recently less was known about the phenotype of *S. aureus* in CF airways. In contrast to the exopolysaccharide-producing *P. aeruginosa* phenotype, *S. aureus* cells were known to produce only small polysaccharide capsules and it remained puzzling why the large number of neutrophils were unable to eliminate these pathogens. Furthermore, *S. aureus* loses its capsular polysaccharide (CP) type 5 (and possibly also other CPs) in the CF air-

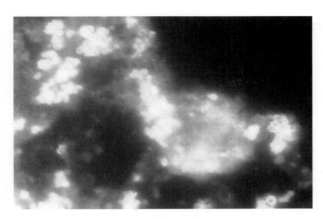

Fig. 6.5 *Production of poly-N-succinyl β-1-6 glucosamine (PNSG) by* S. aureus *in CF airways. Fluorescence micrograph using a rabbit antibody against purified PNSG (Courtesy of Dr. Gerald Pier) and a Cy-3-labeled goat anti-rabbit antibody. White diffuse halo depicts PNSG surrounding multiple* S. aureus *cells.*

ways due to elevated P_{CO_2} (around 4 per cent) compared to normal air (P_{CO_2}: 0.03 per cent)[103]. Without CPs, the major cell wall components of *S. aureus*, protein A and teichoic acid, may play a role in persistence. Protein A, a T-cell independent B-cell mitogen, may bind the Fc part of immunoglobulins, thereby impairing phagocytosis. Teichoic acid also binds immunoglobulins avidly (in the Fab region) and the resulting immune complex may activate complement. Since teichoic acid and protein A can be shed, such an activation may occur far from the bacterial surface without harming the pathogen. However, recently it was shown that *S. aureus* synthesized a large surface polysaccharide designated poly-N-succinyl β-1-6 glucosamine (PNSG) in CF airways, which may explain the persistence of the organism in CF patients[104] (Fig. 6.5).

Whether superantigens of *S. aureus* (mitogens that activate T cells in a Vβ-specific manner) are involved as virulence factors in the host–pathogen relationship in CF lung infection has not yet been investigated. The toxic effect of these superantigens (e.g. staphylococcal enterotoxin B (SEB)) is due to their ability to stimulate tumor necrosis factor α (TNFα) production in T cells[105]. Exogenous IL-10 has been shown to inhibit TNFα production by T cells, thereby protecting animals from SEB toxicity[106]. The observation that endogenous IL-10 production is reduced in CF[11,12], may increase the risk of *S. aureus* toxicity due to its superantigens in CF. In mice, challenge with SEB resulted in acute inflammatory lung injury, characterized by a profound increase in vascular permeability. Inflammation was associated with marked neutrophil infiltration and induction of cell adhesion molecules[107]. All of these signs are present in CF patients infected with *S. aureus*. Thus, as with *P. aeruginosa*, transcript analysis of *S. aureus* genes, expressed during infection, may shed more light on the phenotype of this

pathogen *in vivo*. Recently, a method was developed for direct transcript of *S. aureus* from CF sputum using competitive RT-PCR for three *S. aureus* genes[108]. The results suggested that the global gene regulator *agr* is nonessential in CF[108].

Similarly, factors responsible for the virulence of *B. cepacia* are largely unknown. It has been suggested that its virulence is mainly related to its ability to stimulate a fulminant inflammatory response with deleterious consequences for the host (see Chapter 5). Like *P. aeruginosa* and *S. aureus*, *B. cepacia* attracts and activates neutrophils[109], but at the same time the pathogen is highly resistant to neutrophil phagocytosis[99].

THE HUMORAL IMMUNE RESPONSE: ANTIBODY PRODUCTION AND IMMUNE COMPLEXES

As mentioned earlier, bacterial lung infection in CF is not the result of inadequate antibody production by B cells. *Pseudomonas aeruginosa* infection provokes a rapid production of specific antibodies directed to a large number of *P. aeruginosa* antigens in CF patients, as evidenced by radioimmunoassays and enzyme-linked immunosorbent assays [110–120]. Antibody titers may sometimes differ markedly from patient to patient (Fig. 6.6.) which may not necessarily reflect bacterial strain variation between individual patients but rather the individuality of the immune response. Clearly, antibody production contributes substantially to hypergammaglobulinemia in infected CF patients[121].

In many patients, therefore, prolonged antibody production leads to increased titers of immune complexes, detectable in patients' sputa, bronchial secretions or serum samples (reviewed in ref. [122]). Immune complexes are thought to play an important role in the immunopathology of CF, since they can stimulate phagocytes directly or via bound complement components to release lysosomal enzymes, reactive oxygen species and antimicrobial substances, which may lead to host tissue damage. Therefore, not surprisingly, high immune complex levels (and antibody titers) correlate with poor clinical status of the patients[120, 123–130] (Fig. 6.6) as in other diseases characterized by type III hypersensitivity reactions. During exacerbations, immune complex levels may increase due to elevated production of bacterial virulence factors[131].

In contrast with *P. aeruginosa*, elevated antibody titers against *S. aureus* antigens in CF sera have not been described, suggesting that either *S. aureus* has developed successful strategies for avoiding immunological attack or that major antigens have been overlooked. Thus, until now, no certain correlation has been established between antistaphylococcal antibody titers and the severity of pulmonary disease[132]. Antibody titers to *H. influenzae*[132],

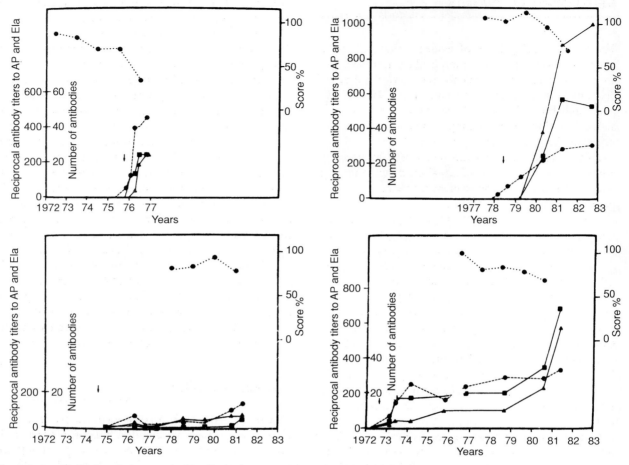

Fig. 6.6 *Longitudinal study (1972–82) of antibody titers to AP, Ela and numbers of precipitins to the St-Ag of* P. aeruginosa *in the sera of four cystic fibrosis patients as determined by radioimmunoassay and crossed immunoelectrophoresis.* ▲—▲ *AP,* ■—■ *Ela,* ●---● *precipitins,* ●·····● *score %. The onset of chronic* P. aeruginosa *infection is indicated by the arrow. (Reproduced with permission from ref. 110.)*

Aspergillus fumigatus[133,134] and *B. cepacia* surface antigens[135,136] have been described.

Some immune complexes formed during the chronic course of the infection do not activate phagocytic cells and rather block this interaction. The antigens involved are polysaccharides of *P. aeruginosa* LPS and alginate (mucoid exopolysaccharide, MEP). Anti-LPS serum IgG antibodies inhibit the phagocytosis of the patient's own *P. aeruginosa* strain by alveolar macrophages[137–140]. Similarly, anti-MEP serum IgG antibodies are nonopsonic[141,142]. These effects are not observed when sera of normal healthy individuals or noninfected CF patients are investigated[137–140]. Based on the results of a longitudinal study[143], the blocking effect tends to increase during the course of the infection. Furthermore, the effect is not specific for CF patients[144,145]. This points to a subclass shift of the respective antibodies during the course of *P. aeruginosa* infection.

Therefore, IgG subclasses of antibodies specific for *P. aeruginosa* LPS (or nonspecific) have been determined in CF sera[146–157]. However, results from subclass determi-

nations differed widely from investigator to investigator and no conclusive evidence has been provided for which IgG subclass is responsible for the blocking effect of CF serum. Some investigators suggested that the blocking effect may be related to the macrophage itself rather than to the opsonizing antibody[158], and receptor expression on alveolar macrophages seems to be critical for functional phagocytosis[159]. The observation that only macrophages but not neutrophils express Fc gamma receptors may explain the sensitivity of macrophages rather than neutrophils to the blocking effect of anti-*P. aeruginosa* antibodies from CF patients[159]. Human alveolar macrophages bind predominantly IgG3[160,161].

Independently of the blocking IgG effect on *P. aeruginosa* phagocytosis by alveolar macrophages, several studies revealed that high levels of the opsonic subclasses IgG2 and IgG3 correlated with poor lung function of the CF patients[150,151,155–157]. Patient-to-patient variation in the degree of lung disease, even in patients homozygous for CFTR ΔF_{508}[162] not only correlated with total IgG titers but also with immunoglobulin allotypes[152].

NEUTROPHIL ACTIVATION

There is a growing body of evidence that the consequences of neutrophil activation in the infected airways are at least partly responsible for respiratory failure and death in CF. Even in adolescents and adults with CF who have mild lung disease and are without symptoms of active infection, there is ample evidence of ongoing inflammation[25]. The inability of the phagocytic cells (i.e. alveolar macrophages or neutrophils) to maintain sterile lungs in CF is not a result of impaired cell function[163]. It rather reflects the capability of microorganisms to persist in an immunocompetent host.

Neutrophils are chemotactically attracted to the site of infection[164]. Chemoattractants responsible for the high neutrophil influx from the vascular space into the tissues are soluble bacterial products resembling N-formylmethionyl-leucyl-phenylalanine[165], activated complement components such as C5a and C5adesArg[166], the product of the lipoxygenase pathway leukotriene B_4 (LTB_4)[167,168], as well as the chemotactic peptide IL-8 (see section on Cytokines, page 123). Other substances with potential importance in this context include the cytokine ENA-78[169], the immunoreactive substance P[170] and the C5a receptor[171]. Up to 10^8 neutrophils per milliliter sputum or BAL fluid may be present in *P. aeruginosa*-infected airways[172,173].

Once the neutrophil has reached the airways it will not return to the circulation and during activation or cell death, lysosomal enzymes may reach the extracellular space. Neutrophils normally die by apoptosis – an active process which prevents release of intracellular contents by surrounding the dying cell with a rigid, cross-linked protein sarcophagus – and the failure of neutrophil apoptosis in the CF airway may result in necrotic cell death with the release of intracellular material. In addition, persistence of the bacterial stimulus contributes to the ongoing release of neutrophil contents and, not surprisingly, several investigators have detected neutrophil enzymes, mainly the serine proteinase elastase, in BAL or sputum samples of CF patients[17,18,24,140,172–177]. Mean values may reach 100 µg neutrophil elastase per mL of sputum supernatant fluid[174]. Due to the local cleavage of the endogenous serine proteinase inhibitors (see below) the major part of the immunologically detectable neutrophil elastase is also enzymatically active. A small amount is bound to the DNA sputum matrix (from decayed neutrophils) and thereby inhibited; this has been demonstrated indirectly by adding DNase to CF sputum *in vitro*[178] and *in vivo*[179,180] and by measuring elastase activity in the presence or absence of DNA[181]. Furthermore, *P. aeruginosa* alginate[182] may bind elastase in CF sputum. Also other neutrophil-derived serine proteinases, cathepsin G[174] and proteinase 3[183], are detectable and display enzymatic activities in the CF airway.

Proteinase inhibitors

The reason why such high levels of active neutrophil elastase are present in the inflamed CF airways is the local inactivation of about 90 per cent of the endogenous α_1-proteinase inhibitor (α_1-PI)[174]. Immunoblots of sputum samples revealed that the majority of the inhibitor was present as low-molecular-mass degradation

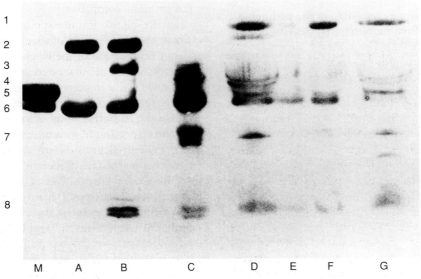

Fig. 6.7 *Immunoblot of cystic fibrosis sputa with specific antibodies against α_1-PI. M, α_1-PI marker; A, B, incubation of $\alpha_1$1-PI with PMN elastase for 30 min at 37°C; A, excess α_1-PI; B, excess PMN elastase; C, sputum sample; D–G, tenfold concentrated sputum; E, 1 : 2 diluted sample D. Molecular weights: 1, 90 000; 2, 78 000; 3, 70 000; 4, 66 000; 5, 54 000; 6, 50 000; 7, 42 000–45 000; 8, 25 000–30 000 Da. (Reproduced with permission from ref. 174.)*

products[24,174], and addition of radiolabeled neutrophil elastase to such samples showed no visible binding of α_1-PI with elastase (Fig. 6.7)[174]. On the other hand, α_1-PI is totally functional in the circulation[174,184].

Most probably, cleavage of α_1-PI is caused by high concentrations of released neutrophil elastase in the CF airways, although proteinases of other, yet unknown, origin have been proposed in this context[185]. If, in addition, the inhibitory function of α_1-PI is further impaired by mutation in the α_1-PI gene (a small subgroup of CF patients carry such risk alleles), such patients might be at higher risk for bacterial lung infections. Indeed, this has been confirmed in one study[186]. This is one example where genes involved in immune regulation may affect the CF phenotype.

Also, the other major serine proteinase inhibitor in the upper respiratory tract, secretory leukocyte proteinase inhibitor (SLPI), initially named bronchial mucosal inhibitor or antileukoprotease[187,188], does not seem to compensate for the inactivation of α_1-PI in vivo. On the contrary, immunoblotting revealed that SLPI was also fragmented and inactive[24,189]. Studies in healthy human individuals revealed that two-thirds of the SPLI recovered from the respiratory epithelium is nonfunctional, and the estimated ratio of functional SLPI to functional α_1-PI was 0.116[189]. Thus, SLPI also plays a minor role in protecting the lower respiratory tract from neutrophil elastase. The same applies to the third important endogenous proteinase inhibitor, α_2-macroglobulin, which does not reach the inflamed airways in sufficient concentrations due to its high molecular mass of 725 000 Da.

Neutrophil elastase and cathepsin G

Neutrophil elastase plays a major role in the pathophysiology of chronic inflammation in CF by cleaving a variety of substrates (Table 6.2). This notion is supported by the detection of elastin-split products (desmosines) in CF urine[190], and cleaved immunoglobulins[140], α_1-PI[174] or

Table 6.2 *Some biological effects of elastase from polymorphonuclear leukocytes*

Substrates	Reference
Elastin	173,190
Proteoglycans	197
Cilia	18
Transferrin	193,194
Fibronectin	16,17
α_2-proteinase inhibitor	174
Immunoglobulins, immune complexes	140,195
Complement components	196,199
Complement receptor 1	191
T lymphocyte cell receptors	192

cell-surface receptors of neutrophil[191] or lymphocyte[192] origin in sputum or BAL fluids. Furthermore, elastase activity[177] or desmosine concentrations[173,190] correlated with the severity of CF lung disease. Additionally, many in vitro experiments showed the broad biological effects of neutrophil elastase, including cleavage of fibronectin[16,17], transferrin[193,194], immune complexes[195], complement components[174,196], proteoglycans[197] and reduction of cilia beat frequency[18]. Thus, as pointed out before, there is a large overlap in the enzymatic activities of neutrophil and P. aeruginosa protease activities (Table 6.2). Hypothetically, addition of neutrophil proteases to P. aeruginosa mutants lacking proteases should substitute for growth retardation of the mutants. Since part of the virulence of P. aeruginosa is provided by the host, I have coined the expression 'mixed virulence' for this situation. Thus, P. aeruginosa, the most successful pathogen in CF, reveals pronounced parasitic or virus-like traits. In this view it is conceivable that P. aeruginosa itself triggers the recruitment of neutrophils to the site of its colonization (via IL-8) and the subsequent activation of these phagocytes, which is accompanied by lysosomal protease release. As is discussed below, the parasite does not have to fear its elimination by opsonophagocytosis.

Successful opsonophagocytosis, mediated by alveolar macrophages, is dependent on intact opsonic immunoglobulins which bind to Fc cell receptors on the phagocytes through the Fc part of the immunoglobulin[159,198]. Neutrophil-mediated phagocytosis is dependent on complement receptors such as CR1 and CR3, the receptors for deposited C3b and C3bi respectively[159]. Thus, intact antibodies and a functional complement system, as well as sufficient receptor expression on the phagocytes, are prerequisites for this process. Neutrophil elastase, as well as cathepsin G, cleaves IgG, IgM and IgG or IgA immune complexes in vitro, leaving the antigen-binding site of the immunoglobulins intact. Cleavage occurs in the hinge region of the immunoglobulins and results in degradation of the Fc portion[195]. This suggests that interaction of the truncated immune complex with a phagocytic cell is impaired. Consequently, neutrophil-elastase-treated immune complexes were not able to stimulate the oxidative burst of neutrophils in vitro[195]. When the Fc portion of immunoglobulins is proteolytically degraded, deposition of activated complement components on the C_H2 domain is also no longer possible. Complement deposition is furthermore directly impaired, since neutrophil elastase cleaves the central complement component of the classic and alternative pathway C3[176], as well as C5[199] and C3bi[196] (but not C3b). Finally, the complement receptor for C3b (CR1) on human neutrophils (but not CR3) is cleaved by neutrophil elastase[191]. Since C3b and CR3 are stable to neutrophil elastase and C3bi and CR1 are labile, the expression 'opsonin–receptor mismatch' was coined[196]. Consequently opsonophagocytosis and killing of P. aeruginosa, as well as other CF-related pathogens such as

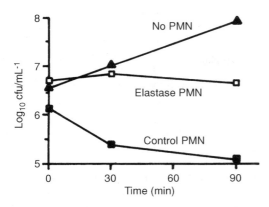

Fig. 6.8 *Killing of opsonized* P. aeruginosa *by elastase-treated and control PMN. Viable* P. aeruginosa, *expressed as log colony forming units (cfu)/mL, increased in the absence of PMN (▲). The effects of PMN pretreated with 10 μg/mL human leukocyte elastase for 30 min are shown by □ and for control PMN preincubated in HBSS-gel alone are shown by ■. Results are for a single representative experiment. (Reproduced with permission from ref. 191.)*

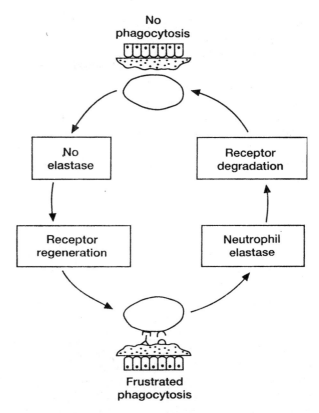

Fig. 6.9 *Cyclical mechanism of elastase release from PMN following frustrated phagocytosis.*

S. aureus, H. influenzae and S. pneumoniae has been shown to be markedly impaired (Fig. 6.8). Bispecific antibodies which cross-link neutrophils via the β-chain of leukocyte integrins (CD18) to bacterial epitopes or C3d on opsonized P. aeruginosa have been developed to overcome this opsonin–receptor mismatch successfully, at least *in vitro*[200]. In summary, neutrophil elastase impairs opsonophagocytosis at the levels of opsonizing immunoglobulins, complement and the complement receptor CR1 on neutrophils.

An important consequence is that free neutrophil elastase levels will decrease in the airway lumen, once the neutrophil cannot be stimulated further due to the damage to CR1, C3bi and Fc-Ig. Oxygen radical production will also be lowered[196]. Since elastase treatment of neutrophils only affects superoxide anion radical responses to stimuli such as opsonized P. aeruginosa, but not those to phorbol myristate acetate or LPS, it is clear that elastase does not interfere with the actual mechanism of superoxide anion radical production by neutrophils but rather with an impairment of surface interaction between the neutrophil and opsonized P. aeruginosa[196].

Therefore, neutrophil elastase has been described as a regulatory enzyme in chronic inflammation. It follows that as soon as neutrophil elastase levels are low, neutrophil stimulation will start again, thus creating fluctuating cycles of neutrophil elastase concentrations in chronic inflammatory states (Fig. 6.9). A longitudinal study of neutrophil elastase and immune complexes in CF sputa indeed revealed such a course[195].

Neutrophil elastase-mediated receptor cleavage on lymphocytes may further inhibit locally the immune defense against the persisting bacteria in the CF airways[192]. In 10 CF sputum samples, 1.0 per cent, 19.1 per cent and 15.7 per cent of all CD3+ T lymphocytes expressed CD4, CD8 and CD2, respectively. Incubation of CF sputum supernatant fluids with peripheral blood T lymphocytes resulted in the total loss of CD4 and CD8 but not of CD2. The addition of α_1-proteinase inhibitor eliminated surface antigen cleavage completely. Purified PMN elastase and cathepsin G cleaved CD2, CD4 and CD8 on peripheral blood T lymphocytes at proteinase concentrations of 0.83–8.3 μM in a dose-dependent manner. Cleaved CD4 and CD8 were re-expressed on the surface of T lymphocytes after 24 h in the absence of PMN elastase. Incubation of a CD4+ T-cell clone with PMN elastase led to a significant reduction of cytotoxicity towards target cells and significantly reduced IL-2 and IL-4 production.

The impairment of opsonophagocytosis and T-cell function by neutrophil serine proteinases may have beneficial and deleterious consequences for the host: temporal downregulation of inflammation on the one hand, and allowance of bacterial survival on the other.

Another trait of neutrophil elastase and cathepsin G with potential beneficial and deleterious consequences for the host is the potent ability of these enzymes to stimulate airway gland secretion[197]. This is especially noteworthy since CF is characterized by gland hypertrophy, hyperplasia and airway obstruction. Mucus hypersecretion may well be regarded as beneficial, since it removes bacterial pathogens from a close contact with airway epithelial cells into the airway lumen (see section on Host factors in bacterial airway colonization, p. 110). The deleterious aspect of this reaction is, however, airway obstruction leading to lung-function impairment.

Other proteinases

Besides neutrophil elastase, other proteinases may act in a destructive way in CF lung inflammation and infection. However, since various inhibitors of metalloproteinases are not able to reduce proteolytic effects in CF sputa or bronchial secretions, damage by this class of proteinases (which includes both *P. aeruginosa* alkaline proteinase and elastase, interstitial collagenase[201], macrophage-derived metalloproteinase[202] and metalloproteinases from neutrophils[203]) must be less pronounced than that due to serine proteinases. However, enzymatic activity due to neutrophil gelatinase (type IV collagenase) has been detected in CF sputa[204] and lung damage, as assessed by increased type IV collagen degradation products in sputum, was significantly correlated with concentrations of a gelatinase[204]. Cysteine proteinases[205] and the mast cell chymase, which is also a potent secretagogue for airway gland serous cells[206], have not been studied in CF airway samples.

Oxygen radicals

Neutrophils respond to stimulation with a burst of oxygen consumption – the respiratory burst – and the production of reactive oxygen species, such as superoxide anion radical, hydrogen peroxide, hydroxyl radical and possibly singlet oxygen[96]. As with lysosomal proteinases, these species are not only released into the phagolysosome but also outside the phagocyte, where they may be toxic to the host. There is indirect evidence that toxic oxygen metabolites produced by stimulated neutrophils contribute to lung injury in CF: high sputum concentrations of extracellular myeloperoxidase (MPO), a PMN-derived enzyme which transforms H_2O_2 into highly reactive oxygen metabolites, have been detected in CF patients[174,177,207,208], and lung function has been inversely correlated with MPO levels[177,207,208]. In addition, increased lipid peroxidation[209], reduced free-radical-trapping capacity[210] and altered plasma antioxidant status[209–211] have been reported to occur in CF patients. Blood neutrophils from CF patients have been shown to release significantly higher amounts of MPO than healthy individuals[208], suggesting that these cells have been primed during the course of the infection. Interestingly, when H_2O_2 concentrations were measured in breath condensates of CF patients, no significant differences were noticed between CF patients and normal individuals[212].

This may be explained by a functional defect of PMNs. As mentioned before, PMNs generate much less

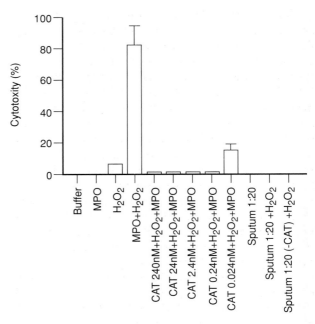

Fig. 6.10 *Cytotoxic effect of hydrogen peroxide (H_2O_2), myeloperoxidase (MPO) and sputum supernatants of seven cystic fibrosis (CF) patients on Chinese hamster ovary cells. Cells were incubated with buffer, purified MPO (33 nM), H_2O_2 (150 µM), MPO/H_2O_2 or supernatants/H_2O_2 for 5 hours. (Reproduced from ref. 212 with permission.)*

superoxide anion radical in the presence of neutrophil elastase[195,196] and activation of adherent PMNs leads to a markedly attenuated release of superoxide anion per cell when neutrophils are activated at high density, in comparison with cells activated at low cell density[213]. Furthermore, MPO may have metabolized H_2O_2 and thus have prevented this reactive oxygen species from being detectable in the exhalate. Such a reaction may lead to considerable tissue damage (Fig. 6.10). However, when CF sputum samples containing high concentrations of MPO were incubated with cell cultures and H_2O_2 was added, cytotoxicity was not observed. This led to the discovery of another scavenger of H_2O_2, catalase (CAT), an enzyme which detoxifies H_2O_2 to oxygen and water, in CF sputum samples[212]. Mean extracellular CAT concentrations of 0.31 µM and activities of 105 units have been detected in 38 CF sputum samples[212].

However, total removal of CAT from sputum samples also did not result in cytotoxicity (Fig. 6.10). This led to the hypothesis that MPO, although present and active in CF sputa, may be prevented from reaching the cell surface. MPO is a highly cationic enzyme at physiological pH, with a pI greater than 10[214] and thus may be complexed by negatively charged mucus glycoproteins (or mucins). Indeed, preincubation of MPO with heparan sulfate or chondroitin sulfate totally inhibited the cytotoxic effect of the MPO in the presence of H_2O_2[212]. These results point to a new protective effect of hypersecretion in the process of inflammation.

Thus, the reported negative correlation of MPO levels and CF lung function[207,208] most probably reflects lung damage caused by PMN-derived lysosomal serine proteinases. However, reactions involving reactive oxygen species may well take place in the sputum of CF patients. DNA from decayed PMN may be oxidized to yield the major reaction product, 8-hydroxydeoxyguanosine, and, indeed, this compound has been detected in urines of CF patients[215]. Since MPO (as well as serine proteinases) may be bound by DNA[212], released from decayed PMN in the sputum, such a reaction may well take place. Likewise, lipids derived from decayed PMN in the sputum, rather than from airway epithelial cells, may also be oxidized. End products such as malondialdehyde may reach the circulation where they are easily detectable[209]. Furthermore, MPO may also oxidize taurine to taurine chloramine which, in turn, may have pathogenic consequences[216]. Although CAT is known to inhibit taurine chloramine formation[216], CF sputum contains high concentrations of long-lived chloramines along with high levels of taurine[217], which may affect endogenous serine proteinase inhibitors (see below). It still remains to be investigated whether MPO/H_2O_2-mediated tissue damage occurs in very young children with CF in an acute stage of infection/inflammation, when sputum is minimal or absent and CAT not present.

BRONCHIAL HYPERREACTIVITY AND ALLERGIC BRONCHOPULMONARY ASPERGILLOSIS (ABPA)

It is not the intention of this chapter to discuss bronchial hyperreactivity and ABPA in CF in detail, since there are already excellent reviews of these topics[218–220]. However, any discussion of the immunopathology associated with CF would be incomplete without at least a brief overview of these two areas.

Wheezing and exercise intolerance have been recognized for many years as pulmonary manifestations of CF. There remains some debate to what extent these are secondary to obstructive airway disease or reflect the autonomic nervous system abnormalities described outside the lung[221]. Nevertheless, there are CF patients who show objective evidence of airway hyperreactivity, judged by short-term improvement with bronchodilators[222] and abnormal responses to methacholine or histamine challenge[223]. This proportion varies between 24 per cent and over 50 per cent of patients in different studies. There is evidence that the proportion may be higher in older patients and in those with worse lung function[224]. Moreover, spirometric indices such as forced vital capacity (FVC) and forced expiratory volume in one second (FEV_1) decline more rapidly in patients with hyperreactive airways[223].

The incidence of airway atopic disease, such as asthma and hay fever, in CF seems to be similar to that in the general population. Following the original description of an association between CF and *Aspergillus fumigatus*[225], this opportunistic pathogen has become increasingly recognized as a significant aeroallergen in CF. The evidence for this is mainly based on immune reactivity at the level of immediate-type skin reactions and IgE and non-IgE antibodies to *A. fumigatus*, detectable in a majority of patients[226,227], the fact that the respiratory tract is colonized with *A. fumigatus* in up to 57 per cent of CF patients[228] and that only about one in five patients shows no clinical or laboratory evidence of *A. fumigatus* reactivity[226]. However, the observation that at least some of the immune reactivities are ephemeral[229] raises doubts about the clinical significance of *A. fumigatus* footprints in CF patients.

Although several studies have reported an incidence of roughly 10 per cent for clinical allergic bronchopulmonary aspergillosis (ABPA), characterized by *A. fumigatus* colonization, IgE and IgG anti-*A. fumigatus* antibodies, pulmonary infiltrates, bronchiectasis and pulmonary fibrosis in CF populations (for example, refs [226,227]), other studies do not support this high percentage[230]. Heterozygosity for a CF mutation has been shown to predispose to ABPA in non-CF patients[231], suggesting that mutant CFTR may be a pathogenic factor in any increased incidence of ABPA in CF patients. Sensitization to *A. fumigatus* in the presence of increased IgE values has been associated with lower lung-function values in children with CF[232], although other studies proved the opposite[233]. In order to increase the discrimination between ABPA and uncomplicated *A. fumigatus* allergy, more specific diagnostic tools are needed[234].

ABPA has also become recognized as a complication in CF lung allograft recipients[235]. One patient developed ABPA both before and after lung transplantation[236]. Since end-stage ABPA is itself associated with bronchiolitis obliterans (reviewed in [237]), studies on the association of *A. fumigatus* markers and the development of bronchiolitis obliterans in CF lung allograft recipients may be of interest.

Little is known regarding T-cell responses and their role in the pathogenesis of ABPA. The majority of T-cell clones isolated from ABPA patients, and specific for the *A. fumigatus* 1 allergen, are IL-4 producing CD4+ cells of the Th2 phenotype[238]. *A. fumigatus* culture filtrates contain antichemotactic and antiphagocytic factors for neutrophils and macrophages[239] and factors that cause damage to human respiratory ciliated epithelium *in vitro*[240]. However, invasive aspergillosis is a rare occurrence in patients with CF with or without ABPA[241]. Not surprisingly in this context, markers of eosinophil recruitment and activation, particularly eosinophil cationic protein and eosinophil protein X, have been detected in CF sputum[208,242].

Although delayed clearance of inhalants, and their correspondingly prolonged exposure to the immune system, may contribute to the frequency of clinical and immunological response to *A. fumigatus*, this mechanism would predict that evidence for atopic responses to other common aeroallergens would also be common. That this is not the case, together with the fact that CF children can also have clinical ABPA, suggests that additional, as yet poorly understood, mechanisms are required to explain the high frequency of mold allergy in CF.

THE LYMPHOCYTE RESPONSE

Most studies on lymphocyte function in CF have been performed on circulating cells, since lavage and especially sequential lavage samples are seldom practicable. The functional activities of circulating cells may not, however, accurately reflect the functions of pulmonary lymphocytes, particularly since antigen-specific lymphocytes will localize to the antigenic foci within the lung and be correspondingly underrepresented in the blood. Care should therefore be taken in extrapolating results of circulating lymphocyte function to that of pulmonary lymphocytes.

Early evidence that CF patients with advanced pulmonary disease might acquire a state of immunosuppression came from *in vitro* studies on the proliferative response of cultured peripheral CF lymphocytes to antibiotic-killed *P. aeruginosa*[243–245]. Lymphocyte proliferation to antigens of *P. aeruginosa* or other Gram-negative bacteria was reduced or absent in hospitalized CF patients with acute exacerbations, and increased when cells were cultured in non-CF serum, after antibiotic therapy and clinical improvement in some, but not all, patients[245]. Possible causes for the reduced lymphocyte proliferation are phenacin pigments of *P. aeruginosa*[246,247], or the excess of circulating suppressor T cells[243]. Local immunosuppression may also be caused by the large amounts of neutrophil elastase activity found in CF sputa, suggesting local functional deficiency of these cells[192] (see section on Neutrophil elastase and cathepsin G, p. 118). Indeed, alveolar macrophages, obtained by *ex vivo* lavage of lungs removed at transplantation from CF, but not non-CF, patients fail to stimulate allogeneic lymphocytes[248]. CF, but not non-CF, cells are also unable to present *A. fumigatus* antigens to autologous lymphocytes. These data are consistent with proteolytic damage to major histocompatibility antigens important in antigen presentation.

Reports that circulating CF lymphocytes produce a lower cytotoxic response when activated with allogenic cells *in vitro* and that this is further compromised during pulmonary exacerbations[249] are difficult to interpret. Although cytotoxic T cells are important for the elimination of *P. aeruginosa* in rabbits[250], the relevance of reduced allogenic activity is obscure. In contrast, T-cell suppressor activity, measured as a reduction in B-cell IgM synthesis, was found to be increased[251]. An increase in T-cell suppression is a common accompaniment of lymphocyte activation, and the finding of increased suppression by CF T cells may simply reflect chronic lymphocyte activation. Indeed, when circulating blood T lymphocytes of infected CF patients were analyzed by flow cytometry, mean CD4/CD8 ratios of 0.56 were found[192], consistent with the proportion of lymphocytes with the CD8 suppressor phenotype being increased.

A major role for T cells in chronic *P. aeruginosa* infection has been excluded by the demonstration that the pathology and mortality are similar in infected intact and athymic nude rats[252]. However, the results may also be interpreted that cellular immunity in normal rats chronically infected with *P. aeruginosa* is suppressed. In *P. aeruginosa*-infected CF patients, T-cell clones have been detected which are predominantly specific for *P. aeruginosa* alkaline proteinase and elastase[253,254].

The question whether T-helper cell subsets (Ths)[255] trigger neutrophil recruitment and which Ths is predominant in CF is not sufficiently settled. A predominant Th1s response is expected to result in enhancement of several cytotoxic mechanisms: γ-interferon (γ-IFN) and lymphotoxin-activate macrophages leading to increased antibody-dependent macrophage cytotoxicity appropriate with intracellular (viral and parasitic) infections. Since neutrophils rather than macrophages dominate the inflammatory cell infiltrate in the inflamed CF airways, one would assume that the immune response in CF is driven by Th2s rather than by Th1s (see section on Anti-inflammatory therapy, p. 126). Preferential activation of Th2s should lead to high general antibody levels, a common finding in CF patients (see section on The humoral immune response, p. 115). IL-4 should cause increased IgE production and increased levels of IgE Fcε receptors on B cells, IL-3 and IL-4 would be expected to result in mucosal mast-cell proliferation and IL-5 would cause proliferation of eosinophils. This may contribute to the bronchial hyperreactivity in CF. However, since the incidence of asthma in CF is no higher than in the general population, clearly there are subtle differences in Ths activation between CF and asthma[256].

T lymphocytes from CF patients have been shown to express mutated CFTR[257] and (as respiratory epithelial cells[12]) to secrete lower concentrations of IL-10 after activation[257], suggesting that T lymphocytes may also contribute to impaired control of inflammation. Greater morbidity and mortality are associated with experimental *P. aeruginosa* infection in transgenic IL-10-deficient mice[258], suggesting that this cytokine is particularly important in the control of *P. aeruginosa* infection. Additionally, mutated CFTR in T cells does not respond to nitric oxide (NO) by increasing chloride currents[259].

It is unclear whether T cells from CF patients chronically infected with *S. aureus* exhibit the phenomenon of anergy (specific unresponsiveness or actual deletion of specific T-cell clones) or whether increased concentrations of specific T-cell clones reactive with *S. aureus* superantigens are present. Preliminary investigations in

31 CF patients showed that responses of peripheral blood lymphocytes of two CF patients to stimulation with SEB were indeed reduced (G. Döring et al., unpublished). Also quantitative differences were seen in Vβ-3, 6a, 8a and 12a chain usage in T-cell clones from CF patients compared with normals.

An interesting observation, though difficult to interpret, is the failure of exogenous glucocorticosteroids to enhance IgG production by CF B lymphocytes cultured with S. aureus and recombinant IL-2[260]. T lymphocytes, however, remained fully responsive to the actions of glucocorticosteroids. CF fibroblasts also differ in their resistance to the cytotoxic effect of glucocorticosteroids[261]. Since CF cells display a normal number of glucocorticosteroids receptors, the authors postulate a postreceptor effect, linked directly to the basic CF abnormality. The finding that steroid hormones modulate chloride channel function in epithelial cells[262] and that B-lymphoblastoid cell lines from CF patients display a cAMP-regulated channel defect[257,263] may support this notion. Nevertheless, expression of CFTR in CF B cells is low. Since glucocorticosteroids reduce T-cell production of IL-2 and the expression of IL-2 receptors in both normal and CF T cells[264], the net effect of steroids would be an overall reduction in antibody production in CF. Since hypergammaglobulinemia is associated with a poor prognosis in CF[121], a reduction in antibody production may be beneficial, and it would be of interest to know whether antibody levels are indeed lower in patients treated with steroids.

Another B-cell defect concerns secreted immunoglobulin which has been reported to be underglycosylated[265]. This observation has yet to be confirmed. Although, therefore, there are several intriguing observations on cellular immune abnormalities in CF, much remains to be done to show whether these are CF-specific or associated with chronic inflammation in general.

CYTOKINES

The inflammatory system in general communicates by a large repertoire of chemical messengers called cytokines. Expression of these is generally increased when the inflammatory system is activated and, not surprisingly, therefore, elevated cytokine levels have been detected in CF patients. As with the lymphocyte response, the local cytokine environment in lavage samples may more truly reflect the inflammatory process within the lung than circulating cytokine levels. However, some cytokines (such as IL-12) may be proteolytically degraded within the CF airway: others (such as IL-8) appear relatively stable. Results of lavage cytokine content should therefore be interpreted with some caution. Many bacterial factors[266–275] as well as host factors [272, 274, 276] stimulate the release of cytokines. Whereas some (but not all) studies show elevated cytokine concentrations in CF sera [130,277,278], BAL samples from CF patients infected with P. aeruginosa contain higher proinflammatory cytokine levels than those from healthy controls[11,276,277,279–281]. Those elevated include TNFα[282], IL-1[283], IL-6 and IL-8[284]. In contrast, pediatric nasal lavage fluids did not contain increased cytokine levels compared to those from non-CF children, suggesting that airway inflammation in early CF is confined to the lower respiratory tract[13]. CF macrophages seem to be primed since they produce substantially higher amounts of proinflammatory cytokines than normal macrophages[11,12,285], possibly due to TNFα which has also been shown to increase levels of the IgA receptor on neutrophils which results in increased superoxide production and phagocytosis of aggregated IgA[286].

If the inflammatory system is chronically activated, persistently high cytokine levels may lead to dramatic consequences for the host. For example, TNFα may cause cachexia[277,282] and osteoporosis[287], and IL-8, the most important chemotactic attractant for neutrophils, may lead to a 'self-perpetuating inflammatory process'[276]. Therefore, control of inflammation is mandatory. Possibly due to the production of autoantibodies to TNFα, which have been detected in 72 per cent of CF patients with chronic P. aeruginosa infections[288], TNFα is undetectable in sera of severely affected CF patients[277]. Locally, at inflammatory sites, neutrophil elastase may block the biological activity of IL-1 and possibly other cytokines by cytokine receptor cleavage[289]. As a result of exposure to high systemic levels of IL-8, CF neutrophils seem to downregulate IL-8 surface receptors[290]. Furthermore, the production of proinflammatory cytokines is regulated by contrainflammatory cytokines such as IL-10, or molecules such as TNF soluble receptor (TNF-sR) and IL-1 receptor antagonist (IL-1Ra). The levels of IL-10 in CF BAL are significantly less than in BAL from normal control individuals, suggesting that control of inflammation in CF is indeed impaired[11,12]. Additionally, as mentioned before, CF T-cell clones produce significantly less IL-10 than T-cell clones from normal individuals[257].

As well as the established cytokines, lymphocytes, alveolar macrophages (AM) and neutrophils can produce hypothalamic and anterior pituitary peptide hormones[291]. For example, activated lymphocytes elaborate a peptide which is functionally equivalent to, though biochemically different from, growth hormone (GH) releasing hormone[292]. This lymphocyte GH releasing hormone increases GH expression by both lymphocytes and pituitary cells. The final common pathway of many of the peripheral actions of GH is insulin-like growth factor 1 (IGF-1), which can be produced by many cell types, including lymphocytes and alveolar macrophages[293]. Both GH and IGF-1 increase free-radical production by activated neutrophils and alveolar macrophages, and may therefore enhance tissue damage from this source[294]. Additionally, IGF-1 is fibrogenic[295]. Rather like excessive production of neutrophil elastase, therefore, overproduction of these inflammatory neurohormones may contribute to lung pathology in CF. This is important to establish, since antagonists such as somatostatin are already available.

NITRIC OXIDE

NO originates from the biotransformation of L-arginine to L-citrulline by an enzyme called NO synthase (NOS)[296]. The inducible isoform of NOS (iNOS) is expressed in the bronchial mucosa of patients with bronchial asthma but not of normal control individuals[297], suggesting the increased levels of NO may result from increased NO production by iNOS. Also eosinophils and alveolar macrophages are sources of NO. The pathophysiological role of increased NO production is not yet known. However, it is clear that NO has effects on immune responses. Using whole-cell patch–clamp recordings, it was shown that NO activates CFTR in normal human (but not CF) cloned T cells by a cGMP-dependent mechanism[259]. Additionally, other chloride channels seem to be regulated by NO[298]. This suggests that an intrinsic immune defect may exist in CF.

NO inhibits both the proliferation of Th1s and their production of IL-2 and γ-IFN, as demonstrated in several infectious disease models[299,300], whereas Th2s are not affected, suggesting that increased amounts of NO may favor a Th2s response[301]. A Th2s-like type of response was proposed for the pathophysiology of CF lung infection (see section on Anti-inflammatory therapy, p. 126). However, NO exhalation was not increased in CF patients[302–306], possibly resulting from the inhibitory effects of inflammatory cytokines on NO synthases in the airways and alveolar epithelial cells and chronic epithelial cell damage[305], or to increased retention in airway secretions [302].

IMMUNOLOGICAL STRATEGIES FOR THERAPY AND PREVENTION

The extensive clinical experience that antibiotics are unable to eradicate bacteria such as *S. aureus* and *P. aeruginosa* from CF airways permanently, the demonstration that antibodies are fragmented in CF sputa and that inappropriate subclasses may predominate, together with evidence that the chronic inflammation does more harm than good, has led to a variety of immunological strategies in the management of CF. These include active immunization with *P. aeruginosa* vaccines, passive intravenous administration with anti-*P. aeruginosa* antibodies, and treatment with steroidal and nonsteroidal anti-inflammatory agents, as well as with proteinase inhibitors. Although none of these approaches has yet provided definite evidence of efficacy, some promising data have already been obtained. Clearly, since inflammation is present very early in CF, these strategies have also to be applied very early[307].

Immunoprophylaxis

P. AERUGINOSA

The historical development of vaccination against *P. aeruginosa* in CF and in other patients has been reviewed[308]. The first study of active immunization used a LPS vaccine[309] and was carried out in patients already infected with *P. aeruginosa*[310]. Most patients in this study, therefore, already had high antibody titers to *P. aeruginosa* which were increased by the immunization. However, *P. aeruginosa* was not eliminated from the airways and the patients even deteriorated clinically. Two possible explanations are:

1. the increased antibody titers resulted in increased immune complex formation with the triggering of further inflammatory reactions; and
2. that the known adverse reactions to the vaccine, which led to febrile responses in 20–40 per cent of the patients, had nonspecifically worsened lung inflammation.

Improvements in the LPS vaccine preparation[311] led to a study in 28 CF patients who were not colonized with *P. aeruginosa*[312]. Again, in this prospective study, neither the acquisition of *P. aeruginosa* nor the course of the disease was changed compared with a nonvaccinated control group, although the vaccine did stimulate specific antibody production. The current explanation for this negative outcome is that parenterally administered vaccines do not provoke sufficiently high antibody levels of the 'right' immunoglobulin class in the secretory immune system of the airways, and that the vaccine does not protect against all different serotypes of *P. aeruginosa*. Unfortunately, the latter hypothesis has not been investigated by analyzing the serotypes of the infecting strains. In this trial the vaccine group also did worse than the control group for several years before the clinical course of both groups became indistinguishable.

Based on observations that both pre-existing antibodies against LPS and exotoxin A improved survival of non-CF patients with episodes of *P. aeruginosa* bacteremia, and anti-LPS antibodies conferred protection in clinical trials, a polysaccharide–exotoxin A conjugate vaccine was developed which, by eliminating the toxic lipid A part of LPS, was shown to be safe and efficient in normal healthy individuals[313]. Thereafter, the vaccine was parenterally administered to CF children who had not been colonized with *P. aeruginosa*[314]. After an observation period of 4 years, 16 patients (61.5 per cent) remained free of infection and 10 (38.5 per cent) became infected.

When compared retrospectively with the rate in a group of age- and gender-matched, nonimmunized, noncolonized patients with CF, the rate at which *P. aeruginosa* infections were acquired was significantly lower ($P \leq 0.02$) among all immunized versus nonimmunized patients during the first 2 years of observation. Subsequently, only those immunized patients who maintained a high-affinity anti-LPS antibody response had a significant reduction ($P \leq 0.014$) in the rate of infection during years 3 and 4[315].

Whether this vaccine elicited significant antibody titers in the airways is not yet known. In view of the fact that most *P. aeruginosa* strains in CF are of mucoid (alginate) phenotype, an alginate–toxin A vaccine has been developed which may circumvent the problem that alginate as antigen is only weakly immunogenic[308]. Interestingly, this vaccine was effective in a chronic *P. aeruginosa* rat lung infection model by switching the Th2s response to infection to a Th1s response[316]. Other vaccines that have been considered for clinical evaluation are composed of *P. aeruginosa* flagella[317,318], outer membrane proteins[319] and whole-cell lysates[320].

Intramuscular application of the *P. aeruginosa* flagella vaccine revealed that specific IgG, IgA and sIA anti-Fla antibodies were elicited in the respiratory tract of healthy human individuals[321] (Fig. 6.11). Based on these encouraging results, a multicenter trial with a bivalent vaccine is currently in progress[322].

VACCINES AGAINST OTHER PATHOGENS

Candidates for a vaccine against *S. aureus* infections are the capsular polysaccharides of *S. aureus* type 5 and type 8[323], based on the hypothesis that the initially colonizing *S. aureus* phenotype is CP-positive (see section on Bacterial phenotypes in acute and chronic lung infec-

tion, p. 113). Animal experiments and *in vitro* phagocytosis studies have provided evidence that a purified capsular polysaccharide protected against infection with a highly encapsulated *S. aureus* strain[324]. However, in the light of the findings that *S. aureus* produces the large polysaccharide PNSG in CF airways, which was shown to be a protective antigen in a rat model of *S. aureus* infection[104] also, PNSG is considered as a new and promising vaccine candidate.

Although a very efficient *H. influenzae* type B vaccine has been developed[325], it will not be helpful in CF patients for protection against *H. influenzae* lung infections, since this pathogen does not produce a capsule in the airways (see Chapter 5), although it will protect against meningitis.

The growing interest in vaccines against certain viruses causing bronchial infection in CF is mainly based on the hypothesis that viral infection of the airways initiates changes of the epithelial cell surface which facilitate colonization by bacterial organisms and aggravate the course of already existing bacterial infection. Thus, adhesion by human PMN to monolayers of primary human tracheal epithelial cells that had been infected with parainfluenza virus type 2 revealed greatly increased PMN adhesion due to increased intercellular adhesion molecule-1 (ICAM-1) expression, a condition which may lead to cytotoxic injury[326]. Respiratory viruses and *Mycoplasma pneumoniae* are the most common causes of lower respiratory tract infections in children[327]. A role for respiratory syncytial virus and other viruses in acquisition of *P. aeruginosa* has been suggested [328–330] and influenza A and other virus infections have been associated with pulmonary deterioration in CF patients[330–332]. However, a 2-year prospective study[333] did not support these findings. No positive association between the frequency of viral infections and a more rapid decline in pulmonary function was found when 19 subjects with CF and their unaffected siblings were studied. However, intercurrently, 18 of the 19 CF patients received a H_3N_2 or H_1N_1 influenza 'split-virus vaccine' during the study period[334]. Unfortunately, the vaccination status of CF patients in the other studies has not been reported. If less pulmonary morbidity from influenza virus infection is, in fact, associated with active influenza immunization, this would strengthen the suggestion of several authors that CF patients should be offered a yearly immunization against influenza (and maybe other viruses) to avoid serious respiratory deterioration or even the onset of bacterial lung infection.

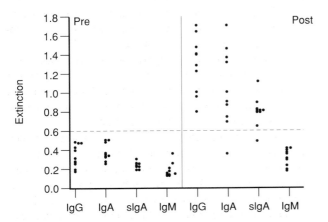

Fig. 6.11 *Extinction values of 1 : 10 concentrated fluids from bronchoalveolar lavage samples in IgG-, IgA-, secretory IgA- (sIgA-) and IgM-specific ELISAs from 10 normal, healthy individuals pre-immunization and post-immunization with a monovalent* P. aeruginosa *flagella vaccine. (Reproduced with permission from ref. 321.)*

Immunotherapy

The availability of hyperimmune globulin preparations enriched more than fivefold over conventional gammaglobulin preparations for *P. aeruginosa* LPS antibodies[335] has promoted studies in CF patients chronically infected with *P. aeruginosa*[336-338]. Although serum anti-*P. aeruginosa* LPS antibody levels increased significantly shortly after administration and remained elevated during the 17-day stay at the clinic, neither a significant decrease of *P. aeruginosa* density nor an increase of circulating immune complexes was seen in treated patients when 500 mg/kg of the hyperimmune preparation was given once. This raises doubts that the transient but significant amelioration of lung function seen in the patients was specifically due to the anti-*P. aeruginosa* antibodies. Basically the same result, i.e. transient lung function improvement during therapy, was obtained in a double-blind study involving a normal gamma globulin preparation[337], supporting the notion that gamma globulins *per se* are effective in improving the clinical state of CF patients, but not in eradicating the pathogens or reducing their numbers. Intravenously administered immunoglobulin was also effective in improving lung function and stabilizing the clinical course in a patient with panhypogammaglobulinemia[338]. As expected, treatment did not affect growth of *P. aeruginosa* or *B. cepacia* in the lungs. Finally, a phase III trial involving a hyperimmune immunoglobulin preparation enriched for opsonizing antibodies specific for the mucoid *P. aeruginosa* exopolysaccharide, which had been shown to be safe in a phase I/II trial[339], was stopped since no significant clinical differences had been noticed between the hyperimmune immunoglobulin treatment group and a nonspecific immunoglobulin treatment group (G. Pier, personal communication).

Anti-inflammatory therapy

The importance of host factors, especially the neutrophil with its lysosomal proteinases, in the progressive pathological processes in the respiratory tract in CF patients has led to the approach of combining anti-inflammatory therapy with effective antibiotic treatment. In 1985, a controlled study of prednisolone in CF revealed a favorable clinical outcome in the treatment group versus the control group, with practically no side-effects of the drug[340]. This prompted a double-blind placebo-controlled multicenter study with 283 CF patients in the USA starting in 1986. Careful examination of the patients revealed impairment of growth and several other complications, including diabetes, in the treatment group, which led to a recommendation to stop the trial for all patients in the high-dose prednisolone group[341]. These results make it unlikely that the use of high-dose steroids will be favored in the long-term treatment of the CF lung infection. Nevertheless, corticosteroids are the treatment of choice for ABPA and short-term oral application has been demonstrated to successfully increase lung function and decrease serum IgG and cytokine concentrations[342].

By inhalation of corticosteroids, side-effects may be prevented. In a short-term study, daily inhalation of budesonide produced small but significant improvements in cough and dyspnea in adult CF patients[343]. Similar positive results have been obtained in another study[344]. However, in a double-blind placebo controlled randomized sequence crossover trial of fluticasone propionate (400 μg/day) in 23 CF children no significant benefit was shown[345]. This was most likely due to failure of the drug to penetrate the viscid mucus lining the airways. Also, no convincing effect of inhaled budesonide dry powder (800 μg/ twice daily)[346] was seen. Thus, larger multicenter trials with higher doses given for a longer time (>3 months) have been suggested.

Nonsteroidal anti-inflammatory drugs with activity against neutrophils, such as piroxicam[347], pentoxifylline[348] and ibuprofen[349,350], have been used in CF patients with some success. A 4-year, randomized, double-blind placebo-controlled ibuprofen study in CF patients with mild lung disease revealed that patients of the treatment group who completed the trial had significantly less decline in pulmonary function. This effect was most pronounced in the youngest patients (13 years)[350]. Interestingly, effects of ibuprofen on inflammation in this study have not been published[350]. Tyloxapol, an alkylaryl polyether alcohol polymer detergent, has been shown *in vitro* to inhibit activation of the transcription factor nuclear factor-κB (NFκB), to reduce the LPS-stimulated release of several cytokines and to scavenge the oxidant hypochlorous acid, and thus may be potentially useful as a new anti-inflammatory drug for CF lung disease[344]. In addition it is mucolytic and could possibly promote clearance of secretions in the CF airway[351]. Finally fish-oil preparations containing ω-3 fatty acids which inhibit LTB$_4$ release by neutrophils have been used in 12 CF patients for 6 weeks without clinical benefit[352]. Based on the observation that CF patients lack this anti-inflammatory fatty acid[353], a 2-year, double-blind, placebo-controlled, multicenter study of fish oil is currently in progress.

Based on the hypothesis that the chronic inflammation in infected CF airways is mainly caused by a Th2s-like response (which would recruit neutrophils), recombinant γ-IFN has been suggested as one way of switching this response to one of a Th1s type[354]. Indeed, in a rat model of chronic *P. aeruginosa* lung infection, intraperitoneal treatment with rat rγ-IFN resulted in a complete shift to an inflammation type dominated by mononuclear leukocytes, although in this study there was no significant difference in lethality between treated and untreated animal groups[354]. However, in another similar study, a protective effect of rγ-IFN was demonstrated[355].

The plausible proteinase pathogenesis hypothesis suggests a strategy of increasing the antiproteinase levels in the lung by supplementation with suitable inhibitors. A wide variety of inhibitors has been developed for neutrophil elastase, but only a few are suitable for human use. Several small-molecular-weight protease inhibitors have been prepared[356-358], and several trials with these are in progress.

Another candidate is recombinant SLPI[359]. Besides inhibition of neutrophil elastase, rSLPI also inhibits mast-cell chymase[360] and histamine[361]. rSLPI aerosol therapy in CF patients caused a marked reduction in IL-8 levels in the epithelial lining fluid[362]. However, the pharmacokinetics of rSLPI aerosolized repeatedly to normal individuals or CF patients showed that rSLPI does not accumulate on the respiratory epithelial surface[363]. At least 100 mg twice daily had to be given to reduce neutrophil elastase levels substantially in CF patients[363]. Recently it has been shown that reaction of SLPI with *N*-chlorotaurine, a major long-lived oxidant generated by activated neutrophils, resulted in oxidation of all four methionine residues in SLPI, associated with substantial diminution in its elastase inhibitory activity[364]. The diminished activity of oxidized SLPI could be almost completely restored by addition of several glycosaminoglycans, including heparin, heparan sulfate or dermatan sulfate. A kinetic analysis revealed that glycosaminoglycans greatly accelerated the association of oxidized SLPI and neutrophil elastase, suggesting that oxidized SLPI is a functionally active form of the inhibitor but that expression of its elastase inhibitory activity is regulated by glycosaminoglycans[364]. However, sulfated polysaccharides, including heparin, also directly bind serine proteinases[365].

A trial with aerosolized α_1-PI in a small number of CF patients for several weeks gave promising results[366]. *In vitro*, the α_1-PI gene has been successfully transferred to CF bronchial epithelial cells where it blocked IL-8 release induced by neutrophil elastase[367]. Interestingly, α_1-PI forms a mixed disulfide with IgA. This complex has a tenfold lower rate constant of inhibition which is, however, still high enough to enable sufficient inhibition of elastase *in vivo*[368]. The use of transgenic α_1-PI produced in the milk of sheep may soon overcome the shortage of the inhibitor for clinical studies[369]. However, what would happen with the aerosolized α_1-PI in the inflammatory environment of the CF airways? MPO present in CF sputa in high concentrations may be capable of oxidizing the methionine residue at amino-acid position 358 (Met358) in the active center of the serine proteinase inhibitor α_1-PI, thereby inactivating the inhibitory capacity of α_1-PI towards elastase[370]. However, complex formation between neutrophil elastase and α_1-PI which renders Met358 inaccessible for MPO-induced oxidation is faster than MPO-induced oxidation of uncomplexed α_1-PI[212]. Thus, aerosolized α_1-PI may complex neutrophil elastase despite the presence of high concentrations and activities of MPO in CF airways. The binding of neutrophil elastase to DNA and alginate also modulates the association rates of elastase with α_1-PI and SLPI. Inhibition of neutrophil serine proteinases may restore neutrophil function, render bacterial survival more difficult and reduce mucus hypersecretion. Decreasing sputum volumes may then enable antibiotics to kill pathogens more effectively. The success of such specific studies and, more importantly, the clinical, bacteriological and inflammatory response, will clarify the true role of neutrophil elastase in the pathogenesis of CF and *Pseudomonas* colonization.

SUMMARY

It is increasingly becoming recognized that much of the lung pathology in CF arises from a normal immune response chronically activated by microorganisms which persist in the inherently abnormal CF airways. The reasons for initial bacterial infection of the lungs are complex and include endogenous factors, such as the abnormal electrolyte transport and the altered cell surfaces of epithelial cells, and exogenous agents such as viral infections. There are only a few major pathogens infecting the lungs of many CF patients, though whether and how prior infection with one predisposes to infection with the next is unclear. Each infective episode or exacerbation not only compromises the gas exchange functions of the lung but adds another cycle of injury to host defense functions such as mucociliary clearance. With each reinfection or exacerbation, bacteria have an opportunity to adapt further to the particular microenvironment of the CF airways. Of special importance in host–parasite interactions is the emergence of pseudomonal microcolonies surrounded by mucoid exopolysaccharide, together with a huge frustrated neutrophil response releasing proteolytic enzymes which hasten the death of the host.

Inhaled gene therapy in the neonatal patient, by reversing the basic CF defect, might prevent the initiation of this vicious cycle. In the older infected patient, in whom a degree of lung damage has already occurred, gene therapy may at best reduce the incidence of infection and slow the rate of deterioration of lung function. In many of these patients, however, inflammation in response to pre-existing lung injury will continue. Management of the older patient in the post-gene-therapy era will continue to be, as now, the management of chronic inflammation.

REFERENCES

1. Shapira, E. and Wilson, G.B. (1984) *Immunological Aspects of Cystic Fibrosis*, CRC Press, Boca Raton.
2. Berger, M. (1990) Inflammation in the lung in cystic fibrosis: a vicious cycle that does more harm than good? in *Cystic Fibrosis. Infection, Immunopathology and Host Response*, (ed. R.B. Moss), Humana Press, Clifton, New Jersey, USA, pp. 119–42.
3. Döring, G. and Dauner, H.-M. (1988) Clearance of *Pseudomonas aeruginosa* in different rat lung infection models. *Am. Rev. Respir. Dis.*, **138**, 1249–1253.

4. Walker, R.I. and Willemze, R. (1980) Neutrophil kinetics and the regulation of granulopoiesis. *Rev. Infect. Dis.*, **2**, 282–292.

5. Savill, J.S., Wyllie, A.H., Henson, J.E., Walport, M.J., Henson, P.M. and Haslett, C. (1989) Macrophage phagocytosis of aging neutrophils in inflammation. Programmed cell death in the neutrophil leads to its recognition by macrophages. *J. Clin. Invest.*, **83**, 865–875.

6. Sturgess, J. and Imrie, J. (1982) Quantitative evaluation of the development of tracheal submucosal glands in infants with cystic fibrosis and control infants. *Am. J. Pathol.*, **106**, 303–311.

7. Lloyd-Still, J.D. (1983) Pulmonary manifestations, in *Textbook of Cystic Fibrosis*, (ed. J.D. Lloyd-Still), John Wright, Boston, pp. 165–198.

8. Khan, T.Z., Wagener, J.S., Bost, T., Martinez, J., Accurso, F.J. and Riches, D.W. (1995) Early pulmonary inflammation in infants with cystic fibrosis. *Am. J. Respir. Crit. Care. Med.*, **151**, 1075–1082.

9. Balough, K., McCubbin, M., Weinberger, M., Smits, W., Ahrens, R. and Fick, R. (1995) The relationship between infection and inflammation in the early stages of lung disease from cystic fibrosis. *Pediatr. Pulmonol.*, **20**, 63–70.

10. Zahm, J.M., Gaillard, D., Dupuit, F., Hinnrasky, J., Porteous, D., Dorin, J.R. and Puchelle, E. (1997) Early alterations in airway mucociliary clearance and inflammation of the lamina propria in CF mice. *Am. J. Physiol.*, **272**, C853–C859.

11. Bonfield, T.L., Panuska, J.R., Konstan, M.W. *et al.* (1995) Inflammatory cytokines in cystic fibrosis lungs. *Am. J. Respir. Crit. Care. Med.*, **152**, 2111–2118.

12. Bonfield, T.L., Konstan, M.W., Burfeind, P., Panuska, J.R., Hilliard, J.B. and Berger, M. (1995) Normal bronchial epithelial cells constitutively produce the anti-inflammatory cytokine interleukin-10, which is downregulated in cystic fibrosis. *Am. J. Respir. Cell. Mol. Biol.*, **13**, 257–261.

13. Noah, T.L., Black, H R., Cheng, P W., Wood, R E. and Leigh, M.W. (1997) Nasal and bronchoalveolar lavage fluid cytokines in early cystic fibrosis. *J. Infect. Dis.*, **175**, 638–647.

14. Meyer, K.C., Sharma, A., Rosenthal, N.S., Peterson, K. and Brennan, L. (1997) Regional variability of lung inflammation in cystic fibrosis. *Am. J. Respir. Crit. Care Med.*, **156**, 1536–1540.

15. Armstrong, D.S., Grimwood, K., Carlin, J.B., Carzino, R., Gutierrez, J.R., Hull, J. *et al.* (1997) Lower airway inflammation in infants and young children with cystic fibrosis. *Am. J. Respir. Crit, Care, Med.*, **156**, 1197–1204.

16. Woods, D.E., Strauss, D.C., Johanson, W.G. Jr and Bass, J.A. (1981) The role of fibronectin in the prevention of adherence of *Pseudomonas aeruginosa* to buccal cells. *J. Infect. Dis.*, **143**, 784–790.

17. Suter, S., Schaad, U.B., Morgenthaler, J.J., Chevallier, I. and Schnebli, H.-P. (1988) Fibronectin-cleaving activity in bronchial secretions of patients with cystic fibrosis. *J. Infect. Dis.*, **158**, 89–100.

18. Smallman, L.A., Hill, S.L. and Stockley, R.A. (1984) Reduction of ciliary beat frequency *in vitro* by sputum from patients with bronchiectasis: A serine proteinase effect. *Thorax*, **39**, 663–667.

19. Niederman, M.S., Merrill, W.W., Polomski, L.M., Reynolds, H.Y. and Gee, J.B.L. (1986) Influence of sputum IgA and elastase on tracheal cell bacterial adherence. *Am. Rev. Respir. Dis.*, **133**, 255–260.

20. Dal Nogare, A.R., Toews, G.B. and Pierce, A.K. (1987) Increased salivary elastase precedes gram-negative bacillary colonization in postoperative patients. *Am. Rev. Respir. Dis.*, **135**, 671–675.

21. Plotkowski, M.C., Beck, G., Tournier, J.M., Bernardo-Filho, M., Marques, E.A. and Puchelle, E. (1989) Adherence of *Pseudomonas aeruginosa* to respiratory epithelium and the effect of leucocyte elastase. *J. Med. Microbiol.*, **30**, 285–293.

22. de Bentzmann, S., Roger, P. and Puchelle, E. (1996) *Pseudomonas aeruginosa* adherence to remodelling respiratory epithelium. *Eur. Respir. J.*, **9**, 2145–2150.

23. Abman, S.H., Ogle, J.W., Harbeck, R.J., Butler-Simon, N., Hammond, K.B. and Accurso, F.J. (1991) Early bacteriologic, immunologic, and clinical courses of young infants with cystic fibrosis identified by neonatal screening. *J. Pediatr.*, **119**, 211–217.

24. Birrer, P., McElvaney, N. G., Rudeberg, A. *et al.* (1994) Protease–antiprotease imbalance in the lungs of children with cystic fibrosis. *Am. J. Respir. Crit. Care Med.*, **150**, 207–213.

25. Konstan, M.W., Hilliard, K.A., Norvell, T.M. and Berger, M. (1994) Bronchoalveolar lavage findings in cystic fibrosis patients with stable, clinically mild lung disease suggest ongoing infection and inflammation. *Am. J. Respir. Crit. Care Med.*, **150**, 448–454 (published erratum appears in *Am. J. Respir. Crit. Care Med.* (1995) **151**, 260.

26. Frates, R.C. Jr, Kaizu, T.T. and Last, J.A. (1983) Mucus glycoproteins secreted by respiratory epithelial tissue from cystic fibrosis patients. *Pediatr. Res.*, **17**, 30–34.

27. Cheng, P.-W., Boat, T.F., Cranfill, K., Yankaskas, J.R. and Boucher, R.C. (1989) Increased sulfatation of glycoconjugates by cultured nasal epithel cells from patients with cystic fibrosis. *J. Clin. Invest.*, **84**, 68–72.

28. Lamblin, G., Aubert, J.P., Perini, J.M. *et al.* (1992) Human respiratory mucins. *Eur. Respir. J.*, **5**, 247–256.

29. Zhang, Y., Doranz, B., Yankaskas, J.R. and Engelhardt, J.F. (1995) Genotypic analysis of respiratory mucous sulfation defects in cystic fibrosis. *J. Clin. Invest.*, **96**, 2997–3004.

30. Schwab, U.E., Thiel, H.-J., Steuhl, K.-P. and Döring, G. (1997) Binding of *Staphylococcus aureus* to fibronectin and glycolipids on corneal surfaces. *German J. Ophthalmol.*, **5**, 417–421.

31. Liang, O.D., Ascencio, F., Franksson, L.-A. and Wadström, T. (1992) Binding of heparan sulfate to *Staphylococcus aureus*. *Infect. Immun.*, **60**, 899–906.

32. Barasch, J., Kiss, B., Prince, A., Saiman, L., Gruenert, D. and al-Awqati, Q. (1991) Defective acidification of

intracellular organelles in cystic fibrosis. *Nature*, **352**, 70–73.

33. Krivan, H.C., Roberts, D.D. and Ginsburg, V. (1988) Many pulmonary pathogenic bacteria bind specifically to the carbohydrate sequence Gal NAcβ1–4Gal found in some glycolipids. *Proc. Natl Acad. Sci. USA*, **85**, 6157–6161.

34. Imundo, L., Barasch, J., Prince, A. and Al-Awqati, Q. (1995) Cystic fibrosis epithelial cells have a receptor for pathogenic bacteria on their apical surface. *Proc. Natl Acad. Sci. USA*, **92**, 3019–3023.

35. de Bentzmann, S., Roger, P., Dupuit, F. *et al*. (1996) Asialo GM1 is a receptor for *Pseudomonas aeruginosa* adherence to regenerating respiratory epithelial cells. *Infect. Immun.*, **64**, 1582–1588.

36. Seksek, O., Biwersi, J. and Verkman, A.S. (1996) Evidence against defective trans-Golgi acidification in cystic fibrosis. *J. Biol. Chem.*, **271**, 15542–15548.

37. Schwab, U.E., Wold, A.E., Carson, J.L. *et al*. (1993) Increased adherence of *Staphylococcus aureus* from cystic fibrosis lungs to airway epithelial cells. *Am. Rev. Respir. Dis.*, **148**, 365–369.

38. Ulrich, M., Herbert, S., Berger, J. *et al*. (1998) Localization of *Staphylococcus aureus* in infected airways of patients with cystic fibrosis and in a cell culture model of *S. aureus* adherence. *Am. J. Respir. Crit. Care Med.*, **18**, 1–9.

39. Plotkowski, M.C., Chevillard, M., Pierrot, D., Altemayer, D. and Puchelle, E. (1992) Epithelial respiratory cells from cystic fibrosis patients do not possess specific *Pseudomonas aeruginosa*-adhesive properties. *J. Med. Microbiol.*, **36**, 104–111.

40. Sanford, BA., Thomas, V.L. and Ramsay, M.A. (1989) Binding of *Staphylococci* to mucus *in vivo* and *in vitro*. *Infect. Immun.*, **57**, 3735–3742.

41. Thomas, V.L., Sanford, B.A. and Ramsay, M.A. (1993) Calcium- and mucin-binding proteins of staphylococci. *J. Gen. Microbiol.*, **139**, 632–639.

42. Shuter, J., Hatcher, V.B. and Lowy, F.D. (1996) *Staphylococcus aureus* binding to human nasal mucin. *Infect. Immun.*, **64**, 310–318.

43. Trivier, D., Houdret, N., Courcol, R.J. *et al*. (1997) The binding of surface proteins from *Staphylococcus aureus* to human bronchial mucins. *Eur. Respir. J.*, **10**, 804–810.

44. Baltimore, R.S., Christie, C.D.C. and Smith, G.W.J. (1989) Immunohistopathologic location of *Pseudomonas aeruginosa* in lungs of patients with cystic fibrosis. *Am. Rev. Respir. Dis.*, **140**, 1650–1661.

45. Scharfman, A., Kroczynski, H., Carnoy, C. *et al*. (1996) Adhesion of *Pseudomonas aeruginosa* to respiratory mucins and expression of mucin-binding proteins are increased by limiting iron during growth. *Infect. Immun.*, **64**, 5417–5420.

46. Sajjan, S.U., Corey, M., Karmali, M.A. and Forstner, J.F. (1992) Binding of *Pseudomonas cepacia* to normal human intestinal mucin and respiratory mucin from patients with cystic fibrosis. *J. Clin. Invest.*, **89**, 648–656.

47. Kubiet, M. and Ramphal, R. (1995) Adhesion of

nontypeable *Haemophilus influenzae* from blood and sputum to human tracheobronchial mucins and lactoferrin. *Infect. Immun.*, **63**, 899–902.

48. Pier, G.B., Grout, M., Zaidi, T.S. *et al*. (1996) Role of mutant CFTR in hypersusceptibility of cystic fibrosis patients to lung infections. *Science*, **271**, 64–67.

49. Pier, G.B., Grout, M. and Zaidi, T.S. (1997) Cystic fibrosis transmembrane conductance regulator is an epithelial cell receptor for clearance of *Pseudomonas aeruginosa* from the lung. *Proc. Natl Acad. Sci USA*, **94**, 12088–12093.

50. Burns, J.L., Jonas, M., Chi, E.Y., Clark, D.K., Berger, A. and Griffith, A. (1996) Invasion of respiratory epithelial cells by *Burkholderia* (*Pseudomonas*) *cepacia*. *Infect. Immun.*, **64**, 4054–4059.

51. Kubesch, P., Dörk, T., Wulbrand, U. *et al*. (1993) Genetic determinants of airways' colonization with *Pseudomonas aeruginosa* in cystic fibrosis. *Lancet*, **341**, 89–193.

52. Smith, J.J., Travis, S.M., Greenberg, E.P. and Welsh, M.J. (1996) Cystic fibrosis airway epithelia fail to kill bacteria because of abnormal airway surface fluid. *Cell*, **85**, 229–236.

53. McCray, P.B. Jr and Bentley, L. (1997) Human airway epithelia express a beta-defensin. *Am. J. Respir. Cell. Mol. Biol.*, **16**, 343–349.

54. Goldman, M.J., Anderson, G.M., Stolzenberg, E.D. *et al*. (1997) Human beta-defensin-1 is a salt-sensitive antibiotic in lung that is inactivated in cystic fibrosis. *Cell*, **88**, 553–560.

55. Smith, J.J., Travis, S.M., Greenberg, E.P. and Welsh, M.J. (1996) Erratum. *Cell*, **87**, 335.

56. Boucher, R.C., Stutts, M.J., Knowles, M.R., Cantley, L. and Gatzy, J.T. (1986) Na^+ transport in cystic fibrosis respiratory epithelia. Abnormal basal rate and response to adenylate cyclase activation. *J. Clin. Invest.*, **78**, 1245–1252.

57. Berger, M. (1990) Complement deficiency and neutrophil dysfunction as risk factors for bacterial infection in newborns and the role of granulocyte transfusion in therapy. *Rev. Infect. Dis.*, **12**, S401–S409.

58. Abughali, N., Berger, M. and Tosi, M.F. (1994) Deficient total cell content of CR3 (CD11b) in neonatal neutrophils. *Blood*, **83**, 1086–1092.

59. Martin, T.R., Rubens, C.E. and Wilson, C.B. (1988) Lung antibacterial defense mechanisms in infant and adult rats: Implications for the pathogenesis of group B streptococcal infections in the neonatal lung. *J. Infect. Dis.*, **157**, 91–100.

60. Sordelli, D.O., Djafari, M., Garcia, V.E., Fontan, P.A. and Döring, G. (1992) Age-dependent pulmonary clearance of *Pseudomonas aeruginosa* in a mouse model: diminished migration of polymorphonuclear leukocytes to N-formyl-methionyl-leucyl-phenylalanine. *Infect. Immun.*, **60**, 1724–1727.

61. Mizgerd, J.P., Kobzik, L., Warner, A.E. and Brain, J.D. (1995) Effects of sodium concentration on human neutrophil bactericidal functions. *Am. J. Physiol.*, **269**, L388–L393.

62. Döring, G., Holder, I.A. and Botzenhart, K. (eds) (1987) *Basic Research and Clinical Aspects of Pseudomonas aeruginosa*, Karger, Basel, pp. 1–311.

63. Høiby, N., Pedersen, S.S., Shand, S.J., Döring, G., and Holder, I.A. (eds) (1989) *Pseudomonas aeruginos Infection*, Karger, Basel, pp. 1–308.

64. Homma, J.Y., Tanimoto, H., Holder, I.A., Høiby, N. and Döring, G. (eds) (1991) *Basic Research and Clinical Aspects of Pseudomonas aeruginosa Infection*, Karger, Basel, pp. 1–250.

65. McClure, C.D. and Schiller, N.L. (1996) Inhibition of macrophage phagocytosis by *Pseudomonas aeruginosa* rhamnolipids *in vitro* and *in vivo. Curr. Microbiol.*, **33**, 109–117.

66. Kownatzki, R., Tümmler, B. and Döring, G. (1987) Rhamnolipid of *Pseudomonas aeruginosa* in sputum of cystic fibrosis patients. *Lancet*, **1**, 1026–1027.

67. Wolz, C., Hohloch, K., Acaktan, A. *et al*. (1994) Iron release from transferrin by pyoverdin and elastase from *Pseudomonas aeruginosa. Infect. Immun.*, **62**, 4021–4027.

68. Muller, M. (1995) Scavenging of neutrophil-derived superoxide anion by 1-hydroxyphenazine, a phenazine derivative associated with chronic *Pseudomonas aeruginosa* infection: relevance to cystic fibrosis. *Biochim. Biophys. Acta*, **1272**, 185–189.

69. Döring, G., Goldstein, W., Röll, W., Schiøtz, P.O., Høiby, N. and Botzenhart, K. (1985) Role of *Pseudomonas aeruginosa* exoenzymes in lung infections of patients with cystic fibrosis. *Infect. Immun.*, **49**, 557–562.

70. Döring, G., Buhl, V., Høiby, N., Schiøtz, P.O. and Botzenhart, K. (1984) Detection of proteases of *Pseudomonas aeruginosa* in immune complexes isolated from the sputum of cystic fibrosis patients. *Acta Pathol. Microbiol.* [C], **92**, 307–311.

71. Döring, G., Obernesser, H.J., Botzenhart, K., Flehmig, B., Høiby, N. and Hofmann, A. (1983) Proteases of *Pseudomonas aeruginosa* in cystic fibrosis. *J. Infect. Dis.*, **147**, 744–750.

72. Li, J.D., Dohrman, A.F., Gallup, M. *et al*. (1997) Transcriptional activation of mucin by *Pseudomonas aeruginosa* lipopolysaccharide in the pathogenesis of cystic fibrosis lung disease. *Proc. Natl Acad. Sci. USA*, **94**, 967–972.

73. Mody, C.H., Buser, D.E., Syme, R.M. and Woods, D.E. (1995) *Pseudomonas aeruginosa* exoenzyme S induces proliferation of human T lymphocytes. *Infect. Immun.*, **63**, 1800–1805.

74. Middlebrook, J.L. and Dorland, R.B. (1984) Bacterial toxins: cellular mechanisms of action. *Microbiol. Rev.*, **48**, 199–221.

75. Döring, G. and Müller, E. (1989) Diffent sensitivity of *Pseudomonas aeruginosa* exotoxin A and diphtheria toxin to enzymes from polymorphonuclear leukocytes. *Microb. Path.*, **6**, 287–295.

76. Raivio, T.L., Ujack, E.E., Rabin, H.R. and Storey, D.G. (1994) Association between transcript levels of the *Pseudomonas aeruginosa* regA, regB, and toxA genes in sputa of cystic fibrosis patients. *Infect. Immun.*, **62**, 3506–3514.

77. Storey, D.G., Ujack, E.E., Mitchell, I. and Rabin, H.R. (1997) Positive correlation of algD transcription to lasB and lasA transcription by populations of *Pseudomonas aeruginosa* in the lungs of patients with cystic fibrosis. *Infect. Immun.*, **65**, 4061–4067.

78. Wang, J., Lory, S., Ramphal, R. and Jin, S. (1996) Isolation and characterization of *Pseudomonas aeruginosa* genes inducible by respiratory mucus derived from cystic fibrosis patients. *Mol. Microbiol.*, **22**, 1005–1012.

79. Govan, J.R. and Deretic, V. (1996) Microbial pathogenesis in cystic fibrosis: mucoid *Pseudomonas aeruginosa* and *Burkholderia cepacia. Microbiol. Rev.*, **60**, 539–574.

80. Lam, J., Chan, R., Lam, K. and Costerton, J.W. (1980) Production of mucoid microcolonies by *Pseudomonas aeruginosa* within infected lungs in cystic fibrosis. *Infect. Immun.*, **28**, 546–556.

81. Martin, D.W., Schurr, M.J., Mudd, M.H., Govan, J.R., Holloway, B.H. and Deretic, V. (1993) Mechanism of conversion to mucoidy in *Pseudomonas aeruginosa* infecting cystic fibrosis patients. *Proc. Natl Acad. Sci. USA*, **90**, 8377–8381.

82. Schurr, M.J. and Deretic, V. (1997) Microbial pathogenesis in cystic fibrosis: co-ordinate regulation of heat-shock response and conversion to mucoidy in *Pseudomonas aeruginosa. Mol. Microbiol.*, **24**, 411–420.

83. Mathee, K., Coifu, O., Sternberg, C. *et al*. (1999) *et al*. Mucoid conversion of *Pseudomonas aeruginosa* by hydrogen peroxide: a mechanism for virulence activation in the cystic fibrosis lung. *Microbiology*, **145**, 1349–1357.

84. Terry, J.M., Pina, S.E. and Mattingly, S.J. (1991) Environmental conditions which influence mucoid conversion *Pseudomonas aeruginosa* PAO1. *Infect. Immun.*, **59**, 471–477.

85. Berry, A., DeVault, J.D. and Chakrabarty, A.M. (1989) High osmolarity is a signal for enhanced algD transcription in mucoid and nonmucoid *Pseudomonas aeruginosa* strains. *J. Bacteriol.*, **171**, 2312–2317.

86. DeVault, J.D., Kimbara, K. and Chakrabarty, A.M. (1990) Pulmonary dehydration and infection in cystic fibrosis: evidence that ethanol activates alginate gene expression and induction of mucoidy in *Pseudomonas aeruginosa. Mol. Microbiol.*, **4**, 737–745.

87. Terry, J.M., Pina, S.E. and Mattingly, S.J. (1992) Role of energy metabolism in conversion of nonmucoid *Pseudomonas aeruginosa* to the mucoid phenotype. *Infect. Immun.*, **60**, 1329–1335.

88. Bayer, A.S., Eftekhar, F., Tu, J., Nast, C.C. and Speert, D.P. (1990) Oxygen-dependent up-regulation of mucoid exopolysaccharide (alginate) production in *Pseudomonas aeruginosa. Infect. Immun.*, **58**, 1344–1349.

89. Krieg, D.P., Bass, J.A. and Mattingly, S.J. (1986) Aeration selects for mucoid phenotype of *Pseudomonas aeruginosa. J. Clin. Microbiol.*, **24**, 986–990.

90. Hassett, D.J. (1996) Anaerobic production of alginate by *Pseudomonas aeruginosa*: alginate restricts diffusion of oxygen. *J. Bacteriol.*, **178**, 7322–7325.

91. Francoeur, C. and Denis, M. (1995) Nitric oxide and

interleukin-8 as inflammatory components of cystic fibrosis. *Inflammation*, **19**, 587–598.

92. Mahenthiralingam, E. and Speert, D.P. (1995) Nonopsonic phagocytosis of *Pseudomonas aeruginosa* by macrophages and polymorphonuclear leukocytes requires the presence of the bacterial flagellum. *Infect. Immun.*, **63**, 4519–4523.

93. Cabral, D.A., Loh, B.A. and Speert, D.P. (1987) Mucoid *Pseudomonas aeruginosa* resists nonopsonic phagocytosis by human neutrophils and macrophages. *Pediatr. Res.*, **22**, 429–431.

94. Boucher, J.C., Yu, H., Mudd, M.H. and Deretic, V. (1997) Mucoid *Pseudomonas aeruginosa* in cystic fibrosis: characterization of muc mutations in clinical isolates and analysis of clearance in a mouse model of respiratory infection. *Infect. Immun.*, **65**, 3838–3846.

95. Henson, P.M. and Johnson, R.B. Jr (1987) Tissue injury in inflammation. Oxidants, proteinases and cationic proteins. *J .Clin. Invest.*, **79**, 669–674.

96. Weiss, S.J. (1989) Tissue destruction by neutrophils. *NEJM*, **320**, 365–376.

97. Ganz, T. and Weiss, J. (1997) Antimicrobial peptides of phagocytes and epithelia. *Semin. Hematol.*, **34**, 343–354.

98. Learn, D.B., Brestel, E.P. and Seethmarama, S. (1987) Hypochlorite scavenging by *Pseudomonas aeruginosa* alginate. *Infect. Immun.*, **55**, 1813–1818.

99. Speert, D.P., Bond, M., Woodman, R.C. and Curnutte, J.T. (1994) Infection with *Pseudomonas cepacia* in chronic granulomatous disease: role of nonoxidative killing by neutrophils in host defense. *J. Infect. Dis.*, **170**, 1524–1531.

100. Döring, G. (1997) The role of proteinases from *Pseudomonas aeruginosa* and polymorphonuclear leukocytes in cystic fibrosis. *Drugs Today*, **33**, 393–403.

101. Barth, A.L. and Pitt, T.L. (1996) The high amino-acid content of sputum from cystic fibrosis patients promotes growth of auxotrophic *Pseudomonas aeruginosa*. *J. Med. Microbiol.*, **45**, 110–119.

102. Mai, G.T., Seow, W.K., Pier, G.B., McCormack, J.G. and Thong, Y.H. (1993) Suppression of lymphocyte and neutrophil functions by *Pseudomonas aeruginosa* mucoid exopolysaccharide (alginate): reversal by physicochemical, alginase, and specific monoclonal antibody treatments. *Infect. Immun.*, **61**, 559–564.

103. Herbert, S., Worlitzsch, D., Dassy, B. *et al.* (1997) Regulation of the *Staphylococcus aureus* capsular polysaccharide type 5: CO_2 inhibition *in vitro* and *in vivo*. *J. Infect. Dis.*, **176**, 431–438.

104. McKenney, D., Tibbetts, K.L., Wang, Y. *et al.* (1999) Broadly-protective vaccine for *Staphylococcus aureus* based on an *in vivo* expressed antigen. *Science*, **284**, 1523–1527.

105. Miethke, T., Wahl, C., Heeg, K., Echtenacher, B., Krammer, P.H. and Wagner, H. (1992) T-cell-mediated lethal shock triggered in mice by the superantigen staphylococcal enterotoxin B: critical role of tumor necrosis factor. *J. Exp. Med.*, **175**, 91–98.

106. Bean, A.G.D., Freiberg, R.A., Andrade, S., Menon, S. and Zlotnik, A. (1993) Interleukin 10 protects mice against staphylococcal enterotoxin B-induced lethal shock. *Infect. Immun.*, **61**, 4937–4939.

107. Neumann, B., Engelhardt, B., Wagner, H. and Holzmann, B. (1997) Induction of acute inflammatory lung injury by staphylococcal enterotoxin B. *J. Immunol.*, **158**, 1862–1871.

108. Goerke, C., Campana, S., Bayer, M.G. *et al.* (2000) Direct quantitative transcript analysis of the *agr* regulon of *Staphylococcus aureus* during human infection in comparison with the expression profile. *Infect. Immun.*, **68**, 1304–1311.

109. Hughes, J.E., Stewart, J., Barclay, G.R. and Govan, J.R. (1997) Priming of neutrophil respiratory burst activity by lipopolysaccharide from *Burkholderia cepacia*. *Infect. Immun.*, **65**, 4281–4287.

110. Döring, G. and Høiby, N. (1983) Longitudinal study of immune response to *Pseudomonas aeruginosa* antigens in cystic fibrosis. *Infect. Immun.*, **42**, 197–201.

111. Döring, G., Goldstein, W., Röll, A., Schiøtz, P.O. and Høiby, N. (1985) Role of *Pseudomonas aeruginosa* exoenzymes in lung infections of patients with cystic fibrosis. *Infect. Immun.*, **49**, 557–561.

112. Anderson, T.R., Montie, T.C., Murphy, M.D. and McCarthy, V.P. (1989) *Pseudomonas aeruginosa* flagellar antibodies in patients with cystic fibrosis. *J. Clin. Microbiol.*, **27**, 2789–2793.

113. Pedersen, S.S., Espersen, F., Høiby, N. and Jensen, T. (1990) Immunoglobulin A and immunoglobulin G antibody respsones to alginates from *Pseudomonas aeruginosa* in patients with cystic fibrosis. *J. Clin. Microbiol.*, **28**, 747–755.

114. Kronberg, G., Fomsgaard, A., Galanos, C., Freudenberg, M.A. and Høiby, N. (1992) Antibody responses to lipid A, core and O sugars of the *Pseudomonas aeruginosa* lipopolysaccharide in chronically infected cystic fibrosis patients. *J. Clin. Microbiol.* **30**, 1848–1855.

115. Johansen, H.K., Norgaard, A., Andersen, L.P., Jensen, P., Nielsen, H. and Høiby, N. (1995) Cross-reactive antigens shared by *Pseudomonas aeruginosa*, *Helicobacter pylori*, *Campylobacter jejuni*, and *Haemophilus influenzae* may cause false-positive titers of antibody to *H. pylori*. *Clin. Diagn. Lab. Immunol.*, **2**, 149–155.

116. Danielsen, L., Westh, H., Balselv, E., Rosdahl, V.T. and Döring, G. (1996) *Pseudomonas aeruginosa* exotoxin A antibodies in rapidly deteriorating chronic leg ulcers. *Lancet*, **347**, 265.

117. Hancock, R.E.W., Movat, E.C.A. and Speert, D.P. (1984) Quantitation and identification of antibodies to outer membrane proteins of *Pseudomonas aeruginosa* in sera of patients with cystic fibrosis. *J. Infect. Dis.*, **149**, 220–226.

118. Pedersen, S.S., Espersen, F. and Høiby, N. (1987) Diagnosis of chronic *Pseudomonas aeruginosa* infection in cystic fibrosis by enzyme-linked immunosorbent assay. *J. Clin. Microbiol.*, **25**, 1830–1836.

119. Thansekaraan, V., Wiseman, M.S., Rayner, R.J., Hiller, E.J. and Shale, D.J. (1989) *Pseudomonas aeruginosa* antibodies

in blood spots from patients with cystic fibrosis. *Arch. Dis. Child.*, **64**, 1599–1603.

120. Granström, M., Ericsson, A., Strandvik, B., Wretlind, B., Pavlovskis, O.R., Berka, R. and Vasil, M.L. (1984) Relation between antibody response to *Pseudomonas aeruginosa* exoproteins and colonization/infection in patients with cystic fibrosis. *Acta Paediatr. Scand.*, **73**, 772–777.

121. Matthews, W.J. Jr, Williams, M., Oliphant, B., Geha, R. and Colton, H.R. (1980) Hypogammaglobulinemia in patients with cystic fibrosis. *NEJM*, **302**, 245–249.

122. Høiby, N., Döring, G. and Schiøtz, P.O. (1986) The role of immune complexes in the pathogenesis of bacterial infections. *Ann. Rev. Microbiol.*, **40**, 29–53.

123. Van Bever, H.P., Gigase, P.L., De Clerck, L.S., Bridts, C.H. and Franckx, H. (1988) Immune complexes and *Pseudomonas aeruginosa* antibodies in cystic fibrosis. *Arch. Dis. Child.*, **63**, 1222–1228.

124. Fomsgaard, A., Dinesen, B., Shand, G.H., Pressler, T. and Høiby, N. (1989) Antilipopolysaccharide antibodies and differential diagnosis of chronic *Pseudomonas aeruginosa* lung infection in cystic fibrosis. *J. Clin. Microbiol.*, **27**, 1222–1229.

125. Schaad, U.B., Lang, A.B., Wedgwood, J., Buehlamm, U. and Fuerer, E. (1990) Serotype-specific serum IgG antibodies to lipopolysaccharides of *Pseudomonas aeruginosa* in cystic fibrosis: correlation to disease, subclass distribution and experimental protective capacity. *Pediatr. Res.*, **27**, 508–513.

126. Winnie, G.B. and Cowan, R.G. (1991) Respiratory tract colonization with *Pseudomonas aeruginosa* in cystic fibrosis: correlation between anti-*Pseudomonas aeruginosa* antibody levels and pulmonary function. *Pediatr. Pulmonol.*, **10**, 92–100.

127. Moss, R.B., Hsu, Y.-P., Lewiston, N. J. *et al.* (1986) Association of specific immune complexes, complement activation and antibodies to *Pseudomonas aeruginosa* lipopolysaccharide and exotoxin A with mortality in cystic fibrosis. *Am. Rev. Respir. Dis.*, **133**, 648–652.

128. Disis, M.L., McDonald, T.L., Colombo, J.L., Kobayashi, R.H., Angle, C.R. and Murray, S. (1986) Circulating immune complexes in cystic fibrosis and their correlation to clinical parameters. *Pediatr. Res.*, **20**, 385–390.

129. Dasgupta, M., Lam, J., Döring, G. *et al.* (1987) Prognostic implications of circulating immune complexes and *Pseudomonas aeruginosa*-specific antibodies in cystic fibrosis. *J. Clin. Lab. Immunol.*, **23**, 25–30.

130. Kronborg, G. (1995) Lipopolysaccharide (LPS), LPS-immune complexes and cytokines as inducers of pulmonary inflammation in patients with cystic fibrosis and chronic *Pseudomonas aeruginosa* lung infection. *APMIS Suppl.*, **50**, 1–30.

131. Grimwood, K., Semple, R.A., Rabin, H.R., Sokol, P.A. and Woods, D.E. (1993) Elevated exoenzyme expression by *Pseudomonas aeruginosa* is correlated with exacerbations of lung disease in cystic fibrosis. *Pediatr. Pulmonol.*, **15**, 135–139.

132. Greenberg, D.P. and Stutman, H.R. (1990) Infection and immunity to *Staphylococcus aureus* and *Haemophilus influenzae*, in *Cystic Fibrosis. Infection, Immunopathology and Host Response*, (ed. R.B. Moss), Humana Press, Clifton, New Jersey, USA, pp. 75–86.

133. Nicolai, T., Arleth, S., Spaeth, A., Bertele-Harms, R.-M. and Harms, H. K. (1990) Correlation of IgE antibody titer to *Aspergillus fumigatus* with decreased lung function in cystic fibrosis. *Pediatr. Pulmonol.*, **8**, 12–15.

134. Knutsen, A.P. and Slavin, R.G. (1990) Allergic bronchopulmonary aspergillosis in patients with cystic fibrosis, in *Cystic Fibrosis. Infection, Immunopathology and Host Response*, (ed. R.B. Moss), Humana Press, Clifton, New Jersey, USA, pp. 103–118.

135. Aronoff, S.C., Quinn F.J. Jr and Stern, R.C. (1991) Longitudinal serum IgG response to *Pseudomonas cepacia* surface antigens in cystic fibrosis. *Pediatr. Pulmonol.*, **11**, 289–293.

136. Lacy, D.E., Smith, A.W., Lambert, P.A. *et al.* (1997) Serum IgG response to an outer membrane porin protein of *Burkholderia cepacia* in patients with cystic fibrosis. *FEMS Immunol. Med. Microbiol.*, **17**, 87–94.

137. Biggar, W.D., Holmes, B. and Good, R.A. (1971) Opsonic defect in patients with cystic fibrosis of the pancreas. *Proc. Natl Acad. Sci. USA*, **68**, 1716–1719.

138. Høiby, N. and Olling, S. (1977) *Pseudomonas aeruginosa* infection in cystic fibrosis. *Acta Pathol. Microbiol. Scand.* [C], **85**, 107–114.

139. Thomassen, M.J., Boxerbaum, B., Demko, C.A., Kuchenbrod, P.J., Dearborn, D.G. and Wood, R.E. (1979) Inhibitory effect of cystic fibrosis serum on *Pseudomonas phagocytosis* by rabbit and human alveolar macrophages. *Pediatr. Res.*, **13**, 1085–1088.

140. Fick, R.B., Naegel, G.P., Squier, S.U., Wood, R.E., Gee, B.L. and Reynolds H.Y. (1984) Proteins of the cystic fibrosis respiratory tract. *J. Clin. Invest.*, **74**, 236–248.

141. Pier, G.B , Saunders, J.M., Ames, P. *et al.* (1987) Opsonophagocytic killing antibody to *Pseudomonas aeruginosa* mucoid exopolysaccharide in older noncolonized patients with cystic fibrosis. *NEJM*, **317**, 793–798.

142. Pier, G.B., Small, G.J. and Warren, H.B. (1990) Protection against mucoid *Pseudomonas aeruginosa* in rodent models of endobronchial infections. *Science*, **249**, 537–540.

143. Tosi, M.F., Zakem-Cloud, H., Demko, C.A. *et al.* (1995) Cross-sectional and longitudinal studies of naturally occurring antibodies to *Pseudomonas aeruginosa* in cystic fibrosis indicate absence of antibody-mediated protection and decline in opsonic quality after infection. *J. Infect. Dis.*, **172**, 453–461 (see comments *J. Infect. Dis.* (1996) Feb., **173**, (2), 513–515).

144. Winnie, G.B., Klinger, J.D., Sherman, J.M. and Thomassen, M.J. (1982) Induction of phagocytic inhibitory activity in cats with chronic *Pseudomonas aeruginosa* pulmonary infection. *Infect. Immun.*, **38**, 1088–1093.

145. Shryock, T.R, Sherman, J.M., Klinger, J.D. and Thomassen, M.J. (1985) Phagocytic inhibitory activity in serum of cats

immunized with *Pseudomonas aeruginosa* lipopolysaccharide. *Curr. Microbiol.*, **12**, 91–96.

146. Eichler, I., Joris, L., Hsu, Y.-P., Van Wye, J., Bram, R. and Moss, R. (1989) Nonopsonic antibodies in cystic fibrosis. *J. Clin. Invest.*, **84**, 1294–1304.

147. Hornick, D.B. and Fick, RB Jr (1990) The immunoglobulin G subclass composition of immune complexes in cystic fibrosis. *J. Clin. Invest.*, **86**, 1285–1292.

148. Moss, R.B., Hsu, Y.-P., Sullivan, M.M. and Lewiston, N.J. (1986) Altered antibody isotype in cystic fibrosis: possible role in opsonic deficiency. *Pediatr. Res.* **20**, 453–459.

149. Shryock, T.R., Moll, J.S., Klinger, J.D. and Thomassen, M.J. (1986) Association with phagocytic inhibition of anti-*Pseudomonas aeruginosa* immunoglobulin G antibody subclass levels in serum from patients with cystic fibrosis. *J. Clin. Microbiol.* **23**, 513–516.

150. Pressler, T., Pedersen, S.S, Espersen, F., Høiby, N. and Koch, C. (1990) IgG subclass antibodies to *Pseudomonas aeruginosa* in sera from patients with chronic *P. aeruginosa* infection investigated by ELISA. *Clin. Exp. Immunol.*, **81**, 428–434.

151. Pressler, T., Mansa, B., Jensen, T., Pedersen, S.S., Høiby, N. and Koch, C. (1988) Increased IgG2 and IgG3 concentration is associated with advanced *Pseudomonas aeruginosa* infection and poor pulmonary function in cystic fibrosis. *Acta Paediatr. Scand.*, **77**, 576–582.

152. Pressler, T., Pandey, J.P., Espersen, F. *et al.* (1992) Immunoglobulin allotypes and IgG subclass antibody response to *Pseudomonas aeruginosa* antigens in chronically infected cystic fibrosis. *Clin. Exp. Immunol.*, **90**, 209–214.

153. Pressler, T., Kronborg, G., Shand, G.H., Mansa, B. and Høiby, N. (1992) Determination of IgG subclass antibodies to *Pseudomonas aeruginosa* outer membrane proteins in cystic fibrosis lung infection using immunoblotting and ELISA. *Med. Microbiol. Immunol.*, **182**, 339–349.

154. Albus, A., Saalmann, M., Tesch, W., Pedersen, S.S. and Döring, G. (1989) Increased levels of IgG subclasses, specific for *Pseudomonas aeruginosa* protein and polysaccharide antigens in chronically infected patients with cystic fibrosis. *Acta. Pathol. Microbiol. Immunol. Scand.*, **97**, 1146–1148.

155. Kronborg, G., Pressler, T., Fomsgaard, A., Koch, C. and Høiby, N. (1993) Specific IgG2 antibodies to *Pseudomonas aeruginosa* lipid A and lipopolysaccharide are early markers of chronic infection in patients with cystic fibrosis. *Infection*, **21**, 297–302.

156. Cowan, R.G. and Winnie, G.B. (1993) Anti-*Pseudomonas aeruginosa* IgG subclass titers in patients with cystic fibrosis: correlations with pulmonary function, neutrophil chemotaxis, and phagocytosis. *J. Clin. Immunol.*, **13**, 359–370.

157. Pressler, T., Jensen, E.T., Espersen, F., Pedersen, S.S. and Høiby, N. (1995) High levels of complement-activation capacity in sera from patients with cystic fibrosis correlate with high levels of IgG3 antibodies to *Pseudomonas*

aeruginosa antigens and poor lung function. *Pediatr. Pulmonol.*, **20**, 71–77.

158. Thomassen, M.J., Demko, C.A., Wood, R.E. and Sherman, J.M. (1982) Phagocytosis of *Pseudomonas aeruginosa* by polymorphonuclear leukocytes and monocytes: effect of cystic fibrosis serum. *Infect. Immun.*, **38**, 802–805.

159. Berger, M., Norvell, T.M., Tosi, M.F., Emancipator, S.N., Konstan, M.W. and Schreiber, J.R. (1994) Tissue-specific Fc gamma and complement receptor expression by alveolar macrophages determines relative importance of IgG and complement in promoting phagocytosis of *Pseudomonas aeruginosa*. *Pediatr. Res.*, **35**, 68–77.

160. Naegel, G.P., Young, K.R. and Reynolds, H.Y. (1984) Receptors for human IgG subclasses on human alveolar macrophages. *Am. Rev. Respir. Dis.*, **129**, 413–418.

161. Hamilton, R.G. (1987) Human IgG subclass measurements in the clinical laboratory. *Clin. Chem.*, **33**, 1707–1725.

162. Krogh-Johansen, H., Nir, M., Høiby, N., Koch, C. and Schwartz, M. (1991) Severity of cystic fibrosis in patients homozygous and heterozygous for delta F508 mutation. *Lancet*, **337**, 631–634.

163. Santos, J.I. and Hill, H.R. (1984) Neutrophil function in cystic fibrosis, in *Immunological Aspects of Cystic Fibrosis*, (eds E. Shapira and G.B. Wilson), CRC Press, Boca Raton.

164. Hann, S. and Holsclaw, D.S. (1976) Interactions of *Pseudomonas aeruginosa* with immunoglobulins and complement in sputum. *Infect. Immun.*, **14**, 114–117.

165. Kharazmi, A., Schiøtz, P.O., Høiby, N., Baek, L. and Döring, G. (1986) Demonstration of neutrophil chemotactic activity in the sputum of cystic fibrosis patients with *Pseudomonas aeruginosa* infection. *Eur. J. Clin. Invest.*, **16**, 143–148.

166. Fick, R.B. Jr, Robbins, R.A., Squier, S.U., Schoderbek, W.E. and Russ, W.D. (1986) Complement activation in cystic fibrosis respiratory fluids: *in vivo* and *in vitro* generation of C5a and chemotactic activity. *Pediatr. Res.*, **20**, 1258–1268.

167. Cromwell, O., Walport, M.J., Morris, H.R. *et al.* (1981) Identification of leukotrienes D and B in sputum from cystic fibrosis patients. *Lancet*, **i**, 164–165.

168. Zakrzewski, J.T., Barnes, N.C., Costello, J.F. and Piper, P.J. (1987) Lipid mediators in cystic fibrosis and chronic obstructive pulmonary disease. *Am. Rev. Respir. Dis.*, **136**, 779–782.

169. Bozic, C.R., Gerard, N.P. and Gerard, C. (1996) Receptor binding specificity and pulmonary gene expression of the neutrophil-activating peptide. *Am. J. Respir. Cell. Mol. Biol.*, **14**, 302–308.

170. Bozic, C.R., Lu, B., Hopken, U.E., Gerard, C. and Gerard, N.P. (1996) Neurogenic amplification of immune complex inflammation. *Science*, **273**, 1722–1725.

171. Hopken, U.E., Lu, B., Gerard, N.P. and Gerard, C. (1996) The C5a chemoattractant receptor mediates mucosal defence to infection. *Nature*, **383**, 86–89.

172. Tournier, J.M., Jacquot, J., Puchelle, E. and Bieth, J.G.

(1985) Evidence that *Pseudomonas aeruginosa* elastase does not inactivate the bronchial inhibitor in the presence of leukocyte elastase. *Am. Rev. Respir. Dis.*, **132**, 524–528.

173. Bruce, M.C., Poncz, L., Klinger, J. D., Stern, R.C., Tomashefski, J.F. Jr and Dearborn, D.G. (1985) Biochemical and pathological evidence for proteolytic destruction of lung connective tissue in cystic fibrosis. *Am. Rev. Respir. Dis.*, **132**, 529–535.

174. Goldstein, W. and Döring, G. (1986) Lysosomal enzymes and proteinase inhibitors in the sputum of patients with cystic fibrosis. *Am. Rev. Respir. Dis.*, **134**, 49–56.

175. Jackson, A.H., Hill, S.L., Afford, S.C. and Stockley, R.A. (1984) Sputum sol-phase proteins and elastase activity in patients with cystic fibrosis. *Eur. J. Respir. Dis.*, **65**, 114–124.

176. Suter, S., Schaad, U.B., Roux, L., Nydegger, U.E. and Waldvogel, F.A. (1984) Granulocyte neutral proteases and *Pseudomonas elastase* as possible causes of airway damage in patients with cystic fibrosis. *J. Infect. Dis.*, **149**, 523–531.

177. Meyer, K.C. and Zimmerman, J. (1993) Neutrophil mediators, *Pseudomonas*, and pulmonary dysfunction in cystic fibrosis. *J. Lab. Clin. Med.*, **121**, 654–661 (see comments *J. Lab. Clin. Med.* (1993) May, **121**, (5), 632–634).

178. Kueppers, F. and Fiel, S.B. (1992) Proteolytic activity of purulent secretions in patients with CF and bronchitis is increased by DNase. *Am. Rev. Respir. Dis.*, **145**, A563.

179. Shah, P.L., Scott, S.F., Knight, R.A., and Hodson, M.E. (1996) The effects of recombinant human DNase on neutrophil elastase activity and interleukin-8 levels in the sputum of patients with cystic fibrosis. *Eur. Respir. J.*, **9**, 531–534.

180. Rochat, T., Dayer-Pastore, F., Schlegel-Haueter, S.E. *et al.* (1996) Aerosolized rhDNase in cystic fibrosis: effect on leukocyte proteases in sputum. *Eur. Respir. J.*, **9**, 2200–2206.

181. Belorgey, D. and Bieth, J.G. (1995) DNA binds neutrophil elastase and mucus proteinase inhibitor and impairs their functional activity. *FEBS Lett.*, **361**, 265–268.

182. Ying, Q.L., Kemme, M. and Simon, S.R. (1996) Alginate, the slime exopolysaccharide of *Pseudomonas aeruginosa*, binds human leukocyte elastase, retards inhibition by alpha 1-proteinase inhibitor, and accelerates inhibition by secretory leukoprotease inhibitor. *Am. J. Respir. Cell. Mol. Biol.*, **15**, 283–291.

183. Schuster, A., Csemok, E., Johnston, T.W. and Groß, W. (1997) Proteinase-3 in cystic fibrosis airways. *Am. J. Respir. Crit. Care Med.*, **155**, A49.

184. Cantin, A.M., Lafrenaye, S. and Begin, R.O. (1991) Antineutrophil elastase activity in cystic fibrosis serum. *Pediatr. Pulmonol.*, **11**, 249–253.

185. Suter, S. and Chevallier, I. (1991) Proteolytic inactivation of α_1-proteinase inhibitor in infected brochial secretions from patients with cystic fibrosis. *Eur. Respir. J.*, **4**, 40–49.

186. Doring, G., Krogh-Johansen, H., Weidinger, S. and Hoiby, N. (1994) Allotypes of alpha 1-antitrypsin in patients with cystic fibrosis, homozygous and heterozygous for deltaF508. *Pediatr. Pulmonol.*, **18**, 3–7.

187. Hochstrasser, K., Reichert, R., Schwartz, S. and Werle, E. (1972) Isolierung und Charakterisierung eines Protease-Inhibitors aus menschlichem Bronchialsekret. *Hoppe-Seyler's Z. Physiol. Chem.*, **353**, 221–226.

188. Dijkman, J.H., Kramps, J.A. and Franken, C. (1986) Antileukoprotease in sputum during bronchial infections. *Chest*, **89**, 731–736.

189. Vogelmeier, C., Hubbard, R.C., Fells, G.A. *et al.* (1991) Anti-neutrophil elastase defense of the normal human respiratory epithelial surface provided by the secretory leukoprotease inhibitor. *J. Clin. Invest.*, **87**, 482–488.

190. Stone, P., Konstan, M.H., Berger, M., Dorkin, H.L., Franzblau, C. and Snider, G.L. (1995) Elastin and collagen degradation products in urine of patients with cystic fibrosis. *Am. J. Respir. Crit. Care Med.*, **152**, 157–162.

191. Berger, M., Sorensen, R.U., Tosi, M.F., Dearborn, D.G. and Döring, G. (1989) Complement receptor expression on neutrophils at an inflammatory site, the *Pseudomonas*-infected lung in cystic fibrosis. *J. Clin. Invest.*, **84**, 1302–1313.

192. Döring, G., Frank, F., Boudier, C., Herbert, S., Fleischer, B. and Bellon, G. (1995) Cleavage of lymphocyte surface antigens CD2, CD4, and CD8 by polymorphonuclear leukocyte elastase and cathepsin G in patients with cystic fibrosis. *J. Immunol.* **154**, 4842-4850.

193. Döring, G., Pfestorf, M., Botzenhart, K. and Abdallah, M. (1988) Impact of proteases on iron uptake of *Pseudomonas aeruginosa* pyoverdin from transferrin and lactoferrin. *Infect. Immun.*, **56**, 291–293.

194. Britigan, B.E., Hayek, M.B., Doebbeling, B.N. and Fick, R.B. Jr (1993) Transferrin and lactoferrin undergo proteolytic cleavage in the *Pseudomonas aeruginosa*-infected lungs of patients with cystic fibrosis. *Infect. Immun.*, **61**, 5049–5055.

195. Döring, G., Goldstein, W., Botzenhart, K., Kharazmi, A., Schiøtz, P.O., Høiby, N. and Dasgupta, M. (1986) Elastase from polymorphonuclear leucocytes – a regulatory enzyme in immune complex disease. *Clin. Exp. Immunol.*, **64**, 597–605.

196. Tosi, M.F., Zakem, H. and Berger, M. (1990) Neutrophil elastase cleaves C3bi on opsonized *Pseudomonas* as well as CR1 on neutrophils to create a functionally important opsonin receptor mismatch. *J. Clin. Invest.*, **86**, 300–308.

197. Sommerhof, C.P., Nadel, J.A., Basbaum, C.B. and Caughey, G.H. (1990) Neutrophil elastase and cathepsin G stimulate secretion from cultured bovine airway gland serous cells. *J. Clin. Invest.*, **85**, 682–689.

198. Leslie, R.G.Y. and Alexander, M.D. (1979) Cytophilic antibodies. *Curr. Top. Microbiol. Immunol.*, **88**, 26–104.

199. Orr, F.W., Varani, J., Kreutzer, D.L., Senior, R.M. and Ward, P.A. (1979) Digestion of the fifth component of complement by leukocyte enzymes. *Am. J. Pathol.*, **94**, 75–84.

200. McCormick, L.L., Karulin, A.Y., Schreiber, J.R. and Greenspan, N.S. (1997) Bispecific antibodies overcome the opsonin-receptor mismatch of cystic fibrosis in vitro: restoration of neutrophil-mediated phagocytosis and killing of *Pseudomonas aeruginosa*. *J. Immunol.*, **158**, 3474–3482.

201. Desrochers, P.E., Jeffrey, J.J. and Weiss, S.J. (1991) Interstitial collagenase (matrix metalloproteinase-1) expresses serpinase activity. *J. Clin. Invest.*, **87**, 2258–2265.

202. Welgus, H.G., Campbell, E.J., Cury, J.D. *et al.* (1990) Neutral metalloproteinases produced by human mononuclear phagocytes. Enzyme profile, regulation and expression during cellular development. *J. Clin. Invest.*, **86**, 1496–1502.

203. Vissers, M.C.M., George, P.M., Bathurst, I.C., Brennan, S.O. and Winterbourn, C.C. (1988) Cleavage and inactivation of α_1-antitrypsin by metalloproteinases released from neutrophils. *J. Clin. Invest.*, **82**, 706–711.

204. Delacourt, C., Le-Bourgeois, M., D'Ortho, M. P. *et al.* (1995) Imbalance between 95 kDa type IV collagenase and tissue inhibitor of metalloproteinases in sputum of patients with cystic fibrosis. *Am. J. Respir. Crit. Care Med.*, **152**, 765–774.

205. Reilly, J.J. Jr, Chen, P., Sailor, L.Z., Mason, R.W. and Chapman, H.A. Jr (1990) Uptake of extracellular enzyme by a novel pathway is a major determinant of cathepsin L levels in human macrophages. *J. Clin. Invest.*, **86**, 176–183.

206. Sommerhoff, C.P., Caughey, G.H., Finkbeiner, W.E., Lazarus, S.C., Basbaum, C.B. and Nadel, J.A. (1989) Mast cell chymase. A potent secretagoge for airway gland serous cells. *J. Immunol.*, **142**, 2450–2456.

207. Regelmann, W.E., Siefferman, C.M., Herron, J.M., Elliott, G.R., Clawson, C.C. and Gray, B.H. (1995) Sputum peroxidase activity correlates with the severity of lung disease in cystic fibrosis. *Pediatr. Pulmonol.*, **19**, 1–9.

208. Koller, D.Y., Urbanek, R. and Gotz, M. (1995) Increased degranulation of eosinophil and neutrophil granulocytes in cystic fibrosis. *Am. J. Respir. Crit. Care. Med.*, **152**, 629–633.

209. Portal, B.C., Richard, M.J., Faure, H.S., Hadjian, A.J. and Favier, A.E. (1995) Altered antioxidant status and increased lipid peroxidation in children with cystic fibrosis. *Am. J. Clin. Nutr.*, **61**, 843–847.

210. Langley, S.C., Brown, R.K. and Kelly, F.J. (1993) Reduced free-radical-trapping capacity and altered plasma antioxidant status in cystic fibrosis. *Pediatr. Res.*, **33**, 247–250.

211. Roum, J.H., Buhl, R., McElvaney, N.G., Borok, Z. and Crystal, R.G. (1993) Systemic deficiency of glutathione in cystic fibrosis. *J. Appl. Physiol.*, **75**, 2419–2424.

212. Worlitzsch, D., Herberth, G., Ulrich, M. and Döring, G. (1998) Catalase, myeloperoxidase and hydrogen peroxide in cystic fibrosis. *Eur. Respir. J.*, **11**, 377–383.

213. Peters, S.P., Cerasoli, F. Jr, Albertine, K.H., Gee, M.H., Berd, D. and Ishihara, Y. (1990) 'Autoregulation' of human neutrophil acitvation *in vitro*: regulation of phorbol myristate acetate-induced neutrophil activation by cell density. *J. Leukoc. Biol.*, **47**, 457–474.

214. Agner, K. (1958) Verdoperoxidase. A ferment isolated from leukocytes. *Acta Physiol Scand.*, **2**, (Suppl. 8), 1–62.

215. Brown, R.K., McBurney, A., Lunec, J. and Kelly, F. J. (1995) Oxidative damage to DNA in patients with cystic fibrosis. *Free. Radic. Biol. Med.*, **18**, 801–806.

216. Weiss, S. J., Klein, R., Slivka, A. and Wei, M. (1982) Chlorination of taurine by human neutrophils. Evidence for hypochlorous acid generation. *J. Clin. Invest.*, **70**, 598–607.

217. Witko-Sarsat, V., Delacourt, C., Rabier, D., Bardet, J., Nguyen, A.T. and Descamps-Latscha, B. (1995) Neutrophil-derived long-lived oxidants in cystic fibrosis sputum. *Am. J. Respir. Crit. Care. Med.*, **152**, 1910–1916.

218. Lewiston, N.J. and Moss, R.B. (1984) Allergic phenomena in cystic fibrosis, in *Immunological Aspects of Cystic Fibrosis*, (ed. E. Shapira and G.B. Wilson), CRC Press, Boca Raton, pp. 126–141.

219. Tepper, R.S. and Eigen, H. (1990) Airway reactivity in cystic fibrosis, in *Cystic Fibrosis. Infection, Immunopathology and Host Response*, (ed. R.B. Moss), Humana Press, Clifton, New Jersey, USA, pp. 159–168.

220. Knutsen, A.P. and Slavin, R.G. (1990) Allergic bronchopulmonary aspergillosis in patients with cystic fibrosis, in *Cystic Fibrosis. Infection, Immunopathology and Host Response*, (ed. R.B. Moss), Humana Press, Clifton, New Jersey, USA, pp. 1031-118.

221. Davis, P.B., Shelhamer, J.R. and Kaliner, C. (1980) Abnormal adrenergic and cholinergic sensitiviy in cystic fibrosis. *NEJM*, **302**, 1453–1456.

222. Larsen, G.L., Barron, R.J., Cotton, E.K. and Brooks, J.G. (1979) A comparative study of inhaled atropine sulphate and isoproterenol hydrochloride in cystic fibrosis. *Am. Rev. Respir. Dis.*, **119**, 399–407.

223. Eggleston, P.A., Rosenstein, B.J., Stackhouse, C.M. and Alexander, M.F. (1988) Airway hyperreactivity in cystic fibrosis. Clinical correlates and possible effects on the course of the disease. *Chest*, **94**, 360–365.

224. Mellis, C.M. and Levison, H. (1978) Bronchial reactivity in cystic fibrosis. *Pediatrics*, **61**, 446–450.

225. Mearns, M., Young, W. and Batten, J. (1965) Transient pulmonary inflitrates in cystic fibrosis due to allergic aspergillus. *Thorax*, **20**, 385–389.

226. Nelson, L.A., Collerame, M.L. and Schwartz, R.J. (1979) Aspergillosis and atopy in cystic fibrosis. *Am. Rev. Respir. Dis.*, **120**, 863–873.

227. Knutsen, A. P., Mueller, K.R., Hutcheson, P.S. and Slavin, R.G. (1994) Serum anti-*Aspergillus fumigatus* antibodies by immunoblot and ELISA in cystic fibrosis with allergic bronchopulmonary aspergillosis. *J. Allergy Clin. Immunol.*, **93**, 926–931.

228. Zeaske, R., Bruns, W.T., Fink, J.N. *et al.* (1988) Immune responses to *Aspergillus* in cystic fibrosis. *J. Allergy Clin. Immunol.*, **82**, 73–77.

229. Hutcheson, P.S., Knutsen, A.P., Rejent, A.J., and Slavin, R.G. (1996) A 12-year longitudinal study of *Aspergillus*

sensitivity in patients with cystic fibrosis. *Chest*, **110**, 363–366.

230. Becker, J.W., Burke, W., McDonald, G., Greenberger, P.A., Henderson, W.R. and Aitken, M.L. (1996) Prevalence of allergic bronchopulmonary aspergillosis and atopy in adult patients with cystic fibrosis. *Chest*, **109**, 1536–1540.

231. Miller, P.W., Hamosh, A., Macek, M. *et al*. (1996) Cystic Fibrosis transmembrane conductance regulator (CFTR) gene mutations in allergic bronchopulmonary aspergillosis. *Am. J. Hum. Genet*., **59**, 45-51.

232. Wojnarowski, C., Eichler, I., Gartner, C. *et al*. (1997) Sensitization to *Aspergillus fumigatus* and lung function in children with cystic fibrosis. *Am. J. Respir. Crit. Care Med*., **155**, 1902–1907.

233. Milla, C.E., Wielinski, C.L. and Regelmann, W.E. (1996) Clinical significance of the recovery of *Aspergillus* species from the respiratory secretions of cystic fibrosis. *Pediatr. Pulmonol*., **21**, 6–10.

234. Little, S.A. and Warner, J.O. (1996) Improved diagnosis of allergic bronchopulmonary aspergillosis with gp66 (formerly antigen 7) of *Aspergillus fumigatus* for specific IgE detection. *J. Allergy. Clin. Immunol*., **98**, 55–63.

235. Egan, J.J., Yonan, N., Carroll, K.B., Deiraniya, A.K., Webb, A.K. and Woodcock A.A. (1996) Allergic brochopulmonary aspergillosis in lung allograft recipients. *Eur. Respir. J*., **9**, 169–171.

236. Fitzsimmons, E. J., Aris, R. and Patterson R. (1997) Recurrence of allergic bronchopulmonary aspergillosis in the posttransplant lungs of a cystic fibrosis patient. *Chest*, **112**, 281–282.

237. Greenberger, P.A. (1997) Immunologic aspects of lung diseases and Cystic Fibrosis. *J. Am. Med. Assoc*., **278**, 1924–1930.

238. Chauhan, B., Knutsen, A.P., Hutcheson, P.S., Slavin, R.G. and Bellone, C.J. (1996) T cell subsets, epitope mapping, and HLA-restriction in patients with allergic bronchopulmonary aspergillosis. *J. Clin. Invest*., **97**, 2324–2331.

239. Murayama, T., Amitani, R., Ikegami, Y., Nawada, R., Lee, W. J. and Kuze, F. (1996) Suppressive effects of *Aspergillus fumigatus* culture filtrates on human alveolar macrophages and polymorphonuclear leucocytes. *Eur. Respir. J*., **9**, 293–300.

240. Amitani, R., Murayama, T., Nawada, R. *et al*. (1995) Aspergillus culture filtrates and sputum sols from patients with pulmonary aspergillosis cause damage to human respiratory ciliated epithelium in vitro. *Eur. Respir. J*., **8**, 1681–1687.

241. Chung, Y., Kraut, J.R., Stone, A.M. and Valaitis, J. (1994) Disseminated aspergillosis in a patient with cystic fibrosis and allergic bronchopulmonary aspergillosis. *Pediatr. Pulmonol*., **17**, 131–134.

242. Koller, D.Y., Nething, I., Otto, J., Urbanek, R. and Eichler, I. (1997) Cytokine concentrations in sputum from patients with cystic fibrosis and their relation to eosinophil activity. *Am. J. Respir. Crit. Care Med*., **155**, 1050–1054.

243. Sorensen, R.U. (1984) Immune responses to *Pseudomonas* and other bacteria, in *Immunological Aspects of Cystic Fibrosis*, (ed. E. Shapira and G.B. Wilson), CRC Press, Boca Raton, pp. 101–123.

244. Høiby, N., Anderson, V. and Bendixen, G. (1975) *Pseudomonas aeruginosa* infection in cystic fibrosis. Humoral and cellular immune responses against *Pseudomonas aeruginosa*. *Acta. Pathol. Microbiol. Scand*. (C), **83**, 459–468.

245. Sorensen, R.U., Sern, R.C., Chase, P.A. and Polmar, S.H. (1981) Changes in lymphocyte reactivity to *Pseudomonas aeruginosa* in hospitalized cystic fibrosis patients. *Am. Rev. Respir. Dis*., **123**, 37–41.

246. Sorensen, R.U. and Klinger, J.D. (1987) Biological effects of *P. aeruginosa* phenacine pigments, in *Basic Research and Clinical Aspects of Pseudomonas aeruginosa*, (eds G. Döring, I.A. Holder and K. Botzenhart). *Antibiot. Chemother*., **39**, 113–124.

247. Sorensen, R.U., Fredricks, D.N. and Waller, R.L. (1991) Inhibiton of normal and malignant cell proliferation by pyocyanine and 1-hydroxyphenzine, in *Pseudomonas aeruginosa in Human Diseases*, (eds J.Y. Homma , H. Tanimoto, I.A. Holder, N. Høiby and G. Döring). *Antibiot Chemother*., **44**, 85–93.

248. Knight, R.A., Kollnberger, S., Madden, B., Yacoub, M., and Hodson, M.E. (1997) Defective antigen presentation by lavage cells from terminal patients with cystic fibrosis. *Clin. Exp. Immunol*., **107**, 542–547.

249. Knutzsen, A.P. and Mueller, K.R. (1990) T cell cytotoxicity in cystic fibrosis: relationship to pulmonary status. *Int. Arch. Allergy Appl. Immunol*., **93**, 54–58.

250. Lahat, N., Rivlin, J. and Iancu, T.C. (1989) Functional immunoregulatory abnormalities in cystic fibrosis patients. *J. Clin. Immunol*., **9**, 287–295.

251. Markham, R.B., Pier, G.B., Goeliner, J.J. and Migel, S.G. (1985) In vitro T-cell-mediated killing of *Pseudomonas aeruginosa*. II. The role of macrophages and T cell subsets in T cell killing. *J. Immunol*., **134**, 4112–4117.

252. Johansen, H.K., Espersen, F., Pedersen, S.S., Hougen, H.P., Rygaard, J. and Høiby, N. (1995) Chronic *Pseudomonas aeruginosa* lung infection in normal and athymic nude rats. *APMIS*, **10**, 207–225.

253. Parmely, M.J. and Horvat, R.T. (1986) Antigenic specificities of *Pseudomonas aeruginosa* alkaline protease and elastase defined by human T cell clones. *J. Immunol*., **137**, 988–994.

254. Parmely, M.J., Iglewski, B.H. and Horvat, R.T. (1984) Identification of the principal T lymphocyte-stimulating antigens of *Pseudomonas* . *J. Exp. Med*., **160**, 1338–1349.

255. Mosmann, T.R. and Coffman, R.L. (1987) TH1 and TH2 cells: different patterns of lymphokine secretion lead to different functional properties. *Ann. Rev. Immunol*., **7**, 145–173.

256. Azzawi, M., Johnston, P.W., Majumdar, S., Kay, A.B. and Jeffery, P.K.T. (1992) Lymphocytes and activated eosinophils in airway mucosa in fatal asthma and cystic fibrosis. *Am. Rev. Respir. Dis*., **145**, 1477–1482.

257. Moss, R.B., Bocian, R.C., Hsu, Y.P. *et al.* (1996) Reduced IL-10 secretion by CD4+ T lymphocytes expressing mutant cystic fibrosis transmembrane conductance regulator (CFTR). *Clin. Exp. Immunol.*, **106**, 374–388.

258. Yu, H., Hanes, M., Chrisp, C.E., Boucher, J.C. and Deretic V. (1998) Microbial pathogenesis in cystic fibrosis: pulmonary clearance of mucoid *Pseudomonas aeruginosa* and inflammation in a mouse model of repeated respiratory challenge. *Infect. Immun.*, **66**, 280–288.

259. Dong, Y.J., Chao, A.C., Kouyama, K. *et al.* (1995) Activation of CFTR chloride current by nitric oxide in human T lymphocytes. *EMBO J.*, **14**, 2700–2707.

260. Emilie, D., Crevon, C., Chicheportiche, R. *et al.* (1990) Cystic fibrosis patients' B-lymphocyte response is resistant to the *in vitro* enhancing effect of corticosteroids. *Eur. J. Clin. Invest.*, **20**, 620–626.

261. Breslow, J.L, Epstein, J., Fontaine, J.H. and Forbes, G.B. (1978) Enhanced dexamethasone resistance in cystic fibrosis cells: potential use for heterozygote detection and prenatal diagnosis. *Science*, **201**, 180–182.

262. Chen, J.H., Schulman, H. and Gardner, P. (1989) A cAMP-regulated chloride channel in lymphocytes that is affected in cystic fibrosis. *Science*, **243**, 657–660.

263. Zeutkubn, P.L., Wagner, M., Markakis, D., Loughlin, G.M. and Guggino, W.B. (1989) Steroid hormones: modulators of Na+ absorption and Cl-secretion in cultured tracheal epithelia. *Proc. Natl Acad. Sci. USA*, **86**, 2502–2505.

264. Efrat, S. and Kaempfer, R. (1984) Control of biologically active interleukin 2 messenger RNA formation in induced human lymphocytes. *Proc. Natl Acad. Sci. USA.*, **81**, 2601–2605.

265. Margolis, R. and Boat, T.F. (1983) The carbohydrate content of IgG from patients with cystic fibrosis. *Pediatr. Res.*, **17**, 931–935.

266. Jorens, P.G., Richman-Eisenstat, J.B., Housset, B.P., Massion, P.P., Ueki, I. and Nadel, J.A. (1994) Pseudomonas-induced neutrophil recruitment in the dog airway in vivo is mediated in part by IL-8 and inhibited by a leumedin. *Eur. Respir. J.*, **7**, 1925–1931.

267. Inoue, H., Hara, M., Massion, P.P. *et al.* (1996) Role of recruited neutrophils in interleukin-8 production in dog trachea after stimulation with *Pseudomonas in vivo*. *Am. J. Respir. Cell. Mol. Biol.*, **13**, 570–577.

268. Massion, P.P., Hebert, C.A., Leong, S. *et al.* (1995) *Staphylococcus aureus* stimulates neutrophil recruitment by stimulating interleukin-8 production in dog trachea. *Am. J. Physiol.*, **268**, L85–L94.

269. Massion, P.P., Inoue, H., Richman-Eisenstat, J. *et al.* (1994) Novel *Pseudomonas* product stimulates interleukin-8 production in airway epithelial cells *in vitro*. *J. Clin. Invest.*, **93**, 26–32.

270. Palfreyman, R.W., Watson, M.L., Eden, C. and Smith, A.W. (1997) Induction of biologically active interleukin-8 from lung epithelial cells by *Burkholderia (Pseudomonas) cepacia* products. *Infect. Immun.*, **65**, 617–622.

271. DiMango, E., Zar, H.J., Bryan, R. and Prince, A. (1995) Diverse *Pseudomonas aeruginosa* gene products stimulate respiratory epithelial cells to produce interleukin-8. *J. Clin. Inves.*, **96**, 2204–2210.

272. Cusumano, V., Tufano, M.A., Mancuso, G. *et al.* (1997) Porins of *Pseudomonas aeruginosa* induce release of tumor necrosis factor alpha and interleukin-6 by human leukocytes. *Infect. Immun.*, **65**, 1683–1687.

273. Miller, E.J., Nagao, S., Carr, F.K., Noble, J.M. and Cohen, A.B. (1996) Interleukin-8 (IL-8) is a major neutrophil chemotaxin from human alveolar macrophages stimulated with staphylococcal enterotoxin A. *Inflamm. Res.*, **45**, 386–392

274. Bedard, M., McClure, C.D., Schiller, N.L., Francoeur, C., Cantin, A. and Denis, M. (1993) Release of interleukin-8, interleukin-6, and colony-stimulating factors by upper airway epithelial cells: implications for cystic fibrosis. *Am. J. Respir. Cell. Mol. Biol.*, **9**, 455–462.

275. Schwartz, D.A., Quinn, T.J., Thorne, P.S., Sayeed, S., Yi, A.K. and Krieg, A.M. (1997) CpG motifs in bacterial DNA cause inflammation in the lower respiratory tract. *J. Clin. Invest.*, **100**, 68–73.

276. Nakamura, H., Yoshimura, K., McElvaney, C. and Crystal, R.G. (1992) Neutrophil elastase in respiratory epithelial lining fluid of individuals with cystic fibrosis induces interleukin-8 gene expression in a human bronchial epithelial cell line. *J. Clin. Invest.*, **89**, 1478–1484.

277. Suter, S., Schaad, U.B., Roux-Lombard, P., Girardin, E., Grau, G. and Dayer, J.-M. (1989) Relation between tumor necrosis factor-α and granulocyte elastase-α1-proteinase inhibitor complexes in plasma of patients with cystic fibrosis. *Am. Rev. Respir. Dis.*, **140**, 1640–1644.

278. Brown, M.A., Morgan, W.J., Finley, P.R. Jr and Scuderi, P. (1991) Circulating levels of tumor necrosis factor and interleukin-1 in cystic fibrosis. *Pediatr. Pulmonol.*, **10**, 86–91.

279. Fick, R.B., Standiford, T.J., Kunkel, S.L. and Strieter, R.M. (1991) Interleukin-8 and neutrophil accumulation in the inflammatory airways disease of cystic fibrosis. *Clin. Res.*, **39**, 292A

280. Salva, P.S., Doyle, N.A., Graham, L., Eigen, H. and Doerschuk, C.M. (1996) TNF-alpha, IL-8, soluble ICAM-1, and neutrophils in sputum of cystic fibrosis patients. *Pediatr. Pulmonol.*, **21**, 11–19.

281. Willmott, R.W., Kassab, J.T., Kilian, P.L., Benjamin, W.R., Douglas, S.D. and Wood, R.E. (1990) Increased levels of interleukin-1 in bronchoalveolar washings from children with bacterial pulmonary infections. *Am. Rev. Respir. Dis.*, **142**, 365–368.

282. Moldawer, L.L. and Lowry, S.F. (1988) Cachectin: its impact on metabolism and nutritional status. *Ann. Rev. Nutr.*, **8**, 585–609.

283. Oppenheim, J.J., Kovacs, E.J., Matsushima, K. and Durum, S.K. (1986) There is more than one interleukin 1. *Immunol. Today.*, **7**, 45.

284. Baggiolini, M., Walz, A. and Kunkel, S.L. (1989) Neutrophil-activating peptide-1/inteukin 8, a novel cytokine that activates neutrophils. *J. Clin. Invest.*, **84**, 1045–1049.

285. Pfeffer, K.D., Huecksteadt, T.P. and Hoidal, J.R. (1993)

Expression and regulation of tumor necrosis factor in macrophages from cystic fibrosis patients. *Am. J. Respir. Cell. Mol. Biol.*, **9**, 511–519.

286. Hostoffer, R.W., Krukovets, I. and Berger, M. (1994) Enhancement by tumor necrosis factor-alpha of Fc alpha receptor expression and IgA-mediated superoxide generation and killing of *Pseudomonas aeruginosa* by polymorphonuclear leukocytes. *J. Infect. Dis.*, **170**, 82–87.

287. Teramoto, S., Matsuse, T. and Ouchi, Y. (1997) Increased production of TNF-alpha may play a role in osteoporosis in cystic fibrosis patients. *Chest*, **112**, 574.

288. Fomsgaard, A., Svenson, M. and Bendtzen, K. (1989) Auto-antibodies to tumor necrosis factor α in healthy humans and patients with inflammatory diseases and gram-negative bacterial infections. *Scand. J. Immunol.*, **30**, 219–223.

289. Döring, G. (1989) Polymorphonuclear leukocyte elastase: its effects on the pathogenesis of *Pseudomonas aeruginosa* infection in cystic fibrosis. *Antibiot. Chemother.*, **42**, 169–176.

290. Dai, Y., Dean, T.P., Church, M.K., Warner, J.O. and Shute, J.K. (1994) Desensitisation of neutrophil responses by systemic interleukin 8 in cystic fibrosis. *Thorax*, **49**, 867–871.

291. Knight, R.A, Sarlis, N. and Stephanou, A. (1992) Interleukins and neurohormones: a common language. *Postgrad. Med. J.*, **68**, 603–605.

292. Stephanou, A., Knight, R.A. and Lightman S.L. (1991) Production of a growth hormone-releasing hormone-like peptide and its mRNA by human lymphocytes. *Neuroendocrinology*, **53**, 628–633.

293. Rom, W.N., Basset, P., Fells, G.A., Nukiwa, T., Trapnell, B.C. and Crystal, R.G. (1988) Alveolar macrophages release an insulin-like growth factor I-type molecule. *J. Clin. Invest.*, **82**, 1685–1693.

294. Fu, Y.K., Arkins, S., Warq, B.S. and Kelley, K.W. (1991) A novel role of growth hormone and insulin-like growth factor I. Priming neutrophils for superoxide anion secretion. *J. Immunol.*, **146**, 1602–1608.

295. Doi, T., Striker, L.J. and Kimana, K. (1991) Glomerulosclerosis in mice transgenic for growth hormone. Increased mesangial extracellular matrix is correlated with kdney mRNA levels. *J. Exp. Med.*, **173**, 1287–1290.

296. Moncada, S. and Higgs, E.A. (1991) Endogenous nitric oxide: physiology, pathology and clinical relevance. *Eur. J. Clin. Invest.*, **21**, 361–374.

297. Barnes, P.J. and Liew, F.Y. (1995) Nitric oxide and asthmatic inflammation. *Immunol. Today*, **16**, 128–130.

298. Kamosinska, B., Radomski, M.W., Duszyk, M., Radomski, A. and Man, S.F. (1997) Nitric oxide activates chloride currents in human lung epithelial cells. *Am. J. Physiol.*, **272**, L1098–L1104.

299. Abrahamson, I.S. and Coffman, R.L. (1995) Cytokine and nitric oxide regulation of the immunosuppression in *Trypanosoma cruzi* infection. *J. Immunol.*, **155**, 3955–3963.

300. Sternberg, J.M. and Mabbott, N.A. (1996) Nitric oxide-mediated suppression of T cell responses during trypanosoma brucei infection: soluble trypanosome products and interferon-γ are synergistic inducers of nitric oxide synthase. *Eur. J. Immunol.*, **26**, 539–543.

301. Taylor-Robinson, A.W., Liew, F.Y., Severn, A. *et al.* (1994) Regulation of the immune response by nitric oxide differentially produced by T helper type 1 and T helper type 2 cells. *Eur. J. Immunol.*, **24**, 980–984.

302. Grasemann, H., Michler, E., Wallot, M. and Ratjen, F. (1997) Decreased concentration of exhaled nitric oxide (NO) in patients with cystic fibrosis. *Pediatr. Pulmonol.*, **24**, 173–177.

303. Lundberg, J.O., Weitzberg, E., Lundberg, J.M. and Alving, K. (1996) Nitric oxide in exhaled air. *Eur. Respir. J.*, **9**, 2671–2680.

304. Lundberg, J.O., Nordvall, S.L., Weitzberg, E., Kollberg, H. and Alving, K. (1996) Exhaled nitric oxide in paediatric asthma and cystic fibrosis. *Arch. Dis. Child.*, **75**, 323–326.

305. Dotsch, J., Demirakca, S., Terbrack, H.G., Huls, G., Rascher, W. and Kuhl, P.G. (1996) Airway nitric oxide in asthmatic children and patients with cystic fibrosis. *Eur. Respir. J.*, **12**, 2537–2540.

306. Balfour-Lynn, I.M., Laverty, A. and Dinwiddie, R. (1996) Reduced upper airway nitric oxide in cystic fibrosis. *Arch. Dis. Child.*, **75**, 319–322.

307. Cantin, A. (1995) Cystic fibrosis lung inflammation: early, sustained and severe. *Am. J. Respir. Crit. Care Med.*, **151**, 939–941.

308. Cryz, S. J. Jr (1991) *Pseudomonas aeruginosa* vaccines, in *Vaccines and Immunotherapy*, (ed. S.J. Cryz Jr), Pergamon Press, New York, pp. 156–165.

309. Fisher, M., Devlin, H.B. and Gnabasik, F. (1969) New immunotype schema for *Pseudomonas aeruginosa* based on protective antigens. *J. Bacteriol.*, **98**, 835–836.

310. Pennington, J.E., Reynolds, H.Y., Wood, R.E., Robinson, R.A. and Levine, A.S. (1975) Use of a *Pseudomonas aeruginosa* vaccine in patients with acute leukemia and cystic fibrosis. *Am. J. Med.*, **58**, 629–636.

311. Miller, J.A., Spilsbury, J.F., Jones, R.J., Roe, E.A. and Lowbury, E.J.L. (1977) A new polyvalent *Pseudomonas aeruginosa* vaccine. *J. Med. Microbiol.*, **10**, 19–27.

312. Langford, D T. and Hiller, J. (1984) Prospective, controlled study of a polyvalent Pseudomonas vaccine in cystic fibrosis – three year results. *Arch. Dis. Child.*, **59**, 1131–1133.

313. Cryz, S. J. Jr, Fürer, E., Cross, A.S., Wegmann, A., Germanier, R. and Sadoff, J.C. (1987) Safety and immunogenicity of a *Pseudomonas aeruginosa* O-polysaccharide-toxin A conjugate vaccine in humans. *J. Clin. Invest.*, **80**, 51–56.

314. Schaad, U.B., Lang, A.B., Wedgewood, J., Ruedeberg, A., Que, J.U., Fürer, E., and Cryz, S. J. Jr (1991) Safety and immunogenicity of *Pseudomonas aeruginosa* conjugate vaccine in cystic fibrosis. *Lancet*, **338**, 1236–1237.

315. Lang, A.B., Schaad, U.B., Rudeberg, A. *et al.* (1995) Effect of high-affinity anti-*Pseudomonas aeruginosa* lipopolysaccharide antibodies induced by immunization

on the rate of *Pseudomonas aeruginosa* infection in patients with cystic fibrosis. *J. Pediatr.*, **127**, 711–717.

316. Johansen, H.K., Hougen, H.P., Cryz, S. J. Jr, Rygaard, J. and Høiby, N. (1995) Vaccination promotes TH1-like inflammation and survival in chronic *Pseudomonas aeruginosa* pneumonia in rats. *Am. J. Respir. Crit. Care Med.*, **152**, 1337–1346.

317. Rotering, H. and Dorner, F. (1989) Studies on a *Pseudomonas aeruginosa* flagella vaccine. *Antibiot. Chemother.*, **42**, 218–228.

318. Crowe, B.A., Enzensberger, O., Schober-Bendixen, S. *et al.* (1991) The first clinical trial of Immuno's experimental *Pseudomonas aeruginosa* flagellar vaccines. *Antibiot. Chemother.*, **44**, 143–156.

319. von Specht, B.-U., Knapp, B., Hungerer, K., Lucking, C., Schmitt, A. and Domdey, C. (1996) Outer membrane proteins of *Pseudomonas aeruginosa* as vaccine candidates. *J. Biotechnol.*, **44**, 145–153.

320. Cripps, A.W., Dunkley, M.L., Clancy, R.L. and Kyd, J. (1997) Vaccine strategies against *Pseudomonas aeruginosa* infection in the lung. *Behring Inst. Mitt.*, **98**, 262–268.

321. Döring, G., Pfeiffer, C., Weber, U., Mohr-Pennert, A. and Dorner, F. (1995) Parenteral application of a *Pseudomonas aeruginosa* flagella vaccine elicits specific anti-flagella antibodies in the airways of healthy individuals. *Am. J. Respir.Crit. Care. Med.*, **151**, 983–985.

322. Döring, G. and Dorner, F. (1997) A multicenter vaccine trial using the *Pseudomonas aeruginosa* flagella vaccine IMMUNO in patients with cystic fibrosis. *Behring Inst. Mitt.*, **98**, 338–344.

323. Fournier, J.-M. (1991) *Staphyloccus aureus*, in *Vaccines and Immunotherapy*, (ed. S. J. Cryz Jr), Pergamon Press, New York, pp. 166–177.

324. Fattom, A.I., Sarwar, J., Ortiz, A. and Naso, R. (1996) A *Staphylococcus aureus* capsular polysaccharide (CP) vaccine and CP-specific antibodies protect mice against bacterial challenge. *Infect. Immun.*, **64**, 1659–1665.

325. Sood, S.K. and Daum, R.S. (1991) *Haemophilus influenzae* type B conjugate vaccine, in *Vaccines and Immunotherapy*, (ed. S.J. Cryz Jr), Pergamon Press, New York, pp. 36–58.

326. Tosi, M.F., Stark, J.M., Hamedani, A., Smith, C.W., Gruenert, D.C. and Huang, Y.T. (1992) Intercellular adhesion molecule-1 (ICAM-1)-dependent and ICAM-1-independent adhesive interactions between polymorphonuclear leukocytes and human airway epithelial cells infected with parainfluenza virus type 2. *J. Immunol.*, **149**, 3345–3349.

327. Murphy, T.F., Henderson, F.W., Clyde, W.A., Collier, W.A., Collier, A.M. and Denny, F.W. (1981) Pneumonia: an eleven year study in pediatric practice. *Am. J. Epidem.*, **113**, 12–21.

328. Petersen, N.T., Høiby, N., Mordhorst, C.H., Lind, K., Flensborg, E.W. and Bruun, B. (1981) Respiratory infections in cystic fibrosis caused by virus, chlamydia and mycoplasma – possible synergism with *Pseudomonas aeruginosa*. *Acta Paediatr. Scand.*, **70**, 623–628.

329. Abman, S.H., Ogle, L.W., Butler S.N., Rumack, C.M. and Accurso, F.J. (1988) Role of respiratory syncitial virus in early hospitalization for respiratoy distress in young infants with cystic fibrosis. *J. Pediatr.*, **113**, 826–830.

330. Johansen, H. K. and Høiby, N. (1992) Seasonal onset of initial colonization and chronic *Pseudomonas aeruginosa* infection in patients with cystic fibrosis in Denmark. *Thorax*, **47**, 109–111.

331. Efthimiou, J., Hodson, M.E., Taylor, P., Taylor, A.G. and Batten, J.C. (1984) Importance of viruses and *Legionella pneumophila* in respiratory exacerbations of young adults with cystic fibrosis. *Thorax*, **39**, 150–154.

332. Wang, E.E.L., Prober, C.G., Manson, B., Corey, M. and Levison, H. (1984) Association of respiratory viral infections with pulmonary deterioration in patients with cystic fibrosis. *NEJM*, **311**, 1653–1658.

333. Conway, S.P., Simmonds, E.J. and Littlewood, J.M. (1992) Acute severe deterioration in cystic fibrosis associated with Influenza A virus infection. *Thorax*, **47**, 112–114.

334. Ramsey, B.W., Gore, E.J., Smith, A.L., Cooney, M.K., Redding, G.J. and Foy, H. (1989) The effect of respiratory viral infections on patients with cystic fibrosis. *Am. J. Dis. Child.*, **143**, 662–668.

335. Collins, M.S. and Roby, R.E. (1984) Protective activity of an intravenous immune globulin (human) enriched in antibody against lipopolysaccharide antigens of *Pseudomonas aeruginosa*. *Am. J. Med.*, **76**, 168–174.

336. Van Wye, J.E., Collins, M.S., Baylor, M. *et al.* (1990) *Pseudomonas* hyperimmune globulin passive immunotherapy for pulmonary exacerbations in cystic fibrosis. *Pediatr. Pulmonol.*, **9**, 7–18.

337. Winnie, G.B., Cowan, R.G. and Wade, N.A. (1989) Intravenous immune globulin treatment of pulmonary exacerbations in cystic fibrosis. *J. Pediatr.*, **114**, 309–314.

338. Bentur, L., McKlusky, I., Levison, H. and Roifman, C.M. (1990) Advanced lung disease in a patient with cystic fibrosis and hypogammaglobulinemia: response to intravenous immune globulin therapy. *J .Pediatr.*, **117**, 741–743.

339. Moss, R., Fink, R., Schroeder, S. *et al.* (1995) Safety and pharmacokinetics of a mucoid *Pseudomonas aeruginosa* immunoglobulin. Intravenous (human) in patients with cystic fibrosis – preliminary results of a phase I/II trial. *Pediatr. Pulmonol.*, **19**, 85.

340. Auerbach, H.S., Williams, M., Kirkpatrick, J.A. and Colton, H.R. (1985) Alternate-day prednisone reduces morbidity and improves pulmonary function in cystic fibrosis. *Lancet*, **2**, 686–688.

341. Rosenstein, B.J. and Eigen, H. (1990) Risks of alternate-day prednisone in patients with cystic fibrosis. *Pediatrics*, **87**, 245–246.

342. Greally, P., Hussain, M.J., Vergani, D. and Price, J.F. (1994) Interleukin-1 alpha, soluble interleukin-2 receptor, and IgG concentrations in cystic fibrosis treated with prednisolone. *Arch. Dis. Child.*, **71**, 35–39.

343. van Haren, E.H., Lammers, J.W., Festen, J., Heijerman, H.G., Groot, C.A. and van Herwaarden, C.L. (1995) The

effects of the inhaled corticosteroid budesonide on lung function and bronchial hyperresponsiveness in adult patients with cystic fibrosis. *Respir. Med.*, **89**, 209–214.

344. Nikolaizik, W.H. and Schoni, M.H. (1996) Pilot study to assess the effect of inhaled corticosteroids on lung function in patients with cystic fibrosis. *J. Pediatr.*, **128**, 271–274.

345. Balfour-Lynn, I.M., Klein, N.J. and Dinwiddie, R. (1997) Randomised controlled trial of inhaled corticosteroids (fluticasone propionate) in cystic fibrosis. *Arch. Dis. Child.*, **77**, 124–130.

346. Bisgaard, H., Pedersen, S.S., Nielsen, K.G. *et al.* (1997) Controlled trial of inhaled budesonide in patients with cystic fibrosis and chronic bronchopulmonary *Pseudomonas aeruginosa* infection. *Am. J. Respir. Crit. Care Med.*, **156**, 1190–1196.

347. Sordelli, D.O., Macri, C.N., Maille, A.J. and Cerquetti, M.C. (1994) A preliminary study on the effect of anti-inflammatory treatment in cystic fibrosis patients with *Pseudomonas aeruginosa* lung infection. *Int. J. Immunopathol. Pharmacol.*, **7**, 109–117.

348. Aronoff, S.C., Quinn, F.J. Jr, Carpenter, L.S. and Novick, W.J. Jr (1994) Effects of pentoxifylline on sputum neutrophil elastase and pulmonary function in patients with cystic fibrosis: preliminary observations. *J. Pediatr.*, **125**, 992–997.

349. Konstan, M.W., Hoppel, C.L., Chai, B.-L. and Davis, P.B. (1991) Ibuprofen in children with cystic fibrosis: pharmacokinetics and adverse effects. *J. Pediatr.*, **118**, 956–964.

350. Konstan, M.W., Byard, P.J., Hoppel, C.L. and Davis, P.B. (1995) Effect of high-dose ibuprofen in patients with cystic fibrosis. *NEJM*, **332**, 848–854.

351. Ghio, A.J., Marshall, B.C., Diaz, J.L. *et al.* (1996) Tyloxapol inhibits NF-kappa B and cytokine release, scavenges HOCl, and reduces viscosity of cystic fibrosis sputum. *Am. J. Respir. Crit. Care. Med.*, **154**, 783–788.

352. Henderson, W.R. Jr, Astley, S.J., McCready, M.M. *et al.* (1994) Oral absorption of omega-3 fatty acids in patients with cystic fibrosis who have pancreatic insufficiency and in healthy control subjects. *J. Pediatr.*, **124**, 400–408.

353. Lloyd-Still, J.D., Bibus, D.M., Powers, C.A., Johnson, S.B. and Holman, R.T. (1996) Essential fatty acid deficiency and predisposition to lung disease in cystic fibrosis. *Acta. Paediatr.*, **85**, 1426–1432.

354. Johansen, H.K., Hougen, H.P., Rygaard, J. and Høiby, N. (1996) Interferon-gamma (IFN-gamma) treatment decreases the inflammatory response in chronic *Pseudomonas aeruginosa* pneumonia in rats. *Clin. Exp. Immunol.*, **103**, 212–218.

355. Pierangeli, S.S., Polk, H.C. Jr, Parmely, M.J. and Sonnenfeld, G. (1993) Murine interferon-gamma enhances resistance to infection with strains of *Pseudomonas aeruginosa* in mice. *Cytokine*, **5**, 230–234.

356. Mumford, R.A., Chabin, R., Chiu, S., *et al.* (1995) A cell-penetrant monocyclic β-lactam inhibitor (MBI) which inactivates elastase within PMN *in vitro* and *in vivo*. *Am. J. Respir. Crit. Care Med.*, **151**, A532.

357. Woods, D.E., Strugnell, T., Kooi, C. and Cantin, A. (1997) Inhibiton of human neutrophil elastase by 2-spirocyclopropyl cephalosporin sulfone derivatives. *Pediatr. Pulmonol.*, (Suppl. 14), A249.

358. Cadene, M., Duranton, J., North, A., Si-Tahar, M., Chignard, M. and Bieth, J.G. (1997) Inhibition of neutrophil serine proteinases by suramin. *J. Biol. Chem.*, **272**, 9950–9955.

359. Rice, W. and Weiss, S. (1991) Regulation of proteolysis at the neutrophil–substrate interface by secretory leukoproetase inhibitor. *Science*, **249**, 178–81.

360. Fink, E., Nettelbeck, R. and Fritz, H. (1986) Inhibition of mast cell chymase by eglin c and antileukoprotease (HUSI-1). *Biol. Chem. Hoppe Seyler*, **367**, 567–571.

361. Dietze, S.C., Sommerhof, C.P. and Fritz, H. (1990) Inhibition of histamine release from human mast cells ex vivo by natural and synthetic chymase inhibitors. *Biol. Chem. Hoppe Seyler*, **371**, S75–S79.

362. McElvaney, N.G., Nakamura, H., Birrer, P. *et al.* (1992) Modulation of airway inflammation in cystic fibrosis. *In vivo* suppression of interleukin-8 levels on the respiratory epithelial surface by aerosolization of recombinant secretory leukoprotease inhibitor. *J. Clin. Invest.*, **90**, 1296–1301.

363. McElvaney, N.G., Doujaiji, B., Moan, M.J., Burnham, M.R., Wu, M.C. and Crystal, R. G. (1993) Pharmacokinetics of recombinant secretory leukoprotease inhibitor aerosolized to normals and individuals with cystic fibrosis. *Am. Rev. Respir. Dis.*, **148**, 1056–1060.

364. Ying, Q.L., Kemme, M., Saunders, D. and Simon, S.R. (1997) Glycosaminoglycans regulate elastase inhibition by oxidized secretory leukoprotease inhibitor. *Am. J. Physiol.*, **272**, L533–L541.

365. Rao, N.V., Kennedy, T.P., Rao, G., Ky, N. and Hoidal, J.R. (1990) Sulfated polysaccharides prevent human leukocyte elastase-induced acute lung injury and emphysema in hamsters. *Am. Rev. Respir. Dis.*, **142**, 407–412.

366. McElvaney, N.G., Hubbard, R.C., Birrer, P. *et al.* (1991) Aerosol α1-antitrypsin treatment for cystic fibrosis. *Lancet*, **337**, 392–394.

367. Canonico, A.E., Brigham, K.L., Carmichael, L.C., Plitman, J.D., King, G.A., Blackwell, T.R. and Christman, J.W. (1996) Plasmid-liposome transfer of the alpha 1 antitrypsin gene to cystic fibrosis bronchial epithelial cells prevents elastase-induced cell detachment and cytokine release. *Am. J. Respir. Cell. Mol. Biol.*, **14**, 348–355.

368. Adam, C. and Bieth, J.G. (1996) Inhibition of neutrophil elastase by the alpha1-proteinase inhibitor-immunoglobulin A complex. *FEBS Lett.*, **385**, 201–204

369. Gershon, D. (1991) Biotechnology. Will milk shake up industry? *Nature*, **353**, 7.

370. Matheson, N.R., Wong, P.S. and Travis, J. (1979) Enzymatic inactivation of human alpha-1-proteinase inhibitor by neutrophil myeloperoxidase. *Biochem. Biophys. Res. Commun.*, **88**, 402–409.

7

The pathology of cystic fibrosis

M. N. SHEPPARD AND A. G. NICHOLSON

Introduction	141	Genitourinary tract	150
Respiratory tract	141	Endocrine system	151
Pleura	147	Muscle, bone and joint changes	151
Heart	147	Skin	151
Gastrointestinal tract	147	Central nervous system	151
Pancreas	148	References	152
Liver and bile ducts	149		

INTRODUCTION

Cystic fibrosis, with its basic defect in ion transport, results in the accumulation of sticky tenacious mucus in relation to epithelial surfaces in many organs, particularly the lungs, gastrointestinal tract, pancreas and liver. The histopathologist is rarely called upon to make the initial diagnosis as cystic fibrosis is usually diagnosed clinically, being characterized by chronic bronchopulmonary infection, malabsorption due to pancreatic insufficiency and a high sweat sodium concentration on sweat testing. Most information concerning both macroscopic and microscopic findings in cystic fibrosis has come from autopsy studies, so the pathological features have often been extreme. However, with increasing survival of patients with cystic fibrosis, we are seeing more subtle changes in other organs and, in addition, more aggressive drug therapy and lung transplantation are bringing with them new disease entities and complications.

RESPIRATORY TRACT

Upper respiratory tract

The upper airway is often involved in cystic fibrosis, with nasal polyps found at all ages, their incidence in children ranges from 6.7 per cent to 20 per cent[1]. Nasal polyps are very rare in childhood outside of patients with cystic fibrosis, so their presence points to the diagnosis in this age group. Histologically, they contain mucous cysts and hyperplastic mucous glands[2], and may be differentiated from non-cystic fibrosis nasal polyps by an absence of basement membrane thickening, few eosinophils and the presence of highly sulfated acidic mucins[3]. The nasal polyps in cystic fibrosis also show greater numbers of mast cells, plasma cells and lymphocytes compared with non-cystic fibrosis cases, the mast cells showing evidence of degranulation[4]. The polyps are often multiple and may cause nasal obstruction with depression and widening of the nasal bridge. Approximately 50 per cent of patients are considered atopic on the basis of allergic symptoms and skin tests[5] but others question its role in the development of polyps[6], believing that chronic mucopurulent discharge may cause irritation of the mucosal lining leading to edema with swelling and resultant polyps.

In adults up to 40 per cent of patients develop polyps, a considerably higher incidence than in children[7]. The presence of nasal polyps bears no relation to the severity of pulmonary involvement in either children or adults. Ultrastructural studies of nasal epithelium reveal that there is disorganization and an irregular stranding pattern of the tight junctions between cells that are involved in the regulation of paracellular permeability[8]. Ciliary abnormalities are also reported, including compound cilia and multiple axonemes, although these changes are believed to be nonspecific and to occur as a result of infection. However, this ciliary disorientation may well perpetuate further damage[9].

Lower respiratory tract

There is widespread variation in pathological processes in the lungs between patients[10], but except for neonatal deaths resulting from meconium ileus, pulmonary complications are responsible for most of the morbidity and mortality in cystic fibrosis. Although infective agents are reviewed elsewhere (Chapter 5), it is worth reviewing them briefly before looking specifically at the airways and parenchyma, as infection is pivotal to pulmonary pathology in cystic fibrosis.

BACTERIAL INFECTION

The main infective agents are bacteria, with *Staphylococcus aureus*, *Haemophilus influenzae* and *Pseudomonas aeruginosa* being the chief pathogens. Repeated cycles of endobronchial and endobronchiolar bacterial infection and inflammation cause chronic damage to the airways, further augmented by impaired ciliary clearance[11]. The role of the inflammatory response, including the cell types involved and their chemical mediators, in propagating further lung damage is well reviewed[12-15]. Defects in host defense with hypogammaglobulinemia[16] and defects in cell-mediated immunity[17] have been implicated in the predisposition to infection in cystic fibrosis, but these reports are few and the majority of patients have no such abnormalities. *Staphylococcus aureus* is associated with infection in the first few years of life. It can be seen in almost 40 per cent of infants within the first 3 months[18]. Chronic *S. aureus* infection usually precedes *P. aeruginosa* infection, and a deterioration in lung function with chronic *S. aureus* infection before colonization by *P. aeruginosa* indicates that often it is the *S. aureus* infection that initiates lung injury[19]. However, it is chronic *P. aeruginosa* infection that is associated with chronic lung injury and reduced survival[20], with *P. aeruginosa* rarely being eradicated. Noncapsulate forms of *H. influenzae* are frequently isolated from the respiratory tract of children with cystic fibrosis, but their role as pathogens remains unknown[21]. In adults, noncapsulate forms of *H. influenzae* are pathogenic and there is a higher isolation rate at the time of a symptomatic respiratory deterioration in patients with cystic fibrosis[22]. Its role may be underestimated as this organism may coexist with *P. aeruginosa* infection in a spheroplast form which is difficult to isolate[23].

Burkholderia cepacia, formerly known as *Pseudomonas cepacia*, has more recently been isolated in older cystic fibrosis patients[24] and its isolation from sputum has been causally associated with a rapid decline in pulmonary function progressing to death[25]. It is now believed that upper airway sites of infection may contribute to perpetuation of lower airway infection[26]. The role of nontuberculous mycobacteria in causing infection and damage in the lungs of patients with cystic fibrosis has also recently been highlighted, with an incidence of isolation in sputum of 3.5 per cent being found, their presence associated with intravenous antibiotic therapy and steroids[27]. However, the significance of sputum isolation has been questioned, since an autopsy report showed granulomatous inflammation in only 2 of 6 cases with repeated positive sputum isolation and in none in cases where only one positive sputum was reported[28]. Chlamydial infection has also been reported in CF[29].

FUNGAL INFECTION

A minority of patients have fungi, usually *Aspergillus fumigatus*, in their sputum and some may develop fungal-precipitating antibodies in their serum[30]. Patients with cystic fibrosis are predisposed to pulmonary fungal colonization because of extensive lung damage and long-term antibiotic therapy, usually within airways but occasionally as intracavity fungal balls[31]. However, the contributory role of fungi in causing lung damage is not well defined.

Allergic bronchopulmonary aspergillosis (ABPA) was first associated with cystic fibrosis in 1965. Its reported incidence varies between 0.6 and 11 per cent[32,33]. There have, in fact, been few studies on the pathology of this condition and numbers of patients have been small[34]. Simple asthma, mucoid impaction, bronchiectasis, bronchocentric granulomatosis and eosinophilic pneumonia have all been described as part of the spectrum of ABPA[35]. Microscopically there may be eosinophilic infiltration of the bronchial wall, desquamation of epithelium, thickening of the basement membrane and mucus plugging, with the mucus containing large numbers of eosinophils and Charcot–Leyden crystals. As an allergic response to inhaled *Aspergillus* spores, fungal elements may be sparse in the mucus plugs (Fig. 7.1). These plugs can have a characteristic appearance. Bands of agglutinated eosinophils alternate with layers of mucus. In cases with coexistent bronchiectasis, there are the characteristic plugs as well as inflammation and destruction of the bronchial walls with a prominent eosinophilic infiltrate. Bronchocentric granulomatosis represents a more profound hypersensitivity reaction, with necrotizing granulomas containing palisading epithelioid cells, Langhans giant cells and many eosinophils surrounding and infiltrating bronchi (Fig. 7.2). When the inflammatory pattern extends into the small airways and alveoli it gives a similar pattern to that of eosinophilic pneumonia. The alveolar infiltrate is thought to be responsible for the fleeting shadows seen on chest radiography. Neither of these entities is characterized by invasion of the lung parenchyma by fungus.

Invasive or disseminated fungal infection was consid-

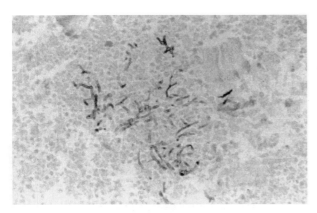

Fig. 7.1 *A small collection of* Aspergillus *hyphae within a dilated bronchus in a cystic fibrosis lung.*

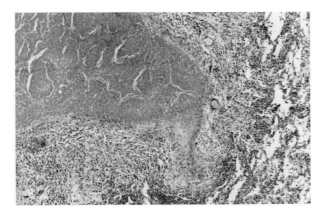

Fig. 7.2 *Lung parenchyma from a cystic fibrosis patient showing a necrotizing granuloma with surrounding multinucleate Langhans-type giant cells.*

ered rare in the cystic fibrosis population prior to the 1980s[36]. Autopsy reports on 156 patients with cystic fibrosis from 1964 to 1982 disclosed only one with disseminated fungal infection. However, in a more recent retrospective study of 63 patients with cystic fibrosis from 1982 to 1987, invasive disease was detected in 13 cases (21 per cent)[37]. The patients with *Candida* infections had foci of acute inflammation and abscess formation, whereas those with *Aspergillus* infection had hemorrhagic foci, with branching hyphae radiating throughout the lung in a 'star-burst' pattern and extensively invading blood vessels. In four of these patients, disseminated extrapulmonary fungal infection was a contributory cause of death. This study also showed that the cellular reaction to fungal infection in cystic fibrosis may be acute with little or no granuloma formation. Therefore, special stains for fungi should be done routinely in any study of cystic fibrosis pathology in the lung[37].

VIRAL INFECTION

The place of viral infection in initiating or promoting lung damage remains controversial. Viral infections can damage mucociliary clearance and encourage secondary bacterial infection[38].

BRONCHI AND BRONCHIOLES

Earlier authors claimed that the lungs were normal at birth[39], but in fetal lungs during the second trimester of pregnancy there is accumulation of mucin in the tracheobronchial glands as compared to controls[40]. Postnatally, histological abnormalities are detectable within the first few days of life[41]. Even before infection becomes clinically detected, there is submucosal gland hypertrophy, duct obstruction and mucous cell hyperplasia of the trachea and major bronchi (Fig. 7.3). These changes have been found in infants who had died from meconium ileus early in the neonatal period, with the lungs showing no evidence of infection[41]. Quantification of the tracheobronchial mucous glands in infants with cystic fibrosis has found a significant increase in luminal volume compared to controls[42]. Mucus hypersecretion is usually seen with florid goblet cell hyperplasia of the bronchial epithelium (Fig. 7.4). The bronchial seromucinous glands are increased in volume, with an elevated gland-to-wall ratio and dilated ducts are filled with inspissated secretions.

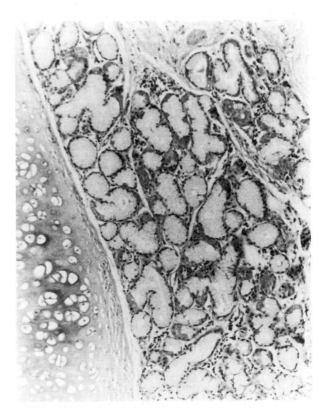

Fig. 7.3 *Bronchial wall showing an increase in seromucous glands in the submucosa inside a cartilage plate.*

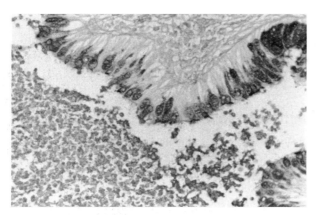

Fig. 7.4 *Bronchial epithelium from a cystic fibrosis patient showing an increase in mucus-containing cells (dark staining) and mucus within the bronchial lumen. Periodic acid–Schiff stain.*

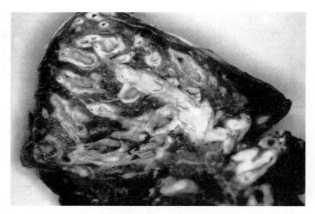

Fig. 7.7 *Cystic fibrosis post-mortem lung with bronchiectasis in the upper lobe. Note dilated thickened bronchi which extend out to the subpleura and contain pus.*

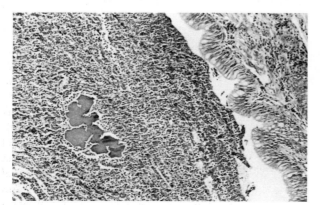

Fig. 7.5 *Bronchial wall showing mucus, proteinaceous debris and polymorphonuclear cells within the lumen.*

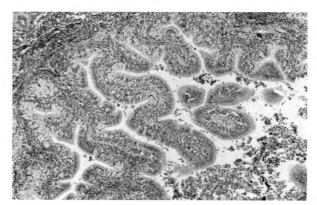

Fig. 7.8 *Bronchial wall showing papillary proliferation of the lining respiratory epithelium and chronic inflammatory cells in the submucosa.*

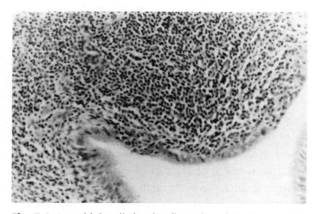

Fig. 7.6 *Bronchial wall showing flattening of the lining epithelium and an increase in chronic inflammatory cells in the submucosa which are infiltrating the overlying epithelium.*

Once infection sets in, the airways are filled with thick, mucopurulent material containing bacterial colonies, neutrophils and thick mucus (Fig. 7.5). The plugging of the bronchi and bronchioles is the earliest macroscopic

finding in the lungs of infants dying of CF[39]. Repeated pulmonary infections cause acute bronchitis, which is found at autopsy in patients with cystic fibrosis dying at more than 1 month of age[43] with *S. aureus* predominating among the pathogens[44]. The bronchitis and bronchiolitis are associated with a mixed cellular infiltrate of acute and chronic inflammatory cells, including neutrophils, histiocytes, lymphocytes and plasma cells, with no difference in the lesions produced by different bacteria (Fig. 7.6). This repeated infection causes ulcerative bronchitis, which commonly leads to irreversible damage of the bronchial wall with resultant bronchiectasis. In patients who survive 6 months, infection with bronchiectasis has been found to be universal in past studies[41], the severity increasing with age[43]. This process affects the proximal airways and the distribution is usually most marked in the upper lobes, right middle lobe, lingula and apical segments of the lower lobes (Fig. 7.7). This pattern of more severe upper lobe inflammation is reflected in lavage specimens[45]. Necrosis and loss of bronchial cartilage may be seen in addition to the inflammatory cell infiltrate[46], as well as papillary prolif-

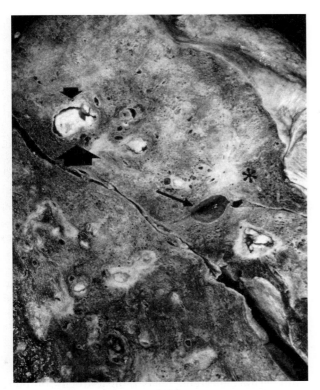

Fig. 7.9 *Cystic fibrosis post-mortem lung showing endo-bronchial abscesses within dilated bronchi. There is also scarring and consolidation of the surrounding lung parenchyma. An intra-pulmonary cyst is also visible.*

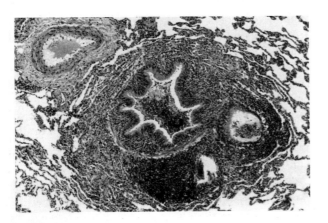

Fig. 7.10 *Lung parenchyma containing a bronchiole with a dense lymphocytic infiltrate within the wall and a lymphoid aggregate. There is also mucus within the lumen.*

eration of the lining epithelium with squamous meta-plasia (Fig. 7.8). Formation of endobronchial abscesses eventually produces saccular spaces within the lung parenchyma (Fig. 7.9) which can result in fibrous scar-ring and lobar collapse. Collapse can also result from impaction of airways by mucus plugging and by enlarged lymph nodes impinging on the bronchi, pre-viously very common in infants[47].

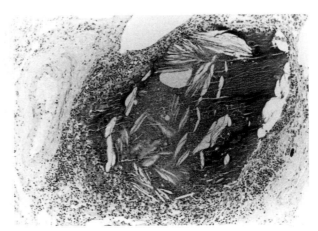

Fig. 7.11 *Bronchiole with destruction of the lining epithelium and filling of lumen by thick mucus-containing cholesterol clefts. There is surrounding chronic inflammation.*

As with the bronchi, bronchiolitis is almost universal in infants[48] with florid mucosal and lumenal inflamma-tion and ulceration. Goblet cells, which are normally not found in bronchioles, proliferate and there is also mucous hypersecretion (Figs 7.10 and 7.11). The lining epithelium undergoes hyperplasia with papillary prolif-eration and squamous metaplasia. Follicular bronchioli-tis with hyperplasia of the mucosa-associated lymphoid tissue is also common (Fig. 7.10). The bronchioles become plugged with cellular debris full of cholesterol clefts and there is destruction of the lining epithelium and bronchiolar wall itself (Fig. 7.11). The inflammation can lead to fibrous obliteration of the airways, resulting in bronchiolitis obliterans which can lead to hyperinfla-tion or collapse, depending on the adequacy of the col-lateral ventilation. This obliteration of small airways tends to occur in older children and adults[10].

LUNG PARENCHYMA

In neonates and infants fulminant necrotizing bronchi-olitis and bronchopneumonia were common before the introduction of appropriate therapy. The bronchioles became filled with thick pus, with subsequent consolida-tion of the surrounding lung parenchyma. Pneumonia tends to be seen at all stages in the evolution of the dis-ease[43] with alveoli filled with neutrophils and/or foci of organization. Although these changes can revert to nor-mal, parenchymal destruction often occurs with repeated infection and *S. aureus* infection is particularly associated with pneumatoceles which result from pul-monary parenchymal necrosis (Fig. 7.12). Distal to obstructed airways there may be an exudate of lipid-filled histiocytes producing endogenous lipoid pneumo-nia. There is also often a chronic inflammatory interstitial infiltrate with lymphocytes, plasma cells and fibrosis of the interstitium, and it has been suggested that these changes could be due to viral infection. Ultrastructural studies of the lung in patients with cystic

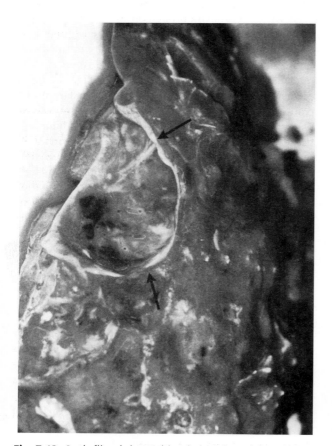

Fig. 7.12 *Cystic fibrosis lung with pale consolidation of the parenchyma and an area of lung destruction with pneumatocele formation (arrow).*

Fig. 7.13 *Cystic fibrosis lung with subpleural cyst (arrows).*

fibrosis show nonspecific changes related to mucus hypersecretion and infection[49].

Cysts can occur within the lung. These are defined as smooth-walled air spaces that are either separate from the bronchial tree or communicate via a small channel. Three types are described. The first and most common is bronchiectatic with direct communication with bronchi.

The second is interstitial with a cystic space located in the visceral pleura or interlobular septae lined by fibrous tissue (Figs 7.9 and 7.13). The third and least common is the emphysematous type, resulting from destruction of alveolar walls with direct continuity into surrounding dilated alveoli. These emphysematous cysts increase with age[43]. All three cyst types are more common in the upper lobes, particularly in the apical and posterior segments.

One of the few evolutionary studies on the pathologic changes over a time period was carried out by Bedrossian[43] who looked at 82 autopsies between 1954 and 1972 and divided them into age groups ranging from birth to 24 years. Bronchial changes and bronchiectasis could be seen from birth and became more common with advancing age and universal by the time patients reached their twenties. Parenchymal changes with pneumonia were also seen from birth and were present in up to 82 per cent of cases by age 24. Emphysema was much less common, being present only from 2 years upwards and reaching 41 per cent in the 10–24 year age group.

PULMONARY VASCULATURE

With airway infection, there is hypertrophy of pulmonary and bronchial arteries, capillaries and bronchial veins[50]. With increasing lung damage, hypoxia occurs which leads to vasoconstrictive pulmonary hypertension. This is initially reversible but with medial hypertrophy and intimal fibrosis caused by the increase in pressure, the hypertension becomes irreversible[51]. Pulmonary hypertension leads to further medial hypertrophy and intimal fibrosis of the pulmonary arterial branches, with medial deposition of mucoid material[52] and calcification of the internal elastic lamina is sometimes seen[41]. There is spread of smooth muscle into the small alveolar arterioles and veins, which normally do not contain muscle, with a reduction in the number of vessels[53]. These changes increase with age and may cause hemoptysis due to rupture of dilated bronchial arteries

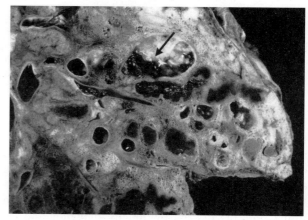

Fig. 7.14 *Cystic fibrosis post-mortem lung with the bronchiectatic cavities filled with fresh blood (arrow).*

or veins through the walls of airways or into bronchiectatic cavities[54]. Direct injury to vessels by infection, an increase in bronchopulmonary arterial anastomoses and loss of elasticity of vessels due to pulmonary hypertension all contribute to the precipitation of bleeding[55], and massive hemoptysis is the terminal event in some patients (Fig. 7.14).

COMPLICATION OF IMPROVED SURVIVAL IN THE LUNGS

The severity of the lung diseases described above increases with age. Hemoptysis and pneumothorax become more common[56]. Pneumothorax contributes significantly to morbidity and mortality in those patients who have prolonged survival. As patients with cystic fibrosis survive longer, pulmonary hypertension and cor pulmonale are more common[53]. Pulmonary amyloidosis can also present with a diffuse interstitial pattern in long-term survivors[57].

COMPLICATIONS OF LUNG TRANSPLANTATION

Heart–lung transplantation is now well established in the management of end-stage respiratory disease in both children and adults with cystic fibrosis[58,59]. As with other allografts, the main complications are lung rejection and infection. In combined heart–lung transplants, the lungs reject earlier and more actively than the heart[60]. Acute lung rejection is characterized by perivascular and peribronchial mononuclear cell infiltrate with extension into the alveoli and interstitium. Lung rejection, like cardiac rejection, is graded according to the severity of the histological changes[60]. Chronic airway rejection results in fibrous obliteration of the bronchioles (obliterative bronchiolitis) and is the main lethal complication in long-term survivors. Chronic vascular rejection associated with fibrointimal thickening of arteries and veins is not as prominent in the lungs as it is in chronic cardiac rejection[60]. Children with cystic fibrosis have an increased incidence of lung rejection compared with cystic fibrosis adults. There is also a higher incidence of tracheal stenosis in children, which could be explained by a less well-developed collateral circulation. Survival in patients with cystic fibrosis has extended up to 10 years on follow-up[59]. However, due to lack of organ donation, 50 per cent of patients die on the waiting list for transplantation.

The lungs are also prone to infection with common bacterial pathogens, and pulmonary infection often coexists with rejection. *Pseudomonas aeruginosa* is the most common isolate[61]. Because of immunosuppression, opportunistic infections are also common. The lung has a much higher opportunistic infection rate than other allografted organs. These opportunistic infections include mycobacteria, cytomegalovirus, herpes simplex virus, aspergillus, *Pneumocystis carinii* and *Toxoplasma*[60].

Lung transplant recipients are also prone to post-transplant lymphoproliferative disorders, mainly of B-cell phenotype and associated with Epstein–Barr virus infection. The spectrum of changes is reviewed extensively elsewhere[62].

PLEURA

As patients survive longer in cystic fibrosis, pneumothorax has emerged as an increasingly common complication. This is related to the spontaneous rupture of apical bullae, which are cysts greater than 1 cm in diameter found commonly in a subpleural location. These bullae can be found in up to 60 per cent of autopsies in cystic fibrosis[56]. Pneumothorax can also follow rupture of pneumatoceles in childhood or rupture of a subpleural abscess. There is little pathological difference between the pleural changes in pneumothorax of non-cystic fibrosis and cystic fibrosis cases. However, columnar cells containing large cytoplasmic vacuoles may line the parietal pleura in patients with cystic fibrosis[63].

HEART

Most changes are secondary to respiratory failure and pulmonary hypertension. As patients survive longer, cor pulmonale frequently occurs late in the course of the disease and carries a poor prognosis[64]. Cor pulmonale is assessed by right ventricular weight, which is best judged by weighing the free wall of the right ventricle compared to the weight of the left ventricle and interventricular septum. The hypertrophy and dilatation can give rise to focal areas of fibrosis within the myocardium[65]. Cardiac fibrosis involving the left ventricle has also been reported in infants with cystic fibrosis without evidence of right-sided cardiac failure and suggested causes include malnourishment and hypovitaminosis[66].

Aortic artherosclerosis is less in patients with cystic fibrosis than in aged-matched controls[67] with a decrease in fatty streaks and fibromusculoelastic lesions[68]. Impaired fat absorption as well as chronic infection has been implicated in this decreased incidence.

GASTROINTESTINAL TRACT

On occasion the pathologist may make a diagnosis of cystic fibrosis in fetal autopsy material, the most obvious changes being found in the gastrointestinal tract where thick meconium plugs can be present from as early as 17 weeks' gestation[69]. Their presence is highly suggestive of cystic fibrosis in the fetus and can occur in the absence of changes in the lung, pancreas or liver. It is a combination of reduction in water content, increase in mucoprotein, absence of proteolytic enzymes and increase in albumin that accounts for the increased viscosity. The plugging can progress to meconium ileus, in which there is mechanical obstruction of the distal ileum, which affects 17 per cent of patients with cystic fibrosis at birth[70]. This shows dense meconium adherent to the intestinal mucosa, with dilatation and obstruction of the lumen. Microscopically there is extensive goblet cell hyperplasia and strongly alcianophilic mucinous material (Fig. 7.15). The villi and crypts are otherwise normal. Obstruction may lead to ischemic necrosis of the ileal wall with perforation and the development of meconium peritonitis[71]. If this occurs early *in utero* there will be an inflammatory reaction with adhesions in the peritoneum and calcification. The perforation is usually sealed by adhesions and although the meconium may be reabsorbed, it can remain in the abdomen and cause perforation that requires surgery in the third trimester or at birth[70,72]. Other associated intestinal abnormalities include volvulus and ileal atresias. While perioperative mortality is high, the patients' later course does not differ from that of patients without these complications[72].

Postnatally, pathology can be found throughout the GI tract. In adults, lesions in the salivary and labial glands can be found, with eosinophilic plugs in ducts causing enlargement[73]. Upper gastrointestinal problems include reflux and esophagitis with peptic ulceration. There is also an increased incidence of Barrett's esophagus and, with increased survival, children with cystic fibrosis may be a high-risk group for Barrett's esophagus and its complications[74]. Esophageal varices associated with portal hypertension occur with cirrhosis due to cystic fibrosis. There have also been occasional case reports of coexistent Crohn's disease and celiac disease[75].

In the small bowel, the characteristic findings of meconium ileus can be one of the earliest features of cystic fibrosis[76]. Some infants present with the 'meconium plug syndrome' in which a hard plug of meconium is present in the colon with abdominal distension. The infant then passes the plug and resumes normal bowel function.

Older patients with cystic fibrosis may develop 'meconium ileus equivalent' or 'distal intestinal obstruction syndrome', especially if oral intake of fluids is inadequate or patients fail to take pancreatic enzyme preparations. The pain of meconium ileus equivalent may mimic appendicitis and the appendix may be removed. Indeed, patients presenting with an acute abdomen offer a diagnostic challenge for the surgeon and appendiceal abscess must be considered as a rare complication of CF[77]. When these occur, microscopic examination of the appendix shows an increase in goblet cells, together with mucus secretion into the crypts and distension of the lumen[78]. Intussusception can also develop in up to 1 per cent of patients with cystic fibrosis, a further differential diagnosis of an acute abdomen[79]. The head of the intussusception is formed by hard masses of stool, which invert into a loop of bowel, causing obstruction and ischemic necrosis.

In recent years colonic strictures, after the use of high-dose pancreatic enzymes, have been reported increasingly[80]. The main histological feature of 'fibrosing colonopathy' is dense fibrosis of the submucosa involving long segments. The pathogenesis is uncertain but a direct toxic effect of the enzymes, low-fiber diet, malabsorbed fat , poor blood supply and abnormal motility may all play a role. Use of laxatives and gastrograffin has also been implicated[81]. Neuropathy with ganglion cell and neural hyperplasia, as well as vascular changes, have also been reported[82].

In the 1950s rectal mucosal prolapse was reported in up to 22 per cent of patients with cystic fibrosis[83], sometimes as the first manifestation of the disease. It often recurs in the first 5 years of life and then spontaneously resolves, often following treatment for pancreatic insufficiency. With modern treatment prolapse is less common.

Patients with cystic fibrosis are at increased risk of developing gastrointestinal adenocarcinoma, although their risk of other cancers is the same as for the general population[84]. Alterations in the expression of the *CFTR* gene, as well as the direct effects of the disease, have all been implicated in this increased risk. Patients with persistent malabsorption are also deficient in the antioxidants selenium and vitamin E, which protect against cancer.

PANCREAS

Prenatally, no changes are seen before 17 weeks[69], but from 20 weeks there may be accumulation of eosinophilic secretions with dilatation of ductules[85]. Quantitative microscopy shows that the volume of acini and duct lumens is greater in cystic fibrosis than in controls.

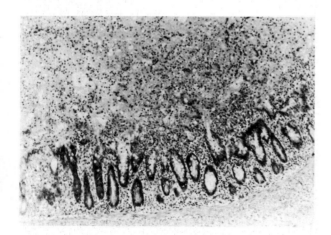

Fig. 7.15 *Cystic fibrosis infant with meconium ileus, showing large intestine with the lumen distended by mucus and marked secretion from lining glands.*

In the postnatal exocrine pancreas, there is tissue damage due to acinar release of lytic enzymes, with loss of acini, fibrosis and fatty replacement. Even in neonates, there may be interstitial fibrosis of the pancreas with inspissation of secretions in the ducts and acini. Four histological grades of severity are described[86]: grade I is accumulation of secretion, grade II exocrine atrophy, grade III atrophy with lipomatosis and grade IV fibrosis with total obliteration of the exocrine glands and ducts with scattered islets of Langerhans. Pancreatic insufficiency results and this often causes the prominent clinical symptoms of cystic fibrosis in infancy and early childhood. About 85 per cent of patients have such severe loss of pancreatic tissue that inadequate secretion of digestive enzymes occurs, causing malabsorption which adversely affects survival. A morphometric analysis in patients with final-stage cystic fibrosis revealed that compared with controls, the proportion of the connective and fatty tissue had increased by about 10 times and 200 times, respectively[87]. The pancreas at autopsy is fibrosed and fatty, with residual dilated ducts filled with secretions at the head (Fig. 7.16). Recurrent pancreatitis can be seen in patients with cystic fibrosis, with or without insufficiency. Presumably the thick secretions block ducts with resultant autodigestion by pancreatic enzymes[88].

In the endocrine pancreas, progressive pancreatic fibrosis ultimately disrupts pancreatic islet function. This used to be rare (1–2 per cent) but has been increasing, presumably as a consequence of increasing survival (8–13 per cent). It is believed that the presence of fibrosis with strangulation of the islet vasculature and subsequent hypoxia is the factor responsible for the disorganization of pancreatic endocrine function and impaired insulin secretion. Examination of the endocrine pancreas reveals that there is a decrease in beta cells and an increase in non-beta cells[87] and at least 30 per cent of patients with pancreatic insufficiency will have an abnormal tolerance to glucose loads. Adenocarcinoma of the pancreas has been reported in cystic fibrosis[89].

LIVER AND BILE DUCTS

Obstructive biliary disease occurs in 15–20 per cent of affected patients. Inspissated secretions can be seen in bile ducts prior to birth, along with bile-duct proliferation, focal chronic inflammation and fibrosis[69,86]. Due to the presence of these inspissated secretions, prolonged jaundice with cholestasis may be seen in neonates[90], as well as with meconium ileus[91]. Excessive mucoid material is noted macroscopically in intra- and extrahepatic bile ducts. This accumulation of mucus leads to the formation of intrahepatic and extrahepatic biliary stones, which can lead to clinical obstruction. These can also calcify and be seen radiologically[92]. In the gallbladder, mucoid material accumulates in the lumen of the gallbladder and multiloculated mucus-containing cysts can be seen in both the epithelium and submucosa[93]. Calculi occur in about 12 per cent of patients due to the production of thick lithogenic bile (Fig. 7.17)[94]. Cholecystitis occurs and microgallbladder is common in cystic fibrosis[91]. With increasing survival, these gallbladder complications are becoming more frequent. Adenocarcinomas of the extrahepatic bile ducts can occur in cystic fibrosis.

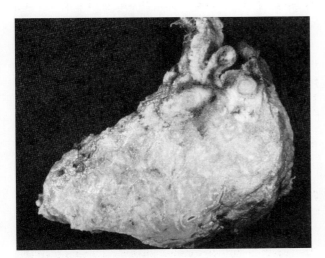

Fig. 7.16 *Head of cystic fibrosis pancreas showing dilated ducts filled with gelatinous material. There is fibrosis and fatty change in the parenchyma.*

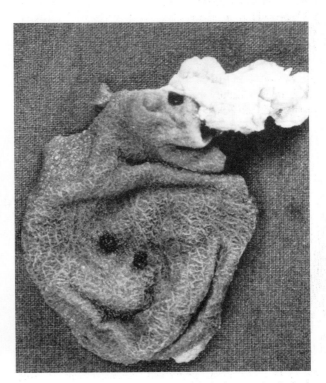

Fig. 7.17 *Cystic fibrosis gallbladder with dark stones in the body and one obstructing the cystic duct.*

Significant histologic liver disease is common in cystic fibrosis, and its exact nature often requires liver biopsy[95]. Within the liver, bile stasis with proliferation of bile ducts and periportal inflammation with fibrosis occurs[41]. These lesions have been called 'focal biliary fibrosis' and are typical of hepatic involvement in up to 25 per cent of patients[96], although such lesions may be asymptomatic and have little clinical significance. Bile-duct stenosis with development of sclerosing cholangitis is also common. There is eventual progression to cirrhosis with the formation of multiple regenerating nodules within the liver (Fig. 7.18). This occurs in a minority of patients (2–5 per cent) and seems to increase with age[91]. This extensive liver pathology is responsible for the development of portal hypertension with esophageal varices and hypersplenism[97]. Fatty infiltration of the liver is common in patients with cystic fibrosis[98]. Giant-cell hepatitis and cytomegalovirus infection of the liver have been reported. Liver as well as heart–lung transplantation has been successful in cystic fibrosis[99].

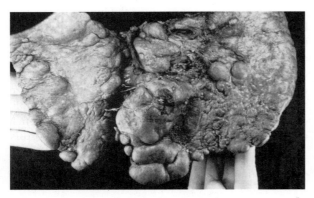

Fig. 7.18 *Cystic fibrosis liver with macronodular cirrhosis.*

GENITOURINARY TRACT

Kidneys

Until recently no abnormality of the kidneys had been reported with cystic fibrosis[86] and glomerular changes were considered to be secondary to diabetes mellitus and hypertension. However, there is an increase in urinary oxalate excretion which is linked to malabsorption in cases with steatorrhea, the patients developing urolithiasis[100], and, recently, a high incidence of microscopic nephrocalcinosis has also been reported. A defect in calcium metabolism has been postulated, but not proven[101].

Female genital tract

Females reach menarche and develop secondary sexual characteristics. Anatomically the female genital tract is normal, but the cervical mucus has reduced water content and may not undergo the normal viscosity change in midcycle that favors sperm penetration[102]. This is one factor contributing to infertility. Chronic pulmonary sepsis also delays menarche and causes menstrual irregularities, but even those with good pulmonary function may have similar problems[103]. Multiple follicular cysts can be found in the ovaries[104]. Cervicitis, cervical erosions and mucous gland hyperplasia are common pathological findings in the cervix, and vaginitis also occurs[105]. However, females can become pregnant with normal delivery of an infant, which is now becoming more frequent as patients survive with good pulmonary function into adulthood.

Male genital tract

Like females, males enter puberty and develop all the secondary sexual characteristics and sexual function is normal. However, there is an anatomical abnormality of the genital tract in nearly all males with cystic fibrosis. The vasa deferentia are atretic or completely absent[106]. The body and tail of the epididymes and seminal vesicles are abnormally dilated or absent (Fig. 7.19)[107]. The abnormalities of these structures cannot be explained simply by obstruction or infection alone and their occurrence remains a mystery. A primarily genital phenotype has been described in otherwise healthy males who have congenital absence of the vas deferens, which is now established as a heterozygous genetic condition, with some cases being heterozygous for ΔF_{508} CFTR while others have no identifiable mutation[108]. It has been suggested that the *CFTR* gene plays a role beyond the normal development of the vas deferens, perhaps being related to spermatogeneseis as well[108]. Thus male patients are generally infertile, but rare patients have a normal

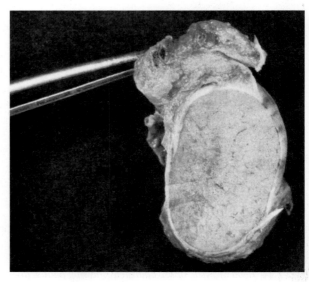

Fig. 7.19 *Cystic fibrosis testis with no identifiable epididymis. Loose fatty tissue is identified. No vas deferens is present.*

genital tract and have fathered children. These are usually patients with good respiratory function.

ENDOCRINE SYSTEM

The carotid bodies are usually enlarged in the late stages of cystic fibrosis due to chronic hypoxia[109] (Fig. 7.20). The female breast shows lobular atrophy[110]. Hyperplasia of the zona glomerulosa of the adrenal gland is described in children and may be related to the loss of salt in sweat[111]. The thyroid can enlarge and become involved by amyloidosis[112] which may lead to hypothyroidism[113].

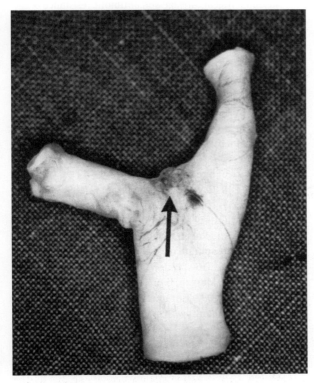

Fig. 7.20 *Hyperplastic carotid body with prominent feeding vessels between internal and external carotid arteries.*

MUSCLE, BONE AND JOINT CHANGES

Many patients suffer malnutrition because of their gastrointestinal pathology, although this is less of a problem than it was formerly. Muscle wasting also occurs. Nearly all patients with cystic fibrosis become clubbed[114]. Hypertrophic pulmonary osteoarthropathy with proliferation of vascular connective tissue beneath the periosteum occurs in both children[115] and adults, but is more common in adults[116]. There are also changes in craniofacial morphology, namely increased mandibular and craniocervical inclination, open bite and decreased posterior facial height, similar in pattern to that of children with nasal obstruction due to enlarged tonsils or adenoids[117]. Patients also develop osteoporosis[118], fractures and kyphosis[119]. Episodic arthropathy is described in adults[120] and children[121] and hip replacement may be required[122].

SKIN

Eccrine glands

The eccrine sweat glands, while providing the invaluable diagnostic clue of excess sodium and chloride concentrations, are usually normal by light microscopy. In normal eccrine sweat glands there is localization of CFTR to the apical membrane of the reabsorptive duct and in the basolateral membranes of the inner layer of cells of the duct. Comparison with patients homozygous for ΔF_{508} showed no membrane staining, whereas the heterozygote carriers had reduced staining[123]. Furthermore, there is increased CFTR staining of cytoplasmic granules in the secretory portion of glands in the cystic fibrosis cases, suggesting abnormal processing of CFTR. A recent study has shown that β-adrenergic-sensitive cells within the sweat gland secretory coil are specifically affected[124].

Apocrine glands

Dilatation with retained secretions are found in up to 33 per cent of post-mortem cases. The changes are more severe in children over the age of 7 years[125].

Other pathologies

Acrodermatitis enteropathica may occur with malabsorption[126].

CENTRAL NERVOUS SYSTEM

In older children, deficiencies of vitamin E with opthalmoplegia, absent reflexes and hand tremors have been reported. Degeneration of fascicular gracilis pathways in the posterior columns of the spinal cord are linked also to vitamin E deficiency[127]. Impaired brainstem auditory potentials[128] and peripheral nerve function have also been reported[129]. Vitamin K deficiency can cause intracerebral bleeding in the neonatal period.

In summary cystic fibrosis is a multiorgan disease, and we are now seeing pathology evolving in organs not previously considered. These changes are associated with increased survival into adulthood and new therapeutic strategies are also altering the progress and evolution of the disease. Clinicians and pathologists must be aware of this changing picture in cystic fibrosis.

REFERENCES

1. Taylor, B., Evans, J.N.G. and Hope, G.A. (1974) Upper respiratory tract in cystic fibrosis. Ear–Nose–Throat survey in children. *Arch. Dis. Child.*, **49**, 133–136.
2. Oppenheimer, E.H. and Rosenstein, B.J. (1979) Differential pathology of nasal polyps in cystic fibrosis and atopy. *Lab. Invest.*, **40**, 445–449.
3. Puchell,e E. (1992) Airway Secretions – New Concepts and Functions. *Eur. Resp. J.*, **5**, 3–4.
4. Henderson, W.R. and Chi, E.Y. (1992) Degranulation of cystic fibrosis nasal polyp mast cells. *J. Pathol.*, **166**, 395–404.
5. Shwachman, H., Kulczycki, L.L., Muller, H.L. *et al.* (1962) Nasal polyposis in patients with cystic fibrosis. *Pediatrics*, **30**, 389–401.
6. Drake-Lee, A.B. and Morgan, D.W. (1989) Nasal polyps and sinusitus in children with cystic fibrosis. *J. Laryngol. Otol.*, **103**, 753–755.
7. Kerrebijn, J.D.F., Poublon, R.M.L. and Overbeek, S.E. (1992) Nasal and paranasal disease in adult cystic fibrosis patients. *Eur. Respir. J.*, **5**, 1239–1242.
8. Carson, J.L., Collier, A.M., Gambling, T.M., Knowles, M.R. and Boucher, R.C. (1990) Ultrastructure of airway epithelial cell membranes among patients with cystic fibrosis. *Hum. Pathol.*, **21**, 640–647.
9. Rayner, C.F., Rutman, A., Dewar, A., Cole, P.J. and Wilson, R. (1995) Ciliary disorientation in patients with chronic upper respiratory tract inflammation. *Am. J. Resp. Crit. Care Med.*, **151**, 800–804.
10. Sobonya, R.E. and Taussig, L.M. (1986) Quantitative aspects of lung pathology in cystic fibrosis. *Am. Rev. Resp. Dis.*, **134**, 290–295.
11. Cole, P.J. (1986) Inflammation: a two-edge sword-the model of bronchiectasis. *Eur. J. Resp. Dis.*, **69**, (Suppl. 147), 6–15.
12. Elborn, J.S. and Shale, D.J. (1990) Cystic fibrosis. 2. Lung injury in cystic fibrosis. *Thorax*, **45**, 970–973.
13. Doring, G. (1996) Mechanisms of airway inflammation in cystic fibrosis. *Pediatr. Allergy Immunol.*, **7**, 63–66.
14. Bonfield, T.L., Panuska, J.R., Konstan, M.W., *et al.* (1995) Inflammatory cytokines in cystic fibrosis lungs. *Am. J. Respir. Crit. Care Med.*, **152**, 2111–2118.
15. Delacourt, C., Le Bourgeois, M., D'Ortho, M.P. *et al.* (1995) Imbalance between 95kD type IV collagenase and tissue inhibitors of metalloproteinases in sputum of patients with cystic fibrosis. *Am. J. Respir. Crit. Care Med.*, **152**, 765–774.
16. Matthews, W.J.J., Williams, M., Oliphant, B., *et al.* (1980) Hypogammaglobulinaemia in patients with cystic fibrosis. *NEJM*, **302**, 245–249.
17. Gibbons, A., Allan, J.D., Holzel, A. *et al.* (1976) Cell-mediated immunity in patients with cystic fibrosis. *BMJ*, **1**, 120–122.
18. Armstrong, D.S., Grimwood, K., Carzino, R., Carlin, J.B., Olinsky, A. and Phelan, P.D. (1995) Lower respiratory infection and inflammation in infants with newly diagnosed cystic fibrosis. *BMJ*, **310**, 1571–1572.
19. Hoiby, N. (1982) Microbiology of lung infections in cystic fibrosis patients. *Acta Paediatr. Scand. Suppl.*, **301**, 33–54.
20. Kerem, E., Corey, M., Gold, R. and Levison, H. (1990) Pulmonary function and clinical course in patients with cystic fibrosis after pulmonary colonization with *Pseudomonas aeruginosa*. *J. Paediatr.*, **116**, 714–719.
21. Howard, A.J., Dunkin, K.T. and Millar, G.W. (1988) Nasopharyngeal carriage and antibiotic resistance of *Haemophilus influenzae* in healthy children. *Epidemiol. Infect.*, **100**, 193–203.
22. Rayner, R.J., Hiller, E.J., Ispahani, P. and Baker, M. (1990) *Haemophilus* infection in cystic fibrosis. *Arch. Dis. Child.*, **65**, 255–258.
23. Roberts, D.E., Higgs, E., Rutman, A. and Cole, P. (1984) Isolation of spheroplastic forms of *Haemophilus influenzae* from sputum in conventionally treated chronic bronchial sepsis using selective medium supplemented with N-acetyl-D-glucosamine: possible reservoir for re-emergence of infection. *BMJ*, **289**, 1409–1412.
24. Taylor, R.F.H., Gaya, H. and Hodson, M.E. (1993) *Pseudomonas cepacia* – pulmonary infection in patients with cystic fibrosis. *Resp. Med.*, **87**, 187–192.
25. Taylor, P.C. and Kalamatianos, C.C. (1995) *Pseudomonas cepacia* in the sputum of cystic fibrosis patients. *Pathology*, **26**, 315–317.
26. Taylor, R.F.H., Morgan, D.W., Nicholson, P.S., Mackay, I.S. and Pitt, T.L. (1992) Extrapulmonary sites of *Pseudomonas aeruginosa* in adults with cystic fibrosis. *Thorax*, **47**, 426–428.
27. Torrens, J.K., Dawkins, P., Conway, S.P. and Moya, E. (1998) Non-tuberculous mycobacteria in cystic fibrosis. *Thorax*, **53**, 182–185.
28. Tomashefski, J.F., Stern, R.C., Demko, C.A. *et al.* (1996) Non tuberculous mycobacteria in cystic fibrosis: an autopsy study. *Am. J. Respir. Crit. Care Med.*, **154**, 523–528.
29. Emre, U., Bernius, M., Roblin, P.M. *et al.* (1996) *Chlamydia pneumoniae* infection in patients with cystic fibrosis. *Clin. Infect. Dis.*, **22**, 819–823.
30. Laufer, P., Fink, J.N., Bruns, W.T. *et al.* (1984) Allergic bronchopulmonary aspergillosis in cystic fibrosis. *J. Allergy Clin. Immunol.*, **73**, 44–48.
31. Maguire, C.P., Hayes, J.P., Hayes, M., Masterson, J. and FitzGerald, M.X. (1995) Three cases of pulmonary aspergilloma in adult patients with cystic fibrosis. *Thorax*, **50**, 805–806.
32. Brueton, M.J., Ormerod, L.P., Shah, K.J. and Anderson, C.M. (1980) Allergic bronchopulmonary aspergillosis complicating cystic fibrosis in childhood. *Arch. Dis. Child.*, **55**, 348–353.

33. Mroueh, S. and Spock, A. (1994) Allergic bronchopulmonary aspergillosis in patients with cystic fibrosis. *Chest*, **105**, 32–36.

34. Slavin, R.G., Bedrossian, C.W. and Hutcheson, P.S. (1988) A pathologic study of allergic bronchopulmonary aspergillosis. *J. Allergy Clin. Immunol.*, **81**, 718–725.

35. Bosken, C.H., Myers, J.L., Greenberger, P.A. and Katzenstein, A.L. (1988) Pathologic features of allergic bronchopulmonary aspergillosis. *Am. J. Surg. Pathol.*, **12**, 216–222.

36. Guidotti, T.L., Luetzeler, J., DiSant'Agnese, P.A. *et al.* (1982) Fatal disseminated aspergillosis in a previously well young adult with cystic fibrosis. *Am. J. Med. Sci.*, **283**, 157–160.

37. Bhargava, V., Tomashefski, J.F.J., Stern, R.C. and Abramowsky, C.R. (1989) The pathology of fungal infection and colonization in patients with cystic fibrosis. *Hum. Pathol.*, **20**, 977–986.

38. Petersen, N.T., Hoiby, N., Mordhorst, C.H., Lind, K., Flensborg, E.W. and Bruun, B. (1981) Respiratory infections in cystic fibrosis patients caused by virus, chlamydia and mycoplasma – possible synergism with *Pseudomonas aeruginosa*. *Acta Paediatr. Scand.*, **70**, 623–628.

39. Zuelzer, W.W. and Newton, W.A. (1949) The pathogenesis of fibrocystic disease of the pancreas. A study of 36 cases with special reference to pulmonary lesions. *Pediatrics*, **4**, 53–69.

40. Ornoy, A., Arnon, J., Katznelson, D., Granat, M., Caspi, B. and Chemke, J. (1987) Pathological confirmation of cystic fibrosis in the fetus following prenatal diagnosis. *Am. J. Med. Genet.*, **28**, 935–947.

41. Oppenheimer, E.H. and Esterly, J.R. (1975) Pathology of cystic fibrosis review of the literature and comparison with 146 autopsied cases. *Perspect. Pediatr. Pathol.*, **2**, 241–278.

42. Sturgess, J. and Imrie, J.R. (1982) Quantitative evaluation of the development of tracheal submucosal glands in infants with cystic fibrosis and control infants. *Am. J. Pathol.*, **106**, 303–311.

43. Bedrossian, C.W., Greenberg, S.D., Singer, D.B., Hansen, J.J. and Rosenberg, H.S. (1976) The lung in cystic fibrosis. A quantitative study including prevalence of pathologic findings among different age groups. *Hum. Pathol.*, **7**, 195–204.

44. Armstrong, D.S., Grimwood, K., Carlin, J.B. *et al.* (1997) Lower airway inflammation in infants and young children with cystic fibrosis. *Am. J. Resp. Crit. Care Med.*, **156**, 1197–1204.

45. Meyer, K.C. and Sharma, A. (1997) Regional variability of lung inflammation in cystic fibrosis. *Am. J. Resp. Crit. Care Med.*, **156**, 1536–1540.

46. Ogrinc, G., Kampalath, B., Tomashefski, J.F. Jr (1998) Destruction and loss of bronchial cartilage in cystic fibrosis. *Hum. Pathol.*, **29**, 65–73.

47. di Sant'Agnese, P.A. (1953) Bronchial obstruction with lobar atelectasis and emphysema in cystic fibrosis of the pancreas. *Pediatrics*, **12**, 178–190.

48. Katznelson, D., Szeinberg, A., Augarten, A. and Yahav, Y. (1997) The critical first six months in cystic fibrosis: a syndrome of severe bronchiolitis. *Pediatr. Pulmonol.*, **24**, 134–136 (discussion 159–161).

49. Dovey, M., Wisseman, C.L., Roggli, V.L., Roomans, G.M., Shelburne, J.D. and Spock, A. (1989) Ultrastructural morphology of the lung in cystic fibrosis. *J. Submicroscop. Cytol. Pathol.*, **21**, 521–534.

50. Wentworth, P., Gough, J. and Wentworth, J.E. (1968) Pulmonary changes and cor pulmonale in mucoviscidosis. *Thorax*, **1968**, 582–586.

51. Goldring, R.M., Fishman, A.P., Turino, G.M. *et al.* (1964) Pulmonary hypertension and cor pulmonale in cystic fibrosis of the pancreas. *J. Pediatr.*, **65**, 501–524.

52. Oppenheimer, E.H. and Esterly, J.R. (1974) Medial mucoid lesions of the pulmonary artery in cystic fibrosis, pulmonary hypertension and other disorders. *Lab. Invest.*, **30**, 411–414.

53. Ryland, D. and Reid, L. (1975) The pulmonary circulation in cystic fibrosis. *Thorax*, **30**, 285–292.

54. Fellows, K.E., Stigol, L., Schuster, S., Khaw, K.T. and Shwachman, H. (1975) Selective bronchial arteriography in patients with cystic fibrosis and massive haemoptysis. *Radiol.*, **114**, 551–555.

55. Holsclaw, D.S., Grand, R.J. and Shwachman, H. (1970) Massive haemoptysis in cystic fibrosis. *J. Pediatr.*, **76**, 829–838.

56. Boat, T.F., di Sant'Agnese, P.A., Warwick, W.J. and Handwerger, S.A. (1969) Pneumothorax in cystic fibrosis. *JAMA*, **209**, 1498–1504.

57. McGlennen, R.C., Burke, B.A. and Dehner, L.P. (1968) Systemic amyloidosis complicating cystic fibrosis. *Arch. Pathol. Lab. Med.*, **110**, 879–884.

58. Hosenpud, J.D., Bennett, L.E., Keck, B.M., Edwards, E.B. and Novick, R.J. (1998) Effect of diagnosis on survival benefit of lung transplantation for end-stage lung disease. *Lancet*, **351**, 24–27.

59. Yacoub, M.H., Gyi, K., Khaghani. A. *et al.* (1997) Analysis of 10-year experience with heart–lung transplantation for cystic fibrosis. *Transplant. Proc.*, **29**, 632.

60. Stewart, S. and Cary, N. (1991) The pathology of heart and heart and lung transplantation – an update. *J. Clin. Pathol.*, **44**, 803–811.

61. Madden, B.P., Hodson, M.E., Tsang, V., Radley-Smith, R., Khaghani, A. and Yacoub, M.Y. (1992) Intermediate-term results of heart–lung transplantation for cystic fibrosis. *Lancet*, **339**, 1583–1587.

62. Swerdlow, S.H. (1992) Post-transplant lymphoproliferative disorders: a morphologic, phenotypic and genotypic spectrum of disease. *Histopathology*, **20**, 373–385.

63. Tomashefski, J.F. Jr, Dahms, B. and Bruce, M. (1985) Pleura in pneumothorax. Comparison of patients with cystic fibrosis and idiopathic spontaneous pneumothorax. *Arch. Pathol. Lab. Med.*, **109**, 910–916.

64. Stern, R.C., Borkat, G. and Hirschfeld, S.S. (1980) Heart failure in cystic fibrosis. *Am. J. Dis. Child.*, **134**, 267–272.

65. McGiven, A.R. (1962) Myocardial fibrosis in fibrocystic disease of the pancreas. *Arch. Dis. Child.*, **37**, 656–660.

66. Wiebicke, W., Artlich, A. and Gerling, I. (1993) Myocardial fibrosis – a rare complication in patients with cystic fibrosis. *Europ. J. Pediatr.*, **152**, 694–696.

67. Holman, R.L., Blanc, W.A. and Andersen, D. (1959) Decreased aortic atherosclerosis in cystic fibrosis of the pancreas. *Pediatrics*, **24**, 34–39.

68. Moss, T.J., Austin, G.E. and Moss, A.J. (1979) Preatherosclerotic aortic lesions in cystic fibrosis. *J. Pediatr.*, **94**, 32–37.

69. Szeifert, G.T., Szabo, M. and Papp, Z. (1985) Morphology of cystic fibrosis at 17 weeks of gestation. *Clin. Genet.*, **28**, 561–565.

70. Murshed, R., Spitz, L., Kiely, E. and Drake, D. (1997) Meconium ileus: a ten-year review of thirty-six patients. *Europ. J. Pediatr. Surg.*, **7**, 275–277.

71. Irish, M.S., Ragi, J.M., Karamanoukian, H., Borowitz, D.S., Schmidt, D. and Glick, P.L. (1997) Prenatal diagnosis of the fetus with cystic fibrosis and meconium ileus. *Pediatr. Surg. Internat.*, **12**, 434–436.

72. Coutts, J.A., Docherty, J.G., Carachi, R. and Evans, T.J. (1997) Clinical course of patients with cystic fibrosis presenting with meconium ileus. *Br. J. Surg.*, **84**, 555.

73. Sweney, L. and Warwick, W.J. (1968) Involvement of the labial salivary gland in patients with cystic fibrosis. 111 ultrastructural changes. *Arch. Pathol.*, **86**, 413–418.

74. Riedel, B.D. (1997) Gastrointestinal manifestations of cystic fibrosis. *Pediatr Annal.*, **26**, 235–241.

75. Eggermont, E. (1996) Gastrointestinal manifestations in cystic fibrosis. *Europ. J. Gastroenterol. Hepatol.*, **8**, 731–738.

76. Oppenheimer, E. and Esterly, J. (1973) Cystic fibrosis of the pancreas, morphologic findings in infants with and without pancreatic lesions. *Arch. Pathol.*, **96**, 149–154.

77. Martens, M., De Boeck, K., Van Der Steen, K. *et al.* (1992) A right lower quadrant mass in cystic fibrosis; a diagnostic challenge. *Eur. J. Paediatr.*, **151**, 329–331.

78. Shwachman, H. and Holsclaw, D.S. (1972) Examination of the appendix at laparotomy as a diagnostic clue in cystic fibrosis. *NEJM*, **286**, 1300–1301.

79. Holsclaw, D.S., Rocmans, L. and Shwachman, H. (1971) Intussusception in patients with cystic fibrosis. *Pediatrics*, **48**, 51–58.

80. Fitzsimmons, S.C., Burkhart, G.A., Borowitz, D., *et al.* (1997) High-dose pancreatic-enzyme supplements and fibrosing colonopathy in children with cystic fibrosis. *NEJM*, **336**, 1283–1289.

81. Dodge, J.A. (1996) The aetiology of fibrosing colonopathy. *Postgrad. Med. J.*, **72**, (Suppl. 2), S52–S55.

82. Collins, M.H., Azzarelli, B., West, K.W., Chong, S.K., Maguiness, K.M. and Stevens, J.C. (1996) Neuropathy and vasculopathy in colonic strictures from children with cystic fibrosis. *J. Pediatr. Surg.*, **31**, 945–950.

83. Kulczycki, L. and Shwachman, H. (1958) Studies in cystic fibrosis of the pancreas, occurence of rectal prolapse. *NEJM*, **259**, 409-412.

84. Neglia, J.P., Fitzsimmons, S.C., Maisonneuve, P. *et al.* (1995) The risk of cancer among patients with cystic fibrosis. *NEJM*, **332**, 494–499.

85. Imrie, J.R., Fagan, D.G. and Sturgess, J.M. (1979) Quantitative evaluation of the development of the exocrine pancreas in cystic fibrosis and control infants. *Am. J. Pathol.*, **95**, 697–707.

86. Vawter, G.F. and Shwachman, H. (1979) Cystic fibrosis in adults: an autopsy study. *Pathol. Ann.*, **14**, (Pt 2), 357–382.

87. Lohr, M., Goertchen, P., Nizze, H. *et al.* (1989) Cystic fibrosis associated islet changes may provide a basis for diabetes. An immunocytochemical and morphometrical study. *Virchows Archiv – A, Pathol. Anat. Histopathol.*, **414**, 179–185.

88. Shwachman, H., Lebenthal, E. and Khaw, K.T. (1975) Recurrent acute pancreatitis in patients with cystic fibrosis with normal pancreatic enzymes. *Pediatrics*, **55**, 86–92.

89. Davis, T.M.E. and Sawicka, E.H. (1985) Adenocarcinoma in cystic fibrosis. *Thorax*, **40**, 199–200.

90. Lykavieris, P., Bernard, O. and Hadchouel, M. (1996) Neonatal cholestasis as the presenting feature in cystic fibrosis. *Arch. Dis. Child.*, **75**, 67–70.

91. Roy, C.C. (1980) Gastrointestinal and hepatobiliary complications: changing pattern with age, in *Perspectives In Cystic Fibrosis*, (ed. J. Sturgess), Imperial Press Ltd. Mississauga, Ontario, p. 197.

92. Lykavieris, P., Guillot, M., Pariente, D., Bernard, O. and Hadchouel, M. (1996) Liver calcifications in cystic fibrosis. *J. Pediatr. Gastroenterol. Nutrit.*, **23**, 565–568.

93. Esterly, J.R. and Oppenheimer, E.H. (1962) Observations in cystic fibrosis of the pancreas. 1. The gallbladder. *Bull. Johns Hopkins Hosp.*, **110**, 247–255.

94. L'heureux, P.R., Isenberg, J.N., Sharp, H.L. *et al.* (1977) Gallbladder disease in cystic fibrosis. *Am. J. Roentgenol.*, **128**, 953–956.

95. Potter, C.J., Fishbein, M., Hammond, S., McCoy, K. and Qualman, S. (1997) Can the histologic changes of cystic fibrosis-associated hepatobiliary disease be predicted by clinical criteria? *J. Pediatr. Gastroenterol. Nutrit.*, **25**, 32–36.

96. di Sant'Agnese, P.A. and Blanc, W.A. (1956) A distinctive type of biliary cirrhosis of the liver associated with cystic fibrosis of the pancreas. *Pediatrics*, **18**, 387–409.

97. Schuster, S.R., Shwachman, H., Toyama, W. *et al.* (1977) The management of portal hypertension in cystic fibrosis. *J. Pediatr. Surg.*, **12**, 201–206.

98. Craig, J.M., Haddad, H. and Shwachman, H. (1957) The pathological changes in the liver in cystic fibrosis of the pancreas. *Am. J. Dis. Child.*, **93**, 357–369.

99. Noble-Jamieson, G., Barnes, N., Jamieson, N., Friend, P. and Calne, R. (1996) Liver transplantation for hepatic cirrhosis in cystic fibrosis. *J. Roy. Soc. Med.*, **89**, (Suppl. 27), 31–37.

100. Chidekel, A.S. and Dolan, T.F. Jr (1996) Cystic fibrosis and calcium oxalate nephrolithiasis. *Yale J. Biol. Med.*, **69**, 317–321.

101. Couper, R., Bentur, L., Kilbourn, J.P. and Wolf, P. (1993) Immunoreactive calmodulin in cystic fibrosis kidneys. *Aust. NZ J. Med.*, **23**, 484–488.

102. Kopito, L.E., Kosasky, H.S. and Shwachman, H. (1973) Water and electrolytes in cervical mucus from patients with cystic fibrosis. *Fertil. Steril.*, **24**, 512–516.

103. Johannesson, M., Gottlieb, C. and Hjelte, L. (1997) Delayed puberty in girls with cystic fibrosis despite good clinical status. *Pediatrics*, **99**, 29–34.

104. Wang, C.I., Reid, B.S., Miller, J.H. *et al*. (1981) Multiple ovarian cysts in female patients with cystic fibrosis. *Cystic Fibrosis Club Abstr.*, **22**, 77.

105. Oppenheimer, E.H. and Esterly, J.R. (1970) Observations on cystic fibrosis of the pancreas. VI. The uterine cervix. *J. Pediatr.*, **77**, 991–995.

106. Anguiano, A., Oates, R.D. and Amos, J.A. (1992) Congenital bilateral absence of the vas deferens: A primary genital form of cystic fibrosis. *JAMA*, **367**, 1794–1797.

107. Holsclaw, D.S., Perlmutter, A.D. and Jockin, H. (1971) Genital abnormalities in male patients with cystic fibrosis. *J. Urol.*, **106**, 568–574.

108. De Braekeleer, M. and Ferec, C. (1996) Mutations in the cystic fibrosis gene in men with congenital bilateral absence of the vas deferens. *Mol. Hum. Repro.*, **2**, 669–677.

109. Lack, E.E., Perez-Atayde, A.R. and Young, J.B. (1985) Carotid body hyperplasia in cystic fibrosis and cyanotic heart disease. A combined morphometric, ultrastructural, and biochemical study. *Am. J. Pathol.*, **119**, 301–314.

110. Ward, A.M. (1972) The structure of the breast in mucoviscidosis. *J. Clin. Pathol.*, **25**, 119–122.

111. Hawkins, E. and Singer, D.B. (1976) The adrenal cortex in cystic fibrosis of the pancreas. *Am. J. Clin. Pathol.*, **66**, 710–714.

112. Samuels, M.H., Thompson, N., Leichty, D. and Ridgway, E.C. (1995) Amyloid goiter in cystic fibrosis. *Thyroid*, **5**, 213–215.

113. Alvarez-Sala, R., Prados, C., Sastre Marcos, J. *et al*. (1995) Amyloid goitre and hypothyroidism secondary to cystic fibrosis. *Postgrad. Med. J.*, **71**, 307–308.

114. di Sant'Agnese, P.A. and Davis, P.B. (1979) Cystic fibrosis in adults: 75 cases and review of 232 cases in the literature. *Am. J. Med.*, **66**, 121–132.

115. Athreya, B.H., Borns, P. and Rosenlund, M.L. (1975) Cystic fibrosis and hypertrophic osteoarthropathy in children. *Am. J. Dis. Child.*, **129**, 634–637.

116. Matthay, M.A., Matthay, R.A. and Mills, D.M. (1976) Hypertrophic osteoarthropathy in adults with cystic fibrosis. *Thorax*, **31**, 572–575.

117. Hellsing, E., Brattstrom, V. and Strandvik, B. (1992) Craniofacial morphology in children with cystic fibrosis. *Europ. J. Orthodont.*, **14**, 147–151.

118. Teramoto, S., Matsuse, T. and Ouchi, Y. (1997) Osteoporosis in lung transplantation candidates with end-stage pulmonary disease. *Am. J. Med.*, **103**, 334–336 [letter; comment].

119. Aris, R.M., Renner, J.B., Winders, A.D. *et al*. (1998) Increased rate of fractures and severe kyphosis: sequelae of living into adulthood with cystic fibrosis. *Ann. Intern. Med.*, **128**, 186–193.

120. Bourke, S., Rooney, M., Fitzgerald, M. and Bresnihan, B. (1987) Episodic arthropathy in adult cystic fibrosis. *Quart. J. Med.*, **64**, 651–659.

121. Newman, A.J. and Ansell, B.M. (1979) Episodic arthritis in children with cystic fibrosis. *J. Pediatr.*, **94**, 594–596.

122. Turner, M.A., Baildam, E., Patel, L. and David, T.J. (1997) Joint disorders in cystic fibrosis. *J. Roy. Soc. Med.*, **90**, (Suppl. 31), 13–20.

123. Kartner, N., Augustinas, O., Jensen, T.J. *et al*. (1992) Mislocalization of F508 CFTR in cystic fibrosis sweat gland. *Nature Genet.*, **1**, 321–327.

124. Reddy, M.M., Bell, C.L. and Quinton, P.M. (1997) Cystic fibrosis affects specific cell type in sweat gland secretory coil. *Am. J. Physiol.*, **273**, C426–C433.

125. Esterly, N.B., Oppenheimer, E.H., and Esterly, J.R. (1972) Observations on cystic fibrosis of the pancreas.The apocrine gland. *Am. J. Dis. Child.*, **123**, 200–203.

126. Ghali, F.E., Steinberg, J.B., Tunnessen, W.W. Jr (1996) Picture of the month. *Acrodermatitis enteropathica*-like rash in cystic fibrosis. *Arch. Pediatr. Adolesc. Med.*, **150**, 99–100.

127. Geller, A., Gilles, F. and Shwachman, H. (1977) Degeneration of fasciculus gracilis in cystic fibrosis. *Neurology*, **27**, 185–187.

128. Vaisman, N., Tabachnik, E., Shahar, E. and Gilai, A. (1996) Impaired brainstem auditory evoked potentials in patients with cystic fibrosis. *Develop. Med. Child Neurol.*, **38**, 59–64.

129. O'Riordan, J.I., Hayes, J., FitzGerald, M.X. and Redmond, J. (1995) Peripheral nerve dysfunction in adult patients with cystic fibrosis. *Irish J. Med. Sci.*, **164**, 207–208.

8

Cardiopulmonary physiology

A. BUSH

Introduction	157	Pulmonary circulation	167
The role of physiological measurements	157	The heart	167
Infant lung-function studies	158	CF physiology under special stresses	168
Airway disease	160	Future research	171
Gas exchange	165	Clinical practice of lung function testing in cystic fibrosis	171
Respiratory mechanics	166	References	172

INTRODUCTION

Despite the fact that CFTR is widely expressed within the fetal lung, the baby with CF has normal lungs at birth. Most will develop chronic bronchopulmonary sepsis, which is the major cause of morbidity and mortality in CF, and hence the main target of therapy, the effects of which, both good and bad, always need to be assessed. There is considerable variation in lung function at a given age, and individual rates of change are almost impossible to predict[1,2]. This chapter first discusses the importance and role of physiological studies in general, and then describes the progressive changes within the cardiopulmonary unit. Infant lung function studies are described first, because they are a separate subject in themselves due to the very different techniques which have to be employed. For simplicity the rest of the chapter is divided into separate but overlapping blocks: 'Airway disease', 'Gas exchange', 'Respiratory mechanics', 'Pulmonary circulation', 'The heart' and 'CF physiology under special stresses'. Finally, areas for future research will be considered.

THE ROLE OF PHYSIOLOGICAL MEASUREMENTS

Before making a measurement in any context, the reasons and the specific question to be addressed should be considered. In general, lung function measurements are made in order to:

- understand the pathophysiology of disease;
- assess the effects of a new therapy in the context of a clinical trial;
- predict prognosis in an individual, particularly when planning lung transplantation;
- guide the requirements for modifying or intensifying treatment in an individual patient;
- follow the response to changes in treatment in an individual.

When assessing how far any particular test is able to deliver the requirements, the limitations of patient and apparatus must be considered, as well as the predictive power of the test. This is well seen in the context of the use of lung function as a surrogate end point in clinical trials and to predict prognosis[3]. In very early disease, lung-function testing is too insensitive to detect improvements with therapy[4]. In late-stage disease, although poor lung function predicts a poor prognosis[5], there is huge variability in lung function in the year before death in CF patients[6]. Physiological measurement is an important tool, but only one tool to be used in clinical management, and must be seen in the context of the whole clinical picture.

A further requirement for understanding the significance of physiological changes is an appreciation of the normal pattern of development and the effects of disease on the growing lung. The bronchial branching pattern is established in the first half of pregnancy but most of the alveolar complement develops in the first 3 years of life. Interference with growth in this crucial period, at least in the contexts in which it has been studied, cannot be compensated for by subsequent catch-up growth[7]. This should be remembered when the results of infant lung function tests are evaluated (below). A further crucial period is puberty, when normals show a spurt in growth in lung size as well as anthropometric variables[8]. Lung function centiles can be used to follow these changes (Fig. 8.1).

INFANT LUNG-FUNCTION STUDIES

It is beyond the scope of this chapter to review all the many techniques available; the interested reader is referred to a recent monograph[9]. The earliest disease in CF lungs is believed to be in the small airways[10], an area that is notoriously difficult to investigate physiologically, in a notoriously difficult age group (not just for physiologists), namely infants and young children.

Conventional pulmonary function testing in infancy is technically very demanding, and the results are difficult to interpret. The most popular techniques involve helium dilution lung volumes; baby plethysmography; the 'squeeze' technique to produce an expiratory flow volume curve, recently modified; and the weighted spirometer method to measure lung compliance. Details of the techniques vary from laboratory to laboratory, making comparison of the results of different centers very difficult. Many studies do not have adequate controls, and it may be difficult to decide even how to find a control for a CF baby who is smaller than normal. When studying the results from these techniques, it is essential to keep a critical, as well as an admiring, mind. It is sad that in the interval between the first and second editions of this book, there have been no large peer-reviewed publications showing the use of these techniques in routine clinical decision making in children with CF.

At the moment, imaging techniques are probably the best clinical surrogate for lung-function testing in infants. We use ventilation scans routinely to assess infants who cannot cooperate with lung function tests[11].

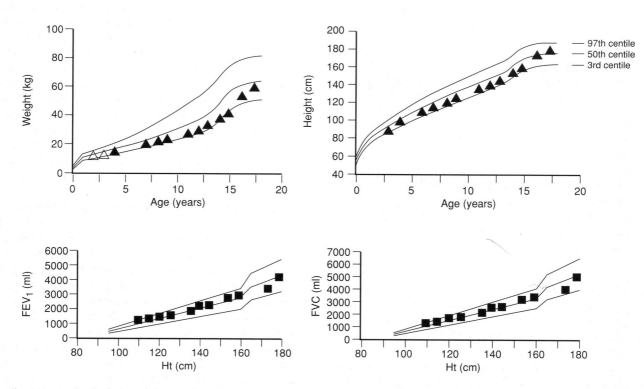

Fig. 8.1 *Longitudinal changes in growth and lung function in an individual with CF. The lung function centiles are generated from reference 8, and the software, in routine use in our department, runs on Paradox for Windows (courtesy Dr R. M. Buchdahl). Note the physiological growth spurt in puberty, mirrored by a spurt in lung function reflecting the changes in chest wall shape and dimensions. This pulmonary growth spurt may not be observed in the severely affected child.*

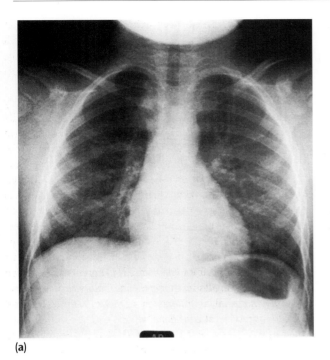

(a)

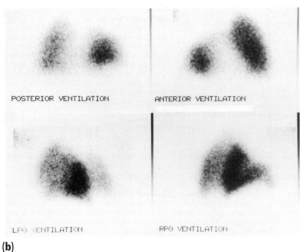

POSTERIOR VENTILATION   ANTERIOR VENTILATION

LPO VENTILATION   RPO VENTILATION

(b)

Fig. 8.2 (a) *Chest radiograph* **(b)** *and isotope ventilation lung scan taken on the same day in a child with CF. There is a large filling defect in the right upper lobe in the ventilation scan. No obvious abnormality was detectable either by clinical examination or the chest radiograph.*

They have the merit of being easy to perform and interpret, with low radiation (equivalent to one-fifth of that of a chest X-ray, CXR). One in seven scans revealed abnormalities not demonstrated by clinical examination or CXR (Fig. 8.2). Scans might also give prognostic information, a normal ventilation scan at presentation was predictive of a normal first second forced expired volume (FEV$_1$) at age seven years[12]. Other scanning techniques include the use of an intravenous isotope such as xenon, which is washed out of the lung, depending on normal perfusion and ventilation; this has the advantage

that one does not have to hold a mask onto a struggling baby, but the drawback of requiring an intravenous line.

In a research context, infant pulmonary function has given us valuable insights. Kraemer[13] used plethysmography, and reported that hyperinflation was present early on in infants with CF. However, he found poor agreement between airway resistance and hyperinflation. It is difficult to understand how one could exist without the other without invoking methodological problems. The volumes measured are so small, and the technical problems so great, that results of plethysmography must be interpreted cautiously in this age group.

Tepper *et al.* measured helium dilution lung volumes and used the weighted spirometer, and hence derived a mixing index (essentially, the number of breaths to equilibration), respiratory system compliance and flow rates in normals and infants with CF[14]. Those presenting with meconium ileus at birth, or isolated failure to thrive with no pulmonary symptoms, had normal lung function. In this study, those who already had respiratory symptoms had impaired gas mixing, lower flow rates, lower compliance and worse oxygen saturation. Alarmingly, the mean age was only 5 months.

The squeeze technique has also caused controversy as to its precise interpretation. This method involves encasing the baby in an airtight jacket, which is very rapidly inflated at the beginning of expiration to produce a maximum squeezed expiratory effort[15]. Flow rates are usually measured at FRC (functional residual capacity), which, for assessment of treatment effects, needs to be measured separately if important changes are not to be missed. The squeeze technique has recently been modified; the baby is rendered transiently apneic by mask ventilation for a few large breaths; the baby is then bagged to total lung capacity and the squeeze applied from that volume rather than at spontaneous end-expiration, the so-called partial forced flow volume curve[16]. This has the advantage of being more readily comparable with flow curves in older children and adults; there are currently no good published data on the clinical relevance of this technique in CF.

There is unfortunately a scarcity of good prospective longitudinal studies. Beardsmore *et al.*[17-19] found that only four of 17 infants had normal lung function at the end of the follow-up period of around 12 months[17]. She found that in many who did have normal lung function in infancy, deterioration had taken place by school age[18]. There was a correlation between thoracic gas volume in infancy and at age 6 years, but not in other indices of lung function. In one of the few studies to apply infant physiology to clinical questions, she also showed that there was no difference in lung function between screened infants who did and did not receive prophylactic antibiotics[19]. Another important longitudinal study[20] using partial flow volume curves and helium dilution lung volumes confirmed that infants presenting with respiratory symptoms had impaired lung function, which did improve over 1 year with therapy, but remained lower than CF infants with non-respiratory presentations. The partial flow volume curves showed better discrimination between those with and without respiratory symptoms than helium dilution lung volumes or the CXR. This study is one of the indirect strands of evidence suggesting that diagnosing CF infants by screening before the onset of respiratory symptoms may be worthwhile.

In summary, however, although studies are conflicting, the balance of evidence is that even in apparently well infants there may be abnormalities in lung function. These abnormalities are worse in those with respiratory symptoms, and will not be appreciated by CXR scoring. This would accord with bronchoscopic studies showing early onset of clinically occult infection and inflammation in CF infants.

AIRWAY DISEASE

The airways can be considered in four parts: the extrathoracic large airway (larynx and first part of trachea); the intrathoracic, extrapulmonary large airway (second part of trachea and first part of main bronchi); the intrapulmonary large airways; and the variably defined small airways. Each section has different possible mechanisms of disease. Early in the course of CF, airway disease is the main problem, with subsequent secondary changes elsewhere. Hence the airways will be considered in detail first.

The intrapulmonary airways

SMALL AIRWAYS

Studies in infants have been covered in the previous section. Small airways disease can be inferred in older subjects by impaired flow at low lung volumes (Figs 8.3 and 8.4), indices of air trapping, or sophisticated methods such as respiratory impedance and multibreath N_2 washout[21]. Long term, the course of the disease is characterized by progressively worsening airflow obstruction; indices of small airway disease such as flow rates at low lung volumes, and a raised residual volume (RV)/total lung capacity (TLC) ratio remain most abnormal[2], but all spirometric variables start to fall progressively in all but those with the most mild disease (Fig. 8.5). As disease progresses, there is flow limitation in large as well as small airways, as shown by improved flow when breathing helium/oxygen mixtures[22]. In terminal CF lung disease, severe airway obstruction is the rule. Even in the severest cases, the rate of progression is unpredictable, and the physiologist is not able to give the accurate prognosis that patient and transplant surgeon would wish.

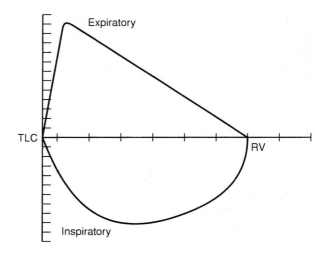

Fig. 8.3 *Normal flow volume loop. The expiratory curve is approximately triangular in shape, the inspiratory curve semicircular, such that peak inspiratory flow = 0.75 × PEFR[132]. TLC, total lung capacity. RV, residual volume.*

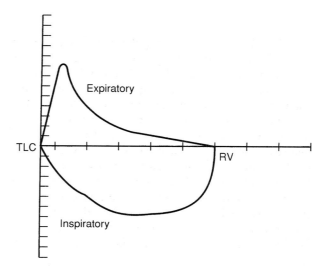

Fig. 8.4 *Flow volume loop of mild small airways disease. The main abnormality is late in expiration, with attenuation of flow at low lung volumes giving a scalloped appearance.*

LARGE AIRWAYS

Initially the large airways are normal. Eventually, destructive changes are found even centrally. The effect of this has been the subject of much physiological investigation. Normally, collapse of intrapulmonary large airways during generation of a positive intrapleural pressure during expiration is prevented by the compliance properties of the wall and the phenomenon of interdependence, the tethering effects of lung connective tissue acting to produce radial traction on the airway

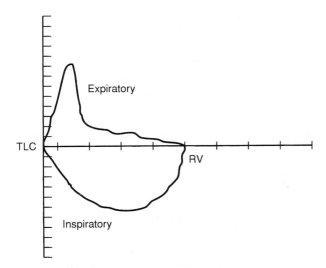

Fig. 8.5 *Flow volume loop of severe airflow obstruction, typical of severe lung disease in CF. There is rapid attenuation of flow early in expiration, and low expiratory flows thereafter.*

wall. The intrathoracic, extrapulmonary large airways rely only upon the wall properties to resist positive pleural pressure. Thus, it is possible that relaxation of airway smooth muscle, leading to an increase in wall compliance, may actually be harmful. This phenomenon was described by Prendiville *et al.*[15] using the technique of squeeze partial flow volume curves. They found that nebulized salbutamol actually worsened flow, and nebulized histamine had the opposite effect in wheezy (not CF) infants. They hypothesized that salbutamol increased airway wall compliance causing airway compression and reduced flow during a forced expiration as the larger airways narrowed more under pressure, with histamine having the converse effects. Similar effects

have been reported in patients with bronchoscopically documented tracheomalacia. Zach *et al.*[23] postulated that progressive airway wall destruction in CF would cause similar effects. Early in expiration, a flow transient would 'escape' the envelope of the flow volume curve, due to air being expelled from the upper airway distended by the previous inspiration (Figs 8.6 and 8.7). Late in expiration, flow would be reduced by dynamic compression of the airway, reducing its caliber. Volume transients of more than 500 mL were recorded. The size of these transients correlated inversely with clinical and radiological score, but not with other lung-function tests. However, there was some correlation with deadspace measurements from nitrogen washout curves. Landau *et al.* modeled transients using a single-compartment lung[24]. This assumes a variable resistor from the equal pressure point to the mouth, and a fixed resistor from the alveoli to the equal pressure point. They found values ranging from 40 to 300 mL, mean 165 mL; interestingly, a patient with forced vital capacity (FVC) 116 per cent predicted had a 225 mL transient, which does not fit with the idea of large transients correlating with severe disease[24].

Are these ideas consistent with the anatomical evidence? Measurements of tracheal anatomy in CF have shown it to be enlarged[25]. Tracheal compliance or, strictly, change in size with lung volume, has been measured with an acoustic reflection technique[25]. In CF, tracheal cross-sectional area was normal at FRC, but increased by a mean of 38 per cent at TLC. This group found no correlation between change in tracheal airway between TLC and FRC, and age or severity of lung-function changes. Normal airway volume is 151 mL to the 14th order, and 194 mL to the 17th (to the level of the respiratory bronchiole)[26]. Assuming a change in area due to CF of 38 per cent all down the airway and no significant change in length, the airway volume figures are increased to 208 mL and 267 mL, respectively. Thus the

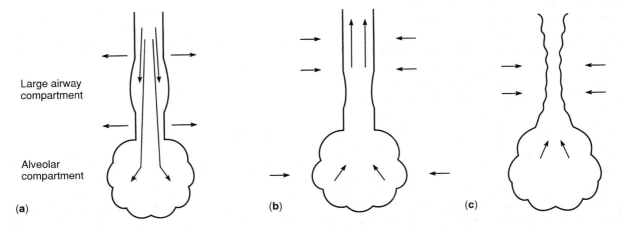

Fig. 8.6 *Two-compartment model lung demonstrating how a compliant upper airway can produce 'flow transients'. (a) End-inspiration with the compliant upper airway compartment and the alveolar compartment full. (b) Early in a forceful expiration, the upper compartment empties rapidly, producing a 'transient'. (c) Late in expiration, the compliant upper compartment is narrowed by further expiratory pressures, impeding the emptying of the alveolar compartment.*

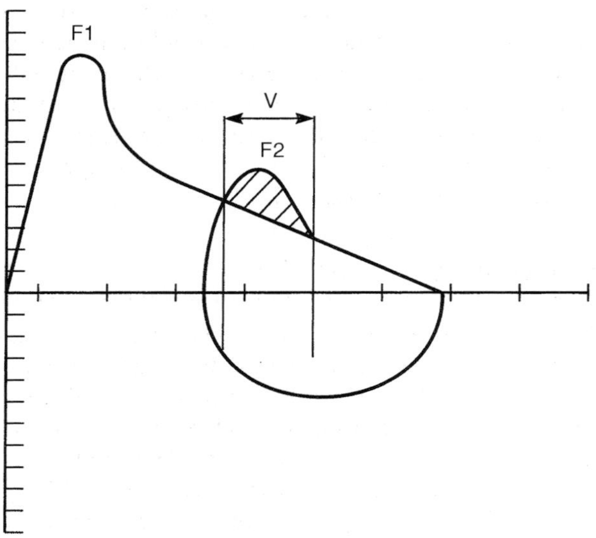

Fig. 8.7 *The use of a partial flow volume curve to demonstrate flow transients. Fl, full expiratory curve; F2, partial expiratory curve, showing the transient 'escaping' from the envelope due to rapid emptying of the upper (airway) compartment. V is the volume of the flow transient.*

tion'), by combining flow and gas analysis measurements.

The debate about airway compliance is relevant to determining what is a beneficial response to bronchodilator therapy, commonly and often uncritically prescribed in CF. Even in asthma, with no suggestion of the rapid upper-airway emptying described in CF, there is considerable debate as to what lung-function variable to measure and how to assess its significance. In asthmatics, it has been thought reasonable to use either an absolute increase in FEV_1 of 190 mL[27] (possibly also in children[28] as well as adults[29]) or normalize to percentage predicted normal FEV_1[30], which seems more logical. The use of peak expiratory flow rate (PEFR) is less satisfactory, but if it has to be relied upon, then reversibility is present with spontaneous swings of 60 liters/min or more. However, PEFR results have a low negative predictive value. In the context of CF, Zach *et al.*[23] have drawn attention to the fact that an increase in FEV_1 could merely be 'wasted gas' expelled from an upper airway made more compliant by bronchodilators, with paradoxical worsening of flow at low lung volumes (Fig. 8.8).

A further important consideration is the coefficient of variation for spirometric variables in CF, which should not be assumed to be the same as in normals, or even in asthmatics. Variability is greater than for normal subjects[30]. For example, the mean change that is likely to be significant (i.e. outside random variation) is 15 per cent for FEV_1, FVC and PEFR; for the least reproducible individuals, it is more than 20 per cent[30]. Plethysmographic measurements may exhibit less variability[31]. Flow rates at low lung volumes are even more variable. It is essential to remember this when assessing alleged improvements in small airways disease. Indeed, the coefficient of variation, often well over 30 per

absolute maximum transient that could be accounted for by upper airway emptying is 267 mL. Thus either the large changes recorded by Zach *et al.*[23] are artefactual or the lower generations are more enlarged than the upper airway to a considerable extent, or some at least of the gas in the flow transient comes from the respiratory bronchiole or below. Part of the debate could be resolved if it was known how much of the flow transient was of the same composition as room air (i.e. 'wasted ventila-

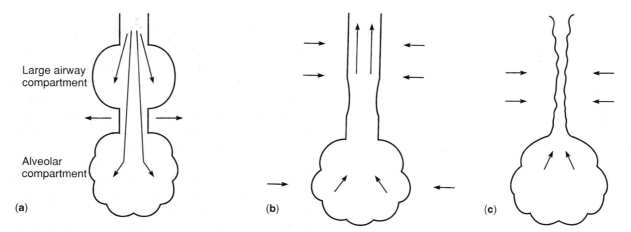

(a) **(b)** **(c)**

Fig. 8.8 *Two-compartment model as in Fig. 8.6 demonstrating how bronchodilators, by relaxing airway smooth muscle, may worsen lung function.* **(a)** *At end-inspiration, the relaxation of smooth muscle increases the compliance of the upper airway compartment, allowing it to fill with a greater volume of gas;* **(b)** *this extra volume empties, increasing the measured FEV_1, but in fact no useful increase in alveolar ventilation has occurred;* **(c)** *the floppier upper airway is now more easily compressed by further expiratory pressure, reducing flow from the alveolar compartment in late expiration. The converse effects may account for benefit seen with bronchoconstrictor challenges such as cold air, exercise or histamine.*

cent, makes small changes likely to be of very dubious significance indeed. The explanation is likely to be that coughing and change in sputum obstruction induced by the maneuvers gives rise to this variability. What then is a beneficial response for the patient? Subjective decrease in morbidity and objective evidence of increased sputum clearance are unarguable benefits. Qualitatively, if the flow volume curve becomes less scalloped and more like the normal triangular shape, this argues for a beneficial response[15]. It is important not to overinterpret small changes in lung function tests. A simple, reproducible test like a 2-minute walk[32] or the step test[32a] may be more useful. Noninvasively measured blood gases are also simple to interpret, but, for strict rigor, they need to be combined with measurement of cardiac output. There is not much real evidence that bronchodilators have caused harm[22], and they are widely prescribed. However, there is pathological evidence that bronchodilators may not be as active in some CF patients as in asthmatics. Autoradiographic studies show reduced β-receptor numbers in CF airways[33], possibly related to pulmonary infection and airway inflammation. The measurement of bronchial hyperreactivity and reversible airway obstruction is discussed in more detail below.

The extrathoracic airway

There is a single case report of vocal cord dysfunction in CF mimicking respiratory deterioration[34]. The cause of breathlessness is tight adduction of the vocal cords, particularly in inspiration. It may be difficult to distinguish this from bronchospasm clinically; clues to the diagnosis are the history of absence of nocturnal symptoms, disproportionate attenuation of the inspiratory curve of the flow volume loop (Fig. 8.9) and (usually but not invariably) normal saturation and blood gases in the presence of a subjective sensation of severe breathlessness. Peak flow measurements are not useful. Treatment is with relaxation techniques or speech therapy and not by intensifying treatment for sepsis or bronchospasm. Another rare cause of large airway compromise described in CF is amyloid goitre[35].

Bronchial hyperreactivity

There is controversy about the prevalence of hyperreactivity and its significance. As in asthma, individual airway hyperreactivity may not be the same to different stimuli. For example, histamine and exercise responsiveness were not correlated in one study[36]. Bronchial hyperreactivity is found in nearly half the children under age 18 years. In adults, hyperreactivity may be even more common. For example, in one study, 14 of 20 showed significant bronchodilatation to either terbutaline or ipratropium[24]. Whether there is any correlation between severity of CF and hyperreactivity is controversial. At least two mechanisms of hyperreactivity have been described, one vagally mediated[37]. Bronchial hyperreactivity can be measured by conventional testing in older, cooperative subjects, and by the squeeze technique in infants[15,38]. A simpler technique in infants is using transcutaneous P_{O_2} as an end point, rather than squeeze spirometry[39]. An important practical point in challenge testing is that a deep inspiration reduces flow in CF, as in asthma[40]. In CF, the mechanism appears to be due to worsening of nonhomogeneous lung emptying. This inhomogeneity may be made worse by bronchodilators, even though they improve flow rates at large lung volumes. The practical message of this paper[40] is to underscore the need to standardize volume history when doing challenge procedures.

HISTAMINE/METHACHOLINE

Bronchial hyperreactivity (BHR) in CF cannot be predicted from a history of wheeze, allergic disease or positive skin-prick tests[41]. However, BHR may be worth determining; acutely, BHR and response to bronchodilator correlate well; and in a long-term study[42], only patients with BHR to methacholine exhibited a favorable response to prolonged bronchodilator therapy. Ackerman et al.[38] studied 14 infants, mean age 16 months, and showed that, compared with controls, CF infants were shorter, had lower baseline flows, and heightened methacholine responsiveness, primarily related to the low baseline. There are many practical points that cause difficulty in interpretation; what dose of methacholine is actually being given to a baby, and how does it compare to an adult dose? What are the effects of (developmentally) small airways appearing artificially reactive because only a very small change is needed to produce marked obstruction? A similar group

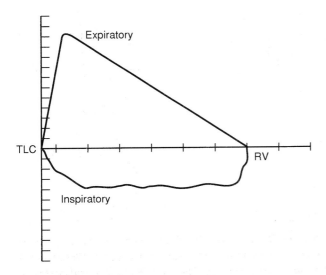

Fig. 8.9 *Flow volume loop of vocal cord dysfunction. The expiratory curve is nearly normal, but there is marked attenuation of the inspiratory curve.*

of infants were shown by the same technique to have low baseline flows which reverted to normal with inhaled metaproterenol; the changes were particularly marked in the presence of acute respiratory symptoms. No paradoxical reductions in flow were seen. Alarmingly, in one study, those with methacholine hyperreactivity had worse lung function and a worse prognosis than nonreactive patients[42]. Both airway obstruction and bronchial hyperreactivity worsened with time. Possible reasons include worse chronic airway inflammation damaging airways and causing concomitant hyperreactivity; possibly atopic, T-cell-driven, eosinophil-mediated airway inflammation, atopy being more common in CF than in normals; autonomic dysfunction and anatomically smaller airways in the hyperreactive group due to lung destruction. Late in the disease, bronchial hyperreactivity becomes more common, and bronchodilators fail to return lung function to normal[22].

EXERCISE

Exercise is a well-known bronchoconstrictor challenge in asthmatics. Macfarlane and Heaf[43] studied 25 CF patients. During exercise, FEV_1 rose, to the greatest extent in those with severest lung disease, confirming the findings of others[44]; after exercise, two patients showed bronchoconstriction, but the lung function of the remainder remained at baseline levels. The bronchodilator response in this group was greatest in the mildly affected patients. It is tempting to speculate that physiotherapy should be preceded by bronchodilators in mild disease, and by exercise in severe disease; however, measurements of expectorated sputum weight and the comparative responses of lung function to exercise and bronchodilators would be needed to address this in each individual case. The possible mechanisms of improvement of lung function on exercise include increased mucus clearance and increased flow transients, accounting for improvement in small airway indices and PEFR, respectively[44].

COLD AIR

Darga et al.[45] studied the response to a cold air challenge in 34 patients with CF. Five patients had the expected reduction in FEV_1 and 13 had reduced flow at low lung volumes. However, paradoxical benefit in these measurements were seen in 10 and 5 patients respectively, particularly in those with more severe disease. The authors speculated that this was the result of the airway instability discussed above.

MISCELLANEOUS

Hypertonic solutions have been shown to cause bronchoconstriction in CF. This should be considered particularly when giving nebulized antibiotics. Ticarcillin caused a fall of more than 10 per cent in 5 of 12 children tested[46]. This can be prevented by pretreatment with nebulized salbutamol. Hypertonic saline has long been used therapeutically to aid expectoration in CF; recently this treatment has been shown to improve mucociliary clearance and lung function to a degree comparable with that obtained by rhDNase. Thus a recent pilot study of the effects on airway function of 10 per cent saline is particularly important[47]; this group documented a very variable response, with 7 patients exhibiting bronchoconstriction and 15 bronchodilatation. If hypertonic saline is to be used therapeutically, then careful monitoring is necessary.

CONCLUSIONS

There is no doubt that bronchial hyperresponsiveness is common in CF but is variable between individuals and within the same individual with time. This may be related to infection. It seems that CF hyperresponsiveness is unrelated to atopy or allergy. There is a trend for those who respond to have more small airways disease and worse baseline lung function. For example, in one study, 80 per cent of those with an FEV_1 of less than 40 per cent predicted were hyperreactive to methacholine, whereas only 40 per cent responded in the group with FEV_1 greater than 80 per cent predicted. As with all treatments, measurement of efficacy should be performed where possible; the practical importance of paradoxical responses (both beneficial to constrictor challenges and harmful to dilator challenges) is still controversial. However, testing the responses to maneuvers is so simple, at least above age 6, that there is no excuse for omitting the investigations. Even in the uncooperative, measurements of saturation and transcutaneous P_{O_2} are a useful guide.

Lung volumes

Measurement of lung volumes in CF is fraught with difficulty, and the technical problems need to be remembered when reviewing results purporting to describe 'restrictive' patterns of physiology. Body plethysmography has been described as the 'gold standard', but for accuracy relies on mouth pressure and alveolar pressure being equal at FRC; in patients with airway obstruction, this is not so, and volumes are overestimated. There are even more formidable problems in infants, and in the presence of severe obstruction and obvious hyperinflation, apparently low lung volumes are measured, for reasons that are unclear[48]. Helium dilution methods are also inaccurate, because equilibration may never be achieved in obstructed compartments with long time constants, underestimating volumes. Indeed, a mixing index has been used to define ventilatory abnormalities in CF based on the number of breaths for helium 'equilibration' to occur[49]. Radiographic methods measure lung gas and tissue volume; if the latter is increased by chronic infection, bronchial wall thickening, etc., then gas volume is overestimated. The difference between plethysmographic and helium total lung capacity has been exploited as an index of airway obstruction[22,50]. None of these three methods should be used interchangeably, and the 95 per cent confidence intervals are large. Attempts have been made to see whether CF with 'restriction' is a sign of more severe disease[51]; there is no evidence for this, and this alleged subgroup may in fact reflect merely methodological artifact. There is no doubt that there is much less increase in TLC for a given degree of airway obstruction in CF than in emphysema. This presumably reflects inflammation, infection and fibrosis limiting the expansion of lung volumes. Of practical interest, measurement of lung volumes from radiographs has shown us how unreliable 'hyperinflation' is as a clinically detectable sign; very often, so-called hyperinflated children (Fig. 8.10) have normal radiographic and plethysmographic lung volumes[52]. This is important, since many 'objective' scores of disease severity include a numerical assessment of 'hyperinflation' from the CXR.

The effect of positive-pressure breathing on lung volumes was assessed in eight CF patients[53]. Positive pressure resulted in recruitment of lung volume, but had no effect on clearance of secretions. At the end of positive-pressure breathing, volumes returned rapidly to baseline.

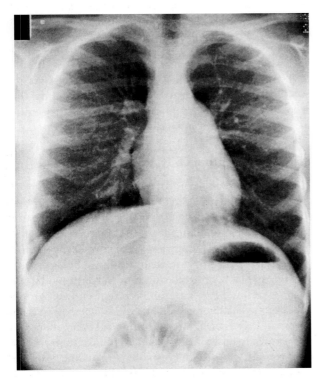

Fig. 8.10 *Chest radiograph showing generalized hyperinflation. However, TLC measured in the plethysmograph was normal. What does 'hyperinflation' mean?*

GAS EXCHANGE

Ventilation inequalities

Airway obstruction and tissue destruction combine to elevate the closing volume into the tidal range in CF. This results in venous admixture and hypoxemia[54]. The physiologic deadspace is increased[55]. In severe CF, nitrogen washout studies suggest a large anatomic deadspace (wasted ventilation)[24]. The elevated ventilatory equivalent for oxygen (below) is further evidence in support of a raised deadspace[56]. Sophisticated multibreath techniques have been used to study inequalities of ventilation[57], but are, at present, restricted to research laboratories.

Carbon monoxide transfer

Although there has been ongoing debate for many years about what is meant by whole lung carbon monoxide transfer (D_LCO), the balance of evidence suggests that it measures the amount of blood (or strictly, hemoglobin) in the pulmonary capillary bed. Early in the course of CF, D_LCO may be elevated because (1) airway obstruction causes increased pleural pressure swings and thus more blood is sucked into the thorax; and (2) small areas of airway occlusion lead to diversion of blood into better-ventilated alveoli, distending the capillary bed; both mechanisms have been described in airway obstruction due to asthma. As bronchiectasis worsens, the bronchial circulation contributes a further blood supply to the lungs, elevating D_LCO. Finally, as cor pulmonale develops, D_LCO may start to fall as the pulmonary capillary bed becomes progressively attenuated. Keens *et al.*[58] measured single-breath D_LCO in 175 patients with CF aged 9–24 years. The results were 122 ± 26 per cent predicted, and correlated inversely with percentage predicted maximal mid-expiratory flow rates. In 10 normals, they showed that inspiratory loading elevated D_LCO by 18 per cent, confirming the importance of airway obstruction in determining the result. However, as lung disease worsens, D_LCO starts to fall, possibly due to a failure of lung growth[59]. D_LCO may correlate with the Shwachman score[60]. It is one of many useful measurements to assess progress, but the factors affecting the result need to be borne in mind.

Circulatory mismatch

The primary disorder of gas exchange is ventilatory, with secondary circulatory consequences. Increased venous admixture is typical[52], mainly due to airway closure during tidal breathing (above). Measurement of shunt fraction by giving the subject 100 per cent oxygen to breathe was described by Kraemer and Sohoni[60]. Mean P_{O_2} on

100 per cent oxygen was 23.9 ± 6.6 kPa, equivalent to a shunt fraction of 25 per cent (normal <5 per cent) in the most severe group. Even in the group with mild disease, the corresponding figures were 38.3 ± 11.2 kPa, shunt fraction 20 per cent. Similar results have been found using the multiple inert gas technique[61]. The anatomic basis of the shunt is presumably blood passing from right to left past totally nonventilated alveoli. Support for this concept comes from studies of intravenous boluses of $^{13}N_2$[62], which demonstrate areas of lung with virtually no airway washout. Hypoxic vasoconstriction can only partly compensate for abnormal ventilation, and failure of complete compensation accounts for the shunt. If hypoxia disproportionate to the severity of lung disease is encountered, the cause may be intrapulmonary shunting secondary to CF liver disease or through a patent foramen ovale. Contrast echocardiography may be diagnostically helpful.

RESPIRATORY MECHANICS

Compliance studies

Lung elastic recoil is abnormal in CF. The weighted spirometer technique involves adding a known weight to the bell of a spirometer in a rebreathing circuit to which the infant is connected. Compliance is calculated from the change in end-expiratory volume divided by the pressure change, and subtracting the compliance of the apparatus[63]. In well infants with CF, this method can detect reduced compliance even before the onset of hyperinflation[13], possibly related to parenchymal changes. In a study of children and young adults[64], lung recoil pressure was reduced in CF compared with controls, and the lung compliance curve was shifted to the left, with some correlation with indices of airflow obstruction. In older subjects, at low lung volume, there is loss of elastic recoil, presumably reflecting tissue destruction; at high volumes there is excessive stiffness, possibly because the lung is at the flat part of the pressure–volume curve[65]. However, the major cause of reduced flows is probably airway obstruction, not compliance change[65].

Mechanics of breathing

Coates et al. used magnetometers to study the relative contributions of rib cage and abdomen in 14 children with CF[66]. As in studies in normals, there was a wide range of ratios, but no trend for a particular abnormality in the CF group. Others have found differences in the use of abdominal muscles in CF, with recruitment at lower loads[67]. However, the number of CF children studied is small.

Respiratory muscles

DIAGNOSTIC STUDIES

Studies on absolute respiratory muscle strength in CF have shown either values of mouth pressure which were normal[68], modestly reduced[69] or increased[70]. In animal models, hyperinflation actually leads to diaphragm hypertrophy and a left shift in the length–tension curve[71]; furthermore, chronic cough and/or the increased work of breathing might 'train' respiratory muscles. Conversely, hyperinflation would be expected to cause a less than optimal length–tension relationship of inspiratory muscles, thus these measurements might underestimate their true power. The main determinant of respiratory muscle strength is probably not hyperinflation but muscle bulk and nutritional status. In general, the changes in respiratory muscle strength in CF are arguably too small to be of clinical significance, although there may be some suggestion that respiratory muscle performance may limit exercise tolerance (below). Interestingly, females appear to preserve respiratory muscle strength better[72]; this is surprising in view of the generally less good prognosis in females of all ages. No effect of posture on respiratory muscle strength has been found.

The oxygen consumption of respiratory muscles was measured by looking at the difference between total oxygen consumption at rest and on exercise under normocapnic and induced hypercapnic conditions[73]. The difference between the oxygen consumptions in normocapnic and hypercapnic states was thought to be the oxygen cost by the respiratory muscles of the extra ventilation. This was only modestly elevated in CF (131 mL/L oxygen supplied at moderate exercise versus 80 mL/L oxygen in normals). The difference, and the absolute oxygen consumption of the respiratory muscles, was not thought to be clinically significant.

RESPIRATORY MUSCLE TRAINING

There is considerable controversy as to whether it is possible to strengthen respiratory muscles in any context. Methods used include voluntary hyperpnea, upper body endurance exercise, biofeedback and periods of breathing through an inspiratory resistance[74]. Keens et al.[74] compared respiratory muscle training by repeated 15 min spells of normocapnic hyperpnea with the changes produced by an exercise program. Each group improved to a similar extent, but with no change in lung function. Inspiratory muscle loading led to small, probably clinically insignificant, changes in inspiratory muscle strength, but with variable effects on exercise performance. There is, on balance, no evidence to suggest that a formal respiratory muscle training program is worthwhile. No comparisons have been carried out to my knowledge between respiratory muscle training, extra exercise, and extra chest physiotherapy as an adjunct to treatment; intuitively, it seems likely that respiratory muscle training is likely neither to be popular nor effective in the long term.

PULMONARY CIRCULATION

Cor pulmonale carries an ominous prognosis in CF, and occurs in up to two-thirds of patients dying of CF. Studies of the pulmonary circulation and heart, and how favorably to manipulate their function, have the potential to be extremely important. However, until useful therapies are developed, their importance is potential only. Siassi *et al.* found that a mean pulmonary artery pressure of 38 mmHg or more correlated with an FEV_1 of less than 1 liter, a Shwachman score of less than 40, a PaO_2 less than 7 kPa and a $PaCO_2$ of more than 6 kPa in 34 CF patients[75]. Initially pulmonary hypertension is reversible with oxygen therapy and treatment of sepsis, implying pulmonary vasoconstriction; later on elevation of PA (pulmonary artery) pressure becomes irreversible, implying structural changes within the pulmonary circulation. The pathological mechanisms are thought to include hypoxic vasoconstriction in areas of poor ventilation, progressing to increased muscularization of small pulmonary arteries and destruction of the vascular bed[76]. The levels of atrial natriuretic peptide are increased, and the main source is thought to be the right atrium[77]. Nifedipine, diltiazem, tolazoline and hydralazine[78] have all been used to try to reduce pulmonary vascular resistance (PVR) in CF, but as in virtually all studies of blood-borne vasodilators, there is no evidence of long-term benefit[78]. Indeed, the risks, including aggravation of hypoxemia, systemic hypotension and worsening pulmonary hypertension, mandate extreme caution in the use of these agents. The possible interactions of the lung complications seen secondary to any primary liver disease ('primary' pulmonary hypertension, multiple diffuse pulmonary arteriovenous fistulas) and the inflammatory lung disease secondary to sepsis and bronchospasm in CF remain to be explored in detail. Clinicians should be aware that the hypoxic CF patient with severe liver disease may not necessarily have severe pulmonary dysfunction. Clues would include hypoxemia or right ventricular hypertrophy disproportionate to the degree of airway obstruction.

THE HEART

Although some workers[79] have postulated that there is early cardiac dysfunction in CF, in general this is not a clinical problem. Rare cases of left ventricular failure due to cardiomyopathy or myocardial infarction in infancy have been reported[80]. Dysfunction occurs secondary to

the vascular and mechanical effects of predominantly late-stage airway disease.

How the lungs affect the heart

There is a huge literature on heart–lung interactions in many pulmonary diseases. In CF, in addition to presenting an increased afterload to the right ventricle, the pressure swings within the pleura affect cardiac function. In the presence of airway obstruction, end-expiratory pressure within the pleural cavity will be supra-atmospheric, so-called auto PEEP (positive end-expiratory pressure) or intrinsic PEEP. This has the same hemodynamic effects as PEEP applied by mechanical ventilation, namely a reduction in venous return and an increase in PVR. That this mechanism may be of more than theoretical importance is demonstrated by a study in which the limitation of the stroke volume response to exercise in CF was partially reversible with improvement of airflow obstruction[81]. This effect was independent of hypoxia. Increased pleural pressure swings also cause abnormal afterload conditions of the left ventricle[82].

Right ventricle

Right ventricular disease is almost invariably secondary to pulmonary vascular disease, itself a consequence of airflow obstruction and tissue destruction. Technical problems make the right ventricle difficult to study. The electrocardiogram is insensitive. The least useless sign is a reduction in voltages in the left chest leads. Transthoracic echocardiography may be impossible in the presence of hyperinflation. Systolic time intervals are too unreliable to be useful, particularly in CF where there are wide respiratory variations in right ventricular preload. If there is pulmonary or tricuspid regurgitation, then mean PA pressure can be estimated using the Bernouilli equation. Failing that, qualitative estimates of right ventricular wall thickness or cavity size have to be relied on. Radionuclide studies are not usually routine procedures, but provide useful information. Matthay *et al.*[83] found reduced right ventricular ejection fraction (RVEF) in 9 of 22 patients, all of whom had PaO_2 less than 8 kPa. Only one hypoxic patient had a normal RVEF. There was some correlation with the Shwachman score. Magnetic resonance imaging overcomes most of the problems of the other techniques, but is time consuming and expensive. In general, cardiac changes in CF are only a feature of advanced pulmonary disease; right ventricular contractility is preserved until late on, when among the benefits of oxygen therapy is the improvement of right ventricular function. However, ejection fraction may be normal even in preterminal lung disease. Attempts to improve cardiac function with digoxin have been a failure[84].

Left ventricle

Left ventricular (LV) changes in CF are usually mild. They may be secondary to right ventricular shape changes, a result of pleural pressure swings, or as a consequence of poor myocardial oxygen supply. Myocardial fibrosis has been seen at autopsy, presumably related to impaired myocardial oxygen delivery and acidosis. Left ventricular ejection fraction is usually normal[83]. Occasional patients have markedly impaired LV function, which may only be apparent on exercise[85]. Echocardiography has demonstrated LV shape changes; the LV is flattened around the abnormally dilated and hypertrophied RV, resulting in impaired LV diastolic function (chamber filling) and systolic function (dyskinetic contractions). Interesting support for the idea that diastolic disease may be present even in mild CF comes from the observation that stroke volume index did not rise normally on going from the upright to the supine position, at rest and on exercise, when venous return would be expected to rise[86]. The alternative explanation, that pleural pressure effects, including auto-PEEP, may not permit venous return to rise, seems unlikely, at least in patients with only mild airflow obstruction. A recent study[87] showed left ventricular perfusion defects not present at rest but appearing on exercise, correlating with poor clinical state. The clinical significance of this observation is not clear. In general, clinical left ventricular disease is not a problem.

CF PHYSIOLOGY UNDER SPECIAL STRESSES

This section covers sleep, exercise, hypoxia, hyperoxia and malnutrition. The effects on the lungs of the special stresses of diabetes and pregnancy are covered elsewhere in this book.

Sleep

Desaturation during sleep is frequent in end-stage CF, and may contribute to the development of hypoxic cor pulmonale. There are a number of important mechanisms to consider in the sleep disorders of CF[88]. Upper airway obstruction by nasal polyps or chronic sepsis is the most easily reversible and should always be excluded. Sleep desaturation due to lung disease cannot be predicted from FEV_1, but is not a clinical problem if resting SaO_2 is above 95 per cent; SaO_2 below 94 per cent is strongly predictive of both significant daytime and night-time desaturation[89]. In general, the worse the lung function at rest, the more likely is sleep or exercise desaturation. Mechanisms postulated include abnormal mechanics during rapid eye movement (REM) sleep, postural worsening of hypoxemia which paradoxically may be greatest in mild disease[90], airway closure in REM

sleep worsening venous admixture, a reduced neuromuscular output during non-REM sleep[91] and a blunted central response to hypercapnia, leading to reduced tidal volume and inspiratory flow rate[92]. The response to hypercapnia in CF relates to the degree of airflow obstruction[66]. Sleep hypoxemia may contribute to the development of cor pulmonale, together with other factors discussed above, but the best management is unclear. Oxygen therapy is discussed below, and can be used to abolish sleep desaturation. Although some investigators have not found deteriorating hypercapnia with low-flow oxygen during sleep, we advise monitoring of blood gases when low-flow oxygen is commenced. Anecdotally, we have used protriptyline if hypercapnia develops, with some success. Sleep quality, in terms of arousals and time spent in each stage of sleep, is not improved by oxygen. Sleep desaturation tends to be more marked than exercise desaturation in the same group of patients[93]. If home monitoring of sleep oxygenation is to be performed, then a pulse oximeter with an 8-hour memory is preferable to the use of transcutaneous electrodes, which in CF tend to drift after about 4 hours.

Other therapies to be considered during sleep are theophylline, which at levels within the conventional therapeutic range may improve oxygenation[94]; nasal continuous positive airway pressure (CPAP)[95], which may improve sleep quality as well as oxygenation; bi-level positive airway pressure (BiPAP)[96]; and intermittent positive-pressure ventilation[97]. Mechanical support has the advantage of not exacerbating hypercapnia in most cases. However, it should be said that little evidence for long-term benefit has accrued; in a small uncontrolled study[98], spirometry and hypercapnia improved slightly after several months' negative pressure ventilation in patients who could tolerate the technique. However, all these treatments should be applied very selectively, according to patient need and short-term benefit in terms of quality of life, rather than in the expectation of long-term benefit. Indeed, in a recent study[97], most patients elected for nocturnal oxygen as preferable to noninvasive ventilatory support.

Exercise

Exercise studies in CF have been diagnostic, to stress the cardiopulmonary unit to determine the level of reserve, the safety of exercise and the cardiopulmonary responses; therapeutic, using exercise to increase fitness, improve lung function or well-being, and to complement or replace physiotherapy; and prognostic. Methods for formal studies include treadmill, exercise bicycle and timed walking tests. More details of exercise in CF are given in Chapter 19. Mild to moderate CF is associated with a reasonably normal exercise performance[99]. There are wide differences between centers in the use made of exercise programs. A questionnaire study highlighted that, although most centers acknowledge the value of exercise, only 44 per cent offered a diagnostic service and 22 per cent a formal exercise program for their patients[100]. Compliance with unsupervised programs is poor, particularly if the patient does not feel that any immediate benefit is accruing.

DIAGNOSTIC EXERCISE STUDIES

Exercise is a severe test of a system which may function adequately at rest. There are numerous possible reasons why would-be athletes stop and retire to their armchairs. The role of the ventilatory system is to blow off CO_2, that of the cardiovascular system to supply oxygen; within the lungs the two systems have to be matched, and within the nervous system, motivation has to be supplied. In CF, resting and exercise oxygen consumption is elevated compared with normals[56]. Oxygen consumption may vary with genotype[101]. Most have a higher ventilatory equivalent for oxygen, presumably reflecting airway, deadspace and compliance changes. Physiological factors limiting exercise may be of respiratory, cardiac or cardiorespiratory matching origin. As in all contexts, motivation is also critical and confounds the interpretation of much exercise testing.

Respiratory factors are likely to be the most important in CF. Total ventilation is a function of respiratory rate and tidal volume, both of which rise in normal exercise. In CF, however, these changes may be impaired. Tidal volume depends in part on inspiratory time and flow rate, and the effective alveolar ventilation depends on the amount of deadspace (wasted) ventilation and new lung recruitment. During normal exercise, end-expiratory lung volume falls (i.e. the chest becomes deflated), so tidal volume can rise. With severe airways obstruction, the opposite is seen. In severe CF, tidal volume is near maximal (i.e. flow limited) at rest and the only available strategy to increase minute volume is to increase respiratory rate. Less severely affected patients can increase tidal volume by up to 40 per cent[102]. The strategy of reducing lung volume during exercise improves the efficiency of the diaphragm, but reduces airway caliber. Inspiratory time must be very short before it becomes limiting. In theory, exercise may be limited purely by ventilation, as it approaches the maximum (flow-limited capacity) of the system. Hypercapnia is certainly a feature of exercise in severe CF, and resting hypercapnia is worsened on exercise[103]. Lactic acidosis fails to stimulate ventilation in CF as it does in normals. Factors leading to hypercapnia include failure to recruit lung volume during exercise; exercise bronchoconstriction; impaired pressure generation by the respiratory muscles as they approach maximum capacity; increased deadspace to tidal volume ratio; and worsening venous admixture with elevation of mixed venous PCO_2. End-tidal CO_2 rises early in exercise, whereas desaturation occurs later. Modeling studies suggest that the effects of collateral ventilation may account for CO_2 retention disproportionate to hypoxemia. This combination of cardiorespiratory changes means that CO_2 must rise, or exercise must stop; the level of tolerable CO_2 depends on central sensitivity, which is disease and age related; it correlates with the ventilatory response to exercise.

An important practical point arises from the impaired CO_2 excretion on exercise. Attempts noninvasively to estimate lactate threshold from ventilatory threshold, but not gas exchange threshold, will result in overestimation of lactate threshold. The protagonists of this method believe that this measurement allows delineation of improved performance at submaximal workloads of cardiac and skeletal muscle, which may not, however, allow increased maximal exercise because of ventilatory impairment[104]. The practical clinical relevance of this may be open to question. However, a point of wider importance is that attempts to apply exercise protocols derived from normal children to those with diseases may lead to false conclusions[105], both in terms of measurement of lactate thresholds and delineating safe levels of exercise (assuming people will stay within 'safe' limits).

Cardiovascular factors may be important in limiting exercise in some cases. Especially if there is exercise desaturation, the myocardium may become ischemic. Exercise cardiac output depends on preload, afterload and myocardial contractility. Preload (venous return) may be impaired by excessive pleural pressure swings; contractility will be discussed below; and afterload may be normal at rest, but the pulmonary circulatory bed may not be able to dilate to accommodate the rise in cardiac output or may even, paradoxically, constrict[106]. The cardiac variables include stroke volume, ejection fraction and heart rate. Cardiac output has been measured on exercise in CF using CO_2 rebreathing and impedance cardiography. We have found the former to be inaccurate even in normals however, and feel these measurements should be interpreted with caution[107]. A recent study[108] showed that even in mildly affected patients, stroke volume was reduced at a given level of exercise and corresponding cardiac output. The theoretical possibility that, in some individuals, cardiac effects disproportionate to lung disease may be important in limiting exercise should always be kept in mind. The lack of correlation of stroke volume response with airway obstruction implies that this may reflect individual variability in the vasoconstrictor response in the pulmonary circulation. Another postulated mechanism is limitation in ventricular diastolic reserve, which becomes unmasked on exercise.

Using the multiple inert gas technique to assess ventilation:perfusion matching and gas exchange, Dantzker et al.[61] showed that matching of ventilation to perfusion actually improves on exercise, but PO_2 does not rise due to the confounding effect of a reduced mixed venous saturation on pulmonary gas exchange. In two patients, shunt fraction also decreased on exercise. Resting saturation of above 94 per cent and CO transfer greater than 84 per cent predicted, predicts normal saturation on exercise and, correspondingly, a lower saturation and CO transfer below 64 per cent predicts desaturation[75]. Desaturation is also likely if FEV_1 is less than 60 per cent. Hypoxia is associated with evidence of cardiac dysfunction on exercise, namely a fall in stroke volume[75].

Why then do patients with CF stop exercising? This cannot be predicted from baseline lung function[109], but in general CF patients with the best lung function tend to have the highest VO_2max (maximum oxygen consumption). For reasons which are not clear, VO_2max is lower in females than males, in absolute terms and when corrected for body size[110]. In the main, exercise ceases because of limitation of ventilation[106]; at extremes of exercise in CF, ventilation approaches resting maximal voluntary ventilation. Ventilation is higher at a given workload and for normal or elevated CO_2 than in normals, implying wasted (deadspace) ventilation[99,106]. Some patients can actually exceed resting 'maximum voluntary ventilation' on exercise; presumably motivation and exercise bronchodilatation (above) are causes for this apparent paradox. This implies that ventilation limits exercise, combined with the lung volume effects described above[102]. By comparison, heart rate does not approach maximum predicted. In a few patients, the failure of an appropriate rise in stroke volume, an abnormal ejection fraction, a failure of the normal rise in cardiac output and an inappropriately high heart rate imply that cardiac factors may also be important.

Attempts have been made to improve exercise tolerance. Of note, it may actually be worsened by salbutamol and theophylline, possibly by worsening physiological deadspace on exercise[111]; it is not improved by breathing a helium–oxygen mixture[112]. CPAP during exercise, particularly in the more severely affected patients, reduces the work of breathing and increases performance[113]. Supplemental oxygen is also beneficial[114].

THERAPEUTIC EXERCISE STUDIES

Exercise may increase well-being, improve lung function, reduce the need for physiotherapy, possibly improve prognosis and have beneficial metabolic and endocrine benefits in CF. Exercise training may diminish the sensation of breathlessness. In eight patients, exercise prior to a session of physiotherapy increased sputum production, but the length of exercise (one hour) makes this strategy of little practical long-term value. It may be that stage of illness is important in determining benefit, if any. The most important practical conclusion from therapeutic exercise studies is that exercise is at best an adjunct to physiotherapy, and cannot replace it. More

details of therapeutic exercise studies are given in Chapter 20.

PROGNOSTIC EXERCISE STUDIES

The limitations of standard lung function tests in assessing prognosis have been discussed above. At the moment, exercise testing cannot be recommended as a better long-term prognostic tool than standard lung function, although improvements in exercise performance may be regarded as a reasonable surrogate end point.

Hypoxia, including altitude

The normal response of the pulmonary vasculature to hypoxia is vasoconstriction. There is marked individual variation in the extent of this response. In cattle, the ability to avoid pulmonary vasoconstriction and peripheral edema at altitude (Brisket disease) is inherited as an autosomal dominant[115]. Chinese babies of families who had lived at sea level and moved to altitude to occupy conquered Tibet died of severe pulmonary hypertension, and had severe plexiform lesions in the pulmonary microcirculation at autopsy; native Tibetan babies tolerated altitude hypoxia with no excess mortality[116]. There is a marked individual variation in response to hypoxic challenge in normal subjects[117] and children with congenital heart disease[118]. Although this has not been studied, there is no reason to doubt that the same variability exists in CF. Hypoxia is also an important cause of bronchoconstriction[119].

This has relevance to CF patients holidaying at altitude or flying in commercial jets (pressurized passenger cabins being equivalent to an altitude of between 6000 and 8000 ft (1800 and 2400 m)). Deterioration in previously stable CF patients during strenuous physical exertion at altitude has been described[120]. Two patients deteriorated irreversibly and required heart–lung transplantation. Although specific 'safe' levels of sea-level PO_2 have been set, this is probably unsound because of the individual variation in circulatory reactivity described above. One approach is to perform a hypoxic challenge at sea level in all children in whom there is doubt as to whether they will become hypoxic in a commercial aeroplane. Breathing 15 per cent oxygen is equivalent to the fractional inspired oxygen concentration (FiO_2) in a pressurized cabin of a commercial jet. This sea-level test, if anything, overestimates the degree of desaturation in flight[121], and can be used to predict the need for in-flight oxygen supplementation to prevent the hypoxia which almost universally elevates pulmonary artery pressure in CF. More recent evidence, however[121a], suggests that FEV_1 less than 50 per cent predicted may be a more useful guide. This test does not mimic the pressure changes in flight or at altitude; although worries of lung rupture have been expressed, due to failure of equilibration of intra-alveolar pressure with the reduced atmospheric pressure in lung compartments with a long time constant, in practice, even in elderly patients with very severe emphysema and bullae, this never seems to happen.

Hyperoxia

There has been one major trial of oxygen therapy in CF. The results were disappointing[122]; 28 patients were enrolled, and there was no difference in outcome between the oxygen and the control groups. There was possibly an improved quality of life in the treatment group. There were no problems with CO_2 retention in this small study. Reasons for the poor response to oxygen therapy may include too few hours per day spent on oxygen compared with the trials in chronic bronchitis. Current recommendations are to reserve oxygen for symptomatic relief; if overnight oxygen is contemplated, then a formal sleep study with measurement of transcutaneous or end-tidal CO_2 is mandatory. Although attempts have been made to predict oxygenation from the flow volume loop[123], it is so simple to measure both indirectly and invasively that prediction hardly seems worthwhile.

Hyperoxia has been shown to reduce PA pressure in the early stages of pulmonary hypertension in CF. Unfortunately, detailed data on the effect of hyperoxia and hypoxia on bronchomotor tone are scanty. Oxygen supplementation may improve exercise performance in patients who desaturate during exercise breathing air, presumably by increasing oxygen delivery to exercising muscles and the myocardium. Other possible mechanisms include relief of hypoxic bronchoconstriction and vasoconstriction. There may be small rises in CO_2 tension during exercise on oxygen in severely affected subjects. Desaturation is abolished by oxygen, and exercise efficiency may be increased.

Malnutrition

There is no question that maintaining good nutrition is valuable for its own sake, and a recent study confirmed that good nutrition correlates with good preservation of lung function[124]. However, there is controversy on the relationship between malnutrition, correction of malnutrition and physiological variables. There can be no doubt that pancreatic sufficiency and better lung function go together[125]. Some of the other studies are confounded by the concomitant use of antibiotics, which are known to improve lung function. Continuous enteral nutrition did not improve lung function or exercise performance[126], and enteral supplements had no significant effect on lung respiratory muscle strength[127]. Total parenteral nutrition did result in some lung-function improvements, but some of these patients were also given antibiotics. Mansell *et al.*[128]

produced small increases in mouth pressures, and maximum breathing capacity by parenteral nutrition, but the changes were of statistical rather than clinical importance. Others have not been able to repeat this work. Malnutrition leads to a reduction in stroke volume on exercise, but not heart rate, and also maximum work, possibly through a direct effect on the myocardium. The data on blood gas changes secondary to different nutritional manipulations are scanty. Two of six patients treated with enteral supplements showed a small increase in arterial Po_2 with no change in spirometry[126]. Parenteral nutrition caused a small fall in arterial saturation (93.5 ± 2.8, falling to 91.5 ± 2.7, $P < 0.005$), presumably due to the effects of intravenous intralipid on ventilation : perfusion matching. There was no change in carbon monoxide transfer or arterial Pco_2[128]. One month after intralipid, saturation had returned to baseline values. The effects of different energy sources on pH and Pco_2 have not been studied in detail. Overall, it is difficult to see how better nutrition can lead to reforming of destroyed airways, but easy to see that the better-nourished patient may deteriorate less quickly.

FUTURE RESEARCH

It seems likely that new and possibly hazardous treatments such as gene therapy will come to be applied at the earliest stage at which one can be reasonably certain that significant deterioration in lung function will occur. The challenge for the physiologist will be to detect early markers of deterioration noninvasively in uncooperative infants, so treatment can be instituted in those who are at risk for deterioration. In other contexts such as emphysema, it has been shown that image processing to quantitate anatomic information is more sensitive than gas exchange methods. Sophisticated techniques such as CT (computed tomography) and MRI (magnetic resonance imaging) are obvious tools with which to do this. CT has the drawback of irradiation risk, but it is likely that single CT slices may contain sufficient information at low risk of radiation. Furthermore, modern scanners require less and less radiation exposure to the subjects. Modern, fast scan-time instruments also obviate the need for anesthesia. Studies to detect early change should be the physiologist's goal. It is not clear whether newer physiological techniques will also be useful (reviewed above). On balance, I believe that quantitative, modern image-processing techniques will be the most effective tool.

CLINICAL PRACTICE OF LUNG FUNCTION TESTING IN CYSTIC FIBROSIS

Classic respiratory physiology is one of the essential clinical tools for monitoring change in clinical state. Spirometry can be used to guide the duration of inpatient treatment as well as outpatient progress. The minimum requirement for the routine clinical assessment is a spirometer, preferably modified[129] to prevent the tiny risk of cross-infection. Alternatively, a disposable filter can be placed in the mouthpiece [130]. Neither of these modifications have any clinically significant effect on the results. Pulse oximetry gives much useful information in uncooperative small children, and overnight saturation studies can be used to monitor the response to intravenous antibiotics[131]. In mildly affected children, postural change in saturation or transcutaneous oxygen tension should be sought[90]. Arterial blood gas analysis adds useful information only if saturation is abnormal. Routine arterial gases are not necessary, and for most purposes venous or capillary samples combined with pulse oximetry are satisfactory. Facilities for histamine challenge, exercise testing, hypoxic challenge and transcutaneous gas measurement for studying infants are desirable in larger centers. Careful and noninvasive monitoring will become ever more important as newer treatments with their attendant risks and benefits become available to our patients.

REFERENCES

1. Corey, M., Levison, H. and Crozier, D. (1976) Five- to seven-year course of pulmonary function in cystic fibrosis. *Am. Rev. Resp. Dis.*, **114**, 1085–1092.

2. Zapletal, A., Houstek, J., Samanek, M., Vavrova, V. and Srajer J. (1979) Lung function abnormalities in cystic fibrosis and changes during lung growth. *Bull. Europ. Physiopath. Resp.*, **15**, 575–592.

3. Bush, A. (1998) Early treatment with Dornase alpha in cystic fibrosis – what are the issues? *Pediatr. Pulmonol.*, **25**, 79–82.

4. Davis, P.B., Byard, P.J. and Konstan, M.W. (1997) Identifying treatments that halt progression of pulmonary disease in cystic fibrosis. *Pediatr. Res.*, **41**, 161–165.

5. Kerem, E., Reisman, J., Corey, M., Canny, G.J. and Levison, H. (1992) Prediction of mortality in patients with cystic fibrosis. *NEJM.*, **326**, 1887–1891.

6. Moorcroft, A.J., Webb, A.K. and Dodd, M.E. (1994) Preterminal disease and dying in adult cysic fibrosis [abstract]. *Thorax*, **49**, 393P.

7. Chan K.N., Wong, Y.C. and Silverman, M. (1990) Relationship between infant lung mechanics and childhood lung function in children of very low birthweight. *Pediatr. Pulmonol.*, **8**, 74–81.

8. Rosenthal, M., Bain, S.H., Cramer, D. *et al.* (1993) Lung function in white children aged 4–19 years: 1 – spirometry. *Thorax*, **48**, 794–802.

9. Stocks, J., Sly, P.D., Tepper, R.S. and Morgan, W.J. (eds) (1996) *Infant Respiratory Function Testing*, John Wiley & Sons, Inc., New York.

10. Lamarre, A., Reilly, B.J., Bryan, C., and Levison, H. (1972) Early detection of pulmonary function abnormalities in cystic fibrosis. *Pediatrics*, **50**, 291–298.

11. Adler, B., Warner, J.O. and Bush, A. (1991) Routine ventilation scanning in cystic fibrosis: is it worthwhile? *Pediatr. Pulmonol. Suppl.*, **6**, 284.

12. Hamutcu, R., Jaffe, A., Adler, B. and Bush, A. (1998) Abnormal ventilation scans in cystic fibrosis: what is the outcome? *Pediatr. Pulmonol. Suppl.,* **17**, 336.

13. Kraemer, R. (1989) Early detection of lung function abnormalities in infants with cystic fibrosis. *J. Roy. Soc. Med.*, **82** (Suppl. 16), 21–25.

14. Tepper, R.S., Hiatt, P., Eigen, H., Scott, P., Grosfeld, J., and Cohen, M. (1988) Infants with cystic fibrosis: pulmonary function at diagnosis. *Pediatr. Pulmonol.*, **5**, 15–18.

15. Prendiville, A., Green, S. and Silverman, M. (1987) Paradoxical response to nebulised salbutamol in wheezy infants, assessed by partial expiratory flow-volume curves. *Thorax*, **42**, 86–91.

16. Feher, A., Castile, R., Kisling, J. *et al*. (1996) Flow limitation in normal infants: a new method for forced expiratory manoeuvers from raised lung volumes. *J. Appl. Physiol.*, **80**, 2019–2025.

17. Beardsmore, C.S., Bar-Yishay, E., Maayan, C., Yahav, Y., Katznelson, D. and Godfrey, S. (1988) Lung function in infants with cystic fibrosis. *Thorax*, **43**, 545–551.

18. Beardsmore, C.S., Thompson, J.R., Williams, A. *et al*. (1994) Pulmonary function in infants with cystic fibrosis: the effect of antibiotic treatment. *Arch. Dis. Child.*, **71**, 133–137.

19. Beardsmore, C.S. (1995) Lung function from infancy to school age in cystic fibrosis. *Arch. Dis. Child.*, **73**, 519–523.

20. Tepper, R.S., Montgomery, G.L., Ackerman, V. and Eigen, H. (1993) Longitudinal evaluation of pulmonary function in infants and very young children with cystic fibrosis. *Pediatr. Pulmonol.*, **16**, 96–100.

21. Lutchen, K.R., Habib, R.H., Dorkin, H.L. and Wall, M.A. (1990) Respiratory impedance and multibreath N2 washout in healthy, asthmatic and cystic fibrosis subjects. *J. Appl. Physiol.*, **68**, 2139–2149.

22. van Haren, E.H.J., Lammers, J.-W.J., Festen, J., and van Herwaarden, C.L.A. (1991) Bronchodilator response in adult patients with cystic fibrosis: effects on large and small airways. *Eur. Respir. J.*, **4**, 301–307.

23. Zach, M.S., Oberwaldner, B., Forche, G. and Polgar, G. (1985) Bronchodilators increase airway instability in cystic fibrosis. *Am. Rev. Respir. Dis.*, **131**, 537–543.

24. Landau, L.I., Taussig, L.M., Macklem, P.T., and Beaudry, P.H. (1975) Contribution of inhomogeneity of lung units to the maximal expiratory flow–volume curve in children with asthma and cystic fibrosis. *Am. Rev. Respir. Dis.*, **111**, 725–731.

25. Brooks, L.J. (1990) Tracheal size and distensibility in patients with cystic fibrosis. *Am. Rev. Respir. Dis.*, **141**, 513–516.

26. Horsfield, K. (1974) The relation between structure and function in the airways of the lung. *Br. J. Dis. Chest.*, **68**, 145–160.

27. Dekker, F.W., Schrier, A.C., Sterk, P.J., and Dijkman, J.H. (1992) Validity of peak expiratory flow measurement in assessing reversibility of airflow obstruction. *Thorax*, **47**, 162–166.

28. Strachan, D.P. (1989) Repeatability of ventilatory function measurements in a population survey of 7 year old children. *Thorax*, **44**, 474–479.

29. Stourk, R.L. and Nugent, K.M. (1983) Bronchodilator testing: confidence intervals derived from placebo inhalations. *Am. Rev. Respir. Dis.*, **128**, 153–157.

30. Nickerson, B.G., Lemen, R.J., Gerdes, C.B., Wegmann, M.J., and Robertson, G. (1980) Within-subject variability and per cent change for significance of spirometry in normal subjects and in patients with cystic fibrosis. *Am. Rev. Respir. Dis.*, **122**, 855–859.

31. Cooper, P.J., Robertson, C.F., Hudson, I.L. and Phelan, P.D. (1990) Variability of pulmonary function tests in cystic fibrosis. *Pediatr. Pulmonol.*, **8**, 16–22.

32. Upton, C.S., Tyrell, J.C. and Hiller, E.J. (1988) Two minute walking distance in cystic fibrosis. *Arch. Dis. Child.*, **63**, 1444–1448.

32a. Balfour-Lynn, I.M., Prasad, S.A., Laverty, A., Whitehead, B.F. and Dinwiddie, R. (1998) A step in the right direction assessing exercise tolerance in cystic fibrosis. *Pediatr. Pulmonol.*, **25**, 278–284.

33. Sharma, R.K. and Jeffery, P.K. (1990) Airway beta-receptor number in cystic fibrosis and asthma. *Clin. Sci.*, **78**, 409–417.

34. Rusakow, L.S., Blager, F.B., Barkin, R.C. and White, C.W. (1991) Acute respiratory distress due to vocal cord dysfunction in cystic fibrosis. *J. Asthma*, **28**, 443–446.

35. Samuels, M.H., Thompson, N., Leichty, D. and Ridgway, E.C. (1995) Amyloid goiter in cystic fibrosis. *Thyroid*, **5**, 213–215.

36. Van Haren, E.H., Lammers, J.W., Festen, J., van Herwaarden, C.L. (1992) Bronchial vagal tone and responsiveness to histamine, exercise and bronchodilators in adult patients with cystic fibrosis. *Eur. Respir. J.*, **5**, 1083–1088.

37. van Asperen, P.P., Manglick, P. and Allen, M. (1988) Mechanisms of bronchial hyperreactivity in cystic fibrosis. *Pediatr. Pulmonol.*, **5**, 139–144.

38. Ackerman, V., Montgomery, G., Eigen, H. and Tepper, R.S. (1991) Assessment of airway responsiveness in infants with cystic fibrosis. *Am. Rev. Respir. Dis.*, **144**, 344–346.

39. Wilts, M., Hop, W.C.J., nan der Heyden, G.H.C., Kerrebijn, K.F. and de Jongste, J.C. (1992) Measurement of bronchial responsiveness in young children: comparison of transcutaneous oxygen tension and functional residual capacity during bronchoconstriction and -dilatation. *Pediatr. Pulmonol.*, **12**, 181–185.

40. Zinman, R., Wohl, M.E.B. and Ingram, R.H. (1991) Nonhomogeneous lung emptying in cystic fibrosis patients. *Am. Rev. Respir. Dis.*, **143**, 1257–1261.

41. Eggleston, P.A., Rosenstein, B.J., Stackbone, C.M. and Alexander, M.F. (1988) Airway hyperreactivity in cystic fibrosis: clinical correlates and possible effects of the disease. *Chest*, **94**, 360–365.

42. Eggleston, P.A., Rosenstein, B.J., Stackhouse, C.M., Mellits, E.D. and Baumgardner, R.A. (1991) A controlled trial of long-term bronchodilator therapy in cystic fibrosis. *Chest*, **99**, 1088–1092.

43. Macfarlane, P.I. and Heaf, D. (1990) Changes in airflow obstruction and oxygen saturation in response to exercise and bronchodilators in cystic fibrosis. *Pediatr. Pulmonol.*, **8**, 4–11.

44. Loughlin, G.M., Cota, K.A. and Taussig, L.M. (1981) The relationship between flow transients and bronchial lability in cystic fibrosis. *Chest*, **79**, 206–210.

45. Darga, L.L., Eason, L.A., Zach, M.S. and Polgar, G. (1986) Cold air provocation of airway hyperreactivity in patients with cystic fibrosis. *Pediatr. Pulmonol.*, **2**, 82–88.

46. Chua, H.L., Collis, G.G. and Le Soeuf, P.N. (1990) Bronchial response to nebulized antibiotics in children with cystic fibrosis. *Eur. Respir. J.*, **3**, 1114–1116.

47. Eng, P.A., Morton, J., Douglass, J.A. *et al.* (1996) Short-term efficacy of ultrasonically nebulized hypertonic saline in cystic fibrosis. *Pediatr. Pulmonol.*, **21**, 77–83.

48. Godfrey, S., Beardsmore, C.S., Maayan, C.H. and Bar-Yishay, E. (1986) Can thoracic gas volume be measured in infants with airways obstruction? *Am. Rev. Respir. Dis.*, **133**, 245–251.

49. Tepper, R.S., Hiatt, P.W., Eigen, H. and Smith, J. (1987) Total respiratory system compliance in asymptomatic infants with cystic fibrosis. *Am. Rev. Respir. Dis.*, **135**, 1075–1079.

50. Desmond, K.J., Coates, A.L., Martin, J.G. and Beaudry, P.H. (1986) Trapped gas and airflow limitation in children with cystic fibrosis and asthma. *Pediatr. Pulmonol.*, **2**, 128–134.

51. Ries, A.L., Sosa, G., Prewitt, L., Friedman, P.J. and Harwood, I.R. (1988) Restricted pulmonary function in cystic fibrosis. *Chest*, **94**, 575–579.

52. Marchant, J.L., Hansell, D. and Bush, A.(1994) Assessment of hyperinflation in cystic fibrosis. *Thorax*, **49**, 1164–1166.

53. Van der Schans, C.P., van der Mark, T.W., de Vries, G. *et al.* (1991) Effect of positive expiratory pressure breathing in patients with cystic fibrosis. *Thorax*, **46**, 252–256.

54. Mansell, A., Dubrovsky, C., Levison, H., Bryan, A.C. and Crozier, D.N. (1974) Lung elastic recoil in cystic fibrosis. *Am. Rev. Respir. Dis.*, **109**, 190–197.

55. Verstegh, F.G.A., Bogaard, J.M., Raatgever, J.W., Stam, H., Neijens, H.J. and Kerrebijn, K.F. (1990) Relationship between airway obstruction, desaturation during exercise and nocturnal hypoxaemia in cystic fibrosis patients. *Eur. Respir. J.*, **3**, 68–73.

174 Cardiopulmonary physiology

56. Hirsch, J.A., Zhang, S.-P., Rudnick, M.P., Cerny, F.J. and Cropp, G.J. (1989) Resting oxygen consumption and ventilation in cystic fibrosis. *Pediatr. Pulmonol.*, **6**, 19–26.

57. Couriel, J.M., Schier, M., App, B., Hutchison, A.A., Phelan, P.D. and Landau, L.I. (1985) Distribution of ventilation in young children with cystic fibrosis. *Pediatr. Pulmonol.*, **1**, 314–318.

58. Keens, T.G., Mansell, A., Krastins, I.R.B. *et al.* (1979) Evaluation of the single breath diffusing capacity in asthma and cystic fibrosis. *Chest*, **76**, 41–44.

59. Cotton, D.J., Graham, B.L., Mink, J.T. and Habbick, B.J. (1985) Reduction in single breath CO diffusing capacity in cystic fibrosis. *Chest*, **87**, 217–222.

60. Kraemer, R. and Sohoni, M.H. (1990) Ventilatory inequalities, pulmonary function and blood oxygenation in advanced states of cystic fibrosis. *Respiration*, **57**, 318–324.

61. Dantzker, D.R., Patten, G.A. and Bower, J.J. (1982) Gas exchange at rest and during exercise in adults with cystic fibrosis. *Am. Rev. Respir. Dis.*, **125**, 400–405.

62. Coates, A.L., Boyce, P., Shaw, D.G., Godfrey, S. and Mearns, M. (1981) The relationship between the chest radiograph, regional lung function studies using $^{13}N_2$, exercise tolerance and clinical condition in children with cystic fibrosis. *Arch. Dis. Child.*, **56**, 106–111.

63. Tepper, R.S., Pagtakhan, R.D. and Taussig, L.M. (1984) Noninvasive determination of total respiratory system compliance in infants by the weighted spirometer method. *Am. Rev. Respir. Dis.*, **130**, 461–466.

64. Zapletal, A., Desmond, K.J., Demizio, D. and Coates, A.L. (1993) Lung recoil and the determination of airflow limitation in cystic fibrosis and asthma. *Pediatr. Pulmonol.*, **15**, 13–18.

65. Mansell, A., Dubrawsky, C., Levison, H. and Crozier, D.N. (1974) Lung elastic recoil in cystic fibrosis. *Am. Rev. Respir. Dis.*, **109**, 190–197.

66. Coates, A.L., Desmond, K.J., Milic-Emili, J. and Beaudry, P.H. (1981) Ventilation, respiratory center output, and contribution of the rib cage and abdominal components to ventilation during CO_2 rebreathing in children with cystic fibrosis. *Am. Rev. Respir. Dis.*, **124**, 526–530.

67. Cerny, F., Armitage, L., Hirsch, J.A. and Bishop, B. (1992) Respiratory and abdominal muscle responses to expiratory threshold loading in cystic fibrosis. *J. Appl. Physiol.*, **72**, 842–850.

68. Mier, A., Redington, A., Brophy, C., Hodson, M. and Green, M. (1990) Respiratory muscle function in cystic fibrosis. *Thorax*, **45**, 750–752.

69. Szeinberg, A., England, S., Mindorff, C., Frazer, I., and Levison, H. (1985) Maximal inspiratory and expiratory pressures are reduced in hyperinflated malnourished young adult male patients with cystic fibrosis. *Am. Rev. Respir. Dis.*, **132**, 766–769.

70. Asher, M.I., Parfy, R.L., Oates, A.L., Thomas, E. and Macklem, P.T. (1982) The effects of inspiratory muscle training in patients with cystic fibrosis. *Am. Rev. Respir. Dis.*, **126**, 855–859.

71. Supinski, G.S. and Kelsen, S.G. (1982) Effect of elastase-induced emphysema on the force generating ability of the diaphragm. *J. Clin. Invest.*, **70**, 978–988.

72. Lands, L.C., Heigenhauser, G.J. and Jones, N.L. (1993) Respiratory and peripheral muscle function in cystic fibrosis. *Am. Rev. Respir. Dis.*, **147**, 865–869.

73. Katsardis, C.V., Desmond, K.J. and Coates, A.L. (1986) Measuring the oxygen cost of breathing in normal adults and patients with cystic fibrosis. *Respir. Physiol.*, **65**, 257–266.

74. Keens, T.G., Krastins, I.R.B., Wannamaker, E.M., Levison, H., Crozier, D.N. and Bryan, A.C. (1977) Ventilatory muscle endurance training in normal subjects and patients with cystic fibrosis. *Am. Rev. Respir. Dis.*, **116**, 853–860.

75. Siassi, B., Moss, A.J. and Dooley, R.R. (1971) Clinical recognition of cor pulmonale in cystic fibrosis. *J. Pediatr.*, **78**, 794–805.

76. Reid, L. (1979) The pulmonary circulation: remodelling in growth and disease – the 1978 J Burns Ambertson lecture. *Am. Rev. Respir. Dis.*, **119**, 531–545.

77. Burghuber, O.C., Hartter, E., Weisseel, M., Woloszczuk, W. and Gotz, M. (1991) Raised circulating plasma levels of atrial natriuretic peptide in adolescent and adult patients with cystic fibrosis and pulmonary artery hypertension. *Lung*, **169**, 291–300.

78. Geggel, R.L., Dozor, A.J., Fyler, D.C. and Reid, L.M. (1985) Effect of vasodilators at rest and during exercise in young adults with cystic fibrosis and cor pulmonale. *Am. Rev. Respir. Dis.*, **131**, 531–536.

79. Moskowitz, W.B., Gewitz, M.H., Heyman, S., Ruddy, R.M. and Scanlin, T.F. (1985) Cardiac involvement in cystic fibrosis: early noninvasive detection and vasodilator therapy. *Pediatr. Pharmacol.*, **5**, 139–148.

80. Aronson, D.C., Heymens, A.S., La Riviere, A.V. and Naeff, M.S. (1990) Nontransmural myocardial infarction as a complication of untreated cystic fibrosis. *J. Pediatr. Gastroenterol. Nutr.*, **10**, 126–130.

81. Hortop, J., Desmond, K.J. and Coates, A.L. (1988) The mechanical effects of expiratory airflow limitation on cardiac performance in cystic fibrosis. *Am. Rev. Respir. Dis.*, **137**, 132–137.

82. Robotham, J.L., Lixfield, W., Molland, L. *et al.* (1978) Effects of respiration on cardiac performance. *J. Appl. Physiol.*, **44**, 703–709.

83. Matthay, R.A., Berger, H.J., Loke, J. *et al.* (1980) Right and left ventricular performance in ambulatory young adults with cystic fibrosis. *Br. Heart J.*, **43**, 474–480.

84. Coates, A.L., Desmond, K., Asher, M.I., and Beaudry, P.H. (1982) The effect of digoxin on exercise capacity and exercising cardiac function in cystic fibrosis. *Chest*, **82**, 543–547.

85. Chipps, B.E., Alderson, P.O., Roland, J.-M.A. *et al.* (1979) Noninvasive evaluation of ventricular function in cystic fibrosis. *J. Pediatr.*, **95**, 379–384.

86. Perrault, H., Coughlan, M., Marcotte, J.-E., Drblik, S.P. and Lamarre, A. (1992) Comparison of cardiac output determinants in response to upright and supine exercise in patients with cystic fibrosis. *Chest*, **101**, 42–51.

87. De Wolf, D., Franken, P., Piepsz, A. and Dab, I. (1998) Left ventricular perfusion defect in patients with cystic fibrosis. *Pediatr. Pulmonol.*, **25**, 93–98.

88. Stokes, D.C., McBride, J.J., Wall, M.A., Erba, G. and Strieder, D.J. (1980) Sleep hypoxemia in young adults with cystic fibrosis. *Am. J. Dis. Child.*, **134**, 734–740.

89. Braggion, C., Pradal, U. and Mastella, G. (1992) Hemoglobin desaturation during sleep and daytime in patients with cystic fibrosis and severe airway obstruction. *Acta Pediatrica*, **81**, 1002–1006.

90. Stokes, D.C., Wohl, M.E.B., Khaw, K.T., and Strieder, D.J. (1985) Postural hypoxaemia in cystic fibrosis. *Chest*, **87**, 785–789.

91. Ballard, R.D., Sutarik, J.M., Clover, C.W. and Suh, B.Y. (1996) Effects of non-REM sleep on ventilation and respiratory mechanics in adults with cystic fibrosis. *Am. J. Respir. Crit. Care Med.*, **153**, 266–271.

92. Tepper, R.S., Skatrud, J.B. and Dempsey, J.A. (1983) Ventilation and oxygenation changes during sleep in cystic fibrosis. *Chest*, **84**, 388–393.

93. Coffey, M.J., Fitzgerald, M.X. and McNicholas, W.T. (1991) Comparison of oxygen desaturation during sleep and exercise in patients with cystic fibrosis. *Chest*, **100**, 659–662.

94. Avital, A., Sanchez, I., Holbrow, J., Kryger, M.. and Chernick, V. (1991) Effect of theophylline on lung function tests, sleep quality, and nighttime SaO_2 in children with cystic fibrosis. *Am. Rev. Respir. Dis.*, **144**, 1245–1249.

95. Regnis, J.A., Piper, A.J., Henke, K.G. *et al.* (1994) Benefits of nocturnal nasal CPAP in patients with cystic fibrosis. *Chest*, **106**, 1717–1724.

96. Padman, R., Lawless, S. and von Nessen, S. (1994) Use of BiPAP by nasal mask in the treatment of respiratory insufficiency in pediatric patients: preliminary investigations. *Pediatr. Pulmonol.*, **17**, 119–123.

97. Gozal, D. (1997) Nocturnal ventilatory support in patients with cystic fibrosis: comparison with supplemental oxygen. *Eur. Respir. J.*, **10**, 1999–2003.

98. Hill, A.T., Edenborough, F.P., Cayton, R.M., and Stableforth, D.E. (1998) Long-term nasal intermittent positive pressure ventilation in patients with cystic fibrosis and hypercapnic respiratory failure. *Respir. Med.*, **92**, 523–526.

99. Cropp, G.J., Pullano, T.P., Cerny, F.J. and Nathanson, I.T. (1982) Exercise tolerance and cardiorespiratory adjustments at peak work capacity in cystic fibrosis. *Am. Rev. Respir. Dis.*, **126**, 211–216.

100. Kaplan, T.A., ZeBranek, J.D. and McKey, R.M. (1991) Use of exercise in the management of cystic fibrosis: short communication about a survey of cystic fibrosis referral centers. *Pediatr. Pulmonol.*, **10**, 205–207.

101. O'Rawe, A., McIntosh, I., Dodge, J.A. *et al.* (1992)

Increased energy expenditure in cystic fibrosis is associated with specific mutations. *Clin. Sci.*, **82**, 71–76.

102. Regnis, J.A., Alison, J.A., Henke, K.G., Donnelly, P.M. and Bye, P.T.P. (1991) Changes in end-expiratory lung volume during exercise in cystic fibrosis relate to severity of lung disease. *Am. Rev. Respir. Dis.*, **144**, 507–512.

103. Kraemer, R., Rudeberg, A., Klay, M. and Rossi, E. (1979) Relationship between clinical conditions, radiographic findings and pulmonary functions in patients with cystic fibrosis. *Helv. Pediatr. Acta*, **34**, 417–428.

104. Casaburi, R., Patessio, A., Ioli, F. *et al.* (1991) Reductions in exercise lactic acidosis and ventilation as a result of exercise training in patients with obstructive lung disease. *Am. Rev. Respir. Dis.*, **143**, 9–18.

105. Nikolaizik, W.H., Knopfil, B., Leister, E. *et al.* (1998) The anaerobic threshold in cystic fibrosis: comparison of V-slope method, lactate turn points, and Conconi test. *Pediatr. Pulmonol.*, **25**, 147–153.

106. Cerny, F.J., Pullano, T.P. and Cropp, G.J.A. (1992) Cardiorespiratory adaptations to exercise in cystic fibrosis. *Am. Rev. Respir. Dis.*, **126**, 217–220.

107. Rosenthal, M., and Bush, A. (1997) The simultaneous comparison of acetylene or carbon dioxide flux as ameasure of effective pulmonary blood flow in children. *Eur. Respir. J.*, **10**, 2586–2590.

108. Pianosi, P. and Pelech, A. (1996) Stroke volume during exercise in cystic fibrosis. *Am. J. Respir. Crit. Care Med.*, **153**, 1105–1109.

109. Freeman, W., Stableforth, D.E., Cayton, R.M. and Morgan, M.D. (1993) Endurance exercise capacity in adults with cystic fibrosis. *Respir. Med.*, **87**, 541–549.

110. Orenstein, D.M. and Nixon, PA. (1991) Exercise performance and breathing patterns in cystic fibrosis: male–female differences and influences of resting pulmonary function. *Pediatr. Pulmonol.*, **10**, 101–105.

111. Kusenbach, G., Friedrichs, F., Skopnik, H. and Heimann, G. (1993) Increased physiological dead space during exercise after bronchodilation in cystic fibrosis. *Pediatr. Pulmonol.*, **15**, 273–278.

112. Martin, D., Day, J., Ward, G., Carter, E. and Chesrown, S. (1994) Effects of breathing a normoxic helium mixture on exercise tolerance of patients with cystic fibrosis. *Pediatr. Pulmonol.*, **18**, 206–210.

113. Henke, K.G., Regnis, J.A. and Bye, P.T. (1993) Benefits of continuous positive pressure during exercise in cystic fibrosis and relationship to disease severity. *Am. Rev. Respir. Dis.*, **148**, 1272–1276.

114. Marcus, C.L., Bader, D., Stabile, M.W. *et al.* (1992) Supplemental oxygen and exercise performance in patients with cystic fibrosis with severe pulmonary disease. *Chest*, **101**, 52–57.

115. Heath, D. (1989) Missing link from Tibet. *Thorax*, **44**, 981–983.

116. Sui, G.J., Liu, Y.H., Cheng, X.S. *et al.* (1988) Subacute infantile mountain sickness. *J. Pathol.*, **155**, 161–170.

117. Rebuck, A.S. and Campbell, E.J.M. (1974) A clinical

method for assessing the ventilatory response to hypoxia. *Am. Rev. Respir. Dis.*, **109**, 345–350.

118. Waldman, J.D., Lamberti, J.J., Mathewson, J.W. *et al.* (1983) Congenital heart disease and pulmonary artery hypertension. 1. Pulmonary vasoreactivity to 15% oxygen before and after surgery. *J. Am. Coll. Cardiol.*, **2**, 1158–1164.

119. Libby, D.M., Briscoe, W.A. and King, T.K. (1981) Relief of hypoxia associated bronchoconstriction by breathing 30% oxygen. *Am. Rev. Respir. Dis.*, **123**, 171–175.

120. Speechly-Dick, M.E., Rimmer, S.J. and Hodson, M.E. (1992) Exacerbations of cystic fibrosis after holidays at high altitude – a cautionary tale. *Respir. Med.*, **86**, 55–56.

121. Oades, P.J., Buchdahl, R.M. and Bush, A. (1994) Prediction of hypoxaemia at high altitude in children with cystic fibrosis. *BMJ*, **308**, 15–18.

121a. Buchdahl, R.M., Frances, J., Bennett, S., Sheehan, D. and Bush, A. (1998) An audit of the fitness to fly test in children with CF. *Pediatr. Pulmonol.*, **117**, 334.

122. Zinman, R., Corey, M., Coates, A.L. *et al.* (1989) Nocturnal home oxygen in the treatment of hypoxemic cystic fibrosis patients. *J. Pediatr.*, **114**, 368–377.

123. Stecenko, A.A., Postotnik, L. and Thomas, R.G. (1989) Predicting arterial oxygen tension from maximum expiratory flow volume curves in cystic fibrosis. *Pediatr. Pulmonol.*, **6**, 27–30.

124. Zemel, B.S., Kawchak, D.A., Cnaan, A. *et al.* (1996) Prospective evaluation of resting energy expenditure, nutritional status, pulmonary function, and genotype in children with cystic fibrosis. *Pediatr. Res.*, **40**, 578–586.

125. Gaslin, K., Gurasitz, D., Durie, P., Corey, M. and Levison, H. (1982) Improved respiratory prognosis in patients with cystic fibrosis and normal fat absorption. *J. Pediatr.*, **100**, 857–862.

126. Bertrand, J.M., Morin, C.L., Lasalle, R., Patrick, J. and Coates, A.L. (1984) Short-term clinical, nutritional, and functional effects of continuous elemental enteral alimentation in children with cystic fibrosis. *J. Pediatr.*, **104**, 41–46.

127. Hanning, R.M., Blimkie, C.J., Bar-Or, O. *et al.* (1993) Relationships among nutritional status and skeletal and respiratory muscle function in cystic fibrosis: does early dietary supplementation make a difference? *Am. J. Clin. Nutr.*, **57**, 580–587.

128. Mansell, A.L., Anderson, J.C., Muttart, C.R. *et al.* (1984) Short-term pulmonary effects of total parenteral nutrition in children with cystic fibrosis. *J. Pediatr.*, **104**, 700–705.

129. Denison, D.M., Cramer, D.S. and Hanson, P.J.V. (1989) Lung function testing and AIDS. *Respir. Med.*, **83**, 133–138.

130. Fuso, L., Accardo, D., Bevignani, G. *et al.* (1995) Effects of a filter at the mouth on pulmonary function tests. *Eur. Respir. J.*, **8**, 314–317.

131. Allen, M.B., Mellon, A.F., Simmonds, E.J., Page, R.L. and Littlewood, J.M. (1993) Changes in nocturnal oximetry after treatments of exacerbations of cystic fibrosis. *Arch. Dis. Child.*, **69**, 197–201.

132. Denison, D.M., du Bois, R. and Sawicka, E. (1983) Pictures in the mind. *Br. J. Dis. Chest*, **77**, 35–50.

9

Diagnostic methods

9a Diagnosis *B. J. Rosenstein*   178
Introduction   178
Criteria for the diagnosis of cystic fibrosis   178

9b Screening *D. J. H. Brock*   189
Neonatal screening   189
Heterozygote screening   193

References   197

9a

Diagnosis

B. J. ROSENSTEIN

INTRODUCTION

It is essential to confirm or exclude the diagnosis of cystic fibrosis (CF) in a timely fashion and with a high degree of accuracy to avoid inappropriate testing; provide appropriate therapies in a timely fashion, prognostic and genetic counseling; and ensure access to specialized medical services. In the majority of cases, the diagnosis is entertained because of the presence of one or more typical clinical features (Table 9.1) and then confirmed by demonstrating an elevated (>60 mmol/L) sweat chloride concentration[1]. Almost all patients have chronic sinopulmonary disease and, in postpubertal males, obstructive azoospermia. Approximately 85–90 per cent of patients have exocrine pancreatic insufficiency, whereas the remainder are pancreatic sufficient[1].

In recent years the ability to detect CF mutations[2] and to measure transepithelial bioelectric properties[3–8] has greatly expanded the CF clinical spectrum. In approximately 2 per cent of patients, there is an 'atypical' phenotype which consists of chronic sinopulmonary disease, pancreatic sufficiency, and either borderline (40–60 mmol/L) or normal (<40 mmol/L) sweat chloride concentrations[9–13]. In addition, there are patients in whom a single clinical feature (e.g. electrolyte abnormalities[14], pancreatitis[15,16], liver disease[17], sinusitis[18] or obstructive azoospermia) predominates[19–23]. In such cases, demonstration of abnormal ion transport across the nasal epithelium and mutation analysis can be used as diagnostic aids.

A CF diagnosis can also be considered in the absence of clinical features. An individual with an affected sibling has a 1 in 4 chance of having the disease. Half-siblings are also at increased risk compared to the general population (Caucasians 1 in 112, African-Americans 1 in 244, and Asian-Americans 1 in 352). These high risks justify careful clinical monitoring and, in appropriate situations, testing of full and half-siblings.

CRITERIA FOR THE DIAGNOSIS OF CYSTIC FIBROSIS

Cystic fibrosis remains a clinical diagnosis based on the presence of one or more characteristic phenotypic (clinical) features (Table 9.1), a history of CF in a sibling, or a positive newborn screening test, *plus* laboratory evidence of a CFTR abnormality as documented by elevated sweat chloride concentrations, identification of two CF mutations, or the *in vivo* demonstration of characteristic abnormalities in ion transport across the nasal epithelium.

Prenatal diagnosis

HIGH-RISK PREGNANCIES

The prenatal diagnosis of CF is usually established in pregnancies known to be at increased risk based on the CF carrier status of the parents[24]. In cases in which the genotype status of the parents is known, either through routine antenatal screening or carrier screening prompted by a positive family history, the diagnosis of CF can be confirmed or excluded with a high degree of accuracy by direct mutation analysis performed on fetal cells obtained by chorionic villus sampling (10 weeks) or cultured amniotic fluid cells (15–18 weeks)[24].

Prenatal testing should always be carried out in conjunction with an experienced geneticist or genetic counselor. It is mandatory to carry out postnasal sweat testing in all cases in which the diagnosis of CF has been made or excluded on the basis of prenatal DNA analysis.

In pregnancies at increased risk, but in which the genotype status of one of both parents is unknown, analysis of amniotic fluid (16–18 weeks' gestation) for concentrations of microvillar intestinal enzymes can be useful[25,26]. If the fetus is affected by CF, there is a reduced concentration of leucine aminopeptidase, alkaline phosphatase, γ-glutamyl transpeptidase and disaccharidases

Table 9.1 *Phenotypic features consistent with a diagnosis of cystic fibrosis*

1. Chronic sinopulmonary disease manifested by:
   (a) persistent colonization/infection with typical CF pathogens including *Staphylococcus aureus*, non-typeable *Haemophilus influenzae*, mucoid and non-mucoid *Pseudomonas aeruginosa*, and *Burkholderia cepacia*
   (b) chronic cough and sputum production
   (c) persistent chest radiograph abnormalities (e.g. bronchiectasis, atelectasis, infiltrates, hyperinflation)
   (d) airway obstruction manifested by wheezing and air trapping
   (e) nasal polyps; radiograph or CT abnormalities of the paranasal sinuses
   (f) digital clubbing
2. Gastrointestinal and nutritional abnormalities, including:
   (a) **intestinal**: meconium ileus; distal intestinal obstruction syndrome (DIOS); rectal prolapse
   (b) **pancreatic**: pancreatic insufficiency; recurrent pancreatitis
   (c) **hepatic**: chronic hepatic disease manifested by clinical or histologic evidence of focal biliary cirrhosis or multilobular cirrhosis
   (d) **nutritional**: failure to thrive (protein—calorie malnutrition); hypoproteinemia and edema; complications secondary to fat-soluble vitamin deficiency
3. Salt loss syndromes: acute salt depletion; chronic metabolic alkalosis
4. Male urogenital abnormalities resulting in obstructive azoospermia

in the amniotic fluid, presumably related to *in utero* intestinal blockage caused by viscus meconium[25,26]. The accuracy of these assays is in the range of 95–98 per cent (false-positive rate 1–4 per cent; false-negative rate 6–8 per cent) when performed on a pregnancy with a 1 in 4 risk of CF. Analysis of microvillar enzymes is not recommended for the detection of CF in routine pregnancies.

Although CF prenatal screening programs have been implemented successfully[27], the role of CF carrier screening in the general population is controversial[28], and widespread implementation has not been recommended[29].

PREIMPLANTATION DIAGNOSIS

An alternative for at-risk couples is the use of preimplantation genetic diagnosis to screen embryos before implantation[30]. After *in vitro* fertilization, a cleavage-stage biopsy is carried out on day 2 or 3, and one or two cells removed for genetic analysis by nested polymerase chain reaction and heteroduplex formation. Normal or carrier embryos are then transferred to establish pregnancy. This procedure can be followed by chorionic villus sampling or amniocentesis to confirm the original diagnosis.

FETAL INTESTINAL OBSTRUCTION

In pregnancies not known to be at increased risk for CF, the diagnosis is sometimes suggested by prenatal ultrasonographic findings, including a hyperechoic fetal bowel pattern suggestive of intestinal obstruction[31,32]. Hyperechoic bowel occurring as a benign variant is distinguished by spontaneous resolution, usually before the third trimester. In pregnancies in which there is evidence of fetal intestinal obstruction, carrier testing for CF mutations can be carried out in the parents. If both parents are carriers of a CF mutation, the diagnosis of CF in the fetus is highly likely and can be confirmed by direct mutation analysis of amniotic fluid cells. Parental CF carrier testing and fetal mutation analysis is also useful in cases of meconium peritonitis detected by prenatal ultrasonography[33].

Postnatal diagnosis

Clinical features which are associated with CF and which should lead to further diagnostic testing are summarized in Table 9.2. Cystic fibrosis is marked by great variability in the frequency and severity of clinical manifestations and complications. The diagnosis should never be discounted because a patient with suggestive clinical findings appears 'too healthy'. Although the incidence of CF is distinctly higher in Caucasians, the diagnosis needs to be considered in patients of diverse racial and ethnic backgrounds[34]. In the majority of cases in the United States, the diagnosis is established by age 1 year[35], but in approximately 10 per cent of patients, the diagnosis is delayed until after the age 10 years, including an increasing number of adults. The subset of patients with pancreatic sufficiency is characterized by a milder clinical course, better nutritional status, better pulmonary function and, consequently, a distinctly later age at diagnosis[36].

SWEAT TEST

The sweat test remains the 'gold standard' for the confirmation or exclusion of the diagnosis of CF[1,37,38]. During the first 24 hours after birth, sweat electrolyte values may be transiently elevated in normal infants[39]. After the first 2 days of life, there is a rapid decline in sweat electrolyte concentrations and an elevated value can be used to confirm the diagnosis of CF. It may be difficult to obtain an

Table 9.2 *Indications for sweat testing*

Pulmonary and upper respiratory tract	Gastrointestinal	Metabolic and miscellaneous
Chronic cough	Meconium ileus	Acrodermatitis enteropathica
Recurrent or chronic pneumonia	Meconium plug syndrome	Family history of CF
Wheezing[a]	Prolonged neonatal jaundice	Failure to thrive
Hyperinflation[a]	Steatorrhea	Salty taste to skin
Tachypnea[a]	Rectal prolapse	Salt crystals on skin
Retractions[a]	Mucoid-impacted appendix	Salt-depletion syndrome
Atelectasis (especially of the right upper lobe)	Late intestinal obstruction	Metabolic alkalosis
Bronchiectasis	Intussusception, recurrent or at an atypical age	Vitamin K deficiency (hypoprothrombinemia and bleeding)
Hemoptysis	Cirrhosis and portal hypertension	Vitamin A deficiency (bulging fontanel, night blindness)
Pseudomonas colonization, especially with a mucoid strain	Recurrent pancreatitis	Vitamin E deficiency (hemolytic anemia)
Nasal polyps		Obstructive azoospermia
Pansinusitis		Absent vas deferens
Digital clubbing		Scrotal calcification
		Hypoproteinemia and edema

[a]If persistent or refractory to usual therapy.

adequate sweat sample during the first 2–3 weeks after birth, especially among preterm infants. Ideally, sweat testing should be carried out at a time when the patient is clinically stable, well hydrated, free of acute illness and not receiving mineralocorticoids.

Methodology

Sweat testing should be carried out in accordance with the guidelines of the National Committee for Clinical Laboratory Standards[40]. It is crucial that testing be carried out by experienced personnel using standardized methodologies in facilities in which adequate numbers of tests are performed to maintain laboratory proficiency and quality control. The only acceptable procedure is the quantitative pilocarpine iontophoresis sweat test[41]. When a physician orders a sweat test, he or she must know the methodology being used[38].

Sample collection

Approved methods of sample collection are the Gibson–Cooke procedure[41] and the Macroduct Sweat Collection System (Wescor, Inc., Logan, Utah, USA; Chemlab Scientific Products, Hornchurch, Essex, UK)[42,43]. In both, localized sweating is stimulated by the iontophoresis of pilocarpine into the skin of the flexor surface of the forearm or thigh. Sweat is then collected on filter paper or gauze (Gibson–Cooke) (Fig. 9.1), or in microbore tubing (Macroduct) (Fig. 9.2), the amount of sweat quantitated, and the sample then analyzed for chloride concentration, sodium concentration or both. The minimum acceptable sweat volume for the Gibson–Cooke procedure is 75 mg and for the Macroduct system 15 μL[40]. When an adequate sweat sample cannot be obtained from one site, collection can be

repeated at another site, but inadequate samples from several sites must never be pooled for analysis.

Sweat should not be stimulated or collected from the head (including forehead), trunk or any area of diffuse inflammation (e.g. eczema), or serous or bloody discharge. Sweat can be collected from a site receiving intravenous fluids as long as good contact between the skin and electrode is possible and the collection technique does not interfere with venous flow. Sweat testing can be carried out while a patient is receiving oxygen by a closed delivery system (i.e. nasal cannula) but not if the patient is receiving oxygen by an open system.

When performed properly, pilocarpine iontophoresis sweat testing has an excellent safety profile, but localized complications can occur[44]. There can be temporary reddening of the skin, reflecting sensitivity to the pilocarpine solution, or blistering, with or without scarring, probably due to acid generated electrolytically during iontophoresis. Frank electrical burns may be produced by high current density over a small skin area, usually as a result of metal contact with the skin. Wescor estimates one burn for every 15 000–20 000 iontophoresis procedures with their equipment[45]. Operator training, use of power units with automatic cut-off features, a moist interface between electrode and skin, and adherence to standardized operating procedures should reduce the risk of injury.

Sample analysis

Electrolytes

While either sodium or chloride can be measured, chloride provides better discrimination between CF patients and unaffected individuals and is usually the analyte of choice[46–48]. Among adults, there may be overlap in sweat sodium concentration between CF patients and unaf-

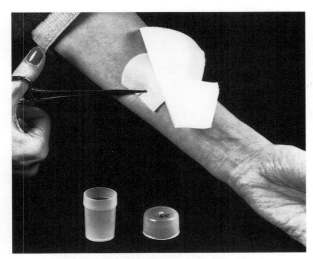

Fig. 9.1 *Quantitative pilocarpine iontophoresis sweat test (Gibson–Cooke). Localized sweating is stimulated by the iontophoresis of pilocarpine; sweat is then collected on filter paper or gauze. (Reproduced from Orenstein, D.M. and Stern, R.C. (1997) Treatment of the Hospitalized Cystic Fibrosis Patient, Marcel Dekker, New York, with permission.)*

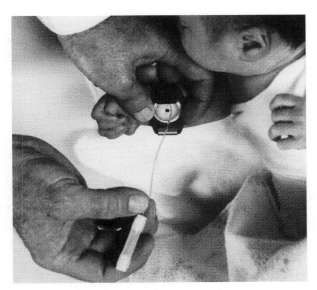

Fig. 9.2 *Macroduct sweat collection system (Wescor Inc., Logan, UT, USA). Localized sweating is stimulated by the iontophoresis of pilocarpine; sweat is then collected in microbore tubing. (Reproduced from Orenstein, D.M. and Stern, R.C. (1997) Treatment of the Hospitalized Cystic Fibrosis Patient, Marcel Dekker, New York, with permission.)*

fected individuals, leading to diagnostic confusion[48,49]. In cases in which there is a borderline sweat sodium concentration, the percentage suppression after administration of a mineralocorticoid has been used to improve diagnostic accuracy; the sweat sodium concentration of CF patients does not decrease, whereas it does in unaffected individuals[49]. However, there is considerable overlap between CF and unaffected individuals, and

interpretation of the results may be difficult. For quality control, it may be helpful to measure the concentration of both sodium and chloride, which should be proportionately increased or decreased[38,40,47,50]. Discordant values can indicate problems with collection or analysis. Sweat chloride or sodium concentrations greater than 160 mmol/L are not physiologically possible[51], and the patient should be retested.

Conductivity

Conductivity represents a nonselective measurement of ions. Sweat conductivity is increased in patients with CF and its measurement has been proposed as a diagnostic test[52]. A conductivity analyzer (Wescor Sweat-Chek) designed specifically for use with the Wescor Macroduct sweat collector has been validated as a screening method. There is excellent correlation between the results of sweat sodium and chloride concentrations and sweat conductivity (Fig. 9.3)[42]. Any conductivity result of 50 mmol/L (equivalent NaCl) or greater is considered positive and should be followed up by a quantitative sweat test.

Osmolality

Osmolality of sweat reflects the total solute concentration in mmol/kg of sweat. It is necessary to use an osmometer capable of measuring undiluted micro-samples of sweat[53]. The reference interval for sweat osmolality in children is approximately 50–150 mmol/kg. Children with CF have sweat osmolality values greater than 200 mmol/kg; values between 150 and 200 mmol/kg are equivocal. Positive and equivocal results should always be followed up by a quantitative sweat test.

Alternative sweat methodology

Alternative sweat-test procedures, such as direct-reading conductivity measurements[54] or a paper patch indicator system[55], are associated with an increased incidence of false-positive and false-negative results, and should never be used as the basis of a definitive CF diagnosis[38,40,56].

Results reporting

The results of quantitative analysis of sweat chloride in patients with CF, unaffected siblings and controls are shown in Fig. 9.4. A chloride concentration greater than 60 mmol/L is consistent with the diagnosis of CF[38,40,57]. However, the results should be interpreted with regard to the patient's age. There are data to suggest that in infants less than 3 months of age, a sweat chloride concentration greater than 40 mmol/L is highly suggestive of a diagnosis of CF[58]. Some unaffected adults can have values above 60 mmol/L, but the sweat test remains the 'gold standard' confirmatory test in adults[59,60]. Borderline sweat chloride concentrations in the range of 40–60 mmol/L occur in approximately 4–5 per cent of all sweat tests. In such cases, repeat testing may yield results that clearly

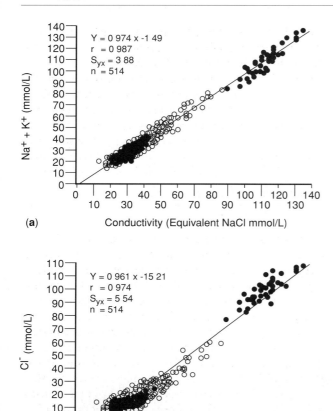

(a)

(b)

Fig. 9.3 *Comparison of conductivity with the sum of sodium and potassium concentrations* (**a**) *and with the chloride concentration* (**b**) *performed on the same sweat samples taken from patients with CF (dark circles) and without CF (clear circles). r, regression coefficient; $S_{y.x}$, standard error of the estimate. (Reproduced, with permission, from ref. 42.)*

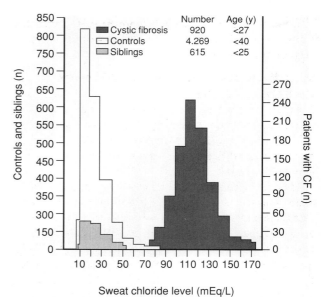

Fig. 9.4 *Chloride concentrations in patients with CF, healthy persons and healthy siblings of patients with CF. (Reproduced, with permission, from ref. 57.)*

fall in the normal or abnormal range. Analysis of the ratio of sodium to chloride also may be helpful. In patients with CF, the chloride concentration is usually higher than the sodium, whereas in normal subjects the reverse usually occurs[47,61]. One exception may be patients who carry less common CF mutations associated with pancreatic sufficiency, in which case the sweat sodium concentration is often higher than the sweat chloride[61].

Diagnostic criteria

Sweat-test results should be interpreted in relation to the patient's clinical picture by a physician knowledgeable about CF. The test results need to be consistent with the clinical picture; no single laboratory result is sufficient to establish or rule out the diagnosis of CF. The diagnosis should be made only if there is an elevated sweat chloride concentration on two separate occasions in a patient with one or more typical phenotypic features, a history of CF in a sibling, or a positive newborn screening test. In 0.1–1.0% of cases, the diagnosis of CF is established

(nasal potential difference measurement, histopathology, mutation analysis) in patients with borderline or normal electrolyte concentrations[9,10,12,13,62]. As more information becomes available concerning the phenotypic expressions of the CF genotype, this number may increase.

Sources of error

The incidence of erroneous sweat-test results is probably in the range of 10–15 per cent[38]. Although most errors represent false-positive results, false-negative results are also a problem[63]. Most errors are caused by the use of unreliable methodology, inadequate sweat collection, technical errors and misinterpretation of results[38,40,64,65].

Technical problems include contamination by salt-containing materials; failure to adequately dry the skin before sweat collection; evaporation of the sweat sample during collection, transfer and transport; failure to include condensate in the sweat sample when using gauze or filter paper; and errors in sample weighing, dilution, elution, electrolyte analysis and result computation.

Duplicate sweat collection and analysis may be useful for quality assurance. There is generally a good correlation between the electrolyte concentrations of sweat collected at different sites[38,40]. Chloride values from two different sites usually agree within 10 mmol/L for values of 60 mmol/L and less, and within 15 mmol/L for values greater than 60 mmol/L.

Errors in interpretation include establishment of a diagnosis of CF on the basis of a single positive test; failure to repeat a borderline test result; and failure to repeat a negative test in a patient with a clinical picture highly suggestive of CF. Transiently negative sweat electrolyte results have been reported in the presence of edema and hypoproteinemia[66]. The test should be repeated after resolution of the edema.

Other diseases associated with elevated sweat electrolyte concentrations

A variety of diseases other than CF may be associated with moderately elevated concentrations of sodium and chloride in sweat (Table 9.3)[38]. However, with few exceptions these conditions do not represent a problem in differential diagnosis.

There is evidence that there may be physiologic variability of sweat electrolyte concentrations over time, and that there may be transient elevation of sweat electrolyte values in unaffected persons[67]. Transient elevations in electrolyte concentrations have also been reported in infants and young children with environmental deprivation (nonorganic failure to thrive)[68] and in adolescents with anorexia nervosa[69]. Repeat testing after medical stabilization is indicated.

When an elevated sweat electrolyte concentration is not consistent with the patient's clinical picture, there is marked variability in electrolyte concentrations on repeat testing, the sweat electrolyte concentration is above a 'physiologically possible' level, or there is a discrepancy among the medical history, examination, laboratory results and response to treatment, it is important to consider the possibility of Münchhausen syndrome by proxy[70].

Indications for repeat sweat testing

1. All positive sweat-test results must be repeated or confirmed by mutation analysis. The diagnosis of CF should never be based on a single positive sweat test.
2. All borderline sweat-test results (chloride concentration 40–60 mmol/L) should be repeated; if results remain in an indeterminate range, additional ancillary tests may be helpful.
3. Sweat testing should be repeated in patients thought to have CF but who do not follow an expected clinical course.

As patients are followed, the clinical, laboratory and chest radiograph findings should be consistent with the diagnosis of CF. It is especially important to re-evaluate those patients in whom the diagnosis was suggested primarily on the basis of failure to thrive or a positive family history; the clinical features prompting the initial sweat test disappear; the patient's course is consistent with asthma without evidence of suppurative lung disease; or there is a normal growth pattern without evidence of digital clubbing, *Pseudomonas* colonization or typical chest radiograph findings.

MUTATION ANALYSIS

In most patients with CF the diagnosis will be confirmed by a positive sweat-test result, but cloning of the gene responsible for CF and identification of disease-producing mutations has raised the possibility that DNA testing may substitute for the sweat test in certain circumstances[2]. The presence of mutations known to cause CF in each *CFTR* gene predicts with a high degree of certainty that an individual has CF. To date, more than 800 putative CF mutations have been described[71]. In Caucasian populations, the ΔF_{508} mutation is found in 68 per cent of CF alleles (Table 9.4). No other mutation accounts for more than 2.4 per cent of CF alleles. Worldwide population variation of common cystic fibrosis mutations is reported periodically by the Cystic Fibrosis Genetic Analysis Consortium[72].

Alterations in the *CFTR* gene designated as CF-causing mutations should fulfill at least one of the following criteria. The mutation has been shown to:

1. cause a change in the amino-acid sequence that severely affects CFTR synthesis and/or function;
2. introduce a premature termination signal (insertion, deletion or nonsense mutations);
3. alter the 'invariant' nucleotides of intron splice sites (the first two or last two nucleotides); or
4. cause a novel amino-acid sequence that does not occur in the normal *CFTR* genes from at least 100 carriers of CF mutations from the patient's ethnic group.

Table 9.3 *Conditions other than cystic fibrosis associated with an elevated sweat electrolyte concentration*

Adrenal insufficiency[a]	Hypogammaglobulinemia
Anorexia nervosa[a]	Hypoparathyroidism, familial[a]
Atopic dermatitis[a]	Hypothyroidism (untreated)[a]
Autonomic dysfunction	Klinefelter syndrome
Celiac disease[a]	Mauriac syndrome
Ectodermal dysplasia	Mucopolysaccharidosis Type I
Environmental deprivation[a]	Malnutrition[a]
Familial cholestasis (Byler's disease)	Nephrogenic diabetes insipidus[a]
Fucosidosis	Nephrosis[a]
Glucose 6-phosphate dehydrogenase deficiency	Prostaglandin E_1 infusion, long-term[a]
Glycogen storage disease Type 1	Protein–calorie malnutrition[a]
	Pseudohypoaldosteronism[a]
	Psychosocial failure to thrive[a]

[a]Sweat test reverts to normal with resolution of underlying condition.

Table 9.4 *Mutations that cause cystic fibrosis*

Mutation	Frequency[a]	Evidence[b]
G85E	0.2	4
R117H[c]	0.3	1
621+1G→T	0.7	1,3
711+1G→T	0.1	1,3
1078delT	0.1	2
R334W	0.1	1
R347P	0.2	1
A455E[c]	0.1	1
ΔI_{507}	0.2	4
ΔF_{508}	66.0	1,4
1717-1G→T	0.6	2
G542X	2.4	3
S549N	0.1	4
G551D	1.6	1,4
R533X	0.7	2
R560T	0.1	4
1898+1G→T	0.1	3
2184delA	0.1	2
2789+5G→A[c]	0.1	1,4
R1162X	0.3	2
3659delC	0.1	3
3849+10kbC→T[c]	0.2	1,4
W1282X	1.2	2
N1303K	1.3	1,4

[a]Caucasian population.

[b](1) Causes a change in the amino-acid sequence that severely affects CFTR synthesis and/or function; (2) introduces a premature termination signal; (3) alters the 'invariant' nucleotides of spliced sites; (4) causes a change in the amino-acid sequence that does not occur in the normal genes from at least 100 carriers of CF mutations from the same ethnic group.

[c]Mutations which may be associated with normal or borderline sweat electrolyte levels.

Mutations that are included in currently available CF mutation panels and that meet one or more of these criteria are shown in Table 9.4. Improvement in DNA technology indicates that CF mutation panels in the future will include a larger number of mutant alleles than shown in Table 9.4. Each additional mutation should meet one or more of the criteria listed above to provide a reasonable degree of certainty that it is disease-producing.

A more complicated situation is presented by the R117H and 5T mutations. Presence of both mutations in the same gene (R117H–5T) is associated with CF[73]. However, neither the R117H mutation alone (i.e. R117H with the common splice variant 7T) nor the 5T mutation alone meets the criteria for a CF mutation. Although these mutations have been associated with male infertility due to CBAVD, diagnosis of CF in patients carrying R117H–7T or 5T will require demonstration of a CFTR abnormality by sweat testing or nasal PD testing.

Confirming the diagnosis of CF based on the presence of two CF-producing mutations is highly specific but not very sensitive. Sensitivity is decreased due to the large number of CF alleles. Current commercially available mutation screening panels detect at most only 80–85 per cent of CF alleles. However, there are CF mutations which occur with increased frequency, or even uniquely, in specific population groups (e.g. Ashkenazi Jewish[2], African-American[74]) and in patients with specific clinical features (e.g. pancreatic sufficiency[75] or normal or borderline sweat electrolyte concentrations[9,10,13]). By customizing mutation panels to match the patient's ethnic background and phenotype, the sensitivity of DNA testing can be enhanced.

Increasing test sensitivity dramatically increases the fraction of CF patients with two mutations identified. However, a substantial fraction of CF patients will carry an unidentified mutation, even when test sensitivity approaches 95 per cent. These patients will have to be diagnosed using other measure of CFTR dysfunction (sweat test or nasal PD testing).

Among patients in whom the diagnosis is confirmed by a positive sweat test result, mutation testing is still helpful. It can provide useful information relative to genetic counseling, pancreatic function status, prognosis and appropriateness for enrolment in trials of new therapies.

Perhaps the most difficult diagnostic situation facing the clinician is the patient with clinical features consistent with CF but a nondiagnostic sweat test and only one identified CF mutation. In such cases, evaluation involves weighing the possibility that the individual is a carrier of a CF mutation against the possibility that the patient has atypical CF. Nasal PD testing and ancillary laboratory tests may be particularly helpful for this group of patients. If CFTR dysfunction cannot be demonstrated by any method (sweat test, mutation analysis or nasal PD), a definitive diagnosis cannot be made and the decision to monitor or treat the patient rests upon the strength of that individual's clinical presentation.

NASAL PD MEASUREMENTS

Sinopulmonary epithelia, including nasal, regulate the composition of fluids that bathe airway surfaces by transport of ions such as sodium (Na⁺) and chloride (Cl⁻). This active transport generates a transepithelial electrical PD which can be measured *in vivo*[76]. Abnormalities of ion transport in respiratory epithelia of patients with CF are associated with a different pattern of nasal PD compared to normal epithelia (Fig. 9.5)[5–7]. This provides a rationale for the use of nasal PD as a diagnostic aid (Fig. 9.6)[3,8,77]. Specifically, there are three features that distinguish CF:

1. higher (raised; more negative) basal PD which reflects enhanced Na⁺ transport across a relatively Cl⁻ impermeable barrier;
2. larger inhibition of PD after nasal perfusion with the Na⁺-channel inhibitor, amiloride, which reflects inhibition of accelerated Na⁺ transport; and
3. little or no change in PD in response to perfusion of the nasal epithelial surface with a Cl⁻ free solution in conjunction with isoproterenol, which reflects an absence of CFTR-mediated Cl⁻ secretion[7].

Although the measurement of nasal PD may assist in the diagnosis or exclusion of CF, there are important variables that need to be addressed to ensure the safety and accuracy of testing.

A schematic representation of the technique used for recording nasal PD is shown in Fig. 9.7. It involves measuring the transepithelial bioelectric PD across various regions of the nasal epithelium, including the anterior tip of the inferior turbinate (squamous epithelium), the medial surface of the inferior turbinate (cuboidal epithelium), and the floor of the nasal cavity and inferior surface of the inferior turbinate (pseudostratified ciliated

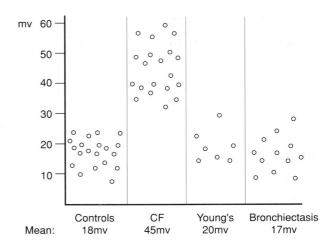

Fig. 9.6 *Nasal potential recordings (in mV, lumen negative) in control subjects and in patients with cystic fibrosis, Young's syndrome and bronchiectasis. (Reproduced, with permission, from ref. 77.)*

epithelium). The measurement of PD uses balanced calomel electrodes and a high impedance voltmeter, an exploring bridge (PE₅₀ tubing) that is perfused with Ringer's solution, and a subcutaneous reference electrode (22-gauge needle filled with a 4 per cent Agar/Ringer's solution).

The basal PD is measured by recording a PD for 5 seconds (or more, until stable) at anatomically defined sites (0.5, 1.0, 1.5, 2.0 and 3.0 cm posterior to the anterior tip of the turbinate) underneath the inferior turbinate. Potential difference values at all 10 sites are averaged to generate a mean basal PD. The PD at the anterior tip of the inferior turbinate is used as an anatomic and physiologic reference point since the PD at that site is usually −5 ± 5 mV.

For studying the response of nasal PD to perfusion of drugs and solutions of differing ion composition, a double-barreled set-up employing two PE₅₀ catheters in parallel is used. The catheters are placed under the inferior turbinate. After a baseline PD is established (±10 per cent change in 30 seconds), the drug or ionic solution of choice is perfused through the second catheter and PD responses recorded.

A modification of the protocol described above, using a solid-state non-perfused exploring electrode and an epicutaneous reference electrode, can be used to measure baseline PD with high reproducibility[4]. However, this technique does not allow for the measurement of responses to perfusion of drugs and ionic solutions.

The technique is safe, provided the PD equipment (high impedance voltmeter) meets appropriate clinical electrical engineering standards, and subcutaneous skin bridges are prepared in an aseptic manner. Technical considerations mandate that nasal anatomy be clearly understood, because the sites of PD measurements are

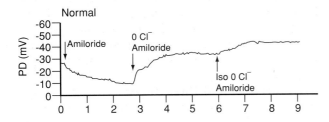

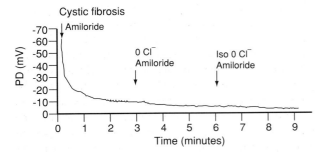

Fig. 9.5 *Nasal PD tracing in a normal subject (top panel) and a CF patient (bottom panel). The tracings illustrate the response of the PD to perfusion with amiloride (10⁻⁴ M), the addition of a Cl⁻ free solution (gluconate buffer) to amiloride, and the addition of isoproterenol (10⁻⁵ M) to the Cl⁻ free solution containing amiloride. (Reproduced, with permission, from ref. 7.)*

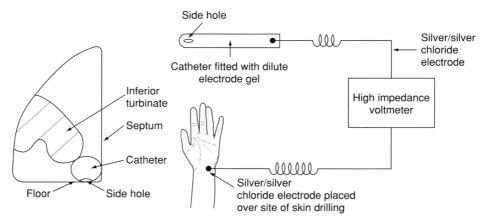

Fig. 9.7 *Schematic representation of equipment for recording nasal PD and anterior view of right nasal cavity showing site of measurement of PD. (Reproduced, with permission, from ref. 3.)*

critical to the accuracy of the measurement. Equipment must be validated and the protocol should be well-defined and standardized. These technical considerations have been described in great detail[7]. Methodologies should be validated and reproducible at any facility that employs this technique for diagnostic purposes. Nasal PD can be measured in patients only a few hours old[78]; older children (age 2–5 years) may require modest sedation. The presence of nasal polyps or inflamed mucosa alters bioelectric properties, and may yield a false-negative result[7].

Interpretation of PD measurements requires understanding of the ion-transport characteristics of the nasal epithelium and the PD responses to perfusion with different agonists and antagonists of ion transport (Fig. 9.5). For example, a raised (more negative) basal nasal PD is strong evidence for the diagnosis of CF. However, the absence of a raised PD does not rule out CF because a false-negative result may occur in the presence of inflamed epithelium. As with any laboratory test that is used to confirm a diagnosis, a raised PD must be duplicated on more than one occasion to be valid as a diagnostic adjunct. It should be emphasized that the absence of a large CFTR-mediated Cl^- conductance (voltage change) in response to perfusion with a low (or zero) Cl^- solution and a β-agonist does not establish the diagnosis of CF, as there are nonspecific effects that inhibit CFTR-mediated Cl^- conductance. However, the presence of a large response to Cl^- free perfusion is strong evidence against CF. Any laboratory planning to establish nasal PD as a clinical diagnostic tool must carry out a large enough number of studies in CF patients with defined mutations, normal subjects, and disease control subjects to establish reference values and to ensure adequate rigor of the technique.

CAVEATS

The most commonly encountered errors regarding the diagnosis of CF are:

1. Failure to consider the diagnosis because the patient is not Caucasian, the patient looks 'too healthy', or pancreatic function is normal.
2. Use of unacceptable sweat-test methodology.
3. Misinterpretation of sweat-test result because of inadequate sweat sample; confusing values for sweat weight, osmolality and electrolyte concentration; failure to repeat positive and borderline results; and failure to repeat a negative sweat test in a patient with a highly suggestive clinical picture.
4. Failure to reconsider the diagnosis in a patient who does not follow the 'usual' or 'expected' clinical course.

EVALUATION OF THE PATIENT WHO PRESENTS WITH AN ATYPICAL PHENOTYPE

In the patient who presents with an atypical phenotype, it is important to carry out a comprehensive clinical, radiographic and laboratory evaluation for features known to be consistent with the CF phenotype or for alternative diagnoses (Table 9.5).

Assessment of exocrine pancreatic function

The exocrine pancreas has a large functional capacity; more than 98 per cent of its capacity to secrete enzyme must be lost before signs and symptoms of malabsorption are evident[79,80]. In infancy, up to 37 per cent of patients with CF have sufficient exocrine pancreatic function to maintain normal fat absorption[81]. However, there is progressive decline in pancreatic function and by late childhood 85–90 per cent of patients have steatorrhea. Even among patients without obvious steatorrhea, there are often subtle abnormalities of pancreatic acinar and ductular function[1,82,83].

Table 9.5 *Clinical evaluation of atypical cases*

Respiratory tract microbiology
Assessment for bronchiectasis
   Plain radiography
   CT
Evaluation of paranasal sinuses
   Plain radiography
   CT
Quantitative assessment of pancreatic function
Male genital tract evaluation
   Semen analysis
   Urologic examination
   Ultrasound
   Scrotal exploration
Exclusion of other diagnoses
   Ciliary structure and function
   Immunologic status
   Allergy
   Infection

A number of direct and indirect (including blood) tests are available to evaluate exocrine pancreatic function[79]. All currently available tests have at least one and, in most cases, several drawbacks. Thus, there is no 'ideal' test. Direct tests are highly specific and capable of evaluating the entire range of pancreatic function. They are of great value for identifying aspects of pancreatic fluid and anion secretion in patients with a questionable diagnosis of CF. However, these tests require special skill to perform and interpret, and their invasive nature precludes their routine use for clinical purposes. Among the indirect tests, fecal fat analysis using a timed pooled stool collection (minimum of 72 hours) is the most widely used and is probably the most informative. However, it does not measure pancreatic reserve. An ELISA assay for the detection of pancreatic elastase 1 in stool is a highly sensitive and specific marker of exocrine pancreatic function that may prove to be useful as an indirect measure of pancreatic function in patients with CF[84,85].

Respiratory tract microbiology

Characterization of the respiratory microbial flora can be diagnostically helpful in the evaluation of patients with atypical features of CF. The unique predilection of *Pseudomonas aeruginosa* to colonize the CF respiratory tract is well known[35,86,87]. The presence of the mucoid phenotype of *P. aeruginosa* in the respiratory tract (bronchoalveolar lavage fluid, sputum, oropharyngeal swab, sinus aspirate), especially if persistent, is highly suggestive of CF. Persistent colonization with other organisms, such as *Staphylococcus aureus*, *Haemophilus influenzae*, and *Burkholderia cepacia*, may support a CF diagnosis[35,87], although each of these pathogens is also found in other conditions.

Evaluation of the paranasal sinuses

Among patients with CF, chronic or recurrent sinusitis[1,88], often in association with nasal polyposis[89,90], is a common clinical feature. Homogeneous opacification of the paranasal sinuses (especially the maxillary) as demonstrated by plain radiography or computed tomography (CT) scans is a constant finding in almost all patients past infancy[88,91,92] and may be diagnostically useful. The CT finding of bilateral medial displacement of the lateral nasal wall and uncinate process demineralization is particularly suggestive of CF[91]. Normal radiographic and CT findings provide strong evidence against a diagnosis of CF.

Chest imaging

While there are no radiographic abnormalities which are diagnostic of CF, there are findings which may be helpful in suggesting the diagnosis. Overaeration and bronchial-wall thickening are the earliest radiographic findings. In infants, segmental or lobar atelectasis, particularly involving the right upper lobe, is highly suggestive of CF. In older patients, typical findings include patchy atelectasis, bronchial-wall thickening, bronchial dilatation, cysts, nonspecific linear shadows, infiltrates, hilar adenopathy and overaeration. Mucoid impaction of the bronchi is highly suggestive of CF[93]. In CF patients with mild lung disease and normal chest radiographs, high-resolution CT often shows evidence of mild bronchiectasis involving the upper lobes[94,95]. The degree of bronchial-wall thickening exceeds lumen dilatation, which is predominantly proximal.

Urogenital evaluation

One of the most consistent features of the CF phenotype in postpubertal males is obstructive azoospermia, a finding present in 98–99 per cent of affected individuals[1,96–98]. Functional sperm and fertility have been reported in males heterozygous or homozygous for the 3849 + 10 kb C→T mutation[10,99]. In the majority of CF patients, azoospermia occurs secondary to absent or rudimentary vas deferens[96,98]. The evaluation of postpubertal males with atypical presentations should include a careful evaluation of urogenital status by urologic examination, semen analysis, ultrasound study of the urogenital structures and, rarely, scrotal exploration.

Individuals who present with CBAVD and other forms of obstructive azoospermia present a particularly difficult diagnostic dilemma. They usually have no evidence of respiratory tract or pancreatic abnormalities but may have CF mutations on one or both *CFTR* genes or an incompletely penetrant mutation (5T) in a noncoding region of CFTR[19–23]. They may have normal, intermediate or elevated sweat chloride concentrations. Individuals presenting with obstructive azoospermia should be assigned a diagnosis of CF only if there is evidence of CFTR dysfunction as documented by elevated sweat chloride concentrations, identification of two CF mutations, or the *in vivo* demonstration of abnormal ion transport across the nasal epithelium. The prognosis for such patients assigned a diagnosis of CF appears to be excellent[100], but it is recommended that they be closely monitored for the development of other CF-related complications.

Post-mortem diagnosis

A patient may die before the diagnosis of CF can be confirmed or ruled out. Making the diagnosis remains important for family knowledge and family planning. Post-mortem diagnosis can sometimes be strongly suggested by the typical histological pattern of the pancreas and intestines[101], particularly the appendix and ileum[102], which show hypereosinophilic secretions overfilling mucous glands.

A one gram section of fresh tissue from any organ, but particularly the liver, can be used for DNA analysis[103,104]. The tissue is best obtained within hours of death, but may suffice even within 72 hours. If the tissue is cut, wrapped in foil, and put in dry ice, it should be usable. DNA analysis can, on occasion, be carried out on paraffin-embedded biopsy or autopsy tissue from years before[105], even – in extenuating circumstances – from autopsy slides. Finding two CF mutations makes the diagnosis likely; finding one or none may modify the estimated likelihood of CF, but does not rule it out.

Screening

D. J. H. BROCK

Two types of screening have been applied to cystic fibrosis (CF). In neonatal screening, the objective is to detect infants affected with the disorder as early in life as possible. In antenatal screening the objective is to find couples where both partners are heterozygous, so that they may be warned of their risk of an affected child and appropriate action taken. Both types of screening have been subjected to detailed and lengthy pilot trials, but with a few exceptions, neither has yet found its way into routine use.

NEONATAL SCREENING

Because CF is not always readily identified in infants or children, there has long been an interest in achieving early diagnosis through newborn screening. This became a practical proposition when Crossley et al.[106] demonstrated that there were increased levels of immunoreactive trypsin (IRT) in blood spots taken from affected infants between 3 and 5 days after birth. The rationale for IRT testing is that when pancreatic ducts are blocked or partially blocked in the newborn there is back-leakage of acinar products, including trypsin and trypsinogen, into the vascular system. Even after the cloning of the cystic fibrosis trans-membrane conductance regulator (CFTR) gene in 1989[107–109], IRT measurement has remained the bedrock of CF screening, although it is increasingly now combined with DNA testing of samples for specific gene mutations.

IRT screening

Since the original description of IRT screening by Crossley et al.[106] and the present, there have been a number of field-trials of the procedure, covering large numbers of infants. In most, the protocol adopted has been very similar. The first sample was tested at between days 1 and 5; any infant with a value above a designated cut-off was retested at about 2–8 weeks, while those with continuing high values were referred for a diagnostic sweat test between 5 and 8 weeks.

Obviously, the two-stage IRT protocol involves a trade-off between false positives and false negatives. If the first IRT cut-off is set too high, there may be a substantial number of false negatives (missed cases of CF). If it is set too low, relatively high proportions of infants will have to be recalled for a second IRT test, with resulting parental anxiety. Furthermore, there is an age-related decline in IRT levels in infants with CF[110], with the rate of decline depending on the measurement method used[111], so that false negatives may also result from the second IRT test.

Methodologies of IRT testing have continued to evolve so that it is difficult to make comparisons between different programs, some of which may have changed the initial cut-off during the survey. There are inherent problems in both sample collection and in sample processing as well as in the assay itself (reviewed in ref. 112). There is a decline in the amount of extractable IRT with age of the sample, and significant differences in median IRT for populations from different areas which seem unlikely to be ethnically determined. It is possible that these derive from slightly earlier times of sample collection in some areas, since it is known that the highest IRT values are found in the first few days of life. Another problem is the question of what exactly is being measured – trypsin, cationic or anionic trypsinogen, trypsin–α_1-antitrypsin complex, or some measure of the four. The answer probably depends on the antibody used and perhaps on the source of radiolabeled trypsin. Different commercial assays give extraordinarily different IRT values. If an infant has meconium ileus the IRT level is usually not raised.

Most of the 'IRT alone' screening trials have chosen an initial cut-off designed to give a fixed percentage recall rate of between 0.3 and 0.7 per cent (113–116)(Table 9.6). By far and away the largest of these is the study of Wilcken et al.[116], who screened more than a million newborns in New South Wales between 1981 and 1992. Using a protocol designed to find the highest 0.6–0.7 per cent of values, they identified 7362 babies (0.73 per cent) in the first screen. Of these 635 (0.063 per cent) had a

Table 9.6 *Results of four large 'IRT alone' screening trials*

Location	Dates	No. screened	Recall rate, %	Detection rate, no. (%)	Ref.
England	1985–90	227 183	0.42	68/78 (87)	113
Colorado	1982–87	279 399	0.32	66/73 (90)	114
Wisconsin	1985–94	220 862	0.17	50/55 (91)	115
New South Wales	1981–92	1 015 000	0.69	359/389 (92)	116

second raised value, while 300 had cystic fibrosis. However, when cases, identified by meconium ileus at birth or because of a family history of the disease leading to sweat testing, were included, Wilcken *et al.* claim that 359 of the 389 infants with cystic fibrosis (92 per cent) received an early diagnosis. If only those identified through screening are considered, the detection rate was 242 out of 272 (89 per cent). This study establishes the benchmark for 'IRT alone' screening.

IRT combined with DNA

Obviously, considerable doubts remain about how to balance the sensitivity and specificity of neonatal IRT screening. With the cloning of the CF gene, alternative strategies became possible. The most obvious of these was to search for a panel of CFTR mutations in the neonatal dried-blood spot specimen. However, because the cost of DNA testing is at least an order of magnitude higher than that of IRT testing, and increases with each mutant allele covered, this was likely to prove far too expensive. Thus was born the idea of combined IRT and DNA testing, with the latter restricted to samples with elevated IRT values.

In the trials of combined testing so far reported, the cut-off level of the initial IRT test has been reduced compared to that of IRT alone testing. In theory this has permitted an improved sensitivity. The larger number of samples from infants with elevated values generated by this policy has then been scanned for the presence of detectable CFTR alleles before any further action is contemplated. In the absence of detectable CFTR alleles, no recall is made and the infant reported as 'cystic fibrosis not indicated'. If the infant is either homozygous for a CFTR allele or compound heterozygous for two CFTR alleles, a definitive diagnosis of cystic fibrosis has been made.

Difficulty arises when only one CFTR allele is detectable in this group of samples. The infant could be either a cystic fibrosis heterozygote (and therefore unaffected) or a compound heterozygote for an unknown allele (and therefore affected). To distinguish between these possibilities a sweat test must be carried out at age 5–8 weeks to confirm or exclude the diagnosis.

One problem in this protocol stems from the heterogeneity of the CFTR gene. Well over 750 different mutations have now been described[117]. Most of these have to be individually assayed for, and costs rise quickly if the net is cast too widely. However, in most European and North American Caucasian populations the ΔF_{508} mutant allele predominates, with a relative frequency ranging from as high as 90 per cent to below 50 per cent. Populations with an ethnic background from northern parts of Europe tend to have higher ΔF_{508} proportions than those from Mediterranean areas[118].

The actual proportion of cases with at least one ΔF_{508} allele is derived from the Hardy–Weinburg equilibrium and given by the formula $p^2 + 2pq$, where p is the relative frequency of ΔF_{508} and q the combined frequency of other mutant alleles in that particular population. Thus if ΔF_{508} represented 90 per cent of mutant alleles, 81 per cent (p^2) of affected cases would be homozygous for this allele and 18 per cent ($2pq$) would be compound heterozygotes for ΔF_{508} and another CFTR allele. Only 1 per cent of affected cases (q^2) would escape detection. On the other hand, at a ΔF_{508} relative frequency of 50 per cent, these figures become 25 per cent, 75 per cent and 25 per cent, respectively. Thus as many as one-quarter of affected cases would be escaping the screen.

In this situation consideration may have to be given to including other CFTR alleles in the assay system. However, no other mutations occur with the type of frequency of ΔF_{508}. In the UK, for example, the other major CFTR alleles are G551D at about 6 per cent, G542X at 5 per cent, R117H at 2 per cent and 1717-1G→A at 1 per

Table 9.7 *Results of combined IRT/DNA screening trials*

Location	Dates	No. screened	Recall rate, %	Detection rate, no. (%)	Ref.
South Australia	1989–93	88 752	0.10	29/29 (100)	120
New South Wales	1993–94	189 000	0.06	61/62 (98.4)	116
Wisconsin	1991–94	104 308	0.13	22/22 (100)	115
Brittany	1993–94	32 300	0.16	13/13 (100)	121
North-east Italy	1993–96	154 637	0.03	58/58 (100)	122

cent[119]. If these were included in the screen, the impact on detection rate would be small. However, the increased costs would not be insignificant.

Combined testing in practice

An illustrative flow chart for combined IRT/DNA testing is shown in Fig. 9.8, applied to a hypothetical population of 1 000 000 newborns in a country with a CF birth prevalence of 1 in 2500. It is assumed that 60 of the 400 cases of CF (15 per cent) would present with meconium ileus and would thus be self-diagnostic. It is also assumed that all of the remaining 340 cases in the primary IRT screen would be above a cut-off at the 99th percentile.

If DNA testing is carried out only for the ΔF_{508} allele, and if this represents 75 per cent of mutant alleles, 191 $\Delta F_{508}/\Delta F_{508}$ CF homozygotes ($340 \times 0.75 \times 0.75$) would be detected at the time of the first report. Of the remaining CF affecteds, 21 ($340 \times 0.25 \times 0.25$) would have no ΔF_{508} on either chromosome and would thus be missed. Another 128 cases ($340 \times 0.75 \times 0.25 \times 2$) would have ΔF_{508} on one chromosome, and another undetected CFTR allele on the other (ΔF/other). These would need to wait until 5–8 weeks of age for their diagnosis to be confirmed. However, this group of 128 would initially be indistinguishable from the genuine ΔF_{508} heterozygotes (ΔF/——) who would also go into the pool to await sweat testing. These can be expected to number about 770, since previous experience has shown that the incidence of ΔF_{508} heterozygotes in the raised IRT group is about twice the population incidence (see below).

It is assumed that sweat chloride levels will be above the 60 mmol/L cut-off in 90 per cent of the 128 ΔF_{508}/other compound heterozygotes, but in none of the 770 heterozygotes. Thus the overall detection rate for the screening program would be 92 per cent (366/400). The recall rate for sweat testing would be 0.09 per cent (128 + 770/10[6]). Thus, although the addition of a layer of DNA testing to the primary IRT test only marginally improves the detection rate (sensitivity), it has a much greater influence on the recall rate, the issue that has most bedeviled neonatal CF screening.

Actual experience[115,116,120–122] is broadly in line with these hypothetical projections for the recall rate after a positive DNA test (0.06–0.16 per cent; see Table 9.7). However, a much better detection rate has been claimed in all five trials reported, with only a single missed case of CF out of 184 being conceded. It is possible that some of the projections made in Fig. 9.8 are too pessimistic; for example, it would seem that in practice sweat testing is picking up more than 90 per cent of the ΔF_{508}/other compound heterozygotes. However, if only ΔF_{508} is being screened for, and if this allele represents 75 per cent of mutant CF alleles, some 6 per cent (0.25×0.25) of cases *must* be missed. Thus it is possible that some of the CF heterozygotes may have been incorrectly scored as affecteds.

Sweat testing

Sweat testing has been the gold standard for the diagnosis of cystic fibrosis since its introduction in 1958[123]. In some ways the cloning of the CFTR gene has added to the importance of the sweat test. It is now customary to refer to CF cases 'with only one detectable CFTR allele' and even to CF cases 'with no detectable CFTR alleles'. That these cases have cystic fibrosis at all usually follows from a sweat chloride value above 60 mmol/L.

However, there are now at least four established 'dominant mild alleles' where individuals who are compound heterozygotes may have equivocal sweat chloride concentrations (40–60 mmol/L) no matter the nature of the other allele. These are R117H[124], A455E[125], 3849 + 10 kb[126,127] and P67L[128]. Thus using the sweat test in IRT/DNA screening to distinguish between affected cases where only one CFTR allele can be detected and genuine heterozygotes must occasionally lead to misclassification.

Detection of heterozygotes

One of the curious features of all IRT/DNA screening programs has been the detection of an excess (over theoretical) of cases with a single mutant CFTR allele, who subsequently had negative sweat tests (Table 9.8). There

Table 9.8 *Actual and expected prevalences of individuals with a single CFTR allele and subsequent negative sweat test detected in screening programs*

Location	Dates	Found	Expected[a]	Ref.
South Australia	1989–93	1 in 17	1 in 32	120
New South Wales	1993–94	1 in 19	1 in 33	116
Wisconsin	1991–94	1 in 18	1 in 48	115
Brittany	1993–94	1 in 10	1 in 25	121
North-east Italy	1993–96	1 in 15	1 in 44	122

[a]Based on birth prevalence of CF and detection rate of DNA testing.

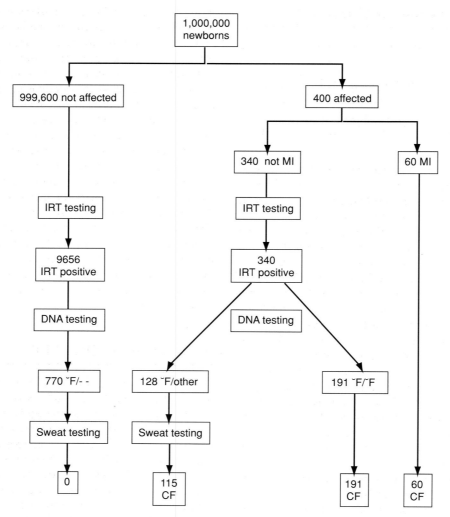

Fig. 9.8 *Illustrative flow chart for combined IRT/DNA testing in a hypothetical newborn population of 1 million (see text for details). ΔF——, ΔF_{508} heterozygotes; ΔF/other, ΔF_{508} compound heterozygotes; ΔF/ΔF, ΔF_{508}/ΔF_{508} homozygotes.*

are a number of possible explanations for this finding. The most likely is that CF heterozygotes have altered pancreatic secretions causing some ductule blockage and a consequent elevation in IRT. However, CF heterozygotes are, in virtually all other respects, clinically and biologically asymptomatic, and it is difficult to see why they should be positive for a marker of pancreatic function. Alternatively, the apparent carriers are in fact compound heterozygotes for an as-yet undetected 'dominant' mild allele, which influences the sweat chloride levels (see above).

Recently, Castellani *et al.*[122] have suggested another explanation. It is known that there is a polymorphism in intron 8 of the *CFTR* gene (the Tn locus) which affects the expression of the gene product[129]. Three alleles have been described, with individuals having 5, 7 or 9 thymidines at a location five base pairs upstream of exon 9. The 5T allele promotes inappropriate splicing of

CFTR mRNA, eliminating exon 9 in a large majority of transcripts, whereas the 7T and 9T alleles are associated with much higher levels of normal-length transcript[130]. Those mRNAs that lack an exon 9 generate a CFTR product that does not mature and therefore will not function as a chloride channel in epithelial cells[131].

Castellani *et al.*[122] found a small excess of 5T alleles in the IRT-positive CF carrier neonates. In four cases they were also able to test the parents of the neonate and to show that the 5T allele was in *trans* (on the opposite chromosome) to a ΔF_{508} allele. This intriguing finding suggested that ΔF_{508}/5T compound heterozygotes might have elevated IRT values and a mild form of cystic fibrosis. However, a later study[132] has shown that the 5T allele in its own right contributes to a raised neonatal IRT. Thus there is still no adequate explanation for the apparent excess of CF heterozygotes in the raised IRT group.

Is neonatal screening for CF justified?

There are two arguments in favor of neonatal screening for CF:

1. that it permits the detection of affected cases early enough to allow counseling of parents before they embark on further pregnancies; and
2. that it allows a favorable alteration in the long-term prognosis for the disease.

The first argument does not stand close scrutiny. In developed countries where neonatal screening is most likely to occur, the average family size is close to 2, and a CF child is as likely to be the second (and final one) as the first. In a neonatal screening program that detected 100 per cent of cases and where all counseled parents availed themselves of antenatal diagnosis and termination of pregnancy, it would still only be possible to prevent recurrences in half the cases. Thus the maximum possible reduction in birth prevalence of CF would be 12.5 per cent. Furthermore, in the absence of neonatal screening, some 10–15 per cent of infants with CF would present at birth with meconium ileus, while some 60–70 per cent would be ascertained clinically in the first year of life. If second pregnancies were not started until a year after the birth of the first child, as many as 80 per cent of heterozygous couples would know that they were at risk. It is therefore probable that a program of neonatal screening would reduce the birth prevalence of the disorder by less than 5 per cent.

The case for screening must therefore rest on whether or not it improves prognosis. Several studies have addressed this point, but as yet with unconvincing results. A trial in the UK, in which screening was carried out on alternate weeks, was followed by assessment of both screened and unscreened groups for the first 4 years of life[113]. CF children detected by screening spent a significantly shorter time in hospital in the first year of life compared to the unscreened group. However, there were no significant differences between the two groups in mean height or mean weight, in Shwachman or Norman–Chrispin scores or in the results of any laboratory tests. This was disappointing in view of the fact that it is often pointed out that nutritional deficiency is a potent indicator of poor prognosis in CF.

A study in The Netherlands[133], again comparing a cohort of infants detected by screening with a group detected clinically, reported less deterioration in lung function in the former group. A similar study in Wisconsin[134] claimed higher height, weight and head circumference percentiles in the screened group, but no difference in Shwachman scores.

All three of the above studies suffer from the same defect. If cystic fibrosis children detected by neonatal screening are compared with those detected clinically, the former will represent a cross-section of severities while the latter will inevitably be weighted towards the more clinically obvious, and therefore, serious cases. Thus any type of case-control study using this format may include a bias towards an apparently improved prognosis for the screened cohort. Given that the observed effects in the three cited studies are so small, it is quite probable that they can be explained by a confounding effect in the study design.

The value of newborn screening for CF, if any, is unlikely to be demonstrated conclusively without sustained follow-up of control trials, using either random assignment or alternative-week methodologies, and starting observations at a point several years after recruitment. It is natural for pediatricians to feel that there *must* be benefits in early detection of this disorder. However, it is dangerous to conclude that the case for screening has been made, and important to resist the pressure for widescale implementation until adequate data on the benefits have been presented. Such a conclusion was recently arrived at by an influential NIH Consensus Panel[135].

HETEROZYGOTE SCREENING

After the CF gene was cloned in 1989, it became possible for the first time to try and reduce the number of affected births through early recognition of parental heterozygosity. CF being inherited as an autosomal recessive disorder, it was natural to see heterozygote screening as aimed at the detection of individuals with a single copy of a mutant CF allele. In parts of Europe and North America this may comprise 5 per cent of the population. However, CF carrier status is harmless and only assumes significance in the context of pregnancy. Then it is the carrier couple who is at risk. Although it is sometimes argued that early knowledge of individual carrier status allows people to choose courses of action that avoid an affected child, the experience with other autosomal recessive disorders suggests that these alternatives are seldom exercised. The response of those who find themselves at risk of bearing a child with a recessive disorder is to stay with their chosen partner and to ask for prenatal diagnosis and a monitored pregnancy.

The probability that CF heterozygote testing would be closely tied to prenatal diagnosis has influenced the discussion of when to perform screening. A prominent school of thought argues that the most effective time is during pregnancy, for only then will it be possible to focus the minds of the general population on the risks of carrier status. An alternative view is that screening during pregnancy places an unacceptable burden of decision-making on a susceptible and captive group, and that attempts must be made to permit individuals to make up their minds about the implications of carrier status before they embark on a pregnancy. In order to try and resolve these issues, several experimental trials of CF carrier screening have been performed and reported.

Allelic heterogeneity

All types of heterozygote screening for CF are confronted by the problem of allelic heterogeneity. Soon after the gene was cloned it was apparent that screening could not be carried out on the gene product, since it was not expressed in any readily accessible tissue. In contrast to the experience with other autosomal recessive disorders, testing would have to be based on genotype rather than phenotype analysis. Centers contemplating screening had therefore to survey their local population for the nature and frequency of CF alleles, and then to calculate how many of these it was possible to cover in laboratory analyses. This in turn was determined by the size of the population to be screened. It is easy to assay for 20 or 30 mutant alleles if the only subjects are a small group of high-risk individuals. With available gene technology it is much more difficult to assay for more than a handful of CF alleles if any substantial through-put of samples is to be achieved.

In most relevant populations it has now been possible to define the majority of segregating CF alleles. For centers that have run trials on screening, there has been acceptance that only 85–90 per cent could realistically be analyzed. Inevitably this creates a problem for couples where one partner carries a mutant allele while the other does not. Such 'positive–negative' couples have a residual risk of bearing a CF child which depends on the proportion of CF alleles detectable and the incidence of the disorder (Table 9.9). For groups with a birth incidence above 1 in 2500, the residual risk for a positive–negative couple only falls below the population risk when over 96 per cent of CF alleles are analyzable. The American Society of Human Genetics took the view that this should be the target detection figure before any population screening programs were initiated[136]. Others felt that this was an impossible precondition[137]. Recently, an NIH Consensus Panel has recommended that CF screening should be offered to all pregnant couples and to those planning pregnancy[135]. It did not advocate heterozygote testing in other segments of the population.

Screening at school-age

Although it makes sense to time the CF carrier test as close to pregnancy as possible, there are also theoretical advantages in directing screening at children of high-school age. Scriver and his colleagues[138,139] had demonstrated that this worked well for Tay–Sachs and β-thalassaemia screening in Montreal schools. The whole concept of genetic risk could be tied into an imaginative program of biology teaching. In a small pilot study aimed at ascertaining CF heterozygotes in Montreal high schools in 1991, they showed a take-up rate of 42 per cent[140]. Response to a questionnaire soliciting participants' attitudes to the project suggested overwhelming (96 per cent) approval of the concept of genetic screening in high schools. However, it was conceded that these were not necessarily typical attitudes, and Scriver and Clow[141] have stated that school-age carrier screening for autosomal recessive disorders would probably not work as well elsewhere. In the UK, for example, a Working Party of the Clinical Genetics Society[142] has recommended against testing children for their carrier status where this would be of purely reproductive significance to the child in the future.

Largely for these reasons, the major pilot programs of CF heterozygosity testing which have been reported have been concerned with adults. The issue has been whether to screen before or during pregnancy.

Screening before pregnancy

In many respects screening young adults at a time when they are beginning to think about their reproductive future is the ideal program. It is the most compatible with the principle of individual autonomy. An identified carrier has a variety of options. She can ignore the information, select an appropriate mating partner, have artificial insemination by a screened donor, forego reproduction or have a pregnancy monitored by prenatal diagnosis. Even when the last option is chosen, there

Table 9.9 *The residual risk of a CF child if one partner tests positive and the other negative compared to the proportion of detectable alleles*

Percentage detectable alleles	Residual risk when population incidence is	
	1/2000	1/2500
70	1/289	1/311
75	1/346	1/388
80	1/431	1/484
85	1/574	1/644
90	1/859	1/964
95	1/1713	1/1924
96	1/2141	1/2404
97	1/2854	1/3204

is time for considered reflection of how to react to an affected pregnancy.

The first pilot trials of CF carrier screening through primary healthcare services were carried out in London and produced some unsettling results. Williamson's group[143] showed that the method of presentation was critical in determining take-up rates. When the offer of screening was made opportunistically and in person by a dedicated member of the research team, between 66 and 87 per cent of those approached agreed to be tested. In contrast, when presentation was by an invitation letter, the take-up rate was only 10 per cent. This was confirmed by Bekker et al.[144] in another study carried out in general practitioner surgeries in London. When there was direct contact between those offering the test and those to whom it was offered, and the possibility of immediate testing, the acceptance rate was 70 per cent. For all other methods of presentation, participation was feeble. Bekker et al.[144] concluded that the most important variable determining participation rates in screening was the personal approach by a professional and the offer of immediate carrier testing.

Similar conclusions have now emerged from a study in the USA. Tambor et al.[145] offered carrier testing to reproductive-age enrollees in a Health Maintenance Organization in the Baltimore area. When letters were sent to the 18–44 age-band, inviting participation in a free trial but also demanding attendance at a pre-testing educational session, the response was 3.7 per cent. In contrast, when counselors approached patients who were already in the waiting room for an appointment, and carried out explanation of the test on the spot, the overall test utilization was 23.5 per cent.

The implications of these three pilot trials (Table 9.10) are obvious. In order to achieve respectable participation rates in individual-directed CF carrier screening programs, some form of personal explanation of the purposes and achievements of screening has to be made. Letters and leaflets will not suffice. The cost conse-quences of this degree of professional staff involvement are considerable. It is no surprise that none of the programs of primary care screening appear to have survived the trial period.

Screening during pregnancy

In many countries most pregnant women attend antenatal clinics during their confinement. Such clinics, whether in hospitals, community centers or private offices, represent 'turnstiles', where the offer of heterozygote testing for CF may be made efficiently. Furthermore, following the success of biochemical screening for the detection of fetal neural tube defects and Down syndrome, pregnancy screening has become a fairly routine aspect of antenatal care. Heterozygote screening may therefore be added to existing programs with minimal input of additional staff.

Two different, but not mutually exclusive, types of screening for CF during pregnancy have been proposed; 'two-step (or sequential)'[146] and 'couple'[147]. In the two-step model the woman is tested first and her partner screened only when she is positive. Although both partners could be screened at the same time, this would almost double the number of tests carried out with consequent cost implications. It is therefore possible, in principle, for a woman to be tested and found to be positive while her partner refuses to participate. In this situation her risk of carrying an affected child would be 1 in 100 and no further practical help could be offered her.

In contrast, in the couple model both partners contract into screening before testing begins. For 96 per cent of couples only one partner need be tested, since a negative result on the first sample means that the couple is not at high risk. For another 3 per cent of couples, the first sample will prove to be positive. thus leading to testing of the second sample. However, where couple screening differs from two-step screening is in the management

Table 9.10 *Take-up rates of CF heterozygote testing in primary care*

Approach to identified target group	Take-up (%)
Watson et al.[143]	
Opportunistic screening, general practice	340/513 (66)
Opportunistic screening, family planning clinics	371/431 (87)
Invitation letter, general practice	87/852 (10)
Bekker et al.[144]	
Letter at beginning of trial in one general practice	59/502 (12)
Letter and booklet	47/496 (9)
Passive opportunistic	81/471 (17)
Active opportunistic – test now	53/649 (70)
Active opportunistic – test at return visit	22/88 (25)
Letter at end of trial	128/2953 (4)
Tambor et al.[145]	
Mailed invitation	101/2713 (4)
On-site invitation	143/608 (24)

of results. In both situations – (1) where only one sample is tested and found negative, and (2) where both samples are tested and only one found positive – the results are regarded as 'couple-negative' and no further action taken.

The initial response to the idea of couple screening was to question its ethical basis. There is something disturbing about the deliberate withholding of genetic information. Discussion on this point was eventually resolved by it being pointed out that there is no moral imperative to disclose a risk situation for which no ameliorating action is possible. Because of the incomplete nature of CF heterozygosity testing, 'positive-negative' couples have a risk of bearing a CF child that is higher than the population risk. However, as there is nothing practical that can be done to reduce this risk, it is in the individual's interest that he or she should not be forced to confront his or her carrier status. If the information is sought, it is freely disclosed; if not sought it is not volunteered.

There are now quite a large number of reported trials[148–160] of both two-step and couple screening, mainly in antenatal clinics, but also in HMOs and one in GP surgeries (Table 9.11). With a few exceptions reported take-ups have been high. However, two-step screening generates moderate anxiety amongst women found to be positive for CF alleles during the period of waiting for their partner's test result. Quantitative measures of this stress, using several different psychological instruments, proved that it was of short duration and did not return later in pregnancy[161]. However, there was a need for specialist counseling during the waiting period and this has cost implications for two-step screening. Furthermore, many obstetricians feel that any additional anxiety generated during pregnancy should be avoided .

The most extensive experience of antenatal screening has been in Edinburgh (Table 9.12) where the numbers are now large enough to begin to answer two critical questions:

1. What proportion of high-risk couples choose prenatal diagnosis? and
2. How many couples carrying an affected pregnancy have a termination of pregnancy?

In Edinburgh 34 of 37 (92 per cent) of couples identified at high risk opted for prenatal diagnosis, and in all 14 of the affected cases the pregnancy was terminated. Amongst this group, five couples came back for a second prenatal diagnosis, one couple for three and two couples for five prenatal diagnoses. The reduction in incidence of CF in the screened group was 70 per cent, close to the theoretical expectation of 72 per cent (obtained by squaring the detection rate of 85 per cent).

In Edinburgh it has been possible to run extended screening trials of both two-step and couple screening in the same hospital. There is no question that couple screening is the mode of delivery preferred by patients, doctors and paramedical staff, and is the form of screening now purchased as service by the three local maternity hospital trusts. However, there are still some[156] who have residual doubts about the nondisclosure aspect of couple screening – 'we feel that it is fundamentally unethical not to divulge the results of any clinical laboratory test to the patient who consented to it' – which suggests that it may be some time before it becomes a generally acceptable model for screening for autosomal recessive disorders.

Cascade testing

In many genetic centers CF heterozygosity testing is now available to the first- and second-degree relatives of an

Table 9.11 *Trials of antenatal CF screening*

Where and when	Mode	No. to whom screening offered	Take-up, %	Ref.
Edinburgh, 1990/2	Two-step	7011	83	148
Copenhagen, 1990/2	Two-step	7400	89	149
East Berlin, 1990/3	Two-step	638	99	150
Aberdeen[a]	Two-step	920	91	151
N. California, 1991/2	Two-step	6617	78	152
Rochester, NY[a]	Two-step	4879	~57	153
Leeds and Hull, 1993	Two-step	6071	62	154
Milan, 1992/4	Two-step	2214	98	155
Los Angeles[a]	Two-step	4739	78	156
Edinburgh, 1992/5	Couple	16571	76	157
Oxford[a]	Couple	810	67	158
Aberdeen[a]	Couple	220	85	151
Maine[a]	Couple	1770	95	159
Manchester, 1992/3	Two-step and couple[b]	623	85	160

[a]Not given.
[b]Randomized trial in GP surgeries.

Table 9.12 *Summary of antenatal CF screening in Edinburgh*

Number of couples to whom screening offered	32 085
Number of couples screened	25 026 (78%)
Heterozygotes identified	941 (1 in 26.6)
Heterozygous couples	37 (1 in 676)
Heterozygous couples opting for prenatal diagnosis	34
Total prenatal diagnoses	48
Affected fetuses	14
Termination of pregnancy, confirmed CF	14
CF cases missed	
Detectable, no prenatal diagnosis	2
Detectable, missed	1
Not detectable	3
Reduction in incidence of CF in screened group	14/20 (70%)

index affected proband. Usually such testing is a response, after counseling, to an individual's request. An alternative and more proactive approach has been proposed by Super *et al.*[162], who suggest taking screening into the wider population by 'cascading' through the relatives of index cases. They argue that there are many advantages to cascade testing: the ratio of carriers detected to people tested will be higher, assays can be restricted to the mutant alleles in the index case, and less anxiety will be generated among the screened population.

In a pilot trial in the Manchester area, Super and colleagues[162] carried out CF heterozygosity testing on 1563 relatives and partners in 129 index families with an affected proband. In this group they identified 15 heterozygous couples, in eight of whom prenatal diagnosis was carried out. By extrapolating to a total of 10 000 relatives and partners, it was suggested that 100 heterozygous couples would be detected and thus 25 affected fetuses found. It was claimed that this is equal to the number of CF children born annually in their region, and that proactive cascade testing was a genuine substitute for population screening.

However, inspection of the data does not support the claim. Among the relatives tested no fewer than 427/1122 (38 per cent) were carriers. Thus the study was obviously concentrating predominantly on first-degree relatives. In the next phase, as the cascade moves to more distant relatives of the index case, the proportion of carriers detected will drop. It is misleading to extrapolate the proportion of heterozygous couples found in the easy part of the program to more difficult parts. Furthermore, it cannot be assumed that all heterozygous couples would be planning pregnancies, or that all would seek prenatal diagnosis and act on the results. In fact, of the 15 heterozygous couples in the study, one had completed their family and another five did not request prenatal diagnosis.

It is impossible to measure the theoretical effectiveness of cascade testing by simple extrapolation. Models need to

be created, with family-size distributions and alternative testing strategies. Our own projections[163], using different models, show that the cascade needs to reach the fourth cousin level to achieve the same cover as population screening. Most people have difficulty in remembering the names and addresses of their first cousins. Even if the cascade is restricted to second cousin level it would only detect between 10 and 25 per cent of heterozygous couples (depending on the model assumed). In contrast, it has been demonstrated that over 50 per cent of heterozygous couples can be detected by either of the two major forms of antenatal screening[157].

There is no doubt that cascade testing is an effective way of identifying large numbers of carriers and carrier couples with a great deal less effort than in any standard population screening. However, it could also be argued that restricting maternal serum α-fetoprotein testing to mothers who had already had a child with a neural tube defect would increase the proportion of positive tests. Neither program would be screening in the conventional sense of the word, nor would either have the necessary impact on the birth incidence of affected cases. Thus cascade testing may be seen as a useful adjunct to population screening but certainly not as a substitute for it.

REFERENCES

Diagnosis

1. Welsh, M.J., Tsui, L.C., Boat, T.F. *et al.* (1995) Cystic fibrosis, in *The Metabolic and Molecular Basis of Inherited Disease*, (7th edn), (eds C.R. Scriver, A.L. Beaudet, W.C. Sly *et al.*), McGraw-Hill, New York, Vol. 3, pp. 3799–3879.
2. Tsui, L.C. (1995) The cystic fibrosis transmembrane conductance regulator gene. *Am. J. Respir. Crit. Care Med.*, **151**, S47–S53.
3. Alton, E.W., Currie, D., Logan-Sinclair, R. *et al.* (1990) Nasal potential difference: a clinical diagnostic test for cystic fibrosis. *Eur. Respir. J.*, **3**, 922–926.
4. Hofmann, T., Bohmer, O., Huls, G. *et al.* (1997) Conventional and modified nasal potential-difference measurement in cystic fibrosis. *Am. J. Respir. Crit. Care Med.*, **155**, 1908–1913.
5. Knowles, M., Gatzy, J. and Boucher, R. (1981) Increased bioelectric potential difference across respiratory epithelia in cystic fibrosis. *NEJM*, **305**, 1489–1495.
6. Knowles, M., Gatzy, J. and Boucher, R. (1983) Relative ion permeability of normal and cystic fibrosis nasal epithelium. *J. Clin. Invest.*, **71**, 1410–1417.
7. Knowles, M.R., Paradiso, A.M. and Boucher, R.C. (1995) In vivo nasal potential difference: techniques and protocols for assessing efficacy of gene transfer in cystic fibrosis. *Hum. Gene Ther.*, **6**, 445–455.
8. Sauder, R.A., Chesrown, S.E. and Loughlin, G.M. (1987)

Clinical application of transepithelial potential difference measurements in cystic fibrosis. *J. Pediatr.*, **111**, 353–358.

9. Augarten, A., Kerem, B.S., Yahav, Y. *et al.* (1993) Mild cystic fibrosis and normal or borderline sweat test in patients with the 3849 + 10 kb C→T mutation. *Lancet*, **342**, 25–26.

10. Highsmith, W.E., Burch, L.H., Zhou, Z. *et al.* (1994) A novel mutation in the cystic fibrosis gene in patients with pulmonary disease but normal sweat chloride concentrations. *NEJM*, **331**, 974–980.

11. Stern, R.C., Boat, T.F., Abramowsky, C.R. *et al.* (1978) Intermediate-range sweat chloride concentration and *Pseudomonas* bronchitis. A cystic fibrosis variant with preservation of exocrine pancreatic function. *JAMA*, **239**, 2676–2680.

12. Stewart, B., Zabner, J., Shuber, A.P. *et al.* (1995) Normal sweat chloride values do not exclude the diagnosis of cystic fibrosis. *Am. J. Respir. Crit. Care Med.*, **151**, 899–903.

13. Strong, T.V., Smit, L.S., Turpin, S.V. *et al.* (1991) Cystic fibrosis gene mutation in two sisters with mild disease and normal sweat electrolyte levels. *NEJM*, **325**, 1630–1634.

14. Leoni, G.B., Pitzalis, S., Podda, R. *et al.* (1995) A specific cystic fibrosis mutation (T3381) associated with the phenotype of isolated hypotonic dehydration. *J. Pediatr.*, **127**, 281–283.

15. Atlas, A.B., Orenstein, S.R. and Orenstein, D.M. (1992) Pancreatitis in young children with cystic fibrosis. *J. Pediatr.*, **120**, 756–759.

16. Shwachman, H., Lebenthal, E. and Khaw, K.T. (1975) Recurrent acute pancreatitis in patients with cystic fibrosis with normal pancreatic enzymes. *Pediatrics*, **55**, 86–95.

17. Stern, R.C., Boat, T.F., Doershuk, C.F. *et al.* (1997) Cystic fibrosis diagnosed after age 13: twenty-five teenage and adult patients including three asymptomatic men. *Ann. Int. Med.*, **87**, 188–191.

18. Wiatrak, B.J., Myer, C.M. and Cotton, R.T. (1993) Cystic fibrosis presenting with sinus disease in children. *Am. J. Dis. Child.*, **147**, 258–260.

19. Anguiano, A., Oates, R.D., Amos, J.A. *et al.* (1992) Congenital bilateral absence of the vas deferens. A primarily genital form of cystic fibrosis. *JAMA*, **267**, 1794–1797.

20. Chillon, M., Casals, T., Mercier, B. *et al.* (1995) Mutations in the cystic fibrosis gene in patients with congenital absence of the vas deferens. *NEJM*, **332**, 1475–1480.

21. Jarvi, K., Zielenski, J., Wilschanski, M. *et al.* (1995) Cystic fibrosis transmembrane conductance regulator and obstructive azoospermia. *Lancet*, **345**, 1578.

22. Osborne, L.R., Lynch, M., Middleton, P.G. *et al.* (1993) Nasal epithelial ion transport and genetic analysis of infertile men with congenital bilateral absence of the vas deferens. *Hum. Mol. Genet.*, **2**, 1605–1609.

23. Patrizio, P., Asch, R.H., Handelin, B. *et al.* (1993) Aetiology of congenital absence of vas deferens: genetic study of three generations. *Hum. Reprod.*, **8**, 215–220.

24. Lemna, W.K., Feldman, G.L., Kerem, B. *et al.* (1990) Mutation analysis for heterozygote detection and the prenatal diagnosis of cystic fibrosis. *NEJM*, **322**, 291–296.

25. Mulivor, R.A., Cook, D., Muller, F. *et al.* (1987) Analysis of fetal intestinal enzymes in amniotic fluid for the prenatal diagnosis of cystic fibrosis. *Am. J. Hum. Genet.*, **40**, 131–146.

26. Szabo, M., Munnich, A., Teichmann, F. *et al.* (1990) Discriminant analysis for assessing the value of amniotic fluid microvillar enzymes in the prenatal diagnosis of cystic fibrosis. *Prenat. Diagn.*, **10**, 761–769.

27. Brock, D.J. (1996) Prenatal screening for cystic fibrosis: 5 years' experience reviewed. *Lancet*, **347**, 148–150.

28. Wilfond, B.S. and Fost, N. (1990) The cystic fibrosis gene: medical and social implications for heterozygote detection. *JAMA*, **263**, 2777–2783.

29. NIH statement (1990) Statement from the National Institutes of Health Workshop on population screening for the cystic fibrosis gene. *NEJM*, **323**, 70–71.

30. Ao, A., Ray, P., Harper, J. *et al.* (1996) Clinical experience with preimplantation genetic diagnosis of cystic fibrosis (delta F508). *Prenat. Diagn.*, **16**, 137–142.

31. Corteville, J.E., Gray, D.L. and Langer, J.C. (1996) Bowel abnormalities in the fetus – correlation of prenatal ultrasonographic findings with outcome. *Am. J. Obstet. Gynecol.*, **175**, 724–729.

32. Muller, F., Dommergues, M., Aubry, M.C. *et al.* (1995) Hyperechogenic fetal bowel: an ultrasonographic marker for adverse fetal and neonatal outcome. *Am. J. Obstet. Gynecol.*, **173**, 508–513.

33. Foster, M.A., Nyberg, D.A., Mahony, B.S. *et al.* (1987) Meconium peritonitis: prenatal sonographic findings and their clinical significance. *Radiology*, **165**, 661–665.

34. Hamosh, A., FitzSimmons, S.C., Macek, M.J. *et al.* (1998) Comparison of the clinical manifestations of cystic fibrosis in Black and White patients. *J. Pediatr.*, **132**, 255–259.

35. FitzSimmons, S.C. (1993) The changing epidemiology of cystic fibrosis. *J. Pediatr.*, **122**, 1–9.

36. Gaskin, K., Gurwitz, D., Durie, P. *et al.* (1982) Improved respiratory prognosis in patients with cystic fibrosis with normal fat absorption. *J. Pediatr.*, **100**, 857–862.

37. di Sant'Agnese, P.A., Darling, R.C., Perera, G.A. *et al.* (1953) Abnormal electrolyte composition of sweat in cystic fibrosis of the pancreas. *Pediatrics*, **12**, 549–562.

38. LeGrys, V.A. (1996) Sweat testing for the diagnosis of cystic fibrosis: practical considerations. *J. Pediatr.*, **129**, 892–897.

39. Hardy, J.D., Davison, S.H., Higgins, M.U. *et al.* (1973) Sweat tests in the newborn period. *Arch. Dis. Child.*, **48**, 316–318.

40. National Committee for Clinical Laboratory Standards (1994) Sweat testing: sample collection and quantitative analysis – approved guideline [Document C34-A], 940 W, Valley Road, Suite 1400, Wayne, PA 19087, The Committee, p. 1.

41. Gibson, L.E. and Cooke, R.E. (1959) A test for

concentration of electrolytes in sweat in cystic fibrosis of the pancreas utilizing pilocarpine by iontophoresis. *Pediatrics*, **23**, 545–549.

42. Hammond, K.B., Turcios, N.L. and Gibson, LE. (1994) Clinical evaluation of the macroduct sweat collection system and conductivity analyzer in the diagnosis of cystic fibrosis. *J. Pediatr.*, **124**, 255–260.

43. Webster, H.L. and Barlow, W.K. (1981) New approach to cystic fibrosis diagnosis by use of an improved sweat-induction/collection system and osmometry. *Clin. Chem.*, **27**, 385–387.

44. Rattenbury, J.M. and Worthy, E. (1996) Is the sweat test safe? Some instances of burns received during pilocarpine iontophoresis. *Ann. Clin. Biochem.*, **33**, 456–458.

45. Chemlab Scientific Products (1994) Wescor Macroduct Manual, Essex, Chemlab Scientific Products.

46. Gleeson, M. and Henry, R.L. (1991) Sweat sodium or chloride? *Clin. Chem.*, **37**, 112.

47. Green, A., Dodds, P. and Pennock, C. (1985) A study of sweat sodium and chloride; criteria for the diagnosis of cystic fibrosis. *Ann. Clin. Biochem.*, **22**, 171–174.

48. Hall, S.K., Stableforth, D.E. and Green, A. (1990) Sweat sodium and chloride concentrations – essential criteria for the diagnosis of cystic fibrosis in adults. *Ann. Clin. Biochem.*, **27**, 318–320.

49. Hodson, M.E., Beldon, I., Power, R. *et al.* (1983) Sweat tests to diagnose cystic fibrosis in adults. *BMJ* (Clin. Res. edn), **286**, 1381–1383.

50. Shwachman, H., Mahmoodian, A. and Neff, R.K. (1981) The sweat test: sodium and chloride values. *J. Pediatr.*, **98**, 576–578.

51. Schulz, I.J. (1969) Micropuncture studies of the sweat formation in cystic fibrosis patients. *J. Clin. Invest.*, **48**, 1470–1477.

52. Shwachman, H., Mahmoodian, A., Kopito, L. *et al.* (1965) A standard procedure for measuring conductivity of sweat as a diagnostic test for cystic fibrosis. *J. Pediatr.*, **66**, 432–434.

53. Barnes, G.L., Vaelioja, L. and McShane, S. (1988) Sweat testing by capillary collection and osmometry: suitability of the Wescor Macroduct System for screening suspected cystic fibrosis patients. *Aust. Paediatr. J.*, **24**, 191–193.

54. Kopito, L. and Shwachman, H. (1969) Studies in cystic fibrosis: determination of sweat electrolytes in situ with direct reading electrodes. *Pediatrics*, **43**, 794–798.

55. Yeung, W.H., Palmer, J., Schidlow, D. *et al.* (1984) Evaluation of a paper-patch test for sweat chloride determination. *Clin. Pediatr.*, **23**, 603–607.

56. Denning, C.R., Huang, N.N., Cuasay, L.R. *et al.* (1980) Cooperative study comparing three methods of performing sweat tests to diagnose cystic fibrosis. *Pediatrics*, **66**, 752–757.

57. Shwachman, H. and Mahmoodian, A. (1967) Pilocarpine iontophoresis sweat testing results of seven years' experience. *Bibl. Paediatr.*, **86**, 158–182.

58. Farrell, P.M. and Koscik, R.E. (1996) Sweat chloride concentrations in infants homozygous or heterozygous for F508 cystic fibrosis. *Pediatrics*, **97**, 524–528.

59. Davis, P.B., Del Rio, S., Muntz, J.A. *et al.* (1983) Sweat chloride concentration in adults with pulmonary diseases. *Am. Rev. Respir. Dis.*, **128**, 34–37.

60. di Sant'Agnese, P.A. and Davis, P.B. (1979) Cystic fibrosis in adults. 75 cases and a review of 232 cases in the literature. *Am. J. Med.*, **66**, 121–132.

61. Augarten, A., Hacham, S., Kerem, E. *et al.* (1995) The significance of sweat Cl/Na ratio in patients with borderline sweat test. *Pediatr. Pulmonol.*, **20**, 369–371.

62. Davis, P.B., Hubbard, V.S., Di Sant'Agnese, P.A. (1980) Low sweat electrolytes in a patient with cystic fibrosis. *Am. J. Med.*, **69**, 643–646.

63. LeGrys, V.A. and Wood, R.E. (1988) Incidence and implications of false-negative sweat test reports in patients with cystic fibrosis. *Pediatr. Pulmonol.*, **4**, 169–172.

64. Rosenstein, B.J., Langbaum, T.S., Gordes, E. *et al.* (1978) Cystic fibrosis. Problems encountered with sweat testing. *JAMA*, **240**, 1987–1988.

65. Shwachman, H. and Mohmoodian, A. (1979) Quality of sweat test performance in the diagnosis of cystic fibrosis. *Clin. Chem.*, **25**, 158–161.

66. Goldman, A.S., Travis, L.B., Dodge, W.F. *et al.* (1961) Falsely negative sweat tests in children with cystic fibrosis complicated by hypoproteinemic edema. *J. Pediatr.*, **59**, 301.

67. Palmer, J., Huang, N.N., Schidlow, D. *et al.* (1984) What is the true incidence and significance of false-positive and false-negative sweat tests in cystic fibrosis? 12 years experience with almost 6,000 tests. *Cystic Fibrosis Club Abstracts*, **25**, 43.

68. Christoffel, K.S., Lloyd-Still, J.D., Brown, G. *et al.* (1985) Environmental deprivation and transient elevation of sweat electrolytes. *J. Pediatr.*, **107**, 231–234.

69. Beck, R., Goldberg, E., Durie, P.R. *et al.* (1986) Elevated sweat chloride levels in anorexia nervosa. *J. Pediatr.*, **108**, 260–262.

70. Orenstein, D.M. and Wasserman, A.L. (1986) Munchausen syndrome by proxy simulating cystic fibrosis. *Pediatrics*, **78**, 621–624.

71. Tsui, L.C. and Durie, P.R. (1997) What is a CF diagnosis? – Genetic heterogeneity. *New Insights into Cystic Fibrosis*, **511**, 5.

72. Cystic Fibrosis Genetic Analysis Consortium (1994) Population variation of common cystic fibrosis mutations. *Hum. Mutat.*, **4**, 167–177.

73. Kiesewetter, S., Macek, M.J., Davis, C. *et al.* (1993) A mutation in CFTR produces different phenotypes depending on chromosomal background. *Nature Genet.*, **5**, 274–278.

74. Macek, M.J., Mackova, A., Hamosh, A. *et al.* (1997) Identification of common cystic fibrosis mutations in African-Americans with cystic fibrosis increases the detection rate to 75%. *Am. J. Hum. Genet.*, **60**, 1122–1127.

75. Kristidis, P., Bozon, D., Corey, M. *et al.* (1992) Genetic

determination of exocrine pancreatic function in cystic fibrosis. *Am. J. Hum. Genet.*, **50**, 1178–1184.

76. Boucher, R.C. (1994) Human airway ion transport. Part two. *Am. J. Respir. Crit. Care Med.*, **150**, 581–593.

77. Alton, E.W., Hay, J.G., Munro, C. *et al.* (1987) Measurement of nasal potential difference in adult cystic fibrosis, Young's syndrome, and bronchiectasis. *Thorax*, **42**, 815–817.

78. Gowen, C.W., Lawson, E.E., Gingras-Leatherman, J. *et al.* (1986) Increased nasal potential difference and amiloride sensitivity in neonates with cystic fibrosis. *J. Pediatr.*, **108**, 517–521.

79. Couper, R.T., Corey, M., Moore, D.J. *et al.* (1992) Decline of exocrine pancreatic function in cystic fibrosis patients with pancreatic sufficiency. *Pediatr. Res.*, **32**, 179–182.

80. Gaskin, K.J., Durie, P.R., Lee, L. *et al.* (1984) Colipase and lipase secretion in childhood-onset pancreatic insufficiency. Delineation of patients with steatorrhea secondary to relative colipase deficiency. *Gastroenterology*, **86**, 1–7.

81. Waters, D.L., Dorney, S.F., Gaskin, K.J. *et al.* (1990) Pancreatic function in infants identified as having cystic fibrosis in a neonatal screening program. *NEJM*, **322**, 303–308.

82. Couper, R. (1995) Pancreatic function tests, in *Pediatric Gastrointestinal Disease. Pathophysiology, Diagnosis, Management*, (2nd edn), (eds W.A. Walker, P.R. Durie, J.R. Hamilton *et al.*), Mosby, St. Louis, p.1621.

83. Kopelman, H., Corey, M., Gaskin, K. *et al.* (1988) Impaired chloride secretion, as well as bicarbonate secretion, underlies the fluid secretory defect in the cystic fibrosis pancreas. *Gastroenterology*, **95**, 349–355.

84. Dominguez-Munoz, J.E., Hieronymus, C., Sauerbruch, T. *et al.* (1995) Fecal elastase test: evaluation of a new noninvasive pancreatic function test. *Am. J. Gastroenterol.*, **90**, 1834–1837.

85. Stein, J., Jung, M., Sziegoleit, A. *et al.* (1996) Immunoreactive elastase I: clinical evaluation of a new noninvasive test of pancreatic function. *Clin. Chem.*, **42**, 222–226.

86. Huang, N.N., Van Loon, E.L. and Sheng, K.T. (1961) The flora of the respiratory tract of patients with cystic fibrosis of the pancreas. *J. Pediatr.*, **59**, 512–521.

87. Thomassen, M.J., Demko, C.A. and Doershuk, C.F. (1987) Cystic fibrosis: a review of pulmonary infections and interventions. *Pediatr. Pulmonol.*, **3**, 334–351.

88. King, V.B. (1991) Upper respiratory disease, sinusitis, and polyposis. *Clin. Rev. Allergy*, **9**, 143–157.

89. Shwachman, H., Kulczycki, L.L. and Mueller, H.L. (1962) Nasal polyposis in patients with cystic fibrosis. *Pediatrics*, **30**, 389–401.

90. Stern, R.C., Boat, T.F., Wood, R.E. *et al.* (1982) Treatment and prognosis of nasal polyps in cystic fibrosis. *Am. J. Dis. Child.*, **136**, 1067–1070.

91. April, M.M., Tunkel, D.E., DeCelie-Germana, J. *et al.* (1995) Computed tomography (CT) scan findings of the paranasal sinuses in cystic fibrosis. *Am. J. Rhinology*, **9**, 277–280.

92. Ledesma-Medina, J., Osman, M.Z. and Girdany, B.R. (1980) Abnormal paranasal sinuses in patients with cystic fibrosis of the pancreas. Radiological findings. *Pediatr. Radiol.*, **9**, 61–64.

93. Waring, W.W., Brunt, C.H. and Hilman, B.C. (1967) Mucoid impaction of the bronchi in cystic fibrosis. *Pediatrics*, **39**,166–175.

94. Hansell, D.M. and Strickland, B. (1989) High-resolution computed tomography in pulmonary cystic fibrosis. *Br. J. Radiol.*, **62**, 1–5.

95. Santis, G., Hodson, M.E. and Strickland, B. (1991) High resolution computed tomography in adult cystic fibrosis patients with mild lung disease. *Clin. Radiol.*, **44**, 20-2-2.

96. Denning, C.R., Sommers, S.C. and Quigley, H.J. (1968) Infertility in male patients with cystic fibrosis. *Pediatrics*, **41**, 7–17.

97. Kaplan, E., Shwachman, H., Perlmutter, A.D. *et al.* (1968) Reproductive failure in males with cystic fibrosis. *NEJM*, **279**, 65–69.

98. Oppenheimer, E.H. and Esterly, J.R. (1969) Observations on cystic fibrosis of the pancreas v. development changes in the male genital system. *J. Pediatr.*, **75**, 806–811.

99. Dreyfus, D.H., Bethel, R. and Gelfand, E.W. (1996) Cystic fibrosis 3849 + 10 kb C→T mutation associated with severe pulmonary disease and male fertility. *Am. J. Respir. Crit. Care Med.*, **153**, 858–860.

100. Colin, A.A., Sawyer, S.M., Mickle, J.E. *et al.* (1996) Pulmonary function and clinical observations in men with congenital bilateral absence of the vas deferens. *Chest*, **110**, 440–445.

101. Rosenstein, B.J., Langbaum, T.S. and Winn, K. (1984) Unexpected diagnosis of cystic fibrosis at autopsy. *South Med. J.*, **77**, 1383–1385.

102. Tomashefski, J.F. Jr, Abramowsky, C.R. and Dahms, B.B. (1993) The pathology of cystic fibrosis, in *Cystic Fibrosis*, (ed. P.B. Davis), Marcel Dekker, New York, p. 467.

103. Ozguc, M., Tekin, A., Erdem, H. *et al.* (1994) Analysis of delta F508 mutation in cystic fibrosis pathology specimens. *Pediatr. Pathol.*, **14**, 491–496.

104. Salcedo, M., Chavez, M., Ridaura, C. *et al.* (1993) Detection of the cystic fibrosis delta-F508 mutation at autopsy by site-directed mutagenesis. *Am. J. Med. Genet.*, **46**, 268–270.

105. Palacios, J., Ezquieta, B., Gamallo, C. *et al.* (1994) Detection of delta F508 cystic fibrosis mutation by polymerase chain reaction from old paraffin-embedded tissues: a retrospective autopsy study. *Mod. Pathol.*, **7**, 392–395.

Screening

106. Crossley, J.R., Elliott, R.B. and Smith, P.A. (1979) Dried-blood spot screening for cystic fibrosis in the newborn. *Lancet*, **i**, 472–474.

107. Rommens, J.M., Iannuzzi, M.C., Kerem, B. *et al.* (1989) Identification of the cystic fibrosis gene; chromosome walking and jumping. *Science*, **245**, 1059–1065.

108. Riordan, J.R., Rommens, J.M., Kerem, B. *et al.* (1989) Identification of the cystic fibrosis gene:cloning and characterization of complementary DNA. *Science*, **245**, 1066–1073.

109. Kerem, B., Rommens, J.M., Buchanan, J.A., *et al.* (1989) Identification of the cystic fibrosis gene: genetic analysis. *Science*, **245**, 1073–1080.

110. Rock, M.J., Mischler, E.H., Farrell, P.M. *et al.* (1990) Newborn screening for cystic fibrosis is complicated by an age-related decline in immunoreactive trypsinogen levels. *Pediatrics*, **85**, 1001–1007.

111. Wilcken, B. and Brown, A. (1989) An analysis of false negative screening tests for cystic fibrosis, in *Current Trends in Infant Screening*, (ed. B.J. Schmidt, A.J. Diament, N.S. Login-Grossa), Excerpta Medica, Amsterdam, p. 19.

112. Ranieri, E., Lewis, B.D., Morris, C.P. and Wilcken, B. (1996) Neonatal screening using combined biochemical and DNA-based techniques, in: *Cystic Fibrosis: Current Topics*, (eds J. Dodge, D.J.H. Brock and J.H. Widdicombe), John Wiley & Sons, Chichester, Vol. III, pp. 181–206.

113. Chatfield, S., Owen, G., Ryley, H.C. *et al.* (1991) Neonatal screening for cystic fibrosis in Wales and the West Midlands: clinical assessment after five years of screening. *Arch. Dis. Child.*, **66**, 29–33.

114. Hammond, K.B., Abman, S.H., Sokol, R.J. and Accurso, F.J. (1991) Efficacy of statewide neonatal screening for cystic fibrosis by assay of trypsinogen concentrations. *NEJM*, **325**, 769–774.

115. Gregg, R.G., Simantel, A., Farrell, P.M. *et al.* (1997) Newborn screening for cystic fibrosis in Wisconsin: comparison of biochemical and molecular methods. *Pediatrics*, **99**, 819–824.

116. Wilcken, B., Wiley, V., Sherry, G. and Bayliss, U. (1995) Neonatal screening for cystic fibrosis: a comparison of two strategies for case detection in 1.2 million babies. *J. Pediatr.*, **127**, 965–970.

117. CF Genetic Analysis Consortium. Newsletter 69, July 30, 1997.

118. The Cystic Fibrosis Genetic Analysis Consortium (1990) Worldwide survey of the ΔF508 mutation. *Am. J. Hum. Genet.*, **47**, 354–359.

119. Schwarz, M.J., Malone, G.M., Hayworth, A. *et al.* (1995) Cystic fibrosis mutation analysis: report from 22 UK regional genetics laboratories. *Hum. Mutat.*, **45**, 326–333.

120. Ranieri, E., Lewis, B.D., Gerace, R.L. *et al.* (1994) Neonatal screening for cystic fibrosis using immunoreactive trypsinogen and direct gene analysis: four year's experience. *BMJ*, **308**, 1469–1472.

121. Ferec, C., Verlingue, C., Parent, P. *et al.* (1995) Neonatal screening for cystic fibrosis: result of a pilot study using both trypsinogen and cystic fibrosis gene mutation analysis. *Hum. Genet.*, **96**, 542–548.

122. Castellani, C., Bonizzatto, A. and Mastella, G. (1997) CFTR mutations and IVS8-5T variant in newborns with hypertrypsinaemia and normal sweat test. *J. Med. Genet.*, **34**, 297–301

123. di Sant'Agnese, P.A., Darling, R.C., Perera, G.A. and Shea, E. (1955) Abnormal electrolyte composition of sweat in cystic fibrosis of the pancreas: clinical significance and relationship to disease. *Pediatrics*, **12**, 549–563.

124. The Cystic Fibrosis Genotype–Phenotype Consortium (1993) Correlation between genotype and phenotype in patients with cystic fibrosis. *NEJM*, **329**, 1308–1313.

125. Gan, K.-H., Veeze, H.J., van den Ouweland, A.M.W. *et al.* (1995) A cystic fibrosis mutation associated with mild lung disease. *NEJM*, **333**, 95–99.

126. Augerten, A., Kerem, B., Yahav, Y. *et al.* (1993) Mild cystic fibrosis and normal or borderline sweat test in patients with the 3849 + 10 kb C-T mutation. *Lancet*, **342**, 25–26.

127. Highsmith, W.E., Burch, L.H., Zhou, Z. *et al.* (1994) A novel mutation in the cystic fibrosis gene in patients with pulmonary disease but normal sweat chloride concentrations. *NEJM*, **331**, 974–980.

128. Gilfillan, A., Warner, J.P., Kirk, J.M. *et al.* (1998) P67L: A cystic fibrosis allele with mild effects found at high frequency in the Scottish population. *J. Med. Genet.*, **35**, 122–125.

129. Chu, C.S., Trapnell, B.C., Curristin, S., Cutting, G.R. and Crystal, R.G. (1993) Genetic basis of variable exon 9 skipping in cystic fibrosis transmembrane conductance regulator mRNA. *Nature Genet.*, **3**, 151–156.

130. Chu, C.S., Trapnell, B.C., Murtagh, J.J. *et al.* (1991) Variable deletion of exon 9 coding sequences in cystic fibrosis transmembrane conductance regulator gene mRNA transcripts in normal bronchial epithelium. *EMBO J.*, **10**, 1355–1363.

131. Delaney, S.J., Rich, D.P., Thomson, S.A., *et al.* (1993) Cystic fibrosis transmembrane conductance regulator splice variants are not conserved and fail to produce chloride channels. *Nature Genet.*, **4**, 426–431.

132. Chin, S., Ranieri, E., Gerace, R.L., Nelson, P.V., and Carey, W.F. (1997) Trequency of intron 8 CFTR polythymidine sequence variant in neonatal blood specimens. *Lancet*, **350**, 1368–1369.

133. Dankert-Roelse, J.E. and te Meerman, G.J. (1995) Long term prognosis of patients with cystic fibrosis in relation to early detection by neonatal screening and treatment in a cystic fibrosis centre. *Thorax*, **50**, 712–718.

134. Farrall, P.M., Kosorok, M.R., Laxova, A. *et al.* (1997) Nutritional benefits of neonatal screening for cystic fibrosis. *NEJM*, **337**, 963–969.

135. National Institutes of Health Consensus Development Statement. Genetic Testing for Cystic Fibrosis. April 16, 1997.

136. Statement of The American Society of Human Genetics on Cystic Fibrosis Carrier Screening (1992). *Am. J. Hum. Genet.*, **51**, 1443–1444.

137. Brock, D.J.H. (1990) Population screening for cystic fibrosis. *Am. J. Hum. Genet.*, **47**, 164–165.

138. Zeesman, S., Clow, C.L., Cartier, L. and Scriver, C.R. (1984) A private view of heterozygosity: Eight year follow study of carriers of the Tay–Sachs gene detected by high-school screening in Montreal. *Am. J. Med. Genet.*, **18**, 769–778.

139. Scriver, C.R., Bardanis, M., Cartier, L. *et al.* (1984) β-

Thalassaemia disease prevention: genetic medicine applied. *Am. J. Hum. Genet.*, **35**, 1024–1038.

140. Kaplin, F., Clow, C., and Scriver, C.R. (1991) Cystic fibrosis carrier screening by DNA analysis: a pilot study of attitudes among participants. *Am. J. Hum. Genet.*, **49**, 240–242.

141. Scriver, C.R. and Clow, C.L. (1991) Carrier screening for Tay–Sachs disease. *Lancet*, **336**, 191.

142. Working Party of the Clinical Genetics Society (UK) (1994) The genetic testing of children. *J. Med. Genet.*, **31**, 785–797.

143. Watson, E.K., Mayall, E., Chappell, J. *et al.* (1991) Screening for carriers of cystic fibrosis through primary health care services. *BMJ*, **303**, 504–507.

144. Bekker, H., Modell, M., Denniss, G. *et al.* (1993) Uptake of cystic fibrosis testing in primary care: supply push or demand pull? *BMJ*, **306**, 1584–1586.

145. Tambor, E.S., Bernhardt, B.A., Chase, G.A. *et al.* (1994) Offering cystic fibrosis screening in an HMO population: factors affecting utilization. *Am. J. Hum. Genet.*, **55**, 626–637.

146. Brock, D.J.H., Shrimpton, A.E., Jones, C. and McIntosh, I. (1991) Cystic fibrosis: the new genetics. *J. Roy. Soc. Med.*, **84**, (Suppl. 18), 2–9.

147. Wald, N.J. (1991) Couple screening for cystic fibrosis. *Lancet*, **338**, 1318–1319.

148. Mennie, M.E., Gilfillan, A., Compton, M. *et al.* (1992) Prenatal screening for cystic fibrosis. *Lancet*, **340**, 214–216.

149. Schwartz, M., Brandt, N.J. and Skovby, F. (1994) Screening for carriers of cystic fibrosis among pregnant women; a pilot study. *Eur. J. Hum. Genet.*, **1**, 239–244.

150. Jung, U., Urner, U., Grade, K. and Coutelle, C. (1994) Acceptability of carrier screening for cystic fibrosis during pregnancy in a German population. *Hum. Genet.*, **94**, 19–24.

151. Miedzybroddzka, Z.H., Hall, M.H., Mollison, J. *et al.* (1995) Antenatal screening for carriers of cystic fibrosis: randomised trial of stepwise v. couple screening. *BMJ*, **310**, 353–357.

152. Witt, D.R., Schaefer, C., Hallam, P. *et al.* (1996) Cystic fibrosis heterozygote screening in 5161 pregnant women. *Am. J. Hum. Genet.*, **58**, 823–825.

153. Loader, S., Caldwell, P., Kozyra, A. *et al.* (1996) Cystic fibrosis carrier population screening in the primary care setting. *Am. J. Hum. Genet.*, **59**, 234–247.

154. Cuckle, H., Quirke, P., Sehmi, I. *et al.* (1996) Antenatal screening for cystic fibrosis. *Br. J. Obstet. Gynaec.*, **103**, 795–799.

155. Brambati, B., Anelli, M.C. and Tului, L. (1996) Prenatal cystic fibrosis screening in a low-risk population undergoing chorionic villus sampling for fetal karyotyping. *Clin. Genet.*, **50**, 23–27.

156. Grody, W.W., Dunkel-Schetter, C., Tatsugawa, Z.H. *et al.* (1997) PCR-based screening for cystic fibrosis carrier mutations in an ethnically diverse pregnant population. *Am. J. Hum. Genet.*, **60**, 935–947.

157. Brock, D.J.H. (1996) Prenatal screening for cystic fibrosis: 5 years' experience reviewed. *Lancet.*, **347**, 148–150.

158. Wald, N.J., George, L., Wald, N. and Mckenzie, I.Z. (1995) Further observations in connection with couple screening for cystic fibrosis. *Prenat. Diagn.*, **15**, 589–590.

159. Doherty, R.A., Palomaki, G.E., Kloza, E.M., Erickson, J.L. and Haddow, J.E. (1996) Couple-based prenatal screening for cystic fibrosis in primary care settings. *Prenat. Diagn.*, **16**, 397–404.

160. Harris, H., Scotcher, D., Hartlie, N. *et al.* (1993) Cystic fibrosis carrier testing in early pregnancy by general practitioners. *BMJ*, **306**, 1580–1583.

161. Mennie, M.E., Compton, M.E., Gilfillan, A. *et al.* (1993) Prenatal screening for cystic fibrosis: psychological effects on carriers and their partners. *J. Med. Genet.*, **30**, 543–548.

162. Super, M., Schwarz, M.J., Malone, G., Roberts, T., Haworth, A. and Dermody, G. (1994) Active cascade testing for carriers of cystic fibrosis gene. *BMJ*, **308**, 1462–1468.

163. Holloway, S.H. and Brock, D.J.H. (1994) Cascade testing for identification of carriers of cystic fibrosis. *J. Med. Screen.*, **1**, 159–164.

10

Respiratory system

10a Pediatrics *S.G. Marshall, M. Rosenfeld and*
B.W. Ramsey 204

Overview 204

Clinical presentation 205

Radiographic and laboratory assessment of the
child with CF 207

Complications 211

Treatment of respiratory disease in children with CF 212

Conclusion 217

10b Adults *M. E. Hodson* 218

Introduction 218

Microbiology 218

Symptoms 219

Physical signs 220

Investigations 220

Treatment 222

Complications 226

Home treatment 229

Terminal care 230

Travel 231

Arranging a system of care 231

Scoring systems 231

References 232

Pediatrics

S. G. MARSHALL, M. ROSENFELD AND B. W. RAMSEY

OVERVIEW

Although cystic fibrosis (CF) is a genetic disorder affecting epithelial cells of multiple organs, it is the respiratory tract which is associated with the most significant morbidity. Ultimately, respiratory failure is the cause of death in over 90 per cent of cases[1,2]. The abnormal gene and its protein product, the cystic fibrosis transmembrane regulator (CFTR) have been identified[3–5]. This protein, which is a cyclic AMP regulated chloride channel[6], is known to be expressed in the apical surface of respiratory epithelial cells, as well as in airway submucosal glands[7]. In patients with CF, the abnormal gene product is associated with relative impermeability of cellular chloride ion flow from epithelial cells, which is felt to lead secondarily to reduced water content in epithelial secretions[8]. It is hypothesized that the 'dehydrated' state of secretions affects the rheologic properties of these secretions, leading to altered mucociliary clearance mechanisms[9]. The altered rheology and clearance do not fully explain the recurrent infections which plague the CF airways. Several hypotheses have emerged in the past 5 years which may begin to explain the pathogenesis of CF lung disease. The propensity for *P. aeruginosa* infection may be explained in part by the observation that this pathogen demonstrates increased binding to cultured airway epithelial cells from patients with CF[10]. This abnormal bacterial binding may be due to the increased concentration of asialoglycoproteins on the surface of CF epithelia due to altered sialylation of exported complex sugars from these cells[11].

A second intriguing observation has been the recent reports by researchers at University of Iowa[12] that an abnormal composition of the airway surface liquid (ASL) or fluid (ASF) covering CF respiratory epithelial cells may inhibit bactericidal activity. These investigators found that normal ASL contains substances, such as β-defensins, lysozyme and lactoferrin, that kill bacterial pathogens in tissue-culture experiments. The difference between normal and CF ASL appears to be the salt concentration; CF ASL has an abnormally high NaCl content. Antimicrobial activity of ASL is inhibited as salt concentration increases. These data could provide a link between the molecular and physiologic abnormalities in CF (i.e. the loss of CFTR chloride channels and airway infections). Future studies are needed to measure the actual salt concentration of ASL *in vivo* and to learn more about how bacterial killing occurs in the complex environment of the airway surface.

Although the abnormal CFTR and ion transport are present at birth[13], the lungs are sterile and normal in appearance, by both gross and microscopic examination[14–16]. The earliest pathologic changes observed are plugging of bronchioles with secretions[17]. Bedrossian *et al.*[18] noted in a retrospective study of autopsy specimens that by 4 months of age, over half of the infants on whom data was collected had mucopurulent plugging, inflammatory infiltrates and epithelial metaplasia. Chow *et al.*[15] also found polymorphonuclear infiltrates in 38 per cent of infants who had died within 21 days of birth. The submucosal glands in the proximal airways demonstrate normal morphology at birth, but become hypertrophied with mucous plugging (Fig. 10.1) over the first months of life.

The changes occur initially in small airways, with progression towards larger, central airways[16]. Mucus plugging and inflammatory infiltrates progress to bronchiolitis and bronchiectasis[19]. Although parenchymal involvement occurs, it is much less important than airway changes[20]. Associated with bronchiectasis is formation of new vessels and bronchopulmonary shunting. In addition, chronic hypoxia leads to pulmonary arterial vasoconstriction and eventually irreversible changes in vessel walls with muscularization of pulmonary vasculature[21].

It is apparent from both our understanding of the basic defect and from pathologic studies that the respiratory manifestations of this disorder frequently begin in infancy, requiring vigilance in identification of new cases and early therapeutic intervention.

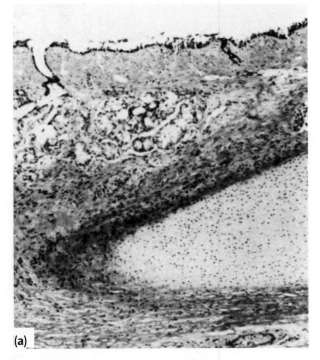
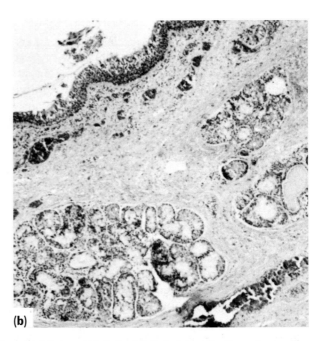

Fig. 10.1 *Light micrographs showing a cross-section of the trachea from* **(a)** *a 1-day-old infant who died of complications of meconium ileus and* **(b)** *an 18-month-old with minimal respiratory symptoms who died of sudden infant death syndrome. Note the relatively normal morphology of the submucosal glands in the neonate* **(a)**, *with the exception of some mucous plugging in the ducts of the gland. By age 18 months* **(b)** *there is hypertrophy of submucosal glands with an increase in mucous plugging.*

CLINICAL PRESENTATION

In a review of the incidence and presentation of cystic fibrosis in Victoria, Australia, over a 24-year period (1955–78) approximately one-third (37 per cent) of 580 children presented with respiratory infections; the majority in the first year of life[22]. Among children diagnosed with cystic fibrosis in the United States, 50.2 per cent presented with respiratory symptoms per the 1996 CF Patient Registry[23]. The most frequent symptoms are cough, tachypnea and wheezing. Infants are frequently diagnosed following recurrent or persistent bronchiolitis[24]. The frequency of wheezing in CF infants is now known. In one study[25], 50 per cent of 28 children (mean age 16 months) with mild respiratory involvement had a history of wheezing, and 43 per cent were responsive to bronchodilator therapy. As children with CF get older, a proportion will continue to have periodic wheezing and a reactive component, but the response to bronchodilators becomes more variable[26].

The most persistent respiratory symptom is cough. The infant or young child may have cough only with intercurrent illnesses (see viral infections, below), but will eventually develop a daily cough usually most prominent in the morning. It is rare for the infant or toddler to expectorate. In a bronchoscopy study done at our institution[27], we found that expectoration more strongly correlated with age rather than the bacterial pathogen colonizing the lower airway. The cough is frequently paroxysmal and in the infant and young child may be associated with emesis. In the small infant it may be misdiagnosed as a pertussis-like syndrome.

Children with CF may experience low-grade fevers with respiratory infections but high fevers are unusual and frequently associated with non-CF-related respiratory infection. Unless severely malnourished, these children have normal systemic immunity[28] and are not at increased risk of bacterial sepsis or meningitis.

Because cystic fibrosis is a life-threatening disease affecting several organ systems, it is recommended by the US Cystic Fibrosis Foundation (CFF) that all patients be evaluated at least quarterly at a regional CF center[29]. Centers are staffed with physicians, nurses, dieticians and social workers, all trained specifically in the nuances of this disease. Patients may be seen by any or all staff, depending on the nature of the visit. A complete clinical evaluation is undertaken, including a review of the nutritional, gastrointestinal, ear/nose/throat, psychosocial and pulmonary aspects of the patient's illness. The remainder of this section will be directed primarily to the respiratory tract examination of the child with CF.

Physical examination of a child with CF should be undertaken with the child as comfortable and calm as possible (frequently on a parent's lap), and undressed so the entire chest can be visualized (Fig. 10.2). The child's respirations should be observed to determine resting respiratory rate, as well as his work of breathing (i.e. use of accessory muscles and intercostal muscle retractions). The degree of hyperinflation (Fig. 10.3) can be assessed by direct visualization or by measuring the mid-inspiration circumference of the chest at the mammary level and comparing this measure with normative values[30]. Calipers may also be used to measure the ratio of anteroposterior (A–P) and transverse chest wall diameters at the mammary level, which is the thoracic index. There is a wide range of normal values[31] so that serial measurements in children are most useful. A thoracic index greater than one is consistent with chronic hyperinflation.

Lung auscultation may be normal in children with mild pulmonary involvement. With increasing airway obstruction, the examiner will note an increased expiratory phase, expiratory polyphonic wheezes and coarse crackles. The breath sounds may be asymmetric, depending on regions of mucous plugging and atelecta-

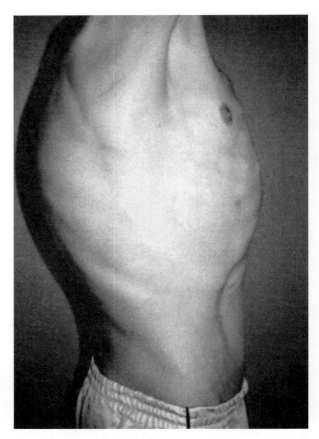

Fig. 10.3 *Lateral view of a 14-year-old male with CF and severe obstructive airway disease, demonstrating a marked increase in apical–posterior diameter, with outward bowing of the sternum and kyphosis of the spine. Also, note the fat and muscle wasting of his upper extremity.*

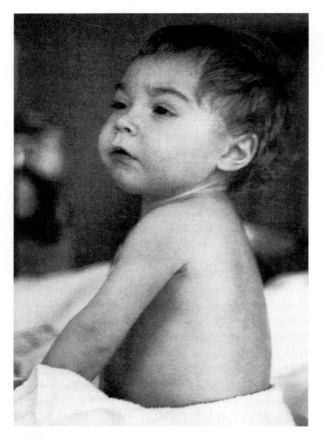

Fig. 10.2 *Photograph of a 2-year-old male with moderate pulmonary disease who already has an increase in apical–posterior diameter of his thorax. He is sitting comfortably with his chest exposed so the examiner may observe his resting respiratory rate, use of accessory respiratory muscles and the presence of intercostal retractions or nasal flaring. (Reproduced with the parents' permission.)*

sis. Because mobilization of airway secretions may significantly change auscultatory findings, it is important to ask the older, cooperative child to cough and clear secretions prior to auscultation. It is also helpful to know the time of the child's last chest physiotherapy.

The nasopharynx and oropharynx of the child with CF should be closely inspected in conjunction with the lung examination. The nares are frequently swollen and erythematous with either clear or purulent discharge. Nasal polyps are rarely seen in the infant but are increasingly common in the preschool and school-age child. There is a common association between sinusitis and nasal polyposis. Presentation of nasal polyps is most common between 5 and 14 years of age[32]. The sinuses are rarely tender to palpation, even though over 90 per cent will be opacified on radiographic examination[33]. Chronic ethmoiditis may lead to broadening of the nasal bridge, which is most evident in the school-age and adolescent patient[34]. Chronic nasal and sinus purulent drainage into the posterior pharynx will produce a cobblestone appearance. Although otitis media can occur in children with CF, it does not occur at a greater frequency than in normal children.

Examination of the extremities for clubbing and cyanosis are useful adjuncts to the assessment of pulmonary status. Clubbing refers to focal enlargement of terminal phalanges of fingers and toes (Fig. 10.4). Although the etiology is unknown, it has been hypothesized that elevated circulating levels of prostaglandins $F_{2\alpha}$ and E may lead to clubbing in these patients[35]. Some clinicians have found it useful to quantify the degree of clubbing[36,37] as a measure of disease progression. For routine clinical practice, it is easiest to assess clubbing by placing the dorsal surfaces of the terminal phalanges of similar fingers together and look for a loss of a 'diamond-shaped' window (Schamroth's sign)[38].

Cyanosis, which refers to blue coloring of the skin and mucous membranes, is the result of reduced hemoglobin in the capillaries. Approximately 4–6 g of reduced hemoglobin per 100 mL of capillary blood are necessary to produce cyanosis[39]. This concentration of reduced hemoglobin is equivalent to a capillary oxygen saturation (Sao_2) of approximately 75 per cent, and is therefore an insensitive measure of hemoglobin desaturation. The presence of cyanosis is also dependent on the rate of blood flow through tissues. Thus, the infant or toddler with cool extremities can appear to have acrocyanosis in the presence of normal oxygen saturation.

Assessment of nutritional status and growth should be an integral part of the pulmonary examination of a child with CF. An appropriate nutritional assessment is outlined in Chapter 11 of this book. The child with chronic respiratory infections and increased work of breathing will require significantly more calories for adequate

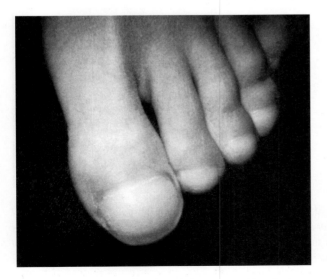

Fig. 10.4 *Pictured is the right foot of the 14-year-old male shown in Fig. 10.3, which displays clubbing or enlargement of the terminal phalanges. The great toes and thumbs frequently demonstrate the most striking changes. In less severe cases, the clinician may assess clubbing by placing the dorsal surfaces of the terminal phalanges of similar fingers together and looking for a loss of a 'diamond-shaped' window (Schamroth's sign)[38].*

growth than a normal child. A sudden fall off in growth in a child with CF who has adequate pancreatic enzyme replacement is frequently a sensitive marker for increased pulmonary disease.

RADIOGRAPHIC AND LABORATORY ASSESSMENT OF THE CHILD WITH CF

Chest imaging techniques

The chest radiograph has been the primary diagnostic method for assessing progression of pulmonary disease during the past 40 years[2,40]. It has been particularly helpful in the child too young to cooperate with pulmonary function testing. The radiographic changes are consistent with progressive, obstructive airway disease[41]. The initial findings are peribronchial thickening (cuffing of end-on bronchi), and irregular aeration with some regions of patchy atelectasis[42]. There is progressive hyperaeration, evidenced by flattening of the diaphragms and increasing A–P diameter (most apparent on lateral examination) and bowing of the sternum (Fig. 10.5). With moderate disease, nodular shadows ranging from 2 to 5 mm in diameter may appear. With more advanced disease, hilar adenopathy, segmental and lobar atelectasis, cyst formation and bronchiectasis become evident (Fig. 10.6).

Several systems exist to quantify the severity of chest radiograph findings in CF patients[43–46]. While the Crispin system is more commonly utilized in Europe and the UK, the Brasfield system is the most widely used in the USA[46]. The Wisconsin scoring system was specifically developed for use in young subjects, and has been shown to be more sensitive than the Brasfield score for mild disease[44]. Pulmonary function has been shown to correlate well with chest radiograph scores in school-age children[47–50] and adults[51,52]. Spirometry seems to be more sensitive than chest radiograph score in detecting small changes in pulmonary status[51]. The relationship of pulmonary function tests to chest radiograph scores in young children has not been assessed systematically.

There are recent reports[53–56] suggesting that the use of high-resolution computed tomography (HRCT) may improve our ability to image pulmonary architectural abnormalities in patients with CF. HRCT better identifies and assesses the type and distribution of bronchial and parenchymal lesions, particularly when chest radiographs are unclear, and may help with clinical management. Further, HRCT correlates well with pulmonary function at time of scanning and at follow-up, and with clinical progress in patients with CF[55]. However, several technical challenges must be overcome before this newer imaging technique is applicable universally in children, including the need for sedation, the cost and increased radiation exposure over time.

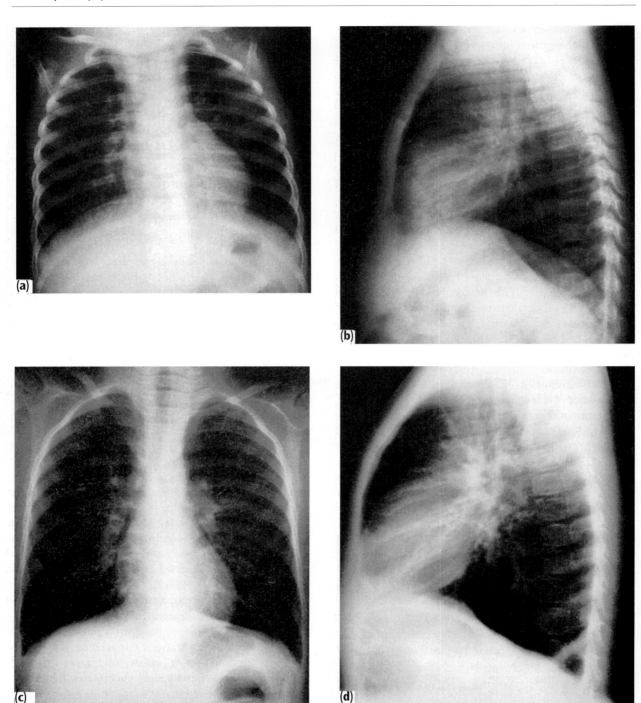

Fig. 10.5 *A 5-month-old girl with CF and persistent tachypnea and wheezing. Frontal (**a**) and lateral (**b**) radiographs show bilateral hyper-aeration. Bronchial-wall thickening is evident as peribronchial cuffing. By age 3 years, the frontal (**c**) and lateral (**d**) radiographs show a progression of hyperaeration, as evidenced by flattening of the diaphragm and outward bowing of the sternum on the lateral view. In addition, thickened bronchi are evident on end in the left perihilar region and are patchy nodular and linear densities.*

Pulmonary function testing

With sufficient training and patience, spirometry can be performed reproducibly in most children of 5 years or older, and plethysmography performed in most school-age children. At accredited CF centers in the US, spiro-metric values are recorded every 3–6 months[29] when the child is stable, and during acute illnesses to assess response to appropriate therapy[57]. Pulmonary function should be tested according to ATS guidelines[58,59]. Because pulmonary function varies physiologically by age, height, and gender, standardization for these factors is

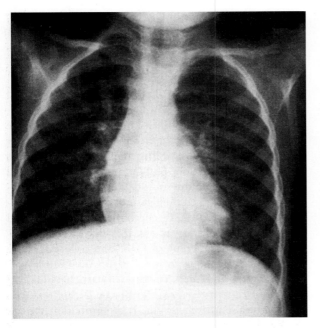

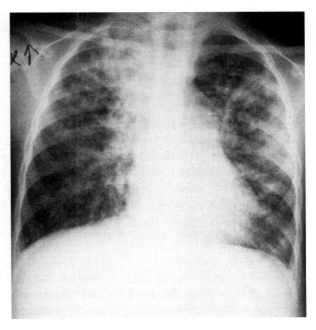

(a)   **(b)**

Fig. 10.6 *The progression of lung disease is displayed in frontal radiographs taken at ages 3 years (**a**) and 6 years (**b**) in a girl with persistent* P. aeruginosa *endobronchial infections. Note the increase in bilateral nodular lesions, interspersed with small cystic lesions which become more prominent over 3 years. She also displays thickened bronchi on end and* en face. *By age 6 (**b**) she had persistent atelectasis in the right upper lobe, and patchy atelectasis in the right lower lobe. She underwent right upper lobectomy 6 months after the second radiograph, which resulted in fewer fevers and improved respiratory symptoms.*

performed in order to allow meaningful comparisons between different subjects, as well as between measures over time in a given subject. Standardization is accomplished by transforming absolute measures to a percentage of predicted for age, height and gender based on data from a comparable reference population[60,61].

The physiologic hallmark of CF lung disease is airway obstruction. Pulmonary function is the clinical measure most highly predictive of mortality[62–64]. The earliest changes in pulmonary function in school-age children with CF are those of small airway obstruction (decline in flows at the midportion of vital capacity, $FEF_{25-75\%}$) and progressive hyperinflation (increased ratio of residual volume to total lung capacity, RV/TLC)[65–67]. The forced expiratory volume in one second (FEV_1) decreases later, and expiratory flows continue to decline over the lifetime of the patient. Progressive airway obstruction eventually causes a decline in forced vital capacity (FVC). $FEF_{25-75\%}$ is the most sensitive measure of early airway obstruction, but it possesses greater intra- and inter-subject variability than FEV_1[68]. FEV_1 and FVC are more stable measures of pulmonary function in patients with moderate to severe disease.

Relative to patients with a normal FEV_1 (>80 per cent predicted), the risk of death 2 years later is 14-fold greater for patients with moderate airway obstruction (95 per cent confidence interval (CI) 8,25), and 57-fold

greater for patients with severe airway obstruction (95 per cent CI, 33,99)[63]. Two-year mortality is about 50 per cent once the FEV_1 reaches 30 per cent of the predicted value[62]. Acquisition of the mucoid phenotype of *P. aeruginosa*[69,70], colonization with *Burkholderia cepacia*[71] and female gender[62,63,69] are risk factors for more rapid decline in FEV_1.

With the advent of new therapeutic modalities, it is increasingly important to have the capability of measuring pulmonary function in patients too young to cooperate with spirometry. In the past decade, innovative new methods for assessing respiratory mechanics in infants and young children have been developed, and older techniques have continued to evolve. Although still used primarily for research purposes, the marketing of commercial devices has increased the availability of these techniques. The procedures are generally performed under sedation (typically with chloral hydrate), they require specialized training and equipment to perform, and testing times are long. Equipment standards and procedural guidelines are being developed[72,73]. Reference values exist for some measurements[74–76]. Infant pulmonary function techniques can generally be carried out in children under the age of 3 years. Few methods are available for subjects between 3 and 5 years of age, who are too old for infant techniques and yet generally not able to perform spirometry. The most widely employed noninvasive methods will be summarized here. The reader is referred to a recent textbook[72] and several excellent reviews[73,77–79] for more detail.

Forced expiratory flows are generally measured in infants using the rapid thoracic compression ('squeeze') technique, first described in 1978 by Adler and Wohl[80] and later modified[81]. In this technique, an inflatable jacket around the thorax and abdomen of the sedated infant is rapidly inflated at the end of a tidal inspiration. The compression of the chest wall by the jacket produces a forced tidal expiration, with exhalation continuing to a point below functional residual capacity (FRC). Flow is measured at the mouth by a pneumotachograph with a face mask, and integrated to obtain volume. With each expiratory maneuver, a partial expiratory flow volume loop is generated, from which flow at FRC can be measured. Compressive pressures are progressively increased until the maximal flow at FRC, V_{max}FRC, is obtained. Partial expiratory flows in CF infants have been shown to be associated with genotype[82], presenting symptoms[83] and pulmonary function at follow-up[84]. Normative data, though limited, are more extensive for V_{max}FRC measurements than for other infant pulmonary function techniques[75,76].

The most significant limitation of partial expiratory flow volume measures is that flow limitation is not produced in all infants. Measurements without true flow limitation are effort-dependent, submaximal and an inaccurate reflection of underlying lung mechanics[79,85]. Flow limitation is more likely to be achieved in infants with underlying obstructive lung disease, but simple, noninvasive methods to assess flow limitation are lacking. Additionally, flows are measured at low lung volumes, where variability is high, and FRC is a volume landmark known to vary with dead space, disease state and sleep state[86,87].

Recent promising modifications of the technique have increased the lung volume range over which expiratory flows are assessed, thereby avoiding the limitations of tidal volume measurements. Turner *et al.* have used a pump to increase lung volumes rapidly prior to a forced expiratory maneuver[88,89]. Castile and colleagues have developed a technique that interrupts spontaneous respiratory muscle activity long enough to perform a raised volume forced expiratory maneuver unimpeded by reflex inspiration[90]. Several sigh-like breaths are delivered in phase with the infant's respiratory cycle, producing a short pause in respiration. Another augmented inflation is then performed, followed by a rapid thoracic compression maneuver. By inhibiting reflex inspiratory effort and extending the lung volume range over which flows can be assessed, their technique allows flow limitation to be achieved in all subjects[90]. Flow–volume curves generated by these new raised-volume techniques appear similar to those produced by standard adult-type spirometry. Raised volume measures appear to have improved sensitivity relative to V_{max}FRC in detecting reduced lung function in CF[88] and chronically wheezy[89] infants.

Functional residual capacity (FRC), the volume of gas in the lungs and airways at end-expiration, can be measured in infants by gas dilution techniques or whole-body plethysmography. The helium dilution and nitrogen washout gas dilution techniques yield comparable results[91]. Because both techniques cannot measure gas trapped in noncommunicating lung regions, they may underestimate true resting lung volume in subjects with airway obstruction. Body plethysmography, based on Boyle's law, measures all the gas in the thorax (thoracic gas volume), including gas not in direct communication with the airways. By combining data from raised volume forced expiratory maneuvers with FRC measurements by plethysmography, Castile and colleagues have developed a technique to measure fractional lung volumes in young children[92]. The ratio of residual volume to total lung capacity (RV/TLC) in young children may prove to be a sensitive measure of hyperinflation and gas trapping, as it is in older subjects[68].

Several techniques exist for measuring compliance and resistance in infants. The most widely used measure of passive compliance, resistance and time constant of the respiratory system is the passive deflation technique. A brief airway occlusion at end-inspiration induces the Hering–Breuer reflex, causing relaxation of expiratory muscles during the deflation following the occlusion. Pressure at the airway opening is measured during the occlusion, and a straight line is fit to the flow–volume curve obtained during the passive deflation, allowing the measurement of resistance and compliance from a single breath. Although these techniques have yielded much information about respiratory physiology in infants, limitations still need to be addressed. The primary limitation of these measures is that the extrathoracic airway is the major component of the total airway resistance, potentially masking changes in lower airway resistance. Additionally, clinically undetectable laryngeal braking (grunting) during expiration may falsely elevate compliance values. There is a paucity of normative data for these techniques and standardization is lacking.

Assessment of arterial oxygen saturation

Ventilatory inhomogeneity and ventilation–perfusion imbalance frequently lead to some degree of hypoxemia even in young children with CF with mild change in pulmonary function[93]. Hypercapnia is usually a later finding in the child with moderate to severe obstructive disease. Quantitation of hypoxemia and hypercapnia is most accurately measured by analysis of the partial pressures of oxygen (P_{O_2}) and carbon dioxide (P_{CO_2}) in arterial blood. Because arterial blood sampling is a painful procedure, pulse oximetry is now widely used as a noninvasive means of estimating arterial oxygen saturation, with capillary blood gas measurements indicating values for pH and $P\text{CO}_2$. With proper usage[94] oximetry is a reproducible and sensitive measure which is useful for routine clinical assessments.

Identification of respiratory pathogens

Chronic colonization of the respiratory tract with bacterial pathogens such as *Pseudomonas aeruginosa* is strongly associated with progression of pulmonary disease[95–99]. Thus, accurate identification of lower airway pathogens is of utmost importance in the clinical management of patients with CF. In subjects old enough to expectorate, sputum specimens are a reliable source for identification of lower airway bacteria[100–102]. The Cystic Fibrosis Foundation recommends complete microbiologic assessment of expectorated sputum, as well as antibiotic susceptibility testing of bacterial pathogens, on an annual basis and during pulmonary exacerbations[103]. In subjects too young to expectorate (generally below 6 years of age), the appropriate source of respiratory cultures remains a dilemma. Oropharyngeal (OP) specimens are frequently utilized as a noninvasive source of respiratory secretions for culture in pre-expectorating patients. Recent studies have evaluated the diagnostic accuracy of oropharyngeal cultures relative to lower airway cultures obtained by bronchoalveolar lavage (BAL). In two studies in children with CF ≤3 years of age, the sensitivity of oropharyngeal cultures for detecting *Pseudomonas aeruginosa* (Pa) in the lower airway was about 50 per cent, while the specificity was about 95 per cent[27,104,105]. Though obviously dependent on the prevalence of Pa, the negative predictive value of oropharyngeal cultures is much higher than the positive predictive value in very young children. Among 141 infants with a mean age of 11 months and a prevalence of Pa in the lower airway of 5 per cent, oropharyngeal cultures had a positive predictive value of 50 per cent and a negative predictive value of 95 per cent[105]. Among 26 subjects with a mean age 4.5 years and a prevalence of Pa in the lower airway of 45 per cent, OP cultures had a positive predictive value of 83 per cent and a negative predictive value of 70 per cent[27]. In summary, in very young children, a negative throat culture may be helpful in ruling out the presence of Pa in the lower respiratory tract, but a positive culture does not reliably rule in the presence of lower airway organisms. The poor predictive value of oropharyngeal cultures has led a growing number of CF centers to incorporate bronchoscopy for lower-airway cultures into the standard care of the infant with CF.

Although the data regarding lower airway bacteriology in infants are limited[104,106–108], it appears that these children are colonized in the first months of life with *H. influenzae* and *S. aureus* and somewhat later by *P. aeruginosa*. Abman *et al.*[106] noted that in 42 infants the mean age for initial isolation for these three pathogens was as follows: *S. aureus*, 12.4 ± 9.5 months; *H. influenzae*, 18.6 ± 12 months; and *P. aeruginosa*, 20.8 ± 10.4 months. *Klebsiella* species have also been noted in younger patients[24,27].

Infants and young children have the highest rates of respiratory viral infection, often at a time of crucial lung growth. Respiratory syncytial virus (RSV) infections are known to cause significant morbidity and mortality in infants with chronic cardiopulmonary disorders[109,110]. Infants with CF are six times more likely than normal infants to require hospitalization during a viral infection[111] and pulmonary function is significantly worse[25]. These infants with RSV infection may have prolonged hospitalization (longer than 22 days) and persistent hypoxemia[112]. Thus, it is important to identify respiratory viral pathogens in acutely ill infants by fluorescent antibody, immunoassay or culture.

In addition to the pathogens discussed above, unusual pathogens and highly antibiotic-resistant organisms, including *Burkholderia cepacia*, *Alcaligenes xylosoxidans* and *Stenotrophomonas maltophilia*, are more frequently recovered from patients with more advanced disease. Fungal species, including *Candida* species and *Aspergillus fumigatus*, and nontuberculosis mycobacterial infections are also of increasing concern in the pediatric as well as the adult population of CF patients, and are discussed at greater length in Chapter 5.

COMPLICATIONS

Chronic endobronchial infection and the secondary inflammatory response eventually lead to airway destruction and progressive bronchiectasis. With improved treatment regimens and prolonged survival, the development of severe bronchiectasis and its sequelae, hemoptysis and rupture of apical bullae leading to pneumothorax, occur predominantly in late adolescence and adulthood. Discussion of these complications is thus included in the subsequent section on pulmonary disease in the adult patient with CF.

There are several complications associated with the respiratory tract which may occur in the younger child:

1. bronchiolitis with or without acute respiratory failure;
2. lobar atelectasis;
3. staphyloccocal pneumonia with pneumatoceles; and
4. gastroesophageal reflux.

Bronchiolitis is a common complication in the first 2 years and, as mentioned previously, is often the presenting symptom at the time of diagnosis[22-24]. RSV is a common etiologic agent which can be readily identified by fluorescent antibody[113]. Initiation of ribavirin within the first 72 hours of infection has been effective in shortening hospitalization and hypoxemia in some infants with RSV and chronic cardiopulmonary disorders[109,110].

Bacterial pathogens, including *S. aureus*, *Klebsiella* and *P. aeruginosa* have been associated with a bronchiolitis presentation as well[24]. It is often difficult to assess whether the bacterial infection is primary or secondary. Some infants with bronchiolitis progress to respiratory failure requiring mechanical ventilation. This presentation was once felt to portend a grave prognosis[24,114,115]. However, improved medical management with better infant ventilators, as well as aggressive use of bronchodilators, appropriate antibiotics and prolonged oxygen supplementation, have significantly improved prognosis for these infants[112,116].

Patchy atelectasis is a common finding, but lobar atelectasis occurs in less than 5 per cent of cases. The right middle lobe in the most common site of prolonged or recurrent atelectasis in the young child. Aggressive use of chest physiotherapy, antibiotics and bronchodilators will frequently resolve the atelectasis and should be attempted prior to bronchoscopic examination and suctioning[2,117]. Even following bronchoscopy, recurrence is common.

Staphylococcal pneumonia was a common cause of death in CF infants in the 1950s and 1960s[118]. The introduction of effective anti-staphylococcal antibiotics and a probable change in the virulence of *S. aureus* during the past 15 years has almost eliminated this complication.

Gastroesophageal reflux is now recognized as a frequent complication of infants and children with cystic fibrosis[119-121]. The probable etiology is increased intra-abdominal pressure and negative intrathoracic pressure associated with coughing and chronic airway obstruction. Although adults will frequently complain of retrosternal chest pain, the infant will usually present with recurrent vomiting, poor weight gain, irritability, as well as increased wheezing and reactive airway disease[122]. Prolonged esophageal pH probe monitoring[123,124] and radionuclide gastroesophagography[125] may be used to aid in diagnosis. Medical treatment with positioning[126], thickening of feeds[127] and H_2-receptor blockers[128] is usually effective and preferable to surgical intervention[129].

TREATMENT OF RESPIRATORY DISEASE IN CHILDREN WITH CF

Introduction

Until therapies become available to treat the underlying genetic abnormality with either gene or protein replacement therapy, the primary goal of the clinician caring for children with cystic fibrosis must be to prevent progressive airway destruction (i.e. bronchiectasis). Because bronchiectasis is the natural sequela of prolonged infection, therapy must be directed towards appropriate treatment of infection with antimicrobial agents as well as optimizing the clearance of airway secretions. There has also been increasing interest in recent years in modulating the host inflammatory response in an attempt to delay airway destruction.

In the following section, several important aspects of pulmonary management in children will be discussed, including:

1. clearance techniques and the role of mucolytics and bronchodilators in mobilization of airway secretions;
2. the use of anti-inflammatory agents; and
3. appropriate antimicrobial therapy for the most common bacterial pathogens.

Enhancement of airway clearance

AIRWAY CLEARANCE TECHNIQUES

Airway clearance techniques (ACTs) are measures used at most stages of CF to improve mucociliary clearance. Chest physiotherapy using percussion and postural drainage, as well as special breathing exercises, are utilized by patients worldwide. Conventional chest physiotherapy utilizes vibration to mobilize entrapped mucus, with clearance enhanced by changes in patient position. Percussion can be accomplished by cupping (or clapping) of the hand, with a mechanical percusser (or vibrator), or with vest/pulse generators. Chest physiotherapy can be time consuming and compliance is a problem. Alternative ACT maneuvers include active cycle of breathing (ACB) technique, positive expiratory pressure (PEP) mask, autogenic drainage, use of an oscillating Flutter® device, and a therapy vest which provides high-frequency chest compression (HFCC). These modalities of therapy are discussed in detail in Chapter 19.

There are limited data documenting short- or long-term effectiveness of airway clearance techniques, and no consensus about which form is ideal for a given clinical scenario[130,131]. However, these techniques are still widely used, and many recommend initiating ACTs at time of diagnosis, even in children where pulmonary disease has not yet been documented.

MUCOLYTIC AGENTS

Purulent airway secretions from patients with cystic fibrosis are highly viscous, impairing proper mucociliary clearance. The abnormal viscoelastic properties of these secretions are primarily due to the highly polymerized, polyanionic deoxyribose nucleic acid (DNA)[132], which is the by-product of degenerating polymorphonuclear neutrophils in the airways[133]. Other factors which have been hypothesized to contribute to the viscosity are the elevated protein content[134] and abnormal hydration[9] and sulfation[135] state of mucopolysaccharides.

For many years, mucolytic agents have been advocated as adjuvant therapy to improve clearance of secretions. Proteolytic agents, such as trypsin, were utilized in the 1950s, but soon fell into disfavor due to airway irritation and allergic reaction[136]. Agents such as *N*-acetyl cysteine, which presumably depolymerizes glycoproteins by cleaving disulfide bonds, have been used empirically for many years. This agent has not been shown to have a significant beneficial effect for patients with CF[137]. In some patients, *N*-acetyl cysteine may be irritating to the tracheobronchial mucosa and impair ciliary function[138].

In recent years, a recombinant human DNase (Pulmozyme®) has been developed which is capable of depolymerizing endogenous human DNA and dramatically reduces the viscosity of CF sputum[139]. Phase I and phase II clinical trials of aerosolized rhDNase (commercially available as dornase alfa) showed that it was both safe and effective[140-143]. Following these studies, a 24-week open-label phase II study of an intermittent, high-dose regimen showed that efficacy of this new mucolytic agent did not diminish with repeated exposure over 6 months, and that maintenance of efficacy was dependent upon regular daily administration[144].

The phase III study was a randomized, placebo-controlled double-blind trial of adults and children which demonstrated that, compared to placebo, those patients receiving rhDNase (dornase alfa) had a decreased overall risk of pulmonary exacerbations, improved FEV_1, improved perception of well-being, reduced CF-related symptoms, experienced fewer days on parenteral antibiotics, fewer days at home ill and fewer days in the hospital[145]. An additional 6-month open-label trial extension followed, and this revealed that more patients in the placebo group experienced exacerbations than in the treatment group, and that improvement in FEV_1 was maintained in the treatment group and became evident in the former placebo group[146].

Adverse events related to drug use were mild and transient and included voice alteration, pharyngitis, laryngitis, rash, chest pain and conjunctivitis. Aerosolized rhDNase has also been studied in patients with more severe lung disease related to CF, and patients receiving the drug exhibited improvement in both FVC and FEV_1[147]. It is currently recommended that patients start aerosolized rhDNase at a relatively early stage of disease and remain on the drug indefinately[148].

BRONCHODILATORS

Airway obstruction and atelectasis with air trapping are characteristic of CF. Studies suggest that 25–50 per cent of patients with CF have evidence of bronchial hyperreactivity when studied with histamine, methacholine or cold air provocation tests[149-151]. Several studies indicate that older children and adolescents show evidence of bronchodilator response[152], as do infants and young children[25].

The use of bronchodilators in patients with CF remains controversial. Some patients clearly benefit from their use, others show no response, and a small group demonstrate worsening pulmonary function[153-155].

A recent study of long-term inhaled albuterol indicates that patients with CF who have bronchial hyperreactivity (as assessed by methacholine challenge) show significant improvement in lung function while on albuterol, whereas those with a negative methacholine challenge show a poor response[156].

Table 10.1 *Selected bronchodilators*

Generic name	Usual dosage	Side-effects
Salbutamol (Albuterol) MDI: 90 µg/dose Rotocap: 200 µg/dose Nebulized solution: 0.5% = 5 mg/mL	MDI:1–2 inhalations Q 4–6 h <12 years: with spacer Rotocaps: inhale contents of capsule up to QID Nebulized solution: ≤12 years: 0.05–0.15 mg/kg/dose in 2–3 mL normal saline Q 4–6 h, with minimum of 1.25 mg/dose and maximum of 2.5 mg/dose (0.5 mL) >12 years: 2.5 mg in 2–3 mL normal saline Q 4–6 h	Nervousness Nausea Vomiting Rapid heart rate Tremor Hyperactivity
Metaproterenol MDI: 900.65 mg/dose Nebulized solution: 5% = 50 mg/mL	MDI: 1–2 inhalations Q 4–6 h <12 years: with spacer Nebulized solution: Newborn–2 years: 0.1 mL in 2–3 mL normal saline Q 4–6 h 2–12 years: 0.1–0.2 mL in 2–3 mL normal saline Q 4–6 h >12 years: 0.2–0.3 mL in 2–3 mL normal saline Q 4–6 h	Nervousness Nausea Vomiting Rapid heart rate Tremor Hyperactivity
Terbutaline MDI: 200 µg/dose Nebulized solution: 1 mg/mL	MDI: 1–2 inhalations Q 4–6 h >12 years Nebulized solution: ≤2 years: 0.5 mL in 2–3 mL normal saline >3 years: 1 mLin 2–3 mL normal saline	Nervousness Nausea Vomiting Rapid heart rate Tremor Hyperactivity

Along with a bronchodilating effect, there are reports which suggest that sympathomimetic agents improve mucociliary function in patients with CF[157]. If this hypothesis is correct, these drugs, prescribed prior to chest physiotherapy, should improve both mucociliary clearance and bronchoconstriction. The use of β-adrenergic agonists in children with CF should be based on clinical response and, if possible, improvement in pulmonary function. Table 10.1 summarizes the most common bronchodilators utilized by CF centers in the United States.

Theophylline use, in general, has become more controversial in recent years, both in acute and long-term management of bronchial hyperreactivity[158]. A 1980 study reported improved lung function in patients with CF treated with aminophylline[159]. In contrast, a more recent study reported that, with the exception of improved peak expiratory flow (PEF), theophylline did not improve pulmonary function findings[154]. Further, this study indicated that theophylline plus a β-adrenergic agent showed no advantage over use of a β-adrenergic agent alone.

Aerosolized ipratropium bromide, an anticholinergic agent with minimal systemic side-effects, acts as a bronchodilator with effectiveness similar to that of β-agonists[160], but this drug has not yet been well studied in patients with CF.

Modulation of inflammatory response

In recent years there has been increased interest in the use of anti-inflammatory agents to decrease inflammation and thereby diminish progressive damage to the CF airway. A preliminary report documented that treatment with every-other-day oral prednisone slowed the decline in pulmonary function in children with CF over a 4-year period[161]. The same study reported reduced morbidity and hospitalization rate in the group receiving 2 mg/kg of prednisone on alternate days. A more recent long-term (4-year) study[162] looked at patients with CF, 6–14 years of age with mild to moderate disease, who were placed on prednisone at 1 mg/kg or 2 mg/kg (to maximum of 60 mg) or placebo every other day. There was some effect on pulmonary function values after 12 months of therapy, but this effect was not sustained. There was no difference between the steroid-treated and placebo groups with respect to clinical score, chest radiography or hospitalizations. There were significant complications, particularly in the high-dose group, including growth retardation, carbohydrate metabolism abnormalities and cataracts. Although there were some modest gains in pulmonary status, these gains appear to be outweighed by side-effects[162]. Long-term alternate-day prednisone is not widely used, but low-dose therapy may be beneficial in a select group of patients. The use of inhaled steroids has increased dramatically for the treatment of asthma, but there are few studies documenting their use in CF. One small study of inhaled budesonide in adult CF patients showed small but significant improvements in cough and dyspnea[163]. Another study of inhaled beclomethasone dipropionate in children with CF showed the drug to be well tolerated, and documented reductions in levels of anti-inflammatory mediators[164]. Clearly, further studies are needed to help elucidate the potential value of inhaled steroids in the CF population.

Cromolyn sodium (sodium cromoglycate) has had a significant impact on the treatment of pediatric asthma in the past decade[165]. Its beneficial effects in patients with CF, even those with bronchial hyperreactivity, continues to be assessed. Earlier studies suggested that cromolyn sodium protected against methacholine-induced bronchial reactivity in selected patients with CF[166,167]. A more recent study considered the use of TID–QID cromolyn over an 8-week period in patients with CF, with bronchial hyperreactivity documented by methacholine challenge[168]. There were no clinical differences between cromolyn and placebo, by PFT evaluation or by change in methacholine response, documented in this study. As with other medications, the clinical and pulmonary function response to cromolyn should be considered on an individual basis.

Ibuprofen, a nonsteroidal anti-inflammatory agent, has been shown to inhibit neutrophil migration and release of lysosomal enzymes, and to reduce lung inflammation[169]. Patients with CF with mild lung disease have been studied over a 4-year period, and those receiving ibuprofen in a dose sufficient to reach peak plasma concentrations of 50–100 mg/mL showed less decline in pulmonary function and chest radiograph scores, better preservation of ideal body weight, and a decrease in number of hospital admissions compared to those receiving placebo[170]. Further studies of ibuprofen in the CF population are ongoing.

Polymorphonuclear leukocytes are present in high numbers in the airway lumen and are likely responsible for generating airway damage via products such as neutrophil elastase and other proteases. Research trials are ongoing to evaluate other new nonsteroidal anti-inflammatory and antiprotease agents, including pentoxifylline, α_1-antitrypsin, secretory leukocyte protease inhibitor (SLPI) and several synthetic inhibitors of elastase and other proteases.

In contrast to regimens which suppress the host response, the use of intravenous immunoglobulin (IVIG) to enhance phagocytosis of *P. aeruginosa* has also been advocated[171]. One study focused on patients with CF (12 years and older) admitted to the hospital with an acute pulmonary exacerbation[172]. All patients received usual therapy with intravenous antibiotics and chest physiotherapy. Those patients randomly assigned to also receive IVIG on days 1, 2, 3 of hospitalization had significant improvement in pulmonary function measurements compared to the placebo group. However, there were no differences in PFTs between the groups by 6 weeks after therapy.

Treatment of pulmonary infection

INTRODUCTION

The primary bacterial pathogens associated with chronic endobronchial infection in children with CF are *S. aureus*, *H. influenzae* and *P. aeruginosa*[173]. In the 1996 Cystic Fibrosis Patient Registry[23] from the US Cystic Fibrosis Foundation, the frequency of these pathogens was as follows: *S. aureus*, 37.5 per cent; *H. influenzae*, 15.4 per cent; and *P. aeruginosa*, 59.9 per cent. The incidence of *P. aeruginosa* increases with age: at 6–10 years, 11–17 years and 18–24 years of age the frequencies of infection are 46.8 per cent, 68 per cent and 78.7 per cent, respectively.

Selection of appropriate antibiotic therapy in children with CF should be based upon isolation of bacterial pathogen(s) from the respiratory tract and determination of the most active antimicrobial agent(s) by *in vitro* antibiotic susceptibility testing. Because multiple bacterial pathogens are frequently isolated simultaneously from respiratory secretions, it is important to choose a combination of antimicrobial activity against all the pathogens. It is also important to monitor serum levels, if available, to minimize potential toxicity while maximizing clinical efficacy. Listed in Table 10.2 are the most common antibiotic agents used in the treatment of CF lung disease, the appropriate dosages for children and the most common adverse effects.

Two antibiotic agents which have potential toxicities unique to the growing child are tetracycline and the quinolones. Tetracycline will stain developing teeth[174] and bones and should not be prescribed until secondary dentition is developed, at approximately age 7 years. The fluoroquinolones, including ciprofloxacin, norfloxacin and ofloxacin, because of their excellent oral absorption and potency against *P. aeruginosa*, have been widely used for adults with cystic fibrosis[175]. Because of possible damage to growing cartilage[176], these oral antibiotics have not been approved (in the US) for use in children. The fluoroquinolones are therefore not recommended for common use in the prepubescent, growing child unless other forms of antibiotic therapy have been ineffective. However, ciprofloxacin has been used on a compassionate basis by over 1000 children, the majority with CF, with no evidence of quinolone-induced arthropathy[177].

ANTIBIOTIC PROPHYLAXIS

There is no current consensus on the use of prophylactic oral antibiotics in the infant and child with CF. Some clinicians prescribe long-term therapy in an effort to delay bacterial colonization, reduce the frequency of pul-

monary exacerbations, and slow progression of airway obstruction. Because *S. aureus* and *H. influenzae* are widely believed to be the most common initial pathogens, oral antibiotic selection is directed towards these pathogens. In some European centers, aggressive anti-staphylococcal therapy at the time of first isolation of this pathogen is initiated. Szaff and Hoiby[178] demonstrated low rates of *S. aureus* respiratory tract colonization and serum precipitants in patients receiving 14 days of oxacillin or dicloxacillin. One American study[179] evaluated the efficacy of chronic suppression antibiotic therapy with the use of oral cephalexin. Although antibiotic administration was associated with decreased hospitalization and acute respiratory infection, there was a disturbing trend towards acquisition of mucoid *P. aeruginosa*.

In a prospective study of newly diagnosed infants with CF in the UK, there was no difference in clinical symptom scores or lung mechanics at age 12 months between infants receiving continuous flucloxacillin and infants receiving antibiotics when clinically indicated[180].

Another multicenter trial of newly diagnosed patients with CF (mean enrollment 16 months) compared children receiving continuous anti-staphylococcal prophylaxis with cephalexin to those receiving placebo for 5–7 years. There were no significant differences between the two groups in pulmonary function, pulmonary exacerbation frequency, nutritional status or chest radiograph scores. Children treated with continuous antibiotics showed decreased colonization with *S. aureus*, but increased colonization with *P. aeruginosa*[181].

Danish physicians have previously advocated routine, quarterly administration of IV antibiotics, reporting a slower decline in lung function and improved survival[182]. However, a subsequent report from the same center described an increased incidence of airway pathogens (principally *P. aeruginosa*) resistant to all common antibiotics[183].

These results suggest the need for ongoing assessment of IV and oral antibiotic suppression, weighing the risks of selecting for antibiotic-resistance with the benefits of decreased pulmonary exacerbations and diminishing the progression of pulmonary disease.

PULMONARY EXACERBATIONS

Patients with CF experience intermittent exacerbations of pulmonary infection, frequently manifested by increased cough, sputum production, shortness of breath, decreased exercise tolerance, decreased appetite and fatigue. *Pseudomonas aeruginosa* is currently the major pathogen associated with pulmonary exacerbation in CF[173]. The standard therapy for a pulmonary exacerbation is a combination of intravenous aminoglycoside and β-lactam antibiotics for a duration of 10–21 days. Combined administration is advocated to decrease antibiotic resistance. Aminoglycosides, includ-

Table 10.2 *Selected antibiotics used to treat lung infections*

Generic name	Usual dosage	Selected side-effects
Penicillins		
Amoxicillin trihydrate plus Clavulanic acid PO	25–45 mg/kg/day TID or BID (max. 1750 mg/day)	Vomiting, diarrhea hives, rash, chills, fever
Ticarcillin IV	300 mg/kg/day Q6 h (max. 12 g/day)	Rash, seizures headache, diarrhea, stomatitis, eosinophilia, leukopenia, hypernatremia, hypokalemia
Ticarcillin plus Clavulanic acid IV	Ticar component as above	
Piperacillin IV	300 mg/kg/day Q4–6 h (max. 24 g/day)	
Meropenem	60 + 120 mg/kg/day Q8 h (max. 6 g/day)	Headache, rash, diarrhea
Cephalosporins		
Cephalexin monohydrate PO	25–50 mg/kg/day BID–QID (max. 2 g/day)	Loss of appetite
Cefaclor PO	20–40 mg/kg/day TID (max. 1.5 g/day)	Diarrhea, loose stools
Ceftazidime IV	150–200 mg/kg/day Q6–8 h (max. 6 g/day)	Serum sickness
Cefixime PO	8 mg/kg/day BID (max. 400 mg/day)	
Aztreonam IV	150–200 mg/kg/day Q6–8 h (max. 6 g/day)	
Cefuroxine IV	100–150 mg/kg/day Q8 h (max. 6 g/day)	Dizziness, headache, rash, nausea
Aminoglycosides		
Amikacin sulfate IV	15–20 mg/kg/day Q8 h (follow blood levels)	Headache, nausea
Gentamicin sulfate IV	7–12 mg/kg/day Q8 h (follow blood levels)	Vomiting, rash
Tobramycin IV	7–12 mg/kg/day Q8 h (follow blood levels)	Hives
Combination		
Trimethoprim–sulfamethoxazole PO/IV[a]	10–20 mgTMP/kg/day BID (max. 320 TMP/1600 SMZ/day) (TID–QID at higher doses)	Nausea, bone marrow suppression, vomiting, diarrhea, headache,
Erthromycin and sulfisoxazole acetyl PO	8–16 kg: 2.5 mL QID 16–24 kg: 5 mL QID 24–45 kg: 7.5 mL QID > 45 kg: 10 mL QID	Loss of appetite, rash, sensitivity to sun
Miscellaneous		
Chloramphenicol IV/PO[b]	50–75 mg/kg/day Q6 h (max. 4 g/day)	Optic neuritis, bone marrow suppression
Ciprofloxacin PO/IV	20–30 mg/kg/day BID (max. PO, 1500 mg/day; max. IV, 800 mg/day)	Restlessness, irritability *joint pain *blood in urine nausea, diarrhea and abdominal discomfort
Azithromycin PO	10–15 mg/kg/day QID (max. 500mg day 1, 250 mg days 2–5)	Headache, rash, diarrhea elevated hepatic enzymes
Clarithromycin PO	15 mg/kg/day Q12 h (max. 1 g/day)	Headache, pruritus, rash, nausea, increased hepatic enzymes

[a]If used for longer than 1 month, do CBC.
[b]Blood levels of drug and laboratory bloods must be monitored.
* Report to physician.

ing gentamicin, tobramycin, amikacin and netilmicin, have the advantage of being active *in vitro* against most strains of *S. aureus*, *H. influenzae* and *P. aeruginosa*. The β-lactams which are most active against *P. aeruginosa* include the ureidopenicillins such as azlocillin, mezlocillin and piperacillin, third-generation cephalosporins such as ceftazidime and cefulodin, a new monobactam, aztreonam, and a combination of ticarcillin and β-lactamase inhibitor, clavulanate acid (Timentin®).

The criteria for initiation of antipseudomonal therapy are not uniform but usually include increased cough, weight loss, decreased exercise tolerance, school absenteeism, change in chest radiograph and decline in pulmonary function. For the young child unable to perform PFTs, respiratory rate, nutritional status and change in chest examination are helpful. Duration of therapy may be based upon improvement in pulmonary function[57], decrease in bacterial density in sputum[184,185] or clinical symptomatology scores[186]. Intravenous therapy should always be initiated in conjunction with aggressive chest physiotherapy and nutrition management.

During the course of intravenous antibiotic therapy, careful drug monitoring should occur. Nephrotoxicity and ototoxicity are primary concerns while patients receive aminoglycosides. Peak blood levels of the aminoglycosides are drawn 30 minutes following the infusion of the third or fourth dose; the trough level is obtained just prior to the subsequent dose. These levels should not be drawn through an indwelling catheter through which the aminoglycoside is administered. A peak tobramycin level of 8–12 μg/mL and a trough of less than 2 μg/mL are optimal. In a child, this dose range for tobramycin is generally achieved by administering 60–80 mg/m²/dose every 8 hours. blood urea nitrogen (BUN), creatinine, urinalysis and aminoglycoside levels should be obtained weekly, and an audiogram is recommended after every 6 weeks of aminoglycoside administration.

Allergic reactions are the major adverse reactions appreciated in patients with CF receiving penicillin derivatives[187]. If a true allergic reaction occurs, the drug must be stopped and appropriate allergic treatment and evaluation performed. Most patients can be switched successfully to another medication. However, if reaction occurs to related antimicrobial agents, desensitization may be necessary.

As an alternative to the expense and disruption to the patient and family when hospitalization is necessary for intravenous therapy, many centers have now set up home intravenous programs[188]. For a subgroup of our patient population, home intravenous therapy is quite successful, but for children in more challenging or chaotic social situations, hospitalization for their intravenous therapy is still mandatory.

INHALED ANTIBIOTICS

Inhaled aminoglycosides are increasingly promising as a means by which to deliver antibiotics in high concentration to the site of infection while decreasing the risk of systemic absorption and toxicity. Several early clinical trials[189–191] found a significant decrease in the number of hospitalizations and need for intravenous antibiotics when patients were maintained on aerosolized aminoglycosides. Smith *et al.*[192] studied the potential toxicity of prolonged aerosol tobramycin use and found no evidence of ototoxicity nor nephrotoxicity, common concerns in patients receiving repeated doses of intravenous aminoglycosides.

Colistin sulfate, colistinethate and polymyxin B have been administered by aerosol to patients with cystic fibrosis[181]. Limited studies have shown that colistin alone or in conjunction with oral ciprofloxacin was associated with a decrease in decline in pulmonary function and in frequency of *P. aeruginosa* isolated from respiratory secretions[193,194]. However, these antibiotics have also precipitated bronchospasm and respiratory failure when inhaled[195].

Tobramycin for inhalation (TOBI™) has been shown to be safe and effective in two randomized, placebo-controlled trials involving 520 patients in the US[196]. Subjects received either 300 mg of inhaled tobramycin or placebo twice daily for four weeks, followed by four weeks with no study drug. Patients received treatment or placebo in three on-off cycles for a total of 24 weeks. The patients treated with inhaled tobramycin had improvements in FEV_1, decreased density of *P. aeruginosa* in sputum, and fewer hospitalizations than patients in the placebo group. There was no detectable ototoxicity or nephrotoxicity. Tobramycin for inhalation is currently the only inhaled antibiotic approved for use by the US Food and Drug Administration.

Other investigational strategies for both children and adults with CF include agents that affect ion transport, modalities enhancing mucus clearance, gene therapy and direct delivery of the CFTR protein into lung epithelial cells. These are all discussed elsewhere in this book.

CONCLUSION

Considering the ever-increasing range of therapeutic modalities available to our patients, children diagnosed with CF in this and the coming decade should have increased survival and an enhanced quality of life, as new therapies and specialized care for children with CF assure them a brighter future.

Adults

M. E. HODSON

INTRODUCTION

Respiratory disease is the major cause of mortality and morbidity in cystic fibrosis (CF)[197]. However, the situation has improved significantly in recent decades. In l938, 70 per cent of babies died within the first year of life[198] but now 50 per cent of patients in the UK survive to 31.5 years[199]. The latest figures from the USA Cystic Fibrosis Foundation show a 50 per cent survival to 30.1 years[200] (data collected differently). In a survey of adolescents and adults, pulmonary disease was responsible for 97 per cent of deaths and three-quarters of hospital admissions. Kerem *et al.* have shown that once the forced expiratory volume in one second is less than 30 per cent of the predicted value, and the partial pressure of arterial oxygen below 55 mmHg or the partial pressure of arterial carbon dioxide above 50 mmHg, the 2-year mortality rates are above 50 per cent[201]. The median life expectancy of children born with cystic fibrosis in 1990 is estimated to be 40 years, double that of 20 years ago[202].

The abnormal CF gene causes primarily an abnormality in sodium and chloride transport. The functionally defective chloride channel in the apical membrane leads secondarily to loss of luminal salt and water in the airways. This predisposes the lung to infection and bronchiectasis. Secondary bacterial colonization leads to excess stimulation of the host's immunological response and excess production of neutrophil, macrophage and lymphocyte factors, predominantly neutrophil elastase, which stimulates more mucus and further damages the airway cells and impairs the immune response (Chapter 6).

The lungs of CF babies may be structurally normal at birth, but thereafter rapidly develop pathological changes[203], probably due to the infection, bronchitis and bronchiolitis commonly found at autopsy, even in young children[204]. As the infection increases and the chronic inflammatory response develops momentum, there is increasing ventilation perfusion imbalance which leads to hypoxia. Ultimately pulmonary hypertension develops and, late in the disease process, cor pulmonale[205]. In older patients massive pulmonary hemorrhage and pneumothorax may occur as the lung disease progresses.

MICROBIOLOGY

This is discussed in detail in Chapter 5. The clinician must consider bacterial, viral and fungal infections. Chronic colonization with *Staphylococcus aureus* is common in children with CF, but intermittent infection also occurs. Infection with *Haemophilus influenzae* is often intermittent and it can cause acute exacerbations of symptoms. The bacteria most commonly isolated from the sputum of CF children and adults is *Pseudomonas aeruginosa*. In adolescents and adults the prevalence of these organisms has been reported as *P. aeruginosa* 83 per cent, *S. aureus* 60 per cent and *H. influenzae* 68 per cent[197]. *Burkholderia cepacia* is becoming an important pathogen and is causing much concern among CF patients and their physicians[206–208]. At a recent study at the Royal Brompton Hospital, the incidence and prevalence rates have been shown to be 1.6–3.1 and 4.1–5.9, respectively[209], although higher rates have been reported in some CF centers in the UK and North America.

Figure 10.7 shows the respiratory microbial colonization rate in patients aged 6–10 years and 25–35 years in the USA[200]. It has been noted that in some patients with *B. cepacia* there is a rapid progression of disease, sometimes with a fatal outcome, whereas other patients appear to have asymptomatic carriage or a slow progressive decline similar to that seen in many patients with *P. aeruginosa*. It should be noted that the prevalence increases with age for *P. aeruginosa*, *B. cepacia*, *Stenotrophonomas maltophilia* (xan-

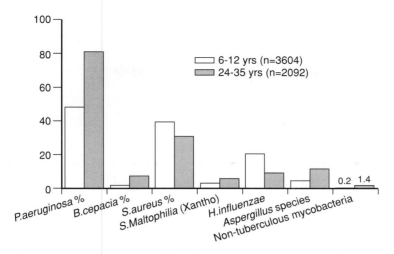

Figure 10.7 *Respiratory microbial colonization rates 1995 for CF patients*

thomonas) aspergillus species and nontuberculous mycobacteria. It decreases significantly for *H. influenzae* and, to a lesser extent, for *S. aureus* and *Stenotrophonomas maltophilia*. There is also increasing concern about the effect of colonization with methicillin-resistant *Staphylococcus aureus* (MRSA) in patients with CF[210].

It is known that the occurrence of viral infections is closely associated with pulmonary deterioration[211]. Infections both with *Mycobacterium tuberculosis* and atypical mycobacteria can complicate the pulmonary disease[212,213]. *Aspergillus fumigatus* is a fungus found in the air which becomes entrapped in the mucus of the respiratory tract. This probably accounts for the high incidence of allergy and precipitins to *A. fumigatus* found in the serum of CF patients (Chapter 6). A proportion of patients develop allergic bronchopulmonary aspergillosis.

Cross-infection

It is not possible to protect noncolonized CF patients from a ubiquitous saprophyte such as *P. aeruginosa*. Reliable typing methods are now available, including pyocin typing and DNA probes to assist with epidemiological surveillance[214]. Evidence so far available does not support cross-infection with *P. aeruginosa*, except rarely between CF siblings. Therefore most clinics do not have strict segregation policies for these patients. The use of single rooms for inpatient care when these are available is advisable as it cuts down the risk of patients acquiring viral infections.

Controlled studies have suggested that the risk of *B.*

cepacia isolation or colonization is increased by: (1) pre-existing severe lung disease; (2) a sibling who is already colonized; and (3) age[215]. It is not certain whether *B. cepacia* infection is just a reflection of patients' surviving longer or if there is a problem with cross-infection[216]. It is essential that laboratories use selective medium to isolate this organism. There is debate as to whether *B. cepacia* can be transmitted from person to person or via equipment or solutions. There does, however, appear to be an increased risk if a sibling is colonized or if there is intimate contact between two patients. There have been clustering of cases in a number of clinics but most patients in these clusterings have contact with one another outside the clinic. Until further evidence is available, it seems advisable to suggest that patients with *B. cepacia*:

1. are nursed in single rooms;
2. do not have intimate social contact with other CF patients;
3. do not share physiotherapy equipment, drinking and eating utensils.

However care should be taken not to allow patients with *B. cepacia* to be treated like 'lepers'. The evidence that cross-infection occurs within the ward or clinic is minimal.

SYMPTOMS

The age of onset of respiratory symptoms is variable[197]. There is no close association between genotype and phenotype. Some patients may be free of respiratory symptoms until they reach their teens or 20s but these are the minority. Other individuals may have marked pulmonary problems as small children and then have a period of quiescence until they reach adult life when major pulmonary problems re-emerge. At the age of 15 years approximately 50 per cent of CF patients will be producing sputum every day and 85 per cent intermittently[197]. In association with the bronchiectasis, hemoptysis is common and is present in over 60 per cent of adults, and in up to 10 per cent there are severe episodes. Many patients complain of chest pain which is often due to overvigorous coughing or physiotherapy, but can be found in association with pneumothorax, pleurisy or allergic bronchopulmonary aspergillosis. Chest pain is a symptom that should always be investigated. Some patients have intermittent or fixed airflow obstruction and wheeze. Exercise tolerance depends on the severity of the pulmonary disease. In some patients with mild disease this may be normal, other patients with severe disease are oxygen dependent and wheelchair bound.

PHYSICAL SIGNS

These depend upon the severity of the disease, and patients with mild disease may have no abnormal physical signs in the lungs. Finger clubbing is very common. As the lungs become overinflated abnormalities of the chest wall may occur in infants, such as bowing of the sternum (pectus carinatum), spinal kyphosis or Harrison's sulci. Hypertrophic pulmonary osteoarthropathy occurs late in the disease and is relative rare. Many patients deny dyspnea even when it can be easily demonstrated if they are asked to perform simple exercise tasks. Severely ill patients are cyanosed. Auscultation of the chest may reveal crepitations over areas of lung damage or retained secretion, and rhonchi due to airflow obstruction.

INVESTIGATIONS

Imaging

In patients with mild disease the chest radiograph may be normal (Fig. 10.8a). In patients with severe disease there may be hyperinflation with bronchial-wall thickening and ill-defined nodular shadows (Fig. 10.9) which are often more prominent in the upper zones. If there is pulmonary hypertension due to hypoxia, the pulmonary artery shadows will be enlarged. Even in patients whose chest radiograph appears normal, there may be evidence of bronchiectasis when a CT scan is performed (Fig.10.8b). In a patient with severe pulmonary disease, the CT (Fig. 10.10) will demonstrate gross bronchiectasis[217]. X-rays may show a large retrosternal space with increasing anterior/posterior diameter of the chest and

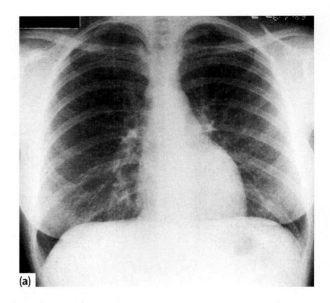

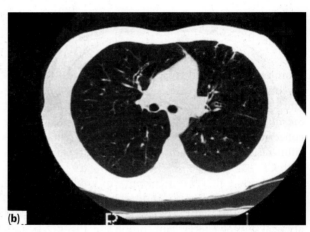

Fig. 10.8 **(a)** *Cystic fibrosis patient with a normal chest radiograph.* **(b)** *Same patient with an abnormal CT scan through the upper lobes, bronchiectatic anterior segmental bronchi.*

flattening of the diaphragm. There may be local areas of collapse and consolidation, with rounded opacities representing small microabscesses or infected bronchiectatic areas. There may be some ring shadows due to cylindrical bronchiectasis and subpleural bleps, which may rupture to produce pneumothoraces (Fig. 10.11). Chest radiographs are not usually helpful in the management of acute exacerbation of infection in adult. Their main value is in excluding complications, such as pneumothorax or atelectasis.

Isotope ventilation scans are quite sensitive in detecting unequal areas of ventilation in subsegmental areas and may be helpful in patients with mild disease[218]. Magnetic resonance imaging has been shown to demonstrate a greater extent of disease than that shown on chest films alone. It clearly demonstrates the peribronchial thickening and mucus impacted in the bronchi[219].

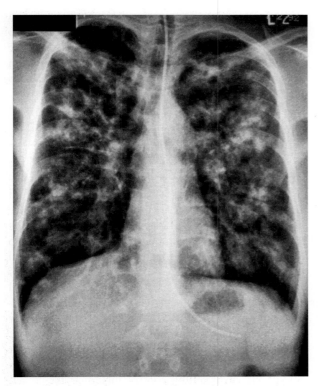

Fig. 10.9 *Chest radiograph of a patient with advanced pulmonary disease; severe changes especially in both upper lobes with a lot of bronchial-wall thickening and diffuse shadowing.*

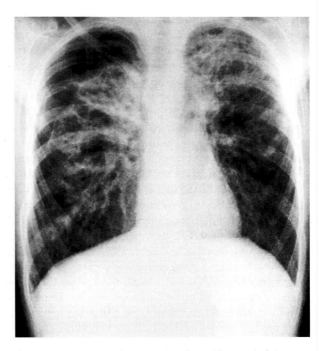

Fig. 10.11 *Chest radiograph showing widespread pulmonary disease and a right-sided pneumothorax.*

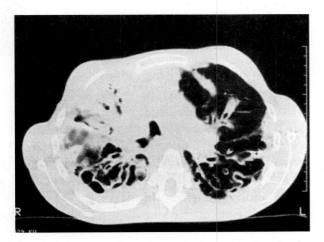

Fig. 10.10 *CT scan section through the upper lobes, showing severe cavitating disease with marked pleural reactions, right more than left, gross bronchiectasis is present.*

Respiratory function

The pulmonary physiology of the CF lung has been reviewed (Chapter 8). Progress of pulmonary disease can be most easily monitored using simple respiratory function tests, such as the forced expiratory volume in one second (FEV_1) and the forced vital capacity (FVC). Oxygen saturation can be performed routinely using an oximeter, and if there is cause for concern, blood gases can be performed to measure PaO_2 and $PaCO_2$. More sophisticated tests include those of small airways, such as the maximum expiratory flow–volume loop or measurement of alveolar–arterial oxygen difference[220].

Bronchial hyperresponsiveness is common but variable in patients with CF and it is not directly related to bronchodilator responsiveness[221]. It is known that some patients deteriorate after use if bronchodilators[222]. It is the author's practice to test each patient with a bronchodilator given by pressurized inhaler or nebulizer before deciding if this medication is indicated. The airway reactivity varies at different stages in the disease and a patient who does not show reversibility to bronchodilator when stable may benefit from this medication during an acute exacerbation.

If long-term oxygen is being prescribed for hypoxic patients, it is important to estimate blood gases before and after breathing oxygen for a long period of time, such as overnight, as some patients may develop significant carbon dioxide retention. They may need to have their dose of oxygen reduced or, in some cases, mild respiratory stimulants such as theophylline or protriptyline may be helpful.

Microbiology

Sputum culture should be taken at regular intervals for microbiological culture. Patients should provide sputum for culture at each outpatient attendance; and during an admission for an acute exacerbation of infection, cultures should be taken at the beginning of treatment, at discharge and at 5-day intervals through the admission. At least once a year all patients should have their sputum cultured for *M. tuberculosis*[212,223]. Appropriate serological tests for viral infections, chlamydia and mycoplasma should be requested when clinically indicated[224]. An appropriate microbiological medium should be used to test for *B. cepacia*[225]. Strategies for culture of respiratory secretions from CF patients have been reviewed extensively by Gilligan[226] (and Chapter 5). Bacteremia is rare in patients with CF; however, certain patients are vulnerable to fungemia, particularly those with implantable venous access systems[227]. Patients with unexplained pyrexia should therefore have blood taken for aerobic, anaerobic and fungal cultures. *P. aeruginosa* can be treated by antibiotics, greatly improving the prognosis for CF patients, but the organism is not permanently eradicated and development of resistance to antibiotics is a problem, particularly to the β-lactams[228,229]. It is important therefore that a laboratory processing sputum from CF patients should perform sensitivity tests to a wide range of commonly used anti-pseudomonal antibiotics. Clinicians are aware, however, of some patients who make a good clinical response when treated with antibiotics to which their organisms show *in vitro* resistance.

Muscles

A number of studies have shown that there is only a relatively small reduction in respiratory muscle strength in CF patients who have not reached the terminal stage of their disease. Routine measurement of respiratory muscles is therefore not indicated[230].

TREATMENT

Prevention

Patients should be encouraged to avoid contact with individuals who have overt respiratory tract infections and should avoid close contact with patients known to be colonized with *B. cepacia*[231], or MRSA. Many clinicians give CF patients a reserve supply of oral antibiotics to take immediately if they develop an upper respiratory tract infection. The reserve supply of antibiotic should be appropriate for the organism in the patient's sputum and *H. influenzae*.

Normal immunization should be administered against pertussis and measles; influenza vaccination should be given as routine, except to those who are allergic to eggs[232]. There is no convincing evidence that vaccination against *P. aeruginosa* is of value and it should not be given, except in clinical trials[233,234]. Good nutrition is clearly imperative as it contributes to the normal immune response (Chapters 6 and 11). No patient with CF should smoke, and the families should be advised to stop smoking. It has been shown that patients who are subject to 'passive smoking' fare less well[235] and children of smoking mothers require significantly longer periods of antibiotic treatment[236].

Physiotherapy

As soon as a patient is diagnosed as having CF both the patient and their relatives should be taught how to perform chest physiotherapy (Chapter 19). Adolescents and adults should be taught to use techniques that make them independent of an assistant, except during acute exacerbations. Many techniques have been developed to aid clearance of bronchial secretions, including postural drainage, autogenic drainage, positive expiratory pressure masks, oral high-frequency oscillation, mechanical percussion, flutter valves, active cycle of breathing techniques, exercise, periodic/continuous positive airway pressure and intermittent positive-pressure breathing[237]. The most effective treatment, for which there is the most scientific justification, is postural drainage using an active cycle of breathing control including the forced expiration technique. Much has been written about the effect of exercise on sputum mobilization and this is fully discussed in Chapter 20. However, it is vitally important that exercise should not be substituted for regular chest physiotherapy in patients with significant sputum production.

Antimicrobial therapy

STAPHYLOCOCCUS AUREUS

Staphylococcus aureus can be treated with oral flucloxacillin, erythromycin, tetracycline, clindamycin with or without the addition of fucidic acid. Teicoplanin or vancomycin may be helpful in severe infections or in patients with MRSA. There has been much debate about the use of anti-staphylococcal drugs to prevent damage and secondary colonization[238]. If patients are colonized with *S. aureus* most clinicians use maintenance oral anti-staphylococcal drugs such as flucloxacillin[239].

HAEMOPHILUS INFLUENZAE

This may be treated with a variety of antibiotics such as ampicillin, amoxycillin, erythromycin, tetracycline (not children), some third-generation cephalosporins or co-trimoxazole. However, 15 per cent of *H. influenzae* organisms are now resistant to amoxycillin. They may, however, be sensitive to amoxycillin with clavulanic acid. The macrolide antibiotics clarithromycin and azithromycin are effective against *H. influenzae* and *S. aureus* but their use in CF remains to be fully evaluated[240,241].

PSEUDOMONAS AERUGINOSA

Oral antibiotics

Oral quinolone antibiotics, such as ciprofloxacin, have been shown to be as effective as intravenous therapy[242]. However, there is increasing evidence that with repeated use the organisms become resistant[243] and the drug should probably not be given more frequently than every 3 months[244]. If used in this way it can replace some of the courses of intravenous antibiotics which would otherwise be necessary for the treatment of acute exacerbations. Due to the development of resistance there is probably no place for long-term administration.

Intravenous antibiotics

It has been claimed that intensive therapy at first colonization might achieve improved prognosis. Some centers give 2 weeks of intravenous antibiotics every 3 months, irrespective of symptoms[245], whereas others choose to treat acute exacerbations with intravenous antibiotics and to use maintenance aerosol antibiotics. It is, however, routine practice to treat acute exacerbations of infection. There are no commonly agreed criteria to define a pulmonary exacerbation, but these are commonly indicated by temperature, increased cough and sputum or breathlessness, together with a deterioration in pulmonary function as measured by FEV_1, FVC or oxygen saturation. The CF Foundation Consensus Conference's definition of a pulmonary exacerbation is shown in Table 10.3[246]. There is usually no change on a chest radiograph. It is essential to treat exacerbations for a minimum of 10–14 days, and drugs may be given in hospital or, if the patient is not severely ill, at home. Antibiotics are given via a cannula, long-line or in some patients with poor venous access via an implanted venous device[247]. Two antibiotics are usually given to take advantage of synergy or to reduce the chances of bacterial resistance.

The currently available preparations include carboxypenicillins (carbenicillin, ticarcillin), ureidopenicillins (mezlocillin, azlocillin, piperacillin), third-generation cephalosporins (ceftazidime, cefsuladin) and other β-lactam antibiotics such as aztreonam or carbapenems, such as imipenem or meropenem[248]. Piperacillin is best avoided in the treatment of CF patients as febrile reactions may follow its use[249] and coagulopathy has also been reported[250]. These are usually given together with an aminoglycoside such as tobramycin, gentamicin, netilmicin or amikacin. The patients frequently need high doses of aminoglycoside and the dose should be adjusted according to peak serum and trough levels to avoid toxicity[251].

Safe peak serum concentrations for gentamicin and tobramycin taken 20 minutes after administration are 8 and 12 mg/liter with a trough of less than 2 mg/liter. The trough and peak levels should be checked at the fifth dose. A large meta-analysis comparing single and multiple doses of aminoglycosides has shown that in patients without renal impairment a single daily dose is as effective, with a lower risk of nephrotoxicity and no greater risk of ototoxicity, than divided doses. There are also benefits of convenience and cost[252]. However, CF patients were not included in these studies. A small study of 29 CF patients showed that twice-daily aminoglycoside was as effective as 8-hourly dosing and may be less toxic[253].

There seems little to choose between various antipseudomonal antibiotics on clinical grounds. Ticarcillin has been compared with carbenicillin[254], azlocillin with carbenicillin[255], tobramycin with gentamicin[256], ceftazidime with carbenicillin and gentamicin[257] and no difference in clinical response was demonstrated. Meropenem produces less nausea than imipenem[248], and it therefore seems sensible to choose the cheapest antibiotic from any group, having excluded any antibiotics to which the patient's organisms are resistant or the patient allergic. It is well recognized that clinical improvement may occur in patients when given an antibiotic which shows in vitro resistance. Monotherapy is not advisable as it may lead to an increase in resistant organisms[258]. The commonly used anti-pseudomonal antibiotics are shown in Table 10.4.

Table 10.3 *Signs and symptoms of pulmonary exacerbations (PE)*

A PE is defined as the presence of at least three of the following 11 new findings or changes in clinical status when compared to the most recent baseline visit:
- Increased cough
- Increased sputum production and/or a change in appearance of expectorated sputum
- Fever (≥38°C for at least 4 hours in a 24-hour period) on more than one occasion in the previous week
- Weight loss ≥1 kg or 5% of body weight associated with anorexia and decreased dietary intake or growth failure in an infant or child
- School or work absenteeism (due to illness) in the previous week
- Increased respiratory rate and/or work of breathing
- New findings on chest examination (e.g. rales, wheezing, crackles)
- Decreased exercise tolerance
- Decrease in forced expiratory volume in one second (FEV_1≥10% from previous baseline study within past 3 months
- Decrease in hemoglobulin saturation (as measured by oximetry) from baseline value within past three months of ≥10%.
- New findings on chest radiograph

CF Foundation Consensus Conference[246].

Table 10.4 *Anti-pseudomonal drugs commonly used for treatment in CF*

Drug	Dose
Azlocillin	Child 300 mg/kg daily in 3 divided doses Adult 5 g t.d.s.
Ceftazidime	Child 150 mg/kg daily in 3 divided doses Adult 2 g daily t.d.s.
Aztreonam	Child 200 mg/kg daily in 4 divided doses Adult 2 g t.d.s.
Gentamicin/tobramycin	Child 2 mg/kg six hourly Adult 5 mg/kg daily in 3 divided doses
Meropenem	Child 4–18 years, 25–40 mg/kg every 8 hours Adult 1–2 g every 8 hours

Aerosol anti-pseudomonal antibiotics

Aerosol carbenicillin and gentamicin has been shown to improve lung function and reduce the frequency of hospital admissions[259,260]. Azlocillin[261], and ceftazidime[262] have produced similar results. Wall *et al.*[263] reported favorable results using ticarcillin and tobramycin, and there have been a number of encouraging reports about the use of tobramycin[264–266]. Extensive reviews of the use of inhaled antibiotics[267,268] and a meta-analysis of benefits and risks[269] concluded they were beneficial. Littlewood and colleagues[270] showed that children have a reduced frequency of positive sputum pseudomonal cultures after inhalation of colistin aerosol. It has also been shown that the early use of oral ciprofloxacin and aerosol colomycin will delay colonization with *P. aeruginosa*[271]. The initial fears that they might lead to sensitization of patients to specific antibiotics or to an increase in drug-resistant organisms have not been realized. Many pediatricians are commencing aerosol antibiotics as soon as *Pseudomonas* is isolated. These are then continued into adolescent and adult life.

In some patients inhaled antibiotics can cause chest tightness[272]. Each patient should have spirometry recorded before and half an hour after a test dose. If a patient bronchoconstricts 10 per cent or more, a bronchodilator should be given, the tonicity of the solution changed or a different antibiotic given. A preservative-free preparation of tobramycin (Tobi™) is now available, which may cause less bronchospasm[272a].

When patients use aerosol antibiotics they should do so twice daily after physiotherapy. It is desirable to choose an air compressor which gives a high flow (6 liters/minute) so that the majority of particles are 2–5 μm and the solution nebulizes quickly. A standard flow compressor (e.g. CR50 or Port-a-Neb) and a breath-enhanced open-vent nebulizer (e.g. Vent Stream or Pari LC+) should be used. The exhaled antibiotic should be absorbed by filters or discharged via the window. The most commonly used inhaled antibiotics are shown in Table 10.5.

BURKHOLDERIA CEPACIA

At initial isolation this organism is usually resistant to aminoglycosides, colomycin, carbenicillin, ticarcillin and the quinolones. It may, however, be susceptible to chloramphenicol, trimethoprim–sulfamethoxazole, ceftazidime and temocillin[273]. Antibiotics should be administered intravenously and by aerosol in accordance with laboratory sensitivity testing. However, some patients have a rapid downhill course in spite of antibiotic therapy (Fig 10.12).

MYCOPLAS MA PNEUMONIAE, CHLAMYDIA TRACHOMATIS AND CHLAMYDIA PNEUMONIAE

These organisms often respond to tetracycline, and, especially when the incidence of *M. pneumoniae* is increased in the community, patients with symptoms should be screened for the presence of this organism.

Table 10.5 *Nebulized drugs*

Antibiotic	Dose	Notes
Colomycin	Child 0.5–2 megaunits b.d. Adult 1–2 megaunits b.d.	1 megaunit + 3.0 mL normal saline 2 megaunits + 4.0 mL normal saline (or sterile water)
Gentamicin	Child 20–80 mg b.d. Adult 80–160 mg b.d.	Use injectable form
Tobramycin	Child 20–80 mg b.d. Adult 80–160 mg b.d.	Use injectable form
Tobramycin	Adult/Child 300 mg b.d. (28 days on, 28 days off)	Preservative free preparation
Amikacin	Adult 500 mg b.d.	Use injectable form

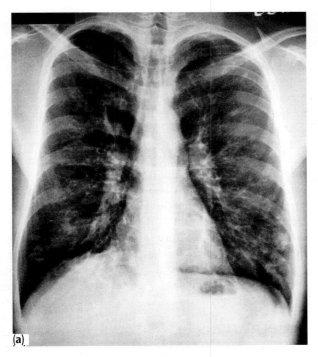 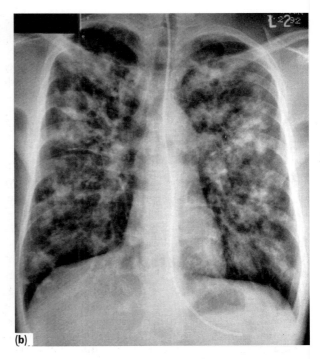

Fig. 10.12 *Chest radiograph* (**a**) *before and* (**b**) *3 months after acquisition of* B. cepacia. *There is a marked increase in interpulmonary shadowing.*

MYCOBACTERIA

Mycobacterium tuberculosis should be treated with conventional chemotherapy using isoniazid, rifampicin, pyrazinamide and ethambutol in most cases. The treatment of atypical mycobacteria infection depends on the sensitivity of the organism.

ANTI-VIRAL AGENTS

An acute deterioration in pulmonary function can be associated with influenza A infection. Once influenza has been contracted, amantadine given in the first 18 hours of the illness may decrease the severity and duration of illness[274, 275].

Mucolytics

The use of mucolytics is controversial and there is little controlled clinical trial evidence that they are of any benefit. However, nebulized hypertonic saline may aid expectoration. In a group of 52 patients with CF, randomly allocated to receive 10 mL of 0.9 per cent saline, or 6 per cent saline, those receiving the hypertonic saline had an increase of 15 per cent in FEV_1, compared to 2.8 per cent for the control group after 2 weeks' treatment. However, many patients find hypertonic saline by nebulizer unpleasant and some show bronchoconstriction[276].

Bronchodilators

It is well recognized that many patients with CF have airways hyperreactivity[277]. Patients should be tested to see if their spirometry improves after a bronchodilator, such as salbutamol, and if it does, this should be administered regularly by pressurized aerosol or nebulizer[278–280]. During acute exacerbations, some patients benefit from intravenous administration of bronchodilators[281]. Some patients appear to benefit from long-acting β-agonists, such as salmeterol. A few patients benefit from theophylline but side-effects can be troublesome.

Corticosteroids

Corticosteroids are indicated for the management of allergic bronchopulmonary aspergillosis and may benefit patients with severe wheezing, and acute exacerbations not responding to antibiotics and physiotherapy. Corticosteroids may increase the sense of well-being of a dying patient.

There is now increasing evidence of immunological hyperresponsiveness contributing to lung damage in CF (Chapter 6). Alternate-day prednisone has been claimed to reduce morbidity and improve pulmonary function in CF[282]; however, later evaluation showed only slight benefit combined with an unacceptable number of side-effects, such as impaired glucose tolerance, cataract formation, fractures and a Cushingoid appearance[283]. Recently, it has been shown that corticosteroids given for 12 weeks improve airflow obstruction[284]. Inhaled corticosteroids have been used in CF but the results are inconclusive[285,285a]. Short-term use of budesonide showed some reduction in bronchial hyperresponsiveness to histamine and improved symptoms[286].

Dornase alfa

Dornase alfa has been shown to decrease viscoelasticity of airway secretions and hence makes it easier for the patient to clear secretions at physiotherapy. Many studies have shown clinical improvement in patients with CF following treatment with dornase alfa. Short-term studies showed an increase in FEV_1 in patients treated with dornase alfa of 10–15 per cent[287,288]. A large multicenter North American study of patients with moderate lung disease showed an improvement of lung function of 5.8 per cent in patients treated with dornase alfa for 6 months compared with the placebo group, who remained at baseline ($P > 0.01$)[289]. Patients with mild pulmonary disease (FVC >85 per cent predicted) or children aged 5–10 years have also been shown to benefit[290]. Patients with severe pulmonary disease have, in two studies, been shown to improve more than patients treated with placebo[291,292]. An uncontrolled, open-labeled study following up patients for 2 years while on treatment with dornase alfa shows that the FEV_1 stabilized about 6 per cent above baseline[293]. These initial studies on dornase alfa are encouraging, suggesting an improvement in pulmonary function and a reduction in the rate of pulmonary exacerbations. It would seem, therefore, appropriate that any patient with cystic fibrosis who has evidence of airway inflammation should have a trial of 3–6 months' treatment with dornase alfa, and the therapeutic end points to be evaluated include pulmonary function, weight, incidence of respiratory-tract infections, breathlessness and patient's objective response. It should be remembered this is a very expensive treatment and, in individual patients, if there is no benefit after 3–6 months, it would be appropriate to stop treatment. More studies on the long-term effectiveness of dornase alfa and the response of children under 5 years are required.

Gamma globulin

In a small group of patients with CF and moderate or severe lung disease, an immunoglobulin infusion was associated with more rapid and greater improvement than infusion of placebo[294]. However, the beneficial effects on pulmonary function did not persist at follow-up. Further studies are warranted, but this treatment could be considered in patients failing to respond to conventional treatment.

New treatments

Drugs that inhibit sodium absorption (e.g. amiloride) and those that stimulate chloride secretion (e.g. uridine triphosphate) are undergoing clinical trials. Other methods of reducing the inflammatory response – such as ibuprofen, which inhibits migration and activation of neutrophils; pentoxifylline which inhibits neutrophil chemotaxis and degranulation; and antiproteases which bind free airways elastase, e.g. α_1-antitrypsin and secretory leukoprotease inhibitors – are also being investigated (Chapter 21). It is hoped that in the near future some of these studies may lead to new and more effective treatment of the pulmonary disease in CF. Gene therapy may be more effective in prophylaxis of lung disease in those patients who are still fairly fit, rather than offering significant improvement in those who already have severe pulmonary damage.

COMPLICATIONS

Atelectasis

Segmental atelectasis or collapse of a whole lobe can occur (Fig. 10.13). It is usually due to a sputum plug and may occur in association with allergic bronchopulmonary aspergillosis. Routine treatment with intensive physiotherapy and antibiotics should be instituted as soon as possible. In resistant cases it may be necessary to use high doses of oral corticosteroids and intermittent positive-pressure breathing techniques to remove the plugs. If medical treatment is unsuccessful, then the patient should be bronchoscoped and as much as possible of the obstructing secretions removed by suction. Gentle lavage should be undertaken and, in some patients, dornase alfa has been instilled with benefit. An atelectatic area may remain, and if the patient has widespread disease it may be best to take no further action. However, there is a small subset of patients where the disease is limited to one lobe who continue to require recurrent admissions to hospital, and for these patients surgical resection of the atelectatic area may be beneficial. This is particularly true of patients who still retain good pulmonary function[295].

Pneumothorax

Pneumothorax (Fig. 10.11) occurs in patients with CF, usually due to rupture of subpleural blebs through the visceral pleura. Occasionally traumatic pneumothorax may occur as a result of the misplacement of a central venous line. Spontaneous pneumothorax is relatively uncommon in childhood but its risk increases in adolescent and adult life. It is more common in males than females, the incidence in adult males being approxi-

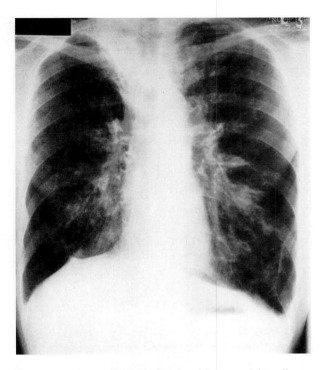

Fig. 10.13 *Chest radiograph showing right upper lobe collapse.*

mately 19 per cent[296]. It has been noted that pneumothorax may be associated with a poor prognosis[297]. A pneumothorax which is small and asymptomatic may be treated conservatively. Larger pneumothoraces require insertion of an intercostal tube. A CT scan may help in assessment in the size of the pneumothorax and in placement. In many cases the lung does not satisfactorily expand, with adhesion of the two layers of pleura. Suction applied to the intercostal tube may resolve the problem in some cases, but otherwise the clinician is left in a dilemma. An extensive pleurodesis, pleurectomy or talc pleurodesis may mean that the patient is unsuitable in the future for transplantation. After these procedures the pleura becomes very difficult to dissect and there may be extensive bleeding at transplantation. The best treatment for a pneumothorax which cannot be treated successfully by conservative means is a limited abrasion surgical pleurodesis. If a patient has had a pneumothorax on two occasions or more, there is such a high risk of recurrence that abrasion pleurodesis is recommended. In patients who would not be suitable for transplantation in the future there may be a role for chemical pleurodesis with talc or bleomycin[298].

Hemoptysis

Minor hemoptysis is common in CF patients, more so in adults than children. Major hemoptysis (>250 mL/24 hours) may occur in up to 7 per cent of older patients. The cause of hemoptysis is the chronic infection causing

granulation tissue and rupture of mucosal vessels by coughing. There may also be proteolytic destruction of bronchial and vascular walls, and major bleeding is almost certainly systemic (bronchial arteries) in origin. Contributing factors may be vitamin K deficiency due to malabsorption and liver disease, drug-induced platelet dysfunction and thrombocytopenia due to hypersplenism[299].

Clinicians should take care to distinguish between hemoptysis and hematemesis. Mild hemoptysis will usually settle with reassurance and appropriate antibiotic therapy. The platelets and prothrombin time should be checked and, if necessary, vitamin K given. Any aspirin-containing drugs should be stopped. Chest physiotherapy should be continued as it will help to clear the clots from the airways. In cases of severe hemoptysis, intervention may be unavoidable and bronchial artery occlusion using gel foam should be performed[300–302] (Fig. 10.14). Some centers bronchoscope these patients first to try and localize the site of bleeding. Conservative management consists of blood transfusion if necessary, correction of impaired clotting, oxygen and positioning the patient head down, lying on the site from which the bleeding originates.

The indications for angiography and embolization have been summarized by Cohen[303] as:

1. One hemorrhage >300 mL/24 hours (major), accompanied by ongoing hemoptysis at a lower daily or near-daily rate.
2. Three or more 100 mL hemorrhages within a week, accompanied by ongoing hemoptysis at a lower daily or near-daily rate.
3. Chronic or slowly increasing hemoptysis interfering with life style.
4. Hemoptysis preventing effective postural drainage or home management.

Patients requiring embolization should be referred to a major center where radiologists expert in the procedure are available.

There have been a number of reports of the successful use of Pitressin® in the management of hemoptysis[304,305] and a report of the successful long-term use of transexamic acid[306]. If these measures fail, bronchial artery ligation or surgical resection may be performed; however, sick patients do not tolerate this procedure well.

Allergic bronchopulmonary aspergillosis

The relationship between *Aspergillus fumigatus* and cystic fibrosis is extremely complex. Low colony counts of *A. fumigatus* can be found in the sputum of up to 50 per cent of patients[307]. The incidence of positive skin tests to *A. fumigatus* has been to be as high as 49 per cent and serum precipitins were found in 27 per cent of patients. *Aspergillus fumigatus* was isolated from

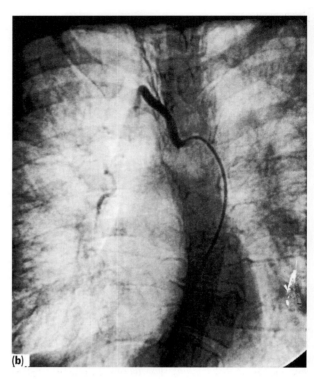

Fig. 10.14 *Selective bronchial arteriogram* **(a)** *showing abnormal bronchial circulation in the right upper zone, and* **(b)** *following embolization when the abnormal vessels have been occluded.*

patients' sputum in 9 per cent of cases in concentrations of 10^3 cfu/mL, and the incidence of allergic bronchopulmonary aspergillosis in CF is approximately 11 per cent[308,309].

Diagnosis of allergic bronchopulmonary aspergillosis should be made when there is transient pulmonary shadowing, a blood eosinophilia and a positive immediate skin test to *A. fumigatus*. The patient may also have serum precipitins, a high IgE and a specific radioallergosorbent test (RAST) to *A. fumigatus*. It is essential that corticosteroids are given so that bronchial plugs can be removed and further damage to the bronchial tree avoided. Patients will require intensive physiotherapy and some, in addition, intermittent positive-pressure breathing. In a few, fibreoptic bronchoscopy and small-volume lavage may be necessary. Treatment will result in a 50–75 per cent drop in total IgE[310]. Maintenance prednisone may be necessary for a considerable period of time. The minimal dose necessary to keep the chest X-ray clear should be given. The use of itraconazole, 200 mg twice daily for up to 4 months, as an adjuvant therapy in allergic bronchopulmonary aspergillosis has been reported, with encouraging results[311], but randomized trials of this agent are warranted to better define its usefulness.

Mycetomas do occur in CF, but only rarely. Invasive *Aspergillus* infection has been reported in CF[312] and increased risk factors include antibiotic and corticosteroid therapy, indwelling intravenous catheters and par-enteral nutrition. Invasive *Aspergillus* can also be a problem in CF patients after transplantation[313].

Cor pulmonale

Patients who have end-stage respiratory disease with severe hypoxia may develop this complication. It is known that patients with significant pulmonary disease will desaturate during sleep and during exercise[314]. Potential mechanisms include hypoventilation and changes in the ventilation perfusion relationships in the diseased lung. Severe hypoxia may lead to the development of pulmonary hypertension and right-sided heart failure. The prognosis of right-sided heart failure in CF is grave[315]. Clinical trials of nocturnal home oxygen in the treatment of hypoxic CF patients have not demonstrated a definite survival advantage[316]. This may be because it was not given for a long enough duration in each 24-hour period. However, as nocturnal oxygen is a considerable imposition on a relatively young patient, it may be appropriate to reserve oxygen therapy for symptom relief rather than use it too early in the disease. Established right-heart failure is treated with oxygen therapy together with diuretics and potassium supplements. Some severely affected CF patients may continue to attend school or go out to work using continuous oxygen therapy given as liquid oxygen or by a concentrator.

Empyema

This is a rare complication of CF. Although most adult CF patients are colonized with *P. aeruginosa* and it is the most important pathogen in acute exacerbations, systemic infection and empyema are rare despite the massive bacterial load in the airways. Empyema has been reported and treated successfully by needle aspiration and intravenous antibiotics[317,318]. If an empyema cannot be managed conservatively, surgical intervention is indicated.

Respiratory failure

Patients may develop hypoxic respiratory failure which leads to pulmonary artery hypertension and cor pulmonale. At the same time, the airflow obstruction reduces the vital capacity and tidal volume, leading to decreased alveolar ventilation. There may be progressive elevation in carbon dioxide and hypercapnic respiratory failure. It is very common for both hypoxemia and hypercapnia to occur together.

Patients should be given the opportunity to be assessed for pulmonary transplantation if appropriate. Immediate management involves the clearance of pulmonary secretions by physiotherapy techniques including, if necessary, intermittent positive-pressure breathing. Appropriate antibiotics should be given intravenously and by aerosol. Anti-inflammatory drugs, including corticosteroids, dornase alfa and bronchodilators, should be given. Hypoxia should be treated by controlled oxygen therapy and some patients, especially those with severe nocturnal hypoxia, may benefit from nasal CPAP[319]. In cases of hypercapnia, the author finds intravenous aminophylline and/or intravenous terbutaline helpful as they act as a respiratory stimulant as well as a bronchodilator. There is little place for submitting a patient with end-stage respiratory failure, who has already had maximal medical treatment, to intubation. The patient should be made comfortable and given symptomatic treatment. However, in occasional circumstances, such as an acute episode of respiratory infection in a patient who is already selected for transplantation, ventilation may be indicated[320]. Classically this was by positive pressure ventilation using an endotracheal tube. It is possible to use nasal ventilation (Fig. 10.15)[321]. Using this technique, the patient can eat, talk and communicate with friends and relatives. It is cost effective as the patient does not use the facilities of the intensive care unit. However, this should only be done when there is a potentially treatable situation, either in an acute episode which will respond to treatment or a realistic hope that an organ for transplantation may become available. It should not be used to prolong the process of dying.

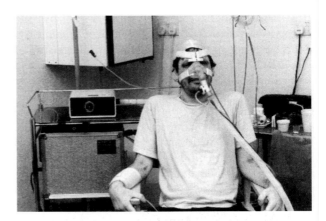

Fig. 10.15 *Patient awaiting heart–lung transplantation using a nasal ventilator.*

HOME TREATMENT

The prognosis for patients with CF has improved significantly in recent years. Many of these patients are colonized by *P. aeruginosa* and require regular treatment with intravenous antibiotics. Periods of hospitalization are disruptive to school, work and family life. They are also very expensive. There is an increasing tendency to use home intravenous antibiotic treatment whenever possible[322]. Patients should be responsible and have been carefully trained in the administration of antibiotics using an aseptic technique. Parents may administer antibiotics at home to children, but adolescents and adults prefer to give their own treatment whenever possible. The first dose of each antibiotic should be given under medical supervision because of the slight risk of anaphylaxis. Antibiotics are usually given via a long line or, in some patients with poor venous access, via an implanted intravenous device[248], as simple cannulas rarely last more than a few days. The use of devices for delivery of premixed antibiotics has also made home treatment easier[323]. In many centers this use of home antibiotics has been made possible by home care nurses who visit the patients in their own home. If patients live a long way from the treatment center, then regular contact can be maintained via telephone, and arrangements are made with the local doctor or hospital to resite a cannula if necessary. In general, the patient should have had at least one previous course of intravenous antibiotics in hospital. It should have been established that the patient has reasonable home conditions. The family should have a telephone. If the family is under particular stress, home intravenous antibiotics may not be suitable. The ward staff train the relatives and the patient to check their drugs, reconstitute and dilute if necessary, and to give by slow bolus infusion. Heparin locks are inserted after administration of drugs. Patients are given careful instructions to look for signs of the cannula blocking, drug leaking from the vein or phlebitis, and are also told to stop using the drugs and inform a doctor immediately if there are any rashes or other symptoms suggestive of anaphylactic reactions. The patient is reviewed at the end of treatment, either at home by the home care nurse or in the outpatient clinic. It is important that respiratory function is measured at the end of treatment to make sure that the maximum improvement has been obtained. It has been shown that home treatment is as effective as hospital treatment and that patients' prefer home treatment[324–326]. The major use of home care services for CF patients is supervising the administration of intravenous antibiotics. However, the home care nurse can visit the families of newly diagnosed CF patients, supervise gastrostomy feeding, oxygen administration and intermittent positive-pressure ventilation at home. Very valuable support can be given to critically sick patients who are awaiting transplantation, and their relatives, by a home visit.

TERMINAL CARE

In any chronic and progressive disease there comes a time when it seems unlikely that further conventional treatment will prolong life for any reasonable length of time. At this stage if one is working in a country with transplant facilities, the patient with cystic fibrosis may be assessed and placed on a transplant waiting list. Other patients who do not wish for transplantation or who are unsuitable for medical, psychological or social reasons, or patients who deteriorate very rapidly will not be suitable for this option. There are also patients who are accepted on to the transplant waiting list whose condition deteriorates and for whom there is no reasonable hope of an organ in time. For these groups of patients it is important that terminal care is given in a kind and efficient manner. It is important that the situation is discussed realistically with both the patient and their next of kin. If the patient is an adolescent or young adult they may well have guessed and be fully conversant with the severity of the situation. In the case of a small child it may only be appropriate to discuss the matter fully with the relatives and only in a more simple way with the patient. Baywater in 1981[327] said that unless something better could be offered, care must be taken not to disturb the defenses of the child. In dealing with a terminal situation Chapman and Goodall[328] emphasize that active treatment is not given up but that active treatment is aimed at relieving troublesome symptoms and no longer at prolonging survival from the disease itself. Frantic activity which has previously surrounded the patient can now be replaced by a more tranquil atmosphere. Physiotherapy is given to relieve symptoms and if the patient is tired, a treatment session can be omitted. It is very important that when a decision to go from 'cure to

care' is made that the senior medical staff discuss all aspects of the patient's management fully with nursing staff, physiotherapists and dieticians, so the family do not get conflicting messages from members of the team. It is important that the roles of doctors, nurses, physiotherapists, dieticians, social workers and chaplains are well coordinated.

During the terminal phase of the disease it would be completely inappropriate to use a ventilator, even nasal ventilation, if this is going to prolong the process of dying with no reasonable hope of survival. There should be completely free visiting for parents and relatives and, if possible, the patient should be cared for in a single room with the next of kin sleeping nearby. Parents and relatives should understand the importance of direct bodily contact and should not be inhibited from holding or comforting their loved one. They should be allowed to help with basic nursing procedures.

The relatives and all members of the 'caring team' have a responsibility to see that the death of a young patient is as dignified and peaceful as possible. The management of terminal disease in CF is similar to that of patients with malignant disease and is extremely well described by Saunders[329]. Good care involves attention to detail. It is important that the patient does not feel guilty because he is not getting better and is given the opportunity to discuss his doubts and fears with those who are caring for him. Older patients should have an opportunity to talk to their senior nurses and doctors without the presence of the next of kin. Sometimes they wish to express anger, but feel unable to do this in the presence of the next of kin as they do not wish to hurt them. Often the biggest worry of the young adults is the effect of their impending death on their relatives. Many of them have seen siblings dying of the same disease and have seen the effect on their parents.

Usually the most distressing symptoms are cough, sputum retention and breathlessness. Gentle physiotherapy, humidification, nebulized bronchodilators and antibiotics can all be helpful. If, in spite of these measures, the patient remains breathless and distressed, then small doses of opiates, such as morphine linctus, initially given in the dose of 2.5 mg 4 hourly, together with prochlorperazine to prevent nausea, can be very helpful. Tranquillizers may relieve anxiety. Antidepressants and steroids can also produce an elevation of mood.

The care of dying patients can be distressing for hospital staff, and it is important that the physician allows time to discuss the impact of caring for a dying patient and their death with nurses, physiotherapists and other members of the team. When a patient dies, if facilities are available, bereavement follow-up by a senior member of the nursing staff or social worker can be very helpful for the family until they adjust to the new situation. Prolonged follow-up is often impractical, but relatives identified as being at risk can be transferred to the care of local social services. Many patients die in hospital because of the necessity of hospital facilities and staff to provide the 24-hour nursing care and medication. However, some parents may wish to nurse the dying patient at home, and when this is their wish everything should be done to make it possible. Liaison with the family doctor and district nurse is then of crucial importance.

TRAVEL

Increasing numbers of adolescents and adults with CF wish to travel. This should be encouraged if their health permits. It is essential that they take out adequate travel insurance and that it covers their cystic fibrosis. They should take with them a list of regular medications in case they need to see a doctor abroad, together with a letter for the local customs officer listing medications and any air compressor, syringes and needles that they are carrying. This can save a lot of delay. Patients should have the appropriate immunizations in most cases, but immunosuppressed transplant patients are normally advised to avoid live vaccines. If patients are going to hot climates, they should take salt supplements. If patients have significant hypoxia they should be advised not to travel unless they have a supply of supplementary oxygen. Commercial aircraft cruise between 10 000 and 60 000 feet above sea level. The air cabin conditions are equivalent to approximately 5000–8000 feet above sea level in aircraft, and the partial pressure of inspired oxygen is reduced to 70–80 per cent of sea-level values. If a patient already has a reduced Pao_2 this will result in significant desaturation. For example a Pao_2 of 9.6 kPa at sea level will drop to 6.3 or less at an altitude of 8000 feet breathing air after 45 minutes[330]. CF patients with a resting Pao_2 of less than 10 kPa should have their need for oxygen during flight carefully assessed before travel.

Recently it has been reported that two patients, unbeknown to their clinicians, went on ski-ing holidays at altitude and developed right ventricular failure[331]. It is certain that more consideration should be given to the risks of exacerbations in patients with severe disease who wish to take holidays at high altitude. Patients with unstable pneumothoraces should not fly. It is advisable that patients attending a CF unit should be encouraged to discuss their holiday arrangements with their medical advisors so that all these issues can be addressed.

ARRANGING A SYSTEM OF CARE

It is part of the pediatrician's responsibility to help the CF adolescent and his or her parents to transfer smoothly from pediatric to adult care. This is usually to the respiratory physician. This can be a difficult time as both the patient and his or her family have usually become very attached to the pediatrician and his team,

who have put so much time and effort into helping the young person survive and live a normal life at school. It is helpful if some joint clinics can be undertaken between the pediatrician and the adult physician, and if some of the other staff, e.g. clinical nurse specialist, physiotherapist, dietician or social worker, can see the patient before transferring.

There is now increasing evidence that care of patients with CF in special centers improves survival[332–335]. It may be that the patient will have to travel some distance to get to a special clinic. In some cases, the patient can be cared for on a shared care basis with a local clinic. In the UK, the Royal College of Physicians[336] has recommended regional centers with teams of specialists to meet the needs of the adolescent and young adult with CF. The team should include a respiratory physician, specialized nurses, physiotherapists, dieticians, medical social workers and chaplains, all with expertise in CF. The respiratory physician will, of course, work closely with colleagues in other specialties, such as gastroenterology, thoracic surgery, abdominal surgery, ENT, gynecology and obstetrics, endocrinology, psychiatry and psychology.

When a patient comes to a CF clinic, he or she should be seen by the physiotherapist, who should check the patient's physiotherapy technique and collect a sputum sample for microbiology. The patient is weighed and his or her diet reviewed by a dietician. The social worker should be available. Patients should be seen by the clinical nurse specialist, and measurements of respiratory function such as peak flow, forced expiratory volume in one second, forced vital capacity and oxygen saturation should be recorded on a flow chart. All aspects of the patient's treatment should be reviewed by the doctor. Routine laboratory tests such as hematology, biochemistry, immunology and radiology should be carried out at least once yearly, with microbiology of the sputum at each visit. The patients should be seen at least every 3 months, and sicker patients at monthly intervals. Patients should be able to make contact with a member of the CF team and be seen at any time should there be an acute change in their condition. It is inappropriate for these patients to be seen in general chest clinics, but they should be seen in special clinics where more time is available for each patient. The family practitioner has an essential role to play in the total care of CF patients. There should be close liaison between the hospital and family doctor and he should be kept informed regularly of the patient's progress.

SCORING SYSTEMS

There are a number of scoring systems, which are valuable for clinical trials and may also assist the clinician in the monitoring of patients with CF. Perhaps the best known is the Shwachman score[337]. This assesses general activity, physical findings, nutritional status and chest radiograph. Twenty-five points are given for each category. A high score indicates a good clinical state: excellent = 100–86; good = 85–71; mild = 70–56; moderate = 55–40; severe = 40 and below.

The Cooperman score 1971[338] is based on five measurements: general activity, chest radiograph, finger clubbing, growth development and complications. The Taussig scoring system[339] is simpler and based predominantly on pulmonary aspects of the disease to which prognosis is closely related. Simple tests of pulmonary function and respiratory complications such as pneumothorax, hemoptysis and cor pulmonale are included. A relatively small proportion of points are related to body weight and activity. Some clinics will score the chest radiograph annually using the Crispin–Norman score[340], Brasfield score[341], Wisconsin score[342] or Northern score[343]. These scoring systems may indeed be very useful in the pediatric age group and in patients with mild disease, but in patients with severe disease it is often more useful to monitor their progress with flow charts recording pulmonary function and oxygen saturation at each visit to the clinic. These scoring systems are valuable for clinical trials and making comparisons between clinics, but are not a substitute for the range of tests needed for monitoring an individual.

REFERENCES

Pediatrics

1. Boat, T.F., Welsh, M.J. and Beaudet, A.L. (1995) Cystic fibrosis, in *The Metabolic Basis of Inherited Disease*, (7th edn), (eds C.R. Scriver, A.L. Beaudet, W.S. Sly and D. Valle), McGraw-Hill, New York.

2. Wood, R.E., Boat, T.F. and Doershuk, C.F. (1976) Cystic fibrosis. *Am. Rev. Respir. Dis*, **113**, 833–878.

3. Rommens, J.M., Ianauzzi, M.C., Kerem, B.T. *et al*. (1989) Identification of the cystic fibrosis gene: Chromosome walking and jumping. *Science*, **245**, 1059–1065.

4. Riordan, J.R., Rommens, J.M., Kerem, B.T. *et al*. (1989) Identification of cystic fibrosis gene: Cloning and characterization of complementary DNA. *Science*, **245**, 1066–1073.

5. Kerem, B.T., Rommens, J.M., Buchanan, J.A. *et al*. (1989) Identification of cystic fibrosis gene: Genetic analysis. *Science*, **245**, 1073–1080.

6. Anderson, M.P., Gregory, R.J., Thompson, S. *et al*. (1991) Demonstration that CFTR is a chloride channel by alteration of its anion selectivity. *Science*, **253**, 202–205.

7. Trapnell, B.C., Chu, E.S., Paakko, P.K. *et al*. (1991) Expression of the cystic fibrosis transmembrane conductance regulator gene in the respiratory tract of normal individuals and individuals with cystic fibrosis. *Proc. Natl Acad. Sci.*, **88**, 6565–6569.

8. Quinton, P.M. (1983) Chloride impermeability in cystic fibrosis. *Nature*, **301**, 421–422.

9. Boucher, R.C. (1992) Drug therapy in the 1990s, what can we expect for cystic fibrosis? *Drugs*, **43**, 431–439.

10. Woods, D.E., Bass, J.A., Johanson, J.W.G. and Straus, D.C. (1980) Role of adherence in the pathogenesis of *Pseudomonas aeruginosa* lung infection in cystic fibrosis patients. *Infect. Immunol.*, **30**, 694.

11. Saiman, L. and Prince, A. (1993) *Pseudomonas aeruginosa* pili bind to asialo GMI, which is increased on the surface of cystic fibrosis epithelial cells. *J. Clin. Invest.*, **92**,1875.

12. Smith, J.J., Travis, S.M., Greenberg, E.P. and Welsh, M.J. (1996) Cystic fibrosis airway epithelia fail to kill bacteria of abnormal airway surface fluid. *Cell*, **85**, 229.

13. Knowles, M., Murray, G., Shallal, J. *et al*. Bioelectric properties and ion flow across excised human bronchi. *J. Appl. Physiol.*, **56**, 868–877.

14. Oppenheimer, E.H. and Esterly, J.R. (1975) Pathology of cystic fibrosis: Review of the literature and comparison with 146 autopsied cases. *Perspect. Pediatr. Pathol.*, **2**, 241–278.

15. Chow, C.W., Landan, L.F. and Taussig, L.M. (1982) Bronchial mucus glands in the newborn with cystic fibrosis. *Eur. J. Pediatr.*, **139**, 240–243.

16. Esterly, J.R. and Oppenheimer, E.H. (1968) Cystic fibrosis of the pancreas: structural changes in peripheral airways. *Thorax*, **23**, 270–275.

17. Zuelzer, W.W. and Newton, W.A. Jr (1949) The pathogenesis of fibrocystic disease of the pancreas. A study of 36 cases with special reference to the pulmonary lesions. *Pediatrics*, **4**, 53–69.

18. Bedrossian, C.W., Greenberg, S.D., Singer, D.B. *et al*. The lung in cystic fibrosis. A quantitative study including prevalence of pathologic findings among different age groups. *Hum. Pathol.*, **7**, 195–204.

19. Tomashefski, J.F., Bruce, M., Goldberg, H.I. and Dearborn, D.G. (1986) Regional distribution of macroscopic lung disease in cystic fibrosis. *Am. Rev. Respir. Dis.*, **133**, 535–540.

20. Sobonya, R.E. and Taussig, L.M. (1986) Quantitative aspects of lung pathology in cystic fibrosis. *Am. Rev. Respir. Dis.*, **134**, 190–195.

21. Reid, L. and de Halley, R. (1964) Lung changes in cystic fibrosis, in *Cystic Fibrosis*, (ed. D. Hubble), The Chest and Heart Association, London, pp. 21–30.

22. Allan, J.L., Robbie, M., Phelan, P.D. and Dorks, D.M. (1980) The incidence and presentation of cystic fibrosis in Victoria 1955–1978. *Austr. Paediatr. J.*, **6**, 270–273.

23. FitzSimmons, S. (1996) Cystic Fibrosis Foundation Patient Registry. Annual Data Report.

24. Lloyd-Still, J.D., Khan, K.T. and Shwachman, H. (1974) Severe respiratory disease in infants with cystic fibrosis. *Pediatrics*, **53**, 678–682.

25. Hiatt, P., Eigen, H., Yu, P. and Tepper, R.S. (1988) Bronchodilator responsiveness in infants and young

children with cystic fibrosis. *Am. Rev. Respir. Dis.*, **137**, 119–122.

26. Landau, L.J. and Phelan, P.D. (1973) The variable effect of a bronchodilating agent on pulmonary function in cystic fibrosis. *J. Pediatr.*, **82**, 863–868.

27. Ramsey, B.W., Wentz, K.R., Smith, A.L. *et al.* (1991) Predictive value of oropharyngeal cultures for identifying lower airway bacteria in cystic fibrosis. *Am. Rev. Respir. Dis.*, **144**, 331–337.

28. Church, J.A., Keens, T.G. and Wang, C.I. (1979) Normal neutrophil and monocyte chemotaxis in patients with cystic fibrosis. *J. Pediatr.*, **95**, 272–274.

29. Schidlow, D. *et al.* (1990) Guidelines for CF care centers. *Am. J. Dis. Child.*, **144**, 1311–1312.

30. Jones, K.L. and Smith, D.W. (1997) *Smith's Recognizable Patterns of Human Malformation*, (5th edn), W.B. Saunders, Philadelphia.

31. Lucas, W.P. and Pryor, H.B. (1935) Range and standard deviations of certain physical measurements in healthy children. *J. Pediatr.*, **6**, 533–545.

32. Stern, R.C., Boat, T.F., Wood, R.E. *et al.* (1982) Treatment and prognosis of nasal polyps in cystic fibrosis. *Am. J. Dis. Child.*, **136**, 1067–1070.

33. Ledesma-Medina, J., Osman, M.Z. and Girdany, B.R. (1980) Abnormal paranasal sinuses in patients with cystic fibrosis of the pancreas. *Pediatr. Radiol.*, **9**, 61–64.

34. Despons, J. and Stoller, F.M. (1965) Nasal polyposis in mucouiscidosis. *Laryngoscopy*, **75**, 475–483.

35. Lemen, R.J., Gates, A.J., Mathe, A.A. *et al.* (1978) Relationships among digital clubbing, disease severity, and serum prostaglandins F_2 and E concentrations in cystic fibrosis patients. *Am. Rev. Respir. Dis.*, **117**, 639–646.

36. Waring, W.W., Wilkinson, R.W., Wiebe, R.A. *et al.* (1971) Quantitation of digital clubbing children. Measurements of casts of the index finger. *Am. Rev. Respir. Dis.*, **104**, 166–174.

37. Bentley, D., Moore, A. and Shwachman, H. (1976) Finger clubbing: A quantitation survey by analysis of the shadowgraph. *Lancet*, **2**, 164–167.

38. Schamroth, L. (1976) Personal experience. *South Afr. Med. J.*, **50**, 297–300.

39. Chernick, V. and Kendig, E. (eds) (1998) *Disorders of the Respiratory Tract*, (6th edn), W.B. Saunders, Philadelphia.

40. Shwachman, H. and Kulczycki, L.L. (1958) Long-term study of 105 patients with cystic fibrosis. *Am. J. Dis. Child.*, **96**, 6–15.

41. Hodson, C.J. and France, N.E. (1962) Pulmonary changes in cystic fibrosis of the pancreas, a radio-pathological study. *Clin. Radiol.*, **13**, 54–61.

42. Amodio, J.B., Berdon, W.E., Abramson, S. and Baker, D. (1987) Cystic fibrosis in childhood: Pulmonary paranasal sinus, and skeletal manifestation. *Semin. Roentgenol.*, **22**, 125–135.

43. Shwachman, H. and Kulczycki, L.L. (1958) Long term study of one hundred five patients with cystic fibrosis. *Am. J. Dis. Child.*, **96**, 6–15.

44. Weatherly, M.R., Palmer, C.G.S., Peters, M.E. *et al.* (1993) Wisconsin cystic fibrosis chest radiograph scoring system. *Pediatrics*, **91**, 488-495.

45. Crispin, A.R. and Norman, A.P. (1974) The systematic evaluation of the chest radiograph in cystic fibrosis. *Pediatr. Radiol.*, **2**, 101–106.

46. Brasfield, D., Hicks, G., Soong, S. *et al.* (1979) The chest roentgenogram in cystic fibrosis: A new scoring system. *Pediatrics*, **63**, 24–29.

47. Brasfield, D., Hicks, G., Soong, S. *et al.* (1980) Evaluation of scoring system of the chest radiograph in cystic fibrosis: A collaborative study. *Am. J. Roentgenol.*, **134**, 1195–1198.

48. Matthew, D.J., Warner, J.O., Crispin, A.R. *et al.* (1977) The relationship between chest radiographic scores and respiratory function tests in children with cystic fibrosis. *Pediatr. Radiol.*, **5**, 198–200.

49. Kraemer, R., Rudeberg, A. and Rossi, E. (1979) Relationship between clinical conditions, chest radiographic findings and respiratory function tests in cystic fibrosis. *Monogr. Paediatr.*, **10**, 61–65.

50. van der Put, J.M., Meradji, M., Danoesastro, D. *et al.* (1982) Chest radiographs in cystic fibrosis. A follow-up study with application of a quantitative system. *Pediatr. Radiol.*, **12**, 57–61.

51. Rosenberg, S.M., Howatt, W.F. and Grum, C.M. (1992) Spirometry and chest roentgenographic appearance in adults with cystic fibrosis. *Chest*, **101**, 961–964.

52. O'Laoide, R.M., Fahy, J., Coffey, M. *et al.* (1991) A chest radiograph scoring system in adult cystic fibrosis: Correlation with pulmonary function. *Clin. Radiol.*, **43**, 308–310.

53. Bhalla, M., Turcios, N., Aponte, V. *et al.* (1991) Cystic fibrosis: scoring system with thin-section CT. *Radiology*, **179**, 783–788.

54. Nathanson, I., Conboy, K., Murphy, S. *et al.* (1991) Ultrafast computerized tomography of the chest in cystic fibrosis: A new scoring system. *Pediatr. Pulmonol.*, **11**, 86.

55. Logan, P.M., O'Laoide, R.M., Mulherin, D., O'Mahony, S., FitzGerald, M.X., and Masterson, J.B. (1996) High resolution computed tomography in cystic fibrosis: correlation with pulmonary function and assessment of prognostic value. *Irish J. Med. Sci.*, **165**, 27–31.

56. Maffessanti, M., Candusso, M., Brizzi, F. and Piovesana, F. (1996) Cystic fibrosis in children: HRCT findings and distribution of disease. *J. Thor. Imag.*, **11**, 27–38.

57. Redding, G.J., Restuccia, R., Cotton, E.K. and Brooks, J.G. (1982) Serial changes in pulmonary functions in children hospitalized in cystic fibrosis. *Am. Rev. Respir. Dis.*, **126**, 31–36.

58. American Thoracic Society (1995) Standardization of spirometry – 1994 update. Statement of the American Thoracic Society. *Am. J. Respir. Crit. Care Med.*, **152**, 1107–1136.

59. Taussig, L.M., Chernick, V., Wood, R. *et al.* (1980) Standardization of lung function testing in children. *J. Pediatr.*, **97**, 668–676.

60. Polgar, E. and Promodhat, V. (1971) *Pulmonary Function Testing in Children: Techniques and Standards*, W.B. Saunders, Philadelphia.

61. Knudsen, R.J., Slatin, R.C., Lebowitz, M.P. *et al*. (1976) The maximal expiratory flow volume curve. Normal standards, variability and effects of age. *Am. Rev. Respir. Dis*., **113**, 587–600.

62. Kerem, E., Reisman, J., Corey, M. *et al*. (1992) Prediction of mortality in patients with cystic fibrosis. *NEJM*, **326**, 1187–1191.

63. Rosenfeld, M., Davis, R., FitzSimmons, S., Pepe, M. and Ramsey, B. (1997) The gender gap in cystic fibrosis mortality. *Am. J. Epidemiol*., **145**, 794–803.

64. Corey, M. and Farewell, V. (1996) Determinants of mortality from cystic fibrosis in Canada, 1970–1989. *Am. J. Epidemiol*., **143**, 1007.

65. Cooper, D.M., Doron, E., Mansell, A.L., Bryan, A.C. and Levison, H. (1974) The relative sensitivity of closing volume in children with asthma and cystic fibrosis. *Am. Rev. Respir. Dis*., **109**, 519.

66. Zapletal, A., Motoyama, E.K., Gibson, L.E. and Bouhuys, A. (1971) Pulmonary mechanics in asthma and cystic fibrosis. *Pediatrics*, **48**, 64.

67. Landau, L.I. and Phelan, P.D. (1973) The spectrum of cystic fibrosis. *Am. Rev. Respir. Dis*., **108**, 593–602.

68. Hilman, B.C. and Allen, J.L. (1993) Clinical applications of pulmonary function testing in children and adolescents, in *Pediatric Respiratory Disease: Diagnosis and Treatment*, (ed. B.C. Hilman), W.B. Saunders, Philadelphia, pp. 98–107.

69. Demko, C.A., Byard, P.J. and Davis, P.B. (1995) Gender differences in cystic fibrosis: *Pseudomonas aeruginosa* infection. *J. Clin. Epidemiol*., **48**, 1041–1049.

70. Pederson, S.S., Høiby, N., Espersen, F. and Koch, C. (1992) Role of alginate in infection with mucoid *Pseudomonas aeruginosa* in cystic fibrosis. *Thorax*, **47**, 6–13.

71. Lewin, L.O., Byard, P.J. and Davis, P.B. (1995) Effect of *Pseudomonas cepacia* colonization on survival and pulmonary function in cystic fibrosis patients. *J. Clin. Epidemiol*., **43**, 125–131.

72. Stocks, J., Sly, P., Tepper, R. and Morgan, J. (eds) (1996) *Infant Respiratory Function Testing*, Wiley-Liss, New York.

73. American Thoracic Society/European Respiratory Society (1993) Respiratory mechanics in infants: physiologic evaluation in health and disease. *Am. Rev. Respir. Dis*., **147**, 474–496.

74. Quanjer, P.H., Stocks, J., Polgar, G., Wise, M., Karlberg, J. and Borsboom, G. (1989) Compilation of reference values for lung function measurements in children. *Eur. Respir. J. Suppl*., **4**, 184S–216S.

75. Tepper, R., Morgan, W., Cota, K., Wright, A. and Taussig, L. (1986) GHMA Pediatricians. Physiologic growth and development of the lung during the first year of life. *Am. Rev. Respir. Dis*., **134**, 513–519.

76. Hanrahan, J.P., Tager, I.B., Castile, R.G., Segal, M.R., Weiss, S.T. and Speizer, F.E. (1990) Pulmonary function

77. Beardsmore, C.S. (1991) Respiratory physiological measurements in infants with cystic fibrosis. *Pediatr. Pulmonol. Suppl*., **7**, 38–41.

78. Morgan, W.J., Geller, D.E., Tepper, R.S., and Taussig, L.M. (1988) Partial expiratory flow–volume curves in infants and young children. *Pediatr. Pulmonol*., **5**, 232–243.

79. England, S.J. (1988) Current techniques for assessing pulmonary function in the newborn and infant: advantages and limitations. *Pediatr. Pulmonol*., **4**, 48–53.

80. Adler, S. and Wohl, M.E.B. (1978) Flow volume relationships at low lung volumes in healthy term newborn infants. *Pediatrics*, **61**, 636–640..

81. Taussig, L.M., Landau, L.I., Godfrey, S. and Arad, I. (1998) Determinants of forced expiratory flow in newborn infants. *J. Appl. Physiol*., **53**, 1220–1227.

82. Mohon, R.T., Wagener, J.S., Abman, S.H., Seltzer, W.K. and Accurso, F.J. (1993) Relationship of genotype to early pulmonary function in infants with cystic fibrosis identified through neonatal screening. *J. Pediatr*., **122**, 550–555.

83. Tepper, R.S., Hiatt, P., Eigen, H., Scott, P., Grosfeld, J. and Cohen, M. (1988) Infants with cystic fibrosis: pulmonary function at diagnosis. *Pediatr. Pulmonol*., **5**, 15–18.

84. Tepper, R.S., Montgomery, G.L., Ackerman, V. and Eigen, H. (1993) Longitudinal evaluation of pulmonary function in infants and very young children with cystic fibrosis. *Pediatr. Pulmonol*., **16**, 96–100.

85. Silverman, M., Prendiville, A. and Green, S. (1986) Partial expiratory flow–volume curves in infancy: technical aspects. *Bull. Eur. Physiopathol. Respir*., **22**, 257–262.

86. LeSouef, P.N., Hughes, D.M. and Landau, L.I. (1988) Shape of forced expiratory flow-volume curves in infants. *Am. Rev. Respir. Dis*., **138**, 590–597.

87. Stark, A.R., Cohlan, B.A., Waggener, T.B., Frantz, I.D. and Kosch, P.C. (1987) Regulation of end-expiratory lung volume during sleep in premature infants. *J. Appl. Physiol*., **62**, 1117–1123.

88. Turner, D.J., Lanteri, C.J., LeSouef, P.N. and Sly, P.D. (1994) Improved detection of abnormal respiratory function using forced expiration from raised lung volume in infants with cystic fibrosis. *Eur. Respir. J*., **7**, 1995–1999.

89. Turner, D.J., Stick, S.M., LeSouef, K.L., Sly, P.D. and LeSouef, P.N. (1995) A new technique to generate and assess forced expiration from raised lung volume in infants. *Am. J. Respir. Crit. Care Med*., **151**, 1441–1450.

90. Feher, A., Castile, R., Kisling, J. *et al*. (1996) Flow limitation in normal infants: a new method for forced expiratory maneuvers from raised lung volumes. *J. Appl. Physiol*., **80**, 2019–2025.

91. Tepper, R.S. and Asdell, S. (1992) Comparison of helium dilution and nitrogen washout measurements of functional residual capacity in infants and very young children. *Pediatr. Pulmonol*., **13**, 250–254.

92. Filburn, D., Castile, R., Flucke, R., Shani, N. and McCoy, K.

measures in healthy infants. *Am. Rev. Respir. Dis*., **141**, 1127–1135.

(1994) Measurement of fractional lung volumes in sedated infants. *Am. J. Respir. Crit. Care Med.*, **149**, 37.

93. Desmond, K.J., Coates, A.L. and Beaudry, P.H. (1984) Relationship between the partial pressure of arterial oxygen and airflow limitation in children with cystic fibrosis. *Can. Med. Assoc. J.*, **131**, 325–326.

94. Powers, S.K., Dodd, S., Freeman, J. *et al*. (1989) Accuracy of pulse oximetry to estimate HbO_2 fraction of total Hb during exercise. *J. Appl. Physiol.*, **67**, 300–304.

95. Wilmott, R.W., Tyson, S.L. and Matthew, D.J. (1985) Cystic fibrosis survival rates: the influences of allergy and *Pseudomonas aeruginosa*. *Am. J. Dis. Child.*, **139**, 669–671.

96. Kerem, E., Corey, M., Gold, R. and Levison, H. (1990) Pulmonary function and clinical course in patients with cystic fibrosis after pulmonary colonization with *Pseudomonas aeruginosa*. *J. Pediatr.*, **116**, 714–719.

97. Winnie, G.B. and Cowan, R.G. (1991) Respiratory tract colonization with *Pseudomonas aeruginosa* in cystic fibrosis: correlations between anti-*Pseudomonas aeruginosa* antibody levels and pulmonary function. *Pediatr. Pulmonol.*, **19**, 92–100.

98. Pamukcu, A., Bush, A. and Buchdahl, R. (1995) Effects of *Pseudomonas aeruginosa* colonization on lung function and anthropometric variables in children with cystic fibrosis. *Pediatr. Pulmonol.*, **19**, 10–15.

99. McCubbin, M.M., Ahrens, R., Kao, S., Seidel, G. and Teresi, M. (1996) *Pseudomonas* infection appears to precede the development of bronchiectasis on chest CT scan in young children with CF. *Pediatr. Pulmonol.*, **13**, 299 (abstract).

100. Thomassen, M.J., Klinger, J.D., Badger, S.J. *et al*. (1984) Cultures of thoracotomy specimens confirm usefulness of sputum cultures in cystic fibrosis. *J. Pediatr.*, **104**, 352–356.

101. Iacocco, V.F., Sibinga, M.S. and Barbero, G.J. (1963) Respiratory tract bacteriology in cystic fibrosis. *Am. J. Dis. Child.*, **106**, 115–124.

102. Huang, N.N., Van Loon, E.L. and Shang, K.T. (1961) The flora of the respiratory tract of patients with cystic fibrosis of the pancreas. *J. Pediatr.*, **59**, 512–521.

103. Cystic Fibrosis Foundation (1997) *Clinical Practice Guidelines for Cystic Fibrosis*, Cystic Fibrosis Foundation.

104. Armstrong, D.S., Grimwood, K., Carlin, J.B., Carzino, R., Olinsky, A., and Phelan, P.D. (1996) Bronchoalveolar lavage or oropharyngeal cultures to identify lower respiratory pathogens in infants with cystic fibrosis. *Pediatr. Pulmonol.*, **21**, 267–275.

105. Rosenfeld, M., Emerson, J., Accurso, F. *et al*. (1999) Diagnostic accuracy of oropharyngeal cultures in infants and young children with cystic fibrosis. *Pediatr. Pulmonol.* **28**, 321–328.

106. Abman, S.H., Ogle, J.W., Harbeck, R.J. *et al*. (1991) Early bacteriology, immunologic, and clinical courses of young infants with cystic fibrosis identified by neonatal screening. *J. Pediatr.*, **119**, 211–217.

107. Kerem, E., Corey, M., Stein, R. *et al*. (1990) Risk factors for *P. aeruginosa* colonization in cystic fibrosis patients. *Pediatr. Infect. Dis. J.*, **9**, 494–498.

108. Khan, T.Z., Wagener, J.S., Bost, T., Martinez, J., Accurso, F. and Riches, D.W.H. (1995) Early pulmonary inflammation in infants with cystic fibrosis. *Am. J. Respir. Crit. Care Med.*, **151**, 1075–1082.

109. Hall, C.B., McBride, J.R., Gala, C.L. *et al*. (1985) Ribavirin treatment of respiratory syncytial viral infection in infants with underlying cardiopulmonary disease. *J. Am. Med. Assoc.*, **254**, 3047.

110. McDonald, N.E., Hall, C.B., Suffin, S.C. *et al*. (1982) Respiratory syncytial virus infants with congenital heart disease. *NEJM*, **307**, 397.

111. Hiatt, P. (1992) The role of viral infections in cystic fibrosis. *Pediatr. Pulmonol. Suppl.*, **8**, 118–119.

112. Abman, S.H., Ogle, J.W., Butler-Simon, N. *et al*. (1988) Role of respiratory syncytial virus in early hospitalizations for respiratory distress of young infants with cystic fibrosis. *J. Pediatr.*, **113**, 826–830.

113. Dennehy, P.H. (1993) New tests for the rapid diagnosis of infection in children. *Adv. Pediatr. Infect. Dis.*, **8**, 91–129.

114. Davis, P. and di Sant'Agnese, P.A. (1978) Assisted ventilation for patients with cystic fibrosis. *J. Am. Med. Assoc.*, **139**, 1851–1854.

115. Stern, R.C., Boat, T.F., Doershuk, C.F. *et al*. (1976) Course of cystic fibrosis in 95 patients. *J. Pediatr.*, **89**, 406–411.

116. Garland, J.S., Chan, Y.M., Kelly, K.J. and Rice, T.B. (1989) Outcome of infants with cystic fibrosis requiring mechanical ventilation for respiratory failure. *Chest*, **96**, 136–138.

117. Stern, R.C., Boat, T.F., Orenstein, D.M. *et al*. (1978) Treatment and prognosis of lobar and segmental atelectasis in cystic fibrosis. *Am. Rev. Respir. Dis.*, **118**, 821–826.

118. Mearns, M.B. (1980) Natural history of pulmonary infection in cystic fibrosis, in *Perspectives in Cystic Fibrosis*, (ed. J.M. Sturgess), Canadian Cystic Fibrosis Foundation, Toronto, pp. 325–335.

119. Feigelson, J., Girault, F. and Pecau, Y. (1987) Gastroesophageal reflux and esophagitis in cystic fibrosis. *Acta Paediatr. Scand.*, **76**, 989–990.

120. Scott, R.B., O'Loughlin, E.V. and Gail, D.G. (1985) Gastroesophageal reflux in patients with cystic fibrosis. *J. Pediatr.*, **106**, 223–227.

121. Thomas, D., Rothberg, R.M. and Lester, L.A. (1985) Cystic fibrosis and gastroesophageal reflux in infancy. *Am. J. Dis. Child.*, **139**, 66–67.

122. Christie, D.L. (1984) Pulmonary complications of esophageal disease. *Pediatr. Clin. North Am.*, **31**, 835–849.

123. Fink, S.M. and McCallum, R.W. (1984) The role of prolonged esophageal pH monitoring in the diagnosis of gastroesophageal reflux. *J. Am. Med. Assoc.*, **252**, 1160–1164.

124. Sondheimer, J.M. and Haase, G.A. (1988) Simultaneous pH recordings from multiple sites in children with and

without distal gastroesophageal reflux. *J. Pediatr. Gastroenterol. Nutr.*, **7**, 46–51.

125. Blumhagen, J.D., Rudd, T.G. and Christie, D.L. (1980) Gastroesophageal reflux in children. Radionuclide gastroesophagography. *Am. J. Roentgenol.*, **135**, 1001–1004.

126. Orenstein, S.R. and Whittington, P.F. (1983) Positioning for prevention of infant gastroesophageal reflux. *J. Pediatr.*, **103**, 534–537.

127. Orenstein, S.R., Magill, H.L. and Brooks, P. (1987) Thickening of infant feedings for therapy of gastroesophageal reflux. *J. Pediatr.*, **110**, 181–186.

128. Orenstein, S.R. and Orenstein, D.M. (1988) Gastroesophageal reflux and respiratory disease in children. *J. Pediatr.*, **112**, 847–858.

129. Wilkinson, J.D., Dudgeon, D.L. and Sondheimer, J.M. (1981) A comparison of medical and surgical treatment of gastroesophageal reflux. *J. Pediatr.*, **99**, 202–205.

130. Reisman, J. (1994) Conventional postural drainage and percussion – is this still the gold standard? – Pro. *Pediatr. Pulmonol. Suppl.*, **10**, 85–86.

131. Lapin, C.D. (1994) Conventional postural drainage and percussion – is this still the gold standard? – Against. *Pediatr. Pulmonol. Suppl.*, **10**, 87–88.

132. Chernick, W.S. and Barbero, G.J. (1959) Composition of transbronchial secretions in cystic fibrosis of the pancreas and bronchiectasis. *Pediatrics*, **24**, 739–745.

133. Potter, J.L., Spector, S., Matthews, L.W. and Lemm, J. Studies on pulmonary secretions: III. The nucleic acids in whole pulmonary secretions from patients with cystic fibrosis, bronchiectasis, and laryngectomy. *Am. Rev. Respir. Dis.*, **99**, 909–916.

134. Farber, S.M., Pharr, S.L., Wood, D.A. and Frost, J.K. (1995) Enzymatic therapy in diseases of the chest. *Lab. Invest.*, **4**, 362–370.

135. Boat, T.F., Cheng, P.W., Iyer, R. *et al.* (1976) Human respiratory tract secretions: Mucus glycoproteins of nonpurulent tracheobronchial secretions and sputum of patients with bronchitis and cystic fibrosis. *Arch. Biochem. Biophys.*, **177**, 95–104.

136. Farber, S.M., Gorman, R.D., Wood, D.A. *et al.* (1954) Enzymatic debridement: particles related to trypsin and deoxyribonuclease in the control of cough and sputum associated with tuberculosis. *J. Thorac. Surg.*, **27**, 45–54.

137. Ratjen, F., Wonne, R., Posselt, H.G. *et al.* (1985) A double-blind placebo controlled trial with oral ambroxol and N-acetylcysteine for mucolytic treatment in cystic fibrosis. *Eur. J. Pediatr.*, **144**, 374–378.

138. Roomans, G.M., Tegner, H. and Toremalm, N.G. (1983) Acetylcysteine and its derivatives: Functional and morphological effects on tracheal mucosa *in vitro*. *Eur. J. Respir. Dis.*, **64**, 416–425.

139. Shak, S., Capon, H., Masters, S.A. and Baker, C.L. (1990) Recombinant human DNase I reduces the viscosity of cystic fibrosis sputum. *Proc. Natl Acad. Sci.*, **87**, 9188–9192.

140. Aitken, M.L., Burke, W., McDonald, G. *et al.* (1992) Recombinant human DNase inhalation in normal subjects and patients with cystic fibrosis: a phase I study. *J. Am. Med. Assoc.*, **267**, 1947–1951.

141. Hubbard, R.C., McElvaney, N.G., Birrer, P. *et al.* (1992) A preliminary study of aerosolized recombinant human deoxyribonuclease I in the treatment of cystic fibrosis. *NEJM*, **326**, 812–815.

142. Ramsey, B.W., Astley, S.J., Aitken, M.L. *et al.* (1993) Efficacy and safety of short-term administration of aerosolized recombinant human deoxyribonuclease in patients with cystic fibrosis. *Am. Rev. Respir. Dis.*, **148**, 145–151.

143. Ranasinha, C., Assoufi, B., Shak, S. *et al.* (1993) Efficacy and safety of short-term administration of aerosolized recombinant human DNase I in adults with stable stage cystic fibrosis. *Lancet*, **342**, 199–202.

144. Eisenberg, J.D., Aitken, M.L., Dorkin, H.L. *et al.* (1997) Safety of repeated intermittent courses of aerosolized recombinant human deoxyribonuclease in patients with cystic fibrosis. *J. Pediatr.*, **131**, 118–124.

145. Fuchs, H.J., Borowitz, D.S., Christiansen, D.H. *et al.* (1994) Effect of aerosolized recombinant human DNase on exacerbations of respiratory symptoms and on pulmonary function in patients with cystic fibrosis. *NEJM*, **331**, 637–642.

146. Hodson, M.E. (1995) Aerosolized dornase alfa (rhDNase) for therapy of cystic fibrosis. *Am. J. Respir. Crit. Care Med.*, **151**, S70–S74.

147. McCoy, K., Hamilton, S. and Johnson, C. (1996) Effects of 12-week administration of dornase alfa in patients with advanced cystic fibrosis lung disease. *Chest*, **110**, 889–895.

148. Ramsey, B.W. and Dorkin, H.L. (1994) Consensus conference: practical application of Pulmozyme. *Pediatr. Pulmonol.*, **17**, 404–408.

149. Mellis, C.M. and Levison, H. (1978) Bronchial hyperreactivity in cystic fibrosis. *Pediatrics*, **61**, 446–450.

150. Mitchell, I., Corey, M., Woenne, R. *et al.* (1978) Bronchial hyperreactivity in cystic fibrosis and asthma. *J. Pediatr.*, **93**, 744–748.

151. Darga, L.L., Eason, L.A., Maximilian, D. *et al.* (1986) Cold air provocation of airway hyperreactivity in patients with cystic fibrosis. *Pediatr. Pulmonol.*, **2**, 82–88.

152. Hordvik, N.L., Konig, P., Morris, D. *et al.* (1985) A longitudinal study of bronchodilator responsiveness in cystic fibrosis. *Am. Rev. Respir. Dis.*, **131**, 889–893.

153. Raeburn, D. (1988) Bronchodilator therapy in cystic fibrosis: for better or worse? *Med. Hypoth.*, **26**, 59–62.

154. Eber, E., Oberwaldner, B. and Zach, M. (1988) Airway obstruction and airway wall instability in cystic fibrosis: The isolated and combined effect of theophylline and sympathomimetics. *Pediatr. Pulmonol.*, **4**, 205–212.

155. Van Asperen, P.P., Manglick, P. and Allen, H. (1988) Mechanisms of bronchial hyperreactivity in cystic fibrosis. *Pediatr. Pulmonol.*, **5**, 139–144.

156. Eggleston, P.A., Rosenstein, B.J., Stackhouse, C.M. *et al.*

(1991) A controlled trial of long term bronchodilator therapy in cystic fibrosis. *Chest*, **99**, 1088–1092.

157. Wood, R.E., Wanner, A., Hirsch, J. and Farrel, P.M. (1975) Tracheal mucociliary transport in cystic fibrosis and its stimulation by terbutaline. *Am. Rev. Respir. Dis.*, **111**, 733–738.

158. Hendeles, L., Weinberger, M., Szefler, S. and Ellis, E. (1992) Safety and efficacy of theophylline in children with asthma. *J. Pediatr.*, **120**, 177–183.

159. Larsen, G.L., Barren, R.J., Landay, R.A. *et al.* (1980) Intravenous aminophylline in patients with cystic fibrosis. *Am. J. Dis. Child.*, **134**, 1143–1148.

160. Summers, Q.A. and Tarala, R.A. (1990) Nebulized ipratropium in the treatment of acute asthma. *Chest*, **97**, 425–429.

161. Auerbach, H.S., Williams, M., Kirkpatrick, J.A. and Colton, H.R. (1985) Alternate-day prednisone reduces morbidity and improves pulmonary function in cystic fibrosis. *Lancet*, **2**, 686–696.

162. Rosenstein, B.J., Eigen, H. and Schidlow, D.V. (1993) Alternate-day prednisone in patients with cystic fibrosis. *Am. Pediatr. Soc./Soc. for Pediatr. Res.*

163. van Haren, E.H.J., Lammers, J.W.J., Festen, J. *et al.* (1995) The effects of the inhaled corticosteroid budesonide on lung function and bronchial hyperresponsiveness in adult patients with cystic fibrosis. *Respir. Med.*, **89**, 209–214.

164. Wojtczak, H.A., Wagener, J.S., Kerby, G. *et al.* (1996) Effect of inhaled beclomethasone dipropionate on airway inflammation in children with cystic fibrosis. *Pediatr. Pulmonol. Suppl.*, 323–324.

165. Bierman, C.W. and Pearlman, D.S. (1998) Asthma, in *Disorders of the Respiratory Tract in Children*, (eds V. Chernick and Kendig Jr), W.B. Saunders, Philadelphia.

166. Mitchell, I. (1985) Sodium cromoglycate-induced changes in the dose–response curve of inhaled methacholine in cystic fibrosis. *Ann. Allergy*, **54**, 233–235.

167. Newth, C.J.L., Eigen, H. and Nickerson, B. (1985) Sodium cromoglycate-induced changes in the dose–response curve of inhaled methacholine in cystic fibrosis. *Pediatr. Res.*, **19**, 1099.

168. Sivan, Y., Acre, P., Eigen, H. *et al.* A double-blind, randomized study of sodium cromoglycate versus placebo in patients with cystic fibrosis and bronchial hyperreactivity. *J. Allergy Clin. Immunol.*, **85**, 649.

169. Konstan, M.W., Vargo, K.M. and Davis, P.B. (1990) Ibuprofen attenuates the inflammatory response to *Pseudomonas aeruginosa* in a rat model of chronic pulmonary infection: implications for anti-inflammatory therapy in cystic fibrosis. *Am. Rev. Respir. Dis.*, **141**, 186–192.

170. Konstan, M.W., Byard, P.J., Hoppel, C.L. *et al.* (1995) Effect of high-dose ibuprofen in patients with cystic fibrosis. *NEJM*, **332**, 848–854.

171. Fick, R.B., Naegel, G.P., Squier, S.U. *et al.* (1984) Proteins of the cystic fibrosis respiratory tract: fragmented immunoglobin G opsonic antibody causing defective opsonophagocytosis. *J. Clin. Invest.*, **74**, 326–348.

172. Winnie, G.B., Cowan, R.W. and Wade, N.A. (1989) Intravenous immune globulin treatment of pulmonary exacerbations in cystic fibrosis. *J. Pediatr.*, **114**, 309–314.

173. Høiby, N. (1982) Microbiology of lung infections in cystic fibrosis patients. *Acta Paediatr. Scand.*, **301**, 33–54.

174. Grossman, E.R., Walchek, A. and Freedman, H. *et al.* (1971) Tetracyclines and permanent teeth: the relation between dose and tooth color. *Pediatrics*, **47**, 567–570.

175. Grenier, B. (1989) Use of the new quinolones in cystic fibrosis. *Rev. Infect. Dis.*, **11**, S1245–S1252.

176. Adam, D. (1989) Use of quinolones in pediatric patients. *Rev. Infect. Dis.*, **11**, S1113–S1116.

177. Chysky, V., Kapila, K., Hullmann, R. *et al.* (1991) Safey of ciprofloxacin in children; worldwide clinical experience based on compassionate use: emphasis on joint evaluation. *Infection*, **19**, 289–296.

178. Szaff, M. and Høiby, N. (1982) Antibiotic treatment of *Staphylococcus aureus* infection in cystic fibrosis. *Acta Paediatr. Scand.*, **71**, 821–826.

179. Loening-Baucke, V.A., Mischler, E., Myers, M.G. (1979) A placebo-controlled trial of cephalexin therapy in the ambulatory management of patients with cystic fibrosis. *J. Pediatr.*, **95**, 630–637.

180. Beardsmore, C.S., Thompson, J.R., Williams, A. *et al.* (1994) Pulmonary function in infants with cystic fibrosis: the effect of antibiotic treatment. *Arch. Dis. Child.*, **71**, 133–137.

181. Ramsey, B.W. (1996) Management of pulmonary disease in patients with cystic fibrosis. *NEJM*, **335**, 179–188.

182. Szaff, M., Høiby, N. and Flensborg, E.W. (1983) Frequent antibiotic therapy improves survival of cystic fibrosis patients with chronic *Pseudomonas aeruginosa* infection. *Acta Pediatr. Scand.*, **72**, 651–657.

183. Jensen, T., Pederson, S.S., Hoiby, N., Koch, C. and Flensborg, E.W. (1989) Use of antibiotics in cystic fibrosis: the Danish approach. *Antibiot. Chemother.*, **42**, 237–246.

184. McLoughlin, F.J., Matthew, W.J., Strieder, D.J. and Goldman, D.A. (1983) Clinical and bacteriological responses to three antibiotoc regimens for acute exacerbation of cystic fibrosis. Ticarcillin–tobramycin, azlocillin–tobramycin and azlocillin–placebo. *J. Infect. Dis.*, **147**, 559–567.

185. Smith, A.L., Redding, G.J., and Doershuk, C.F. (1988) Sputum changes associated with therapy for endobronchial exacerbations in cystic fibrosis. *J. Pediatr.*, **112**, 547–554.

186. Mastella, G. (1983) Alternative antibiotics for the treatment of *Pseudomonas* infections in cystic fibrosis. *J. Antimicrob. Chemother.*, **12**, 297–311.

187. Moss, R.B., Babin, S., Hsu, Y.P. *et al.* (1984) Allergy to semisynthetic penicillins in cystic fibrosis. *J. Pediatr.*, **104**, 460–465.

188. Kuzenko, J.A. (1988) Home treatment of pulmonary infections in cystic fibrosis. *Chest*, **94**, 162S.

189. Hodson, M.E., Penketh, A.R.L. and Batten, J.C. (1981) Aerosol carbenicillin and gentamicin treatment of *Pseudomonas aeruginosa* infection in patients with cystic fibrosis. *Lancet*, **2**, 1137–1139.

190. Stead, R.J., Hodson, M.E. and Batten, J.C. (1984) Inhaled ceftazidine compared with gentamicin and carbenicillin in older patients with cystic fibrosis infected with *P. aeruginosa*. *Br. J. Dis. Chest*, **81**, 272–279.

191. Wall, M.A., Terry, A.B., Eisenberg, J. and McNamara, M. (1983) Inhaled antibiotics in cystic fibrosis. *Lancet*, **1**, 1325.

192. Smith, A.L., Ramsey, B.W., Hedges, D.L. *et al.* (1989) Safety of aerosol tobramycin administration for 3 months in patients with cystic fibrosis. *Pediatr. Pulmonol.*, **7**, 271.

193. Jensen, T., Pederson, S.S., Garne, S. *et al.* (1987) Colistin inhalation therapy in cystic fibrosis patients with chronic *Pseudomonas aeruginosa* lung infection. *J. Antimicrob. Chemother.*, **19**, 831–838.

194. Valerius, N.H., Koch, C. and Høiby, N. (1991) Prevention of chronic *Pseudomonas aeruginosa* colonization in cystic fibrosis by early treatment. *Lancet*, **338**, 725–726.

195. Wilson, F.E. (1981) Acute respiratory failure secondary to polymyxin-B inhalation. *Chest*, **79**, 237–239.

196. Ramsey, B.W., Pepe, M.S., Quan, J.M. *et al.* (1999) Efficacy and safety of chronic administration of inhaled tobramycin in patients with cystic fibrosis. *NEJM*, **340**, 23–30.

Adults

197. Penketh, A.R., Wise, A., Mearns, M.B., Hodson, M.E. and Batten, J.C. (1987) Cystic fibrosis in adolescents and adults. *Thorax*, **42**, (7), 526–532.

198. Andersen, D.H. (1938) Cystic fibrosis of the pancreas and its relation to celiac disease. A clinical and pathological study. *Am. J. Dis. Child.*, **56**, 344–399.

199. Dodge, J.A., Morison, S., Lewis, P.A. *et al.* (1997) Incidence, population and survival of cystic fibrosis in the UK 1968–95. *Arch. Dis. Child.*, **77**, 493–496.

200. FitzSimmons, S.C. (l996) Cystic Fibrosis Foundation, Patient Registry Annual Data Report 1995, Bethesda, MD, USA.

201. Kerem, E., Reisman, J., Corey, M., Canny, G.J. and Levison, H. (1992) Prediction of mortality in patients with cystic fibrosis. *NEJM*, **326**, (18), 1187–1191.

202. Elborn, J.S., Shale, D.J. and Britton, J.R. (1991) Cystic fibrosis: current survival and population estimates to the year 2000. *Thorax*, **46**, (12), 881–885.

203. Girod, S., Galabert, C., Lecuire, A., Zahm, J.M. and Puchelle, E. (1992) Phospholipid composition and surface active properties of tracheobronchial secretions from patients with cystic fibrosis and chronic obstructive pulmonary diseases. *Paediatr. Pulmonol.*, **13**, (1), 22–27.

204. Bedrossian, C.W., Greenberg, S.D., Singer, D.B., Hansen, J.J. and Rosenberg, H.S. (1976) The lung in cystic fibrosis. A quantitative study including prevalence of pathologic findings among different age groups. *Hum. Pathol.*, **7**, (2), 195–204.

205. Ryland, D. and Reid, L. (1975) The pulmonary circulation in cystic fibrosis. *Thorax*, **30**, (3), 285–292.

206. Isles, A., Maclusky, I., Corey, M. *et al.* (1984) *Pseudomonas cepacia* infection in cystic fibrosis: an emerging problem. *J. Pediatr.*, **104**, (2), 206–210.

207. Thomassen, M.J., Demko, C.A., Klinger, J.D. and Stern, R.C. (1985) *Pseudomonas cepacia* colonisation among patients with cystic fibrosis. A new opportunist. *Am. Rev. Respir. Dis.*, **131**, (5), 791–796.

208. Tablan, O.C., Martone, W.J., Doershuk, C.F. *et al.* (1987) Colonisation of the respiratory tract with *Pseudomonas cepacia* in cystic fibrosis. Risk factors and outcomes. *Chest*, **91**, (4), 527–532.

209. Taylor, R.F.H., Gaya, H. and Hodson, M.E. (1993) *Pseudomonas cepacia*; pulmonary infection in patients with cystic fibrosis. *Resp. Med.*, **87**, 187–192

210. Branger, C., Fournier, J. and Loulergue, J. (1994) Epidemiology of *Staphylococcus aureus* in patients with cystic fibrosis. *Epidemiol. Infect.*, **112**, (3), 489–500.

211. Efthimiou, J., Hodson, M.E., Taylor, P., Taylor, A.J. and Batten, J.C. (1984) Importance of viruses and *Legionella pneumophila* in respiratory exacerbations of young adults with cystic fibrosis. *Thorax*, **39**, (2), 150–154.

212. Smith, M.J., Efthimiou, J., Hodson, M.E. and Batten, J.C. (1984) Mycobacterial isolations in young adults with cystic fibrosis. *Thorax*, **39**, (5), 369–375.

213. Hjelt, K., Høiby, N., Howitz, P. *et al.* (1994) The role of mycobacteria other than tuberculosis (MOTT) in patients with cystic fibrosis. *Scand. J. Infect. Dis.*, **26**, 569–576.

214. Govan, J.R.W. and Nelson, J.W. (1992) Microbiology of lung infection in cystic fibrosis. *Br. Med. Bull.*, **48**, (4), 912–930.

215. Tablan, O.C., Martone, W.J., Doershuk, C.F. *et al.* (1987) Colonisation of the respiratory tract with *Pseudomonas cepacia* in cystic fibrosis. Risk factors and outcomes. *Chest*, **91**, (4), 527–532.

216. LiPuma. J.J., Dasen, S.E., Nielson, D.W., Stern, R.C. and Stull, T.L. (1990) Person-to-person transmission of *Pseudomonas cepacia* between patients with cystic fibrosis. *Lancet*, **336**, 1094–1096.

217. Santis, G., Hodson, M.E. and Strickland, B. (1991) High resolution computed tomography in adult cystic fibrosis patients with mild lung disease. *Clin. Radiol.*, **44**, (1), 20–22.

218. Ronchetti, R., Stocks, J., Freedman, N., Glass, H. and Godfrey, S. (1975) Clinical application of regional lung function studies in infants and small children using $_{13}$N. *Arch. Dis. Child.*, **50**, (8), 595–603.

219. Kinsella, D., Hamilton, A., Goddard, P., Duncan, A. and Carswell, F. (1991) The role of magnetic resonance imaging in cystic fibrosis. *Clin. Radiol.*, **44**, (1), 23–26.

220. Zach, M.S. (1990) Lung disease in cystic fibrosis – an updated concept. *Pediatr. Pulmonol.*, **8**, (3), 188–202.

221. Zach, M.S., Oberwaldn, B., Forche, G. and Polgar, G.

(1985) Bronchodilators increase airway instability in cystic fibrosis. *Am. Rev. Respir. Dis.*, **131**, (4), 537–543.

222. Landau, L.I. and Phelan, P.D. (1973) The variable effect of a bronchodilating agent on pulmonary function in cystic fibrosis. *J. Pediatr.*, **82**, (5), 863–868.

223. Hjelte, L., Petrini, B., Kallenius, G. and Strandvik, B. (1990) Prospective study of mycobacterial infections in patients with cystic fibrosis. *Thorax*, **45**, (5), 397–400.

224. Petersen, N.T., Høiby, H., Mordhorst, G.H., Lind, K., Flensborg, E.W. and Bruun, B. (1981) Respiratory infections in cystic fibrosis patients caused by virus; chlamydia and mycoplasma – possible synergism with *Pseudomonas aeruginosa*. *Acta Paediatr. Scand.*, **70**, (5), 623–628.

225. Gilligan, P.H., Gage, P.A., Bradshaw, L.M., Schidlow, D.V. and DeCicco, B.T. (1985) Isolation medium for the recovery of *Pseudomonas cepacia* from respiratory secretions of patients with cystic fibrosis. *J. Clin. Micro.*, **22**, (1), 5–8.

226. Gilligan, P.H. (1991) Microbiology of airway disease in patients with cystic fibrosis. *Clin. Microbiol. Rev.*, **4**, (1), 35–51.

227. Fahy, J.V., Keoghan, M.T., Crummy, E.J. and FitzGerald, M.X. (1991) Bacteraemia and fungaemia in adults with cystic fibrosis. *J. Infect.*, **22**, (3), 241–245.

228. Høiby, N., Friis, B., Jensen, K., Koch, C., Moller, M.E. and Stovring, S. (1982) Antimicrobial chemotherapy in cystic fibrosis patients. *Acta Paediatr. Scand. Suppl.*, **301**, 75–100.

229. Szaff, M., Høiby, N. and Flensborg, E.W. (1983) Frequent antibiotic therapy improves survival of cystic fibrosis patients with chronic *Pseudomonas aeruginosa* infection. *Acta Paediatr. Scand.*, **72**, (5), 651–657.

230. Mier, A., Redington, A., Brophy, C., Hodson, M. and Green, M. (1990) Respiratory muscle function in cystic fibrosis. *Thorax*, **45**, 750–752.

231. Pegues, D.A., Carson, L.A., Tabler, O.C. *et al.* (1994) Acquisition of *Pseudomonas cepacia* at summer camps for patients with cystic fibrosis. *J. Pediatr.*, **124** (5 Pt 1), 694–702.

232. Ong, E.L., Bilton, D., Abbott, J., Webb, A.K., McCartney, R.A. and Caul, E.O. (1991) Influenza vaccination in adults with cystic fibrosis. *BMJ*, **303**, (6802), 557.

233. Langford, D.T. and Hiller, J. (1984) Prospective, controlled study of a polyvalent pseudomonas vaccine in cystic fibrosis – three year results. *Arch. Dis. Child.*, **59**, (12), 1131–1134.

234. Schaad, U.B., Lang, A.B., Wedgwood, J. *et al.* (1991) Safety and immunogenicity of *Pseudomonas aeruginosa* conjugate. A vaccine in cystic fibrosis. *Lancet*, **338**, (8777), 1236–1237.

235. Gilljam, H., Stenlund, C., Ericsson-Hollsing, A. and Strandvik, B. (1990) Passive smoking in cystic fibrosis. *Resp. Med.*, **84**, (4), 289–291.

236. Campbell, P.W., Parker, R.A., Roberts, B.T., Krishnamani, M.R.S. and Phillips, J.A. (1992) Association of poor clinical status and heavy exposure to tobacco smoke in patients with cystic fibrosis who are homozygous for the F508 deletion. *J. Paediatr.*, **120**, 261–264.

237. Pryor, J.A. and Webber, B.A. (1992) Physiotherapy in cystic fibrosis – which technique? *Physiotherapy*, **78**, 105–108.

238. Lawson, D. and Porter, J. (1976) Serum precipitins against respiratory tract pathogens in 522 'normal' children and 48 cases of cystic fibrosis treated with cloxacillin. *Arch. Dis. Child.*, **51**, (11), 890–891.

239. Weaver, L.T., Green, M.G., Nicholson, K. *et al.* (1994) Prognosis in cystic fibrosis treatment with continuous flucloxacillin from the neonatal period. *Arch. Dis. Child.*, **70**, 84–89.

240. Aldons, P.M. (1991) A comparison of clarithromycin with ampicillin in the treatment of out-patients with acute bacterial exacerbations of chronic bronchitis. *J. Antimicrob. Chemother.*, **27**, (Suppl. A), 101–108.

241. Daniel, R. (1991) Simplied treatment of acute lower respiratory tract infection with azithromycin: a comparison with erythromycin and amoxycillin. European Axithromycin Study group. *J. Intl Med. Res.*, **19**, (5), 373–383.

242. Hodson, M.E., Roberts, C.M., Butland, R.J., Smith, M.J. and Batten, J.C. (1987) Oral ciprofloxacin compared with conventional intravenous treatment for *Pseudomonas aeruginosa*, infection in adults with cystic fibrosis. *Lancet*, **1**, (8527), 235–237.

243. Campbell, I.A., Jenkins, J. and Prescott, R.J. (1989) Intermittent ciprofloxacin in adults with cystic fibrosis and chronic *Pseudomonas* pulmonary infection. *Med. Sci. Res.*, **17**, 797–798.

244. Dostal, R.E., Seale, J.P. and Yan, B.J. (1992) Resistance to ciprofloxacin of respiratory pathogens in patients with cystic fibrosis. *Med. J. Aust.*, **156**, (1), 20–24.

245. Szaff, M., Høiby, N. and Flensborg, E.W. (1983) Frequent antibiotic therapy improves survival of cystic fibrosis patients with chronic *Pseudomonas aeruginosa* infection. *Acta Paediatr. Scand.*, **72**, (5), 651–657.

246. Cystic Fibrosis Foundation (l994) *Consensus Conferences – Concepts in Care*, Vol. V, Section 1, Cystic Fibrosis Foundation, Bethesda, Maryland.

247. Stead, R.J., Davidson, T.I., Duncan, F.R., Hodson, M.E. and Batten, J.C. (1987) Use of a totally implantable system for venous access in cystic fibrosis. *Thorax*, **42**, (2), 149–150.

248. Byrne, S., Maddison, J., Connor, P. *et al.* (1995) Clinical evaluation of meropenem versus ceftazidime for the treatment of *Pseudomonas* spp. infections in cystic fibrosis patients. *J. Antimicrob. Chemother.*, Suppl A, 135–143.

249. Stead, R.J., Kennedy, H.G., Hodson, M.E. and Batten, J.C. (1985) Adverse reactions to piperacillin in adults with cystic fibrosis. *Thorax*, **40**, (3), 184–186.

250. Rye, P. J., Roberts, G., Staugas, R.E.M. and Martin, A.J. (1994) Coagulopathy with piperacillin administration in cystic fibrosis: two case reports. *J. Paediatr. Child Hlth.*, **30**, 278–279.

251. Hsu, M.C., Aguila, H.A., Schmidt, V.L. et al. (1984) Individualisation of tobramycin dosage in patients with cystic fibrosis. Pediatr. Infect. Dis., 3, (6), 526–529.

252. Barza, M., Ioannidis, J.P.A., Cappelleri, J.C. and Lau, J. (1996) Single or multiple daily doses of aminoglycosides: a meta-analysis. BMJ, 312, 338–345.

253. Wood, P.J., Ioannides-Demos, L.L., Shu Chi et al. (1996) Minimisation of aminoglycoside toxicity in patients with cystic fibrosis. Thorax, 51, 369–373.

254. Penketh, A.R.L., Hodson, M.E. and Batten, J.C. (1983) Ticarcillin compared with carbenicillin in the treatment of exacerbations of bronchopulmonary infection in cystic fibrosis. Br. J. Dis. Chest, 77, (2), 179–184.

255. Penketh, A.R.L., Hodson, M.E., Gaya, H. and Batten, J.C. (1984) Azlocillin compared with carbenicillin in the treatment of bronchopulmonary infection due to Pseudomonas aeruginosa in cystic fibrosis. Thorax, 39, (4), 299–304.

256. Hodson, M.E., Wingfield, H.J. and Batten, J.C. (1983) Tobramycin and carbenicillin compared with gentamicin and carbenicillin in the treatment of infection with Pseudomonas aeruginosa in adult patients with cystic fibrosis. Br. J. Dis. Chest, 77, (1), 71–77.

257. British Thoracic Society Research Committee (1985) Ceftazidime compared with gentamicin and carbenicillin in patients with cystic fibrosis, pulmonary pseudomonas infection, and an exacerbation of respiratory symptoms. Thorax, 40, (5), 358–363.

258. Cheng, K.C., Smyth, R.L. and Govan, J.R.W. (1996) Spread of β-lactam-resistant Pseudomonas aeruginosa in a cystic fibrosis clinic. Lancet, 348, 639–642.

259. Hodson, M.E. (1988) Antibiotic treatment: aerosol therapy. Chest, 94, (Suppl. 2), 156–162.

260. Hodson, M.E., Penketh, A.R. and Batten, J.C. (1981) Aerosol carbenicillin and gentamicin treatment of Pseudomonas aeruginosa infections in patients with cystic fibrosis. Lancet, 2, (8256), 1137–1139.

261. Stroobant, J., Heaf, D.P., Tyson, S. and Matthew, D.J. (1985) Effect of inhaled azlocillin, mistabron and combination therapy in children with cystic fibrosis. Paediatr. Res., 19, (10), 1099.

262. Stead, R.J., Hodson, M.E. and Batten, J.C. (1987) Inhaled ceftazidime compared with gentamicin and carbenicillin in older patients with cystic fibrosis infected with P. aeruginosa. Br. J. Dis. Chest, 81, (3), 272–279.

263. Wall, M.A., Terry, A.B., Eisenberg, J., McNamara, M. and Cohen, R. (1983) Inhaled antibiotics in cystic fibrosis. Lancet, 1, (8337), 1325.

264. Maclusky, I.B., Gold, R., Corey, M. and Levison, H. (1989) Long-term effects of inhaled tobramycin in patients with cystic fibrosis colonised with Pseudomonas aeruginosa. Paediatr. Pulmonol., 7, (1), 42–48.

265. Ramsey, B.W., Dorkin, H.L., Eisenberg, J.D. et al. (1993) Efficacy of aerosolised tobramycin in patients with cystic fibrosis. NEJM, 328, 1740–1746.

266. Ramsey, B., Burns, J. and Smith, A. (1997) Safety and efficacy of tobramycin solution for inhalation in patients with cystic fibrosis. Pediatr. Pulmonol. Suppl., 14, 137–138.

267. Touw, D.J., Brimicombe, R.W., Hodson, M.E., Heijermen, H.G.M. and Bakker, W. (1995) Inhalation of antibiotics in cystic fibrosis. Eur. Respir. J., 8, 1594–1604.

268. Campbell, P.W. and Saiman, L. (chairpersons) (1999) Use of aerosolised antibiotics in patients with cystic fibrosis. Chest, 116, 775–788.

269. Mukhopadhyay, S., Singh, M., Cater, J.I., Ogston, S., Franklin, M. and Oliver, R.E. (1996) Nebulised antipseudomonal antibiotics therapy in cystic fibrosis: a meta-analysis of benefits and risks. Thorax, 51, 364–368.

270. Littlewood, J.M., Miller, M.G., Ghoneim, A.T. and Ramsden, C.H. (1985) Nebulised colomycin for early pseudomonas colonisation in cystic fibrosis. Lancet, 1, (8433), 865.

271. Valerius, N.H., Koch, C. and Høiby, N. (1991) Prevention of chronic Pseudomonas aeruginosa colonisation in cystic fibrosis by early treatment. Lancet, 338, (8769), 725–726.

272. Maddison, J., Dodd, M. and Webb, A.K. (1994) Nebulised colistin causes chest tightness in adults with cystic fibrosis. Resp. Med., 88, 145–147.

272a. Ramsey, B.W., Pepe, M.S., Quan, J.M. et al. (1999) Intermittent administration of inhaled tobramycin in patients with cystic fibrosis. NEJM, 340, 25–30.

273. Taylor, R.F., Gaya, H. and Hodson, M.E. (1992) Temocillin and cystic fibrosis: outcome of intravenous administration in patients infected with Pseudomonas cepacia. J. Antimicrob. Chemother., 29, (3), 341–344.

274. Douglas, R.G. Jr (1990) Prophylaxis and treatment of influenza. NEJM, 332, (7), 443–450.

275. Conway, S.P., Simmonds, E.J. and Littlewood, J.M. (1992) Acute severe deterioration in cystic fibrosis associated with influenza A virus infection. Thorax, 47, (2), 112–114.

276. Eng, P.A., Morton, J., Douglas, J.A., Riedler, J., Wilson, J. and Robertson, C.F. (1996) Short-term efficacy of ultrasonically nebulised hypertonic saline in cystic fibrosis. Pediatr. Pulmonol., 21, 77–83.

277. Eggleston, P.A., Rosentein, B.J., Stackhouse, C.M. et al. (1988) Airways hyper-reactivity in cystic fibrosis. Chest, 94, 360–365.

278. Ormerod, L.P., Thomson, R.A., Anderson, C.M. and Stableforth, D.E. (1980) Reversible airway obstruction in cystic fibrosis. Thorax, 35, (10), 768–772.

279. Avital, A., Sanchez, I. and Chernick, V. (1992) Efficacy of salbutamol and ipratropium bromide in decreasing bronchial hyperreactivity in children with cystic fibrosis. Pediatr. Pulmonol., 13, (1), 34–37.

280. Van Haren, E.H.J., Lammers, J.W.J. and Fester, J. et al. (1991) Bronchodilator response in adult patients with cystic fibrosis; effects on large and small airways. Eur. Respir. J., 4, 301–307.

281. Finnegan, M.J., Hughes, D.V. and Hodson, M.E. (1992) Comparison of nebulised and intravenous terbutaline

during acute exacerbations of pulmonary infection in patients with cystic fibrosis. *Eur. Respir. J.*, **5**, 1089–1091.

282. Auerbach, H.S., Williams, M., Kirkpatrick, J.A. and Colten, H.R. (1985) Alternate day prednisone reduces morbidity and improves pulmonary function in cystic fibrosis. *Lancet*, **2**, (8457), 686–688.

283. Rosenstein, B.J. and Eigen, H. (1991) Risks of alternate day prednisone in patients with cystic fibrosis. *Pediatrics*, **87**, (2), 245–246.

284. Greally, P., Sampson, A.J., Piper, P.J. and Price, J.F. (1992) Effect of prednisolone on airways obstruction in patients with cystic fibrosis. *Eur. Resp. J.*, **5**, (Suppl. 15), 259.

285. Bisgaard, H., Pedersen, S.S. and Nielsen, K.G. *et al.* (1997) Controlled trial of inhaled Budesomide in patients with cystic fibrosis and chronic bronchopulmonary pseudomonas aeruginosa infection. *Am. J. Respir. Crit. Care Med.* **156**, 1190–1196.

285a. Balfour-Lynn, I.M., Klein, N.H. and Dinwiddie, R. (1997) Randomized controlled trial of inhaled corticosteroids (Fluticasone propionate) in cystic fibrosis. *Arch. Dis. Child.*, **77**, 124–130.

286. Harem, E.H.J., Lammers, J.W.J., Fester, J., Heijerman, H.G.M., Groot, C.A.R. and Van Herwaarder, D.L.A. (1995) The effects of the inhaled corticosteroid budesonide on lung function and bronchial hyperresponsiveness in adult patients with cystic fibrosis. *Resp. Med.*, **89**, 209–214.

287. Ranasinha, C., Assoufi, B., Shak, S. *et al.* (1993) Efficiacy and safety of short-term administration of aerosolised recombinant human DNase I in adults with stable stage cystic fibrosis. *Lancet*, **342**, 199–202.

288. Ramsey, B.W., Astley, S.J., Aitken, M.L. *et al.* (1993) Efficacy and safety of short-term administration of aerosolised recombinant human deoxyribonuclease in patients with cystic fibrosis. *Am. Rev. Respir. Dis.*, **148**, 145–151.

289. Fuchs, H.J., Borowitz, D.S., Christiansen, D.H. *et al.* (1994) Effect of aerosolised recombinant human DNase on exacerbations of respiratory symptoms and on pulmonary function in patients with cystic fibrosis. *NEJM*, **331**, 637–642.

290. Accurso, F.J. (1995) Aerosolised dornase alfa in cystic fibrosis patients with clinically mild lung disease. *Dornase alfa Clinical Series*, **2**, (1), 1–6.

291. Shah, P.L., Bush, A., Canny, G.J. *et al.* (1995) Recombinant human DNase 1 (rhDNase) in cystic fibrosis patients with severe pulmonary disease; a short-term double-blind study followed by six months open-label treatment. *Eur. Respir. J.*, **8**, 954–958.

292. McCoy, K., Hamilton, S. and Johnson, C. for the Pulmozyme Study Group (1996) Effects of 12 week administration of dornase alfa in patients with advanced cystic fibrosis lung disease. *Chest*, **110**, 889–895.

293. Shah, P.L., Scott, S.F., Geddes, D.M. and Hodson, M.E. (1995) Two years experience with recombinant human DNase I in the treatment of pulmonary disease in cystic fibrosis. *Respir. Med.*, **89**, 499–502.

294. Winnie, G.B., Cowan, R.G. and Wade, N.A. (1989) Intravenous immune globulin treatment of pulmonary exacerbations in cystic fibrosis. *J. Pediatr.*, **114**, (2), 309–314.

295. Smith, M.B., Hardin, W.D., Dressel, D.A., Beckerman, R.C. and Moynihan, P.C. (1991) Predicting outcome following pulmonary resection in cystic fibrosis patients. *J. Pediatr. Surg.*, **26**, (6), 655–659.

296. Penketh, A.R., Knight, R.K., Hodson, M.E. and Batten, J.C. (1982) Management of pneumothorax in adults. *Thorax*, **37**, (11), 850–853.

297. Spector, M.L. and Stern, R.C. (1989) Pneumothorax in cystic fibrosis; a 26 year experience. *Ann. Thorac. Surg.*, **47**, (2), 204–207.

298. Egan, T.M. (1992) Treatment of pneumothorax in the context of lung transplantation. *Pediatr. Pulmonol. Suppl.*, **8**, 80–81.

299. Wood, R.E. (1992) Haemoptysis in cystic fibrosis. *Pediatr. Pulmonol. Suppl.*, **8**, 82–84.

300. Fairfax, A.J., Ball, J., Batten, J.C. and Heard, B.E. (1980) A pathological study following bronchial artery embolisation for haemoptysis in cystic fibrosis. *Br. J. Dis. Chest*, **74**, (4), 345–352.

301. Sweezey, N.B. and Fellows, K.E. (1990) Bronchial artery embolisation for severe haemoptysis in cystic fibrosis. *Chest*, **97**, (6), 1322–1326.

302. Stern, R.C., Wood, R.E., Boat, T.F. *et al.* (1978) Treatment and prognosis of massive haemoptysis in cystic fibrosis. *Am. Rev. Respir. Dis.*, **117**, (5), 825–828.

303. Cohen, A.M.. (1992) Haemoptysis – role of angiography and embolisation. *Pediatr. Pulmonol. Suppl.*, **8**, 85–86.

304. Magee, G. and Williams, M.H. Jr (1982) Treatment of massive haemoptysis with intravenous pitressin. *Lung*, **160**, (3), 165–169.

305. Bilton, D., Webb, A.K., Foster, H., Mulvenna, P. and Dodd, M. (1990) Life threatening haemoptysis in cystic fibrosis: an alternative therapeutic approach. *Thorax*, **45**, 975–976.

306. Wong, L.T.K., Lillquist, Y.P., Culham, G., DeJong, B.P. and Davidson, A.G.F. (1996) Treatment of recurrent haemoptysis in a child with cystic fibrosis by repeated bronchial artery embolisation and long-term transexamic acid. *Pediatr. Pulmonol.*, **22**, 275–279.

307. Nelson, L.A., Callerame, M.L. and Schwartz, R.H. (1979) Aspergillosis and atopy in cystic fibrosis. *Am. Rev. Respir. Dis.*, **120**, (4), 863–873.

308. Brueton, M.J., Ormerod, L.P., Shah, K.I. and Anderson, C.M. (1980) Allergic bronchopulmonary aspergillosis complicating cystic fibrosis in childhood. *Arch. Dis. Child.*, **55**, (5), 348–353.

309. Hiller, E.J. (1990) Pathogenesis and management of aspergillosis in cystic fibrosis. *Arch. Dis. Child.*, **65**, (4), 397–398.

310. Patterson, R., Greenberger, P.A. and Roberts, M. (1992) Allergic bronchopulmonary aspergillosis. *Pediatr. Pulmonol. Suppl.*, **8**, 120–122.

311. Denning, D.W., Van Wye, J.E., Lewiston, N.J. and Stevens,

D.A. (1991) Adjunctive therapy of allergic bronchopulmonary aspergillosis with itraconazole. *Chest*, **100**, (3), 813–819.

312. Bhargava, V., Tomashefski, J.F., Stern, R.C. and Abramowsky, C.R. (1989) The pathology of fungal infection and colonization in patients with cystic fibrosis. *Hum. Pathol.*, **20**, (10), 977–986.

313. Madden, B.P., Chan, C.M., Kamalvand, K., Siddiqi, A.J., Vuddanalay, P. and Hodson, M.E. (1993) Aspergillus infection in patients with cystic fibrosis following lung transplantation, in *Clinical Ecology of Cystic Fibrosis*, Elsevier Science Publications.

314. Coffey, M.J., FitzGerald, M.X. and McNicholas, W.T. (1991) Comparison of oxygen desaturation during sleep and exercise in patients with cystic fibrosis. *Chest*, **100**, (3), 659–662.

315. Stern, R.C., Borkat, G., Hirschfeld, S.S. *et al.* (1980) Heart failure in cystic fibrosis. treatment and prognosis of cor pulmonale with failure of the right side of the heart. *Am. J. Dis. Child.*, **134**, 267–272.

316. Zinman, R., Coates, A.L., Carry, G.J. *et al.* (1989) Nocturnal home oxygen in the treatment of hypoxaemic cystic fibrosis patients. *J. Pediatr.*, **114**, (3), 368–377.

317. Mestitz, H. and Bowes, G. (1990) *Pseudomonas aeruginosa* empyema in an adult with cystic fibrosis. *Chest*, **98**, (2), 485–487.

318. Taussig, L.M., Belmonte, M.M. and Beaudry, P.H. (1974) *Staphylococcus aureus* empyema in cystic fibrosis. *J. Pediatr.*, **84**, (5), 724–727.

319. Regnis, J.A., Piper, A.J., Henke, K.G., Parker, S., Bye, P.T.P. and Sullivan, C.E. (1994) Benefits of nocturnal nasal CPAP in patients with cystic fibrosis. *Chest*, **106**, 1717–1724.

320. Yankaskas, J.R. (1992) Respiratory failure in CF. Pathophysiology and treatment, including the role of mechanical ventilation. *Pediatr. Pulmonol. Suppl.*, **8**, 87–88.

321. Hodson, M.E., Madden, B.P., Steven, M.H., Tsang, V.T. and Yacoub, M.H. (1991) Non-invasive mechanical ventilation for cystic fibrosis patients – a potential bridge to transplantation. *Eur. Respir. J.*, **4**, (5), 524–527.

322. Kuzemko, J.A. (1988) Home treatment of pulmonary infection in cystic fibrosis. *Chest*, **94**, (Suppl. 2), 162–166.

323. Bramwell, E.C., Halpin, D.M., Duncan-Skingle, F., Hodson, M.E. and Geddes, D.M. (1995) Home treatment in patients with cystic fibrosis using the 'Intermate' – the first year's experience. *J. Adv. Nurs.*, **22**, (6), 1063–1067.

324. Gilbert, J., Robinson, T. and Littlewood, J.M. (1988) Home intravenous antibiotic treatment in cystic fibrosis. *Arch. Dis. Child.*, **63**, (5), 512–517.

325. Donati, M.A., Guenette, G. and Auerbach, H. (1987) Prospective controlled study of home and hospital therapy of cystic fibrosis pulmonary disease. *J. Pediatr.*, **111**, (1), 28–33.

326. Pond, M.N., Newport, M., Joanes, D. and Conway, S.P. (1994) Home versus hospital intravenous antibiotic therapy in the treatment of young adults with cystic fibrosis. *Eur. Respir. J.*, **7**, 1640–1644.

327. Bywater, E.M. (1981) Adolescents with cystic fibrosis: psychosocial adjustment. *Arch. Dis. Child.*, **56**, (7), 538–543.

328. Chapman, J.A. and Goodall, J. (1980) Helping a child to live whilst dying. *Lancet*, **1**, (8171), 753–756.

329. Saunders, C. (ed.) (1978) *The management of terminal disease*, Edward Arnold, London.

330. Dillard, T.A., Berg, B.W., Rajagopal, K.R., Dooley, J.W. and Mehm, W.J. (1989) Hypoxaemia during air travel in patients with chronic obstructive pulmonary disease. *Ann. Int. Med.*, **111**, (5), 362–367.

331. Speechley-Dick, M.E., Rimmer, S.J. and Hodson, M.E. (1992) Exacerbations of cystic fibrosis after holidays at high altitude – a cautionary tale. *Respir. Med.*, **86**, (1), 55–56.

332. Phelan, P. and Hey, E. (1984) Cystic fibrosis mortality in England and Wales and in Victoria, Australia 1976–80. *Arch. Dis. Child.*, **59**, (1), 71–73.

333. Høiby, N. (1982) Microbiology of lung infections in cystic fibrosis patients. *Acta Paediatr. Scand.*, **301**, 35–54.

334. Cystic Fibrosis Foundation (1978) Report of the Patient Registry.

335. Mahadeva, R., Webb, K., Westerbeck, R.C. *et al.* (1998) Clinical outcome in relation to care in centres specialising in cystic fibrosis: cross sectional study. *BMJ*, **316**, 1771–1775.

336. Royal College of Physicians of London (1990) *Cystic Fibrosis in Adults: Recommendations for care in the UK*, Report of the Royal College of Physicians.

337. Shwachman, H. and Kulczycki, L.L. (1958) Long-term study of 105 patients with cystic fibrosis: studies made over a 5–14 year period. *Am. J. Dis. Child.*, **96**, (1), 6–15.

338. Cooperman, E.M., Park, M., McKee, J. and Assad, J.P. (1971) A simplified cystic fibrosis scoring system, (a preliminary report). *Can. Med. Ass. J.*, **105**, (6), 580–582.

339. Taussig, L.M., Kattwinkel, J., Friedewald, W.T. and Di Sant'Agnese, P.A. (1973) A new prognostic score and clinical evaluation system for cystic fibrosis. *J. Pediatr.*, **82**, (3), 380–390.

340. Chrispin, A.R. and Norman, A.P. (1974) The systematic evaluation of the chest radiograph in cystic fibrosis. *Pediatr. Radiol.*, **2**, 101–106.

341. Brasfield, D., Hicks, G., Soong, S.J., Peters, J. and Tiller, R. (1980) Evaluation of scoring system of the chest radiograph in cystic fibrosis. *AJR*, **134**, 1195–1196.

342. Weatherly, M.R., Palmer, C.G., Peters, M.E. *et al.* (1993) Wisconsin cystic fibrosis chest radiograph scoring system. *Pediatrics*, **91**, (2), 488–495.

343. Conway, S.P., Pond, M.N., Bowler, I. *et al.* (1994) The chest radiograph in cystic fibosis: a new scoring system compared with the Chrispin–Norman and Brasfield scores. *Thorax*, **49**, (9), 860–862.

11

Growth, development and nutrition

J. M. LITTLEWOOD AND S. P. WOLFE

Introduction	243	Nutrition and growth of CF individuals	248
Effect of the nutritional state on prognosis	243	Factors that influence the growth and nutritional state	250
Evaluation of nutrition and growth	244	Feeding and growth of CF infants	252
Chest infection is a common cause of short-term		Conclusion	254
suboptimal weight gain	244	References	254
Measuring growth and the nutritional state	244		

INTRODUCTION

Until relatively recently many children who had cystic fibrosis (CF) were of below normal weight and height and had a delayed puberty[1-3]. The minority who survived to adulthood were ultimately below average weight and of relatively short stature[4,5]. Thus, even nowadays, many CF adults are below average in weight and height, which is a significant psychological problem for some of them[6].

The steadily more effective treatment of the respiratory infection and more intensive nutritional support over the past 10 or 15 years have resulted in an impressive and continuing improvement in both the physical condition and survival of many individuals who have cystic fibrosis[7,8]. Certainly most children and young people who have cystic fibrosis should now be adequately nourished, grow and enter puberty normally and ultimately have weights and heights distributed normally within the reference range for their population. However, growth and nutrition are closely dependent on the treatment the patient receives[9], both for the chest infection and the intestinal malabsorption. Not all patients have benefited, nor are benefiting, to the same extent from recent advances in treatment; nutritional state, ultimate size and even survival still vary between clinics and countries[10,11].

EFFECT OF THE NUTRITIONAL STATE ON PROGNOSIS

It has been recognized for some time that a better nutritional state is associated with a better prognosis[12]. The nutritional management was suggested as a major factor in the difference in survival between two established specialist CF centers[10]. Both these reports described patients prior to the introduction of more intensive intravenous and nebulized antibiotic treatments and the availability of the more effective acid-resistant pancreatic enzymes. Whether the improved survival is a direct result of better nutrition, or the nutrition is maintained because the respiratory infection is more effectively treated and controlled, is not entirely clear, probably both factors are relevant. The sequence of infection, malnutrition and depressed immunologic response, resulting in further increase in infection, is a well-established progression in other clinical situations. Certainly the nutritional state, respiratory function and prognosis are better in the few patients who have sufficient residual pancreatic function to achieve normal fat absorption (so-called 'pancreatic-sufficient' patients). Although this advantage was described before the acid-resistant enzymes became generally available[13], recent data from the US CF Foundation Registry in 1995 is just as impressive, with a median survival of 56 years among pancreatic-sufficient patients but only 29 years among those with pancreatic insufficiency. Presumably the combined effect of a better nutritional state and less severe physico-chemical abnormalities within the airways associated with the presence of one of the so-called mild mutations (e.g. R117H, R334W, R347P, A445E; see Chapter 12) both contribute to the better survival of these pancreatic-sufficient patients.

EVALUATION OF NUTRITION AND GROWTH

Infants should be seen every 2 weeks until thriving, then every 4 weeks; older children should attend every 4–8 weeks if they are well and in a stable state. Ideally, adult patients whose condition is stable should attend the CF clinic every 2–3 months. As the condition of the chest is so closely related to the nutritional state they are always considered together, i.e. the 'whole patient' is considered. The patient should see an experienced doctor at every visit and the dietitian at most clinic visits, and always if weight progress is unsatisfactory[14]. The information listed in Table 11.1 is essential for assessment and monitoring of the nutritional state at every clinic visit.

CHEST INFECTION IS A COMMON CAUSE OF SHORT-TERM SUBOPTIMAL WEIGHT GAIN

The condition of the chest is carefully evaluated by the presence of symptoms, particularly cough and sputum production, or in young children, who swallow sputum, whether the cough sounds productive. Clinical examination, respiratory cultures and respiratory function tests are done at every clinic visit – spirometry in children over 6 years, peak expiratory flow rates in younger patients and pulse oximetry on all. More detailed monitoring of the respiratory tract is described in Chapter 10.

MEASURING GROWTH AND THE NUTRITIONAL STATE

These data are an important indicator of progress and techniques for making the measurements correctly in the clinic and normal values are well described[16]. It is important that measurements are made accurately by regular clinic staff who are familiar with the techniques of measuring height and weight, and that they appreciate the importance of the information in monitoring CF patients.

Table 11.1 *Information necessary for assessment of the patient's nutritional state*

History	
Energy intake	Appetite, food intake, energy supplementation and other nutritional support, e.g. enteral feeding. Ideally an accurate assessment of nutrient intake every year. This is mandatory if the nutritional state is abnormal (Chapter 14)
Abdominal symptoms	Pain and distension should not affect more than 10 per cent of patients if the control of their intestinal absorption is adequate[15]
Bowels	Frequency and characteristics of the stools
Pancreatic enzymes	Type, dose, method and timing of administration
Vitamins	Dose and type of supplements
Compliance	Failure to adhere to treatment may account for symptoms and/or nutritional problems and must always be considered in every patient
Physical examination	
Abdominal contour	Fullness suggests inadequate control of the malabsorption
Abdominal masses	Presence suggests constipation and/or colonic overloading
Liver and spleen	Liver – firmness or enlargement. Presence and enlargement of the spleen
Urine	Tested periodically for glucose. Over 10 years old an annual glucose tolerance test is required to identify glucose intolerance and diabetes mellitus

Caution should be exercised in making interclinic and international comparisons of the calculated growth status, for this is influenced by the standards that are used[17]. A recent study compared the use of the anthropometric standards of the US National Center for Health Statistics, the British Tanner and Whitehouse standards and a new British composite (UK 90) in the interpretation of Canadian CF Registry data for 1994; even ideal weight was not free from bias[18].

Weight and height

These should be measured at each clinic attendance, as they are a valuable objective measurement of progress. The values are compared to those of the normal population and charted to assess progress[16,19,20]. Values are expressed either as (per) centiles, as percentage of the normal values for age[21] or as standard deviation scores (SD or Z scores). All these values give some idea of how the patient compares to apparently healthy individuals of the same age, and they are widely used to interpret weight and height measurements[22]. Percentages weight for height and weight and height for age are often used when expressing the nutritional status of children in preference to body mass index (BMI). The measurements are calculated either by using the Cole's growth assessment slide rule[21] or from a standard equation:

$$\frac{\text{Current weight (kg)} \times 100}{\text{Weight (kg) equivalent to current height percentile}}$$

Although the measurement is simple to perform and easy to undertake in routine clinical practice, care must be taken as a high degree of inaccuracy in the calculation has been reported[23]. For a population whose values are normally distributed, the relationship of percentiles and SD scores are as follows: −3.0 SD (0.13th centile), −2.0 SD (2.28th centile), −1.0 SD (15.87th centile), 0 SD (50th centile), +1.0 SD (84.13th centile), +2.0 SD (97.72nd centile), +3.0 SD (99.87th centile)[16].

The body mass index

The body mass index (BMI) is derived by dividing the weight in kilograms by the square of the height in meters. It has only recently been validated for UK children[24], and values for UK CF individuals have been reported[6] (Figs 11.1 and 11. 2). It is a measure of a person's fatness relatively independent of height, which can be a disadvantage in assessing the nutritional state of children whose height may have been adversely affected by chronic malnutrition, i.e. who are stunted and/or who have delayed puberty. The BMI is already widely used as a convenient measure of the nutritional state of adults, more often as a means of measuring obesity than malnutrition. However, many adult CF clinics now use BMI as a convenient measure of nutritional state in their

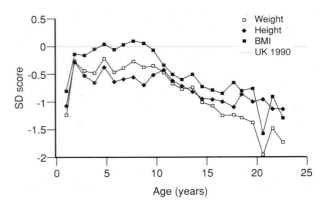

Fig. 11.1 *Mean weight, height and BMI by age in UK male patients with cystic fibrosis, expressed as SD scores relative to the British 1990 growth standards[6]. (With permission of the BMJ Publishing Group.)*

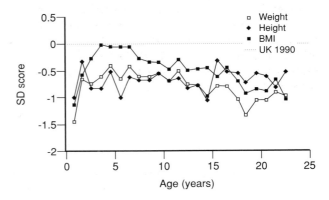

Fig. 11.2 *Mean weight, height and BMI by age in UK female patients with cystic fibrosis, expressed as SD scores relative to the British 1990 growth standards[6]. (With permission of the BMJ Publishing Group.)*

patients whose growth has ceased. Recently BMI categories for adults have been redefined as follows: underweight, less than 18.5; ideal, 18.5–24.9; pre-obese, 25.0–29.9; obese Class I, 30.0–34.9; obese Class II 35.0–39.9; and obese Class III greater than 40.0 kg/m^2 [25]. These fixed classifications of BMI are considered to be inappropriate for children as the 50th centile for BMI shows marked changes from birth through early childhood. The value must be interpreted on the basis of the centile charts[26]. As the normal standards are derived from cross-sectional data, as with other anthropomorphic measurements, an individual child's values will not adhere to the same centile through puberty, as the age at which maximal pubertal growth occurs varies. A low BMI without deficient fatness will be found in patients with proportionately long limbs and a short trunk, where there is poor musculature or in adolescents with delayed puberty[16].

The mid upper-arm circumference and skinfold measurements

The mid upper-arm circumference (MUAC) and skinfold measurements are useful simple clinical measurements of nutritional status, but are inappropriate for the detailed monitoring required in cystic fibrosis[27]. There is conflicting evidence regarding the reliability of the use of skinfold thickness to estimate fat-free mass in CF[28–31]. Direct methods of body composition analysis allow more accurate measurement of body composition.

Pubertal status

Noting the stages of breast, pubic hair and genital development and recording the age of the menarche in girls are important as a measure of the stage of development[19]. Assessment of the stage of sexual development is essential for the correct interpretation of changes in weight and height gain during adolescence. Children with early puberty will accelerate in height growth and weight gain, moving to higher centiles during their period of rapid growth; conversely those who are late developers will lose centiles, usually height and weight moving to a similar degree, but will catch up when their growth eventually accelerates. Thus after the age of 10 years or so, serial values of both weight and height and knowledge of the pubertal state are required to adequately assess growth and nutrition. This should include estimation of the skeletal age, preferably using the Tanner and Whitehouse (TW2) method[32]. Skeletal age estimated from a hand X-ray corresponds with the stage of puberty in adolescents and, in practice, adds little to the management of prepubertal children, being normal or only mildly retarded for age in the majority. Although some delay in puberty has usually been attributed to malnutrition, in one series of Swedish female CF patients, pubertal delay of approximately 2 years was present despite good clinical status. The delay was most marked in those patients homozygous for ΔF_{508} and those with evidence of glucose intolerance[33].

Bone mineral density

Osteopenia and osteoporosis have been desribed in both adults and children with cystic fibrosis[34,35]. Bone mineral density (BMD) is assessed by dual energy X-ray absorptiometry (DEXA). Although expensive, because of increasing evidence of reduced BMD, DEXA scans, which can be carried out at most major CF units, should be considered as part of the nutritional assessment in all patients over the age of 10 years.

Rate of weight gain and growth

Regular charting of height and weight on an appropriate growth chart at every clinic attendance is essential (UK, Child Growth Foundation, 2 Mayfield Avenue, London W4 1PW, UK). It is also helpful to use a Cole Rule to calculate the percentage weight for height[21]. Standards for charting height and weight velocity are available but charting height and weight on a standard growth chart usually provides adequate information. Any slowing of weight gain or rate of growth (fall in centiles) or fall in the percentage weight for height (or BMI) is carefully evaluated, both from the gastrointestinal and respiratory aspects, by the clinician (Fig. 11.3). The dietitian should always be involved to assess the adequacy of the energy intake and general nutritional management.

The weight for height should remain above 90 per cent and ideally should be over 95 per cent. Oral energy supplements are usually advised if the weight for height is between 85 and 90 per cent and enteral tube feeding if it falls below 85 per cent (Chapter 19b).

A normal nutritional state and rate of growth are now attainable goals in the majority of CF patients if they are prepared to accept the often invasive methods of nutritional support. It is important to consider other causes of abnormal nutrition and growth, either gastrointestinal, such as food intolerance, celiac disease or inflammatory bowel disease[15], or even endocrine[36]. The slowing of height gain in the presence of apparently normal or excessive weight gain from high-dose oral steroid treatment is usually obvious but may be less obvious when it is the result of long-term inhaled steroids, which are now widely used in CF patients, often in substantial doses[37,38].

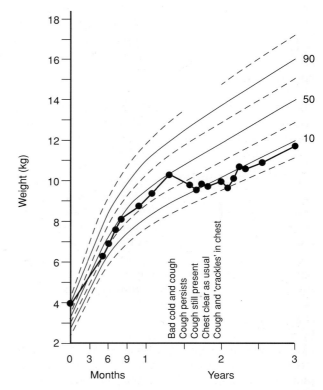

Fig. 11.3 *Slowing of weight gain due to respiratory infection in a pancreatic-sufficient CF patient, screened in the 1970s.*

Unexpected loss of height is usually due to a measuring error, except for the rare instance where vertebral collapse results from severe osteoporosis.

Laboratory investigations

A variety of investigations are helpful in the assessment of the patient's nutritional state and are performed in most CF units as part of the patient's annual assessment[7,39]. These include hemoglobin, total white cell and neutrophil count, plasma viscosity, erythrocyte sedimentation rate, C-reactive protein, immunoglobulins and *Pseudomonas* antibodies, serum albumin and/or pre-albumin. Urea and electrolytes should be checked whenever clinical progress is not entirely satisfactory, to identify salt depletion and pseudo-Bartter's syndrome, which may cause significant growth failure[40]. Liver function tests should be checked and many units arrange an ultrasound examination of the liver and upper abdomen. Fasting plasma fat-soluble vitamin A, D and E levels should be measured annually.

VITAMIN A

Clinical evidence of vitamin A deficiency is rarely recognized, but has been reported as causing abnormal dark adaptation, conjunctival xerosis[41], xerophthalmia[42] and raised intracranial pressure[43], which has also been reported with excessive doses of vitamin A[44]. In our experience, correction of vitamin A deficiency is associated with an improved general condition and clinical course[45]. With regular vitamin A supplementation and annual monitoring to achieve normal plasma levels, dark adaptation is normal[46].

VITAMIN D

Clinical evidence of vitamin D deficiency is rare, although both rickets[47] and osteomalacia[48] have been reported. Low levels of vitamin D metabolites are well documented, particularly in older patients[49]; also low normal values of 25-hydroxy vitamin D may be associated with abnormally low values of 1,25-dihydroxy vitamin D[34]. In contrast to rickets, osteoporosis is common in CF patients[50,51], particularly after transplantation operations[52]. However, in one series of well-nourished young CF patients, bone mineral content and body composition were normal, suggesting that the osteoporosis reported in CF was nutritional and therefore preventable if early nutrition was appropriate[53].

VITAMIN K

The initial presentation of CF may be with bleeding due to vitamin K deficiency[54]. In the past, as coagulation studies are usually normal, regular vitamin K supplements were given only if prothrombin levels were low and to patients with liver disease. However, having observed a tendency to excessive postoperative bleeding, it has been our practice to give water-soluble vitamin K (phytomenadione, 10 mg daily) to all CF patients for some days before surgery. Although plasma vitamin K levels have been reported as normal[55], recent work, using PIVKA II levels (prothrombin induced in vitamin K absence), has revealed subclinical vitamin K deficiency in many CF children who have pancreatic insufficiency. This work suggests that routine supplements should be given to all CF patients[56,57].

VITAMIN E

Plasma vitamin E levels of CF infants identified by neonatal screening fall in the first weeks of life prior to starting treatment[58,59]. Early and severe hemolytic anemia has been reported in CF infants[60]. Neurological complications in CF adults associated with vitamin E deficiency are well documented but rare, and include loss of tendon reflexes, muscle weakness, reduced vibration and proprioceptive sensation[61,62]. Vitamin E is also a powerful antioxidant (see below).

WATER-SOLUBLE VITAMINS

These are all well absorbed, and regular supplements are unnecessary[63,64]. Folate and vitamin B_{12} status may be compromised in patients who have had extensive small intestinal resections, usually for meconium ileus, but are usually normal. The role of vitamin C and β-carotene as antioxidants is under investigation.

MINERALS AND TRACE ELEMENTS

Plasma levels are usually normal[65]. There are isolated reports of malabsorption and deficiencies of trace elements, even when taking regular pancreatic enzyme supplements[66]. Although symptomatic zinc deficiency has been described in an adult[67] and in newly-diagnosed infants[68], plasma levels are usually normal[65,69]. Hypomagnesemia has been reported as a complication of N-acetyl cysteine treatment of distal intestinal obstruction[70] and aminoglycoside treatment[71].

ESSENTIAL FATTY ACIDS

Essential fatty acid (EFA) deficiency, as evidenced by abnormal triene:tetraene ratio values, occurred in 27 per cent of young CF infants identified by neonatal screening[72]. Clinical evidence of EFA deficiency is very rare in treated patients although abnormalities of blood lipids are common[73,74]. The role of EFA and their precursors the ω-3 fatty acids, eicosapentaenoic acid and docosahexaenoic acid, and the significance of their deficiency in CF are under investigation[75–77]. Recent evidence has suggested that an imbalance of essential fatty acids in the cell membrane may play a role in the phenotypic expression of CF[78].

ANTIOXIDANTS

There is increasing interest in the role of antioxidants in protecting against oxidative damage caused to the lungs by reactive oxygen species. Vitamins C and E, β-carotene and selenium (precursor of glutathione) are the main dietary forms of antioxidants. Requirements for vitamin C have been found to increase as lung disease progresses[79]. In its capacity as an antioxidant, vitamin C scavenges oxygen free radicals interrupting the inflammatory process[79]. β-carotene levels have also been shown to be low in CF[80,81] and oral supplementation has been shown to correct deficiency[82]. The role of glutathionone and value of selenium supplementation in lung defence is also under investigation[83].

NUTRITION AND GROWTH OF CF INDIVIDUALS

Birth weight

The birth weight of CF individuals has been reported as below normal[3,84,85]. Mearns recorded the gestation and birth weights of 257 of her 288 patients. The mean birth weights for males (3.18 kg) and females (3.04 kg) were below that of unaffected infants (3.37 kg and 3.25 kg, respectively)[3]. Others have failed to confirm the lower birth weights[86,87]. A recent report, in addition to reporting that CF infants had a significantly lower length (−1.24 SD) and weight (−0.72 SD), also noted a smaller head circumference (−1.82 SD) than in controls[88]. However, in this series, infants presenting with meconium ileus were overrepresented (34.6 per cent) which could have been associated with their poor intrauterine growth. By 4 years, although their length had improved to −0.15 SD and weight to −0.53 SD, the head circumference remained significantly low at −1.05 SD.

Subsequent growth of CF infants

The subsequent early growth pattern of CF infants is dependent on both the age of diagnosis and the subsequent treatment they receive. The majority have pancreatic insufficiency and experience early gastrointestinal symptoms and subnormal weight gain. Even some infants diagnosed by neonatal screening have subnormal growth throughout the first year if the start of treatment is delayed more than a few weeks. In one large series of screened Wisconsin CF infants, the mean age of diagnosis was 12 weeks, when the SD score for weight was already −0.5 and for height −0.2. There was suboptimal growth in the second half of the first year[59]; a feature also described in the Colorado screened CF infants[89]. However, when the diagnosis is made within 2 or 3 weeks of birth, the mid-year fall off of weight gain and suboptimal growth is avoided[87] (Fig. 11.4). Subsequent growth of these infants is normal provided that both the chest infection is prevented or treated aggressively and the intestinal malabsorption is adequately treated[86,87].

Growth and nutrition after infancy

Aggressive nutritional treatment has always been encouraged in Toronto and even in 1979 the heights of their patients conformed to the normal distribution, the medians being well above the 25th centile. The weights were more often distributed in the lower centiles but, even then, very few weights were below 3rd centile

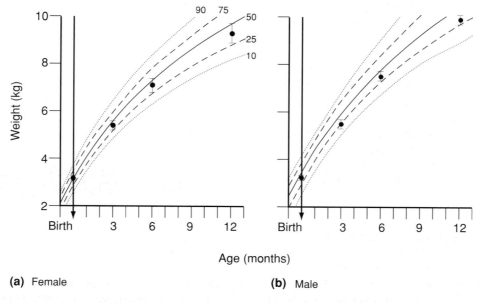

(a) Female

(b) Male

Fig. 11.4 *Normal growth in a series of screened CF infants, adapted from ref. 87. (Mean ± s.e).*

(approximately 3.5 per cent of males and 11.4 per cent of females)[90]. More recently it was reported that almost normal growth and weight gain could be maintained throughout childhood in the Toronto patients[10].

In Sweden, 51 CF children were studied during their first 8 years. The mean age of diagnosis was 0.4 years (0.0–6.1 years). Their height fell to −1.3 SD over the first 0.25 years and remained subnormal for the first year, but thereafter catch-up occurred, reaching almost normal (mean −0.3 SD) by 5 years of age. Height gain was normal between 5 and 8 years. The authors conclude that subnormal growth in infancy is compensated for by supernormal growth thereafter[91].

In an Australian series growth, weight and respiratory function were better at age of 10 years in a group of screened patients than in those born before screening was introduced[92].

In 1998 the American Cystic Fibrosis Foundation (CFF) reported that 12.7 per cent of children and 21.6 per cent of adults respectively were below 85 per cent weight for height[93]. In 1996, the CFF reported that 33.6 per cent of all USA patients had a weight below the 10th centile (by National Center for Health Statistics standards) and 24.4 per cent of patients were below the 5th centile; the mean weight centile for all patients was 29.5 (SD 25.8). For height, 28.3 per cent were less than the 10th centile and 19.8 per cent were below the 5th centile; the mean height centile of the CF patients was 32.9 (SD 26.8)[94]. In 1993 20 per cent of all children on the US CFF Registry were less than 5th centile for height or weight for age. The mean and median height and weight for age were at the 30th and 20th centiles. Malnutrition (height or weight for age less than the 5th centile) was particularly pronounced in infants (47 per cent) and adolescents (34 per cent) and newly diagnosed patients (44 per cent). The children's mean weight centile was 32.8 (SD 26.5) and the adults' 23.1 (SD 23.1); the children's mean height centile was 30.5 (SD 25.9), compared to the adults' 37.5 (SD 27.9)[95].

In a recent comparison between the growth status of children with CF in the US and Canada, using data from their respective CF registries, comparable median centile values for Canadian and US patients were for height, 28 and 21; weight, 27 and 22; but both were 103 per cent of ideal weight for height. Also more US patients were below the 5th centile for height (22 versus 16 per cent) and weight (20 versus 16 per cent). In 7 per cent of both groups the ideal weight for height was below the 5th centile[11].

Growth and nutrition of UK patients

During 1994 and 1995 height and weight data were obtained on 3056 patients (1604 males, 1452 females) registered with the UK CF Survey. They were attending 33 different CF clinics and represented almost half (48.5

per cent) of the UK CF population. Data from the 2883 of these patients who were under 30 years were analyzed and compared with normal values[20,24]. Only 23 per cent of UK infants are screened for CF and there were substantial nutritional deficits in the first year. Most of the catch-up growth, which followed the introduction of treatment, was completed within 2 years. The mean weight SD scores of the males were between −0.25 and −0.5 until the age of 10 years, after which they declined, as did the body mass index (BMI). The mean weight SD scores of females were approximately −0.5 but they had a declining BMI after the age of 5 years[6] (Figs 11.1 and 11.2). The pattern of growth in this cross-sectional study was disappointingly similar, but less severe, to that described in 1975[96], when the weight and height SD scores had fallen to between −1.0 and −1.5 by the time of diagnosis. In the recent series[6], the phase of 'catch-up' growth continued for 2 years or so, followed by a plateau during mid-childhood with the weight SD score around −0.5 (−1.0 in the 1975 series); after 10 years there was a progressive decline in SD scores for both height and weight. This deterioration in SD scores after the age of 10 years could be explained by some delay in the onset of puberty, but was more likely a reflection of an overall deterioration associated with an increase in the severity of the pulmonary disease.

It is increasingly apparent that the condition of the patients is closely related to the treatment they receive, and patients may be in a better nutritional state in clinics where regular attention is paid to nutrition and growth. It is encouraging that the nutritional state of new CF patients referred to our unit from other hospitals has steadily improved over the years[97] (Fig. 11.5), as has the nutrition of patients currently attending our clinic (Figs. 11.6 and 11.7).

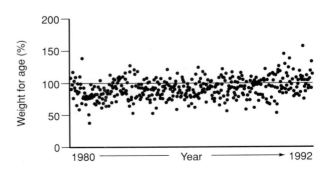

Fig. 11.5 *Significant improvement in percentage weight for age of 380 new patients at the time of referral to the Leeds Regional Paediatric CF Unit. (Adapted from ref. 97).*

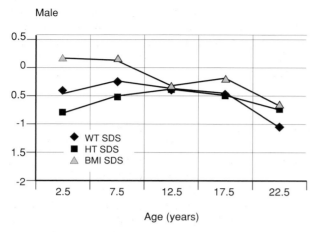

Fig. 11.6 *Mean weight, height and BMI by age of males attending the Leeds Regional CF Units, expressed as SD scores relative to the British 1990 growth standards.*

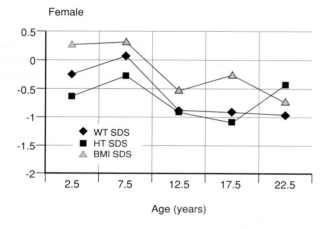

Fig. 11.7 *Mean weight, height and BMI by age of females attending the Leeds Regional CF Units, expressed as SD scores relative to the British 1990 growth standards.*

Delayed puberty and growth spurt

There is delay in the onset of puberty and menarche in CF patients who have significant nutritional problems[98]; even in well-nourished females some delay has been reported[33]. The anatomical abnormalities of the vas deferens, although responsible for the infertility affecting virtually all CF men, do not appear to influence the onset or the anatomic and endocrine changes associated with puberty (Chapter 14). The growth spurt in one recent series was delayed by an average of 0.8 years and was about 1 cm/year slower at its peak in CF patients compared to normal controls[99]. Surprisingly, the delay in skeletal maturation is modest in CF patients; in one series 20 per cent had a delay of skeletal maturation of greater than 1 year but only 6 per cent more than 2 years. The delay in skeletal maturity seemed to increase with age as pulmonary problems became more severe[3].

Body composition in cystic fibrosis

More sophisticated methods of measuring body composition offer more accurate assessment of nutritional status and growth response to nutritional therapy. These methods include total body potassium (TBK)[100], total body electrical conductivity (TOBEC)[101], bioelectrical impedance analysis (BIA)[102], total body water by isotope dilution[103] and dual-energy X-ray absorptiometry (DEXA)[31,104]. Total body potassium (TBK) measurements have shown a reduced body cell mass (BCM) at the time of diagnosis in screened infants[105]. With instigation of nutritional therapy, TBK levels improved to normal between 3 and 9 months and by 12 months children seemed to have normal weight, height and BCM but reduced body fat stores. This pattern may suggest that some weight gain is made up of water and therefore there may be subclinical nutritional disturbances, indicating that nutritional management should aim to normalize body fat stores. Total body potassium measurements have also shown a reduction in BCM with increasing age, and that malnourished children show a significant improvement in BCM with long-term nutritional rehabilitation[99]. DEXA studies in older CF patients have also shown variable deficits of fat body mass (FBM) but uniform reduction in bone body mass (BBM) and lean body mass (LBM) was also seen[106].

FACTORS THAT INFLUENCE THE GROWTH AND NUTRITIONAL STATE

The nutritional state of individuals who have CF is largely determined by the adequacy of their treatment. There is commonly an impressive improvement in the nutritional state when appropriate treatment is given to patients transferred from a general hospital clinic to a specialized CF center[9,107]. Also patients referred to adult CF centers from specialized pediatric CF clinics are in better condition than those referred from general pediatric clinics[108].

Factors which contribute to the poor nutritional state of many CF patients include an inadequate energy intake, the often severe and rarely completely controlled intestinal malabsorption, the increased energy demands resulting from chest infection and a variable intrinsic increase in resting energy expenditure (REE), even in those who appear to have little or no chest involvement[109,110]. It has been suggested that the presence of the CF mutation itself results in increased energy expenditure, being particularly marked in those who are homozygous for the ΔF_{508} mutation[111]. These factors will be discussed in more detail particularly as to their effect on nutritional state and growth.

Energy intake

The poor energy intake of many CF individuals has been well documented in the past[112,113]. Although intakes in excess of 120 per cent of the estimated average requirement (EAR) are commonly advised, when the actual energy intake is measured it is often considerably less than this[107,114–116]. In addition, female patients have also been documented to have poorer energy intakes than male patients[117]. The mean energy intake of patients attending our pediatric CF unit in Leeds in 1995 for full care was: for the 0–5-year-olds, 122 per cent; 5–l0 years, 127 per cent; and for the 10–15-year-olds, 133 per cent of the estimated average requirement for age (Department of Health, 1991). The many reasons for the poor energy intake and their management are discussed in Chapter 19b.

Malabsorption (see also Chapter 12)

The majority of CF infants detected by neonatal screening have pancreatic insufficiency from the time of diagnosis, although some may have adequate function to prevent malabsorption for a few months[118]. Pancreatic insufficiency was present in 79 per cent of one series of screened CF infants at 6 months, and 92 per cent at 1 year[119]. The pancreatic damage is present to some extent at birth in all infants and thereafter is progressive[120]. The majority of patients therefore require pancreatic enzyme replacement therapy and, with adequate treatment, between 85 and 95 per cent fat absorption should be achieved[121].

There are factors other than pancreatic enzyme deficiencies that contribute to the intestinal malabsorption and these are discussed in Chapter 12. As the patient becomes older, other factors may have an adverse effect on metabolism, nutrition and growth: diabetes mellitus (DM) and liver disease are of particular importance.

Diabetes mellitus (see also Chapter 15)

Estimates of prevalence of diabetes mellitus (DM) in CF vary from 2.5 to 12 per cent of patients, increasing with age. In the Copenhagen clinic 32 per cent developed DM by the age of 25 years[122], which is the experience of most large CF clinics. Of the 184 patients (87 males; 97 females) attending the Regional Adult CF Clinic in Leeds for all their care (i.e. excluding 'shared-care' patients), 32.6 per cent have DM (28.7 per cent of males; 36.1 per cent of females). For some years before the onset of clinical DM (a 2-hour glucose of more than 12.2 mmol/L during a glucose tolerance test), the presence of glucose intolerance (a 2-hour glucose of 8.8–12.2 mmol/L), as distinct from clinical diabetes, has an adverse effect on the patient's respiratory and nutritional state[123]. Treatment of the glucose intolerance with oral hypoglycemic agents before the development of clinical DM offers a potential therapeutic approach which is usually not taken, but which requires further investigation[124,125].

Liver disease (see also Chapter 13)

Some 20 per cent of CF individuals eventually have biochemical, ultrasound or clinical evidence of liver disease, and 5 per cent have clinical liver disease, rising from 0.3 per cent in the under 5-year-olds to 9 per cent in those over 16 years old[126]. Although it is difficult to identify a significant impact of the relatively frequent subclinical liver involvement on nutrition and growth[127], increased resting energy expenditure has been described in non-CF individuals who have chronic liver disease[128]. Also CF patients with overt clinical liver disease commonly have serious nutritional problems, both with general nutrition and also with specific macronutrients, fat-soluble vitamins and clotting factors[129]. The observation that the nutritional state of CF patients with liver disease improved with ursodeoxycholic acid[130] was not confirmed in a controlled trial[131]. However, a subsequent study showed that both biochemical tests and liver histology improved with ursodeoxycholic acid therapy[132]. Liver transplantation in CF patients with severe liver disease does have an impressive effect on their nutritional state[133].

Endocrine abnormalities

Diminished concentrations of insulin-like growth factor 1 and a correlation with the height score have been described in CF patients[134,135]. Insulin-like growth factor 1 (IGF-1) is an anabolic hormone and an important marker of nutritional status, liver function and linear growth. A weak correlation with BMI suggested that malnutrition was not the prime cause of the lowered IGF-1 levels; recurrent infection, impaired liver function and insulin deficiency may all contribute[134]. Although IGF-1 deficiency may be a secondary phenomenon, it does correlate both with the Shwachman score and respiratory function. The reduced IGF-1 levels and reduced insulin secretion may both contribute to the common persisting abnormalities of weight for height[135]. There is some preliminary data indicating that growth hormone therapy may be beneficial in improving growth[136,137].

Recent work on leptins, which are involved in controlling body weight and energy expenditure, suggests that these recently described proteins may prove to have considerable relevance to the nutritional problems of CF patients[138].

Increased energy expenditure, chest infection and genotype

The importance of the chronic inflammation associated with the respiratory infection in increasing energy expenditure and contributing to malnutrition and growth problems cannot be overemphasized. Initial observations on the increased energy expenditure in undernourished CF adolescents and adults[139] led to further studies, using indirect calorimetry, which demonstrated increased resting energy expenditure (REE) even in patients with mild chest disease[109] and also in infants[140–142]. Many subsequent studies have confirmed REE is increased in CF[110,111,143], as is the total energy expenditure during periods of recovery from mild exercise[144]. This is presumably due to the increased work of breathing consistent with higher ventilatory requirements. In many patients, the increase in the REE is related to the severity of the chest infection and is significantly reduced during treatment with an appropriate course of antibiotics[145, 146]. REE has been reported to be higher in patients colonized with *Pseudomonas* species in comparison to those who are not[147].

There is discussion as to the relative importance of the type of CF mutation and the severity of the chest infection[111,142,148]. Whether the increased REE observed in patients who appear to have little or even no chest infection is related to subclinical infection or to the basic abnormality in CFTR function, has not been determined[141]. Certainly, many patients who have little or no clinical evidence of chest infection have uniformly raised inflammatory markers[149]. Thus the chronic respiratory infection, present in so many CF individuals, seems to be the major cause of the increased REE and is the major factor responsible for the poor nutritional state of most patients who have significant chest involvement. In our pediatric clinic, those patients with relatively mild chest involvement (FEV_1 > 80 per cent predicted) had a mean weight for age of 98.4 per cent and a mean energy intake of 126 per cent of their EAR, but those with more severe chest involvement (FEV_1 < 60 per cent predicted) had a mean weight for age of only 88.7 per cent despite a mean energy intake of 136 per cent of their EAR[150]. The increased energy requirement does not appear to be due to increased energy expenditure during the various activities of daily living, as it was found to be increased to the same extent during two levels of activity in CF patients and controls[151]. However, there may be a partial compensation for the increased resting energy expenditure by a reduction in spontaneous physical activity during courses of treatment[152,153]. These findings support the practice of assessing each patient's individual energy requirements according to their general clinical condition, their nutritional state and growth rate for children, rather than aiming for an arbitrary increased intake in every patient.

Pregnancy (see also Chapter 14)

Pregnancy represents a particular and significant nutritional stress for the woman who has CF. However, an increasing number of women who have CF are having babies[154,155]. Even though the patient may appear to have relatively mild CF at the beginning of the pregnancy, it is essential that she be referred to a CF center early in the pregnancy, if not already attending a specialized clinic. Both the chest and the major nutritional problems of the pregnant patient who has CF will require all the expertise of the combined CF center medical and obstetric teams. Detailed nutritional management is discussed in Chapters 14 and 19b.

FEEDING AND GROWTH OF CF INFANTS

The preferred method of infant feeding in CF has been the subject of debate. Infants fed on a predigested formula containing medium-chain triglycerides (MCT) e.g. Pregestimil® (Mead Johnson) achieve normal weight gain and growth by the age of 1 year[156], as will those fed on human milk[86] and normal infant formulae[87]. Infants who receive a feed containing adequate energy should thrive satisfactorily irrespective of the type of milk[86,157]. However, a predigested MCT-containing formula may be of benefit to infants who have undergone extensive small bowel resection for meconium ileus or those who have coexisting intolerance to cows' milk[158].

Whatever the type of milk used, pancreatic-insufficient infants will require enzyme supplements even with predigested formulae[159]. A standard enteric-coated microsphere preparation should always be used at a starting dose of one-third of a capsule per feed, equivalent to approximately 3300 IU lipase for Creon® 10 000 (Solvay Health Care, Ltd.). Most infants should thrive providing they are taking sufficient quantities of milk (usually 200 mL/kg/day) and adequate pancreatic supplements. Occasionally, if weight gain is poor, additional energy supplements may be added to the feed. CF infants are usually weaned between 4 and 6 months of age. A normal to high-fat weaning diet is recommended, depending on the infant's growth, and the enzyme supplementation is adjusted accordingly. Dietetic support at this time should include advice on coping with food and enzyme refusal, both of which are common problems.

The first 2 years is a period of very rapid growth and it is therefore important that the treatment, general condition, nutritional state and growth rate of the CF infant is monitored every 2–4 weeks in the clinic until the treatment regime is firmly established, the parents are confident and the weight gain is at least normal – often there is catch-up growth, even in screened infants. Persisting

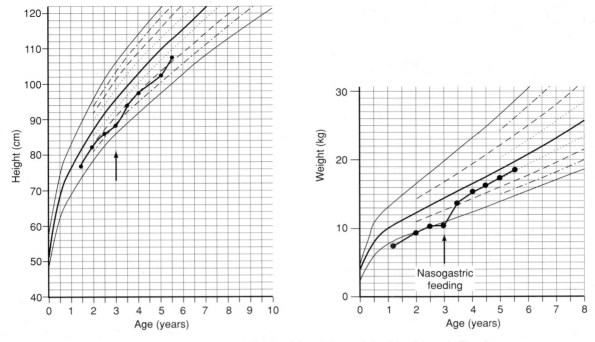

Fig. 11.8 *Persisting catch-up growth with treatment following delayed diagnosis in girls with cystic fibrosis.*

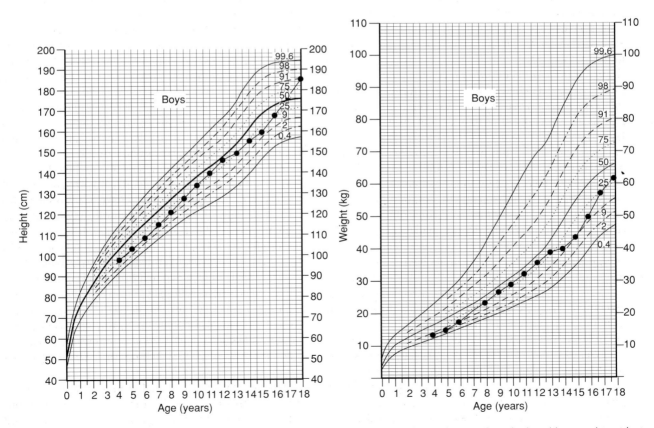

Fig. 11.9 *Some improvement in growth and weight gain during childhood following early gastrointestinal problems and transient* Pseudomonas *infection. From 12 years there is an apparent slowing of growth with loss of centiles due to the delayed onset of puberty. Accelerating growth and weight gain are seen from 15 years following the onset of the puberty growth spurt, with eventual height and weight being above average.*

suboptimal weight gain at this stage should prompt detailed investigation of both the respiratory and gastrointestinal systems and, if necessary, admission to hospital. If the poor weight gain is related to chest infection, which may not be obvious, irreparable pulmonary damage may occur if this is not identified and treated (Fig. 11.3).

CONCLUSION

The nutritional and growth consequences of untreated CF are severe. However, with present-day treatments, many introduced over the past decade, gastrointestinal symptom and signs should be controlled in over 90 per cent of CF patients, and their nutritional state and growth should be normal. Of particular importance has been the realization that many patients have a poor dietary energy intake and raised resting energy expenditure and that expert dietary advice, if necessary with enteral feeding, can restore and maintain a good nutritional state and growth rate, even in patients with advanced chest disease. It is important that these techniques are made available to all CF patients who require them. Intestinal malabsorption can be well controlled in the majority with modern acid-resistant pancreatic enzyme preparations, and fat-soluble vitamin deficiency is avoided if daily supplements sufficient to normalize plasma levels are taken.

As the CF population becomes older, the potential for chronic nutritional deficiencies increases, diabetes mellitus and chronic liver disease become major problems, and more invasive measures may be needed to combat the nutritional consequences of the chronic chest infection. The increased resting energy expenditure and its relationship to both the type of CF mutation present and the chest infection are areas of intense interest.

With particular regard to growth, some but not all authors report that CF infants have some interference with their intrauterine growth, as evidenced by the reduced birth weight, length and head circumference. In the absence of treatment, most infants have subnormal growth from early infancy and serious nutritional deficiencies are described even by the time screened infants are diagnosed[58]. After diagnosis, following improved absorption with pancreatic enzymes, the increase in absorbable energy exceeds the increased expenditure, resulting in catch-up growth. A stable plateau is followed by reasonably normal growth through mid childhood. The progressive chest infection, which affects increasing numbers of children during adolescence, becomes more severe, so that dietary energy intake is often insufficient to maintain weight and sustain normal growth and pubertal development.

It is now well established that by providing a sufficient energy intake to redress the balance, often by enteral feeding regimes (Fig. 11.8), even patients with severe chest involvement and high energy requirements can be returned to positive energy balance, improving their weight and growth. The normal growth and development of an increasing proportion of patients, who have avoided significant chest infection and whose absorption has been adequately controlled, suggests that the growth potential of the majority of CF individuals is normal provided these adverse factors are controlled (Fig. 11.9).

REFERENCES

1. Shwachman, H. and Kulczycki, L.L. (1958) Long term study of one hundred and five patients with cystic fibrosis. *Am. J. Dis. Child.*, **96**, 6–15.
2. Sproul, A. and Huang, N. (1964) Growth patterns in children with cystic fibrosis. *J. Pediatr.*, **65**, 664.
3. Mearns, M.B. (1983) Growth and development, in *Cystic Fibrosis*, (eds M.E. Hodson, A.P. Norman and J.C. Batten), Baillière Tindall, London, pp. 183–196.
4. Mitchell-Heggs, P., Mearns, M. and Batten, J.C. (1976) Cystic fibrosis in adolescents and adults. *Q. J. Med. (New Series)*, **45**, 479–504.
5. Penketh, A.R., Wise, A., Mearns, M.B., Hodson, M.E. and Batten, J.C. (1987) Cystic fibrosis in adolescents and adults. *Thorax*, **42**, 526–532.
6. Morison, S., Dodge, J.A., Cole, T.J. *et al*. (1997) Height and weight in cystic fibrosis: a cross sectional study. *Arch. Dis. Child.*, **77**, 497–500.
7. Littlewood, J.M. (1993) Value of comprehensive assessment and investigation in the management of cystic fibrosis, in *Clinical Ecology of Cystic Fibrosis*, (ed. H. Escobar, L. Basquero and L. Suarez), Elsevier, pp. 181–187.
8. Dodge, J.A., Morison, S., Lewis, P.A., *et al*. (1997) Incidence, population, and survival of cystic fibrosis in the UK, 1968–95. *Arch. Dis. Child.*, **77**, 493–496.
9. Collins, C.E., MacDonald-Wicks, L., Rowe, S., O'Loughlin, E.O. and Henty, R.L. (1999) Normal growth in cystic fibrosis associated with a specialist centre. *Arch. Dis. Child.*, **81**, 241–246.
10. Corey, M., McLaughlin, F.J., Williams, M. and Levison, H. (1988) A comparison of survival, growth and pulmonary function in patients with cystic fibrosis in Boston and Toronto. *J. Clin. Epidemiol.*, **41**, 583–591.
11. Lai, H.C., Corey, M., FitzSimmons, S., Kosorok, M.R. and Farrell, P.M. (1999) Comparison of growth status of patients with cystic fibrosis between the United States and Canada. *Am. J. Clin. Nutr.*, **69**, 531–538.
12. Kraemer, R., Rudeberg, A., Hadorn, B. and Rossi, E. (1978) Relative underweight in cystic fibrosis and its prognostic value. *Acta Paediatr. Scand.*, **67**, 33–37.
13. Gaskin, K., Gurwitz, D., Durie, P.R., Corey, M., Levison, H. and Forstner, G.G. (1982) Improved respiratory prognosis in patients with cystic fibrosis with normal fat absorption. *J. Pediatr.*, **100**, 857–862.

14. Ramsey, B.W., Farrell, P.M. and Pencharz, P. (1992) Nutritional assessment and management in cystic fibrosis: a consensus report. The Consensus Committee. *Am. J. Clin. Nutr.*, **55**, 108–116.

15. Littlewood, J.M. (1992) Gastrointestinal complications of cystic fibrosis. *J. Roy. Soc. Med.*, **85**, (Suppl. 19), 13–19.

16. Buckler, J.M.H. (1997) *A Reference Manual of Growth and Development*, (2nd edn), Blackwell Science, Oxford.

17. Lai, H.C., Kosorok, M.R., Sondel, S.A. *et al.* (1998) Growth status in children with cystic fibrosis based on the National Cystic Fibrosis Patient Registry data: Evaluation of various criteria used to identify malnutrition. *J. Pediatr.*, **132**, 478–485.

18. Shin, J., Corey, M., Kalnins, D. and Pencharz, P. (1997) A comparison of anthropomorphic standards for evaluation of CF patients. *Pediatr. Pulmonol. Suppl.*, **14**, 312.

19. Tanner, J.M. and Whitehouse, R.H. (1976) Clinical longitudinal standards for height, weight, height velocity, weight velocity and the stages of puberty. *Arch. Dis. Child.*, **51**, 1170–1179.

20. Freeman, J.V., Cole, T.J., Chinn, S., Jones, P.R.M., White, E.M., and Preece, M.A. (1995) Cross-sectional stature and weight reference curves for the UK, 1990. *Arch. Dis. Child.*, **73**, 17–24.

21. Cole, T.J., Donnett, M.L. and Stanfield, J.P. (1981) Weight for height indices to assess nutritional status – a new index on a slide rule. *Am. J. Clin. Nutr.*, **34**, 1935.

22. Smith, D.E. and Booth, I.W. (1989) Nutritional assessment of children: guidelines on collecting and interpreting anthropometric data. *J. Hum. Nutr. Diet*, **2**, 217–224.

23. Poustie, V.J., Watling, R.M., Ashby, D. and Smyth, R.L. (1999) Is percentage ideal weight for height a reliable measure of nutritional status in children with cystic fibrosis? *The Netherlands J. Med.*, **54**, (1), S3–S8.

24. Cole, T.J., Freeman, J.V. and Preece, M.A. (1995) Body mass index reference curves for the UK, 1990. *Arch. Dis. Child.*, **73**, 25–29.

25. International Obesity Task Force (1998) *Obesity; preventing and managing the global epidemic*, Report of the WHO consultation on obesity, Geneva, 3–5 June 1998. WHO, Geneva.

26. Prentice, A.M. (1998) Body mass index standards for children. *BMJ*, **317**, 1401–1402.

27. Frisancho, A.R. (1981) New norms of upper limb fat and muscle areas for assessment of nutritional status. *Am. J. Clin. Nutr.*, **34**, 2540–2545.

28. Johnston, J.L., Leong, M.S., Checkland, E.G., Zuberbuhler, P.C. and Conger, P.R. (1988) Body fat assessed from body density and estimated from skinfold thickness in normal children and children with cystic fibrosis. *Am. J. Clin. Nutr.*, **48**, 1362–1366.

29. Newby, M.J., Kiem, N.L. and Brown, D.L. (1990) Body composition of adult cystic fibrosis patients and control subjects as determined by densitometry, bioelectrical impedance, total electrical body conductivity, skinfold measurements and deuterium oxide dilution. *Am. J. Clin. Nutr.*, **52**, 209–213.

30. De Meer, K., Gulmans, V.A., Westerterp, K.R., Houwen, R.H. and Berger, R. (1999) Skinfold measurements in children with cystic fibrosis: monitoring fat free mass and exercise effects. *Eur. J. Pediatr.*, **158**, (10), 800–806.

31. Tomezsko, J.L., Scanlin, T.F. and Stallings, V.A. (1994) Body composition of children with cystic fibrosis with mild clinical manifestations comapred with normal children. *Am. J. Clin. Nutr.*, **59**, 123–128.

32. Bull, R.K.., Edwards, P.D., Kemp, P.M., Fry, S. and Hughes, I.A. (1999) Bone age assessment: a large scale comparison of Greulich and Pyle, and Tanner and Whitehouse (TW2) methods. *Arch. Dis. Child.* **81**, 172–173.

33. Johannesson, M., Gottlieb, C. and Hjelte, L. (1997) Delayed puberty in girls with cystic fibrosis despite good clinical status. *Pediatrics*, **99**, 29–34.

34. Henderson, R.C. and Madsen, C.D. (1996) Bone mineral density in children and adults with cystic fibrosis. *J. Pediatr.*, **128**, (1), 28–34.

35. Haworth, C.S., Selby, P.L., Webb, A.K. *et al* (1999) Low bone mineral density in adults with cystic fibrosis. *Thorax*, **54**, 961–967.

36. Mullins, P.E., Liechti-Gallati, S., Di Silvio, L., Brook, C.G. and Paes-Alves, A.F. (1991) Short stature in a patient with cystic fibrosis caused by a 6.7-kb human growth hormone deletion. *Horm. Res.*, **36**, 4–8.

37. Littlewood, J.M., Johnson, A.W., Edwards, P.A. and Littlewood, A.E. (1988) Growth retardation in asthmatic children treated with inhaled beclomethasone dipropionate. *Lancet*, **i**, 115–116.

38. Shaw, N.J., Fraser, N.C. and Weller, P.H. (1997) Asthma treatment and growth. *Arch. Dis. Child.*, **77**, 284–286.

39. Carr, S.B. and Dinwiddie, R. (1996) Annual review or continuous assessment? *J. Roy. Soc. Med.*, **89**, (Suppl. 27), 3–7.

40. Kennedy, J.D., Dinwiddie, R., Daman-Williams, C., Dillon, M.J. and Matthew, D.J. (1990) Pseudo Bartter's syndrome in cystic fibrosis. *Arch. Dis. Child.*, **65**, 786–787.

41. Rayner, R.J., Tyrell, J.C., Hiller, E.J. *et al.* (1989) Night blindness and conjunctival xerosis due to vitamin A deficiency in cystic fibrosis. *Arch. Dis. Child.*, **64**, 1151–1156.

42. Campbell, D.C., Tole, D.M., Doran, R.M.L. and Conway, S.P. (1998) Vitamin A deficiency in cystic fibrosis resulting in xerophthalmia. *J. Hum. Nutr. Diet*, **11**, 529–532.

43. Abernathy, R.S. (1976) Bulging fontanelle as presenting sign in cystic fibrosis. *Am. J. Dis. Child.*, **130**, 1360–1362.

44. Eid, N.S., Shoemaker, L.R. and Samiec, T.D. (1990) Vitamin A in cystic fibrosis case report and review of the literature. *J. Pediatr. Gastroenterol. Nutr.*, **10**, 265–269.

45. Rayner, R.J. and Littlewood, J.M. (1992) Vitamin A status as a marker of prognosis in cystic fibrosis, 11th International Cystic Fibrosis Congress, Dublin, Poster MP73.

46. Ansari, E., Sahni, K., Etherington, C. *et al.* (1999) Ocular signs and symptoms and vitamin A status in patients with

cystic fibrosis treated with daily vitamin A supplements, *B. J. Ophthalmol.*, **83**, 688–691.

47. Scott, J., Elias, E., Moutt, P.J.A., Barnes, S. and Wills, M.R. (1977) Rickets in adult cystic fibrosis with myopathy, pancreatic insufficiency and proximal renal tubular acidosis. *Am. J. Med.*, **63**, 488–492.

48. Friedman, H.Z., Ingman, C.B. and Favus, M.J. (1985) Vitamin D metabolism and osteomalacia in cystic fibrosis. *Gastroenterology*, **88**, 808–813.

49. Stead, R.J., Houlder, S., Agnew, J., Thomas, M., Hodson, M.E. and Batten, J.C. (1987) Vitamin D and parathyroid hormone and bone mineralisation in adults with cystic fibrosis. *Thorax*, **43**, 190–194.

50. Stamp, T.C.B. and Geddes, D.M. (1993) Osteoporosis and cystic fibrosis. *Thorax*, **48**, 585–586.

51. Bhudhikanok, G.S., Lim, J., Marcus, R., Harkins, A., Moss, R.B. and Bachrach, L.K. (1997) Correlates of osteopenia on patients with cystic fibrosis. *Pediatrics*, **97**, 103–111.

52. Ferrari, S.L., Nicod, L.P., Hamacher, J. *et al.* (1996) Osteoporosis in patients undergoing lung transplantation. *Eur. Respir. J.*, **9**, 2378–2382.

53. Salamoni, F., Roulet, M., Gudinchet, F., Pilet, M., Thiebaud, D. and Burckhardt, P. (1996) Bone mineral content in cystic fibrosis patients: correlation with free fat mass. *Arch. Dis. Child.*, **74**, 314–318.

54. Walters, T.R. and Koch, H.F. (1972) Heamorrhagic diathesis and cystic fibrosis in infancy. *Am. J. Dis. Child.*, **124**, 641–647.

55. Choonara, I.A., Winn, M.J., Park, B.K. and Littlewood, J.M. (1989) Plasma vitamin K concentration in cystic fibrosis. *Arch. Dis. Child.*, **64**, 732–734.

56. Rashid, M., Durie, P., Kalins, D. *et al.* (1996) Prevalence of vitamin K deficiency in children with cystic fibrosis. *Pediatr. Pulmonol. Suppl.*, **13**, 313 (Poster 377).

57. Beker, L.T., Ahrens, R.A., Fink, R.J. *et al.* (1997) Effect of vitamin K1 supplementation on vitamin K status in cystic fibrosis patients. *J. Pediatr. Gastroenterol. Nutr.*, **24**, 512–517.

58. Sokol, R.J., Reardon, M.C., Accurso, F.J., Stall, C., Narkewicz, M. and Abman, S.H. (1989) Fat soluble vitamin status during the first year of life in infants with cystic fibrosis identified by screening newborns. *Am. J. Clin. Nutr.*, **50**, 1064–1071.

59. Farrell, P.M., Kosorok, M.R., Laxova, A. *et al.* (1997) Nutritional benefits of neonatal screening for cystic fibrosis. *NEJM*, **337**, 963–969.

60. Wilfond, B.S., Farrell, P.M., Laxova, A. and Mischler, E. (1994) Severe hemolytic anaemia associated with vitamin E deficiency in infants with cystic fibrosis. *Clin. Pediatr.*, **33**, 2–7.

61. Sitrin, M.D., Lieberman, F., Jensen, W.E., Noronha, A., Milburn, C. and Addington, W. (1987) Vitamin E deficiency and neurologic disease in adults with cystic fibrosis. *Ann. Int. Med.*, **107**, 51–54.

62. Cynamon, H.A., Milov, D.E., Valenstein, E. and Wagner, M. (1988) Effect of vitamin E deficiency on neurological function in patients with cystic fibrosis. *J. Pediatr.*, **113**, 637–640.

63. Congdon, P.J., Bruce, G., Rothburn, M.M. *et al.* (1981) Vitamin status in treated patients with cystic fibrosis. *Arch. Dis. Child.*, **56**, 708–714.

64. Peters, S.A. and Rolles, C.J. (1993) Vitamin therapy in cystic fibrosis. A review and rationale. *J. Clin. Pharm. Therapeut.*, **18**, 33–38.

65. Kelleher, J., Goode, H.F., Field, H.P., Walker, B.E., Miller, M.G. and Littlewood, J.M. (1986) Essential element status in cystic fibrosis. *Hum. Nutr.: Appl. Nutr.*, **40A**, 79–84.

66. Aggett, P.J., Thorn, J.M., Delves, H.T., Harries, J.T. and Clayton, B.E. (1979) Trace element malabsorption in exocrine pancreatic insufficiency. *Monogr. Paediatr.*, **10**, 8–11.

67. Dodge, J.A. and Yassa, J.G. (1978) Zinc deficiency syndrome in a British youth with cystic fibrosis. *BMJ*, **i**, 411.

68. Krebs, N.F., Sontag, M., Accurso, F.J. and Hambidge, K.M. (1998) Low plasma zinc concentrations in young infants with cystic fibrosis. *J. Pediatr.*, **133**, (6), 761–764.

69. Solomons, N.W., Reiger, C.H.L., Jacob, R.A., Rothberg, R. and Sandstead, H.H. (1981) Zinc nutrient and taste activity in patients with cystic fibrosis. *Nutrit. Res.*, **1**, 13–24.

70. Godson, C., Ryan, M.P., Brady, H.R., Bourke, S. and Fitzgerald, M.X. (1988) Acute hypomagnesaemia complicating the treatment of meconium ileus equivalent in cystic fibrosis. *Scan. J. Gastroenterol. Suppl.*, **143**, 148–158.

71. Makker, H., Edenborough, F., Jones, A. and Stableforth, D. (1996) Symptomatic hypomagnesaemia in cystic fibrosis. *Pediatr. Pulmonol. Suppl.*, **13**, 320 (Poster 402).

72. Marcus, M.S., Sondel, S.A., Farrell, P.M., Carey, P.M. and Langhough, R. (1991) Nutritional status of infants with cystic fibrosis associated with early diagnosis and intervention. *Am. J. Clin. Nutr.*, **54**, 578–585.

73. Farrell, P.M., Mischler, E.H., Engle, M.J., Brown, D.J. and Lau, S. (1985) Fatty acid abnormalities in cystic fibrosis. *Pediatr. Res.*, **19**, 104–109.

74. Benabdeslam, H., Garcia, I., Bellon, G., Gilly, R. and Revol, A. (1998) Biochemical assessment of the nutrional status of cystic fibrosis patients treated with pancreatic enzyme extracts. *Am. J. Clin. Nutr.*, **67**, (5), 912–918.

75. Henderson, W.R. Jr, Astley, S.J., McCready, M.M., Kushmerick, P., Casey, S. and Ramsey, B.W. (1994) Oral absorption of omega-3 fatty acids in patients with cystic fibrosis who have pancreatic insufficiency and healthy control subjects. *J. Pediatr.*, **124**, 400–408.

76. Burdge, G.C., Goodale, A.J., Hill, C.M., Halford, P.J., Lambert, E.J. and Postle, A.D. (1994) Plasma lipid concentrations in children with cystic fibrosis: the value of a high fat diet and pancreatic supplementation. *Br. J. Nutr.*, **71**, 959–964.

77. Van Egmond, A.W., Kosorok, M.R., Koscik, R., Laxova, A. and Farrell, P.M. (1996) Effect of linoleic acid intake on growth of infants with cystic fibrosis. *Am. J. Clin. Nutr.*, **63**, (5), 746–752.

78. Freedman, S.D., Katz, M.H., Parker, E.M., Laposata, M., Urman, M.Y. and Alvarez, J.G. (1999) A membrane lipid imbalance plays a role in the phenotypic expression of cystic fibrosis in CFTR -/- mice. *PNAS*, **96**, (24) 13995–14000.

79. Winklhofer-Roob, B.M., Ellemunter, H., Fruhwirth, M., Schlegel-Hauter, S.E., Khoschsorur, G., van't Hof, M.A. and Shmerling, D.H. (1997) Plasma vitamin C concentrations in patients with cystic fibrosis: evidence of association with lung inflammation. *Am. J. Clin. Nutr.*, **65**, 1858–1866.

80. Kawchak, D.A., Sowell, A.L., Hofley, P.M., Zemel, B.S., Scanlin, T.F. and Stallings, V.A. (1999) Longitudinal analysis shows serum carotenoid concentrations are low in children with cystic fibrosis. *J. Am. Diet Assoc.*, **99**, (12), 1569–1572.

81. Collins, C.E., Quaggiotto, P., Wood, L., O'Loughlin, E.V., Henry, R.L. and Garg, M.L. (1999) Elevated plasma levels of F2 alpha isoprostane in cystic fibrosis. *Lipids*, **34**, (6), 551–556.

82. Rust, P., Eichler, I., Renner, S. and Elmadfa, I. (1998) Effects of long term oral beta-carotene supplementation on lipid peroxidation in patients with cystic fibrosis. *Int. J. Vit. Nutr. Res.*, **68**, (2), 83–87.

83. Kelly, F.J. (1999) Glutathione: in defense of the lung. *Food Chem. Toxicol.*, **37**, (9–10), 963–966.

84. Hsai, D. (1959) Birth weight in cystic fibrosis of the pancreas. *Ann. Hum. Genet.*, **23**, 289–299.

85. Dodge, J.A. and Yassa, J.G. (1980) Food intake and supplementary feeding programmes, in *Perspectives in Cystic Fibrosis*, (ed. J.M. Sturgess), Proceedings of the 8th International Cystic Fibrosis Congress, Canadian Cystic Fibrosis Association, Toronto, pp. 125–136.

86. Holliday, K. and Allen, J. (1991) Growth of human milk-fed and formula-fed infants with cystic fibrosis. *J. Pediatr.*, **118**, 77–79.

87. Simmonds, E.J., Wall, C.R., Wolfe, S.P. and Littlewood, J.M. (1994) A review of infant feeding practices at a regional cystic fibrosis unit. *J. Hum. Nutr. Diet*, **7**, 31–38.

88. Ghosal, S., Taylor, C.J., Pickering, M. *et al.* (1995) Disproportionate head growth retardation in cystic fibrosis. *Arch. Dis. Child.*, **72**, 150–152.

89. Sontag, M.K., Drescher, A.A., Accurso, F.J. and Krebs, N.F. (1997) Longitudinal characterization of growth and growth tracking in infants and toddlers with cystic fibrosis identified by newborn screening. *Pediatr. Pulmonol. Suppl.*, **14**, 304 (Poster 357).

90. Corey, M.L. (1980) Longitudinal studies in cystic fibrosis, in *Perspectives in Cystic Fibrosis*, (ed. J.M. Sturgess), Proceedings of the 8th International Cystic Fibrosis Congress, Canadian CF Association, Toronto, pp. 246–255.

91. Karlberg, J., Kjellmer, I. and Kristiansson, B. (1991) Linear growth in children with cystic fibrosis. *Acta Paediatr. Scand.*, **80**, 508–514.

92. Waters, D.L., Wilcken, B., Irwig, L. *et al.* (1999) Clinical outcomes of newborn screening for cystic fibrosis. *Arch. Dis. Child.*, **80**, F1–F7.

93. Cystic Fibrosis Patient Registry (1999) *Annual Data Report 1998.* Cystic Fibrosis Foundation, Bethesda, Maryland, USA.

94. FitzSimmons, S.C. (1997) *Cystic Fibrosis Patient Registry Annual Report, 1996.* Cystic Fibrosis Foundation.

95. Hui-Chuan Lai, Kosorok, M.R., Sondel, S.A. *et al.* (1998) Growth status in children with cystic fibrosis based on the National Cystic Fibrosis Patient Registry data: Evaluation of various criteria used to identify malnutrition. *J. Pediatr.*, **132**, 478–485.

96. Berry, H.K., Kellog, F.W., Hunt, M.H., Ingberg, R.L., Richter, L. and Gutjahr, C. (1975) Dietary supplement and nutrition in children with cystic fibrosis. *Am. J. Dis. Child.*, **129**, 165–171.

97. Littlewood, J.M. and Wolfe, S.P. (1994) Nutrition in cystic fibrosis, in *Consensus in Clinical Nutrition*, (eds R.V. Heatley, J.H. Green and M.S. Losowsky), Cambridge University Press, Cambridge, pp. 388–419.

98. Weltman, E.A., Stern, R.C., Doershuk, C.F., Moir, R.N., Palmer, K. and Jaffe, A.C. (1990) Weight and menstrual function in patients with eating disorders and cystic fibrosis. *Pediatrics*, **85**, 282–287.

99. Byard, P.J. (1994) The adolescent growth spurt in cystic fibrosis. *Ann. Hum. Biol.*, **21**, 229–240.

100. Shepherd, R.W., Holt, T.L., Greer, R., Cleghorn, G.J. and Thomas, B.J. (1989) Total body potassium in cystic fibrosis. *J. Pediatr. Gastroenterol. Nutr.*, **9**, 200–205.

101. Pichard, C., Kyle, U.G. and Slosman, D.O. (1999) Fat-free mass in chronic illness: comparison of bioelectrical impedance and dual-energy x-ray absorptiometry in 480 chronically ill and healthy subjects. *Nutrition*, **15**, (9), 668–676.

102. Quirk, P.C., Ward, L.C., Thomas, B.J., Holt, T.L., Shepherd, R.W. and Cornish, B.H. (1997) Evaluation of bioelectrical impedance for prospective nutritional assessment in cystic fibrosis. *Nutrition*, **13**, (5), 412–416.

103. Azcue, M., Fried, M. and Pencharz, P.B. (1993) Use of bioelectrical impedance analysis to measure total body water in patients with cystic fibrosis. *J. Pediatr. Gastroenterol. Nutr.*, **16**, 440–445.

104. Slosman, D.O., Casez, J.P., Pichard, C. *et al.* (1992) Assessment of whole body composition with dual-energy X-ray absorptiometry. *Radiology*, **185**, 593–598.

105. Greer, R., Shepherd, R., Cleghorn, G., Bowling, F.G. and Holt, T. (1991) Evaluation of growth and changes in body composition following neonatal diagnosis of cystic fibrosis. *J. Pediatr. Gastroenterol. Nutr.*, **13**, 52–58.

106. Rochat, T., Slosman, D.O., Pichard, C. and Belli, D.C. (1994) Body composition analysis by dual-energy X-ray absorptiometry in adults with cystic fibrosis. *Chest*, **106**, 800–805.

107. Littlewood, J.M., Kelleher, J., Rawson, I., Gilbert, J., Firth, J., Morton, S. and Wall, C. (1988) Comprehensive assessment at a CF centre identifies suboptimal treatment and improves management, symptoms and condition. 10th International Cystic Fibrosis Congress, Sydney. Excerpta Medica Asia Pacific Congress 1988, Series 74, 89 (Poster R(a)18).

108. Mahadeva, R., Webb, K., Westerbeek, R., Carroll, N., Bilton, D. and Lomas, D. (1997) Clinical outcome in patients with cystic fibrosis in the UK is improved by CF centre care, 21st European Cystic Fibrosis Conference, Davos, Poster 164.

109. Vaisman, N., Pencharz, P., Corey, M., Canny, G.J. and Hahn, E. (1987) Energy expenditure in patients with cystic fibrosis. *J. Pediatr.*, **11**, 496–500.

110. Buchdahl, R.M., Cox, M., Fulleylove, C. *et al.* (1988) Increased energy expenditure in cystic fibrosis. *J. Appl. Physiol.*, **64**, (5), 1810–1816

111. O'Rawe, A., McIntosh, I., Dodge, J.A. *et al.* (1992) Increased energy expenditure in cystic fibrosis is associated with specific mutations. *Clin. Sci.*, **82**, 71–76.

112. Chase, H.P., Long, M.A. and Lavin, M.H. (1979) Cystic fibrosis and malnutrition. *J. Pediatr.*, **95**, 337–347.

113. Hubbard, V.S. (1985) Nutritional considerations in cystic fibrosis. *Semin. Respir. Med.*, **6**, 308–313.

114. Buchdahl, R.M., Fullylove, C., Marchant, J.L., Warner, J.O. and Brueton, M.J. (1989) Energy and nutrient intakes in cystic fibrosis. *Arch. Dis. Child.*, **64**, 373–378.

115. Ellis, J.A., Bond, S.A. and Wootton, S.A. (1992) Energy and protein intakes of patients with cystic fibrosis. *J. Hum. Nutr. Diet.*, **5**, 333–342.

116. Morrison, J.M., O'Rawe, A., McCracken, K.J., Redmond, A.O.B. and Dodge, J.A. (1994) Energy intakes and losses in cystic fibrosis. *J. Hum. Nutr. Diet.*, **7**, 39–46.

117. Collins, C.E., O'Loughlin, E.V. and Henry, R. (1998) Discrepancies between males and females with cystic fibrosis in dietary intake and pancreatic enzyme use. *J. Pediatr. Gastroenterol. Nutr.,* **26**, (3), 258–262.

118. Waters, D.L., Dorney, S.F., Gaskin, K.J., Gruca, M.A., O'Halloran, M. and Wilken, B. (1990) Pancreatic function in infants identified as having cystic fibrosis in a neonatal screening program. *NEJM*, **332**, 303–338.

119. Bronstein, M.N., Sokel, R.J., Abman, S.H. *et al.* (1992) Pancreatic insufficiency, growth, and nutrition in infants identified by newborn screening as having cystic fibrosis. *J. Pediatr.*, **120**, 533–540.

120. Couper, R.T., Corey, M., Moore, D.J., Fisher, L.J., Forstner Durie, P.R. (1992) Decline of exocrine pancreatic function in cystic fibrosis patients with pancreatic sufficiency. *Pediatr. Res.*, **32**, 179–182.

121. Littlewood, J.M. (1996) Management of malabsorption in cystic fibrosis: influence of recent developments on clinical practice. *Postgrad. Med. J.*, **72**, (Suppl. 2), S56–S62.

122. Lanng, S. Thorsteinsson, B., Nerup, J. and Koch, C. (1991) Glucose tolerance in cystic fibrosis. *Arch. Dis. Child.*, **66**, 612–616.

123. Lanng, S., Thorsteinsson, B., Nerup, J. and Koch, C. (1992) Influence of the development of diabetes mellitus on clinical status in patients with cystic fibrosis. *Eur. J. Paediatr.*, **151**, 684–687.

124. Zipf, W.B., Kein, C.L., Horswill, C.A., McCoy, K.S., O'Dorsio, T. and Pinyerd, B.L. (1991) Effects of tolbutamide on growth and body composition of non-diabetic children with cystic fibrosis. *Pediatr. Res.*, **30**, 309–314.

125. Culler, F.L., McKean, L.P., Buchanan, C.N., Caplan, D.B. and Meacham, L.R. (1994) Glipizide treatment of patient with cystic fibrosis and impaired glucose tolerance. *J. Pediatr. Gastroenterol. Nutr.*, **18**, 375–378.

126. Scott-Jupp, R., Lama, M. and Tanner, M.S. (1991) Prevalence of liver disease in cystic fibrosis. *Arch. Dis. Child.*, **66**, 698–701.

127. Ling, S.C., Wilkinson, J.D., Hollman, J., McColl, J., Evans, T.J. and Paton, J.Y. (1999) The evolution of liver disease in cystic fibrosis. *Arch. Dis. Child.,* **81**, 129–132.

128. Green, J.H., Bramley, P.N. and Losowsky, M.S. (1991) Are patients with primary biliary cirrhosis hypermetabolic? A comparison between patients before and after liver transplantation and controls. *Hepatology*, **14**, 464–472.

129. Sokol, R.J. and Durie, P.R. (1999) for the Cystic Fibrosis Foundation Hepatobiliary Disease Consensus Group. *J. Pediatr. Gastroentrol. Nutr.,* **28**, S1–S13.

130. Cotting, J., Lentze, M.J. and Reichen, J. (1990) Effects of ursodeoxycholic acid treatment on nutrition and liver function in patients with cystic fibrosis and long-standing cholestasis. *Gut*, **31**, 918–921.

131. Merli, M., Bertasi, S., Servi, R. *et al.* (1994) Effect of a medium dose of ursodeoxycholic acid with or without taurine supplementation on the nutritional status of patients with cystic fibrosis: a randomized, placebo controlled, crossover trial. *J. Pediatr. Gastroenterol. Nutr.*, **19**, 198–203.

132. Wong, L.T.K., Davidson, A.G.F., Jevon, G., Jameison, D., Peacock, D. and Schmidt, J. (1997) Hepatobiliary disease in cystic fibrosis: enzymatic and histopathologic response to ursodeoxycholic acid therapy. *Pediatr. Pulmonol. Suppl.*, **14**, 303. Poster 356.

133. Noble-Jamieson, G., Barnes, N., Jamieson, N., Friend, P. and Calne, R. (1996) Liver transplantation for hepatic cirrhosis in cystic fibrosis. *J. Roy. Soc. Med.*, **89**, (Suppl. 27), 31–37.

134. Laursen, E.M., Juul, A., Lanng, S. *et al.* (1995) Diminished concentrations of insulin-like growth factor I in cystic fibrosis. *Arch. Dis. Child.*, **72**, 494–497.

135. Taylor, A.M., Bush, A., Thomson, A. *et al.* (1997) Relation between insulin like growth factor-1, body mass index, and clinical status in cystic fibrosis. *Arch. Dis. Child.*, **76**, (4), 304–309.

136. Hardin, D.S., Stratton, R., Kramer, J.C., Reyes de al Rocha, S., Govaerts, K. and Wilson, D.P. (1998) Growth hormone improves weight velocity and height velocity in prepubertal children with cystic fibrosis. *Horm. Metab. Res.*, **30**, (10), 636–641.

137. Hardin, D.S. and Sy, J.P. (1997) Effects of growth hormone treatment in children with cystic fibrosis: the National Cooperative Growth Study experience. *J. Pediatr.,* **131**, (1 pt 2), S65–S69.

138. Auwerx, J. and Staels, B. (1998) Leptin. Review article. *Lancet*, **351**, 737–742.

139. Pencharz, P., Hill, R., Archibald, E., Levy, L. and Newth, C. (1984) Energy needs and nutritional rehabilitation in undernourished adolescents and adults with cystic

fibrosis. *J. Pediatr. Gastroenterol. Nutr.*, Suppl. 1, S147–153.

140. Shepherd, R. (1997) Energy expenditure in infants in health and disease. *Can. J. Gastroenterol.*, **11**, (1), 101–104.

141. Giradet, J.P., Tounian, P., Sardet, A., Veinberg, F., Grimfield, A. and Tournier, G. (1994) Resting energy expenditure in infants with cystic fibrosis. *J. Pediatr. Gastroenterol. Nutr.*, **18**, 214–219.

142. Thomson, M.A., Wilmott, R.W., Wainwright, C., Masters, B., Francis, P.J. and Shepherd, R.W. (1996) Resting energy expenditure, pulmonary inflammation, and genotype in the early course of cystic fibrosis. *J. Pediatr.*, **129**, (3), 367–373.

143. Bowler, I.M., Green, J.H., Wolfe, S.P. and Littlewood, J.M. (1993) Resting energy expenditure and substrate oxidation rates in cystic fibrosis. *Arch. Dis. Child.*, **68**, 754–759.

144. Ward, S.A., Tomezsko, J.L., Holsclaw, D.S. and Paolone, A.M. (1999) Energy expenditure and substrate utilization in adults with cystic fibrosis and diabetes mellitus. *Am. J. Clin. Nutr.*, **69**, 913–919.

145. Steinkamp, G., Drommer, A. and von der Hardt, H. (1993) Resting energy expenditure before and after treatment for *Pseudomonas aeruginosa* infection in patients with cystic fibrosis. *Am. J. Clin. Nutr.*, **57**, 685–689.

146. Peckham, D., Leonard, C., Range, S. and Knox, A. (1996) Nutritional status and pulmonary function in patients with cystic fibrosis with and without *Burkholderia cepacia* colonisation: role of specialist dietetic support. *J. Hum. Nutr. Diet*, **9**, 173–179.

147. Vinton, N.E., Padman, R., Davis, M. and Harcke, H.T. (1999) Effects of *Pseudomonas* colonisation on body composition and resting energy expenditure in children with cystic fibrosis. *JPEN*, **23**, (4), 233–236.

148. Fried, M.D., Durie, P.R., Lap-Chee Tsui, Corey, M., Levison, H. and Pencharz, P.B. (1991) The cystic fibrosis gene and resting energy expenditure. *J. Pediatr.*, **119**, 913–916.

149. Dagli, E., Warner, J.A., Besley, C.R. and Warner, J.O. (1992)

Raised serum soluble interleukin-2 receptor concentrations in cystic fibrosis patients with and without evidence of lung disease. *Arch. Dis. Child.*, **67**, 479–481.

150. Wolfe, S.P., Littlewood, J.M. and Littlewood, A.E. (1995) Chest involvement as a determinant of energy requirement for cystic fibrosis patients, 20th European Cystic Fibrosis Conference. Brussels, O4.

151. Grunow, J.E., Azcue, M.P., Berall, G. and Pencharz, P.B. (1993) Energy expenditure in cystic fibrosis during activities of daily living. *J. Pediatr.*, **122**, 243–246.

152. Spicher, V., Roulet, M. and Schutz, Y. (1991) Assessment of total energy expenditure in free-living patients with cystic fibrosis. *J. Pediatr.*, **118**, 865–872.

153. Elborn, J.S., Cordon, S.M., Western, P.J., MacDonald, I.A. and Shale, D.J. (1993) Tumour necrosis factor-α, energy expenditure and cachexia in cystic fibrosis. *Clin. Sci.*, **85**, 563–568.

154. Edenborough, F.P., Stableforth, D.E., Webb, A.K., Mackenzie, W.E. and Smith, D.L. (1995) Outcome of pregnancy in women with cystic fibrosis. *Thorax*, **50**, 170–174.

155. Fiel, S.B. and FitzSimmons, S. (1995) Pregnancy in patients with cystic fibrosis. *Pediatr. Pulmonol. Suppl.*, **12**, S4.2.

156. Farrell, P., Mischler, E.H., Sondel, S. *et al.* (1987) Predigested formula for infants with cystic fibrosis. *J. Am. Diet. Assoc.*, **93**, 1353–1356.

157. Ellis, L., Kalnins, D., Corey, M., Brennan, J., Pencharz, P. and Durie, P. (1998) Do infants with cystic fibrosis need a protein hydrolysate formula? A prospective, randomized, comparative study. *J. Pediatr.*, **132**, 270–276.

158. Hill, S.M., Phillips, A.D., Mearns, M. and Walker-Smith, J.A. (1989) Cows' milk sensitive enteropathy in cystic fibrosis. *Arch. Dis. Child.*, **64**, 1251–1255.

159. Durie, P.R., Newth, C.J., Forstner, G.G. and Gall, D.G. (1980) Malabsorption of medium-chain triglycerides in infants with cystic fibrosis. Correction with pancreatic enzyme supplements. *J. Pediatr.*, **96**, 862–864.

12

Gastrointestinal and pancreatic disease in cystic fibrosis

A. G. F. DAVIDSON

The pancreas in cystic fibrosis	261	References		283
Gastrointestinal tract in cystic fibrosis	271			

THE PANCREAS IN CYSTIC FIBROSIS

Introduction

The importance of the pancreatic lesions in cystic fibrosis (CF) was emphasized by Dorothy Andersen in 1938[1] when she named the disorder 'cystic fibrosis of the pancreas', and building on the work of Fanconi and others, established that CF was a separate entity distinct from other causes of the 'celiac syndrome'. The presence of gastrointestinal symptoms and the demonstration of pancreatic exocrine insufficiency formed the basis for the diagnosis of CF until the discovery of the sweat electrolyte abnormalities in 1953 by di Sant'Agnese et al. and the development by Gibson and Cooke of a reliable sweat test.

Modern therapy can ameliorate many of the pancreatic, hepatobiliary and intestinal manifestations of CF. However, abnormalities affecting these systems still contribute significantly to the overall morbidity and mortality of CF as well as affecting nutrition, which is itself an important factor affecting prognosis[2].

Pathology and pathophysiology

Changes in the pancreas have been detected early in intrauterine life; and complications, i.e. meconium ileus (see below), demonstrated by ultrasound from early in the second trimester of gestation[3-5]. The severity of the pancreatic histological and functional disorder in CF is variable; it tends to increase with age and appears to be influenced by genotype[3,6-11]. The pathological changes in the CF pancreas include obstruction of the proximal ductules, poor development and destruction of acinar cells, fibrosis, fatty change and microcyst formation with, eventually, destruction of functioning pancreatic exocrine tissue. Stenosis of the large ducts and stone formation can also occur and calcification may be prominent[3,6,7].

The pathophysiology of the pancreatic abnormality in CF can be related to the abnormal CF gene product, the cystic fibrosis transmembrane conductance regulator protein (CFTR), which affects transmembrane fluid and electrolyte movement. Inadequate ion and fluid influx into the pancreatic zymogen granules after fusion with the acinar cell apical membrane prior to secretion, leads to decreased enzyme output. The CFTR-modulated abnormality in chloride and fluid transport leads to decreased pancreatic fluid secretion and decreased bicarbonate exchange from acinar and ductal cells[12-16]. The resulting concentrated pancreatic secretions lead, in turn, to microductal and ductal obstruction and the typical progressive destructive pancreatic lesions and pancreatic exocrine insufficiency of CF. The thick, sticky, pancreatic secretions typical of CF are low in fluid and bicarbonate and (in 80–85 per cent of CF patients) enzymes are absent or low. When pancreatic enzymes are present, their concentration tends to be paradoxically high, due to the relatively greater deficiency of water[13-16].

The balance between the destructive and obstructive

lesions inherent in the CF pancreas is reflected by the level of circulating (serum) immunoreactive trypsinogen (IRT)[17]. IRT has been shown to be pancreatic in origin, and the elevation in circulating levels appears to reflect an obstruction (whether metabolic or physical) to secretion, typical of, but not unique to, CF. Increased circulating IRT continues as long as sufficient pancreatic enzyme secreting tissue remains. In essentially all CF newborn infants, sufficient enzyme-secreting tissue is present to result in high levels of circulating IRT. This phenomenon in CF infants forms the basis of successful newborn screening programs for CF[18] and, perhaps, also offers a rationale to stimulate research towards preserving pancreatic exocrine function in CF infants. In CF individuals whose pancreas retains the ability to secrete enzymes, IRT remains elevated[17]; however, in the 80–85 per cent of CF infants who are pancreatic insufficient, the blood IRT levels fall through normal to subnormal within the first year of life. Another marker of the destructive process affecting the pancreas, the 'pancreatitis-associated protein' (PAP), which reflects pancreatic injury, may also be elevated in CF, and has also been suggested as potentially useful in newborn screening[19].

CF genotype–pancreatic phenotype correlation

The genetic, metabolic nature of the pancreatic disorder in CF was presaged by Sir Archibald Garrod in 1912. The discovery of the CF gene and its abnormal gene product (CFTR) by Tsui, Reardon and Collins in 1989 provided a basis upon which to explain the phenotypic abnormalities of CF. However, attempts to demonstrate a reliable correlation between CFTR mutation and CF phenotype have generally not been successful; a notable exception being pancreatic function, where correlation, though not absolute, has been supported by several clinical studies (Fig. 12.1)[8–11]. In one study for example, only 2 of 199 patients homozygous for ΔF_{508} were pancreatic sufficient (PS); whereas of 25 patients with other alleles, 16 were PS[11]. ΔF_{508} was therefore termed 'severe' (with regard to pancreatic status). The same group suggested that PS was a dominant trait associated with mutations such as R117H, R334W, R347P, A455E and P574H which were termed 'mild'. In general, 'missense' or 'splice' mutations may be 'mild' or 'severe' and other mutations 'severe'. Although the common ΔF_{508} mutation is considered 'severe'[8,9], this association is not absolute, perhaps reflecting the influence of environmental factors or other 'modifier' genes. Although the terms 'mild' and 'severe' are in common usage among professionals and are supportable on a population basis, they can be misleading and erroneous when applied to an individual patient. For this reason, we believe these terms would be better not used, particularly in counseling affected patients.

Pancreatic sufficiency and insufficiency

The most common clinical manifestation of pancreatic disease in CF is exocrine pancreatic insufficiency. In

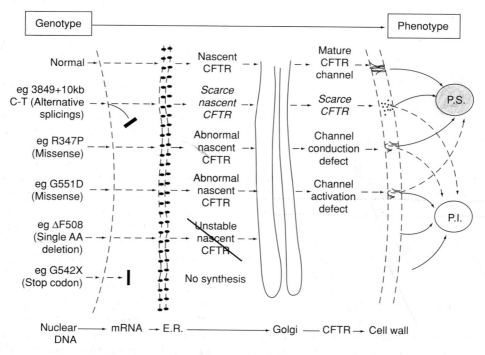

Fig. 12.1 *Genetic basis for pancreatic sufficiency or insufficiency in cystic fibrosis: pancreatic function remains the best example of genotype–phenotype correlation in CF. (Modified, after refs 8 and 9.)*

about 85 per cent of CF patients, this is present from neonatal life. These 'pancreatic-insufficient' (PI) patients secrete insufficient pancreatic lipolytic enzymes (e.g. lipase, colipase) or proteolytic enzymes (e.g. trypsin, chymotrypsin) and bicarbonate for normal fat and protein digestion and absorption. In non-CF adults with pancreatic disease, steatorrhea due to pancreatic insufficiency has been shown to occur when pancreatic enzyme output falls below 10 per cent of normal, while studies in CF suggest that 98 per cent or more of pancreatic secretory capacity must be lost before clinical evidence of malabsorption is evident[20].

In approximately 15 per cent of CF individuals, pancreatic changes are less severe. Sufficient functional pancreatic exocrine tissue remains beyond the neonatal period in such PS individuals to allow normal fat and protein digestion. IRT levels tend to remain elevated in CF patients who are PS[17]. Although PS CF individuals retain the ability to secrete enzymes, abnormalities of pancreatic function can usually still be demonstrated if fluid and bicarbonate secretion, total enzyme output or IRT response to pancreatic stimulation are considered[13–17,21]. Although even these parameters may fall within the normal range in some patients, detailed measurement of pancreatic function (i.e. secretin–pancreozymin/cholecystokinin test) can be helpful in patients with equivocal sweat tests and in whom DNA analysis does not resolve the issue of diagnosis. With increasing age, PS individuals may eventually become PI, particularly if they have 'severe' mutations such as ΔF_{508}[9,10].

CF patients who are PS have been reported to have better nutrition and an improved prognosis with regard to the development of respiratory disease[2]. It is important to remember, however, that the differentiation between PS and PI is not absolute but represents two ends of a spectrum of exocrine pancreatic functional capacity in CF, and any relationship to other clinical parameters must still be considered to be only a generalization.

CLINICAL PRESENTATION OF PANCREATIC INSUFFICIENCY

The clinical effects of pancreatic dysfunction in CF are shown in Table 12.1. Pancreatic insufficiency may present dramatically, as in the edematous pale infant with diarrhea. The edema is caused by hypoalbuminemia and the pallor is due to hemolytic anemia as a result of vitamin E deficiency. Malnutrition, failure to thrive, abdominal pain, bloating with foul flatus, foul, fatty, oily, bulky diarrhea stools and rectal prolapse are also frequent and prominent symptoms. The triad of ravenous appetite, foul, bulky stools and malnutrition or failure to thrive in an infant or young child is highly suggestive of CF with PI. Diagnostic sweat test is mandatory in such patients. It should be noted, however, that particularly in early infancy, CF infants with PI or PS may initially appear

Table 12.1 *Clinical effects of pancreatic dysfunction in cystic fibrosis*

1. Mainly or exclusively in PI patients
   Meconium ileus
   Diarrhea/steatorrhea
   Fat-soluble vitamin deficiencies
   Hemolytic anemia (infant)
   Edema (hypoalbuminemia)
   Malnutrition
   Growth failure
   Rectal prolapse
   DIOS
   Intussusception
   Volvulus
2. Mainly in PS patients
   Pancreatitis
3. In PS or PI patients
   Pancreatic cysts, stones

well nourished. This may be at least in part because pre-duodenal ('lingual' or 'gastric') lipase is present in young infants even if PI, and breast-fed infants may also benefit from lipases present in human milk[22,23]. Nevertheless, even presymptomatic CF infants detected by newborn screening may have significant nutritional deficiencies. In one study of such infants detected by IRT screening, deficiencies of fat-soluble vitamins such as vitamin D (35 per cent), vitamin E (38 per cent) and vitamin A (21 per cent), and low serum albumin (36 per cent) were present by 3 months of age[24]. These deficiencies correct in most patients when adequate pancreatic enzyme replacement therapy and vitamin supplementation are given.

LABORATORY ASSESSMENT OF PANCREATIC FUNCTION

Laboratory investigations for the assessment of pancreatic function are shown in Table 12.2 and discussed in Chapter 9. Non-specific evidence of fat malabsorption is provided by demonstration of increased numbers of unsplit fat globules on stool smear or increased 3-day fecal fat excretion; or by evidence of fat-soluble vitamin deficiency, such as prolonged prothrombin time, increased PIVKA ('protein in vitamin K absence'), or decreased vitamin A, D or E levels. Subnormal IRT in a patient known to have CF suggests PI, whereas elevated fasting or postprandial levels beyond the first year of life are in keeping with PS. Stool chymotrypsin assay, when specific substrate is used[25], is a useful screening test for pancreatic insufficiency. Recently, elastase measurement in stool has been shown to be highly sensitive and specific for pancreatic insufficiency. Elastase has the advantage over stool chymotrypsin of not being affected by concurrent administration of pancreatic enzyme supplements[26], and it correlates well with the definitive secretin-cholecystokinin test[26a].

Table 12.2 *Assessment of pancreatic function in CF*

1. Blood
   Serum amylase
   Serum lipase
   Immunoreactive trypsin(ogen) (IRT)
   Fat-soluble vitamins (ADE)
   Prothrombin time (vitamin K) PIVKA
   Carotene
   Albumin, pre-albumin, retinol binding protein
2. Meconium
   Albumin
   Lactase
3. Stool
   Fat (microscopy)
   3-day fat excretion
   Chymotrypsin, elastase
4. Urine (indirect) tests
   Bentiromide, Pancreolauryl
5. Duodenal aspirate
   Secretin-cholecystokinin (pancreozymin) stimulation
   Lundh meal

The definitive test of exocrine pancreatic function remains the secretin–pancreozymin (cholecystokinin), stimulation test and extensive experience has been reported in CF patients[13–16]. The Lundh test meal provides similar information on pancreatic secretion, as well as on the integrity of the endogenous mechanism for pancreatic stimulation. So-called 'tubeless' tests of pancreatic function such as the Chymex (bentiromide) or pancreolauryl (fluorescein dilaurate) tests are relatively simple to perform and noninvasive, but are less reliable and less informative than the secretin pancreozymin test.

THERAPY OF PANCREATIC INSUFFICIENCY

Therapy of pancreatic insufficiency in CF patients is based on oral replacement pancreatic enzyme preparations. The first enzyme supplements were relatively crude extracts of (porcine) pancreas, with low enzyme (lipase, trypsin, chymotrypsin, amylase) potency. Large dosages were required because of the low potency of the preparation and their acid denaturation in the stomach. The relative impurity of the extracts and the high dosages required led to problems with hyperuricemia and hyperuricosuria, in part related to nucleic acid contaminants in the enzyme preparations[27]. The development of higher-potency enzyme preparations protected from stomach acid denaturation by enteric coating of granules, microspheres or microtablets represented a major advance in the therapy of CF. More effective control of steatorrhea can be obtained with lower dosage and less risk of hyperuricemia, although the latter may still occur with excessive enzyme dosage or for reasons unrelated to enzyme therapy[27]. However, despite their advantages, these preparations have inherent characteristics which may affect their efficacy in some patients.

For example, particle size affects rate of passage through the pylorus[28], and this may differ from the rate of passage of chyme (food)[28a,28b]. In addition, the enteric coating is designed to prevent enzyme release at low pH, as may often be the case in the upper small intestine of CF patients.

The aim of pancreatic replacement enzyme therapy is to achieve normal or near-normal fat and protein digestion. From this should naturally follow normal nutrition, growth and development, and a normal or near-normal stooling pattern. However, achievement of these goals may be limited by factors other than pancreatic enzyme insufficiency affecting the gastrointestinal milieu. These factors include gastrointestinal dysmotility, decreased bicarbonate secretion, and other abnormalities including a possible decrease in intestinal solubilization or absorption of long-chain fatty acids[28c]. Furthermore, determining and adjusting the pancreatic enzyme dosage required to achieve the best possible result, and monitoring efficacy of therapy present practical problems. Ideally, fecal fat and protein balance studies should be done and enzyme dosage adjusted accordingly, but these tests are not practical in routine clinical use. Usually, therefore, initial enzyme dosage is calculated and then individually adjusted on clinical grounds to achieve a normal or near normal stool pattern with formed, nongreasy stools with normal odor, and absence of abdominal pain or excessive and malodorous flatus. Stool microscopy for fat globules may be helpful to monitor efficacy of therapy and adjust enzyme dosage on an outpatient basis[29].

Unfortunately, the increased potency of modern enteric-coated pancreatic enzyme preparations has also encouraged the use of greatly increased enzyme doses in some patients, and this has been linked to the emergence of an unexpected, previously undescribed, severe, complication – fibrosing colonopathy[30,31]. For this reason, unlimited increases in enzyme dosage in an attempt to completely abolish steatorrhea or intestinal symptoms should be avoided, and guidelines with upper limits for replacement pancreatic enzyme dosage have recently been recommended[32–35].

INITIATION AND ADJUSTMENT OF ENZYME THERAPY

The first prerequisite of pancreatic enzyme replacement therapy in CF is to establish that such therapy is required. This is most accurately determined by measurement of 72-hour fecal fat excretion. Specific pancreatic function tests (secretin–cholecystokinin stimulation, fecal chymotrypsin or elastase assay) are also useful in this regard. Initiation and adjustment of enzyme dosage is the responsibility of the physician and dietitian; the patient or family should be taught guidelines within which to adjust dosage, but should not be expected to do this without regular supervision. Discussion and evaluation of enzyme therapy should be part of all CF clinic visits.

Once the need for pancreatic enzyme therapy is established, a standard enteric-coated pancreatic enzyme preparation should be started. Enzymes are required with each fat- or protein-containing meal or snack, and for fat- or protein-containing drinks such as milk, but not for juices or fruit. It is often advised that enzymes be administered both at the beginning and during the meal to ensure thorough 'mixing'. We prefer the simpler approach of giving enzymes at the start of the meal, as this is simpler to remember, and less likely to provoke social comment (which may be important for adherence to therapy in sensitive patients). There is also evidence that enteric-coated preparations are more effective when given at the start of a meal[36]. Although it may be considered 'ideal' to calculate enzyme dosage daily for each individual meal based on that meal's actual fat and protein content, this approach is seldom practical and patients or parents have difficulty predicting and calculating enzyme requirements on this basis. It is generally more satisfactory to calculate enzyme dosage initially by body weight, or on fat content of an average meal, and then adjust dosage as discussed below.

For the newly diagnosed CF patient over 1 year of age, an initial dose of 500 U lipase/kg body weight/meal and 250 U/kg/snack can be given. Initial dosage should be calculated per average (for that patient) meal; if some of the day's meals are consistently larger and substantially higher in fat content, the enzyme dosage for those meals should be greater; but continued variation in dosage based on day-to-day variation in meal size is not advised. For young children who cannot yet swallow capsules, these may be opened and given in a teaspoon of apple sauce or similar medium. Care must be taken to ensure that the child does not chew and break the microspheres.

Once enzymes have been started, dosage is then gradually adjusted at 3–4-day intervals to achieve normal or near-normal stool pattern and fat or protein absorption, or until dosage of enzymes has reached the maximum recommended dose of 2500 U/kg/meal or 10 000 U lipase/kg/day[32–34]. An alternative method for calculation of maximal enzyme dosage is to base it on fat intake, using 4000 U lipase/g dietary fat as the upper limit[35]. Dosages above these limits are not recommended because of the risk of development of fibrosing colonopathy (FC). If dosages above those recommended are thought to be required because of poor growth, steatorrhea or refractory abdominal symptoms, careful investigation into compliance or other complicating factors should first be carried out (Table 12.3, Fig. 12.2), and response to a different distribution of enzyme dosage between each meal or snack, use of a different enzyme preparation or use of adjuvants should be assessed as discussed below. Only if this approach is unsuccessful, should an increase in enzyme dosage even be contemplated. Under such circumstances, a small increase in dosage may be considered, but only if

Table 12.3 *Diagnostic evaluation of refractory gastrointestinal symptoms in cystic fibrosis patients: useful clinical and laboratory investigations*

1. Clinical history and physical examination
2. Diet review
3. Stool
   Microscopy
   Chymotrypsin assay
   Culture, ova and parasites
   Fecal fat excretion (3-day)
4. Urinalysis, culture
5. Blood
   Complete blood count
   Erythrocyte sedimentation rate
   Vitamin A, D, E levels
   Prothrombin time, PIVKA (protein in vitamin K absence)
   BUN, creatinine
   Serum electrolytes
   Bilirubin, liver enzymes
   Amylase, immunoreactive trypsinogen
   Immunoglobulins, IgE, milk precipitins or RAST
   Helicobacter pylori antibodies, *Yersinia* antibodies
   Antigliadin antibodies, antiendomysial antibodies
6. Lactose tolerance test, breath hydrogen test
7. Diagnostic imaging
   Plain radiograph of abdomen
   Abdominal ultrasound (kidney, liver, gallbladder, pancreas, bowel, ovaries)
   Gastric emptying (technecium-99) (solid phase, with enzymes)
   Gastroesophageal reflux scan (technecium-99)
   Barium swallow and follow-through
8. 24-hour esophageal pH monitoring
9. Endoscopy and biopsy (esophagus, stomach, duodenum, colon, rectum)
10. Detailed psychological assessment

documented by 3-day fecal fat excretion to significantly improve fat malabsorption, and only under close, continuing, supervision[43].

Initiation of enzyme supplementation therapy in the newly diagnosed CF infant requires special care. In this age group, the number of feeds per day will change as the infant grows, and the nutritional requirements for growth and development will increase. Therefore not only must enzyme intake be frequently adjusted to cover the increasing nutrient needs for growth, but also to accommodate changes in meal patterns. Some authorities still recommend use of powdered enzyme preparations for infants up to 1 year of age[35], but we prefer to use an enteric-coated preparation. The enteric-coated microspheres or microtablets should be emptied from the capsule, divided equally (by inspection, not by counting), and given in a small amount of apple sauce immediately before each feed. The same regimen can be used for breast-fed CF infants, since the enteric coating prevents the damage to mother's nipple, which occurs, and which inhibits breast-feeding when powdered preparations are used. (Breast-fed infants should also receive a salt supplement of 2-4 meg/kg/day). When an infant's next feed occurs within 1–2 hours of receiving its previous enzyme dose, it is generally not necessary to repeat the dose. Care must be taken to ensure that the infant does not chew and break the microspheres.

A suitable initial dose for a full-term CF infant is ⅛-¼ capsule per feed of an 8000 U lipase/capsule enteric-coated preparation. This usually approximates 250–500 U lipase per kg body weight per feed or 1500–4000 U/kg body weight/day. This initial dosage will require revision upwards at 3-4 day intervals until normal growth is attained and stooling pattern is normalized. As the infant grows and gets older, the number of feeds per day will naturally decrease, while the nutritional intake per feed will increase; hence an increased enzyme dosage per feed will be required. By 1 year of age, the infant is usually taking 3 meals and 2 snacks per day, and required enzyme dosage is usually in the range of 500–2000 U lipase/kg/meal and half that per snack. Total daily enzyme dose should not exceed 10 000 U lipase per kg per day, and in our experience, requirements are usually below this. Failure to achieve growth and control of gastrointestinal symptoms at dosages within the recommended range, should be the signal for careful reassessment of the patient (Fig 12.2) as previously discussed.

Malnourished infants in particular may suffer from excoriation of the buttocks and perianal area when enzymes are started. Protective 'barrier' cream should be used until this problem resolves and care should be taken to ensure that the enzyme dose is not excessive. Infants also have a relative propensity to develop watery diarrhea, crampy abdominal pain or colic, and perianal excoriation when excessive enzyme dosage is given. These may resemble the signs of pancreatic insufficiency, and can be misconstrued by the inexperienced observer as due to inadequate, rather than excessive, enzyme intake; care should therefore be taken that enzyme dosage is not mistakenly increased in such a situation.

In some instances, CF patients may require tube feeding via a nasogastric tube, gastrostomy or jejunostomy. Pancreatic enzyme therapy during tube feeding can pose a challenge since enteric-coated enzymes cannot be administered down small tubes. To circumvent this problem, an 'elemental', low-fat formula can be used, in which case, enzymes are not necessary. In this case, fat should be supplied parenterally or by concomitant oral fat-containing feeds with appropriate oral dosage of enzymes. Alternatively, when fat- or protein-containing tube feeds are used, enteric-coated enzymes can be swallowed at intervals during the tube feed or if the patient wakens during the night[35]. Our preference is to use

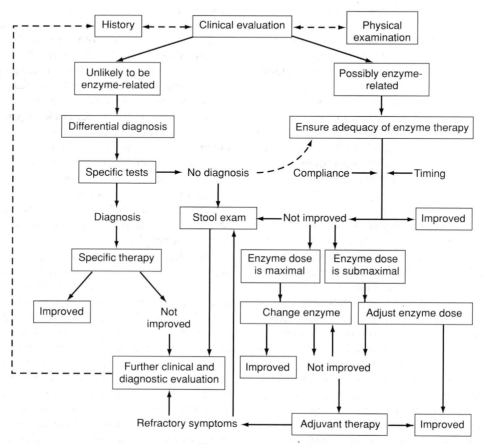

Fig. 12.2 *Diagnostic evaluation of refractory gastroenteric complaints or poor response to pancreatic enzyme therapy in cystic fibrosis.*

instead a powdered enzyme preparation at an initial dose range of 1000–2000 U lipase/g fat (maximum 4000 U/g fat), dissolved and mixed with the tube feed before administration.

There is currently insufficient data to guide rigidly the adjustment of enzyme dosage for adult CF patients. As adolescent growth is left behind and calorie requirements decrease into adulthood, it is likely that dosage expressed on a per kg basis will be less useful. At this time, the use of an upper limit, based on fat intake (as discussed above), may be preferable.

INADEQUATE THERAPEUTIC RESPONSE

Despite prescription of adequate enzyme dosage, 10 per cent or more of CF patients may continue to have significant fat malabsorption, abdominal complaints or poor growth[34]. There may be many reasons for this (Fig. 12.2), but the most common cause of inadequate response to enzyme therapy is noncompliance or nonadherence, such as may particularly occur on social occasions, at school or at work. Often this may be a sign that the patient or family has failed to come to terms with the implications of having CF. If careful explanation and discussion does not improve the situation, such patients (and families) may require extensive psychological or psychiatric counseling.

The efficacy of the enzyme preparation should also be considered. Substandard potency and inadequate dissolution characteristics have been reported with some generic or alternative-brand enzyme preparations[27]. Since pancreatic enzymes are biological products; faulty or prolonged storage may result in significant loss of activity and inadequate therapeutic response (it is more likely, however, that the actual potency of the preparation exceeds the manufacturer's advertised strength, at least in fresh preparations)[27]. If there is any question about potency or dissolution characteristics of a product, these should either be assayed, or a new supply obtained and response to its use assessed before progressing to further investigation.

Poor response to enzyme replacement may occur in spite of full compliance and use of appropriate doses of an active enzyme preparation. For these patients, a careful clinical history and physical examination should be done, all possible causes of the symptoms considered, and any diagnostic leads followed up (see Fig. 12.2 and Table 12.3). Initial testing should include stool examination for parasites or infection. Consideration should be given to trial of a different type of enteric-coated enzyme preparation since the emptying of enteric-coated enzyme granules, microspheres or minitablets from the stomach and the release of enzymes from their enteric coating is a complex process affected by gastric emptying, particle size and dissolution characteristics, small bowel pH and bile salt concentration[27,28,28a,28b,38]. Because of these differences between the various commercial enzyme preparations, it may be worthwhile assessing the effectiveness of a different preparation, before proceeding to more intensive measures and investigations.

Allergy to pancreatic enzyme preparations has been reported[38a]. Desensitization was successfully accomplished.

ADJUVANTS TO PANCREATIC ENZYME THERAPY

Various therapeutic adjuncts have been found to be helpful in CF patients with a poor response to standard enzyme therapy. These may be classified as strategies to protect or enhance the activity or the release from enteric coating of replacement pancreatic enzymes; agents which improve bile salt solubility and micellar formation; or measures to bypass the need for enzymes by utilizing alternative pathways of absorption.

Strategies to protect or enhance the activity and release of replacement pancreatic enzymes are based on the fact that pancreatic enzymes are sensitive to denaturation by acidic conditions and their activity and release from enteric coating is also pH dependent. For this reason, medications to alter gastric or duodenal pH may be quite helpful in patients with persisting severe steatorrhea despite appropriate pancreatic enzyme dosage. The administration of sodium bicarbonate with the oral enzyme preparation is well tolerated, economical and often effective in dosage ranging from 5 to 15 g/m²/day in divided doses taken with enzymes[39–41]. Other antacids such as aluminum hydroxide may also be effective, but magnesium- or calcium-based antacids should not be used as they have been reported to interact with glycine-conjugated bile salts[39]. Suppression of gastric acid production with agents such as cimetidine, ranitidine or omeprazole have yielded conflicting results with regard to fat absorption but may be helpful in some situations[27,42]. In a placebo-controlled double-blind trial, misoprostol, a prostaglandin analog which is said to increase duodenal pH, decreased fecal fat loss in CF patients who had continued to have fat malabsorption despite enzyme therapy[43].

The effectiveness of pancreatic enzymes is also dependent on bile salt concentration reaching the critical level for micellar formation. Bile salts in CF tend to be glycine- rather than taurine-conjugated because of ileal malabsorption of bile salts and the differential rate of synthesis of glycine over taurine conjugates. Glycine-conjugated bile salts tend to precipitate more readily in an acidic milieu. The net effect is that critical micellar concentrations may not be achieved in some CF patients. Agents that improve bile-salt solubility and micellar formation may be useful in such situations. On this basis, addition of taurine to the diet increases the bile salt taurine : glycine conjugate ratio and was initially found to improve essential fatty acid absorption in CF patients with steatorrhea. However further study has questioned the efficacy of taurine in this regard[44]. Initial studies with ursodeoxycholic acid suggested that nutrition was improved, but this has not been borne out by further study[45]. Nonspecific bile-salt preparations may actually worsen steatorrhea, perhaps due to the effect of unconjugated bile salts contaminating these preparations.

Use of medium chain triglycerides (MCT) as a fat source which utilizes alternative absorptive pathways has also been advocated. MCT is water soluble and can be absorbed without first undergoing lipolysis, although absorption is improved by the presence of pancreatic enzymes. MCT has been shown to be effective in short-term studies, but benefits of longer-term use were less convincing[46].

Meconium ileus

Meconium ileus (MI) is the earliest clinical manifestation of cystic fibrosis, occurring in approximately 10–15 per cent of CF neonates[7]. It presents as a bowel obstruction associated with abnormally viscid meconium. The association between MI and pancreatic disease was first described by Landsteiner in 1905, long before CF was recognized as a distinct clinical entity. The majority of infants born with MI have CF; in one recent series CF was proven in 36 of 44 cases of MI[47]. However, when *in utero* diagnoses are included, CF appears to be the cause less often; in a recent collaborative study of 102 neonates, stillbirths and abortuses with MI, intestinal atresia, stenosis or meconium peritonitis, only 20 were due to CF[5]. Those with CF had uncomplicated MI (15/38), or jejunal atresia and meconium peritonitis (5/13). Non-CF causes of MI included intrauterine viral or bacterial infection, chromosomal abnormalities and fetal blood swallowing. MI also occurs in association with pancreatic abnormalities not related to CF, such as pancreatic duct stenosis, and partial pancreatic aplasia. It has also been reported in Niemann–Pick C disease, as well as for no known cause[5,47,48]. For these reasons, MI suspected on the basis of *in utero* ultrasound appearance requires careful diagnostic evaluation (Fig. 12.3).

PATHOPHYSIOLOGY

There is evidence to suggest that abnormal function of the small intestine also contributes to the development of MI [7,49,50], but in CF it is almost always associated with pancreatic exocrine insufficiency and appears to correlate with ΔF_{508}, G542X and other mutations which are 'severe' with respect to pancreatic phenotype[51]. MI in CF most commonly develops in the second trimester of pregnancy, with thick, viscid meconium obstructing the lumen of the small intestine. In about 40 per cent of cases, complications such as volvulus and perforation may occur and meconium peritonitis develops. Small-

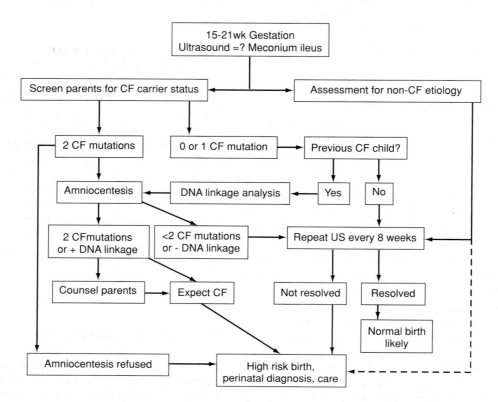

Fig 12.3 *Algorithm for investigation of prenatal ultrasound examination suggestive of meconium ileus. (Modified from ref. 4, see also ref. 5.)*

bowel ischemia due to volvulus or damage to the bowel wall may lead to jejunal atresia, which usually appears in the third trimester[5], and to calcification which is usually intramural. Less commonly, perforation and resulting chemical peritonitis may lead to the rapid development of serosal calcification[52].

CLINICAL PRESENTATION AND DIAGNOSIS

MI can be detected *in utero* by ultrasound early in the second trimester[4,53]. Hyperechoic or dilated fetal bowel presenting early in the second trimester and persisting after 20 weeks' gestation is suggestive of CF and MI, but is not specific. Such a result mandates a careful diagnostic evaluation[4,5,48,52] for which a useful algorithm has been published[5] (see also Fig. 12.3). The usual clinical presentation is postnatal as a bowel obstruction within 48 hours of birth, or earlier if perforation and meconium peritonitis are present. History may reveal polyhydramnios and failure to pass meconium, although occasionally small amounts may be passed[47,47a]. Emesis may be bile stained. Abdominal distension and dilated bowel loops are usually apparent on inspection and palpation, and there may be a right lower quadrant or pelvic mass. Rectal examination produces only a small amount of sticky meconium or a dry mucous plug. Abdominal radiograph may demonstrate calcification in about a quarter of cases of CF and MI[52]. The classic right lower quadrant speckled 'ground-glass' or 'soap-bubble' appearance on X-ray is seen in about one-third to half of patients (Fig. 12.4); and distended bowel loops are typical, usually with no air–fluid levels[47,53]. Contrast enema may show microcolon.

THERAPY

Therapy of MI involves decompression and relief of obstruction. In uncomplicated cases, this can often be accomplished by use of a gastrografin enema[54]. Surgery may be necessary if perforation, gangrene or volvulus are suspected, but every effort should be made to preserve as much bowel as possible. Gastrografin or *N*-acetylcysteine irrigation of the obstructed segment to remove inspissated meconium, and construction of a temporary ileostomy to allow a microcolon time to enlarge, may ensure that the maximum amount of bowel is spared[55].

Use of hypertonic contrast agents such as gastrografin may irritate the bowel mucosa, and deaths from necrotizing enterocolitis following use of gastrografin or renografin for MI have been reported[53]. Nonionic, less hyperosmolar, contrast agents or dilute ionic contrast agents mixed with *N*-acetylcyteine may be safer. With early detection and appropriate therapy[4,47,47a,53], it is now uncommon for infants to die of this complication and long-term outcome equals that of other CF patients[56]. Stagnant-loop syndrome has been reported as a late sequel to ileostomy for MI[57].

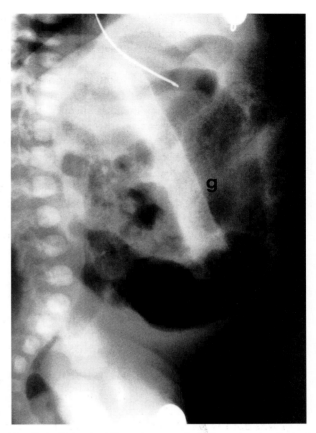

Fig 12.4 *Abdominal X-ray in meconium ileus showing typical 'ground-glass' or 'soap-bubble' appearance (g).*

Meconium plug syndrome

The meconium plug syndrome may often be confused with MI, but is a separate and distinct entity. Affected infants have mild abdominal distension and fail to pass meconium at birth. Rectal exam reveals a 'tight' anal canal. Radiographic exam (enema) reveals distal colonic obstruction by meconium[53]. The meconium plug is often expelled, with relief of symptoms, after rectal exam or enema. The majority of infants with meconium plug syndrome do not have CF, although in one series, 6 of 24 infants were found to have CF[58]. In some cases the meconium plug may be associated with a small left colon – the 'small left colon syndrome' which is a functional disorder sometimes seen in infants of diabetic mothers or mothers with substance abuse[53]. There is one case report suggestive of small left colon syndrome in a CF infant[53].

Pancreatitis in cystic fibrosis

Pancreatitis is probably a more common occurrence in CF than is usually recognized. Shwachman[59] first drew attention to this problem when he reported 10 adolescent and young adult CF patients with recurrent acute pancreatitis. It can also occur in younger CF children[60].

In two of Shwachman's patients, pancreatitis was diagnosed before CF, and diagnosis of CF in the others had been delayed because they did not have pancreatic insufficiency, although pancreatic function testing showed decreased bicarbonate output. The viscid, concentrated pancreatic secretions typical of CF patients, even if PS, are likely factors in the development of this problem.

Pancreatitis typically occurs in CF patients who are PS, with up to 15 per cent of such patients suffering an attack at some time. There have been several reports of acute and chronic pancreatitis in CF patients who are thought to be PI on the basis of steatorrhea, but pancreatic function tests or stool enzyme results in keeping with premorbid PI in these individuals have been lacking. It is also worth noting that recurrent attacks of pancreatitis in PS CF patients may precipitate the development of PI.

There have been several recent publications drawing attention to an association between idiopathic pancreatitis and the carrier state for CF mutations[60a].

CLINICAL PRESENTATION AND DIAGNOSIS

Pancreatitis in CF may present as a severe acute attack or as chronic recurrent abdominal pain. It should be suspected in any CF patient with unexplained abdominal pain, particularly if the patient is PS. The profound systemic effects of acute pancreatitis seen in non-CF patients are not so prominent, perhaps because of the decreased functional capacity and scarring of the exocrine pancreas, even in PS CF patients.

Typically the pain of acute pancreatitis is severe and constant, epigastric, penetrating to the back or radiating to the substernal area or flank. Leaning forward or lying on the side with hips flexed may bring partial relief. Vomiting is frequent. Physical examination may show abdominal distension and mid-epigastric tenderness or mass. Periumbilical or costovertebral angle bluish or hemorrhagic discoloration (Cullen's or Gray–Turner's signs) may be present. Laboratory tests may show elevated serum or urinary amylase or lipase, or elevated circulating IRT. Abdominal imaging using ultrasound or CT is often diagnostic and its use has recently been reviewed[61]. MRI or PET are not indicated. Abdominal X-ray may show pancreatic calcification , dilated transverse colon, or isolated dilated 'sentinel' loop of small bowel in the upper mid or left abdomen. ERCP may sometimes be helpful after the acute attack has subsided, to rule out an obstructive etiology.

In non-CF patients, profound pulmonary effects of acute pancreatitis include pulmonary edema, atelectasis, pulmonary effusion (typically left sided) and diffuse pulmonary infiltrates. These have not generally been noted in CF, but it cannot be entirely discounted that these may occur in CF patients but not be recognized as the effects of pancreatitis.

THERAPY

Therapy of a severe attack of pancreatitis requires bowel rest with nasogastric drainage and use of H_2 blockers or proton pump inhibitors. Systemic resuscitation and support with intravenous fluids may be necessary, and parenteral nutrition is indicated until symptoms and serum enzymes subside. This may be followed by use of a low-fat elemental diet given via continuous nasogastric or nasoduodenal infusion, before starting regular diet. Addition of supplemental pancreatic enzymes in an attempt to suppress pancreatic secretion is common practice, although objective evidence of efficacy in this regard is lacking. Pulmonary disease should be treated aggressively with antibiotics and physiotherapy. Conventional percussion and drainage chest physiotherapy may not be well tolerated because of pain, and the positive expiratory pressure technique may be preferable.

Pancreatic microcysts, cysts and stones

MICROCYSTS

Multiple microscopic or small macroscopic pancreatic retention cysts are classic features of the pathology of cystic fibrosis. These cysts probably develop as a result of ductal obstruction from viscid secretions leading to ductal ectasia and epithelial-lined cysts. These cysts are typically 1–3 mm in diameter, rarely larger than 1 cm, and are usually asymptomatic, except as markers of the generalized pancreatic disease of CF. Multiple cystosis occasionally occurs in CF as an asymptomatic process with an inflammatory component[62]. The process can extend to virtually complete replacement of the pancreas by multiple macroscopic cysts. The development of cysts implies the presence of secreting pancreatic tissue, and cyst contents typically include IRT. Nevertheless, CF patients who are clinically PI with gross steatorrhea may still develop symptomatic cysts.

GIANT PANCREATIC CYSTS

Large isolated macrocysts occur rarely in CF[63,64]. These may be asymptomatic or may present as an upper abdominal mass, or with severe abdominal pain and distention. These must be differentiated from pancreatic pseudocysts, which are often traumatic or postpancreatitis in origin; do not have an epithelial-cell-lined wall; and are not a feature of CF. Diagnosis is apparent on abdominal imaging with ultrasound or CT[61]. If treatment is necessary because of symptoms, surgical drainage has been reported as successful[63]. We have had experience with 'skinny needle' aspiration under ultrasound guidance, resulting in dramatic relief of symptoms and resolution of the cyst.

PANCREATIC STONES

Pancreatic stones can be seen in the CF pancreas at autopsy or on computed tomography, but are rarely symptomatic. However, severe chronic abdominal pain with pancreatitis and stones in the pancreatic duct visualized during ERCP has been reported in CF. Symptoms were relieved by lithotripsy[65].

GASTROINTESTINAL TRACT IN CYSTIC FIBROSIS

Introduction

Involvement of the gastrointestinal tract has been recognized since the first studies in CF. Farber demonstrated inspissated mucus in dilated glands in the duodenum and esophagus, and eosinophilic plugs in salivary glands similar to those demonstrable in the pancreas[66]. Bodian commented upon the abnormal mucus secreted by the intestinal glands, and attributed this to be the cause of meconium ileus[50]. Freye *et al.* demonstrated (using periodic acid–Schiff reagent) a thick mucinous layer overlying the intestinal mucosa, supporting the suggestion that abnormal intestinal mucus contributed to the absorption defect in CF[67], although later studies failed to confirm this as a general pathogenetic mechanism. There has been a lack of consensus regarding intestinal mucosal abnormalities[67a], but studies using electron microscopy have described abnormalities involving goblet cells[67a], as well as the tight junctions (between epithelial cells), mitochondria and the Golgi apparatus[68]. Discovery of the CF gene and evolving knowledge of the function of the gene product (CFTR) has tended to focus attention away from these earlier studies, while at the same time confirming involvement of the intestinal tract, since CFTR is expressed throughout the alimentary tract in the apical membrane of epithelial cells, from salivary glands to colon. CFTR expression in the intestine is higher in crypts than in villi, where the multi-drug-resistant transporter becomes more prominent[69–71].

Observed functional defects of the intestinal tract include abnormalities of secretion, absorption, paracellular permeability, enzyme activity, gut hormone secretion and motility [49,69,70,72–74]. CF intestinal mucins have been studied extensively, often with conflicting results[75,76]. Suggested abnormalities in these macromolecules include differences in side-chain length and constitution, leading to differences in three-dimensional conformation, which can be expected to affect receptor sites and function, as well as possibly affecting diffusion characteristics in the unstirred water layer overlying the intestinal absorptive surfaces[69,75–77]. There are conflicting reports whether gastric acid secretion is normal in CF, but basal and postprandial gastric pH is normal, as are gastrin levels[69,70]. Abnormal ion transport in the intestine reflects the generalized CFTR-mediated abnormalities in CF, and is associated with decreased intestinal fluid (water) and electrolyte transport, absent secretory response, thick, viscid secretions, and decreased duodenal pH[57,70,78,79]. Although Cl⁻ secretion is absent, reflecting lack of chloride-channel activity, active transport mediated absorption of glucose and alanine is increased[57]. The net effect of this is to transfer solute out of the intestinal lumen, further contributing to dehydration of intestinal content and clinical problems such as the distal intestinal obstruction syndrome (DIOS). With regard to enzyme abnormalities, studies suggest increased pharyngeal lipase secretion, while gastric lipase is probably normal; but the whole question of preduodenal lipase activity needs further study[22,23]. Abnormal enzyme levels in the intestine include increased enterokinase levels in the small bowel brush border[69]. It is not clear if intestinal disaccharidase activity is affected; or whether this might be a secondary effect of the acidic duodenal milieu[69,80]. Absorption of disaccharides such as sucrose, lactose, lactulose or cellobiose is increased via the paracellular route, suggesting altered intestinal permeability, although this may, at least in part, be secondary to PI[72,77,81,82]. Absorption and turnover of essential fatty acids (EFA) is not normal, even in pancreatic-sufficient CF patients, and may in turn cause systemic and pulmonary, as well as hepatic, pancreatic and intestinal effects[83,84]. These EFA effects may be mediated through changes in cell-membrane fluidity, chloride-channel function, or abnormalities in prostaglandins, leukotrienes or other EFA metabolites. A specific defect in retinol handling in CF appears to be present and results in increased fecal losses of vitamin A[85]. There is some disagreement as to whether bile salt malabsorption is present in the terminal ileum, contributing to abnormal bile salt metabolism[86–88]. Gut hormone abnormalities arise as a result of the altered intestinal milieu and include gut motility regulatory peptides as well as other biochemical regulators[83,89,94]; and may, at least in part, explain the abnormalities of gastrointestinal motility demonstrable in many CF patients.

Salivary glands and oropharynx

Involvement of the salivary glands in CF is generally considered of limited clinical significance, which may be more an indication of our limited understanding of the importance of salivary secretions, than of absolute knowledge. CFTR is expressed in salivary ductal cells and histological changes, such as eosinophilic mucus plugs, are demonstrable[66,95]. Salivary secretions in CF show decreased water content and increased concentrations of calcium[96]. Extensive investigations have failed to confirm other abnormalities consistently, although there is evidence that mucins may be oversulfated or have increased fucosylation or decreased sialylation, perhaps due to abnormal CFTR-related function of the Golgi apparatus[69,75,76]. Salivary amylase is elevated in serum, although total serum amylase tends to be normal because of a decreased pancreatic fraction. Lingual (pharyngeal) lipase secretion appears to be increased in CF infants and may be an important factor in fat digestion in this age group[22,23]. On physical examination, asymptomatic enlargement of the submaxillary gland is evident in most CF patients[97].

Gastrointestinal dysmotility in CF

The clinically most important abnormalities of the gastrointestinal tract in CF involve disorders of motility. These cause significant problems. In addition to upper gastrointestinal dysmotility manifesting as gastroesophageal reflux (GER), there is evidence to suggest abnormalities in gastric emptying, small intestinal transit time and motility of the large bowel in CF[7,72,73,89,98]. Evidence for small bowel bacterial overgrowth, which can result from dysmotility, has also been documented[99]. Although these conditions have been considered separately with regard to symptomatology, causation, diagnosis and therapy, it is logical to consider them as separate manifestations of a generalized gastrointestinal dysmotility syndrome (GDS) in CF. When the underlying cause of these disorders is determined, it is likely that common etiological and pathophysiological factors will be found which may lead to better understanding and more effective therapy.

Control of motor activity of the esophagus, stomach and intestines is complex and not fully understood. Normal physiological homeostatic mechanisms regulate and integrate motility with secretory, digestive and absorptive functions of the gastrointestinal tract. This regulation and integration is achieved via a complex interplay between intrinsic muscle activity and neurocrine, endocrine and paracrine systems and through the mediation of a variety of biological chemicals[100]. These systems are responsive to intestinal and extraintestinal stimuli and sensitive to changes in the intestinal milieu. In CF, abnormal CFTR has major effects on the intestinal milieu, digestive and absorptive function. It is therefore to be expected that gastrointestinal motility will also be affected.

Abnormal levels of a variety of biochemical agents with the potential to act as gastrointestinal motility regulators have been found in CF. Gut regulatory peptides such as motilin, enteroglucagon, neurotensin and peptide YY, which are associated with altered intestinal motility in non-CF subjects, are increased in CF[89,92,93]. Although the physiological role of these and other gut hormones is not fully understood, it has been shown that gastrin and motilin can increase lower esophageal sphincter (LES) pressure, whereas secretin, glucagon and cholecystokinin (CCK) decrease it, and intestinal transit may be slowed by elevated levels of enteroglucagon[93]. Abnormal essential fatty acid and eicosanoid (prostaglandin) metabolism in CF may affect motility and the LES; it has been shown, for example, that prostaglandin E_1 affects LES pressure. Dopamine is also known to decrease LES pressure and is elevated in CF[90]. Pharmacologic agents used in the treatment of CF may also affect gastrointestinal motility; examples including isoproteronol, salbutamol and theophylline, which cause relaxation of the LES, and macrolide antibiotics (e.g. erythromycin) which have prokinetic properties.

Various factors may be responsible for the abnormal levels of these biochemical regulatory compounds. These include pancreatic insufficiency leading to unabsorbed products of (mal)digestion and (mal)absorption in the intestine, decreased duodenal pH, and other CFTR-related disturbances of intestinal function; all of which may affect duodenal or ileal receptors and derange normal physiological homeostatic mechanisms, such as, for example, in the 'ileal brake' phenomenon[91]. Although there is as yet insufficient knowledge upon which to base a complete explanation for the disturbances of gastrointestinal motility in CF, nor for that matter is there complete understanding of the extent and full implications of these disturbances of motility, it is clear that the abnormal internal milieu of the CF patient is a major contributing factor. Further study is needed to achieve a better understanding of the pathophysiology involved in CF gastrointestinal dysmotility, and allow the development of more rational and effective therapy.

GASTROESOPHAGEAL REFLUX

Gastroesophageal reflux (GER) is defined as an abnormal increased frequency or duration of regurgitation of gastric content into the esophagus. This gastric content may contain duodenal biliary secretions. The presence of acidic gastric content in the esophagus may lead to transient inappropriate relaxation of the upper esophageal sphincter and facilitate aspiration into the lungs, leading to respiratory disease. GER in CF patients was first reported in 1975[101] but the significance of this association and its importance as a cause of morbidity in CF has been largely ignored until relatively recently. This is, at least in part, because many of the signs and symptoms of GER are also 'typical' of CF (Table 12.4) and hence readily ignored. The true prevalence of GER in CF is not known, but where its presence has been carefully considered, it has been found to occur frequently[102]. In one study, 76 per cent of all CF patients under 5 years of age were found to have GER[102].

Etiology and pathogenesis of gastroesophageal reflux in CF

The etiology of GER in CF appears to be multifactorial (Fig. 12.5). Although obstructive pulmonary disease may predispose to reflux through flattening of the diaphragm, increased sterno-vertebral angle or increased

Table 12.4 *Clinical features of gastroesophageal reflux which are also 'typical of CF'*

Pulmonary
  Cough
  Apneic episodes (infant)
  Wheezing
  Obstructive airway disease (bronchodilator responsive)
  Lower respiratory infections, bronchopneumonia
  Atelectasis
  Bronchiectasis
  Digital clubbing
Gastrointestinal
  Nausea
  Regurgitation or vomiting
  Abdominal pain (epigastric)
  Dyspepsia
  Anorexia or poor feeding (infant)
Other
  Malnutrition
  Unhappy, crying, infant
  Halitosis
  Anemia

causative factors. The therapeutic use of agents known to relax the lower esophageal sphincter (e.g. aminophylline, salbutamol or isoproteronol) or the adoption of head-down positions during chest physiotherapy can also contribute to reflux[103–105]. Regardless of the cause, repeated or prolonged regurgitation into the esophagus eventually leads to mucosal injury and esophagitis of varying degree. In severe or prolonged GER, damaged esophageal squamous epithelial cells are replaced by metaplastic columnar epithelial cells, defining the pre-malignant condition termed Barrett's esophagus which occurs in CF as well as non-CF patients[106].

Pulmonary disease, physiotherapy and gastroesophageal reflux in CF

The pulmonary lesions associated with GER in non-CF individuals bear a striking similarity to pulmonary disease in CF patients (Table 12.4). Although direct proof of reflux-induced pulmonary aspiration is lacking in CF, it is now generally accepted that GER can contribute to the progression of lung disease (Fig 12.6). It has now also been demonstrated that chest physiotherapy (CPT) can induce reflux episodes, particularly in the head down positions, even in CF infants not identified as having severe GER[104]. This has important implications if confirmed, because of the widespread use of postural

intra-abdominal pressure during cough, GER is frequently present in CF patients who have only minor pulmonary involvement and clearly there must be other

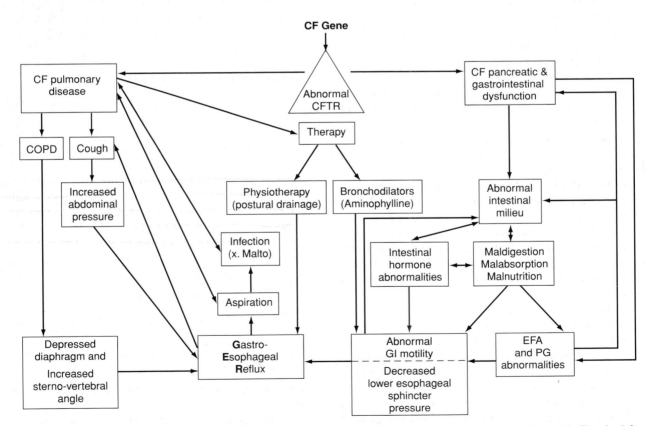

Fig. 12.5 *Hypothesis relating gastroesophageal reflux, gastrointestinal dysfunction and pulmonary disease in cystic fibrosis. (After Davidson and Wong (1991) Pediatr. Pulmonol. Suppl.,* **2***, 99.) CFTR, cystic fibrosis transmembrane conductance regulator protein; COPD, chronic obstructive pulmonary disease; EFA, essential fatty acid; PG, prostaglandin.*

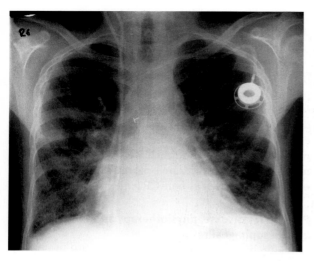

Fig. 12.6 *Aspiration damage to transplanted lung in a cystic fibrosis patient with gastroesophageal reflux. Note patchy subsegmental atelectasis and interstitial changes.*

drainage with head-down positions during CPT in CF, and has led to discussion as to whether these positions should be avoided[104,105].

Clinical presentation of gastroesophageal reflux in CF

GER may be asymptomatic or may present with a variety of symptoms, such as overt vomiting or retrosternal pain ('heartburn'). The signs and symptoms of GER are shown in Table 12.4. Many of these are also 'classic' symptoms or signs of CF. The possibility of GER should particularly be considered in the CF patient who has significant problems with abdominal pain, poor appetite or poor nutrition; or progressive pulmonary disease despite compliance with appropriate CF therapy. It is also worth emphasizing that in many cases, CF patients may not complain of symptoms, even with severe complications of GER such as Barrett's esophagus[106].

Diagnosis and therapy of gastroesophageal reflux

The approach to diagnosis of GER in CF is similar to that for non-CF patients. Other causes of vomiting must be excluded by appropriate tests, and a barium cine-swallow and follow-through examination must be done to ensure that reflux is not secondary to a gastric or intestinal obstructive lesion. The most sensitive and reliable test for GER is 24-hour intra-esophageal pH monitoring. Other tests such as barium cine-swallow or ^{99}Tc-labeled swallow are less invasive and better tolerated, but false-negative or false-positive results are more frequent. Electrical impedance tomography has also been used[107]. Esophageal manometry is useful in determining whether LES pressure is decreased, but reflux may be associated with inappropriate relaxation of the sphincter rather than constant decreased pressure[108]. Confirmation of the presence and degree of complications of GER, such as esophagitis or Barrett's esophagus, requires esophagoscopy and biopsy (Fig. 12.7). There are no sensitive or reliable tests suitable

for routine clinical use, to confirm aspiration or pulmonary damage occurring during, or as a consequence of, GER.

'Traditional' therapy employed, often with very little success, elevation of the head of the bed and (in infants) use of thickened feeds and/or avoidance of 'acid' or spicy foods. Current therapy involves use of prokinetic agents and/or gastric acid suppressants, and can be very effective in some but not all patients. Cisapride appears to be the most effective prokinetic drug currently available, with effects both on LES and gastric emptying. In some patients, use of cisapride is dramatically effective, but in others symptoms may persist[108].

Careful assessment and supervision is required when cisapride is used because of its potential effect on the cardiac QT interval, and potentiation of this effect by interaction with other medications (eg erythromycin, itraconazole). A recent 'Medical Position Statement' of the European Society of Pediatric Gastroenterology, Hepatology and Nutrition[108a] discusses the use of cisapride and precautions required. No special safety procedures regarding potential cardiac adverse events were recommended when there is medical justification for cisapride use in an otherwise healthy individual and dosage does not exceed 0.8 mg/kg/day (maximum 40 mg/day)[108a]. However if the patient is known or suspected to be at risk for drug-associated increases in QTc interval, or if doses greater than those recommended above are used, ECG monitoring should be performed before initiation of therapy and after 3 days of cisapride use. If a prolonged QTc is found, the drug should be discontinued or dose reduced until the ECG normalizes[108a].

In several trials in non-CF patients, combined therapy using cimetidine or ranitidine and cisapride has been shown to be more effective in promoting healing of esophagitis than use of either drug alone[109,110]. Proton pump inhibitors such as omeprazole or pantoprazole show promise in reducing symptoms and in treatment of severe esophagitis or Barrett's esophagus[106], but the safety of their long-term use has not been established. Published experience with surgical correction of GER in CF is limited and reported successes are few. Our limited experience with Nissen fundoplication in CF GER has been discouraging, with rapid failure of the repair. This is perhaps due to chronic cough which is recognized as a major risk factor in failure of surgical antireflux procedures in non-CF GER patients[110]. The presence of delayed gastric emptying (DGE) also contributes to failure of fundoplication procedures, hence gastric drainage procedures (pyloroplasty or pyloromyotomy) should be considered in patients with GER and DGE not responding to medical management[109,111,112,115].

GASTRIC EMPTYING IN CF

The normal process of gastric emptying is subject to the same system of complex control and integration that

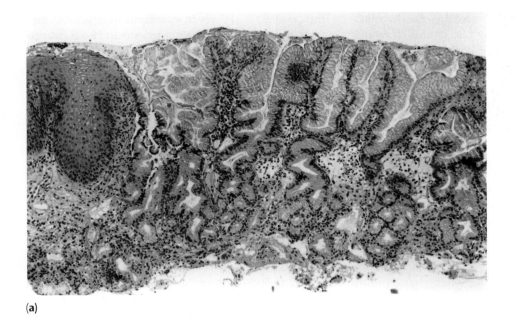

(a)

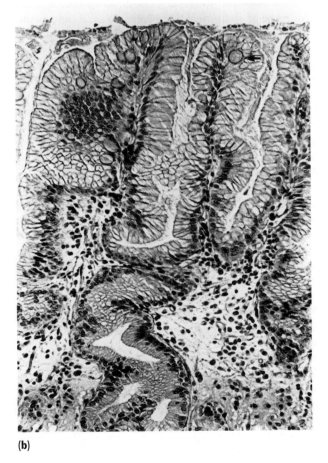

(b)

Fig. 12.7 *Barrett's esophagus in a patient with cystic fibrosis and gastroesophageal reflux. Distal squamocolumnar junction of esophagus. (a) Photomicrograph ×40 showing specialized epithelium of metaplasia (Barrett's); (b) photomicrograph ×100 showing villus architecture and goblet cells (arrow). (Photos courtesy of Dr J. Dimmick.)*

operates throughout the gastrointestinal tract, and therefore is also vulnerable to the altered internal milieu of CF. In the normal situation, as food enters the stomach, reflex neural and hormonal responses coordinate the gastric functions of storage, secretion and mixing to form chyme; and prepare the pancreas and intestine to receive the stomach content. As chyme enters the duodenum, the rate of gastric emptying and intestinal motility is coordinated with intestinal digestive and absorptive processes. The signals that coordinate these actions arise from receptor responses to the volume, acidity and osmolality of chyme and its carbohydrate, protein and fat composition. The system controlling gastric emptying is sufficiently discriminatory to control separately the emptying of solid and liquid constituents of the gastric content[113].

Pancreatic insufficiency affects gastric emptying because the balance between digestion and absorption, and feedback from pancreatic secretions, are affected. In CF, the signals controlling gastric motility are additionally impacted by the low duodenal pH, decreased or absent bicarbonate secretion, and intestinal dysfunction. Use of pancreatic enzyme therapy in CF introduces a further set of variables, such as enzyme dosage, time to appear in the intestine, dissolution characteristics, as well as enzyme activity consequent to the effects of duodenal pH. All combine to affect digestion, site of digestion, absorption and intraluminal concentrations of nutrients and digestion products, such as fats, fatty acids, proteins, amino acids or peptides. These changes in the internal milieu in turn affect receptors throughout the intestinal tract. It is presumably the net effect of these potentially opposing factors that results in the abnormal levels of CCK, secretin and other gut regulatory chemicals which have been documented in CF. Since these substances may have motor regulatory function, it is therefore to be expected that gastric motility in CF will be affected, but there is insufficient knowledge of the detailed pathophysiology involved to allow a priori conclusions regarding the net clinical effect on the patient.

A variety of clinical observations suggest that gastric emptying may be delayed in CF. Complaints of undigested food or enzymes present in gastric content vomited many hours after a meal, are relatively frequent in CF. Poor appetite or early satiety are also frequently voiced concerns of CF patients or parents, and are symptoms that could be due to delayed gastric emptying (DGE). Delayed small bowel transit has been reported in CF, and it has been suggested that DGE may have contributed to this. GER is now known to be common in CF, and it is well recognized that DGE occurs in as many as 50 per cent of non-CF patients who have GER[112].

There are significant technical and methodological problems involved in measuring gastric emptying[114]. Nevertheless, several studies have investigated gastric emptying in CF patients. Tests performed without administration of supplemental enzymes, found emptying to be rapid. This is not surprising and is in keeping with results for patients with pancreatic insufficiency not due to CF. However, rapid gastric emptying of liquids has also been found in CF, even when pancreatic enzymes were administered. Studies of solid-phase emptying in CF have yielded conflicting results and the situation is further complicated because the rate of emptying of the pancreatic enzyme preparation may be different from that of food[28a,28b]. A study using $^{99}Tc^m$-macroalbumin-labeled pancakes taken with pancreatic enzymes found gastric emptying to be more rapid in CF patients, than in non-CF controls (53 min versus 72.2

min, $P < 0.05$)[114]. However, measurement of gastric emptying using real-time ultrasonography in 29 CF patients found significantly ($P < 0.01$) prolonged emptying time at 60 and 90 minutes in 26 patients, as well as exaggerated antral distention after feeding[115]. Using $^{99}Tc_m$ tracer incorporated into cooked egg, we have also found that gastric emptying is commonly delayed in CF. We have found DGE ($t_{1/2} > 90$ min) in 34 of 70 CF patients who were studied because of suggestive clinical symptoms or the presence of GER, out of a CF pediatric clinic population of 135. Of those patients with DGE, nine had $t_{1/2} = 90-120$ minutes, six patients had $t_{1/2} = 120-150$ minutes, and 19 had $t_{1/2} < 120$ minutes.

MECONIUM ILEUS EQUIVALENT OR DISTAL INTESTINAL OBSTRUCTION SYNDROME

Jensen in 1961 first used the term 'meconium ileus equivalent' (MIE)[116] to describe intestinal obstruction with inspissated intestinal contents occurring in CF patients after the neonatal period. More recently, the syndrome of abdominal pain, palpable cecal masses and partial or complete intestinal obstruction with abnormally viscid mucofeculent material in the terminal ileum or right colon has been called the 'distal intestinal obstruction syndrome' (DIOS)[7].

The reported incidence of DIOS varies widely. It may occur at any time after the neonatal period and appears to increase with age and be more common in adolescent or adult patients[7,98]. Estimates range from less than 2 per cent of CF patients under age 5 years, to 27 per cent of those over age 30 years, and 7–15 per cent of all CF patients beyond the neonatal period[7,74,98,117]. If the occurrence of partial manifestations or complications is included, the incidence of DIOS is further increased with one retrospective review documenting one or more of constipation, palpable cecal masses, intussusception, volvulus and intestinal obstruction in 26 of 63 (41 per cent) CF patients[74].

Pathophysiology

The pathophysiology of DIOS is not fully understood. It was first believed that infants with meconium ileus might be more likely to develop MIE in later life, but this has not been supported by further study. Rapid increase in pancreatic enzyme dosage may precipitate an attack, but a clear relationship to enzyme dosage has not been established. Dehydration, which may occur with the development of diabetes mellitus, can also precipitate DIOS[118]. Intestinal abnormalities in CF related to CFTR expression have received relatively little attention with respect to causation of DIOS, but it is likely that abnormalities of intestinal secretion and perhaps of motility contribute significantly[69]. It is noteworthy in this regard that DIOS has also been reported, though uncommonly, in CF patients with PS[119,120].

In view of current information, it seems likely that multiple factors, including dehydration, pancreatic dysfunction with decreased pancreatic fluid and bicarbonate output, rapid increase in enzyme dosage, viscid intestinal secretions, disturbed intestinal fluid and electrolyte transport, decreased duodenal pH, and abnormal intestinal motility, may all play a role in the development of DIOS.

Clinical presentation and diagnosis

Patients typically present with crampy abdominal pain, which is usually referred to the right lower quadrant and may be exacerbated by eating. Symptoms may be chronic and recurring. Firm or hard, irregular masses can often be palpated in the right ileal fossa. Distended bowel loops with visible peristalsis may be present. Usually the obstruction is partial but intussusception or volvulus may complicate the syndrome[7], or there may be complete bowel obstruction with classic signs such as severe pain, abdominal distension and bile-stained vomiting. Even with chronic partial obstruction, symptoms may be of sufficient severity to lead to surgery in the mistaken belief that appendicitis or other acute surgical condition is present. DIOS mistakenly diagnosed as appendicitis may present before the patient is recognized to have CF, and the diagnosis of CF only be made after pathological examination of the surgically removed appendix[121,122].

DIOS is usually the prime diagnosis suspected in CF patients presenting with abdominal cramps, with or without abdominal mass or vomiting. However, these patients are not immune to other causes of such symptoms, which may need prompt and accurate diagnosis and treatment[74,123]. Differential diagnosis includes other causes of abdominal pain; particularly 'simple' constipation, appendicitis, intussusception or volvulus, inflammatory bowel disease, fibrosing colonopathy, gastrointestinal malignancy, pancreatitis, biliary tract or gallbladder disease and ovarian disease (e.g. dermoid cyst). It can be extremely difficult to identify other conditions in the differential diagnosis and careful diagnostic work-up is essential (Fig. 12.2, Table 12.3)[74,123]. In one study, eight of 32 patients thought to have DIOS had other pathology, including Crohn's disease (1), small bowel volvulus (2), and one each of small bowel fistula, appendiceal abscess and ovarian dermoid[74].

Laboratory investigations in a patient known to have CF should include white blood count, serum amylase, liver enzymes, urinalysis and stool examination for fat globules and enteric pathogens. Abdominal ultrasound[123], and erect and supine abdominal radiograph are helpful, with dilated small bowel loops and 'bubbly' ileocecal soft-tissue mass often demonstrable on X-ray[53]. Contrast enema studies not only help to define the mass, but may also be therapeutic by relieving obstruction and mobilizing the tenacious feculent material[53]. CT scan can aid diagnosis or monitor the effect of therapy.

Therapy

In some cases, adjustment of pancreatic enzyme dosage, adequate dietary fiber, and adequate hydration may be sufficient to relieve symptoms. Use of mineral oil has been advocated, but we have not found its efficacy sufficient to warrant the esthetic objections to its use. Lactulose or other stool softener and/or a prokinetic agent may be very helpful in minimizing or preventing recurrent episodes. Oral N-acetylcysteine given as granules, or 10 mL or more of 20 per cent solution diluted in cola beverage or juice three times daily can be very effective in relieving pain[124]. Oral gastrografin can also be used in a dose of 100 mL in 400 mL water or juice (for adults) or 50 mL in 200 mL (for children under 8 years) for 1 or 2 weeks.

When significant inspissated fecal masses are present, the most effective measure is the use of a balanced intestinal lavage solution (Golytely®)[125], administered via nasogastric tube at a rate of up to 750–1000 mL/h and a total volume of 4–6 liters. Some very stoic individuals manage to drink, without recourse to a nasogastric tube, sufficient volume to achieve the desired effect. Enemas of gastrografin 100 mL twice or three times a day, or 50 mL of a 20 per cent solution of N-acetylcysteine in 50 mL water or saline, may also be effective, but magnesium levels should be monitored[126]. Irrigation during colonoscopy may also be used to clear inspissated material.

CONSTIPATION

'Simple' constipation may occur in the CF patient as in any individual and may evolve into a chronic and/or severe problem[117]. Causes may be similar to that seen in the non-CF population, or may be related to the pathophysiology of CF. Too rapid an increase in pancreatic enzyme dosage may also lead to symptoms of constipation. Presentation in the CF patient may be relatively silent, with few symptoms or signs beyond a 'loaded' colon on plain abdominal radiograph or ultrasound. In severe cases, abdominal pain may be prominent. More severe cases should be considered as part of the spectrum of DIOS and treated accordingly.

Management of constipation in CF entails careful adjustment of enzyme dosage, high-fiber diet (in patients over 3 years of age), adequate fluid intake, and establishment of regular bowel habit. Lactulose may be useful as stool softener, and a prokinetic agent can be helpful in refractory cases. When constipation occurs as a symptom after (too) rapid advancement of pancreatic enzyme dosage, it may be necessary to add lactulose or to temporarily decrease enzyme dosage and then advance it more gradually.

Appendicitis

Appendicitis is not uncommon in cystic fibrosis and the diagnosis should be considered in any CF patient with suggestive symptoms, or right iliac fossa mass, especially if barium enema shows extrinsic compression of the cecum. An extensive review reported 4.9 per cent of 1220

CF patients had had an appendectomy[127]. The spectrum of disease ranged from simple mucus distension causing pain, to acute appendicitis with perforation. Presentation may be acute 'classical'; or atypical with chronic, intermittent, right lower quadrant pain and tenderness. An association between intussusception, recurring abdominal pain and appendiceal distention has been reported. Other CF conditions, particularly DIOS, may mimic appendicitis, hence diagnosis can be difficult and delays in diagnosis are frequent, even in the presence of a right iliac fossa mass or a perforation[127].

Appendicitis can be the presenting feature of CF. Histological examination of the removed appendix may indicate the underlying diagnosis of CF in an otherwise asymptomatic, previously undiagnosed patient[121,122].

Gastritis, peptic ulcer disease and *Helicobacter* infection in CF

Peptic ulcer disease may often be suspected in CF because of abdominal or epigastric pain, nausea or anorexia. However, the symptoms are more likely due to gastroesophageal reflux and reports do not indicate an increased likelihood of gastric or duodenal ulcers in CF. One frequently quoted autopsy series recorded peptic ulcer in 8 per cent of 146 CF patients[6], but many of these were likely terminal events. Barium studies of the duodenum and small bowel may show thickened nodular mucosal folds[53], and can be readily misinterpreted as demonstrating 'duodenitis', but the appearance is due to abnormal mucus secretions, perhaps with accompanying muscle spasm due to acid stimulation, and does not represent any other complication. Conversely, these mucosal abnormalities may mask appearance of true peptic ulcer disease, and consideration should be given to endoscopic examination and biopsy if significant unexplained symptoms persist[53].

Helicobacter pylori infection occurs in CF with similar or slightly lower frequency than in the general population[128]. It is often asymptomatic, but infection with this microbe is the major causal factor in non-CF individuals in the development of chronic active (type B) gastritis and peptic ulcer disease affecting stomach and duodenum. Chronic *Helicobacter* infection is also considered a risk factor for gastric adenocarcinoma and lymphoma and it has been declared a type I carcinogen by an IARC working group of the World Health Organization. Its presence may be suspected from serum antibodies and confirmed by gastric biopsy. It should be noted that *Helicobacter pylori* shares cross-reacting antigens with *Pseudomonas aeruginosa*, *Campylobacter jejuni* and *Hemophilus influenzae*, making interpretation of high 'H. pylori' immunoglobulin G antibodies impossible without special immunoglobulin adsorption studies[129]. A promising breath test has been recently developed based on urea release by *H. pylori*[129a].

Intussusception

Intussusception is a relatively infrequent complication of CF in children and adults. Early experience suggested a frequency of 1 per cent of CF patients[130] and a mean age of onset of 9 years, which is much later than in the non-CF population, in whom 75 per cent of cases present before the age of 2 years. Presentation may be acute or chronic with pain and obstructive symptoms, and may be very difficult to differentiate from uncomplicated DIOS or appendicitis with abscess.

The diagnosis is easily missed because presentation in CF is usually at an older age, bloody stool less common, and symptoms usually milder as compared to the non-CF population. The diagnosis should always be considered in any CF patient with colicky abdominal pain, right iliac fossa mass or bowel obstruction, including patients with previously diagnosed DIOS. Typical clinical features in addition to the pain are abdominal mass (usually in the right iliac fossa), abdominal distension and vomiting. Only about 25 per cent of patients have rectal bleeding. The intussusception may be ileo-colic, ileo-ileal or colo-colic, with thick sticky feculent matter at the lead point. Distended appendix has also been reported at the lead point[127]. Radiological features are the same as in the non-CF population. Abdominal plain film may show a soft-tissue mass with abnormal gas pattern in about 50 per cent of patients, with an additional 25 per cent showing features of a small bowel obstruction[53]. Ultrasonography shows a 'doughnut' sign on transverse scans, while CT shows a similar 'target' configuration[53].

A contrast enema under fluoroscopic control may be both diagnostic and therapeutic, but there is some debate regarding the most appropriate technique[131,132]. Laparotomy should be considered if the intussusception cannot be reduced by enemas or the patient's condition deteriorates. Intussusception can be simply and effectively treated if diagnosed promptly, but delay may be fatal.

Volvulus

In the CF fetus or newborn, volvulus may complicate meconium ileus and lead to perforation and meconium peritonitis. This may be detectable *in utero* by ultrasound, or postnatally during investigation for neonatal bowel obstruction. In later life, volvulus may be associated with adhesions due to previous surgery or with DIOS.

The clinical presentation and symptoms of volvulus are those of small bowel obstruction and may be indistinguishable from uncomplicated meconium ileus in the infant, or from DIOS in the older individual[74]. It is therefore essential that all patients with DIOS be carefully assessed for other possible disorders, including volvulus, and have at least an abdominal ultrasound performed.

Therapy at any age requires surgical relief of the volvulus and any other obstruction, excision of gangrenous bowel and construction of a temporary ostomy if required.

Cows' milk intolerance in cystic fibrosis

Intolerance of cows' milk or milk-based formulas may occur as a result of deficient intestinal lactase activity leading to lactose intolerance, or because of an allergic reaction leading to cows' milk enteropathy (CME). In CF, both of these conditions have been reported, and both may give rise to somewhat similar symptoms[80,133]. These symptoms may readily be falsely attributed to 'CF' and failure to recognize CME or lactose intolerance in a CF patient may lead to significant, avoidable morbidity[133].

LACTOSE INTOLERANCE

Intolerance to lactose, the disaccharide found in mammalian milk, is an important and common cause of gastrointestinal symptoms. Lactose intolerance occurs when intestinal brush-border lactase enzyme activity is insufficient to hydrolyze dietary lactose to its constituents (glucose and galactose), as is necessary before absorption can occur. The unabsorbed sugar ferments to cause intestinal gas and an acidic intestinal content which, together with the osmotic effect of unabsorbed sugar, leads to gastrointestinal symptoms. In younger patients, these symptoms are likely to be watery, frothy, gassy, acidic diarrhea, often causing severe perianal erythematous rash, and abdominal pain or colic. In older children or adults, the most prominent symptoms may be increased abdominal gas, bloating and cramping pain, with little or no diarrhoea. In CF, initial reports suggested an increased incidence of lactose intolerance, but further study indicated that its incidence is no higher than in the non-CF population[80].

Lactose intolerance is a clinical diagnosis which implies loss of intestinal brush-border lactase activity. However, loss of intestinal lactase activity and lactose intolerance are not synonymous, since not all individuals with low lactase activity are clinically lactose intolerant. Loss of intestinal lactase activity, may be primary or secondary, and it is important to understand the difference between these two entities. Primary loss of intestinal brush-border lactase activity is an irreversible natural phenomenon under genetic control, occurring after puberty in up to one-third of Caucasians, and earlier in most non-Caucasians. Persistence of lactase activity beyond puberty is inherited as an autosomal dominant trait.

Secondary loss of lactase activity leading to lactose intolerance may occur at any age, due to any condition damaging the small bowel mucosa, such as viral, bacterial, or protozoal infections, bacterial overgrowth (blind loop) syndrome, celiac disease or allergic enteropathy (e.g. due to CME). Secondary lactose intolerance is potentially reversible if the underlying cause is treated. So-called 'congenital' lactose intolerance, which is often (mis)diagnosed in infancy, is due to secondary loss of lactase activity.

Diagnosis of lactose intolerance may be made by breath test, lactose tolerance tests or stool assay for increased fecal reducing substances. Definitive diagnosis of lactase deficiency can be made by biopsy and duodenal mucosal (lactase) disaccharidase assay, but is not usually done. Therapy is usually symptomatic, unless a readily treatable underlying cause of secondary lactose intolerance (e.g. giardiasis or allergy) is present. Symptoms of lactose intolerance, whether primary or secondary, respond to restriction of lactose-containing foods (e.g. cows' milk) and/or use of lactase enzyme preparations (e.g. Lactaid). If relief of symptoms requires complete exclusion, rather than simple restriction, of all cows' milk products, the patient is likely to be suffering from an underlying problem such as CME or an enteropathy due to another cause.

In breast-fed infants, lactose intolerance may be misdiagnosed frequently due to the (normal) appearance of lactose or reducing substances in infant's stools[134], or because of loose stools, gas or colicy symptoms arising as a result of incorrect breast-feeding practices[135]. The presence of lactose or reducing substances in stools from a breast-fed infant is not an indication to stop breast-feeding or to investigate for other pathology, but rather to ensure that proper breast-feeding technique is followed.

COWS' MILK ALLERGY (ENTEROPATHY)

Cows' milk allergy or enteropathy (CME) occurs as a result of an allergic reaction to one or more of the proteins in cows' milk (usually casein, lactalbumin or lactoglobulin). It may cause vomiting, mimicking gastroesophageal reflux[136]. Other prominent symptoms include diarrhea, which may be watery due to secondary lactose intolerance; abdominal pain or colic, malnutrition and failure to thrive. There may be an associated protein-losing enteropathy and intestinal loss of blood. In severely affected infants, bloody diarrhea may occur, indicating a severe colitis, and symptoms of anaphylaxis can result from administration of even small amounts of cows' milk. CME in infants may also be associated with atopic symptoms of eczema or asthma. Diagnosis may be based on small-bowel biopsy changes, and clinical or histological response to strict milk exclusion. Patients may also have positive allergen-specific RAST tests to milk, elevated IgE, eosinophilia, or positive skin tests. Anemia, decreased IgA levels and hypoalbuminemia are frequent. A similar problem due to soy allergy may occur with soy-based formulas. Allergy to human breast milk does not occur.

It has been suggested that there is an increased incidence of CME in CF, and that it might be the underlying cause of some of the previously reported cases of lactose intolerance in CF[133].

Therapy of CME requires strict exclusion of all products based on cows' milk from the diet. Infants with CME may be able to tolerate cows' milk after 12–24 months of age, but because of the risk of anaphylaxis, the initial reintroduction of milk should be carried out under close medical supervision.

Inflammatory bowel disease (Crohn's disease, ulcerative colitis)

Inflammatory bowel disease, particularly Crohn's disease has been reported with increasing frequency in patients with cystic fibrosis. It is not clear whether this is due to increasing recognition or increasing incidence, perhaps related to longer survival of CF patients[57,137]. Estimates of the prevalence of Crohn's disease in CF are very variable and range up to 1 per cent[137].

The signs and symptoms of Crohn's disease in CF appear similar to those in non-CF patients. Classical symptoms include recurrent abdominal pain, diarrhea and weight loss or growth failure, often accompanied by significant malaise, lethargy and anorexia with or without nausea and vomiting. Diarrhea may be urgent, bloody, nocturnal and may be accompanied by tenesmus. Other manifestations indicating the systemic nature of the illness include pyrexia, arthritis or arthralgia, uveitis or conjunctivitis, and skin manifestations such as erythema nodosum or pyoderma gangrenosum. Anemia and hypoalbuminemia with edema may develop due to enteric losses and malnutrition. Physical examination may reveal aphthous ulceration, cheilosis; abdominal mass (often right iliac), tenderness or guarding; perianal abscess, skin tags or fistulas. Some of these signs and symptoms are indistinguishable from those due to CF or its complications, such as DIOS, which must be included in the differential diagnosis[74]. The presence of physical stigmata suggestive of Crohn's disease, such as perianal fistula, abscess or anal tags, makes further investigation of the CF patient mandatory. Differential diagnosis is similar in CF and non-CF patients; except that in CF, fibrosing colonopathy due to high pancreatic enzyme dosage must also be considered[138].

Results of standard investigations include low hemoglobin and elevated erythrocyte sedimentation rate. Serum albumin may be low due to the associated protein-losing enteropathy. Enteric protein loss can be documented by ^{51}Cr tagged albumin or fecal α_1-antitrypsin clearance studies. X-ray contrast studies, endoscopy and biopsy must be carried out for diagnosis and to delineate the extent of the disease. The presence of noncaseating granulomata in biopsies is considered confirmatory evidence for Crohn's disease, but is not always demonstrable.

Standard medical therapy of Crohn's disease is appropriate even when this condition coexists with CF. In patients with active disease, elemental diet therapy by continuous nasogastric infusion should be considered early, both for reversal of malnutrition as well as induction of remission. The indications for surgery in CF patients with Crohn's disease are similar to those in non-CF patients (e.g. growth failure, severe pain, intestinal obstruction, not responding to medical therapy).

Celiac disease

Celiac disease (CD, gluten-induced enteropathy) is a serious, life-long gastrointestinal disorder that can cause a wide spectrum of clinical symptoms, not all confined to the gastrointestinal tract, and many indistinguishable from the symptoms of CF. This is hardly surprising, since CD and CF were two of the major constituents of the now archaic 'celiac syndrome'. Of interest, the classical description of CD in 1888 by Samuel Gee could equally be describing a patient with CF. Whereas CF was separated from the celiac syndrome in 1938 through the work of Dorothy Andersen, CD remained part of the syndrome until the 1950s, when the causal role of dietary gluten and therapeutic effect of gluten-free diet was discovered, and the ability to diagnose CD in life from typical lesions demonstrable in small-bowel biopsies was recognized.

The coexistence of CD and CF was first reported by Hide and Burman[139] and there have been several reports since. Valletta and Mastella[140] assessed 1100 CF patients and, on the basis of clinical and biochemical evidence of malnutrition and malabsorption, persisting despite adequate pancreatic enzyme therapy, found five CF patients with CD proven by small bowel biopsy. This prevalence of CD in CF patients (i.e. 1 : 220) is significantly higher than that generally accepted for the non-CF population in western Europe (i.e. approximately 1 : 1100), but close to that previously reported for the general population of the west of Ireland (1 : 300) and to that reported in an increasing number of European studies using antibody screening followed by biopsy to prove the diagnosis[141].

SCREENING AND DIAGNOSIS OF CELIAC DISEASE

Because the clinical symptoms of CD are so similar to those of CF, it is difficult to determine by clinical assessment alone whether a given CF patient may have CD. However, the possibility of CD should be considered in any CF patient with unexplained gastrointestinal, growth or nutritional problems or with a first-degree relative with biopsy-proven CD. Nonspecific tests used in the evaluation of failure to thrive and malabsorption (e.g. serum carotene, folate, xylose tolerance or fecal fat assay) are unreliable, insensitive and unhelpful in evaluating CF patients for the presence of CD. Serum antibody tests, particularly the IgA antigliadin antibody test

(IgA-AGA, or IgG-AGA for IgA-deficient individuals), the antiendomysial or antireticulin antibody tests, and tTG (tissue trans-glutaminase) are now well established as screening tests for CD[141]. These tests can be used readily to screen CF patients for CD, with small bowel biopsy used to confirm the diagnosis in screening-positive patients.

Specific criteria for the diagnosis of CD have been developed, revised and simplified by the European Society for Pediatric Gastroenterology and Nutrition[142]. Diagnosis requires small-bowel biopsy (Fig. 12.8), which should be done for any patient where clinical suspicion of CD is high or antibody screening yields positive results. Gluten-containing foods should never be removed from the diet before biopsy has confirmed the diagnosis, since this will invalidate the tests and give false-negative results.

Therapy of CF patients with CD requires a lifelong, strict gluten-free diet (GFD) which, as originally developed, avoids wheat, rye, barley and oats, and their derivatives. Recent studies have suggested that oats may be allowed, at least for older patients, but further, longer-term studies are needed to confirm this. It is important that the high nutrient needs of the CF patient are recognized in planning gluten-free diet for the patient with both CF and CD, and that the importance of lifelong adherence to GFD be emphasized.

Enteric infection/infestation

It has long been speculated that the frequency of the CF gene in Caucasians reflects a heterozygote advantage due to resistance to certain enteric infections or enterotoxins. There is some support for this hypothesis, such as the recent demonstration that CFTR mutant mice are relatively resistant to infection with *Salmonella typhi*[143]. Nevertheless, CF patients can develop a variety of enteric infections and infestations, diagnosis of which may be

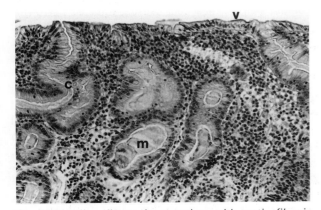

Fig. 12.8 *Celiac disease in a patient with cystic fibrosis. Duodenal mucosa from area of ligament of Treitz showing villus atrophy (v); crypt hyperplasia (c) and inflammatory infiltrate typical of CD, plus mucus inspissation (m) typical of CF. (Photomicrograph ×100, courtesy of Dr J. Dimmick.)*

delayed because of failure to recognize that gastrointestinal symptoms, malabsorption or weight loss in CF patients may be due to infectious bacterial or parasitic causes, and that these diseases may lead to significant morbidity or mortality if not diagnosed quickly and treated appropriately.

CLOSTRIDIUM DIFFICILE COLITIS

Clostridium difficile-associated colitis in non-CF patients typically presents with diarrhea, crampy abdominal pain and tenderness precipitated by antibiotic use. Toxin can be demonstrated in stool, and anaerobic culture shows presence of the organism. There is usually an associated fever and leukocytosis. The disease is often fulminant with development of toxic megacolon and a high mortality.

Because of the frequent use of antibiotics in CF, it could be expected that diarrhea or colitis due to *C. difficile* would be common. However, there have been very few published cases of severe disease in CF[144,145]. Although studies have shown a high rate of recovery of the organism and its toxin from stools of CF patients, most patients were without symptoms[145]. It has been speculated that relative unresponsiveness to *C. difficile* toxin (as well as to cholera or *E. coli* enterotoxins) may occur in CF as a result of CFTR-mediated chloride channel unresponsiveness and decreased receptor activity.

Nevertheless, severe *C. difficile*-associated disease may not be as rare in CF as previously supposed. Fulminant *C. difficile*-associated colitis was described in four CF children from three geographically distinct CF treatment centers, of whom two died[144]. We are also aware of three further (unpublished) fulminant cases with one death, from two other centers. Another report has described atypical presentation with abdominal distension and decreased stooling in five cases of *C. difficile* enteritis who had extensive pancolitis demonstrated by CT[145a]. Two of these five patients died from the disease. Whether relative susceptibility to *C. difficile* disease is genetically determined in CF needs to be further examined, since of the series of four reported fulminant cases, three had an unusual (N1303K/?) genotype, and two of the three unpublished fulminant cases were ΔF_{508}/? genotype.

Therapy requires supportive measures, oral and/or iv antibiotics (metronidazole, vancomycin), and in some cases, colectomy.

GIARDIASIS

Patients with CF appear to be at increased risk from infestation with the protozoan parasite *Giardia lamblia* which typically causes nausea, vomiting, diarrhea, malabsorption and weight loss accompanied by abdominal distension[57,146]. In one study, ELISA antibody tests showed 28 per cent of CF samples were positive for *Giardia*, compared to 6 per cent of controls[146]. Giardiasis should be suspected and stool specimens examined in any CF patient with abdominal discomfort, nausea, vomiting, weight loss or with diarrhea persisting despite adequate enzyme dosage. Therapy with metronidazole is usually effective, though it may be necessary to repeat treatment and treat close contacts (family members, playschool mates) to prevent re-infection.

STAGNANT LOOP (SMALL-BOWEL BACTERIAL OVERGROWTH) SYNDROME

Small-bowel bacterial overgrowth syndrome is an uncommon but significant cause of diarrhea, abdominal pain and malabsorption, usually related to disorders of intestinal anatomy, immunity or motility. Increased urinary excretion of p-hydroxyphenylacetic acid, due to bacterial metabolism of unabsorbed amino acids in the gut, is a marker of the contaminated small-bowel syndrome in non-CF patients[147]. It has been recognized for some time that CF patients also excrete this compound[148]. However, reports of clinically significant small bowel bacterial overgrowth syndrome in CF are few, although a case of stagnant loop syndrome centered upon the previous site of an ileostomy after meconium ileus surgery has been reported[57].

Rectal prolapse

Rectal prolapse is usually a complication affecting untreated or inadequately treated CF PI patients. It occurs in as many as 20 per cent of untreated CF patients under 5 years of age[149]. Contributing factors include frequent stools, sticky tenacious intestinal residue, diminished muscle tone and loss of perianal tissue due to malnutrition; and increased intra-abdominal pressure from pulmonary hyperinflation and coughing. Not all patients with rectal prolapse have CF, however, with one series finding CF in only 11 per cent. Nevertheless, sweat test should be performed in any patient presenting with this complaint. Immediate therapy involves manual replacement of prolapsed mucosa. In most cases, the problem resolves after initiation of adequate pancreatic enzyme therapy, high-fiber diet and improved nutrition. Intractable cases may respond to elemental diet or oral N-acetylcysteine. Surgery or injection therapy[149a] is now rarely, if ever, required.

Fibrosing colonopathy

Fibrosing colonopathy (FC) is a newly described complication of CF, first reported in 1994[30,31]. It was first recognized as causing intestinal obstruction or abdominal pain due to a thickened and narrowed segment of colon. Epidemiological studies have found a strong association between FC and use of very high doses of pancreatic enzymes[37,150]. FC appears to be a disease affecting children, with most cases being under the age of 14 years[150]. The highest risk appears to be in the younger patient receiving an enzyme dose exceeding 6000 U lipase/kg/meal for more than 6 months[33].

The etiology and pathogenesis of FC has still not been definitely established. The first cases involved patients using 'high strength' enzyme preparations[30,31,138], but it has subsequently been reported in patients receiving large doses of 'standard' strength preparations[37,151]. Current evidence, therefore, strongly favors high dosage of pancreatic enzymes rather than 'high strength' preparations per se as leading to the problem. It has not been established, however, whether the pathological changes are due to the action of specific toxic component(s) of the enzyme preparations, or as a result of the interaction of high enzyme doses, particle size and/or dissolution characteristics of the enzyme preparations and CF abnormalities of intestinal pH or motility, leading to release of potentially damaging amounts of active ingredients at inappropriate and sensitive sites[32,138]. Concern has also been expressed that indomethacin may increase intestinal permeability and act synergistically with pancreatic enzymes to cause intestinal damage[138a].

Clinical presentation is nonspecific. Onset may be slow and insidious over many months, coming to attention only when bowel obstruction develops, or symptoms may develop abruptly in a matter of days. Symptoms can mimic DIOS, with abdominal pain, distension, vomiting, constipation; or can mimic an inflammatory colitis with bloody, mucusy diarrhea, abdominal pain, anorexia, distension and ascites[138]. In the younger child, diarrhea can be watery[32].

Patients presenting with suggestive symptoms should have a plain X-ray of the abdomen and abdominal ultrasound. If either investigation shows thickened colonic wall (e.g. >2 mm), decreased peristalsis or free fluid, a contrast study should be done[138]. Contrast studies may show focal or long segment involvement, usually of the right colon, but may extend to the distal colon[152]. The colonic wall is thickened, causing lumenal narrowing ranging from mild stenosis to complete occlusion and obstruction, and there may be loss of haustral markings, decreased peristalsis, loss of distensibility and colonic shortening. Lumenal narrowing occurs without significant reduction in external colonic diameter. Mucosal abnormality may be evident and there may be signs of more extensive inflammation with marked mucosal irregularity, nodular thickening and spiculation[32,33,53,138,152]. Endoscopy in acute cases may show erythema, nodular irregular mucosa, edema and friable mucosa or superficial ulceration[153].

Diagnosis is histopathological, but since biopsies should be full thickness to show fibrosis of the lamina propria, endoscopic biopsies are often unsatisfactory and therefore this confirmation of diagnosis is frequently not obtained[32,33,138,152]. In established cases, the epithelium may be intact with little inflammatory change, except for mild chronic inflammatory infiltrate in the submucosa centered about blood vessels, or evidence of mucosal injury and repair. Submucosal thickening by fibrous connective tissue causes stenoses, which may be long-segment, and there may be fatty infiltration. Fibrosis of the lamina propria, inflammation with eosinophils, focal neutrophilic cryptitis and apoptosis have been reported as possibly representing prestenotic lesions[33].

The first line of therapy is prevention, by ensuring pancreatic enzyme dosage is within current recommendations[32–35]. For established disease, conservative treatment with reduction of enzyme dosage to recommended levels, close clinical monitoring and regular ultrasound assessment of bowel appears to give best results[138]. Patients with more rapid onset and active inflammatory response but less submucosal fibrosis may represent a prestricture state, and here also conservative therapy should be tried[153]. If bowel obstruction develops, surgery with removal of the constricted area is necessary, and has also been required for patients with intractable diarrhea, fecal incontinence, severe anorexia or weight loss. Attempts to preserve bowel by use of defunctioning ostomy have not given good results and may make later surgery more difficult[138].

Pneumatosis intestinalis

Pneumatosis intestinalis describes intestinal submucosal or subserosal blebs or cysts or linear intramural gas[53]. In non-CF individuals it may be associated with serious disease, but in CF it has been reported as a clinically silent, incidental X-ray finding[53]. It may be more common in CF than generally believed. An extensive post-mortem series found mural air in the colon in 21 of 441 patients. Although usually clinically silent, it correlates with the development of obstructive pulmonary disease and probably results from infradiaphragmatic dissection of air along perivascular tissue planes[154].

Malignant disease in cystic fibrosis

A retrospective cohort study of over 38 000 CF patients in North America and Europe has established that the overall risk of malignancy in CF is similar to that in the non-CF population. However, there is an increased risk for cancers of the digestive tract in CF[155]. These malignancies included cancers of the esophagus, stomach, small and large intestine, liver, biliary tract, pancreas and rectum. The odds ratio for these malignancies of the digestive tract was greater than 6 in both the European and North American samples, and was also increased for myeloma and for endocrine tumors. The odds ratio was most increased for the 20–29 year age group. There was no significant increase over expected in the broad group of lymphatic and hematopoietic neoplasms. Extra-abdominal malignancy has also been reported, including leukaemias, neuroblastoma, seminoma, astrocytoma, retinoblastoma and Wilm's tumors, but no increased odds ratio for these was found in the larger series.

Various possibilities have been suggested as explanations for the observed increase in malignancy of the digestive tract in CF. These possibilities include a relationship to CFTR expression. However, for the patients in whom genetic data was available, the frequency of the ΔF_{508} mutation was similar to that in the cancer-free CF patients[155]. Other possible but unproven causes of increased cancer risk in CF include antioxidant deficiency (selenium or vitamin E), increased intestinal permeability or a relationship between the CF gene and an oncogene. It is not known whether the coexistence in CF of conditions with premalignant potential such as Barrett's esophagus, CD, inflammatory bowel disease, *H. pylori* infection, or even delayed intestinal transit time may also contribute. As the longevity of CF patients increases, malignant disease may assume greater significance, and continual surveillance is indicated.

REFERENCES

1. Andersen, D.H. (1938) Cystic fibrosis of the pancreas and its relation to celiac disease. *Am. J. Dis. Child.*, **56**, 344–399.
2. Gaskin, K., Gurwitz, D., Durie, P., Corey, M., Levison, H. and Forstner, G. (1982) Improved respiratory prognosis in patients with cystic fibrosis with normal fat absorption. *J. Pediatr.*, **100**, 857–862.
3. Imrie, J., Fagan, D. and Sturgess, J. (1975) Quantitative evaluation of the development of the exocrine pancreas in cystic fibrosis and controlled subjects. *Am. J. Pathol.*, **95**, 697–708.
4. Irish, M.S., Ragi, J.M., Karamanoukian, H., Borowitz, D.S., Schmidt, D. and Glick, P.L. (1997) Prenatal diagnosis of the fetus with cystic fibrosis and meconium ileus. *Pediatr. Surg. Int.*, **12**, (5–6), 434–436.
5. Gaillard, D., Bouvier, R., Scheiner, C. *et al.* (1996) Meconium ileus and intestinal atresia in fetuses and neonates. *Pediatr. Pathol. Lab. Med.*, **16**, (1), 25–40.
6. Oppenheimer, E.H. and Esterley, J.R. (1975) Pathology of cystic fibrosis: review of literature and comparison of 146 autopsy cases. *Perspect. Pediatr. Pathol.*, **2**, 241–278.
7. Park, R.W. and Grand, R.J. (1981) Gastrointestinal manifestations in cystic fibrosis: a review. *Gastroenterology*, **81**, 1143–1161.
8. Kristidis, P., Bozon, D., Corey, M. *et al.* (1992) Genetic determination of exocrine pancreatic function in cystic fibrosis. *Am. J. Hum. Genet.*, **50**, 1178–1184.
9. Tsui, L. and Durie, P. (1997) Genotype and phenotype in cystic fibrosis. *Hosp. Pract.*, June, 115–142.

10. Guy-Crotte, O., Carrere, J. and Figarella, C. (1996) Exocrine pancreatic function in cystic fibrosis. *Europ. J. Gastroenterol. Hepatol.*, **8**, 755–759.

11. Kerem, E., Corey, M., Kerem, B.-S. *et al*. (1990) The relationship between genotype and phenotype in cystic fibrosis. Analysis of the most common mutation (ΔF_{508}). *NEJM*, **323**, 1517–1522.

12. McIntosh, I. and Cutting, G.R. (1992) Cystic fibrosis transmembrane conductance regulator and the etiology and pathogenesis of cystic fibrosis. *FASEB J.*, **6**, 2775–2782.

13. Rick, W. (1963) Untersuchung zur exokrinen funktion des pankreas bei zystischer pankreasfibrose. *Med. Welt.*, **42**, 2158.

14. Hadorn, B., Johansen, P.G. and Anderson, C.M. (1968) Pancreozymin secretin test of exocrine pancreatic function in cystic fibrosis and the significance of the result for the pathogenesis of the disease. *Can. Med. Assoc. J.*, **98**, 377–385.

15. Wong, L.T.K., Turtle, S. and Davidson, A.G.F. (1982) Secretin pancreozymin stimulation test and confirmation of the diagnosis of cystic fibrosis. *Gut*, **23**, 744–750.

16. Gaskin, K.J., Durie, P., Corey, M., Wei, P. and Forstner, G.G. (1982) Evidence of a primary defect of bicarbonate secretion in cystic fibrosis. *Pediatr. Res.*, **16**, 554–557.

17. Davidson, A.G.F., Wong, L.T.K., Kirby, L.T. and Applegarth, D.A. (1984) Immunoreactive trypsin in cystic fibrosis. *J. Pediatr. Gastroenterol. Nutr.*, **3**, (Suppl. 1), 79–87.

18. Crossley, J.A., Elliott, R.P. and Smith, P.A. (1979) Dried blood spot screening for cystic fibrosis in the newborn. *Lancet*, **i**, 472–474.

19. Sarles, J., Barthellemy. S., Ferec. C. *et al*. (1999) Blood concentrations of pancreatitis associated protein in neonates: relevance to neonatal screening for cystic fibrosis. *Arch. Dis. Child. Fetal & Neonatal Edition*, **80**, F118–122.

20. Durie, P. (1997) Inherited causes of exocrine pancreatic dysfunction. *Pediatr Gastroenterol*, **11**, (2), 145–153.

21. Davidson, A.G.F, Wong, L.T.K, Applegarth, D.A. *et al*. (1981) Plasma immunoreactive trypsin levels after secretin pancreozymin stimulation, in *1000 years of Cystic Fibrosis*, (ed. W. J. Warwick), University of Minnesota Press, pp. 292–293.

22. Manson, W. and Weaver, L. (1997) Fat digestion in the neonate. *Arch. Dis. Child.*, **76**, F206–F211.

23. Abrams, C.K., Hamosh, M., Hubbard, V.S., Dutta, S.K. and Hamosh, P. (1984) Lingual lipase in cystic fibrosis. Quantitation of enzyme activity in the upper small intestine of patients with exocrine pancreatic insufficiency. *J. Clin. Invest.*, **73**, 374–382.

24. Sokol, R.J., Reardon, M.C., Accurso, F.J., Stall, C., Narkewicz, M., Abman, S.H. and Hammond, K.B. (1989) Fat-soluble-vitamin status during the first year of life in infants with cystic fibrosis identified by screening of newborns. *Am. J. Clin. Nutr.*, **50**, 1064–1071.

25. Smith, J.S., Ediss, J., Mullinger, M.A. and Bogoch, A. (1971) Fecal chymotrypsin and trypsin determinations. *Can. Med. Assoc. J.*, **104**, 691–695.

26. Gullo, L., Graziano, L., Babbini, S., Battistini, A., Lazzari, R. and Pezzilli, R. (1997) Faecal elastase 1 in children with cystic fibrosis. *Europ. J. Pediatr.*, **156**, (10), 770–772.

26a. Walkowiak, J., Cichy, W.K. and Herzig, K.H. (1999) Comparison of fecal elastase-1 determination with the secretin-cholecystokinin test in patients with cystic fibrosis. *Scand. J. Gastro.*, **34**, 202–207.

27. Kraisinger, M., Hochhaus, G., Stecenko, A., Bowser, E. and Hendeles, L. (1994) Clinical pharmacology of pancreatic enzymes in patients with cystic fibrosis and *in vitro* performance of microencapsulated formulations. *J. Clin. Pharmacol.*, **34**, 158–166.

28. Meyer J.H., Elashoff J., Porter-Fink, Dressman J. and Amidon G.L. (1988) Human postprandial gastric emptying of 1–3 millimeter spheres. *Gastroenterology*, **94**, 1315–1325.

28a. Meyer, J.H. and Lake, R. (1997) Mismatch of duodenal deliveries of dietary fat and pancreatin from enterically coated microspheres. *Pancreas*, **15**, 226–235.

28b. Taylor, C.J., Hillel, P.G., Ghosal, S. *et al*. (1999) Gastric emptying and intestinal transit of pancreatic enzyme supplements in cystic fibrosis. *Arch. Dis. Child.*, **80**, 149–152.

28c. Kalivianakis, M., Minich, D.M., Bijleveld, C.M. *et al*. (1999) Fat malabsorption in cystic fibrosis patients receiving enzyme replacement therapy is due to impaired intestinal uptake of long-chain fatty acids. *Am. J. Clin. Nutrition*, **69**, 127–134.

29. Walters, M.P., Kelleher, J., Gilbert, J. and Littlewood, J.M. (1990) Clinical monitoring of steatorrhea in cystic fibrosis. *Arch. Dis. Child.*, **65**, 99–102.

30. Smyth, R.L., van Velzen, D. and Smyth, A.R. (1994) Strictures of ascending colon in CF and high strength pancreatic enzymes. *Lancet*, **343**, 85–86.

31. Sharp, D. (1994) High lipase pancreatin. *Lancet*, **343**, 108.

32. Dodge, J. (1995) Fibrosing colonopathy: recent advances. *J. Roy. Soc. Med.*, **27**, (89), 19–23.

33. Borowitz, D., Grand, R., Durie, P. and the Consensus Committee (1995) Use of pancreatic enzyme supplements for patients with cystic fibrosis in the context of fibrosing colonopathy. *J. Pediatr.*, **127**, 681–684.

34. Littlewood, J.M. (1996) Implications of the committee on safety of medicines 10 000 IU lipase/kg/day recommendation for use of pancreatic enzymes in cystic fibrosis. *Arch. Dis. Child.*, **74**, 466–468.

35. Anthony, H., Collins, C.E., Davidson, G. *et al*. (1999) Pancreatic enzyme replacement therapy in cystic fibrosis: Australian guidelines. *J. Ped. Child. Health*, **35**, 125–129.

36. Brady, M.S., Rickard, K., Yu, P.L. and Eigen, H. (1992)

Effectiveness of enteric coated pancreatic enzymes given before meals in reducing steatorrhea in children with cystic fibrosis. *J. Am. Diet. Assoc.*, **92**, 813–817.

37. Freiman, J. and FitzSimmons, C. (1996) Colonic strictures in patients with cystic fibrosis: results of a survey of 114 cystic fibrosis care centers in the United States. *J. Pediatr. Gastroenterol. Nutr.*, **22**, 153–156.

38. Robinson, P.J., Smith, A.L., and Sly, P.D. (1990) Duodenal pH in cystic fibrosis and its relationship to fat malabsorption. *Dig. Dis. Sci.,* **35**, 1299–1304.

38a. Chamarthy, L.M., Reinstein, L.J., Schnapf, B., Good, R.A. and Bahna, S.L. (1998) Desensitization to pancreatic enzyme intolerance in a child with cystic fibrosis. *Pediatrics*, **102**, e13.

39. Graham, D. (1982) Pancreatic enzyme replacement. The effect of antacids or cimetidine. *Dig. Dis. Sci.*, **27**, 485–490.

40. Braggion, C., Borgo, G., Faggionato, P. and Mastella, G. (1987) Influence of antacid and formulation on effectiveness of pancreatic enzyme supplementation in cystic fibrosis. *Arch. Dis. Child.*, **62**, 349–356,

41. Durie, P.R., Bell, L., Linton, W., Corey, M.L. and Forstner, G.G. (1980) Effect of cimetidine and sodium bicarbonate on pancreatic replacement therapy in cystic fibrosis. *Gut*, **21**, 778–786 .

42. Heijerman, H.G.M., Lamers, C.B., Bakker, W. and Dijkman, J.H. (1993) Improvement of fecal fat excretion after addition of omeprazole to pancrease in cystic fibrosis is related to residual exocrine function of the pancreas. *Dig. Dis. Sci.*, **38**, 1–6.

43. Robinson, P. and Sly, P.D. (1990) Placebo-controlled trial of Misoprostol in cystic fibrosis. *J. Pediatr. Gastroenterol. Nutr.*, **11**, 37–40.

44. De Curtis, M., Santamaria, F., Ercolini, P. and Vittoria, L. (1992) Effect of taurine supplementation on fat and energy absorption in cystic fibrosis. *Arch. Dis. Child.*, **67**, 1082–1085.

45. Merli, M., Bertasi, S., Servi, R. *et al.* (1994) Effect of a medium dose of ursodeoxycholic acid with or without taurine supplementation on the nutritional status of patients with cystic fibrosis: a randomized, placebo-controlled crossover trial. *J. Pediatr. Gastroenterol. Nutr.*, **19**, 198–203.

46. Gracey, M., Burke, V. and Anderson, C.M. (1969) Assessment of medium-chain triglyceride feeding in infants with cystic fibrosis. *Arch. Dis. Child.*, **44**, 401–403.

47. Murshed, R., Spitz, L., Kiely, E. and Drake D. (1997) Meconium ileus: a ten-year review of thirty-six patients. *Europ. J. Pediatr. Surg.*, **7**, 275–277.

47a. Mushtaq, I., Wright, V.M., Drake, D.P., Mearns, M.B. and Wood, C.B. (1998) Meconium ileus secondary to cystic fibrosis. The East London experience. *Pediatr. Surg. Internat.*, **13**, 365–369.

48. Gaillard, D. (1997) Diagnosis of meconium ileus. *Ann. Patholog*, **17**, (4), 306–308.

49. Eggermont, E. (1985) The role of the small intestine in

cystic fibrosis patients. *Acta Paediatr. Scand. Suppl.*, **317**, 16–21.

50. Bodian, M. (1952) *Fibrocystic disease of the pancreas. A congenital disorder of mucus production – mucosis.* William Heineman Medical Books, London.

51. Tsui, L.C. (1992) The spectrum of mutations in cystic fibrosis. *Reviews*, **8**, 392–398.

52. Lang, I. Daneman, A., Cutz, E., Hagen, P. and Shandling, B. (1997) Abdominal calcification in cystic fibrosis with meconium ileus: radiologic-pathologic correlation. *Pediatr. Radiol.*, **27**, 523–527.

53. Agrons, G.A., Corse, W.R., Markowitz, R.I., Suarez, E.S. and Perry, D.R. (1996) Gastrointestinal manifestations of cystic fibrosis: radiologic–pathologic correlation. *Radiographics*, **16**, 871–893.

54. Noblett, H. (1969) Treatment of uncomplicated meconium ileus by gastrografin enema: a preliminary report. *J. Pediatr. Surg.*, **4**, 190–197.

55. Waggett, H., Bishop, H.C. and Koop, C.E. (1970) Experience with gastrografin enema in the treatment of meconium ileus. *J. Pediatr. Surg.*, **5**, 649–654.

56. Coutts, J.A., Docherty, J.G., Carachi, R. and Evans, T.J. (1997) Clinical course of patients with cystic fibrosis presenting with meconium ileus. *Br. J. Surg.*, **84**, 555.

57. Baxter, P.S., Dickson, J.A.S., Variend, S. and Taylor, C.J. (1988) Intestinal disease in cystic fibrosis. *Arch. Dis. Child.*, **63**, 1496–1497.

58. Ellis, D.G. and Clatworthy, H.W. (1966) The meconium plug syndrome revisited. *J. Pediatr. Surg.*, **1**, 54–61.

59. Shwachman, H., Lebenthal, E. and Khaw, P.-T. (1975) Recurrent acute pancreatitis in patients with cystic fibrosis with normal pancreatic enzymes. *Pediatrics*, **55**, 86–94.

60. Atlas, A.B., Orenstein, S.R. and Orenstein, D.M. (1992) Pancreatitis in young children with cystic fibrosis. *J. Pediatr.*, **120**, 756–759.

60a. Choudari, C.P., Lehman, G.A. and Sherman, S. (1999) Pancreatitis and cystic fibrosis gene mutations. *Gastro. Clin. North Am.,* **28**, 543–549.

61. Keogan, M.T. and Baker, M.E. (1995) Computed tomography and magnetic resonance imaging in the assessment of pancreatic disease. *Gastrointest. Endosc. Clin. North Am.*, **5**, (1), 31–59.

62. Hernanz-Schulman M., Teele, R.L., Perez-Atayde, A. *et al*. (1986) Pancreatic cystosis in cystic fibrosis. *Radiology*, **158**, 629–631.

80. Toth, I.R. and Lang, J.N. (1986) Giant pancreatic retention cyst in cystic fibrosis: a case report. *Pediatr. Pathol.*, **6**, 103–110.

64. Liu, P., Daneman, A. and Stringer, D. (1986) Pancreatic cysts and calcification in cystic fibrosis. *J. Can. Assoc. Radiol.*, **37**, 279–282.

65. Weiss, A.A., Greig, J.M. and Fache, S. (1991) Lithotripsy of pancreatic stones in a patient with cystic fibrosis: successful treatment of abdominal pain. *Can. J. Gastroenterol.*, **6**, 25–28.

66. Farber, S. (1944) Pancreatic function and disease in

early life. V. Pathologic changes associated with pancreatic insufficiency in early life. *Arch. Pathol.*, **37**, 238–250.

67. Freye, H.B., Kurtz, S.M. and Spock, A. *et al.* (1964) Light and electron microscopic examination of the small bowel of children with cystic fibrosis. *J. Pediatr.*, **64**, 575–579.

67a. Sbarbati, A., Bertini, M., Catassi, C., Gagliardini, R. and Osculati, F. (1998) Ultrastructural lesions in the small bowel of patients with cystic fibrosis. *Ped. Res., **43**, 234–239.

68. Gosden, C.M. and Gosden, J.R. (1984) Fetal abnormalities in cystic fibrosis suggest a deficiency in proteolysis of cholecystokinin. *Lancet*, **ii**, 541–546.

69. Eggermont, E. (1996) Gastrointestinal manifestations in cystic fibrosis. *Europ. J. Gastroenterol. Hepatol.*, **8**, 731–738.

70. Gregory, P.C. (1996) Gastrointestinal pH, motility/transit and permeability in cystic fibrosis. *J. Pediatr. Gastroenterol. Nutrit.*, **23**, 513–523.

71. Strong, T., Boehm, K. and Collins, F. (1994) Localization of cystic fibrosis transmembrane conductance regulator mRNA in the human gastrointestinal tract by in situ hybridization. *J. Clin. Invest.*, **93**, 347–354.

72. Escobar, H., Perdomo, M., Vasconez, F., Camarero C., del Olmo, M.T. and Suarez, L. (1992) Intestinal permeability to ^{51}Cr-EDTA and orocecal transit time in cystic fibrosis. *J. Pediatr. Gastroenterol. Nutr.*, **14**, 204–207.

73. Dalzell, A.M., Freestone, N.S., Billington, D. and Heaf, D.P. (1990) Small intestinal permeability and orocaecal transit time in cystic fibrosis. *Arch. Dis. Child.*, **65**, 585–588.

74. Dalzell, A.M., Heaf, D.P. and Carty, H. (1990) Pathology mimicking distal intestinal obstruction syndrome in cystic fibrosis. *Arch. Dis. Child.*, **65**, 540–541.

75. Wesley, A., Forstner, J.I., Qureshi, R., Mantle, M. and Forstner, G. (1983) Human intestinal mucin in cystic fibrosis. *Pediatr. Res.*, **17**, 65–69.

76. Mantle, M. and Stewart, G. (1989) Intestinal mucins from normal subjects and patients with cystic fibrosis. *Biochem. J.*, **259**, 243–253.

77. Baxter, P., Goldhill, J., Hardcastle, J., Hardcastle, P.T. and Taylor, C.J. (1990) Enhanced intestinal glucose and alanine transport in cystic fibrosis. *Gut*, **31**, 817–820.

78. Berschneider, H.M., Knowles, M.R., Azizkhan, R.G. *et al.* (1988) Altered intestinal chloride transport in cystic fibrosis. *FASEB J.*, **2**, 2625–2629.

79. Taylor, C.J., Baxter, P.S., Hardcastle, J. and Hardcastle, P.T. (1987) Absence of secretory response in jejunal biopsy samples from children with cystic fibrosis. *Lancet*, **ii**, 107–108.

80. Antonowicz, I., Lebenthal, E. and Shwachman, H. (1978) Disaccharidase activities in small intestinal mucosa in patients with cystic fibrosis. *J. Pediatr.*, **92**, 214–219.

81. Gibbons, I.S.E. (1969) Disaccharides and cystic fibrosis of the pancreas. *Arch. Dis. Child.*, **44**, 63–68.

82. Mack, D.R., Flick, J.A., Durie, P.R., Rosenstein, B.J., Ellis, L.E. and Perman, J.A. (1992) Correlation of intestinal lactulose permeability with exocrine pancreatic dysfunction. *J. Pediatr.*, **120**, 696–671.

83. Strandvik, B. (1989) Relation between essential fatty acid metabolism and gastrointestinal symptoms in cystic fibrosis. *Acta Pediatr. Scand. Suppl.*, **363**, 58–65.

84. Lloyd-Still, J.D., Bibus, D.M. Powers, C.A., Johnson, S.B. and Holman, R.T. (1996) Essential fatty acid deficiency and predisposition to lung disease in cystic fibrosis. *Acta Paediatr.*, **85**, 1426–1432.

85. Ahmed, F., Ellis, J., Murphy, J., Wootton, S. and Jackson, A.A. (1990) Excessive faecal losses of vitamin A (retinol) in cystic fibrosis. *Arch. Dis. Child.*, **65**, 598–593.

86. Weber, A.M. and Roy C.C. (1985) Bile acid metabolism in children with cystic fibrosis. *Acta Paediatr. Scand. Suppl.*, **317**, 9–15.

87. Fondacaro, J.D., Heubi, J.E. and Kellog, F.W. (1982) Intestinal bile acid malabsorption in cystic fibrosis: a primary mucosal cell defect. *Pediatr. Res.*, **16**, 494–498.

88. Thompson, G.N. and Davidson, G.P. (1988) In vivo bile acid uptake from terminal ileum in cystic fibrosis. *Pediatr. Res.*, **23**, 323–328.

89. Bali, A., Stabelforth, D.E. and Asquith, P. (1983) Prolonged small intestinal transit time in cystic fibrosis. *BMJ*, **287**, 1011–1013.

90. Schoni, M.H., Turler, K., Kaser, H. and Kraemer, R. (1985) Plasma and urinary catecholamines in patients with cystic fibrosis. *Ped. Res.*, **19**, 1947–1952.

91. Spiller, R.C., Trotman, I.F., Adrian, T.E., Bloom, S.R., Misiewicz, J.J. and Silk, D.B.A. (1988) Further characterisation of the 'ileal brake' reflex in man: effect of ileal infusion of partial digests of fat, protein and starch on jejunal motility and release of neurotensin, enteroglucagon, and PYY. *Gut*, **29**, 1042–1051

92. Murphy, M.S., Brunetto, A.L., Pearson, A.D.J. *et al.* (1992) Gut hormones and gastrointestinal motility in children with cystic fibrosis. *Dig. Dis. Sci.*, **37**, 187–192.

93. Adrian, T.E., McKiernan, J., Johnstone, D.I. *et al.* (1980) Hormonal abnormalities of the pancreas and gut in cystic fibrosis. *Gastroenterology*, **79**, 460–465.

94. Allen, J.M., Penketh, A.R.L., Adrian, T.E. *et al.* (1983) Adult cystic fibrosis: postprandial response of gut regulatory peptides. *Gastroenterology*, **85**, 1379–1383.

95. Sweney, L. and Warwick, W.J. (1968) Involvement of labial salivary gland in patients with cystic fibrosis. III. Ultrastructural changes. *Arch. Pathol.*, **86**, 413–418.

96. Gugler, E., Pallavicini, J.C., Swerdlow, H. and di Sant'Agnese, P.A. (1967) The role of calcium in submaxillary saliva of patients with cystic fibrosis. *J. Pediatr.*, **71**, 585.

97. Barbero, G.J. and Sibinga, M.S. (1962) Enlargement of the salivary gland in cystic fibrosis. *Pediatrics*, **29**, 788–793.

98. Rosenstein, B.J. and Langbaum, T.S. (1983) Incidence of distal intestinal obstruction syndrome in cystic fibrosis. *J. Pediatr. Gastroenterol. Nutr.*, **2**, 299–301.

99. Bali, A., Stableforth, D.E. and Asquith, P. (1984) Evidence for bacterial contamination of the small intestine in adults with cystic fibrosis, in *Cystic Fibrosis: Horizons*, (ed. D. Lawson), John Wiley and Sons, Chichester, p. 323.

100. Weisbrodt, N.W. (1992) The regulation of gastrointestinal motility, in *Motility Disorders of the Gastrointestinal Tract*, (ed. F. Anuras), Raven Press, New York, pp. 27–48.

101. Feigelsen, J. and Sauvegrain, J. (1975) Reflux gastroesophagien dans la mucovisidose. *N. Press. Med.*, **4**, 2729–2730.

102. Vic, P., Tassin, E., Turck, D., Gottrand, F., Vaunay, V. and Farriaux, J.P. (1995) Frequence du reflux gastrooesophagien chez le nourrisson et le jeune enfant atteints de mucoviscidose. *Arch. Pediatr.*, **2**, 742–746.

103. Vandenplas, Y., Diericx, A., Blecker, U., Lanciers, S. and Denayer, M. (1991) Esophageal pH monitoring data during chest physiotherapy. *J. Pediatr. Gastroenterol. Nutr.*, **13**, 23–26.

104. Button, B., Heine, R., Catto-Smith, A., Phelan, P. and Olinsky, A. (1997) Postural drainage and gastro-oesophageal reflux in infants with cystic fibrosis. *Arch. Dis. Child.*, **76**, 148–150.

105. Taylor, C.J. and Threlfall, D. (1997) Postural drainage techniques and gastro-oesophageal reflux in cystic fibrosis. *Lancet*, **349**, (9065), 1567–1568.

106. Hassall, E., Israel, D.M., Davidson, A.G.F. and Wong, L.T.K. (1993) Barrett's esophagus in children with cystic fibrosis: not a coincidental association. *Am. J. Gastroenterol.*, **88**, 1974–1978.

106a. Ledson, M.J., Wilson, G.E., Tran, J. and Walshaw, M.J. (1998) Tracheal microaspiration in adult cystic fibrosis. *J. Roy. Soc. Med.*, **91**, 10–12.

107. Ravelli, A.M. and Milla, P.J. (1994) Detection of gastroesophageal reflux by electrical impedance tomography. *J. Pediatr. Gastroenterol. Nutr.*, **18**, 205–213.

108. Cucchiara, S., Santamaria, F., Andreotti, M.R. et al. (1991) Mechanisms of gastroesophageal reflux in cystic fibrosis. *Arch. Dis. Child.*, **66**, 617–622.

108a. Vandenplas, Y., Belle, D.C., Benatar, A. *et al.* (1999) The role of Cisapride in the treatment of pediatric gastroesophageal reflux. *J.Pediatr. Gastroenterol. Nutr.*, **28**, 518–528.

109. Wiseman, L. and Faulds, D. (1994) Cisapride: An updated review of its pharmacology and therapeutic efficacy as a prokinetic agent in gastrointestinal motility disorders. *Drugs*, **47**, (1), 116–152.

110. Taylor, L., Weiner, T., Lacey, S. and Azizkhan, G. (1994) Chronic lung disease is the leading risk factor correlating with the failure (wrap disruption) of antireflux procedures in children. (1994) *J. Pediatr. Surg.*, **29**, 161–166.

111. Okuyama, H., Urao, M., Starr, G., Drongowski, R., Coran, A. and Hirschi, R. (1997) A comparison of the efficacy of pyloromyotomy and plyoroplasty in patients with gastroesophageal reflux and delayed gastric emptying. *J. Pediatr. Surg.*, **32**, (2), 316–320.

112. Fonkalsrud, E., Ellis, D., Shaw, A. *et al.* (1995) A combined hospital experience with fundoplication and gastric emptying procedure for gastroesophageal reflux in children. *J. Am. Coll. Surg.*, **180**, 449–455.

113. Moffett, D., Moffett, S. and Schauf, C. (eds) (1993) *Regulation of Gastrointestinal Function. Human Physiology*, (2nd edn), pp. 643–650.

114. Collins, C., Francis, J., Thomas, P., Henry, R. and O'Loughlin, E. (1997) Gastric emptying time is faster in cystic fibrosis. *J. Pediatr. Gastroenterol. Nutr.*, **25**, 492–498.

115. Cucchiara, S., Raia, V., Minella, R., Frezza, T., De Vizia, B. and De Ritis, G. (1996) Ultrasound measurement of gastric emptying time in patients with cystic fibrosis and effect of ranitidine on delayed gastric emptying. *J. Pediatr.*, **128**, (4), 485–488.

116. Jensen, K. (1962) Meconium ileus equivalent in a fifteen year old patient with mucoviscidosis. *Acta Paediatr. Scand.*, **51**, 344–348.

117. Rubinstein, S., Moss, R. and Lewiston, N. (1986) Constipation and meconium ileus equivalent in patients with cystic fibrosis. *Pediatrics*, **78**, 473–479.

118. Hodson, M.E., Mearns, M.B. and Batten, J.C. (1976) Meconium ileus equivalent in adults with cystic fibrosis of the pancreas: a report of six cases. *BMJ*, **2**, 790–791.

119. Davidson, A.C., Harrison, K., Steinfort, C.L. and Geddes, E.M. (1987) Distal intestinal obstruction syndrome in cystic fibrosis treated by oral intestinal lavage and a case of recurrent obstruction despite normal pancreatic function. *Thorax*, **42**, 538–541.

120. Millar-Jones, L. and Goodchild, M.C. (1995) Cystic fibrosis, pancreatic sufficiency and distal intestinal obstruction syndrome: a report of four cases. *Acta Paediatr.*, **84**, (5), 577–578.

121. Shwachman, H. and Holsclaw, D. (1972) Examination of the appendix at laparotomy as a diagnostic clue in cystic fibrosis. *NEJM*, **286**, 1300–1301.

122. Avioli, L, Parigi, G.B., Fasani, R. and Verga, G. (1997) Fortuitous diagnosis of cystic fibrosis at laparotomy for acute appendicitis. *Pediatr. Surg. Internat.*, **12**, (5–6), 441–442.

123. Dik, H., Nicolai, J.J., Schipper, J., Heijerman, H.G. and Bakker W. (1995) Erroneous diagnosis of distal intestinal obstruction syndrome in cystic fibrosis: clinical impact of abdominal ultrasonography. *Europ. J. Gastroenterol. Hepatol.*, **7**, 279–281.

124. Gracey, M., Burke, V. and Anderson, C.M. (1969) Treatment of abdominal pain in cystic fibrosis by oral administration of N-acetyl cysteine. *Arch. Dis. Child.*, **44**, 404–405.

125. Cleghorn, G.J., Stringer, D.A., Forstner, G.G. and Durie, P.R. (1986) Treatment of distal intestinal obstruction syndrome in cystic fibrosis with a balanced intestinal lavage solution. *Lancet*, **i**, 8–11.

126. Godson, C., Ryan, M.P., Brady, H.R., Bourke, S. and FitzGerald, M.X. (1988) Acute hypomagnesaemia complicating the treatment of meconium ileus

equivalent in cystic fibrosis. *Scand. J. Gastroenterol.*, **S.143**, 148–150.

127. Coughlin, J.P., Gauderer, M.W., Stern, R.C., Doershuk, C.F., Izant, R.J. Jr and Zollinger, R.M. Jr (1990) The spectrum of appendiceal disease in cystic fibrosis. *J. Pediatr. Surg.*, **25**, 835–839.

128. Przyklenk, B., Bauerfeind, A., Bertele-Harms, R.M. and Harms, K.H. (1991) *The significance of* Helicobacter pyloridis *in patients with cystic fibrosis*. Proceedings, 17th European CF Conference, p. 85.

129. Johansen, H.K., Norgaard, A., Andersen, L.P., Jensen, P., Nielsen, H. and Hoiby, N. (1995) Cross-reactive antigens shared by *Pseudomonas aeruginosa*, *Helicobacter pylori*, *Campylobacter jejuni*, and *Haemophilus influenzae* may cause false-positive titers of antibody to *H. pylori*. *Clin. Diag. Lab. Immunol.*, **2**, (2), 149–155.

129a. Fallone, C.A., Veldhuyzen van Zanten, S.J.O. and Chiba, N. (2000) The urea breath test for *Helicobacter pylori* infection: taking the wind out of the sails of endoscopy. *Can. Med. Assoc. J.*, **162**, 371–372.

130. Holsclaw, D.S., Rocmans, C. and Shwachman, H. (1971) Intussusception in patients with cystic fibrosis. *Pediatrics*, **48**, 51–58.

131. Kirks, D.R. (1995) Air intussusception reduction: 'the winds of change'. *Pediatr Radiol.*, **25**, 89–91.

132. Poznanski, A.K. (1995) Why I still use barium for intussusception. *Pediatr. Radiol.*, **25**, 92–93.

133. Hill, S.M., Phillips, A.D., Mearns, M. and Walker-Smith, J.A. (1989) Cows' milk sensitive enteropathy in cystic fbrosis. *Arch. Dis. Child.*, **64**, 1251–1255.

134. Davidson, A.G.F. and Mullinger, M.M. (1970) Reducing substances in neonatal stool detected by clinitest. *Pediatrics*, **46**, 632–635.

135. Woolridge, M.W. and Fisher, C. (1988) Colic, 'overfeeding', and symptoms of lactose malabsorption in the breast-fed baby: a possible artifact of feed management? *Lancet*, **2**, 382–384.

136. Cavataio, F., Iacono, G., Montalto, G., Soresi, M., Tumminello, M. and Carroccio, A. (1996) Clinical and pH-metric characteristics of gastro-oesophageal reflux secondary to cow's milk protein allergy. *Arch. Dis. Child.*, **75**, 51–56.

137. Lloyd-Still, J.D. (1990) Cystic fibrosis, Crohn's Disease, biliary abnormalities, and cancer. *J. Pediatr. Gastroenterol. Nutr.*, **11**, 434–437.

138. Smyth, R. (1996) Fibrosing colonopathy in cystic fibrosis. *Arch. Dis. Child.*, **74**, 464–468.

138a. Kimura, R.E., Arango, V. and Lloyd-Still, J. (1998) Indomethacin and pancreatic enzymes synergistically damage intestine of rats. *Dig. Dis. Sci.,* **43**, 2322–2332.

139. Hide, D.W. and Burman, D. (1969) An infant with both cystic fibrosis and coeliac disease. *Arch. Dis. Child.*, **44**, 533–535.

140. Valletta, E.A. and Mastella, G. (1989) Incidence of celiac disease in a cystic fibrosis population. *Acta. Paediatr. Scand.*, **78**, 784–785.

141. Davidson, A.G.F. and Hassall, E. (1997) Screening for celiac disease. *Can. Med. Assoc. J.*, **157**, 547.

142. Walker-Smith, J.A., Guandalini, S., Schmitz, J., Shmerling, D.H. and Visakorpi, J.K. (1990) Revised criteria for diagnosis of coeliac disease: Report of working group of European Society of Paediatric Gastroenterology and Nutrition. *Arch. Dis. Child.*, **63**, 909–911.

143. Pier, G.B., Grout, M., Zaidi, T. *et al.* (1998) Salmonella typhi uses CFTR to enter intestinal epithelial cells. *Nature*, **393**, (6680), 79–82.

144. Rivlin, J., Lerner, A., Augarten, A., Wilschanski, M., Kerem, E., and Ephros, M. (1998) Severe *Clostridium difficile*-associated colitis in young patients with cystic fibrosis. *J. Pediatr.*, **132**, 177–179.

145. Welkon, C., Long, S., Murry Thompson C. Jr and Gilligan, H. (1985) *Clostridium difficile* in patients with cystic fibrosis. *AJDC*, **139**, 805–808.

145a. Binkovitz, L.A., Allen, E., Bloom, D. *et al.* (1999) Atypical presentation of *clostridium difficile* colitis in patients with cystic fibrosis. *Am. J. Roentgenol.,* **172**, 517–521.

146. Roberts, D.M., Craft, J.C., Mather, F.J., Davis, S.H. and Wright, J.A. Jr (1988) Prevalence of giardiasis in patients with cystic fibrosis. *J. Pediatr.*, **112**, 555–559.

147. Chalmers, R.A., Valman, H.B. and Liberman, M.M. (1979) Measurement of 4-hydroxyphenylacetic aciduria as a screening test for small-bowel disease. *Clin. Chem.*, **25**, 1791-1794.

148. Gibbons, I.S.E., Seakins, J.W.T. and Ersser, R.S. (1967) Tyrosine metabolism and faecal amino acids in cystic fibrosis of the pancreas. *Lancet*, **I**, 877–878.

149. Stern, R.C., Izant, R.J., Boat, T.F., Wood, R.E., Matthews, L.W. and Doershuk, C.F. (1982) Treatment and prognosis of rectal prolapse in cystic fibrosis. *Gastroenterology*, **82**, 707–710.

149a. Chan, W.K., Kay, S.M., Laberge, J.M., Gallucci, J.G., Bensoussan, A.L. and Yazbeck, S. (1998) Injection sclerotherapy in the treatment of rectal prolapse in infants and children. *J. Pediatr. Surg.,* **33**, 255–258.

150. Smyth, R.L., Ashby, D., O'Hea, U. *et al.* (1995) Fibrosing colonopathy in cystic fibrosis. Results of a case control study. *Lancet*, **346**, 1247–1251.

151. Taylor, C.J. and Steiner, G.M. (1995) Fibrosing colonopathy in a child on low-dose pancreatin. *Lancet*, **346**, 1106–1107.

152. Crisci, K., Greenberg, S., Wolfson, B., Geller, E. and Vinocur, C. (1997) Contrast enema findings of fibrosing colonopathy. *Pediatr. Radiol.*, **27**, 315–316.

153. Ablin, D.S. and Ziegler, M. (1995) Ulcerative type of colitis associated with the use of high strength pancreatic enzyme supplements in cystic fibrosis. *Pediatr. Radiol.*, **25**, 113–116.

154. Hernanz-Schulman, M., Kirkpatrick, J. Jr, Shwachman, H., Schulman, H. and Vawter, G.F. (1986) Pneumatosis intestinalis in cystic fibrosis. *Radiology*, **160**, 497–499.

155. Neglia, J., FitzSimmons, S., Maisonneuve, P. *et al.* and the Cystic Fibrosis and Cancer Study Group (1995) The risk of cancer among patients with cystic fibrosis. *NEJM*, **332**, 494–499.

13

Liver and biliary disease in cystic fibrosis

D. WESTABY

Introduction	289		The management of liver disease in cystic fibrosis	294
Pathogenesis of chronic liver disease	289		Management of the complications of liver disease	
Clinical features	291		in cystic fibrosis	295
Chronic liver disease as a prognostic factor in cystic			Extrahepatic biliary disease in cystic fibrosis	297
fibrosis	291		References	298
Investigations	292			

INTRODUCTION

Liver involvement in cystic fibrosis (CF) has been recognized for over 50 years[1], predominantly based on post-mortem studies. Symptomatic liver disease is an uncommon complication, reported in less than 5 per cent of cases and the cause of death in 2 per cent [2]. These data markedly underestimate the incidence of liver abnormalities. The typical biliary cirrhosis associated with CF has been reported in up to 50 per cent of post-mortem studies[3,4] and in approximately 25 per cent of adult CF populations studied prospectively to detect this abnormality[5,6]. This emphasizes the clinically occult nature of much liver involvement. There is evidence to suggest that the prevalence increases with age[2]; however, a recent large study including 1100 children and adults with CF observed a decline in the prevalence of liver disease in the third decade[7]. Such a 'fall-off' raises the possibility of premature mortality in those with chronic liver disease which the study was not designed to detect. This has recently been supported by a time-dependent multiple regression analysis of risk factors in CF, which has confirmed liver disease as an important predictor of mortality (see below). With the vast improvements in the care of pulmonary complications of CF, as well as the availability of cardiopulmonary transplantation, it might be anticipated that the prevalence of chronic liver disease will further increase, particularly in the second decade of life.

PATHOGENESIS OF CHRONIC LIVER DISEASE

The characteristic hepatic lesion in cystic fibrosis is a focal biliary fibrosis with edema, chronic inflammatory cell infiltration and bile duct proliferation with patchy accumulation of an eosinophilic PAS-positive diastase-resistant material in the intrahepatic ducts. Such pathological changes are consistent with those seen in partial biliary obstruction. The plugging of intrahepatic bile ducts has been compared to that seen within the pancreatic ducts of patients with cystic fibrosis[8]. Recent work has confirmed the localization of the cystic fibrosis transmembrane conductance regulator (CFTR) to the apical membrane of intrahepatic bile duct cells[9]. There is no evidence of the CFTR being expressed in hepatocytes. The abnormalities of chloride transport secondary to a mutation of the *CFTR* gene account for the failure to adequately hydrate the canalicular-produced bile, resulting in increased bile viscosity. There is also recent evidence to suggest that the intrahepatic biliary epithelial cells in cystic fibrosis produce excessive mucus predominantly composed of proteoglycans[10]. This will further enhance the viscosity of bile and the tendency to form biliary plugs.

Whether biliary duct obstruction is alone sufficient to account for the observed cirrhosis of CF is a matter of controversy. A recent light- and electron-microscopic study of liver disease in CF reported no signs of cholestasis, such as ductal plugs or intracellular bile pigments[11]. Dilatation of bile canaliculi was only infrequently observed. The most prominent feature was evidence of bile duct destruction and associated collagen deposition. The authors suggest a bile-related toxin as a most likely explanation for these findings. Elevations and changes in components of the serum bile acid pool have previously been implicated[2,12]. Although available studies have shown no significant difference in the serum bile acid profile between those with and without evidence of liver disease[5], these crude levels may not accurately reflect the exposure of the hepatocyte to potentially hepatotoxic bile acids. In the absence of advanced liver disease, bile salt output remains normal or modestly reduced, but in the presence of the CFTR defect the total volume of bile is significantly decreased[12,13]. Thus a high concentration of bile acids is generated within the intrahepatic bile ducts. If there is plugging of these ducts, it could be speculated that bile acid reflux will occur, exposing the hepatocytes to a high local concentration of potentially toxic lipophilic bile acids, either primary (chenodeoxycholic acid) or secondary (deoxycholic acid and lithocholic acid). The extent to which such reflux and retention causes hepatocyte injury will depend upon the cell's uptake rate, intracellular binding and ability to detoxify by sulfation or glucuronidation (Fig. 13.1).

There has been some evidence to suggest that obstruction of the common bile duct as it passes through the diseased pancreas in CF may also contribute to the pathogenesis of the observed biliary cirrhosis[5]. Using both hepatobiliary scintigraphy and cholangiography, evidence of distal bile duct obstruction was recorded in 48 of 50 patients with CF-related chronic liver disease. Of the 29 undergoing cholangiography, 27 showed a distal common bile duct stricture. In an otherwise comparable group of patients with CF without liver disease such a stricture was not observed. The authors of this

paper speculated that common bile duct obstruction was the common denominator accounting for the progression from a focal biliary lesion to multilobular biliary cirrhosis. However, two subsequent studies which employed both biliary scintigraphy and endoscopic retrograde cholangiography failed to identify distal common bile duct strictures in similar patients with chronic liver disease[6,14]. Abnormalities of isotope excretion were common in both investigations, but this was by no means restricted to the distal common bile duct. Stricturing of the common bile duct as it passed through the pancreas was only observed in 15 per cent of cases (Fig. 13.2). Caliber irregularities of the intrahepatic ducts were an almost uniform finding in the patients with chronic liver disease (Fig. 1.3.3). Therefore, the balance of these studies would be in favor of a diffuse intrahepatic biliary lesion with distal common bile duct obstruction, perhaps of relevance in a very small proportion of patients.

Although the above provides a possible etiological basis for chronic liver disease in CF, it does not account for the absence of liver involvement in a sizeable proportion of patients and a wide spectrum of severity in those in whom this does occur. The high prevalence of chronic liver disease in post-mortem studies in adults with CF provides some support for the view that with extended

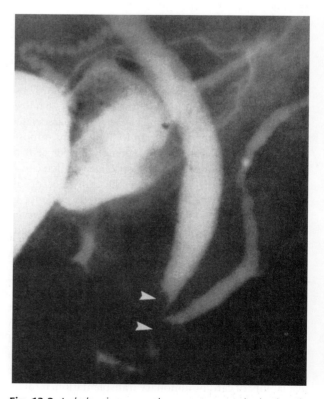

Fig. 13.2 *A cholangiogram and pancreatogram obtained at the time of ERCP. A short stricture of the distal common bile duct is observed (arrowheads) in close proximity to the pancreatic duct. The common bile duct is dilated proximally.*

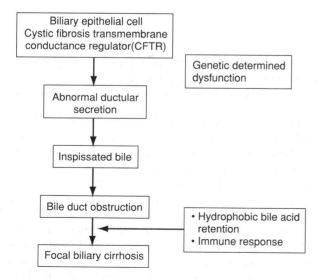

Fig. 13.1 *Pathogenesis of chronic liver disease in cystic fibrosis.*

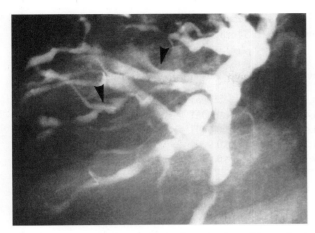

Fig. 13.3 *A cholangiogram obtained at the time of ERC, showing the abnormal intrahepatic ducts (arrowheads). The ducts are somewhat dilated with irregularities of calibre, typical of that seen in established chronic liver disease in the presence of CF.*

survival a much higher proportion of patients would develop liver involvement. However, other factors are required to explain the timing of development and subsequent severity of disease. The possible association of chronic liver disease with a specific gene defect has been investigated but not identified.

There was no significant difference in the frequencies of the ΔF_{508}, G551 or R553X cystic fibrosis gene mutations in those with and without liver involvement[15]. However, the high familial concordance of liver disease suggests that genes outside a CF locus, or possibly environmental factors, may be involved in its pathogenesis. One study has suggested an almost 3 : 1 male to female bias in those with liver disease, although this has not been supported by others[7]. Further evidence of a genetic influence has come from HLA studies which have shown an increased frequency of A2, B7, DR2 (DRw15) and DQw6 in those with established liver disease[16]. The relative risk of chronic liver disease increased from the HLA A2 to the DQ position, suggesting that a disease-associated allele may lie near the DQB locus. The presence of a subpopulation of lymphocytes, cytotoxic to hepatocytes and directed towards the liver-specific lipoprotein, suggests that immune mechanisms might also be involved in the pathogenesis[17]. It is likely that such immune mechanisms are a secondary phenomenon to the obstructive biliary lesions, but may be important in determining the extent of damage observed.

CLINICAL FEATURES

Although the characteristic liver lesion of CF is a focal or multilobular biliary cirrhosis, other manifestations may occur, particularly in early infancy. Deep cholestasis secondary to common bile duct obstruction with inspissated bile may be the earliest manifestation of CF[18,19]. Fatty infiltration of the liver is also a recognized feature, which may be so gross as to present with massive abdominal distension and may be complicated by hypoglycemia[2]. This has been associated closely with malnutrition, but may occur in its absence. Carnitine deficiency has been reported as a possible contributing factor. Neonatal hepatitis with giant-cell infiltration is an exceptionally rare manifestation of CF[20].

Features of biliary cirrhosis may appear at any time from infancy to adult life. Established chronic liver disease is infrequently the presenting feature of CF. It is usually detected on the basis of hepatosplenomegaly in a patient under surveillance. Abnormal liver function tests alone may be the only indicator. Evidence of decompensation in the form of jaundice, ascites or encephalopathy are uncommon, either as presenting features or as part of the natural history of the disease. Similarly, variceal hemorrhage is a rare complication of CF but may occur in up to 30 per cent of patients with established local or diffuse cirrhosis (a figure similar to cirrhotides of other etiologies)[21]. Variceal bleeding may be the presenting feature of underlying liver disease and occurs in the absence of any other signs of decompensation. Such early presentation with complications or portal hypertension may reflect the presinusoidal component of portal vascular resistance, which is well recognized in biliary cirrhosis and can occur in the precirrhotic phase of the disease[21]. Overall, the clinical picture is one of a very slowly progressive liver disease, the natural history of which is usually interrupted by premature mortality related to the pulmonary disease. The long natural history of the cirrhosis associated with CF is not dissimilar from that seen in other biliary cirrhotides, such as primary biliary cirrhosis and primary sclerosing cholangitis[22,23].

CHRONIC LIVER DISEASE AS A PROGNOSTIC FACTOR IN CYSTIC FIBROSIS

There is evidence that liver disease may have an adverse effect on prognosis in CF which cannot be accounted for by hepatic decompensation alone. To investigate this further, we have recently carried out a time-dependent regression analysis to evaluate risk factors for mortality in 403 adult patients with CF, followed over a median of 7 years. This confirmed that chronic liver disease (based on the presence of hepatomegaly) was an important predictor of outcome, with similar importance to the severity of lung disease and nutritional status[24]. Clinical detection of hepatomegaly as a marker of chronic liver disease may have some limitations, particularly with respect to interobserver variation. It is also well recog-

Table 13.1 *Significant variables correlating with survival in CF derived from a time-dependent regression analysis. Using this model a predictive index (PI) was calculated (See Fig. 13.4). PI = (0.99 × hepatomegaly) – (3.41 × height) – (0.038 × % PFVC) – (0.0590 × % PFEV$_1$) + (0.090 × WBC)*

Variable	Coefficient	SE	Coef/SE	*P* value	Relative risk
Height (m)	−3.41	0.828	−4.12	<0.0001	0.033
Hepmeg. (0,1)	0.99	0.154	6.48	<0.0001	2.69
% Pred. FEV	−0.059	0.013	−4.46	<0.0001	0.943
% Pred. FVC	−0.038	0.009	−3.27	<0.0001	0.963
WBC × 10⁹ per liter	0.090	0.014	6.40	<0.0001	1.095

Hepatomegaly: presence, 1; absence, 0.
WBC, white blood cell count.

nized that in the late stages of CF-related liver disease the liver may become small in size (although the left lobe is almost always prominent). However, the use of hepatomegaly as a predictive factor is supported by data from other biliary cirrhotides[22]. Based on this regression analysis, it proved possible to calculate a predictive index (Table 13.1; Fig. 13.4) which appears to provide considerable predictive accuracy for survival over a period of up to 7 years. The most relevant part of information is the predictive value over 12–18 months, when its application could be used to predict and therefore prepare for those requiring organ transplantation.

The means by which the presence of liver disease determines premature mortality has not been fully explained. In a recent publication we have documented the marked abnormalities of systemic hemodynamics in those patients with underlying cirrhosis as compared to those without liver disease[25]. It might be speculated that this increased cardiac output might have an adverse effect upon cardiopulmonary status if maintained in the long term. A second observation was the incidence of significant intrapulmonary shunts in those patients with CF-related liver disease. Approximately 15 per cent of

patients studied had shunting in excess of 10 per cent, which was absent in the group of patients without underlying liver disease. In the presence of deteriorating pulmonary function such shunting might have a detrimental affect upon survival.

INVESTIGATIONS

Standard laboratory liver-related tests have proved disappointing as predictive factors for liver disease. It is well recognized that a small proportion of patients with established cirrhosis will have entirely normal liver biochemistry[5,7]. Modest elevations in the aminotransferase levels are frequently observed in CF patients with no significant correlation with established liver disease. This has been attributed to many different factors, including chronic infection, hypoxemia and secondary to drug ingestion. Similarly, minor elevations of the liver isoenzyme of alkaline phosphatase as well as γ-glutamyl-transpeptidase have little specificity. However, elevation of these enzymes above four times the normal level is almost always associated with some degree of biliary-related liver disease. The crude assessment of serum bile acids is also nondiscriminatory[5].

Imaging of the liver appears to offer the greatest potential for accurately identifying underlying chronic liver disease. The availability of real-time ultrasound has enabled detection of multilobular cirrhosis with considerable accuracy[26]. The recognition of more focal disease will depend very much on its extent. A dilated portal vein, splenomegaly and collateral vessels are all important markers of portal hypertension[26]. The use of Doppler ultrasound allows the close mapping of the portal and splenic veins, which may identify venous thrombosis occurring in the presence of CF-related chronic pancreatitis[27]. In a recent study we have utilized real-time ultrasound to provide a grading system for the presence or absence of underlying liver disease[28]. This scoring system depends upon the detection of three ultrasound

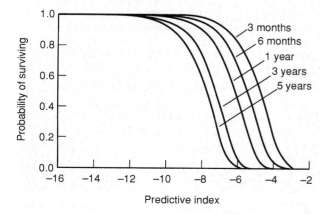

Fig. 13.4 *Survival curves for patients with cystic fibrosis, in relationship to the predictive index (see Table 13.1).*

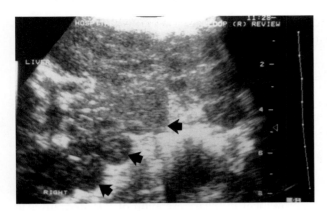

Fig 13.5 *Hepatic ultrasound scan showing marked nodularity (arrows) diagnostic of underlying cirrhosis.*

characteristics which previously have been associated with chronic liver disease: parenchymal irregularity, periportal fibrosis (increased periportal echoes) and irregularity of the liver edge consistent with the macro-nodular pattern of cirrhosis (Fig. 13.5; Table 13.2).

Initial evaluation of this scoring system appeared to confirm its accuracy in differentiating between established cirrhosis and a normal underlying liver parenchyma. There was also some suggestion that the scoring was able to identify a group of patients with evidence of liver disease but in a pre-cirrhotic phase. Such detailed characterization of the underlying liver status may have considerable clinical relevance but still requires prospective evaluation.

Cholangiography, most frequently using the endoscopic approach, has produced important diagnostic information and is sometimes required for the therapy of choledocholithiasis (see below)[5,6]. Caliber irregularities of the intrahepatic ducts appear to be specific for established chronic liver disease in CF. These intrahepatic ductular changes almost certainly reflect damage to the biliary radicals and are not dissimilar from those observed in primary sclerosing cholangitis, but do not provide any specific information as to their pathogenesis. Cholangiography also provides the means of detecting the small proportion of patients with a significant distal common bile duct stricture secondary to the pancreatic disease. However, as a more general investigation of patients with CF, endoscopic retrograde cholangiopancreatography is disadvantaged by its invasive nature. In a recent study we have evaluated magnetic resonance

imaging (MRI) and, in particular, magnetic resonance cholangio-pancreatography as a noninvasive means of assessing the liver disease in CF. MRI has provided excellent definition of the hepatic parenchyma as well as the portal and splenic vascular bed (Fig. 13.6). The extra-hepatic biliary tree was well defined by the MRI technique, but resolution of the intrahepatic ducts (Fig. 13.7) has not always been sufficient for identification of the characteristic caliber abnormalities seen on endoscopic cholangiography.

Radionuclide imaging using derivatives of iminodiacetic acid (IDA) labeled with technetium-99m provides an alternative means of assessing the biliary tree[29]. IDA is taken up by the hepatocytes and then cleared rapidly in the bile. A number of recent studies have utilized these derivatives as a means of assessing biliary function and

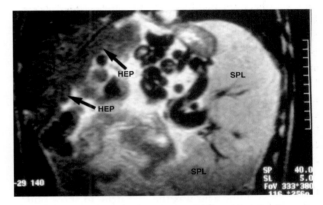

Fig 13.6 *A T2W abdominal MRI scan with fast spin echo. A small cirrhotic liver (Hep) identified with gross splenomegaly (spl). Large collaterals can be seen to arise from the splenetic hilum.*

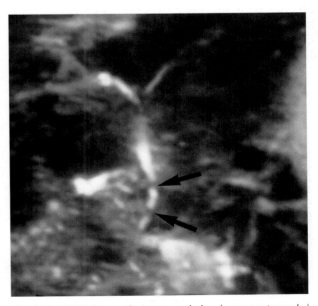

Fig 13.7 *A MRCP (magnetic resonance cholangio-pancreatography) sequence. Two small calculi are seen in the common bile duct (arrows). These are confirmed at ERCP and removed.*

Table 13.2 *The ultrasound scoring system*

Score	1	2	3
Characteristic			
Hepatic parenchyma	Normal	Coarse	Irregular
Liver edge	Smooth	–	Nodular
Periportal fibrosis	None	Moderate	Severe

have confirmed impaired drainage in patients with chronic liver disease. Delay of excretion was documented in both intra- and extrahepatic sites, in keeping with delayed bile flow, rather than a single site of obstruction[5,6,14]. The introduction of quantitative IDA imaging may allow an objective means of documenting deterioration in liver disease or response to therapy.

Histological assessment forms a fundamental basis for most aspects of hepatology. However, in CF liver disease the focal nature of the early changes results in sampling error. Ultrasound-guided biopsy may reduce this risk, if focal lesions are detectable. There has been an understandable reluctance to carry out liver biopsy in patients with CF, on the basis that management was seldom changed. The imaging techniques described above, carried out in experienced hands, may well provide sufficient diagnostic information for most patients. It is unlikely that such imaging techniques will be able to define an ultrastructural response to a therapeutic agent, so histological assessment may still be required in the setting of therapeutic trials.

THE MANAGEMENT OF LIVER DISEASE IN CYSTIC FIBROSIS

Bile acid therapy

Ursodeoxycholic acid was the first drug to show potential as treatment for the underlying liver disease. This bile acid is known to increase bile flow[30] and it is believed to protect the hepatocyte from the toxicity of hydrophobic bile acids[31]. Ursodeoxycholic acid taken by mouth has not been shown to change the pool size of the hydrophobic bile acids (chenodeoxycholate and deoxycholic acid) but does, by expanding the overall pool size, diminish the relative concentration of these toxic bile acids[32]. There is also some evidence that this drug has an immunoregulatory effect[33], although this remains to be confirmed. Evidence of a beneficial effect in primary biliary cirrhosis and primary sclerosing cholangitis[34,35] prompted the use of this drug in CF-related liver disease. A number of uncontrolled studies demonstrated both biochemical and clinical improvement in response to ursodeoxycholic acid[36,37]. The dose of ursodeoxycholic acid used in the early studies varied between 10 and 15 mg/kg, although it was speculated that bile salt malabsorption in CF may require a higher oral dosage. Two studies have specifically investigated the dose response to this drug[38,39] and suggest that the optimum dose with respect to the biliary management with ursodeoxycholic acid and the biochemical response varies between 15 and 20 mg/kg/day.

Attention has also been paid to the need for taurine supplementation as part of ursodeoxycholic acid therapy. Taurine deficiency is frequently observed in patients

with CF and ongoing malabsorption secondary to the faecal loss of taurine-conjugated bile salts. Such taurine deficiency increases the proportion of glyco-conjugated bile acids, which are potentially more hepatotoxic. Evidence to date suggests that taurine supplementation as part of ursodeoxycholic acid therapy has no effect on the biochemical features of liver disease but may have a nutritional benefit, perhaps by improving the micellar solubilization of lipolytic products and reducing malabsorption[40].

A small, unblinded controlled trial was first reported in 1992, showing benefit in liver biochemistry as well as improvement in biliary excretion of IDA derivatives in those taking ursodeoxycholic acid[41]. A much larger, placebo-based controlled trial has confirmed the improvement in liver biochemistry as well as benefits with respect to a general illness score (Shwachman–Kulczycki score)[40]. However, neither of these two controlled trials has been of sufficient power or duration to comment upon important end points, such as the development of complications of liver disease or associated mortality. Furthermore, there was no attempt to assess the histological response to ursodeoxycholic acid.

Despite the concerns with respect to sampling error (see above), two recent studies have attempted to evaluate the histological response to ursodeoxycholic acid[42,43]. In both studies liver biopsy was taken before and 1 or 2 years after starting treatment with ursodeoxycholic acid. The liver biopsies were assessed blind to the clinical information and a scoring system was used to assess the degree of bile duct proliferation, fibrosis and inspissation of bile as well as inflammatory changes. Using the scoring system, and despite the small numbers, in both studies there was clear evidence of histological benefit.

The accumulated evidence would suggest a beneficial effect of ursodeoxycholic acid in established chronic liver disease associated with CF. The most encouraging evidence is that pointing to histological benefits over a 12–24-month period.

There must be some concerns that appropriate studies to revaluate the possible long-term benefit of this drug, both with respect to the complications of cirrhosis and mortality, will not be undertaken because of a reluctance to incorporate a control group in the light of the current evidence in favor of using this drug. This is particularly the case because of the very low toxicity of ursodeoxycholic acid. In primary biliary cirrhosis there is evidence of benefit of ursodeoxycholic acid in patients with early liver disease[34] and it would be timely to set up appropriate controlled trials of this drug in patients with minimal or no evidence of liver involvement in CF.

Liver transplantation

Liver transplantation has been widely adopted as the definitive management for many different types of chronic liver disease. This has proved highly beneficial in biliary cirrhotides such a primary biliary cirrhosis and primary sclerosing cholangitis. Initially, the use of liver transplantation in CF had few protagonists because of concerns that the underlying pulmonary disease would preclude such surgery, and that if there was survival into the postoperative period, then the required immunosuppression would increase the risk of overwhelming pulmonary infection. However, several, published, small series of patients undergoing liver transplantation have encouraged a more aggressive approach to decompensated liver disease in CF[44,45].

The criteria for inclusion of patients for liver transplantation in CF have gradually expanded with increasing experience. As for other types of chronic liver disease, features of advanced liver decompensation are standard, including encephalopathy, poorly controlled ascites and, in the case of biliary cirrhosis, progressive jaundice in the absence of bile duct obstruction. The importance of portal hypertension and variceal bleeding as a factor indicating liver transplantation is somewhat controversial. In the Cambridge series[44] an episode of variceal bleeding was the highest-scoring factor determining referral for liver transplantation, whereas others[45] have considered this only to be of importance if the bleeding has failed to respond to available methods (see below).

This latter approach would appear to be most appropriate as variceal bleeding may occur very early in the natural history of liver disease in CF, when all other parameters point to well-compensated disease. The major impetus to liver transplantation came with recognition that in many patients pulmonary function improved postoperatively and there were very few examples of overwhelming pulmonary infection when immunosuppression was in place[44,45]. There are several potential explanations for the improvement in respiratory function in these patients: first, in the presence of cirrhosis there may be diaphragmatic splinting secondary to hepatosplenomegaly; second, intrapulmonary shunting has been identified as an important complication of portal hypertension; and third, malnutrition is frequently associated with cirrhosis and, in turn, might adversely effect diaphragmatic and intercostal muscle function. All these factors might improve after successful liver transplantation. To date the most dramatic improvement in pulmonary function has been seen in those patients with significant preoperative intrapulmonary shunts.

However, a number of pulmonary contraindications to liver transplantation remain, including severely compromised lung function or frequent exacerbations of pulmonary infection, colonization with *Pseudomonas cepacia* or other multiresistant organisms and a raised resting arterial P_{CO_2} as a consequence of ventilatory failure. Evidence of severe pulmonary hypertension (a recognized complication of cirrhosis) would also represent an absolute contra indication.

The two largest series[44,45] of liver transplantation in CF have reported nine and eight patients, respectively. Of the Cambridge series[44] all nine patients were alive 4–55 months postoperatively, with a mean survival period of 30 months. In the Nebraska series[45] six of eight patients survived the operative period and all six were still alive at the time of publication, representing a mean survival of 4.1 years.

There remains a small but important group of patients with CF who have advanced liver disease as well as pulmonary disease of such severity that liver transplantation alone would not be feasible. There is now a growing, number of reports of such patients being managed by heart, lung, liver or lung–liver transplantation[46,47]. With a shortage of donated organs there has been considerable reluctance to use those available in such a high-risk undertaking. However, the largest series to date, of 10 patients[46], reported a 70 per cent 1-year survival, which remained unchanged after 3 years. Such results would justify a guarded expansion of this approach.

Gene therapy

The identification and cloning of a CF gene opens the way for the development of gene therapy for this condition. Mostly this approach has been directed towards pulmonary disease, but there is recent evidence to suggest that it might be applied to the prevention or treatment of hepatic disease in CF.

Recombinant adenoviruses expressing the human *CFTR* gene have been infused in a retrograde fashion into the biliary tract of a rat model[48]. Recombinant gene expression was achieved in virtually all the cells of the intrahepatic bile ducts. Expression persisted in the smaller bile ducts for the duration of the experiment, which was 21 days. These studies suggest that it may be feasible to treat or prevent CF liver disease by genetically reconstituting *CFTR* gene expression in the biliary tract by retrograde biliary infusion of an appropriate vector.

MANAGEMENT OF THE COMPLICATIONS OF LIVER DISEASE IN CYSTIC FIBROSIS

Despite progress in the management of the underlying liver disorder, described above, the majority of patients with CF-related liver disease have their management directed towards treating specific complications. The protein–calorie requirements are frequently increased in the prescence of established cirrhosis and careful monitoring is required[49].

Deficiencies in fats and soluble vitamins may occur, particularly with established cholestasis. However, vitamin A should be supplemented with caution, as complications have been documented in the absence of overt overdosage[50].

Jaundice

Jaundice as a consequence of CF-related chronic liver disease is infrequent and usually a late event. In one published series only 20 per cent of patients with established chronic liver disease had a history of jaundice[6]. The onset of jaundice requires detailed investigation to detect or exclude other treatable causes. An ultrasound scan is essential to exclude bile duct obstruction (manifest by bile duct dilatation), either as a consequence of choledocholithiasis or, less frequently, a distal common bile duct stricture. Other possible contributing factors to the development of jaundice include sepsis, drug toxicity or hemolysis. For those patients in which jaundice represents the advanced stage of chronic liver disease, ursodeoxycholic acid has been shown to improve cholestasis, although long-term benefits require confirmation.

Variceal hemorrhage

Variceal hemorrhage represents the most frequent serious complication of chronic liver disease. The approach to management is standard, as applied to patients with portal hypertension or other etiologies[51]. At the time of active variceal bleeding there is a critical need to protect the airway and prevent aspiration pneumonia, one of the common causes of death during any episode of bleeding, but particularly important in the presence of pre-existing pulmonary disease. Endoscopic techniques, such as injection sclerotherapy[52] or band ligation[53], represent the current treatment of choice for an episode of bleeding and can be integrated into mandatory diagnostic endoscopy.

In the absence of appropriate endoscopic expertise, it is usual to use conservative measures, such as balloon tamponade or vasoconstrictor drugs, to provide initial hemostasis and allow time for the appropriate resources for further treatment to be mobilized. However, in the presence of pulmonary disease, balloon tamponade may be poorly tolerated and associated with a high risk of complications[54]. Furthermore, the cardiovascular side-effects of vasoconstrictor drugs, such as vasopressin and Glypressin[*55], should lead to dosage caution in their use for patients with CF and evidence of right-sided heart disease. Such side-effects may be minimized by the addition of a vasodilator in the form of nitroglycerin[55], most conveniently applied as skin patches[56]. Somatostatin or its analog, octreotide, has few cardiovascular side-effects but may not be as effective as Glypressin[*] in controlling acute hemorrhage[57].

In a small proportion of patients, the technique of transjugular intrahepatic portal systemic shunt (TIPPS) may offer a valuable alternative treatment[58]. After a first episode of variceal bleeding there is a high risk of further recurrence (60–80 per cent over 2 years) unless long-term measures are employed. Endoscopic, surgical and pharmacological methods to prevent rebleeding have been evaluated. In patients with CF each of these approaches may have serious drawbacks. Repeated endoscopic techniques expose the patient to pulmonary complications, although with meticulous care these can be minimized. There is evidence to suggest that the introduction of newer techniques, such as band ligation[53], may reduce the number of sessions of treatment required to obliterate esophageal varices.

Surgical techniques, in particular the portal systemic shunt operation, are highly successful in preventing rebleeding, but are poorly tolerated in the presence of significant respiratory disease. Here again the TIPPS procedure[58], which is carried out entirely via the transjugular route, may provide a means of controlling bleeding in the long term without exposing the patient to the risk of a prolonged surgical procedure. Nonselective β-receptor blocking agents have been shown to influence long-term rebleeding[59], but the risk of bronchoconstriction in patients with CF may preclude widespread use.

Treatment to prevent the first variceal hemorrhage (prophylaxis) has been widely advocated, even in patients with CF[60]. However, increasing evidence from controlled trials has confirmed that prophylactic therapy has no influence upon survival and may be detrimental[61]. The risk of a detrimental outcome must be significantly increased in the presence of the pulmonary disease of CF and there is therefore no justification to consider prophylaxis a therapeutic option.

Ascites

In contrast to variceal bleeding, which may occur in patients with well-compensated CF-related liver disease, ascites is always accompanied by other features of decompensation, such as jaundice and poor liver synthetic function. The management of ascites should not differ from that applied to cirrhosis of other etiologies[62]. The majority of cases (80–90 per cent) may be managed by the implementation of a 40 mmol, restricted sodium diet, as well as the judicious use of diuretics. The sodium restriction should be implemented by a dietitian, with considerable attention being paid to maintaining a high protein–calorie intake. The diuretics of choice are those that act on the distal convoluted tubule and collecting ducts, including spironolactone, amiloride and triamterene. These diuretics avoid the major fluid and electrolyte shifts that may occur with the loop diuretics, which are frequently detrimental to renal function in patients with cirrhosis. The dosage of diuretics should be increased slowly over several days, with the aim of losing between 500 and 750 mg in weight per 24 hours. Low doses of loop diuretics may be added if there is a poor response to the distal convoluted tubule diuretics alone.

The use of paracentesis, either by repeated small-volume or total-volume removal, has been shown to be safe in patients with maintained renal function[63]. Tense ascites may cause additional ventilatory impairment and justifies urgent removal of 3–4 liters of ascites, which can almost always be carried out without risk of renal impairment. For larger-volume paracentesis, vascular support is necessary in the form of volume expanders to prevent the inevitable hypovolemia that occurs with paracentesis[64]. In a small proportion of patients both diuretics and paracentesis are poorly tolerated, leading to renal impairment. In such cases the peritoneovenous shunt represents an alternative approach, allowing the ascites to drain back into the central circulation, thus maintaining central blood volume and renal perfusion[65]. Problems with this approach are not infrequent, including shunt occlusion, sepsis, disseminated intravascular coagulation, as well as precipitating variceal hemorrhage. There are very few circumstances where this more invasive approach has a role in patients with CF.

Encephalopathy

Hepatic encephalopathy is an extremely infrequent complication of CF-related liver disease. This may develop in patients with advanced disease as a consequence of other complicating factors such as ventilatory failure, sepsis, gastrointestinal hemorrhage or constipation. Under such circumstances the encephalopathy will usually regress when the precipitating factor is corrected. Specific treatment is aimed at preventing absorption of nitrogenous compounds from the gut, using nonabsorbable disaccharides such as lactulose or lactitol[66,67]. The use of these compounds should be titrated to effect a soft bowel action two to three times daily. Oral neomycin, via its action on gut flora, has also been shown to reduce the absorption of potential nitrogenous toxins but there are well-documented risks of renal toxicity associated with use of the aminoglycoside[68].

A protein-restricted diet is a commonly used measure to manage encephalopathy, but in many instances is unnecessary. This is particularly important in patients with CF, where there may be pre-existing malnutrition. The response to a regulated protein intake should be carefully documented by objective measurements of encephalopathy, using measures such as number connection tests. The oral protein intake need only be reduced if sensitivity is confirmed. The use of feeds enriched with branched-chain amino acids may offer a more readily assimilated amino-acid source for those who show sensitivity to whole protein[69].

Splenomegaly and hypersplenism

Gross splenomegaly with left upper quadrant pain is an infrequent complication of portal hypertension[70]. The majority of patients can be managed by simple analgesia alone. In a very small proportion of patients the severity of symptoms justifies splenectomy. Hypersplenism is a frequently incidental observation in patients with splenomegaly but the low white cell and platelet count is almost always without clinical significance and is not an indication for splenectomy or portal systemic shunt surgery.

The influence of liver disease on organ transplantation

To date there has been no systematic study assessing the influence of established liver disease on lung transplantation. Most transplant programs have excluded patients with overt complications of liver disease, such as variceal bleeding, jaundice or ascites. However, the frequently occult nature of much CF liver disease has inevitably resulted in patients with established focal or diffuse cirrhosis undergoing heart–lung transplantation. Prospective evaluation of such patients during and after transplantation is lacking, but in the Brompton–Harefield series identification of those with evidence of liver disease has not shown postoperative liver decompensation. Of those undergoing heart–lung transplantation, 28 had abnormal liver function tests prior to the procedure. None of these patients were known to have established cirrhosis prior to transplantation and none have been jaundiced. Until further evidence becomes available, it would seem justified to exclude from transplantation patients with persistent jaundice, ascites or encephalopathy. Previous variceal bleeding independent of other signs of decompensation may in itself not represent an absolute contraindication.

EXTRAHEPATIC BILIARY DISEASE IN CYSTIC FIBROSIS

Abnormalities of the extrahepatic biliary system are commonly observed in CF, the pathogenesis of which may be indivisible from that of the biliary liver disease discussed above. Approximately 25 per cent of patients have nonfunctioning gallbladders, and at post-mortem 30 per cent have micro-gallbladders (defined as less than 1.5 cm in length and less than 0.5 cm in width)[26].

Stenosis or atresia of the cystic duct is also common. At post-mortem, 24 per cent of adult CF patients were found to have gallstones[71]. A reduced prevalence in younger patients suggests increasing risk with age. These stones are almost always radiolucent and initial studies suggested that they were of cholesterol origin[72]. It was postulated that bile salt loss in stool, secondary to malabsorption, resulted in bile salt deficiency and supersaturation of bile. This, however, has now been challenged, both on the grounds that bile salt deficiency is unusual, and that analysis of bile in CF shows no evidence of cholesterol supersaturation[73]. Analysis of stones removed from patients with CF has shown the predominant constituents to be calcium bilirubinate and proteinaceous material. The most likely stimulus for stone formation is the low-volume, high-viscosity composition of the bile, although the specific mechanisms involved are unknown.

Complications of cholelithiasis, including biliary colic, cholecystitis and bile-duct obstruction, are well recognized in CF, although they appear to be less frequent than might be predicted from the overall prevalence of gallstones. The management of cholelithiasis should follow current standard procedures[73]. The laparoscopic approach to cholecystectomy may be a less exacting technique than open surgery, particularly in those patients with poor respiratory reserve. The endoscopic approach offers a minimally invasive means of managing choledocholithiasis (Fig. 13.8). This may also be the optimal approach to the management of the small proportion of patients with a distal common bile duct stricture, secondary to chronic pancreatitis. Whether the choloretic effect of ursodeoxycholic acid may have a role in the prevention or management of cholelithiasis has not been formally investigated.

We have recently diagnosed a gallbladder cancer in a man of 40 who presented with biliary colic (in the presence of gallbladder calculi). This provides further evidence in support of the increased risk of gut-related malignancies in patients with CF[74].

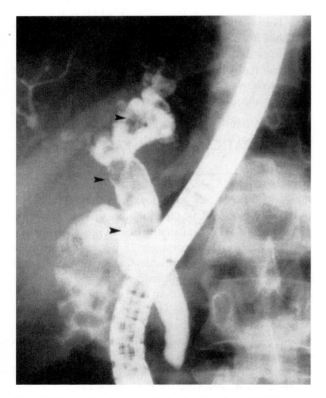

Fig. 13.8 *A cholangiogram obtained at the time of ERCP, showing multiple stones within the common bile duct, common hepatic and intrahepatic ducts (arrowheads). There are also multiple stones within the gallbladder.*

REFERENCES

1. Andersen, D.H. (1938) Cystic fibrosis of pancreas and its relation to coeliac disease. *Am. J. Dis. Child.*, **56**, 344–349 .
2. Roy, C.C., Weber, A.M., Morin, C.C. *et al.* (1982) Hepatobiliary disease in cystic fibrosis: a survery of current issues and concepts. *J. Pediatr. Gastroenterol. Nutr.*, **1**, 469–478.
3. di Sant'Agnese, P.A. and Blanc, W.A. (1956) A distinctive type of biliary cirrhosis associated with cystic fibrosis of the pancreas. *Paediatrics*, **18**, 387–409.
4. Oppenheimer, E.H. and Esterly, J.R. (1975) Hepatic changes in young infants with cystic fibrosis: possible relation to focal biliary cirrhosis. *J. Paediatr.*, **86**, 683–689.
5. Gaskin, K.J., Water, D.L.M., Howman-Giles, R.N. *et al.* (1988) Liver disease and common bile duct stenosis in cystic fibrosis. *NEJM*, **318**, 340–346.
6. Nagel, R.A., Westaby, D., Javaid, A. *et al.* (1989) Liver disease and bile duct abnormalities in adults with cystic fibrosis. *Lancet*, **ii**, 1422–1425.
7. Scott-Jupp, R., Lama, M. and Tanner, M.S. (1991) Prevalence of liver disease in cystic fibrosis. *Arch. Dis. Child.*, **66**, 698–701.
8. Marino, C.R. and Gorelick, F.S. (1992) Scientific advances in cystic fibrosis. *Gastroenterology*, **103**, 681–693.
9. Cohn, J.A., Strong, T.V., Picciotto, M.R., Nairn, A.C., Collins, F.S. and Fitz, J.G. (1993) Localisation of the cystic fibrosis transmembrane conductance regulator in human bile duct epithelial cells. *Gastroenterology*, **105**, 1857–1864.
10. Bhaskar, K.R., Turner, B.S., Grubnian, S.A., Jefferson, D.M. and Lamont, J.T. (1998) Dysregulation of proteoglycan production by intrahepatic biliary epithelial cells bearing defective (Delta-F508) cystic fibrosis transmembrane conductance regulator. *Hepatology*, **27**, 7–14.
11. Linblad, A., Hultcrantz, R. and Strandvik, B. (1992) Bile duct destruction and collagen deposition: a prominent ultrastructural feature of the liver in cystic fibrosis. *Hepatology*, **16**, 372–381.
12. Robb, T.A., Davidson, G.P. and Kirubakaran, C. (1985) Conjugated bile acids in scrum and secretions in response to cholecystokinin secretin stimulation in children with cystic fibrosis. *Gut*, **26**, 1246–1256.
13. Weizman, Z., Durie, P.R. and Kopeinian, H.R. *et al.* (1986) Bile acid secretion in cystic fibrosis: evidence for a defect unrelated to fat malabsorption. *Gut*, **27**, 1043–1048.
14. O'Brien, S., Keogan, M., Caseu, M. *et al.* (1992) Biliary complications of cystic fibrosis. *Gut*, **33**, 387–391.
15. Duthie, A., Doherty, D.G., Williams, C. *et al.* (1992) Genotype analysis for delta F508, G551D and R553X mutations in children and young adults with cystic

fibrosis with and without chronic liver disease. *Hepatology*, **15**, 660–664.

16. Duthie, A., Doherty, D.G., Donaldson, P.T. *et al.* (1990) HLA phenotype and genotype in children and young adults with cystic fibrosis with and without liver disease. *Hepatology*, **12**, 218–223.

17. Miele-Vergani, G., Psacharopoulos, H.T., Nicholson, A.M. *et al.* (1980) *Arch. Dis. Child.*, **55**, 696–701.

18. Furuya, K.N., Roberts, E.A., Canny, G.J. and Philips, M.J. (1991) Neonatal hepatitis syndrome with paucity of interlobular bile ducts in cystic fibrosis. *J. Pediatr. Gastroenterol. Nutr.*, **12**, 127–130.

19. Vaiman, H., France, N. and Wallis, P. (1971) Prolonged neonatal jaundice in cystic fibrosis. *Arch. Dis. Child.*, **46**, 805–809.

20. Treem, W.R. and Stanley, C.A. (1989) Massive hepatomegaly, steatosis and secondary carnitine deficiency in an infant with cystic fibrosis. *Paediatrics*, **83**, 993–997.

21. Navasa, M., Pares, A., Bruguera, M. *et al.* (1987) Portal hypertension in primary biliary cirrhosis. Relationship with histological features. *J. Hepatol.*, **5**, 292–298.

22. Farrant, J.M., Hayllar, K.M., Wilkinson, M.L. *et al.* (1991) Natural history and prognostic variables in primary sclerosing cholangitis. *Gastroenterology*, **100**, 1710–1717.

23. Dickson, E.R., Grambsch, P.M., Flemming, J.R. *et al.* (1989) Prognosis in primary biliary cirrhosis: Model for decision making. *Hepatology*, **10**, 1–7.

24. Hayllar, K.M., Williams, S.G.J., Wise, A.E. *et al.* (1997) A prognostic model for the prediction of survival in cystic fibrosis. *Thorax*, **52**, 313–317.

25. Williams, S.G.J., Samways, J., Innes, J.A. *et al.* (1996) Systemic haemodynamics in patients with cystic fibrosis at rest and during exercise: an adverse effect of underlying liver disease. *J. Hepatol.* **25**, 900–908.

26. McHugo, J.M., McKeown, C., Brown, M.T. *et al.* (1987) Ultrasound findings in children with cystic fibrosis. *Br. J. Radiol.*, **60**, 137–141.

27. Vergesslich, K.A., Gotz, M., Mostbeek, G. *et al.* (1989) Portal venous blood flow in cystic fibrosis: assessment by Duplex Doppler sonography. *Pediatr. Radiol.*, **19**, 371–374.

28. Williams, S.G.J., Evanson, J.E., Barrett, N., Hodson, M.E., Boultbee, J. and Westaby, D. (1995) An ultrasound scoring system for the diagnosis of liver disease in cystic fibrosis. *J. Hepatol.*, **225**, 513–521.

29. Klingensmith, W.C., Fitzberg, A.R., Spitzer, V.M. *et al.* (1980) Clinical comparison of 99m Tc-diethyl-IDA and 99m Tc PIPIDA for evaluation of the hepatobiliary system. *Radiology*, **134**, 195–199.

30. Renner, E.L., Lake, J.R., Cragoe, E.J. *et al.* (1980) Urosdeoxycholic acid choleresis: relationship to biliary HCO_3 and effects of $Na^+ H^+$ exchange inhibitors. *Am. J. Physiol.*, **254**, G232–G241.

31. Hoffman, A.F. (1990) Bile acid hepatotoxicity and the rationale of UCDA therapy in chronic cholestatic liver disease: some hypotheses, in *Strategies for the Treatment of Hepatobiliary Diseases*, (eds G. Paumgartner *et al.*), Kluwer Academic, Dordrecht, The Netherlands, pp. 13–33.

32. Beuers, U., Spengler, U., Zwiebel, F.M. *et al.* (1992) Effect of ursodeoxycholic acid on kinetics of the major hydrophobic bile acids in health and in chronic cholestatic liver disease. *Hepatology*, **15**, 603–608.

33. Yoshikawa, M., Tsijii, T., Matsumura, K. *et al.* (1992) Immunomodulatory effects of ursodeoxycholic acid on immune responses. *Hepatology*, **16**, 358–364.

34. Poupon, R.E., Lindor, K.D., Cauch-Dudek, K., Dickson, E.R., Poupon, R. and Heathcote, E.J. (1997) Combined analysis of randomised controlled trials of ursodeoxycholic acid in primary biliary cirrhosis. *Gastroenterology*, **113**, 884–890.

35. Stiehi, A., Walker, S., Stiehl, L., Rudolph, G., Hofmann, W.J. and Thielmann, L. (1994) Effect of ursodeoxycholic acid on liver and bile duct disease in primary sclerosing cholangitis: a 3 year pilot study with a placebo-controlled period. *J. Hepatol.*, **20**, 57–64.

36. Colombo, C., Setchell, K.D.R., Podda, M. *et al.* (1990) The effects of ursodeoxycholic acid therapy in liver disease associated with cystic fibrosis. *J. Paediatr.*, **117**, 482–489.

37. Cotting, J., Lentze, M. and Reichen, J. (1990) Effects of ursodeoxycholic acid treatment on nutrition and liver function in patients with cystic fibrosis and longstanding cholestasis. *Gut*, **31**, 918–921.

38. Colombo, C., Grosignani, A., Assaiso, M. *et al.* (1992) Ursodeoxycholic acid therapy in cystic fibrosis-associated liver disease: a dose–response study. *Hepatology*, **16**, 924–930.

39. Van De Meeberg, P.C., Houwen, R.H.J., Sinaasappel, M., Heijerman, H.G.M., Bijleveld, C.H.M.A. and Vanberge-Henegouwen, G.P. (1997) Low dose versus high dose ursodeoxycholic acid in cystic fibrosis related cholestatic liver disease. *Scand. J. Gastroenterology*, **32**, 369–373.

40. Colombo, C., Battezzati, P.M., Padda, M., Bettinardi, N. and Giunta, A. (1996) Ursodeoxycholic acid for liver disease associated with cystic fibrosis: A double blind multi-centre trial. *Hepatology*, **23**, 1484–1490.

41. O'Brien, S, Fitzgerald, M.X. and Hegarty, J.E. (1992) A controlled trial of ursodeoxycholic acid treatment in cystic fibrosis related liver disease. *Eur. J. Gastroenterol. Hepatol.*, **4**, 857–863.

42. Linblad, A., Glaumann, H. and Strandvik, B. (1998) A two-year prospective study of the effect of ursodeoxycholic acid on urinary bile acid excretion and liver morphology in cystic fibrosis-associated liver disease. *Hepatology*, **27**, 166–174.

43. Davidson, A.G.F., Wong, L.T.K., Peacock, D., Jamieson, D. and Gravelle, A. (1997) Liver biopsy and evaluation of ursodeoxycholic acid therapy in cystic fibrosis. Proceedings of the 21st EWGCF.

44. Noble-Jamieson, G., Barnes, N., Jamieson, N., Friend, P. and Calne, R. (1996) Liver transplantation for hepatic cirrhosis in cystic fibrosis. *J. Roy. Soc. Med.*, **89**, (Suppl. 27), 31–37.

45. Mack, D.R., Traystman, M.D., Colombo, J.L. *et al*. (1995) Clinical denouement and mutation analysis of patients with cystic fibrosis undergoing liver transplantation for biliary cirrhosis. *J. Pediatr*., **127**, 881–887.

46. Couetil, J.P., Houssin, D.P., Soubrane, O. *et al*. (1995) Combined lung and liver transplantation in patients with cystic fibrosis A 4[half] year experience. *J. Thorac. Cardiovasc. Surg*., **110**, 1415–1422.

47. Dennis, C.M., McNeil, K.D., Dunning, J. *et al*. (1996) Heart–lung–liver transplantation. *J. Heart Lung Transp.*, **15**, 536–538.

48. Yang, Y., Raper, S.E., Cohn, J.A., Engelhardt, J.F. and Wilson, J.M. (1993) An approach for treating the hepatobiliary disease of cystic fibrosis by somatic gene transfer. *Proc. Natl Acad. Sci. USA*, **90**, 4601–4605.

49. Mamadden, Morgan M.Y. (1999) Resting energy expenditure should be measured in patients with cirrhosis not predicted. *Hepatology*, **30**, 655–664.

50. Eid, N.S., Shoemaker, L.R. and Samiec, T.D. (1990) Vitamin A in cystic fibrosis: case report and review of the literature. *J. Pediatr. Gastroenterol. Nutr*., **10**, 265–269, 340–346.

51. Westaby, D. (ed.) (1992) Variceal bleeding. W.B. Saunders, Philadelphia.

52. Westaby, D., Hayes, P., Ginison, A. *et al*. (1989) Controlled clinical trial of injection sclerotherapy for active variceal bleeding. *Hepatology*, **9**, 276–277.

53. Stiegmann, G.Y., Goff, J.S., Sun, J.H. *et al*. (1989) Endoscopic elastic band ligation for active variceal haemorrhage. *Am. Surg*., **55**, 124–128.

54. Vlavianos, P., Gimson, A.E.S., Westaby, D. and Williams, R. (1989) Balloon tamponade for the management of variceal bleeding: uses and misuses. *BMJ*, **298**, 1158.

55. Groszmann, R.J., Kravetz, D., Bosch, J. *et al*. (1982) Nitroglycerin improves the haemodynamic reponse to vasopressin in portal hypertension. *Hepatology*, **2**, 757–762.

56. Bosch, J., Groszmann, R.J., Garcia Pagan, J.C. *et al*. (1989) Association of transdermal nitroglycerin to vasopressin infusion in the treatment of variceal haemorrhage: a placebo controlled clinical trial. *Hepatology*, **10**, 962–968.

57. Ferayorni, L., Polio, J. and Groszmann, R.J. (1996) Drug therapy for portal hypertension: a 5 year review, in *Portal Hypertension*, (ed. R. De Franchis), Blackwell Science, Oxford, pp. 68–99.

58. Conn, H.O. (1993) Transjugular intrahepatic portal systemic shunts: the state of the art. *Hepatology*, **17**, 148–155.

59. Lebrec, D., Poynard, T., Vernau, J. *et al*. (1984) Randomised control study of propranolol for prevention of recurrent gastrointestinal bleeding in patients with cirrhosis: a final report. *Hepatology*, **4**, 355–358.

60. Schuster, S., Shwachman, H., Toyama, W. *et al*. (1977) The management of portal hypertension in cystic fibrosis. *J. Pediatr. Surg*., **12**, 201–206.

61. McCormick, P.A. and Burroughs, A.K. (1992) Prophylaxis for variceal haemorrhage, in *Variceal Bleeding*, (ed. D.Westaby), Saunders, Philadelphia, pp. 167–182.

62. Moore, K., Wilkinson, S. and Williams, R. (1992) Ascites and renal dysfunction in liver disease, in *Wright's Liver and Biliary Disease*, Vol. 11, (eds Millward-Sadler and A.Wright), Saunders, London, pp. 1346–1366.

63. Gines, P., Arroyo, V., Quintero, E. *et al*. (1987) Comparison of paracentesis and diuretics in the treatment of cirrhotics with tense ascites. Results of a randomised study. *Gastroenterology*, **93**, 234–241.

64. Panos, M., Moore, K.P., Vlavianos, V. *et al*. (1990). Single, total paracentesis for tense ascites: sequential haemodynamic changes and right atrial size. *Hepatology*, **11**, 662–667.

65. Arroyo, V., Epstein, M., Gallus, G. *et al*. (1989) Refractory ascites in cirrhosis: mechanism and treatment. *Gastroenterology Int*., **2**, 195–207.

66. Elkington, S.G., Floch, M.U. and Conn, H.O. (1969) Lactulose in the treatment of chronic portal-systemic encephalopathy: A double blind clinical trial. *NEJM*, **281**, 408–413.

67. Morgan, M.Y., Alonso, M. and Stanger, L.C. (1989) Lactitol and lactulose for the treatment of sub-clinical hepatic encephalopathy in cirrhotic patients. *J. Hepatol*., **8**, 208–217.

68. Berk, D.P. and Chalmers, T. (1970) Deafness complicating antibiotic therapy of hepatic encephalopathy. *Ann. Intern. Med*., **73**, 393–396.

69. Horst, D., Grace, N.D., Conn, H.O. *et al*. (1984) Comparison of dietary protein with an oral branched chain enriched amino acid supplement in chronic portal-systemic encephalopathy: a randomised controlled study. *Hepatology*, **4**, 279–287.

70. Psacharopoulos, H.T., Howard, E.R., Portmann, B. *et al*. (1981) Hepatic complications of cystic fibrosis. *Lancet*, **ii**, 78–80.

71. Roy, C.C., Weber, A.M., McRin, C.C. *et al*. (1977) Abnormal biliary lipid composition in cystic fibrosis: effect of pancreatic enzymes. *NEJM*, **297**, 1301–1305.

72. Angelico, M., Gandin, C., Canussi, P. *et al*. (1991) Gallstones in cystic fibrosis: a critical reappraisal. *Hepatology*, **14**, 768–775.

73. Kozarek, R.A. (ed.) (1991) Endoscopic approach to biliary stones. W.B. Saunders, Philadelphia.

74. Neglia, J.P., Fitzsimmons, S.C., Maisonneuve, P., Schoni, M.A., Schoni-Affolter, F. and Lowenfels, A.B. (1995) The risk of cancer among patients with cystic fibrosis. *NEJM*, **332**, (8), 494–499.

Reproductive and sexual health

14

S. M. SAWYER

Introduction	301	Relationships and sexual function	309
Growth and pubertal delay in adolescence	301	Parenting decision making	309
Male reproductive and sexual health	303	Summary	310
Female reproductive and sexual health	305	References	310

INTRODUCTION

An important result of improving survival in people with cystic fibrosis (CF) is that the significance of particular CF-related issues or complications differs physiologically as well as psychologically as children become adolescents and mature as adults. In most large CF centers today, the majority of children are expected to survive through adolescence to face the array of sexual and reproductive health issues negotiated by healthy young people as they mature. Additionally, however, there are significant reproductive and sexual health complications of CF itself. Improved survival in CF now results in reproductive and sexual health issues being of greater significance to a greater proportion of people with CF, with wide-ranging repercussions for individuals with CF, their families and their healthcare professionals.

People with CF risk not being fully informed about reproductive and sexual health issues for a range of reasons. Participation in a specialty CF clinic may be at the expense of primary-care involvement[1] which reduces opportunities for access to universally important reproductive and sexual health education and screening opportunities (e.g. safe sex, PAP smears). Recent studies suggest that young people with CF are not optimally informed about the specific reproductive and sexual health issues affected by CF[2,3]. This may reflect the fact that the attention and expertise of health professionals is on promoting disease stability and survival. However, an integral part of CF management is to ensure that young people are informed of the various impacts of CF at developmentally appropriate times. While there are many unanswered questions deserving further research in this area, the difficulty that health professionals have in discussing reproductive and sexual health topics is another reason why young people are not fully informed[4]. Reliable clinical information and strong communication skills are equally important components of reproductive and sexual health discussions.

GROWTH AND PUBERTAL DELAY IN ADOLESCENCE

Growth has long been recognized to be affected by CF[5-7]. The impressive improvement in growth statistics over the past few decades no doubt reflects improvements in healthcare at many levels. Despite these improvements, however, poor growth continues to be a problem in many adolescents with CF[8-10]. The adolescent growth spurt is delayed by an average of 0.8 years and is about 1 cm/year slower at its peak in young people with CF than in controls[10]. There are significant correlations between pulmonary function and growth parameters, with poor pulmonary function associated with lower growth velocity[10,11]. The US 1990 CF Foundation Data Registry reported that the mean height centile in the 10–24-year age bracket was only 17, and the mean

Table 14.1 *Adolescent male and female height- and weight-for-age percentiles and Z-scores*[13]

Sex	Height-for-age percentile Mean (SD)	Height-for-age Z-score Mean (SD)	Weight-for-age percentile Mean (SD)	Weight-for-age Z-score Mean (SD)
Male	24.6 (22.1)	−0.94 (0.95)	18.3 (17.9)	−1.12 (0.87)
Female	34.5 (27.6)	−0.52 (1.07)	28.6 (23.8)	−0.79 (0.91)
Total	29.1 (25.1)	−0.75 (1.02)	23.0 (21.4)	−0.97 (0.90)

weight centile was 20[12]. Growth data from a representative study of 114 Australian adolescents aged from 10 to 18 years is presented in Table 14.1[13].

Pubertal delay was previously a frequent occurrence in both males and females. While the extent and severity of pubertal delay in contemporary adolescents is less than previously, as with growth delay, pubertal delay is still common. In one contemporary study of adolescents with CF, boys were delayed by a mean of 1.6 years at each Tanner stage of genital development and delayed by 1.1 years for each Tanner stage of pubic hair development[13]. Girls were delayed by a mean of 2.0 years and 2.4 years, respectively[13]. Age of menarche is a reliable indicator of pubertal development and may be delayed in girls with CF. The mean age of menarche was reported as 14.5 years[14], a delay of nearly 2 years from the US norm. Recent studies are more reassuring, with menarche at 13.8 years being less than 1 year delayed from Australian norms[13]. However, 23 per cent of these 22 girls had menarchal delay greater than 2 standard deviations from the mean. Normal adult hormonal function is expected upon maturation.

The association of growth delay with poor respiratory function makes all aspects of growth important to monitor, especially as there are some suggestions that disease progression may be reflected in poor growth several years before major declines in pulmonary function[10]. The promotion of normal growth is also important because of the impact that poor growth and delayed puberty has on bone density, which has greater significance as survival increases. Cross-sectional studies document reduced bone mineral density in children and adolescents with CF, and predictors of reduced bone density include age, pubertal status, body mass, energy expenditure, illness severity, glucocorticoid therapy and gonadal dysfunction[15,16].

The psychological significance of pubertal delay is also known to be highly relevant for the adolescent. General physical appearance shapes human interactions, and the timing of developmental changes in body shape and size in young people are determinants of perceived age, adult care-giving responses and adjustment during the adolescent years[17,18]. The additional burden of pubertal delay for adolescents with chronic illness is not well established. It may be thought that girls with growth delay will be less troubled than boys, as girls with CF who are thin conform to the socially acceptable body shape for women in Western cultures, in contrast to boys, for whom the male physical ideal of body size and strength is less easily achieved. However, pubertal delay negatively affects both males and females with CF[19].

Attention to respiratory and nutritional status is an integral part of CF management at all ages, with regular monitoring of growth and pubertal development an essential component of outpatient review. Meticulous efforts to optimize respiratory function and promote normal growth and pubertal development should be made in both males and females. In addition to strategies to improve respiratory status, consideration should be given to a range of methods to increase caloric input, such as supplementary or gastrostomy feeds. Aggressive nutritional interventions can result in weight gain, and declining respiratory function can at least be stabilized[20,21].

If respiratory and nutritional interventions fail to improve growth, the judicious use of sex steroids in boys with delayed puberty can promote growth and pubertal development, the attainment of peak bone mass and muscle bulk, and improve self-esteem and self-confidence[22,23]. Pubertal delay and delayed virilization are usually cause for complaint in boys by 14 years of age. A range of different testosterone regimens can be used to promote successfully the induction of puberty. Oral androgens have variable absorption but are highly satisfactory for careful and slow induction if the prime indication is for improvement of growth velocity with some virilization. Low-dose (20–40 mg) testosterone undecanoate (Andriol®) can be used daily for 6 months, gradually increasing to 80 mg daily. A stronger androgen is recommended once the bone age reaches 14.5 years if spontaneous pubertal progress has not occurred. Oxandrolone is a weak androgen that has a greater effect on height velocity than on virilization. It is potentially hepatotoxic. While still used to promote growth in short boys, it cannot be recommended.

Puberty can also be induced using 125–250 mg testosterone enanthate intramuscularly (Primoteston Depot®) followed by two further 250 mg injections 3 weeks apart. Hypothalamic–pituitary priming is usually induced by this brief regimen and no further treatment is indicated in the majority of boys. If there has been no ongoing pubertal progress 6–12 months after the initial treatment, continuing treatment of 250 mg at 2-weekly intervals will provide adequate adult levels of testosterone and promote the completion of virilization. These injections cause significant local pain at the injection site. They are also commonly associated with gynecomastia. Subcutaneous crystalline testosterone can satisfactorily complete virilization and is generally preferred over intramuscular injections[23]. A regimen of 300 mg every 6 months is recommended for a bone age from 14.5 to 15.5 years, with the adult dose of 600 mg at 6-monthly intervals thereafter. However, long-term treatment is very infrequently required.

In girls with significant pubertal delay, hormone replacement with continuous daily oral estrogen, initially using 2.5 µg ethinyl estradiol and gradually increasing to 20 µg over 2–3 years, can be used. Abnormal nipple and breast shape can result if the dose is increased too rapidly. The addition of cyclical progestogen at the time of vaginal bleeding, or when the ethinyl estradiol dose reaches 15 µg/day is recommended. Cyclical progesterone is essential once adult estrogen doses are reached to ensure regular endometrial shedding.

Apart from determining the effect that CF has on puberty, the question of what effect puberty has on CF is equally relevant. The deteriorating survival of females relative to males, which is strikingly noted in some CF centers, is most marked during adolescence[24,25]. Whether psychosocial, hormonal, or other biological factors are responsible is not known, but this warrants more extensive research.

MALE REPRODUCTIVE AND SEXUAL HEALTH

Men with CF are azoospermic due to the absence of the vas deferens[26–28]. Most males with CF, regardless of the severity of their respiratory or gastrointestinal disease, have aberrant development of the reproductive portion of the mesonephric (wolffian) duct, accounting for absence or atrophy of the vas deferens, seminal vesicle, ejaculatory duct and body and tail of the epididymis (Fig. 14.1)[29]. There can be variability in the clinical findings: in some men the epididymes are entire and the scrotal portion of one or both of the vasa may be present. Dysfunction (and often absence) of the seminal vesicles accounts for the low volume and acidic ejaculate in men with CF. Testicular histology is normal and active spermatogenesis occurs. Occasionally sperm antibodies develop. Sexual potency is not affected by these abnormalities. However, acute and chronic ill health can impair testicular function and coincidental defective spermatogenesis is relatively common.

Little is known about the reproductive and sexual health knowledge of men with CF, the significance of infertility in adolescent and adult life, or the use of and attitudes toward modern reproductive technologies. Early studies suggested widespread lack of awareness of

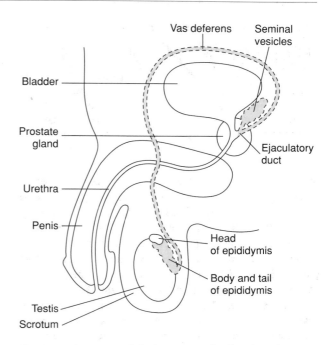

Fig. 14.1 *The mesonephric duct system develops into the ureter and renal pelvis, as well as the seminal vesicles, vas deferens and the body and tail of the epididymis. In cystic fibrosis the general parts of the mesonephric ducts are usually absent (shaded).*

male infertility among both adolescent and adult males and parents[30,31], which suggested widespread lack of communication about male infertility. In a more recent study, 90 per cent of adult males and 60 per cent of adolescent males, but only 50 per cent of parents, knew of male infertility[3]. In an interview survey of the attitudes and practices of 32 CF health professionals about their approaches to discussing male infertility, 68 per cent reported they informed parents soon after diagnosis, 22 per cent waited until later childhood and 10 per cent waited until adolescence to inform parents of infertility[4].

While contemporary health professionals report talking to male adolescents about likely infertility, there are still many barriers to more complete and timely discussions. These include physician and patient embarrassment, insufficient time and insufficient training. Detailed discussion may also be deferred because of concerns of the negative impact of this information[4]. Physicians are encouraged to discuss these issues with adolescents, as the majority of male adolescents report they were not particularly distressed when they first heard about infertility during adolescence[3]. The greater significance of infertility with increasing maturity confirms that, as with all aspects of CF care, these issues need to be revisited on more than one occasion. This is reinforced by a number of misunderstandings that have been reported, such as confusing the meaning of infertility with impotence or the lack of need for contraception with the lack of protection from sexually transmitted diseases[3]. Reassuringly, there is no evidence that the known negative psychological effects of infertility[32] are compounded when known prospectively.

Small-volume ejaculates in men with CF are well described, being generally less than 1.5 mL in comparison to 3.5 mL in healthy controls[26,27]. Many males with CF do not experience nocturnal emissions[3], presumably a consequence of variably reduced semen volume from atretic seminal vesicles. Even in the absence of medical explanation, many males with CF know they have a small-volume ejaculate[3]. Because some are worried about this, an explanation of reduced volume or absent ejaculate should be a routine part of reproductive and sexual health discussions.

Infertility is thought to occur in approximately 98 per cent of men with CF. Bilateral absence of the vas is an easy clinical diagnosis to make, as the normal epididymis and vas are palpable. Retroversion of the testis, in which the epididymis and vas are anterior to the testis instead of posterior, is relatively common and may cause confusion. Semen analysis will confirm azoospermia or identify the small number of men with CF who are

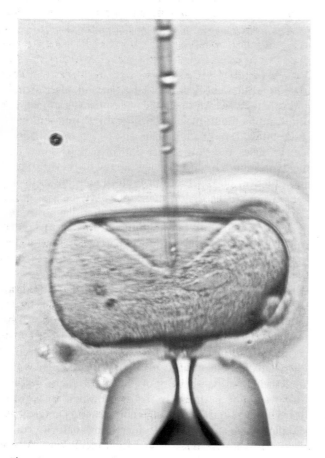

Fig. 14.2 *Intracytoplasmic sperm injection (ICSI). This figure shows the human oocyte being held on a holding pipette and being pierced by a glass pipette containg a single sperm. A single sperm is injected into each oocyte during the process of ICSI and the egg then cultured in a test tube.*

Table 14.2 *Appropriate age to first be told about male infertility, compared with the actual age when this information was given (reproduced with permission from the publishers of Pediatric Pulmonology from Sawyer, S.M., Tully, M.A., Dovey, M. and Colin, A.A. (1998) Reproductive health in males with cystic fibrosis: Knowledge, attitudes, and experiences of patients and their parents. Pediatr. Pulmonol., 25, 226–230; ref.3)*

	No.	Appropriate age	Actual age
Adult males	40	14.2 ± 2.6	16.0 ± 4.7*
Adolescent males	10	–	13.9 ± 1.6
Parents	10	13.9 ± 2.6**	–

*, $P < 0.001$, Wilcoxon matched-pair signed rank sum test;
**, $P = 0.76$, Student's t-test.

potentially fertile. This is more likely in men with particular genotypes such as the 3849 +10 kb C→T mutation[33,34]. Only a minority of men are offered semen analysis through CF clinics. In one study, half of the men offered semen analysis were tested. However, an additional 17 per cent were tested without medical recommendation[3], suggesting the value of this information for some males. The most appropriate time for semen analysis is unknown, but the value of the test appears to be independent of current relationship status. There are no normative data for boys less than 18 years old. Also, testing should not be within a few months of serious illness as usual sperm production is affected by illness. The embarrassment of obtaining a specimen and the sadness and disappointment of the likely negative result suggests that sensitive discussion is required both prior to the test as well as after azoospermia is confirmed.

When is the right age to talk to boys about infertility? Parents should know of likely male infertility so that they can discuss this with their sons at an appropriate time. Health professionals, parents and young people themselves are in general agreement that mid-adolescence is an appropriate time to talk to boys about these issues[3,4] (Table 14.2). Recommended topics to discuss include infertility (including differentiating infertility from impotence, encouraging safe sex practices, and the role of semen analysis), small-volume ejaculates and reproductive options.

The current reproductive options to facilitate parenthood for men with CF, if they and their partner want to have children, are adoption, artificial insemination by donor sperm and microscopic epididymal sperm aspiration (MESA). Most adoption agencies will not accept parents with illnesses likely to reduce their life span. In other countries, long waiting lists for adoption agencies may limit the appropriateness of adoption. There may be advantages in short-term fostering for some individuals and couples. It is not known how frequently these options are utilized.

The assisted reproductive technology known as MESA is a surgical technique to retrieve epididymal and testicular spermatozoa. Use of aspiration techniques to yield epididymal spermatozoa is the preferred method because the large numbers of spermatozoa obtained can be easily frozen and used in subsequent cycles. MESA is usually performed under general anesthesia and the risk of anesthesia and CF needs to be considered. If motile epididymal spermatozoa are not retrievable, testicular biopsy using a fine-needle technique under local anesthesia can be used. There is a minimal risk of intratesticular bleeding and infection following fine-needle biopsy.

Most centers had very poor results with MESA and standard *in vitro* fertilization for congenital bilateral absence of the vas deferens. The newer technique of intracytoplasmic sperm injection (ICSI) involves microinjection of either epididymal or testicular sperm directly into the oocyte[35,36,37]. Significantly higher rates of fertilization have been achieved using ICSI when compared to previous conventional *in vitro* fertilization techniques[37]. Neither CF genotype nor sperm morphology has an adverse effect on fertilization or pregnancy rates using ICSI[38]. A prospective study of 904 pregnancies conceived using ICSI techniques in men with obstructed vas for a variety of causes reported 877 live births (465 singletons, 379 twins and 33 triplets)[39]. An abnormal karyotype was identified in 1.2 per cent of the offspring. All were familial structural aberrations transmitted by the father. Major malformations were observed in 2.6 per cent of live births, within the expected range for children born using assisted reproductive techniques. Between 15 and 40 per cent of ICSI treatments in men with congenital bilateral absence of the vas will result in a live birth[40].

Because of the increased risk of CF in the offspring, both partners should be screened for CFTR mutations. If the female partner is positive for a CFTR mutation, a good outcome can be achieved when MESA–ICSI is coupled with preimplantation embryo diagnosis, with transfer of embryos that are either free of the mutation or carriers[41–43]. However, misdiagnosis is known to have occurred in some cases and preimplantation genetic diagnosis remains a technical challenge.

Congenital bilateral absence of the vas deferens

In contrast to male infertility as fundamental to the clinical picture of CF, congenital bilateral absence of the vas deferens (CBAVD) can occur in otherwise healthy men without coexistent pulmonary or gastrointestinal disease. CBAVD accounts for up to a quarter of men with obstructive azoospermia, which itself accounts for 1–2 per cent of male infertility[44]. Once thought to be a distinct clinical entity, the genetic link between men with CF and those with CBAVD that was first postulated by Holsclaw *et al.*[45] has been confirmed. Genetic similarities between the two conditions, excluding men with CBAVD and renal agenesis, are now well described[46–50]. A small proportion of men with obstructive azoospermia will be found to have the more complete clinical phenotype of CF on more thorough assessment, although the majority of otherwise healthy men with CBAVD have no clinical evidence of CF apart from infertility[51].

The genetic similarities between CF and CBAVD suggest that CFTR mutations are important in the etiology of infertility in both conditions. CFTR mRNA is present in the male genital tract from 18 weeks' gestation, with variable expression in different anatomical regions[52–54]. The pathogenesis of genital tract abnormalities in CBAVD and CF remains unclear and there is currently no explanation of how dysfunctional CFTR causes aberrant duct development in males with CF. What is clear from recent research[55,56] is that there will be far more complex regulation or modulation of currently known CFTR alleles and other unknown alleles than is currently understood.

In this widening spectrum of CFTR-associated disease, a dichotomy is emerging between the perspective of the scientist and that of the clinician and patient. While it is highly appropriate for the scientist to consider CBAVD as part of the spectrum of CFTR-related disorders, it is important to make distinctions between etiology, nosology and the clinical interface. The clinically relevant question is whether CBAVD as an isolated finding should be classified within the spectrum of CF disease or defined as CFTR-associated but distinguishable from clinical CF. While the importance of genetic studies in this area cannot be overstated, caution is advocated in describing CBAVD alone as a mild version of CF in the clinical setting[51].

FEMALE REPRODUCTIVE AND SEXUAL HEALTH

Women with CF have anatomically normal reproductive tracts[57] but abnormalities of cervical mucus have been described[58]. The water content of cervical mucus is reduced in comparison to control subjects, resulting in the formation of thick, tenacious cervical mucus without cyclic variation with ovulation, which may reduce sperm penetration. The success of intrauterine insemination suggests that cervical mucus abnormalities may contribute to infertility in some women[59]. However, while it was widely reported that women with CF have reduced fertility[60,61], the basis of the original report of fertility rates as low as 20 per cent of normal is obscure[58] and there are no systematic studies of fertility rates in women with CF.

Apart from the effect of cervical mucus, women with CF who have very poor nutritional status and severe respiratory disease are likely to have secondary amenorrhea and anovulatory cycles. The combination of improved respiratory function, better nutrition and longer survival means that contemporary young women with CF will have higher fertility rates than previous generations of women. Indeed, the annual number of pregnancies reported to the CF Foundation Data Registry in the United States doubled between 1986 and 1990[62] and included a significant number of unplanned pregnancies.

Adolescents and young women with CF commence sexual activity at the same age as otherwise healthy young women[2]. However, a number of sexually active young women erroneously believe that they have reduced fertility and therefore do not need to use contraception. Women with CF should be considered fertile and contraception should be offered to all sexually active women who do not want to become pregnant.

The range of available contraceptive devices is wider now than ever before, but different factors will determine the most appropriate contraceptive agent for each woman. Barrier methods are safe and effective in motivated patients but are associated with high failure rates in the adolescent population. Tubal ligation is an option to consider for those women who have decided against pregnancy. The oral contraceptive pill is the most common method of contraception in women with CF[2]. Depot progesterone may also suit some women.

There are theoretical concerns about using the oral contraceptive pill in women with CF if complicated by diabetes, cholelithiasis, liver disease, poorly controlled malabsorption or indwelling intravenous access[63]. However, avoiding unplanned pregnancy is a priority, and the risks of contraception need to be balanced with the physiological and psychosocial risks of unplanned pregnancy. Higher pill failure occurs with both short- and long-term antibiotic use[64] although pill failure through this mechanism has not been reported in CF. Malabsorption, ileal resection, active liver disease and poor adherence can all be associated with reduced serum steroid levels and reduced contraceptive reliability. These factors, together with the altered pharmacokinetics of CF, raise concerns that low-dose estrogen preparations will be less reliable in some patients[65]. Estrogen preparations of 50 μgm should provide more reliable contraception.

High rates of symptoms consistent with vaginal yeast infections are reported in women with CF[66], which is likely to reflect the combination of frequently changing systemic antibiotics and the higher than normal prevalence of diabetes mellitus in adult women. It may also reflect an intrinsic alteration of vaginal flora. Inquiring about the frequency of vaginal symptoms prior to changing antibiotics is recommended, as is the concurrent prescription of topical treatment for yeast infections for those women who commonly suffer from vaginal yeast infections with a change in antibiotics. Nebulized antibiotics may be an appropriate alternative for women who suffer from frequent infections.

Women with CF may also suffer from stress incontinence due to frequent coughing, although this has not been reported. It may also be expected that women with CF, especially those with severe disease who are anovulatory, will have hypoestrogenized vaginal epithelium and be at greater risk of dyspareunia. The use of lubricant gels may assist, as might topical and systemic estrogens.

Pregnancy

There have been many single reports of pregnancy in women with CF following the first case report in 1960[67]. Two large series described 129 pregnancies from many centers[68] and 38 pregnancies from a single center[69], and there have been a number of smaller case series reported from single centers[70–74].

The high rates of spontaneous abortion (21 per cent), pre-term delivery (27 per cent) and maternal death (10 per cent) reported in early series[68,70,72] raised serious concerns about the safety of pregnancy for both women and their offspring. The accumulated clinical experience is that pregnancy is generally well tolerated by women with mild disease (FEV_1 > 70 per cent predicted), but that maternal and fetal outcomes are more guarded for those with moderate (FEV_1 50–69 per cent predicted) to severe (FEV_1 <50 per cent predicted) disease. Increasing numbers of women with CF are becoming pregnant, and over 100 pregnancies are reported annually to the US Cystic Fibrosis Data Registry.

A review of 111 pregnancies reported to the Cystic Fibrosis Data Registry in 1990 revealed that 48 per cent of pregnancies were completed, 22 per cent of pregnancies ended in termination and 31 per cent were continuing at that time[62]. Pregnant women represented all severities of lung function. Thirty-seven per cent had mild lung function with FEV_1 > 70 per cent predicted, 26 per cent had more moderate disease, with FEV_1 50–69 per cent predicted and 36 per cent had severe disease with FEV_1 <50 per cent predicted. Women who delivered a live birth at term had the highest level of lung function. Approximately one-quarter of completed pregnancies resulted in a preterm delivery. Women with moderate to severe lung disease were more likely to deliver prematurely or to terminate pregnancy. The outcome of pregnancies reported to the National (US) Patient Data Registry for the 5-year period from 1990 to 1994 is presented in Table 14.3[75]. It is noteworthy that in 1994, 29 per cent of pregnancies reported to the Cystic Fibrosis Foundation's Registry ended in termination of pregnancy.

A number of specific recommendations have been made in regard to pregnancy and CF, but these are all based on the experiences of small numbers of women and have not been validated prospectively[69,72,76]. It is generally accepted that pregnancy is less hazardous in those with milder disease. These women can be reassured that they should tolerate pregnancy relatively well, although the potential for pregnancy to affect significantly the

Table 14.3 *Pregnancy outcomes among pregnant women with CF, 1990–94 (modified from ref. 75)*

	1990	1991	1992	1993	1994
Number of reported pregnancies	114	127	119	133	140
Number of completed pregnancies	70	99	74	99	87
Pregnant and live birth (%*)	45 (64)	72 (73)	54 (73)	74 (75)	62 (71)
Pregnant and still birth (%)	1 (1)	10 (10)	7 (9)	2 (2)	0 (0)
Pregnant and termination (%)	24 (34)	17 (17)	13 (18)	23 (23)	25 (29)
Pregnancy continuing	35	28	39	31	50
Pregnancy outcome uncertain	9	0	6	3	3

* Percentage of completed pregnancies.

health of any women with CF, even for those with mild disease, needs to be understood[77]. It is worrying that a significant proportion of young women with CF do not know that pregnancy has the potential to affect their respiratory status detrimentally[2]. Pregnancy cannot be recommended for those with severe lung disease, especially those with pulmonary hypertension, significant liver disease, poor nutritional status or diabetes. Despite this, a significant proportion of pregnancies occur in those with severe respiratory disease[62]. In this situation, or if there is a worrying deterioration in respiratory status as the pregnancy progresses, careful consideration should be given to therapeutic termination of pregnancy to protect the mother's health[78].

An important issue is whether pregnancy affects adversely the longer-term course of illness in the mother. A large prospective study matched pregnant with non-pregnant women 1 year prior to the year of pregnancy[79]. A total of 372 pregnancies were reported, with 271 live births, 29 still births and 72 terminations. Evaluation of women with a live birth showed that the rate of decline in FEV₁ 2 years after pregnancy was not significantly greater in pregnant than in non-pregnant women with CF. General survival was worse for all women with CF and poor nutritional or pulmonary status, whether they had been pregnant or not, and the 3-year survival rate for pregnant women was 94 per cent compared to survival in the control group of 91 per cent[79]. This is a very important study and the follow-up results will be of great significance for those counseling women with CF about the risks of pregnancy.

Pregnancy in women with CF is best managed when it is a planned event and where there is close collaboration between the medical and obstetric teams. A strong emphasis needs to be placed on achieving the best possible respiratory and nutritional status prior to pregnancy. Pregnancy counseling should include genetic counseling and carrier screening. If the women's partner is not a known CF carrier, the risk of an affected child is 1 in 50, with all unaffected children being carriers. If her partner is a known CF carrier, the risk of a child with CF is 1 in 2. Antenatal screening using chorionic villus sampling can be performed at 8–12 weeks' gestation. In addition to genetic counseling, topics to discuss include the

increased risks to the mother, the increased risks to the fetus, and the complex short- and longer-term issues surrounding parenthood in CF.

Regular monitoring and early treatment of complications will help minimize the risks of pregnancy for both the mother and fetus. Monitoring of pulmonary status should include serial pulmonary function tests, with close monitoring of cardiovascular status. Different approaches to physiotherapy may be required as the pregnancy progresses. A woman's usual exercise regimen may need modifying during pregnancy, with increasing reliance on specific physiotherapy techniques. Increased gastroesophageal reflux is expected in pregnancy generally, which will have repercussions for any physiotherapy regimen involving positioning.

Close involvement with an experienced nutritionist before, during and after pregnancy is recommended for all women with CF considering pregnancy. Close attention should be paid to maternal weight gain. Women with CF are advised to reach 90 per cent of their ideal body weight prior to pregnancy and a weight gain during pregnancy of 12.5 kg is recommended[75]. Consideration should be given to nutritional supplementation for poor weight gain during pregnancy. Nasogastric feeds are better tolerated early rather than later in pregnancy, and women better tolerate continuous rather than bolus feeds[75]. Close monitoring of fetal growth is also required. In addition to regular monitoring of maternal weight gain, close monitoring of endocrine pancreatic function is particularly recommended during pregnancy.

Hospital admission may be required for a range of reasons, including management of hyperemesis, respiratory infection, nutritional supplementation or rest. Consideration of the teratogenic effects of maternal drug use, especially systemic antibiotics, will result in the avoidance of particular drugs during pregnancy if at all possible, although the priority needs to be the mother's health. Review of all medications with an appropriate reference text is recommended (see Table 14.4)[80]. The β-lactam class of antibiotics is generally considered safe during pregnancy. There are no controlled studies of the safety of gentamicin in pregnancy, although there are few concerning case reports. Intravenous gentamicin is safer than some other aminoglycosides, although aerosolized

Table 14.4 *Drug safety in pregnancy (adapted from ref. 80)*

Drug category	Drug name or type	Fetal risk category[a]
Antibiotics	Aztreonam	B
	Cephalosporins	B
	Chloramphenicol	C
	Clavulanate potassium	B
	Gentamicin	C
	Penicillins	B
	Quinolones	C
	Tetracyclines	D
	Tobramycin	C
	Trimethoprim	C
	Vancomycin	C
Antifungals	Amphotericin B	B
	Clotrimazole	B
	Ketoconazole	C
	Nystatin	B
Nonsteroidal anti-inflammatory drugs	Ibuprofen	B (risk category D if used in third trimester)
	Indomethacin	B (risk category D if used for longer than 48 hours, after 34 weeks' gestation or close to delivery)
Sedatives	Chloral hydrate	C
	Diazepam	D
	Ethanol	D (risk category X if used in large amounts)
	Temazepam	X
Antisecretory agents	Cimetidine	B
	Ranitidine	B
Gastrointestinal stimulant	Cisapride	C
Adrenal steroids	Prednisolone	B
	Dexamethasone	C
Bronchodilators	Salbuterol	C
	Theophylline	C
Antidiabetic agents	Insulin	B
Immunosuppressive agents	Cyclosporin	C
	Azathioprine	D
Vitamins	Vitamin A	A (risk category X if taken above recommended daily allowance)
	Vitamin E	A (risk category C if taken above recommended daily allowance)
Pancreatic supplementation		(Not reported in text, but the enteric coating, diethylphthalate, is known to be teratogenic in rats)

[a]Category A: controlled studies in women fail to demonstrate a risk to the fetus in the first trimester (and there is no evidence of risk in later trimesters) and the possibility of fetal harm appears remote.

Category B: either animal-reproduction studies have not demonstrated a fetal risk but there are no controlled studies in pregnant women, or animal-reproduction studies have shown an adverse effect (other than a decrease in fertility) that was not confirmed in controlled studies in women in the first trimester (and there is no evidence of a risk in later trimesters).

Category C: either studies in animals have revealed adverse effects on the fetus (teratogenic or embryocidal or other) and there are no controlled studies in women, or controlled studies in women and animals are not available. Drugs should be given only if the potential benefit justifies the potential risk to the fetus.

Category D: there is positive evidence of human fetal risk but the benefits from use in pregnant women may be acceptable despite the risk.

Category X: studies in animals or humans have demonstrated fetal abnormalities or there is evidence of fetal risk based on human experience, or both, and the risk of the drug in pregnant women clearly outweighs any possible benefit. The drug is contraindicated in women who are, or may become, pregnant.

antibiotics will be safer than intravenous administration due to reduced systemic availability. Less safety data are available concerning vancomycin and ciprofloxacin, although they have been associated with good fetal outcomes.

Close monitoring of the mother is recommended during labor with a low threshold for supplemental oxygen. A vaginal delivery is actively encouraged.

The first analysis of breast milk from a mother with CF was found to be hypernatremic[81] and led to the widespread but erroneous belief that this was a universal finding. The amount of sodium and protein is in fact normal[82–84]. Although a low–normal lipid content has been reported[83,85], analysis of the specific lipid content of milk from six women with CF revealed that in all cases they supplied the energy needs of nursing infants[85]. Breast-feeding in women with CF is generally able to supply sufficient infant energy without a deleterious effect on maternal nutritional status[86], although the additional energy requirements imposed by breast-feeding may be difficult to achieve for some women. Possible drug transmission through breast milk needs to be considered when prescribing medication for the breast-feeding mother, and review of all medications with an appropriate reference text is recommended[80].

RELATIONSHIPS AND SEXUAL FUNCTION

Young people with chronic illness such as CF are at increased risk of low emotional and social well-being, with body image, family connectedness and concern about peer relations being salient explanatory variables[87]. The physical burdens of CF, such as prominent coughing, growth and pubertal delay, surgical scars, and the visibility of permanent intravenous access ports may complicate the development of relationships, or the perception of physical attractiveness and self-worth. Both physical and emotional factors may result in young people being less well connected to a peer group than otherwise healthy young people, with less opportunity for the development of social skills. Family and personal expectations about survival, relationships and children, whether real or perceived, realistic or not, are also likely to be influential factors.

There is no difference in the proportion of young people with chronic illness ever having intercourse or the age of onset of sexual activity when compared to those without CF or other chronic disease[2,3,88]. It is noteworthy that a significantly greater proportion of girls and boys with invisible conditions such as CF report a history of sexual abuse than in those without chronic illness[88].

As respiratory illness progresses and exercise capacity declines, it is normal for interest in sexual activity as well as sexual function to be reduced, at least to some extent. Greater planning and preparation for sexual activity may reduce the spontaneity but increase the enjoyment. Consideration of different sexual position (because of pain or the effect of their partner's body weight, for example), optimizing the time of day to when the person with CF is least fatigued, as well as the use of supplemental oxygen may all improve the enjoyment of sexual activity as well as improving sexual function. While sexual function may decline, the need for intimacy does not. This provides a challenge for individuals with CF and their partners, but particularly for those without partners.

PARENTING DECISION MAKING

Decisions about reproductive options may come more easily to some individuals and couples than to others. A proportion will elect to conceive regardless of any potential health risks; others will try to conceive having made an informed decision. For some, a decision against parenting may be made independently of CF; for others the lack of a partner (which may be due, at least in part, to CF) will reduce the chance of parenthood. However, for many couples living with CF, the added challenge that CF brings to daily life will result in a decision against parenthood. A decision against parenthood will not necessarily alter the sadness associated with known infertility for many men, or the sadness that many women experience knowing they will never be well enough to parent children.

Any decision to proceed with a pregnancy rests with the patient and their partner, not the health professional. However, it is important that the array of issues surrounding conception, antenatal screening, pregnancy and parenting is discussed explicitly and sensitively. Topics need to include the amount of time and energy required to parent children, a frank discussion of likely survival in the face of CF and the implications for the partner and child following the premature death of a parent. These topics are probably as difficult for health professionals to discuss as they are for couples affected by CF.

Health professionals are encouraged to discuss the range of reproductive options in a balanced manner. It is important to ensure that patients are fully informed of new technologies. However, there is a risk that discussion of a newly available technical intervention such as MESA subtly changes the focus from a complex and emotional discussion of infertility and its consequences to a more typical medical consultation, where information is provided to 'fix a problem'. We should recognize that in the very situation where we most want patients to reflect maturely and realistically on the personal risks of parenthood and the future of those children, our own (professional) need to offer technological solutions (that we may find easier to discuss and that may reduce our personal level of discomfort) may also reduce the opportunities for people with CF, both men and women, to start to come to terms with the reality that they may not be well enough to parent children for very long.

SUMMARY

CF has both specific and broad impacts upon the reproductive and sexual health of individuals. The significance of these issues to individuals, as well as the impact on parents, partners and families, changes as the person matures. A single discussion about any of these issues is therefore insufficient. Rather, as with other aspects of CF care, reviewing these topics and tailoring the content to the individual's life stage and level of maturation is an integral component of complete CF care. As young people with CF face the same range of reproductive and sexual health issues as other people, it is important that sexuality education is comprehensive of the range of issues faced by young people.

Discussions about many of these issues are as difficult for physicians as they are for patients and their families. It is important that physicians are themselves fully informed of the reproductive and sexual health issues that affect people with CF. It is, however, equally important that these issues are communicated to young people in an appropriate manner. Sensitivity, empathy and confidentiality should be key components of these consultations.

REFERENCES

1. Carroll, G., Massarelli, E., Opzoomer, A., *et al.* (1983) Adolescents with chronic disease. Are they receiving comprehensive health care? *J. Adolesc. Hlth Care*, **4**, 261–265.
2. Sawyer, S.M., Bowes, G. and Phelan, P.D. (1995) Reproductive health in young women with cystic fibrosis: Knowledge, attitudes and behaviour. *J. Adolesc. Hlth*, **17**, 46–50.
3. Sawyer, S.M., Tully, M.A., Dovey, M. and Colin, A.A. (1998) Reproductive health in males with cystic fibrosis: Knowledge, attitudes, and experiences of patients and their parents. *Pediatr. Pulmonol.*, **25**, 226–230.
4. Sawyer, S.M., Tully, M.A., Dovey, M. and Colin, A.A. (1995) Reproductive health in males with CF. A questionnaire study of the practice and attitudes of CF physicians. North American Cystic Fibrosis Conference. *Pediatr. Pulmonol. Suppl.*, **12**, 389.
5. Shwachman, H. and Kulczycki, L. (1958) Long term study of 105 patients with cystic fibrosis. *Am. J. Dis. Child.*, **96**, 6–15.
6. Sproul, A. and Huang, N. (1964) Growth patterns in children with cystic fibrosis. *J. Pediatr.*, **65**, 664–676.
7. Mitchell-Heggs, P., Mearns, M. and Batten, J. (1976) Cystic fibrosis in adolescents and adults. *Quart. J. Med.*, **179**, 479–504.
8. Soutter, V.L., Kristidis, P., Gruca, M.A. and Gaskin, K.J. (1986) Chronic undernutrition/growth retardation in cystic fibrosis. *Clin. Gastroenterol.*, **15**, 137–155.
9. Haeusler, G., Frisch, H., Waldor, T. and Gotz, M. (1994) Perspectives of longitudinal growth in cystic fibrosis from birth to adult life. *Eur. J. Paediatr.*, **153**, 158–163.
10. Byard, P.J. (1994) The adolescent growth spurt in children with cystic fibrosis. *Ann. Hum. Biol.*, **21**, 229–240.
11. Neijens, H.J., Duiverman, E.J., Kerrebijn, K.F. and Sinaasappel (1986). Influence of respiratory exacerbations on lung function variables and nutritional status in CF patients. *Acta Paediatr. Scand. (Suppl.)*, **317**, 38–41.
12. FitzSimmons, S.C. (1993) The changing epidemiology of cystic fibrosis. *J. Pediatr.*, **122**, 1–9.
13. Sawyer, S.M. (1994) Young people with cystic fibrosis: a re-evaluation of morbity and outcome. Doctorate of Medicine thesis, University of Melbourne.
14. Stead, R.J., Hodson, M.E., Batten, J.C. *et al.* (1987) Amenorrhoea in cystic fibrosis. *Clin. Endocrinol.*, **26**, 187–195.
15. Bhudhikanok, G., Lim, J., Marcus, R., *et al.* (1996) Correlates of osteopenia in patients with cystic fibrosis. *J. Pediatr.*, **97**, 103–111.
16. Henderson, R. and Madsen, C. (1996) Bone density in children and adolescents with cystic fibrosis. *J. Pediatr.*, **128**, 28–34.
17. Alley, T.R. (1983). Growth produced changes in body shape and size as determinants of perceived age and adult caregiving. *Child Dev.*, **4**, 241–248.
18. Petersen, A.C. and Crockett, L. (1985) Pubertal timing and grade effects on adjustment. *J. Youth Adolesc.*, **14**, 191–206.
19. Sawyer, S.M., Rosier, M., Phelan, P.D. and Bowes, G. (1995) Self-image in adolescents with cystic fibrosis. *J. Adolesc. Hlth*, **16**, 204–208.
20. Levy, L., Durie, P., Pencharz, P. and Corey, M. (1985) Effects of long term nutritional supplementation on body composition and clinical status in malnourished children and adolescence with cystic fibrosis. *J. Pediatr.*, **107**, 225–230.
21. Shepherd, R., Holt, T., Thomas, B. *et al.* (1986) Nutritional rehabilitation in cystic fibrosis: controlled studies on effects on nutritional growth retardation, body protein turnover and course of pulmonary disease. *J. Pediatr.*, **109**, 788–794.
22. Landon, C. and Rosenfeld, R.G. (1987) Short stature and pubertal delay in cystic fibrosis. *Pediatrician*, **14**, 253–260.
23. Zacharin, M.R. and Warne, G.L. (1997) Treatment of hypogonadal adolescent boys with long acting subcutaneous testosterone pellets. *Arch. Dis. Child.*, **76**, 495–499.

24. The Australian Cystic Fibrosis Associations Federation National Data Registry (1994) Annual Data Report.

25. Kerem, E., Reisman, J., Corey, M. *et al.* (1992) Prediction of mortality in patients with cystic fibrosis. *NEJM*, **326**, 1187–1190.

26. Denning, C.R., Sommers, S.C., and Quigley, H.J. (1968) Infertility in male patients with cystic fibrosis. *Pediatrics*, **41**, 7–17.

27. Kaplan, E., Shwachman, H., Perlmutter, A.D. *et al.* (1968). Reproductive failure in males with cystic fibrosis. *NEJM*, **279**, 65–69.

28. Landing, B.H., Wells, T.R. and Wang, C.-I. (1969) Abnormality of the epididymis and vas deferens in cystic fibrosis. *Arch. Pathol.*, **88**, 569–580.

29. Oppenheimer, E.H. and Esterley, J.R. (1969) Observations on cystic fibrosis of the pancreas V. Developmental changes in the male genital system. *J. Pediatr.*, **75**, 806–811.

30. Hames, A., Beesley, J. and Nelson, R. (1991) Cystic fibrosis: what do patients know and what else would they like to know? *Respir. Med.*, **85**, 389–392.

31. Nolan, T., Desmond, K., Herlich, R. and Hardy, S. (1986) Knowledge of cystic fibrosis in patients and their parents. *Pediatrics*, **77**, 229–235.

32. Mahlstedt, P.P. (1985) The psychological component of infertility. *Fertil. Steril.*, **43**, 335–346.

33. Stern, R.C., Doershuck, C.F. and Drumm, M. (1995) 3849+10kb C–T mutation and disease severity in cystic fibrosis. *Lancet*, **346**, 274–276.

34. Dreyfus, D.H., Bethel, R. and Gelfand, E.W. (1996) Cystic fibrosis 3849 +10kb C–T mutation associated with severe pulmonary disease and male fertility. *Am. J. Resp. Crit. Care Med.*, **153**, 858–860.

35. Palermo, G., Joris, H., Devroey, P. and Van Steirteghem, A. (1992) Pregnancies after intracytoplasmic injection of single spermatozoon into an oocyte. *Lancet*, **340**, 17–18.

36. Palermo, G., Joris, H., Derde, M. *et al.* (1993) Sperm characteristics and outcome of human assisted fertilization by subzonal insemination and intracytoplasmic sperm injection. *Fertil. Steril.*, **59**, 826–835.

37. Van Steirteghem, A.C., Nagy, Z., Joris, H. *et al.* (1993) High fertilization and implantation rates after intracytoplasmic sperm injection. *Hum. Reprod.*, **8**, 1061–1066.

38. Schlegel, P.N., Cohen, J., Goldstein, M. *et al.* (1995) Cystic fibrosis gene mutations do not affect sperm function during *in vitro* fertilisation with micromanipulation for men with bilateral congenital absence of vas deferens. *Fertil. Steril.*, **64**, 421–426.

39. Bonduelle, M., Wilikens, A., Buysse, A. *et al.* (1996) Prospective follow-up study of 877 children born after intracytoplasmic sperm injection (ICSI), with ejaculated epididymal and testicular spermatozoa and after replacement of cryopreserved embryos obtained after ICSI. *Hum. Reprod.*, **11**, (Suppl. 4), 131–155.

40. Harari, O., Bourne, H., McDonald, M. *et al.* (1995) Intracytoplasmic sperm injection: a major advance in the management of severe male subfertility. *Fertil. Steril.*, **64**, 360–368.

41. Harper, J.C. and Handyside, A.H. (1994) The current status of preimplantation diagnosis. *Curr. Obstet. Gynecol.*, **4**, 143–149.

42. Handyside, A.H., Lesko, J.G., Tarin, J.J., Winston, R.M. and Hughes, M.R. (1992) Birth of a normal girl after *in vitro* fertilization and preimplantation diagnostic testing for cystic fibrosis. *NEJM*, **327**, 905–909.

43. Liu, J., Lissens, W., Silber, S.J. *et al.* (1994) Birth after preimplantation diagnosis of the cystic fibrosis ΔF508 mutation by polymerase chain reaction in human embryos resulting from intracytoplasmic sperm injection with epididymal sperm. *J. Am. Med. Assoc.*, **23**, 1858–1860.

44. Hull, M.G.R., Glazener, C.M.A., Kelly, N.J. *et al.* (1985) Population study of causes, treatment and outcome of infertility. *BMJ*, **291**, 1693–1697.

45. Holsclaw, D.S., Perlmutter, A.D., Jockin, H. and Shwachman, H. (1971) Congenital abnormalities in male patients with cystic fibrosis. *J. Urol.*, **106**, 568–574.

46. Dumur, V., Gervais, R., Rigot, J.M. *et al.* (1990) Abnormal distribution of CF deltaF508 allele in azoospermic men with congenital aplasia of epididymis and vas deferens. *Lancet*, **336**, 512.

47. Rigot, J.M., Lafitte, J.J., Dumur, V. *et al.* (1991) Cystic fibrosis and congenital absence of the vas deferens. *NEJM*, **325**, 64–65.

48. Anguiano, A., Oates, R.D., Amos, J.A. *et al.* (1992) Congenital bilateral absence of the vas deferens. A primarily genital form of cystic fibrosis. *J. Am. Med. Assoc.*, **267**, 1794–1797.

49. Oates, R.D. and Amos, J.A. (1994) The genetic basis of congenital bilateral absence of the vas deferens. *J. Androl.*, **15**, 1–8.

50. Osborne, L.R., Lynch, M., Middleton, P.G. *et al.* (1993) Nasal epithelial ion transport and genetic analysis of infertile men with congenital bilateral absence of the vas deferens. *Hum. Mol. Genet.*, **2**, 1605–1609.

51. Colin, A.A., Sawyer, S.M., Mickel, J.E. *et al.* (1996) Pulmonary function and clinical observations in males with congenital bilateral absence of the vas deferens. *Chest*, **110**, 440–445.

52. Tizzano, E.F., Chitayat, D. and Buchwald, M. (1993) Cell-specific localization of CFTR mRNA shows developmentally regulated expression in human fetal tissues. *Hum. Mol. Genet.*, **2**, 219–224.

53. Trezise, A.E., Chambers, J.A., Wardle, C.J. *et al.* (1993) Expression of the cystic fibrosis gene in human foetal tissues. *Hum. Mol. Genet.*, **2**, 213–218.

54. Tizzano, E.F., Silver, M.M., Chitayat, D. *et al.* (1994) Differential cellular expression of cystic fibrosis transmembrane regulator in human reproductive tissues. Clues for the infertility in patients with cystic fibrosis. *Am. J. Pathol.*, **144**, 906–914.

55. Kiesewetter, S., Macek, M. Jr, Davis, C. *et al.* (1995) A

mutation in CFTR produces different phenotypes depending on chromosomal background. *Nature Genet.*, **5**, 274–278.

56. Chillon, M., Casals, T., Mercier, B. *et al*. (1995) Mutations in the cystic fibrosis gene in patients with congenital absence of the vas deferens. *NEJM*, **332**, 1475–1480.

57. Oppenheimer, E.H. and Esterly, J.R. (1970) Observations on cystic fibrosis of the pancreas.VI. The uterine cervix. *J. Pediatr.*, **77**, 991–995.

58. Kopito, L.E., Kosasky, H.J. and Shwachman, H. (1973) Water and electrolytes in cervical mucus from patients with cystic fibrosis. *Fertil. Steril.*, **24**, 512–516.

59. Kredentser, J.V., Pokrant, C. and McCoshen, J.A. (1996) Intrauterine insemination for infertility due to cystic fibrosis. *Fertil. Steril.*, **45**, 425–426.

60. Brugman, S.M. and Taussig, L.M. (1984) The reproductive system, in *Cystic fibrosis*, (ed. L.M. Taussig), Thième-Stratton, New York, pp. 323–337.

61. Stern, R.C. (1993) Cystic fibrosis and the reproductive system, in *Cystic Fibrosis*, (ed. P.B. Davis), Marcel Dekker, New York, pp. 381–400.

62. Kotloff, R.M., FitzSimmons, S.C. and Fiel, S.B. (1992) Fertility and pregnancy in patients with cystic fibrosis. *Clin. Chest Med.*, **13**, 623–635.

63. FitzPatrick, S.B., Stokes, D.C., Rosenstein, B.J. *et al*. (1984) Use of oral contraceptives in women with cystic fibrosis. *Chest*, **86**, 863–867.

64. Hughes, B.R. and Cunliffe, W.J.(1990) Interactions between the oral contraceptive pill and antibiotics. *Br. J. Dermatol.*, **122**, 717–718.

65. Stead, R.J., Grimmer, S.F.M., Rogers, S.M. *et al*. (1987) Pharmacokinetics of contraceptive steroids in patients with cystic fibrosis. *Thorax*, **42**, 59–64.

66. Sawyer, S.M., Bowes, G. and Phelan, P.D. (1994) Vulvovaginal candidiasis in young women with cystic fibrosis. *BMJ*, **308**, 1690.

67. Siegal, B. and Siegal, S. (1960) Pregnancy and delivery in a patient with cystic fibrosis of the pancreas. *Obstet. Gynecol.*, **16**, 438–440.

68. Cohen, L.F., di Sant'Agnese, P.A. and Friedlander, J. (1980) Cystic fibrosis and pregnancy. A national survey. *Lancet*, **2**, 842–844.

69. Canny, G.J., Corey, M., Livingstone, R.A. *et al*. (1991) Pregnancy and cystic fibrosis. *Obstet. Gynecol.*, **77**, 850–853.

70. Grand, R.J., Talamo, R.C., di Sant'Agnese, P.A. and Shwartz, R.H. (1966) Pregnancy in cystic fibrosis of the pancreas. *J. Am. Med. Assoc.*, **195**, 993–1000.

71. Corkey, C.W.B., Newth, C.J.L., Corey, M. and Levison, H. (1981) Pregnancy in patients with cystic fibrosis: A better prognosis in patients with pancreatic function? *Am. J. Obstet. Gynecol.*, **140**, 737–742.

72. Palmer, J., Dillon-Baker, C., Tecklin, J.S. *et al*. (1983) Pregnancy in patients with cystic fibrosis. *Ann. Int. Med.*, **99**, 596–600.

73. Metz, O. and Metz, S. (1991) Cystic fibrosis and pregnancy. *Monatsschrift Kinderheilkunde*, **139**, 409–412.

74. Jankelson, D., Robinson, M., Parsons, S. *et al*. (1998) Cystic fibrosis and pregnancy. *Aust. NZ J. Obstet. Gynecol.* **38**, (2), 180–184.

75. Hilman, B.C., Aitken, M.L. and Constantinescu, M. (1996) Pregnancy in patients with cystic fibrosis. *Clin. Obstet. Gynecol.*, **39**, 70–86.

76. Larson, J.W. (1972) Cystic fibrosis and pregnancy. *Obstet. Gynecol.*, **39**, 880–883.

77. Frangolias, D.D., Nakielna, E.M. and Wilcox, P.G. (1997) Pregnancy and cystic fibrosis: A case-controlled study. *Chest*, **111**, 963–969.

78. Bose, D., Yentis, S.M. and Fauvel, N.J. (1997) Caesarian section in a parturient with respiratory failure caused by cystic fibrosis. *Anaesthesia*, **52**, 578–582.

79. Fiel, S.B. and FitzSimmons, S. (1995) Pregnancy in patients with cystic fibrosis. *Pediatr. Pulmonol. Suppl.*, **12**, S4.2.

80. Briggs, G.E., Freeman, R.K. and Yaffe, S.J. (1998) *Drugs in pregnancy and lactation. A reference guide to fetal and neonatal risk*, (5th edn), Williams and Wilkins.

81. Whitelaw, A. and Butterfield, A. (1977) High breast milk sodium in cystic fibrosis. *Lancet*, **2**, 1288.

82. Alpert, S.E. and Cormier, A.D. (1983) Normal electrolyte and protein content in milk from mothers with cystic fibrosis: an explanation for the initial report of elevated milk sodium concentration. *J. Pediatr.*, **102**, 77–80.

83. Welch, M.J., Phelps, D.L. and Osher, A.B. (1981) Breast-feeding by a mother with cystic fibrosis. *Pediatrics*, **67**, 664–666.

84. Shiffman, M.L., Seale, T.W., Flux, M. *et al*. (1989) Breast-milk composition in women with cystic fibrosis: report of two cases and a review of the literature. *Am. J. Clin. Nutr.*, **49**, 612–617.

85. Bitman, J., Hamosh, M., Wood, D.L. *et al*. (1987) Lipid composition of milk from mothers with cystic fibrosis. *Pediatrics*, **80**, 927–932.

86. Michel, S.H. and Mueller, D.H. (1994) Impact of lactation on women with cystic fibrosis and their infants: a review of five cases. *J. Am. Diet. Assoc.*, **95**, 159–165.

87. Wolman, C., Resnick, M.D., Harris, L.J. and Blum, R.W. (1994) Emotional well-being among adolescents with and without chronic conditions. *J. Adolesc. Hlth*, **15**, 199–204.

88. Suris, J.C., Resnick, M.D., Cassuto, N. and Blum, R.W. (1996) Sexual behavior of adolescents with chronic disease and disability. *J. Adolesc. Hlth*, **19**, 124–131

15

Other organ systems

15a Other organ systems C. Koch and S. Lanng	314
Diabetes mellitus	314
Nasal polyps and sinusitis	323
Arthropathy, arthritis and vasculitis	324
Amyloidosis	325
Thyroid gland	326
The kidney	327

15b Osteoporosis S. L. Elkin	329
Introduction	329
Bone physiology and measurement of bone mineral density	329
Prevalence of low bone mass in CF	330
Clinical relevance	330
Risk factors	330
Management of bone disease	332
Conclusion	332
References	332

Other organ systems

C. KOCH AND S. LANNG

DIABETES MELLITUS

Incidence and prevalence

Changes in glucose metabolism in patients with cystic fibrosis (CF) were described in 1938 and 1949[1,2] but the association between CF and diabetes mellitus (DM) was first recognized in 1955[3]. In the ensuing years a number of studies reported varying prevalence of impaired glucose tolerance (IGT), ranging between 21 and 75 per cent and that of DM between 0 and 24 per cent[4–32]. The large variations in incidence and prevalence could be due to differences in diagnostic criteria for the diagnosis of IGT and DM and to differences in selection, size and age distribution of the CF population studied. Many earlier studies were surveys of the number of patients with an established diagnosis of diabetes in larger patient populations where actual tolerance tests were not performed in all patients[7,11,12,19,22,23,25,26,29,31]. Most important, however, is the age distribution of the patient populations studied. Many previous publications have drawn attention to the fact that IGT and DM become more frequent with age, the mean age of onset of DM being approximately 20 years[18,22,26,29,31,32].

Two nationwide studies of the prevalence of DM in CF have been published[29,30]. In the study from the Cystic Fibrosis Foundation in the USA, including 15 569 patients (with an unknown ascertainment rate), 4.1 per cent of the patients were diabetic, all treated with insulin[30] but the diagnostic criteria for DM were not stated. In the Danish study, including 278 patients, all tested with the oral glucose tolerance test (OGTT; Table 15.1), with an estimated ascertainment rate above 98 per cent, glucose intolerance was detected in 28.4 per cent of the patients, IGT in 13.7 per cent and DM in 14.7 per cent[29]; 68 per cent of the Danish diabetic CF patients were treated with insulin. The difference in the prevalence of DM between American and Danish CF patients is probably due to the diagnostic criteria used. Thus, in

the USA the OGTT is not used routinely, and since the development of DM in CF is insidious and symptomless, 'diabetes may frequently be underdiagnosed or undetected; the prevalence of diabetes may therefore be higher' in the USA[30].

The Danish study found a prevalence of DM in CF patients aged 10, 20 and 30 years of 1.5 per cent, 13 per cent and 50 per cent, respectively[29] (Fig. 15.1). In parallel, from the age of 15 to 30 years the percentage of patients with normal glucose tolerance (NGT) decreased almost linearly; within this age span the proportion of patients with NGT was reduced by roughly 5 per cent per year among the remaining patients. Thus, 86 per cent of the

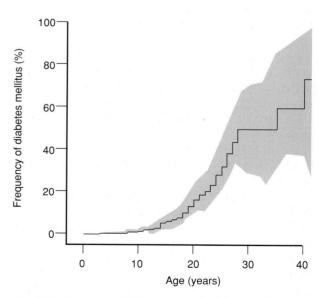

Fig. 15.1 *Percentage of CF patients with diabetes mellitus plotted against age. Based on life-table analysis with 311 CF patients: 278 patients with known glucose tolerance, including 41 diabetics, and 33 patients with unknown glucose tolerance. The shaded area indicates the 95 per cent confidence interval. (Based on data in ref. 29, with permission of the publishers.)*

patients had NGT at the age of 15 years, whereas only 35 per cent had NGT at the age of 25 years[26].

The incidence of DM was studied in a 5-year prospective study of 191 Danish CF patients[31]. The patients, aged 14 years at entry (range 2–40 years), were tested annually with OGTTs. During the 5-year study period, the prevalence of DM increased from 11 per cent to 24 per cent in the study population, with an average annual incidence rate of 3.8 per cent[31]. As expected, the incidence rate of DM increased with age. In patients aged ≥10 years and 20 years or more, the annual incidence rates of DM were 5.0 per cent and 9.3 per cent, respectively, and 12 per cent of the patients aged 10–19 years had developed DM during the 5-year study period, versus 46 per cent of the patients aged 20 years or more[31].

The important conclusion to be drawn from these studies is that abnormal glucose tolerance is not an 'all or none' phenomenon, but that it appears that there is a gradual transition with age of the patient from NGT, through IGT, and further progression to DM.

Diagnosis of diabetes mellitus

It is highly characteristic that diabetic CF patients are often asymptomatic and unlikely to present with ketoacidosis[4,5,8,11,12,18,20,26,29,33] which thereby clearly separates this type of DM from type 1 (insulin-dependent diabetes mellitus, IDDM). It must, however, be emphasized that the diagnosis of DM in CF patients must be based upon criteria universally accepted to be adequate when dealing with type 1 (IDDM), as well as type 2 (non-insulin-dependent diabetes mellitus, NIDDM) diabetes[34].

In the Danish 5-year prospective study of glucose tolerance, DM was suspected on clinical grounds (polyuria, polydipsia, loss in weight, blurred vision) in only 33 per cent of the patients, and only 4 per cent of the patients had ketonuria (without acidosis) at the time of diagnosis of DM[31].

Unless DM has been confirmed by the presence of clear-cut hyperglycemic symptoms and a random capillary plasma glucose concentration of 12.2 mmol/L or greater, or repeated fasting capillary plasma glucose levels of 7.8 mmol/L or more, the diagnosis in all types of DM should be based on an OGTT[34]. According to WHO criteria, the blood glucose concentration measured 2 hours after an oral glucose load is used to classify the degree of glucose tolerance (Table 15.1). The requirement for diagnostic confirmation in the asymptomatic patient with a blood glucose value found to be just above the diagnostic cut-off value will differ from that for a patient presenting with severe symptoms and gross hyperglycemia. For the asymptomatic patient, at least one additional OGTT with a value in the diabetic range is desirable[34].

Table 15.1 *Classification of glucose tolerance*

Oral glucose tolerance test (WHO 1985)[34]: 1.75 g glucose monohydrate/kg body weight, max. 75 g
Classification of glucose tolerance according to capillary plasma glucose concentration (mmol/L) 2 hours after the glucose load:
normal glucose tolerance (NGT) : ≤8.8
impaired glucose tolerance (IGT) : 8.9–12.2
diabetes mellitus (DM) : ≥12.2

Although the OGTT is recommended as the standard diagnostic test for the diagnosis of DM in CF patients with equivocal or no symptoms of DM, the test is relatively laborious. Therefore, simpler screening procedures, i.e. testing for glycosuria, fasting blood glucose concentration or glycated hemoglobin level, have been suggested for use in CF patients[13,20,27,33,35].

The reliability of the use of glycosuria as a diagnostic criterion for DM has not been evaluated systematically in CF patients. However, urine glucose testing, both fasting and postprandially, is not sufficiently sensitive to diagnose patients with IDDM and NIDDM[34].

Interpretation of fasting blood glucose concentration requires care because true fasting cannot be assured, which may lead to the false positive diagnosis of DM[34]. Moreover, a normal fasting blood glucose concentration does not ensure a nondiabetic oral glucose tolerance. Thus, the fasting plasma glucose concentration at the diagnosis of DM was 6.7 mmol/L (4.1–9.0 mmol/L) in the Danish diabetic CF patients[31]; only 16 per cent of the newly diagnosed diabetic patients had fasting plasma glucose values above the upper normal limit of 7.8 mmol/L[34]. The positive and negative predictive values of a fasting plasma glucose of 7.8 mmol/L or more on the day of the OGTT diagnosed as diabetic were 33 per cent and 96 per cent, respectively. Two other groups have also found that measurement of the fasting blood glucose level is not a reliable marker of DM in CF patients[20,28].

Glycated hemoglobin levels provide an integrated index of glycemia 4–6 weeks in retrospect. WHO, however, advises against the use of HbA_{1c} measurements as a screening test for DM, because of inadequate standardization with the risk of substantial misclassification compared to the OGTT[34]. In the Danish prospective study, the HbA_{1c} level at the diagnosis of DM was 5.8 per cent (4.8–9.3 per cent; normal range 4.1–6.4 per cent) and the ranges of HbA_{1c} values greatly overlapped between the groups with NGT, IGT and DM[31]; only 16 per cent of the newly diagnosed diabetic patients had HbA_{1c} levels above the upper normal limit. The positive and negative predictive values of a HbA_{1c} level greater than 6.4 per cent on the day of the OGTT were 50 and 96 per cent, respectively. Other groups have also reported the measurement of HbA_{1c} to be of limited value, if any, in the diagnosis of DM in CF[22,27,28].

Although we, the authors, have confirmed the use of annual OGTT, some CF centers find it time-consuming for the patient and inconvenient for a patient who is traveling a long distance to have to go fasting. These centers recommend HbA_{1c} measurements together with either random or fasting blood glucose and assessment of hyperglycemic symptoms and proceed to an OGTT only when one of the previous three are abnormal. We believe that these screening procedures postpone or even miss the DM diagnosis.

In conclusion, screening for glycosuria, fasting hyperglycemia, or increased HbA_{1c} levels cannot reliably identify CF patients with DM. The OGTT is therefore mandatory as a screening test for DM in the CF population. When the OGTT is diabetic, the diagnosis can only be accepted in patients with symptoms of hyperglycemia[34]. When the OGTT is diabetic in a patient without symptoms of hyperglycemia, one additional OGTT is required in order to confirm the diagnosis of DM, according to WHO[34]. Since only two of the 46 Danish diabetic CF patients developed DM before the age of 10 years, and since both presented with frank symptoms of hyperglycemia and ketonuria, annual OGTTs are now performed in all CF patients aged 10 years or more in the Danish CF clinic.

Finally, it should be added that in 1997 an expert committee, sponsored by the American Diabetes Association (ADA), has suggested new lower fasting criteria for DM (fasting capillary plasma glucose of ≥ 7.0 mmol/L, as opposed to ≥ 7.8 mmol/L in the WHO criteria[34])[36]. Moreover, for screening purposes, an intermediate group of subjects has been suggested. who, although not meeting the criteria for DM, have impaired fasting glucose levels of 6.1–6.9 mmol/L.

These new criteria, suggested by ADA, have not been validated in CF patients, and they are not yet universally adopted, but are under consideration by WHO. Since the most recent studies of glucose tolerance in CF are based upon 2 hours' post-glucose load values (which are similar in the WHO criteria and the ADA suggestion), estimates of incidence and prevalence are unchanged.

Etiology and pathogenesis

Since the discovery and cloning of the *CFTR* gene, it has been possible to search for expression at the mRNA level and at the gene product level in various tissues. The evidence today suggests that CFTR mRNA in the pancreas is present in the centroacinar cells of the intercalated duct but not in the surrounding serous acini or in the islets of Langerhans[37]. Correspondingly, the CFTR gene product is detectable in the centroacinar epithelial cells and intralobular cells lining the small ducts but not in the acinar cells[38,39].

The pathogenesis underlying the gradual development of insulinopenia in CF is generally believed to be due to gradual loss of beta-cell mass. The vast majority of CF patients have exocrine pancreatic insufficiency, and in these patients essentially all functional exocrine pancreatic tissue is eventually destroyed so that the ratio of endocrine cells versus exocrine parenchyma is increased from 1:20 to 1:5[40]. In very young patients, the gross appearance of the pancreas may be nearly normal, while the pancreas in older patients is usually smaller, thinner and firmer than normal and sometimes with visible cyst formation[41]. The early microscopic changes reveal dilatation of the acini and ductules, which contain an amorphous eosinophilic material, with flattening of the epithelium; small cysts are common and represent ducts or ductules[42]. The islets of Langerhans seem to be preserved for some time but later in life there is loss of acinar tissue and the islets exist in more or less fragmented clusters separated by fibrous and fatty tissue[5,43]. Apparently, decreased islet-cell function results primarily from loss of both beta and later alpha cells, but abnormal endocrine function may also be caused in part by impairment of blood supply, as well as by slight inflammatory infiltration, often with predominance of eosinophils, and, hypothetically, disturbed paracrine function between the islet cells[41,43].

DM in CF patients is invariably associated with widespread pathohistological changes in the exocrine pancreas and occurs against a background of exocrine pancreatic insufficiency[14,44]. A number of studies have been carried out in order to establish the relationship between genotype and phenotype in CF patients. CF patients homozygous for the ΔF_{508} mutation have a more severe clinical course, including a greater frequency of exocrine pancreatic insufficiency, than do compound heterozygous patients with only one copy of ΔF_{508}[45–49]. If the exocrine dysfunction causes the endocrine dysfunction, a higher frequency of DM would be expected in CF patients homozygous for ΔF_{508}. However, in the Danish CF population, in which 76 per cent of 211 CF patients were homozygous and 22 per cent were compound heterozygous for ΔF_{508}, exocrine (as judged by the intake of pancreatic enzyme capsules) but not endocrine (as judged by the OGTT[34]) pancreatic insufficiency was more pronounced in the homozygous than in the compound heterozygous patients, and the age at diagnosis of DM was similar in homozygous and compound heterozygous patients[49]. The ΔF_{508} mutation is only one of many severe mutations leading to exocrine pancreatic insufficiency, and further studies are needed to reveal a possible relationship between a specific CF genotype and the development of DM. DM in CF is not characterized by a positive family history of DM[32].

The progressive pancreatic destruction contributes to disposition to DM in CF, but cannot solely explain the development of DM, because more than the 50 per cent reduction in beta-cell mass seen in diabetic CF patients is needed to produce clinical disease in IDDM.

Not all CF patients with exocrine pancreatic insufficiency develop DM, so availability of a genetic and/or an immunological marker for DM in CF would be highly desirable, in order to identify patients at risk of DM. The major histocompatibility genes HLA-DR3, -DR4 and -DR3/4 within the HLA class II region normally confer susceptibility and HLA-DR2 normally confers resistance to the development of IDDM[50]. Earlier studies disagree about involvement of HLA genes in the pathogenesis of DM in CF[28,51–53]. In 34 Danish diabetic CF patients, the distribution of the IDDM-related HLA-DR types did not differ from those in matched CF patients without DM and in normal subjects, whereas the distribution of the HLA-DR types in both patient groups differed significantly from that in IDDM patients[54]. In another study, the HLA class II gene HLA-DQB1*0201 (Asp57⁻) was found to be more frequent in 26 insulin-treated diabetic CF patients from one clinic (69 per cent) than in 41 nonmatched, apparently nondiabetic CF patients from another clinic (48 per cent) and in control subjects (50 per cent)[55].

Islet-cell cytoplasmic antibodies (ICCA) are detectable in 60–85 per cent of newly diagnosed IDDM patients[34], and are present for years before the clinical onset of IDDM[56]. The role of autoimmunity in DM associated with CF is disputed. Some groups have reported the presence of ICCA in 15–18 per cent of their diabetic CF patients, particularly in patients with HLA-DR3 or HLA-DR4 genes[51,52], while others have failed to detect ICCA in any of their diabetic CF patients[27,28,57–59]. One study has compared ICCA in diabetic CF patients with that in nondiabetic CF patients, 5 years and 1 year before and at the time of diagnosis of DM in the index cases and 1 year after the diagnosis of DM. Of 236 sera tested for ICCA, only two (0.8 per cent) were slightly positive, so this finding strongly argues against a role of autoimmunity in the development of DM in CF[54]. Insulin autoantibodies (IAA) have only been measured in one study in CF patients, none of the 21 patients (including two with DM) had IAA[58].

Subjects who develop DM may pass through a phase of IGT, which describes a nondiabetic condition of glucose tolerance outside the normal range that can only be detected by an OGTT. IGT is a risk marker for the development of DM in CF because the odds ratio for the development of DM was 5.6 compared to NGT[31]; 21 out of the 25 patients who developed DM during a 5-year prospective study, had at least one previous IGT. However, 58 per cent of OGTTs showing IGT in CF patients were normalized at the following OGTT, whereas only 14 per cent had deteriorated to DM. Thus, IGT is a risk marker for the development of DM in CF, but the usefulness of the IGT class is limited by the variability of the response to an oral glucose load[32].

Pathophysiology

Several factors may be of importance for the abnormal development of glucose homeostasis in CF patients:

1. impaired function of the beta cells (insulin, C peptide, proinsulin);
2. impaired function of other islets cells, such as alpha cells (pancreatic glucagon) and pancreatic polypeptide (PP) cells;
3. impaired secretion of insulinotropic gut hormones (glucagon-like peptide-1 7–36 amide (GLP-1), gastric inhibitory polypeptide (GIP) and enteroglucagon) normally released from the small intestine following the ingestion of food (entero-insular axis);
4. changes in insulin sensitivity; and
5. changes in insulin clearance rate.

BETA-CELL FUNCTION

The insulin response to OGTT, intravenous glucose, intravenous glucagon, intravenous arginine, intravenous tolbutamide, test meal and milk becomes increasingly impaired – delayed as well as blunted – with decreasing glucose tolerance in CF patients[5,9,10,14–16,21,27,44,59–71]. Most studies were carried out in CF patients with NGT, and even in these patients, insulin secretion is blunted and delayed[5,10,15,16,68,71] or delayed only[9,14,21,27,44,59,67,70]. After an oral glucose load, the incremental insulin area above baseline decreases with decreasing glucose tolerance (on average 88 per cent, 87 per cent and 45 per cent of normal in CF patients with NGT, IGT and DM, respectively), and the time to peak insulin concentration is increasingly delayed from around 30–60 min in healthy subjects to around 90–120 min in diabetic CF patients[68] (Fig. 15.2).

In response to intravenous glucagon, the incremental insulin area above baseline also decreases with decreasing glucose tolerance, while the time to peak insulin levels does not differ between CF patients with NGT, IGT or DM and normal subjects[68].

The initial insulin and C-peptide responses to oral glucose (incremental areas over the first 30 min postload) decrease proportionately with decreasing glucose tolerance, and are positively correlated with the 6-min postglucagon C-peptide concentration[68]. Therefore, the 6-min postglucagon C-peptide concentration gives a valid estimate of residual beta-cell function in CF patients, as is the case in patients with IDDM and NIDDM[72].

The first-phase insulin and C-peptide responses to intravenous glucose in CF patients with NGT are reported to be normal[14,70] or impaired[9,44,59,71], and are always impaired in diabetic CF patients[9,14,44,70]. Unlike patients with NIDDM, diabetic CF patients have no enhancement in the first-phase insulin and C-peptide responses to intravenous glucose when their fasting glucose levels are normalized by an overnight exogenous insulin infusion[44]. These findings argue against a glucoreceptor abnormality, but favor the importance of the loss and disorganization of beta cells in the pathophysiology of glucose intolerance in CF, as does the fact that delayed and blunted insulin responses to oral glucose

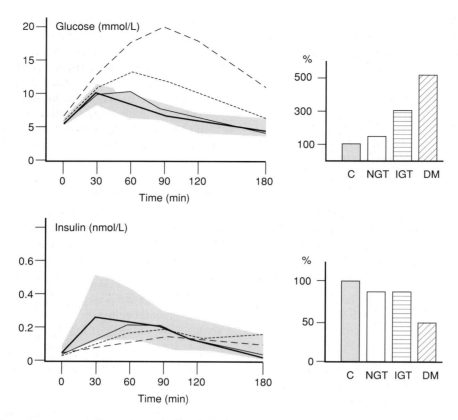

Fig. 15.2 *Insulin response to oral glucose in cystic fibrosis patients with normal glucose tolerance (NGT; thin, solid lines; N = 14), impaired glucose tolerance (IGT; dotted lines, N = 4), diabetes mellitus (DM; broken lines; N = 12) and in normal subjects (C; thick, solid lines; N = 10). Left: median values with normal range (shaded areas). Right: relative incremental areas abone baseline with normal subject set as 100 per cent. (Based on data in ref. 32.)*

have also been observed in patients with DM secondary to chronic pancreatitis[73] and in hemipancreatectomized healthy humans[74].

ALPHA-CELL FUNCTION

Most authors have found normal fasting glucagon concentrations in CF patients with NGT and DM[10,15,44,62,64,68]. Arginine infusion stimulates glucagon secretion in normal subjects, and this response is exaggerated in IDDM and NIDDM[75]. The arginine-stimulated glucagon response has been found to be normal[10,15] or decreased[44,60,61] in CF patients with NGT, and normal[15] or decreased[10,44,60,61,69] in diabetic CF patients. The glucagon response to insulin-induced hypoglycemia is decreased in CF patients with NGT as well as with DM[44].

Oral glucose normally suppresses glucagon secretion, but this suppressibility is impaired or absent in IDDM and NIDDM[76]. Following oral glucose, the decremental glucagon area below baseline decreases with decreasing glucose tolerance in CF patients (on average 68 per cent, 30 per cent and 14 per cent of normal in CF patients with NGT, IGT and DM, respectively)[68]. Other groups also reported impaired suppressibility of glucagon after

oral glucose in CF patients, but not significantly so compared to controls[10,15]. It may be suggested that the presence of insulinopenia together with an impaired glucagon secretion might maintain glucose tolerance, and, for a while, delay DM in CF.

PP CELL FUNCTION

A remarkable feature of endocrine function in CF is the low basal PP level in CF patients with exocrine pancreatic insufficiency, whether diabetic or not[44,62,64–66]. Following various stimuli, PP responses are also absent in these patients[44,62,64–66,68]. In contrast, CF patients with exocrine pancreatic sufficiency have normal basal PP levels and normal or slightly blunted stimulated PP responses[44,55]. Since the number of PP cells in the islets of Langerhans in CF patients is apparently normal[40], the dichotomy between complete absence of stimulated PP responses in CF patients with exocrine pancreatic insufficiency, whether NGT, IGT or DM[68], and presence of almost normal PP responses in CF patients with exocrine pancreatic sufficiency[44,65] may suggest a CF gene-related defect in PP cells. To our knowledge, however, there are no published data on *CFTR* gene expression in PP cells. In both nondiabetic and diabetic patients with chronic pancreatitis (without CF), PP secretion is also severely impaired, but in these patients the impairment has been ascribed to the progressive loss of PP cells[77,78].

THE ENTERO-INSULAR AXIS

Disturbances in the 'entero-insular axis', through which gut hormones (incretins) are released into the circulation during glucose absorption, are postulated to influence insulin secretion and could be involved in the pathogenesis of glucose intolerance in CF. The major incretins are believed to be GIP and GLP-1, with the latter considered the most potent[79]. Fasting GIP levels have been found to be normal[14,63,64,68] or increased[14,62] in CF patients with NGT, and normal[68] or increased[14] in diabetic CF patients. In CF patients with NGT, the GIP response to oral glucose is either normal[14,68] or increased[63], while GIP levels following a test meal[64] or milk ingestion[62] are decreased. In diabetic CF patients, GIP responses after oral glucose are normal[68] or increased[14].

In a study of GLP-1 in CF patients, no differences in GLP-1 concentrations were observed between healthy subjects and CF patients with NGT, IGT or DM, neither fasting nor following an oral glucose load[68].

INSULIN SENSITIVITY

Insulin sensitivity is an important determinant of glucose tolerance, particularly in NIDDM patients. Results of studies of insulin sensitivity in CF patients are divergent. Earlier studies, applying OGTT, various insulin/glucose ratios, continuous glucose infusion (CIGMA)[80] or intravenous glucose (Bergman's minimal model)[81] as markers of insulin sensitivity, have reported increased[5,9,10,16], normal[68,80] or decreased[62,81,82] insulin sensitivity in CF patients with NGT, and decreased insulin sensitivity in diabetic CF patients[68,81]. The method most widely accepted and used to study insulin sensitivity is the hyperinsulinemic normoglycemic glucose clamp technique[83]. By this method, insulin sensitivity has been found to be normal[59,84,85], increased[86,87] or decreased in CF patients with NGT[88], and normal[84,85] or decreased in diabetic CF patients[87,88].

Several reasons for the divergent results of glucose clamp-derived measures of insulin sensitivity in CF exist. But when insulin sensitivity, indicated as the M/I ratio corrected for body weight, was compared in adult CF patients with well-defined glucose tolerance (NGT and DM, WHO criteria) and in healthy subjects, clamped at a blood glucose level sufficiently low to suppress endogenous insulin secretion and hepatic glucose production, it was normal in CF patients, whether NGT or DM[85]. Using a very similar design, Ahmad and coworkers observed an increased insulin sensitivity in a group of younger CF patients who were heterogeneous in terms of glucose intolerance[86].

Therefore, insulin resistance seems not to be of primary pathophysiological importance for the development of DM in CF. However, as in poorly controlled IDDM and NIDDM patients, whose insulin sensitivity can be improved by near-normalization of the glycemic level, diabetic CF patients may be insulin resistant secondary to their level of glycemic control. Thus diabetic CF patients with HbA_{1c} levels of 6.0 per cent or more had lower insulin sensitivity than those with HbA_{1c} below 6.0 per cent[85].

INSULIN CLEARANCE RATE

Studies of insulin kinetics have shown that the insulin clearance rate (MCR_{ins}) is increased by 30–40 per cent in CF patients[85,86], by equal amounts in diabetic and nondiabetic patients[85], and after correction for lean body mass[86]. Insulin degradation is at least partially receptor mediated. The number of insulin receptors on monocytes has been shown to be normal[59] or increased[82,89] in nondiabetic CF patients. An increased number of insulin receptors, if present, could result in an increased receptor-mediated insulin degradation and hence partly explain the insulinopenia seen in CF, even in patients with NGT.

In conclusion, the diabetic condition in CF is characterized by impaired and delayed insulin secretion and impaired glucagon suppression after oral glucose, by increased insulin clearance rate and probably by normal insulin sensitivity. Even in nondiabetic CF patients, insulin secretion is impaired and the insulin clearance rate is increased, so that changes in insulin secretion and insulin clearance rate precede the development of DM. Whether the impaired insulin secretion precedes the increase in insulin clearance rate, or vice versa, remains to be established. The entero-insular axis is intact, and the PP response is absent in CF patients with exocrine pancreatic insufficiency, whether diabetic or not.

Clinical features

DM in CF patients mostly develops insidiously, without symptoms and is unlikely to present with ketoacidosis, either at the time of diagnosis of DM or in the course of DM[4,5,8,11,12,18,20,26,33]. Symptoms of hyperglycemia such as polyuria, polydipsia, loss of weight, marked fatigue and blurred vision are only present at the diagnosis of DM in about one-third of the patients[31].

The median age at diagnosis of DM is approximately 20 years[18,22,25,31,33]. Data from some groups indicate that females develop DM at a younger age than males[18,22,33], while others do not find any statistically significant difference[31].

Precipitating factors for the development of DM in CF patients are severe lung infections[18,22,32], treatment with corticosteroids[31,33,35] and hyperalimentation, either administered parenterally or by gastric tubes[33,35].

CYSTIC FIBROSIS CLINICAL STATUS IN PREDIABETES

Whether diabetic or not, the overall clinical status of CF patients gradually declines with age, including lung function and liver involvement. It is debated whether the prediabetic condition accentuates the decline in overall clinical status over years.

Progressive clinical deterioration in CF patients with prediabetes has been reported by some groups[22,90], but was not detected by others[18,25]. Rodman and coworkers compared clinical status on two occasions (5 years before and at the diagnosis of DM) in prediabetic CF patients with those in two groups of patients with NGT and IGT[18]. They were unable to detect any differences between the three groups in the rate of deterioration of the clinical scores, lung function and the number of lung infections with *Pseudomonas aeruginosa*, *Staphylococcus aureus*, *Haemophilus influenzae* and *Streptococcus pneumoniae*. Reisman and coworkers were also unable to detect any differences in FEV$_1$ between 31 'insulin-dependent' diabetic and 31 matched nondiabetic patients tested on two occasions, 5 years before and at the diagnosis of DM[25]. Finkelstein and coworkers reported a progressive decrease over 10 years of the clinical score in 'insulin-dependent' diabetic CF patients compared to a matched control group[22]. The difference in clinical scores between their groups reached statistical significance 2 years prior to the diagnosis of DM.

Lanng and coworkers compared the impact of the prediabetic condition on clinical status in 38 diabetic CF patients and in 38 CF patients with NGT[34], carefully matched in pairs according to sex, age and presence of chronic *P. aeruginosa* lung infection at the diagnosis of DM in the index case[90]. Clinical parameters (height, weight, body mass index (BMI), FEV$_1$, FVC and lung infections) were retrospectively studied quarterly for 6 years prior to the diagnosis of DM in the index cases. Neither at entry nor at any point in time during the study period or at the diagnosis of DM did the clinical parameters differ significantly between the prediabetic and the control patients. Over the 6 years, however, BMI, lung function and intake of pancreatic enzymes deviated significantly in the prediabetic group from those in the control group. Statistically significant differences in weight, BMI, FEV$_1$, FVC and intake in pancreatic enzymes between the two groups emerged 4, 4, 1.25, 3, and 4.5 years prior to the diagnosis of DM, respectively. All these changes indicate that an insidious decline in CF clinical status precedes the development of DM by several years. The decline in clinical status in prediabetic patients was not due to worsening in the number of lung infections, because the percentages of sputum cultures positive for *S. aureus*, *H. influenzae* and *S. pneumoniae*

and the precipitins against *P. aeruginosa* were similar in the two study groups[90].

EFFECT OF INSULIN THERAPY ON CLINICAL STATUS IN DIABETIC CYSTIC FIBROSIS PATIENTS

Is the clinical deterioration in the prediabetic CF patients, which was reported by two[22,90] of four groups including matched control groups[18,22,25,90], a result of deterioration in CF clinical status leading to DM, or a result of the prediabetic condition leading to deterioration in the CF clinical status?

Three groups have studied CF clinical status after the diagnosis of DM[18,25,91]. Rodman and coworkers and Reisman and coworkers were unable to detect any differences in clinical status between their groups, when tested at, and 5 years after, the diagnosis of DM[18,25]. However, the data of Reisman and coworkers show that FEV$_1$, measured 5 years after the diagnosis of DM in the insulin-treated patients, was similar to that measured at the diagnosis of DM, whereas FEV$_1$ in the control patients had decreased further to the level of the diabetic patients, indicating a postponement of clinical deterioration during insulin therapy.

Lanng *et al.* compared 18 diabetic CF patients, who had been treated with insulin for at least 2 years, with 18 CF patients with NGT, matched in pairs according to age, sex and presence of chronic *P. aeruginosa* lung infection at the time of diagnosis of DM. Parameters of CF clinical status were collected for 6 years prior to 2 years after the onset of insulin therapy. During the 6 years before onset of insulin therapy, BMI and FVC, but not FEV$_1$ in the (pre-) diabetic patients deviated increasingly from those in the control group. Sharp decreases in BMI and lung function during the last 3 months before onset of insulin therapy were reverted within 3 months of insulin therapy. From 3 months to 2 years after onset of insulin therapy, the differences in BMI, FEV$_1$ and FVC diminished between diabetic and control patients. After 2 years of insulin therapy, BMI was similar in the two groups and the percentage differences in FEV$_1$ and FVC between the two groups were similar to those found 6 years before the onset of insulin therapy[91] (Fig. 15.3). Further, after onset of insulin therapy, the percentages of sputum samples positive for *H. influenzae* and *S. pneumoniae* decreased in the diabetic patients, whereas the levels of organisms causing the more severe lung infections, *S. aureus* and *P. aeruginosa*, remained unchanged[91].

SURVIVAL IN DIABETIC CYSTIC FIBROSIS PATIENTS

The survival rate of diabetic CF patients has been calculated as survival from birth or survival from the time of diagnosis of DM. Survival from birth in CF patients developing DM has been described as unaffected[18,25] or reduced[22] as compared to nondiabetic CF patients. Analysis of survival from birth in CF patients with DM

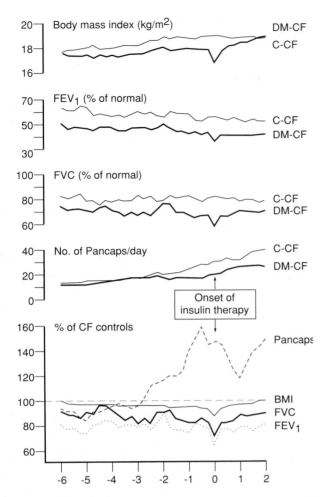

Fig. 15.3 *Top: body mass index (BMI), lung function (FEV₁ and FVC) and daily intake of pancreatic enzyme capsules during 6 years before and 2 years after onset of insulin therapy in 18 diabetic CF patients (DM-CF) and 18 matched, non-diabetic CF patients (C-CF). Bottom: BMI, FEV₁, FVC and daily intake of pancreatic enzyme capsules in the diabetic CF patients in per cent of the same parameters in control CF patients. Mean values. (Based on data in ref. 32.)*

has limitations, because the prevalence of DM in CF increases with age, so that those who died at young ages in the nondiabetic group may have become diabetic had they lived long enough. Moreover, in all three survival studies[18,22,25] CF patients, both in the diabetic and the nondiabetic groups, were not proven to be so based on an OGTT.

Reisman *et al.* also investigated survival rates in matched groups of diabetic and nondiabetic patients from the time of DM diagnosis and did not observe any difference between the two groups[25]. However, their data are difficult to interpret because the event (DM) develops late and follow-up is relatively short. Besides, some of the patients in the nondiabetic group may later develop DM.

In conclusion, since insulin therapy can improve BMI

and lung function and reduce the percentage of sputum samples positive for *H. influenzae* and *S. pneumoniae* in diabetic CF patients, screening for DM with OGTT is mandatory in CF patients above the age of 10 years, and insulin therapy should most probably be initiated when DM is diagnosed.

Late diabetic complications

In IDDM and NIDDM, the duration of DM and the level of glycemic control are important determinants of late diabetic complications.

DM in CF has often been considered mild and unlikely to result in the development of late diabetic complications[5,12,19,20,92]. However, these authors only looked for obvious clinical signs without using specified measurements to identify patients with late diabetic complications. The management of DM in CF has therefore tended to focus on symptomatic relief, on the assumption that aggressive treatment was unnecessary because life expectancy in CF was too short for the microvascular complications of DM to develop.

Reports of diabetic CF patients beginning to exhibit microvascular complications have now been published[18,29,33,93,94]. These patients had a median duration of DM of 14 years(range 1–28 years), were often poorly compliant in their medical care and had poor glycemic control (high HbA₁c levels).

It thus appears that diabetic CF patients may be equally prone to develop late diabetic complications as are patients with other types of DM of similar duration and similar glycemic control. Therefore, late diabetic complications should be screened for annually from the diagnosis of DM. This examination should include ophthalmoscopy, measurement of blood pressure, urinary albumin excretion rate and plasma creatinine concentration, and an assessment of peripheral neuropathy with inspection of feet and measurement of tendon reflexes and vibration sensation.

Treatment of diabetes mellitus in cystic fibrosis

The treatment goal in diabetic CF patients is to achieve and maintain a metabolic state as normal as possible in order to secure an optimal nutritional and clinical status, and to avoid or postpone the development of late diabetic complications. Suggested guidelines for treatment of diabetes in CF are given in Table 15.2.

NUTRITIONAL MANAGEMENT

The goal of nutritional management in CF is to restore and maintain optimal nutritional well-being. The nutritional status is usually more impaired by CF than by DM. Therefore, the nutritional strategy in diabetic CF

Table 15.2 *Guidelines for treatment of diabetes in CF*

Treat cystic fibrosis before diabetes mellitus
Energy requirements = 150% of normal: 40% fat, 20% protein,
    40% carbohydrates
Adjust the insulin regimen to the diet – not opposite
Eat as often and as much as possible: 3 meals and 3 snacks
    should be evenly distributed throughout the day
Every meal should contain a balance of protein, fat and
    carbohydrate; 'simple sugars' are allowed if planned and
    balanced
Pancreatic enzyme replacements at every meal and snack
Modify the diet according to the individual patient needs –
    make compromises
Make self-care education programs in order to enable the
    patients to adjust diet and insulin dose themselves

Table 15.3 *Recommendations for the OGTT and blood glucose measurements*

OGTT at least once a year in patients above 10 years of age
Repeat OGTT in case of weight loss and/or clinical instability,
    especially in patients with IGT
24-hour blood glucose profile in patients with DM and not yet
    on insulin
24-hour blood glucose profile in control of patients with DM
    on insulin substitution, and HbA$_{1c}$ every third month

patients is to treat CF before DM. A normal balanced diet is recommended for all CF patients, diabetic or non-diabetic; however, quantitatively containing 50 per cent more calories (E% = 150 per cent) than generally recommended for IDDM patients.

The total energy requirement recommended is divided into: 35–40 per cent as lipids (compared to 30 per cent or less in IDDM), 20 per cent as protein (IDDM, 15 per cent) and 40–45 per cent as carbohydrates (IDDM, 50–55 per cent), the latter corresponding to approximately 60 E% on a 150 E% diet; about 10 per cent simple sugar is allowed. In order to achieve this high energy intake and to diminish the postprandial blood glucose peaks, the diabetic CF patients are recommended to take at least six meals (three main meals and three snacks), containing a balance of lipids, protein and carbohydrates, evenly distributed throughout the day, and with pancreatic enzyme replacement with every meal.

MEDICAL THERAPY

Diabetic CF patients cannot be managed on a (hypocaloric) DM diet alone because they will invariably lose further weight. Pharmacological treatment is also needed. It is still debated whether the initial medical treatment in newly diagnosed diabetic CF patients should be insulin or oral hypoglycemic agents (sulfonylureas). Since DM in CF is an insulinopenic condition, most prefer insulin therapy to sulfonylureas.

The decision to start insulin therapy is normally based on clinical grounds (symptoms of hyperglycemia, growth retardation, malnutrition, exacerbations of lung infections, deteriorating lung function) and the prevailing glycemic level, detected by blood glucose profiles (Table 15.3), with measurements before and 90 minutes after each main meal and at bedtime. The glucagon test gives valid estimates of beta-cell function in CF patients[68]. Measurements of 6 min postglucagon C-peptide concentrations may therefore be useful to predict insulin dependency.

The insulin supply should be scaled to the patients' increased energy requirement, but insulin treatment is often complicated by the inconstant intake of food in CF patients due to nausea, anorexia and emesis. Initially, a daily dose of intermediate-acting insulin of 0.1–0.3 IU/kg body weight is administered subcutaneously as a single injection in the morning. After some time, it is often necessary to increase the dose and to give intermediate-acting insulin twice daily in the morning and before bedtime. Very few patients need additional regular insulin. Once glycemia is stabilized, the insulin dose is adjusted according to HbA$_{1c}$ and blood glucose profiles. Blood glucose levels of 4–8 mmol/L before meals, 4–12 mmol/L 90 minutes after meals, and 6–10 mmol/L before bedtime are considered optimal. Special attention is given to patients on prednisone treatment, during exacerbation of lung infection and during surgery.

Two groups studied the effect of stimulating insulin secretion with the sulfonylurea agents tolbutamide[95] and glipizide[96] in nondiabetic CF patients. From a study of 12 CF patients with NGT studied before, during and after 4 months of 750 mg tolbutamide daily the authors concluded that short-term tolbutamide treatment increases linear growth and lean body mass in slowly growing CF patients, probably by a direct effect of tolbutamide or an enhanced insulin action in the peripheral tissue[95]. Culler *et al.* studied six CF patients with 2 hour post-load blood glucose levels ranging from 9.8 to 15.5 mmol/L, treated with glipizide for 3 months[96]. They found no increase in weight or BMI, but an increase in the first-phase insulin secretion after intravenous glucose, and less glycosuria was seen. Their results suggest that glipizide may be considered for CF patients with IGT, but the authors recommend insulin therapy in patients with DM[96]. Bertele-Harms and Harms have treated 28 diabetic CF patients with glibenclamide 2.5–7.5 mg as one morning dose. They found that in 65 per cent of the patients the elevated HbA$_{1c}$ values declined into the normal range, in 20 per cent HbA$_{1c}$ were still slightly elevated and in 15 per cent the improvement was insufficient, so the patients had to switch to insulin therapy after a mean of 8 months. In the 85 per cent of patients on successful glibenclamide therapy, this was effective for a limited period of a mean of 2.5 years.

All diabetic CF patients treated with insulin or oral hypoglycemic agents should be instructed to be aware of, to prevent and to treat hypoglycemic symptoms, and always to carry simple sugar. So far, no studies have dealt with the frequency of hypoglycemic reactions in diabetic CF patients treated with insulin or oral hypoglycemic agents. Theoretically, diabetic CF patients should be at an increased risk of hypoglycemia due to an impaired ability to counter-regulate with glucagon, but glucose recovery from insulin-induced hypoglycemia was reportedly normal in CF patients, whether diabetic or not[44], and severe hypoglycemia with unconsciousness is apparently rare[18].

In order to fulfil the recommended 150 E% energy intake, diabetic CF patients have to eat as much and as often as possible. They must learn (self-care) to adjust the insulin dosage according to the diet and not the opposite. Generally, insulin is considered the therapy of choice in the insulinopenic condition of DM in CF; it has, however, not been studied systematically whether oral hypoglycemic agents, at least temporarily, are of use in diabetic CF patients. The treatment regimen should be individualized and be as simple as possible. In patients burdened by both CF and DM, self-care, modifications and compromises are often necessary in order to obtain a life as normal as possible.

NASAL POLYPS AND SINUSITIS

Nasal polyps are found frequently in patients with CF, the incidence ranging from 10 per cent to 32 per cent in various reports[97-102]. The histology shows mucus retention cysts, degeneration of glandular epithelium, and ductal dilatation containing inspissated eosinophilic material[103], but although these features are found more often than in patients with allergic polyposis, none are specific to CF. The most consistent feature distinguishing nasal polyps in the two diseases is the infiltration with eosinophilic cells which is much less pronounced in CF nasal polyps[104-106]. Many cases are asymptomatic and spontaneous regression can occur[99] but is less frequent than in other conditions[107]. Nasal obstruction is the most common symptom and indication for removal, but recurrence is frequent and polypectomy must often be repeated[99,107-110]. Recurrence may be less frequent when polypectomy is combined with ethmoidectomy and Caldwell–Luc operation[109,111]. In the opinion of the authors, routine examination by otologist and simple polypectomy, also in recurrent cases, will prevent the need for more extensive surgery. Complications to polypectomy are extremely rare[110].

Medical treatment with systemic or local corticosteroids, antihistamines and decongestants has, in general, met with limited success[97,100,101,108,109,111]. This probably reflects the fact that polyps in CF are primarily a direct consequence of intrinsic glandular and epithelial cell dysfunction due to CFTR mutations, although the recent finding that HLA class II antigens are expressed in the epithelial cells of nasal polyps in CF indicates that immune reactions may be involved[112]. Complicating local allergic reactions should, however, be ruled out by appropriate examinations since a subgroup of patients with this complication may experience symptomatic relief from steroid treatment[97,100,101]. Local bacterial infection may be a more common complicating factor and the intensive antimicrobial treatment regimens, received by most patients for pulmonary infections, may have an additional beneficial effect on polyps, as well as sinusitis, and possibly also prevent an otherwise more frequent occurrence of cellulitis and osteomyelitis[97,111].

The sinuses are affected in more than 90 per cent of patients with CF[97,103,113,114], involving primarily the maxillary and ethmoid sinuses. Findings on plain radiograph range from thickening of the mucosa lining the sinuses to completely uniform opacity (Fig. 15.4), probably due to accumulation of secretions, and in rare patients mucocele has been reported[115] (Fig. 15.5). Using modern CT scans mucosal swelling is an ubiquitous finding in

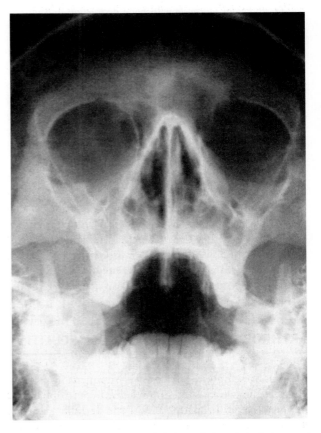

Fig. 15.4 *The margin of the left frontal sinus is indistinct and sclerotic, consistent with chronic sinusitis. The maxillary antra are opacified due to mucosal thickening.*

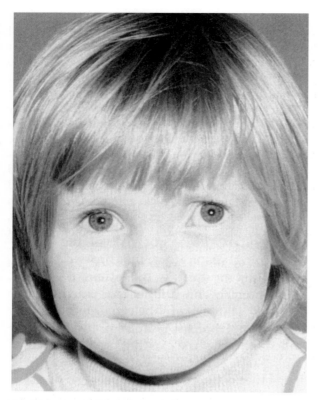

Fig. 15.5 *Lateral dislocation and slight protrusion of the left eye due to ethmoidal mucocele with bone destruction and intraorbital expansion. (Reproduced with the parents' permission.)*

children with CF. Most cases are asymptomatic, and acute purulent sinusitis is relatively uncommon. There have been reports of increased frequency of secretory otitis and conductive hearing loss but others have found no differences from patients without CF[99].

Recently, two independent studies have shown that the presence of nasal polyps appears to be inversely correlated with the course of the lung disease[116,117]. One study[116] suggested a link to type of CFTR mutation but it is also possible that genetic factors outside the CFTR locus may modify electrolyte transport abnormalities, leading to a greater degree of nasal polyposis and milder lung disease[117].

ARTHROPATHY, ARTHRITIS AND VASCULITIS

Rheumatic symptoms are relatively frequent in patients with CF, the two most common being hypertrophic pulmonary osteoarthropathy (HPO) and periodic arthritis, both seen in 2–9 per cent of patients[118]. The well-known clubbing of the fingers and toes has been considered a form of HPO[119], the degree of clubbing being primarily linked to the degree of pulmonary disease[120], and marked

regression is seen after successful heart–lung transplantation. The classic HPO is a condition which, like clubbing, can also be seen in other diseases of the chest, typically involving the distal parts and adjoining joints of the tibia, fibula, femur and sometimes also the long bones of the arms[12,121–123]. There is pain, swelling and warmth of the involved areas, and occasionally small joint effusions. There are characteristic radiological findings in affected areas, often revealing discrete layers of periosteal new-bone formation, seen most frequently at the distal end of the tibia and fibula sometimes together with evidence of osteoporosis[124]. In contrast to clubbing, which can occur rapidly in children with pulmonary disease, this classic presentation of HPO is seen mostly in older patients[119].

A more transient or episodic form of acute or subacute arthritis is also seen frequently in patients with CF[125–130]. According to some studies, this form of joint involvement is not as closely linked to severe pulmonary disease as HPO[127,128]. A subgroup of patients with episodic arthritis may go on to develop persistent synovitis with progressive erosive disease[127]. Further, some patients have symptoms of rheumatic disease which cannot be classified as HPO or episodic arthritis[128,129]. There have also been isolated reports of the concurrence of arthritis, psoriasis and CF[131] and of sarcoid arthropathy and CF[132] where a causal connection has not been established.

Rheumatoid factor, and less often antinuclear antibodies, have been identified in only some of the patients[126–130] but, interestingly, patients with cystic fibrosis with bacterial infection at time of study had elevated IgM and IgA antibodies to Fab fragments of IgG and elevated IgA antibodies to Fc fragments, a pattern different from that found in a number of other infectious diseases and in rheumatoid arthritis and systemic lupus erythematosus[133]. Circulating immune complexes can frequently be detected in patients with CF and arthritis[130] predominantly in patients with chronic *P. aeruginosa* infection[126,134] and synovial biopsy reveals mild and nonspecific synovitis[129] with scanty lymphocytic infiltrates and deposits of IgM, IgG and complement[130]. The information obtained from these studies might indicate that massive formation of complexes of microbial antigens and specific antimicrobial antibodies in the lower respiratory tract might reach the circulation and lead to systemic deposition, giving rise to 'nonspecific' extrapulmonary inflammatory lesions.

A role of autoantibodies cannot be excluded, and antibodies against two human antigens have been detected in sera from patients with CF: IgG antibodies against the 60 kDa heat-shock protein (HSP60)[135], and IgG as well as IgA antibodies against bactericidal/permeability-increasing protein (BPI)[136]. Heat-shock proteins are found in procaryotic as well as eucaryotic organisms and there is some sequence homology between bacterial and human heat-shock proteins. IgG anti-HSP60 has been detected in sera from patients with juvenile chronic arthritis and from children with systemic lupus erythematosus, but in even higher titers in sera from patients with CF, which is certainly interesting in view of the recurrent and chronic bacterial infections in patients with CF[135]. The connection between bacterial infections and anti-human HSP60 antibodies and the possible consequences of the presence of these antibodies in patients with CF remains to be explored in detail. Anti-bactericidal/permeability-increasing protein (BPI) antibodies are detected by indirect immunofluorescence as an antineutrophil cytoplasmic autoantibody (c-ANCA) and IgG as well as IgA antibodies against BPI have been found in a majority of sera from patients with CF, in particular patients with secondary vasculitis[136]. It was also shown that anti-BPI levels were inversely correlated with FEV$_1$ and FVC.

The episodic arthritis is often associated with fever and skin lesions presenting as erythema nodosum[126–128] and other forms of nodular skin lesions[127], as well as purpura, usually located distally on the legs (Fig. 15.6), around the ankles, and on the dorsum of the feet[126,137–140]. In a report of a series of 12 patients with vasculitis, proven by biopsy in seven, two had manifestations of systemic vasculitis[139]. There was no evidence of autoimmune disease but antineutrophil cytoplasmic antibodies were present in 40 per cent of the patients, as compared to none of 61 control patients without vasculitis[136]. From this report, as well as from our experience, it appears that this very characteristic complication is often associated

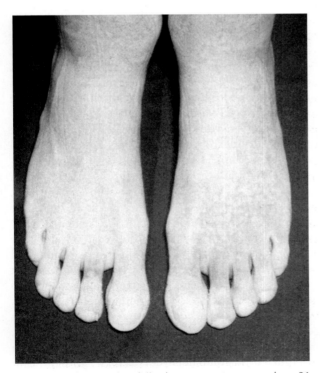

Fig. 15.6 *Pigmentation following recurrent purpura in a 21-year-old female CF patient with advanced lung disease and marked hypergammaglobulinemia. The patient died 1 year later.*

with a severe progressive course of the pulmonary infections, often being chronic *P. aeruginosa* infection, and that it is associated with poor prognosis. Whether it is a consequence of a massive presence in the lungs of antigen–antibody complexes with 'spill-over' into the peripheral blood is unknown. Circulating immune complexes can be demonstrated[139,140] but it has proved difficult to detect the presence of specific bacterial antigens in biopsies[139]. As mentioned above, autoantibodies against bactericidal/permeability-increasing protein are particularly frequent in patients with CF and secondary vasculitis[136]. The vasculitis is leukocytoclastic and deposits of complement C3 and immunoglobulins are found[139,140]. Neither HPO nor episodic arthritis has been linked to any particular HLA type[126,134,141].

AMYLOIDOSIS

Systemic secondary amyloidosis is a complication of long-standing chronic inflammatory diseases due to infections, autoimmune diseases and malignancies. Given the increased longevity in spite of the presence of chronic *P. aeruginosa* lung infection, it seems surprising that only around 20–30 cases of secondary amyloidosis have been reported[142–148]. The mean age of diagnosis was 20 years with a range of 6–33 years[148] and there seems to be a preponderance of males over females[142]. Most reported patients have died from chronic respiratory failure, often with complicating chronic renal failure[142,147]. Autopsies have shown that frequently involved organs are the spleen, liver, kidneys, adrenal glands, heart and bowel[142–144,147] but it is interesting that the thyroid gland has been involved in seven patients[144,148]. Clinical suspicion of amyloidosis has mostly been based on the presence of nephrotic syndrome or isolated proteinuria, but in some patients on thyroid gland enlargement or hepatosplenomegaly[142,144,146–148], and the diagnosis has been confirmed by renal, rectal, hepatic or thyroid biopsy[142–144,146–148] and in one patient by biopsy of abdominal subcutaneous fat[142].

Amyloid fibrils have been analyzed in one cystic fibrosis patient with secondary amyloidosis and been shown to be of the secondary amyloid A (AA) type[144]. The protein was amino-acid sequenced and showed minor heterogeneity when compared to that of amyloid fibrils from patients with juvenile rheumatoid arthritis and rheumatoid arthritis[144]. Amyloid A fibril protein is the product of a larger serum amyloid A (SAA) protein, which is an acute-phase protein produced in the liver in response to inflammation and tissue destruction, possibly via stimulation of hepatocytes by cytokines[144,145]. The levels of SAA and C-reactive protein (CRP) are positively correlated to an increase in pulmonary inflammation, with SAA possibly being a more sensitive parameter than CRP[145]. The reason for the low incidence of amyloidosis in CF may, therefore, be improved control of chronic inflammation by early treatment of infectious exacerbations through improved antimicrobial therapy, leading to only a few patients going through prolonged periods of uncontrolled inflammation.

A recent autopsy study including 41 patients with CF, showed that islet amyloidosis was present in approximately 70 per cent of patients with diabetes, and in 20 per cent of borderline diabetic patients, as opposed to none of the nondiabetic patients[149]. The principal subunit of islet amyloid is a 37-amino-acid protein (islet amyloid polypeptide) which is almost exclusively expressed in beta cells, and islet amyloidosis is also seen in type 2 diabetes, but whether islet amyloidosis is secondary to beta-cell stress, or plays a direct role in the pathogenesis of diabetes in CF is unknown[149].

THYROID GLAND

The thyroid gland has received much less attention than other organs, although an unexpectedly high incidence of goiter in patients being treated with iodide as expectorant was reported by Dolan et al. more than 20 years ago[150]. The recent demonstration of expression of CFTR both at mRNA and at protein level in thyroid follicular cells has renewed interest in this gland in CF[151]. The original work by Dolan and Gibson[150] was a retrospective study of 110 patients with cystic fibrosis, of whom 55 had received daily iodide therapy for at least 1 year, and 55 nontreated control patients. Forty-seven of the 55 patients (85 per cent) receiving iodide developed goiter, as opposed to none of the 55 patients not treated. In the patients with goiter, the thyroid gland was visibly enlarged, diffusely symmetric, non-nodular and occasionally tender. Goiter could already be seen 3 months after onset of iodide treatment, but the usual time interval was 2–3 years[150]. Fourteen patients had laboratory or clinical evidence of hypothyroidism, and clinical cases ($N = 8$) all responded promptly to thyroid extract treatment[150].

Subsequent studies by Azizi et al.[152] of 41 patients with CF, aged 6–24 years, all clinically well, euthyroid and without goiter, revealed normal serum thyroxine (T_4) but significantly reduced serum triiodothyronine (T_3) and significantly increased serum thyroid stimulating hormone (TSH) as compared to age- and sex-matched normal controls. Eighteen of the patients were then put on 5 drops of a saturated solution of potassium iodide three times daily. Treatment was discontinued if goiter or evidence of hypothyroidism developed and the treatment period ranged from 77 to 265 days[152]. Goiter developed in 8 of the 18 patients, there was a highly significant decrease in serum T_4 and clinical evidence of mild hypothyroidism was seen in a few patients and one developed frank myxedema.

Baran et al.[153] studied 32 patients aged 3 months to 18 years, none of whom had received iodides, and 36 age-matched normal controls. In contrast to Azizi et al. [152], they found normal basal levels of serum T_4, T_3, TSH and thyrotropin-releasing hormone (TRH). However, in response to intravenous bolus injection of 200 µg synthetic TRH there was a significantly higher output of TSH in the older children ($N = 26$) with the same trend in younger (<2 years, $N = 6$), which led the authors to conclude that the reserve of pituitary TSH was increased in CF, suggesting the occurrence of compensated hypothyroidism[153]. Segall-Blank et al.[154] could not confirm the findings of Baran et al.[153] of increased release of TSH in response to TRH, but argued that the dose employed by Baran et al. was higher per kg body weight than the dose they used. They did, however, confirm the previous finding of normal serum T_4 but decreased T_3 concentrations in the patients, and suggested that there is, in CF, a state of decreased peripheral conversion of T_4 to T_3 (decreased peripheral outer-ring monodeiodination of T_4 to T_3) which can be observed in other nonthyroid illnesses[154]. The authors concluded that the results of their studies did not delineate the reason(s) for the observed proneness of CF patients to develop iodide-induced hypothyroidism. In a subsequent study by De Luca et al.[155] of 10 iodide-untreated children with CF compared to 84 controls, the results revealed slightly decreased serum T_4 but normal T_3, but they confirmed the finding by Baran et al.[153] of a significantly exaggerated increase in serum TSH in response to intravenous injection of TRH, indicating subclinical hypothyroidism in CF[155].

The general picture from these studies (though not all[156]) is that the thyroid gland has an abnormally increased propensity to development of goiter and hypothyroidism in response to treatment with iodide, and that even in patients not receiving iodide, there is a state of compensated hypothyroidism. This could be secondary to CF disease manifestations, i.e. malnutrition and/or infections. Borel and Reddy[157] studied the thyroid gland from autopsied patients and found excessive accumulation of lipofuscin, a feature commonly found in other organ systems in patients with a wide range of diseases associated with malnutrition, and possibly related to chronic vitamin E deficiency leading to auto-oxidation of lipids[157]. Rosenlund et al.[158] administered essential fatty acids as corn oil orally for 1 year to a small group of patients with CF and found a small though significant decrease in serum T_3, but not T_4 after treatment, and interestingly, they also found a decrease in sweat sodium concentration[158]. Finally Kauf et al.[159] administered peroral sodium selenite therapy to 32 patients with CF for 3 months, leading to a significant increase in serum selenium, a significant malondialdehyde decrease, a significant increase in serum vitamin E, and also an increase in serum T_3 and a highly significant decrease in the serum T_4/T_3 ratio. The authors argued that selenium therapy might improve peripheral $T_4 \rightarrow T_3$ conversion by type-1 iodothyronine-5'-deiodinase, which is a specific selenoenzyme[159]. Finally, subclinical hypothyroidism[153,155] could be due to decreased reabsorption of thyroxine secondary to pancreatic insufficiency and/or changes in intestinal transit[155].

The finding of expression of CFTR in the human thyroid epithelium by Devuyst *et al.* clearly puts the focus on an intrinsic abnormality in the thyroid glandular cells and the possibility that changes in the metabolic activities of the thyroid follicular cells led to alterations in colloid secretion[151]. Using immunocytochemistry, CFTR protein was found to be present in approximately two-thirds of the thyroid follicles but only 16 per cent of the follicular cells were positive per follicle, suggesting phase-specific expression of CFTR[151]. The function of CFTR in thyroid epithelial cells is unknown and could involve iodide secretion into the thyroid follicles as well as regulation of transport of electrolytes and fluid, either directly by virtue of CFTR chloride-channel activity or by regulation of other electrolyte channels by CFTR[151]. CFTR might also be involved in acidification of Golgi vesicles, leading to a sialylation defect with hyposialylation of thyroglobulin[151,160].

It is quite unknown whether the continued presence of a state of compensated hypothyroidism is of any clinical importance, but present knowledge warrants increased awareness of the possibility of hypothyroidism in individual patients, and prospective studies in large patient groups should be carried out.

THE KIDNEY

Following the characterization of the *CFTR* gene and gene product it became possible to study mRNA and protein expression in different organs and different cells. Immunocytochemical studies by Crawford *et al.* showed that CFTR protein was abundantly present in the epithelium lining the kidney tubules, in fact expression was even more pronounced than in bronchial surface epithelium[161]. The CFTR protein was detected in the apical region of epithelial cells in the proximal as well as in the distal renal tubules and expression was most pronounced in the first part of the proximal tubules, while it was not detected in the glomeruli or in the collecting ducts[161]. Subsequent studies by the same group confirmed the differential expression in various nephron segments, most pronounced in outer medulla and cortex probably as a result of abundant expression in proximal tubules[162]. A recent review summarizes the results of studies using immunocytochemistry, mRNA expression and patch–clamp techniques, showing that mRNA expression has been detected in all parts of the nephron from the proximal tubule, and that the protein has been detected in the proximal tubule, the thin limbs of the loop of Henle, the distal tubule, the principal cells of cortical collecting ducts, and the inner medullary collecting duct[163].

The pronounced expression of CFTR protein in the kidney was somewhat surprising since the presence of mutated CFTR appears to have no clinical consequences. Physiological studies *in vivo* have, however, indicated decreased ability to excrete a salt load, decreased ability to dilute and concentrate urine, and increased proximal tubule sodium absorption[163–165]. In contrast to tubular function, most studies have indicated that glomerular filtration rate (GFR) is normal in patients with CF[166], with the possible exception of one[164]; however, that same group also reported that correction of abnormal fatty acid status by active supplementation resulted in normalization of GFR[167]. In the kidney, CFTR is likely to function primarily as a chloride channel and the activities of other chloride channels may, to a large extent, compensate for a mutated, nonfunctioning CFTR[163]. The role of CFTR in the kidney may, however, not be limited to chloride transport, since CFTR may interact with both sodium and potassium channels, as is the situation in other epithelia[160] – thus CFTR has recently been shown to regulate the activity of a specific renal potassium channel, as shown in studies where both channels were coexpressed in *Xenopus* oocytes[168].

It has recently been shown that CFTR is present in epithelial cells lining the cysts in patients with autosomal dominant polycystic kidney disease (ADPKD)[169–171] and that CFTR was present at the apical cell surface of cyst epithelial cells that had been stimulated to secretion by forskolin, but was present intracellularly in nonstimulated cells[171]. CFTR seems to be active in the secretion of fluid and electrolytes into the cysts, and cultures of epithelial cells from patients with ADPKD may prove to be an important tool for studying CFTR function(s) in the kidney.

Katz *et al.*[72] did autopsy studies of kidney tissue in 38 patients with CF and found microscopic nephrocalcinosis in 35 (92 per cent). This was apparently not secondary to disease manifestations outside the kidney, since nephrocalcinosis was detected in six patients below 1 year of age, including two neonatal patients and one stillborn, leading the authors to conclude that there might be a primary abnormality of calcium metabolism in the kidney in CF patients[173]. They also did 24-hour urinary calcium determination in 14 patients and 15 controls and found an increase in the ratio of calcium to creatinine urinary output in five of the patients (36 per cent) with a normal ratio in all of the controls. Bentur *et al.*[73] could not confirm these findings. Thirty out of 34 patients with CF had normal urinary calcium excretion, while only four had hypercalciuria, which was believed to be secondary to immobilization, increased sodium load or steroid treatment. Ultrasonic examination of 17 patients was without evidence of renal calcinosis[173].

Autopsy studies in 14 patients revealed sparse renal calcinosis in 5, but this was also detected in 6 of 12 autopsied patients with other diseases[173].

Strandvik and Hjelte performed a retrospective study of 140 patients with CF and found five with nephrolithiasis[174]. Similarly Chidekel and Dolan studied 140 patients and found a cumulative incidence of nephrolithiasis of 5.7 per cent (eight patients, of whom seven had calcium oxalate stones)[175]. An additional six patients had incidences of calcium oxalate crystaluria[175]. All of the afflicted patients were pancreatic insufficient with fat malabsorption, and the authors reviewed the literature showing that hyperoxaluria is frequently observed in other gastrointestinal diseases, in particular those associated with fat malabsorption ('enteric' hyperoxaluria)[175].

Several mechanisms by which fat malabsorption can lead to an increased load of oxalate on the nephrons are discussed[175].

The pharmacokinetics of a number of antibiotics are changed in patients with CF, and increased clearance leading to lower serum concentrations has been reported for aminoglycosides, β-lactam antibiotics and quinolones[166]. The mechanism is uncertain but it is argued – on the basis of an extensive review of studies of renal function – that this can hardly be ascribed to changes in GFR or in renal plasma flow (RPF) and it would appear that for most drugs the increased renal clearance must be due to impaired tubular reabsorption, and thus directly linked to alterations in tubular ion-transport mechanisms[166].

15b

Osteoporosis

S. L. ELKIN

INTRODUCTION

Osteoporosis is a systemic skeletal disease characterized by low bone mass and microarchitectural deterioration of bone tissue, with a consequent increase in bone fragility and susceptibility to fracture risk[176]. Over the past decade low bone mass has been recognized as a complication in both children and adults with CF. However, skeletal health is largely ignored by clinicians in the field despite the fact that bone loss and fracture could further decrease the quality of life of these patients. Physicians should now have a basic understanding of skeletal health to help prevent occurrence of these problems.

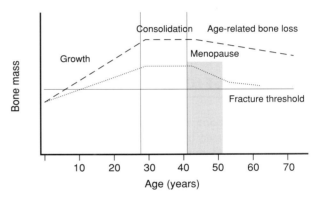

Fig. 15.7 *Age-related changes in bone mass.*

BONE PHYSIOLOGY AND MEASUREMENT OF BONE MINERAL DENSITY

Bone is a living tissue that undergoes constant remodeling throughout life. This process serves to maintain the mechanical integrity of the skeleton and to provide a means by which calcium homeostasis may be maintained. Bone remodeling occurs at discrete sites termed bone remodeling units and consists of the removal by osteoclasts of a quantum of bone followed by the formation of a similar amount of new bone by the osteoblasts[177]. Under normal circumstances this is a balanced process. Bone loss in osteoporosis may occur as a result of remodeling imbalance. This occurs when the amount of bone formed is less than that resorbed. In the general population during growth, bone formation exceeds resorption up to a peak bone mass, which is reached between 25 and 30 years of age. There is then a period of stabilization before age-related bone loss occurs in both sexes, with bone resorption exceeding formation (Fig. 15.7). There is a phase of accelerated loss in women around the menopause.

Measurement of bone density

Several techniques are now available for assessment of bone mineral density (BMD), including dual-energy X-ray absorptiometry (DXA), quantitative computed tomography (QCT) and broad-band ultrasound attenuation. DXA is the most commonly used as it is noninvasive, quick, highly reproducible and delivers an extremely low dose of radiation (less than daily natural background levels). It can measure bone mass at both axial and appendicular sites[178]. Bone density values are usually expressed in relation to reference data as standard deviation scores. A Z score represents the number of standard deviations above or below the age- and sex-matched mean reference value. A T score is similarly expressed in relation to reference values for young adults who have achieved their peak bone mass. When assessing bone density in younger patients with CF, Z scores are potentially more useful as peak bone mass has often yet to be reached.

There are a few points that need to be realized when

using DXA scanning for assessment of bone density in CF patients.

1. The technique should be used with caution in smaller individuals, such as children who are below average height, as the measurements are areal (2-dimensional) not volumetric. However, it has been shown that bone mineral is still significantly low in CF patients even when corrected for body size[179] and that in adults similar BMD values are given by DXA and QCT[182].

2. Both osteomalacia and osteoporosis give low bone mineral density results. The treatments for these two conditions are quite different. Until data from bone histomorphometry is available, we cannot be certain of the bone pathology.

3. Different manufacturers use different reference ranges, so the same measured value might give a different result. If longitudinal data are to be looked at, all measurements should ideally be from the same machine.

PREVALENCE OF LOW BONE MASS IN CF

In children, low bone mineral density has been found to occur when assessed by QCT and by DXA. Gibbens et al.[180] found bone density to be reduced by 10 per cent in 57 patients (mean age 12 years). This finding was confirmed by DXA scanning in a study by Henderson et al.[181] who investigated 62 patients (mean age 10.7 years). They found BMD to be reduced with mean Z scores of −1.03 at the lumbar spine and −0.71 at the femoral neck. Both studies found that BMD values correlated with disease severity.

Several studies have found low bone mass in adults with CF. These studies have tended to investigate small numbers or concentrate on patients with end-stage pulmonary disease. Two more informative studies were conducted by Haworth et al.[182] from the UK and Aris et al.[183] from the USA. The former investigated 151 adults aged 15–52 years with both DXA and QCT and found mean BMD Z scores of −1.21 at the lumbar spine and −1.25 at the femoral neck when measured by DXA and −0.56 at the lumbar spine when measured by QCT. Thirty four per cent of patients had Z scores of −2 or less at one or more skeletal site. Body mass index, percentage predicted forced expiratory volume in one second and physical activity were all positively related to the mean BMD score. The latter studied 60 adult CF patients who had been referred for lung transplantation. They found mean BMD Z scores of −2.17 at the lumbar spine and −2.02 at the femoral neck. Body mass index and cumulative glucocorticoid dosage were the strongest predictors of low BMD.

CLINICAL RELEVANCE

In view of the inverse relationship between bone mineral density and fracture risk that has been demonstrated in population-based studies[184], the increased prevalence of low bone mineral density in children and adults with CF may predispose to fracture.

To date, there are very few data available on fractures in CF. Henderson et al.[185] sent questionnaires to 143 children with CF and found 36 to have sustained a fracture. This was not statistically greater than the normal population. Aris et al.[186] investigated 70 patients awaiting lung transplantation and reported a significant increase in fractures in adolescent females and older males. A significant increase in rib and vertebral fractures was found. A significant increase in the rate of rib fracture has also been found in adults at the Royal Brompton Hospital (UK)[187]. The finding of a high rate of rib fractures is of particular importance, in view of the severe pain associated with these fractures and the resulting adverse consequences for chest physiotherapy and disease control.

Osteoporosis also occurs as a result of lung transplantation[188], which is being carried out with increasing frequency for patients with end-stage CF. Lung transplantation may further increase bone loss and fracture risk in these patients and it is therefore important to have an optimal peak bone mass prior to operation.

RISK FACTORS

These are summarized in Table 15.4.

Malabsorption

The majority of patients with CF secrete insufficient enzymes for normal fat and protein absorption, leading to steatorrhea, malnutrition and deficiencies of fat-soluble vitamins (D, E, A and K). These problems can be

Table 15.4 *Risk factors for osteoporosis in patients with cystic fibrosis*

Malabsorption
  Vitamin D
  Calcium
Low body weight
Decreased physical activity
Delayed puberty
Male hypogonadism
Amenorrhea
Glucocorticoid usage
Diabetes
Chronic infection – increased cytokines
Transplantation

avoided in the majority of patients with adequate pancreatic enzyme replacement therapy and vitamin supplementation. Vitamin D is important to bone health, deficiency leading to osteomalacia, while subclinical deficiency can lead to osteoporosis by increasing bone turnover via secondary hyperparathyroidism. Hypovitaminosis D can usually be avoided by adequate exposure to sunlight and vitamin intake.

Although 1,25-hydroxylated vitamin D is the active form, the 25-OH vitamin D gives a better measure of vitamin D stores, having a longer half-life of 3–4 weeks. It is difficult to say what a normal level of serum 25-OH vitamin D should be as the range is large due to differences in latitude and season. Most textbooks quote optimum serum levels as being between 50 and 150 nmol/L[189]. Hypovitaminosis D has been reported as a common occurrence in patients with CF despite vitamin supplementation of 600–900 IU/day. Levels are lower in areas of lower sun exposure. Ott and Aitken[190] in Washington, USA, found average values of 18.9 ng/L, with 63 per cent of the 87 patients having levels below 20 ng/L, and in a recent study in the UK, 69 per cent of 233 patients were found to have levels below 50 nmol/L (<20 ng/mL)[191]. There have also been reports from areas with higher sun exposure, such as California[186], with 20 per cent of patients having subnormal 25-OH vitamin D levels (mean 20.9 ng/L). These low vitamin levels must be contributing to the decreased bone mass found in this population by increasing bone turnover. Levels should be checked regularly and corrected.

Low serum calcium can also lead to lower bone mass, especially if intake is low during the time of bone acquisition[192]. It is important to ensure that patients with CF, especially adolescents, receive enough dairy produce and that enzymes are adequately replaced to ensure optimal absorption. It is recommended that healthy adolescents and young adults receive 1200-1500 mg/day of calcium[193]. CF patients should receive at least this.

Low body mass

Body mass may influence bone mineral by the force it exerts on the skeleton. In patients with CF it may also represent an indirect measure of nutritional status and disease severity. Many studies have found a correlation between low bone mineral density and low body mass[180–182]. Maintenance of body mass therefore appears highly important for maintenance of bone mass. This is yet another reason why nutritional support is paramount in this population.

Decreased physical activity

Physical activity and weight-bearing exercise are essential for the acquisition and maintenance of skeletal mass. It is well known that immobilization leads to bone loss due to increased resorption and decreased bone formation. Although few studies have assessed the benefits to the skeletal system of exercise in CF patients, it seems sensible to advise weight-bearing activity (with varying strains), especially in children while bone is being acquired. Older patients should be encouraged to carry out weight-bearing activity such as walking and weight training to the best of their ability. This will help improve balance and maintain muscle and bone mass.

Delayed puberty and hypogonadism

It is known that adolescents with CF can be late to enter puberty and this is usually linked to malnutrition and low BMI. As nutritional status improves, so should skeletal and sexual maturation. Testosterone replacement therapy can be given to males with delayed puberty; however, it should not be given too early as it can encourage epiphyseal closure and thus prevent further growth. In women, estrogen can be given if still without menstrual periods at the age of 17.

Hypogonadism is often seen in adults with CF and is probably under-recognized. In males, low testosterone levels can occur with normal gonadotropins(central hypogonadism). In studies to date, the low levels have not correlated with low bone mineral density; however, hypogonadism is likely to be contributing to bone loss in males as well as being detrimental to muscle and sexual health. Replacement therapy should be considered if serum levels are consistently below 10 nmol/L in a morning sample.

Glucocorticoid therapy

Glucocorticoids decrease bone formation and increase bone resorption by:

- decreasing intestinal calcium absorption;
- increasing renal calcium excretion;
- increasing parathyroid hormone concentrations;
- depressing gonadal function;
- decreasing osteoblast number.

In the general population administration of glucocorticoids is the most common cause of secondary osteoporosis, the extent of the bone loss depending on the underlying condition, total dose and duration of the steroids. Most loss is thought to occur in the first 3–6 months of therapy. Aris found the cumulative dose of steroids to be a predictor of bone mineral density in patients awaiting transplantation[194], other studies have found no correlation. Although more evidence is needed as to the effect of steroids on bone in patients with CF, common sense tells us to give the lowest dose symptoms allow and to ensure that the diet contains adequate calcium and vitamin D.

MANAGEMENT OF BONE DISEASE

It is important to remember that bone loss in patients with CF is multifactorial and it is therefore difficult to make general recommendations. The plan below should help to prevent bone loss and the treatment should be individualized as necessary.

1. If possible, bone density scans should be carried out on any patient with risk factors, especially those awaiting lung transplantation or on long-term glucocorticoids. If the T or Z score is below −1, measures to prevent further loss should be instigated and the scan should be repeated in a year to ensure no further loss.
2. Adequate nutritional support is essential to maintain a good body weight. Where possible, a dietitian should be involved.
3. Check vitamin D levels regularly and ensure adequate replacement therapy (at least 800 IU/day), keeping serum levels between 50 and 150 nmol/L (20–60 ng/L).
4. Ensure that diet contains *at least* the recommended daily intake of calcium.
5. Encourage weight-bearing exercise, especially in periods of fast growth (puberty).
6. Encourage adequate sunlight exposure if there are no contraindications, such as ciprofloxacin therapy which can cause photosensitive rash.
7. Check pubertal stage in adolescents and, if delayed, consider hormone replacement with either testosterone or estrogen.
8. Check testosterone levels in adult males and consider correction of low levels with replacement therapy if less than 10 nmol/L in a morning sample.
9. Use glucocorticoids only when necessary and at the lowest dose possible.

There are at present inadequate data on the use of bisphosphonates in patients with CF. Although cyclical etidronate is sometimes used when patients are on oral steroids, it should be remembered that bisphosphonates are poorly absorbed in a normal population, can cause esophageal erosions and osteomalacia and the safety in children is not yet established. To date, their use in patients with CF cannot be recommended, especially in light of the findings of Haworth *et al*[195]. This group found that on administration of the intravenous bisphosphonate, Pamidronate, a significant proportion of patients experienced severe bone pain when compared to the control group. The reason for this is as yet undecided, although an increase in cytokines may be contributing. Further information is needed from treatment trials to provide evidence of efficacy in this group of patients.

CONCLUSION

Patients with CF are at high risk for the development of low bone mineral density. As the life expectancy increases in these patients, poor skeletal health could add to the morbidity in early adulthood and should be avoided. An increased awareness of this possible problem by careworkers in both pediatric and adult CF care, together with increased information from ongoing research, should help minimize osteopenia in the future.

REFERENCES

Other organ systems

1. Andersen, D.H. (1938) Cystic fibrosis of the pancreas and its relation to celiac disease. *Am. J. Dis. Child.*, **56**, 344–399.
2. Lowe, C.U., May, C.D. and Reed, S.C. (1949) Fibrosis of the pancreas in infants and children. *Am. J. Dis. Child.*, **78**, 349–374.
3. Shwachman, H., Uubner, H. and Catzel, P. (1955) Mucoviscidosis. *Adv. Pediatr.*, **7**, 249–323.
4. Rosan, R.C., Shwachman, H. and Kulczycki, L.L. (1962) Diabetes mellitus and cystic fibrosis of the pancreas. *Am. J. Dis. Child.*, **104**, 625–634.
5. Handwerker, S., Roth, J., Gorden, P. *et al.* (1969) Glucose intolerance in cystic fibrosis. *NEJM*, **281**, 451–461.
6. Gracey, M. and Andersen, C.M. (1969) Cystic fibrosis of the pancreas in adolescents and adulthood. *Aust. Ann. Med.*, **18**, 91–101.
7. Milner, A.D. (1969) Blood glucose and serum insulin levels in children with cystic fibrosis. *Arch. Dis. Child.*, **44**, 351–355.
8. Mitchell-Heggs, P., Mearns, M. and Batten, J.C. (1976) Cystic fibrosis in adolescents and adults. *Q. J. Med.*, **45**, 479–504.
9. Wilmshurst, E.G., Soeldner, J.S., Holsclaw, D.S. *et al.* (1975) Endogenous and erogenous insulin responses in patients with cystic fibrosis. *Pediatrics*, **55**, 75–82.
10. Lippe, B.M., Sperling, M.A. and Dooley, R.R. (1977) Pancreatic alpha and beta cell functions in cystic fibrosis. *J. Pediatr.*, **90**, 751–755.
11. Shwachman, H., Kowalski, M. and Khaw, K.T. (1977) Cystic fibrosis: a new outlook. *Medicine*, **56**, 129–149.
12. di Sant'Agnese, P.A. and Davis, P.B. (1979) Cystic fibrosis in adults: 75 cases and a review of 232 cases in the litterature. *Am. J. Med.*, **66**, 121–132.
13. Bistritzer, T., Sack, J., Eskol, A. and Katznelson, D. (1983) Hemoglobin A1 and pancreatic beta-cell function in cystic fibrosis. *Isr. J. Med. Sci.*, **19**, 600–603.
14. Geffner, M.E., Lippe, B.M., Kaplan, S.A. *et al.* (1984)

Carbohydrate tolerance in cystic fibrosis is closely linked to pancreatic exocrine function. *Pediatr. Res.*, **18**, 1107–1111.

15. Knöpfle, G. (1985) Endokrine Pankreasfunktion bei Mukoviszidose. *Klin. Pädiat.*, **197**, 13–20.

16. Mohan, V., Alagappan, V. and Snehalatha, C. *et al.* (1985) Insulin and C-peptide responses to glucose load in cystic fibrosis. *Diab. Metab.*, **1**, 376–379.

17. Berkin, K.E., Alcock, S.R. and Stack, B.H. (1985) Cystic fibrosis – a review of 26 adolescents and adult patients. *Eur. J. Respir. Dis.*, **67**, 103–111.

18. Rodman, H.M., Doershuk, C.F. and Roland, J.M. (1986) The interaction of two diseases: diabetes mellitus and cystic fibrosis. *Medicine*, **65**, 389–397.

19. Penketh, A.R.L., Wise, A., Mearns, M.B. *et al.* (1987) Cystic fibrosis in adolescents and adults. *Thorax*, **42**, 526–532.

20. Stutchfield, P.R., O'Halloran, S., Teale, J.D. *et al.* (1987) Glycosylated haemoglobin and glucose intolerance in cystic fibrosis. *Arch. Dis. Child.*, **62**, 805–810.

21. Hartling, S.G., Garne, S., Binder, C. *et al.* (1988) Proinsulin, insulin, and C-peptide in cystic fibrosis after an oral glucose tolerance test. *Diabetes Res.*, **7**, 165–169.

22. Finkelstein, S.M., Wielinski, C.L., Elliott, G.R. *et al.* (1988) Diabetes mellitus associated with cystic fibrosis. *J. Pediatr.*, **112**, 373–377.

23. Nagel, R.A., Westaby, D., Javaid, A. *et al.* Liver disease and bileduct abnortalities in adults with cystic fibrosis. *Lancet*, **ii**, 1422–1425.

24. Schwartz, R.H. and Milner, M.R. (1984) Other manifestations and organ involvement, in *Cystic Fibrosis*, (ed. L.M. Taussig), Thième-Stratton, Inc., New York, pp. 376–407.

25. Reisman, J., Corey, M., Canny, G. and Levison, H. (1990) Diabetes mellitus in patients with cystic fibrosis: effect on survival. *Pediatrics*, **86**, 374–377.

26. Lanng, S., Thorsteinsson, B., Erichsen, G. *et al.* (1991) Glucose tolerance in cystic fibrosis. *Arch. Dis. Child.*, **66**, 612–616.

27. De Luca, F., Arrigo, T., Nibali, S.C., *et al.* (1991) Insulin secretion, glycosylated haemoglobin and islet cell antibodies in cystic fibrosis children and adolescents with different degrees of glucose tolerance. *Horm. Metab. Res.*, **23**, 495–498.

28. Robert, J.J., Grasset, E., De Montalembert, M. *et al.* (1992) Recherche de facteurs d'intolrance au glucose dans la mucoviscidose. *Arch. Fr. Pediatr.*, **49**, 17–22.

29. Lanng, S., Thorsteinsson, B., Lund-Andersen, C., Nerup, J., Schiøtz, P.O. and Koch, C. (1994) Diabetes mellitus in Danish cystic fibrosis patients: prevalence and late diabetic complications. *Acta Paediatr.*, **83**, 72–77.

30. FitzSimmons, S.C. (1993) The changing epidemiology of cystic fibrosis. *J. Pediatr.*, **122**, 1–9.

31. Lanng, S., Hansen, A., Thorsteinsson, B., Nerup, J. and Koch, C. (1995) Glucose tolerance in patients with cystic fibrosis: a five-year prospective study. *BMJ*, **311**, 655–658.

32. Lanng, S. (1997) Glucose intolerance in cystic fibrosis. *Dan. Med. Bull.*, **44**, 23–39.

33. Sullivan, M.M. and Denning, C.R. (1989) Diabetic microangiopathy in patients with cystic fibrosis. *Pediatrics*, **84**, 642–647.

34. WHO Study Group (1985) Diabetes mellitus. *WHO Techn. Rep. Ser.*, **727**, 1–113.

35. Dodge, J.A. and Morrison, G. (1992) Diabetes mellitus in cystic fibrosis: a review. *J. R. Soc. Med.*, **85**, (Suppl. 19), 25–28.

36. The Expert Committee on the Diagnosis and Classification of Diabetes Mellitus (1997) Report of the Expert Committee on the Diagnosis and Classification of Diabetes Mellitus. *Diabetes Care*, **20**, 1183–1197.

37. Trezise, A.E.O. and Buchwald, M. (1991) *In vivo* cell-specific expression of the cystic fibrosis transmembrane conductance regulator. *Nature*, **353**, 434–437.

38. Crawford, I., Maloney, P.C., Zeitlin, P.L. *et al.* (1991) Immunocytochemical localization of the cystic fibrosis gene product CFTR. *Proc. Natl Acad. Sci. USA*, **88**, 9262–9266.

39. Marino, C.R., Matovcik, L.M., Gorelick, F.S. and Cohn, J.A. (1991) Localization of the cystic fibrosis transmembrane conductance regulator in pancreas. *J. Clin. Invest.*, **88**, 712–716.

40. Löhr, M., Goertchen, P., Nizze, H. *et al.*, (1989) Cystic fibrosis associated islets changes may provide a basis for diabetes. *Virchows Archiv. Pathol. Anat.*, **414**, 179–185.

41. di Sant'Agnese, P.A. and Hubbbard, V.S. (1984) The pancreas, in *Cystic Fibrosis*, (ed. L.N. Taussig), Thième-Stratton, New York, pp. 230–295.

42. Oppenheimer, E.H. and Esterly, J.R. (1975) Pathology of cystic fibrosis: review of the literature and comparison with 146 autopsied cases, in *Perspectives in Pediatric Pathology*, (eds H.S. Rosenberg and R.P. Bolande), Vol. 2, Year Book Medical Publishers, Chicago, pp. 241–278.

43. Buchanan, K.D., Kerr, J.I., Johnston, C.F. *et al.* (1983) The diffuse endocrine system in cystic fibrosis. *Scand. J. Gastroenterol.*, **19**, 600–603.

44. Moran, A., Diem, P., Klein, D.J. *et al.* (1991) Pancreatic endocrine function in cystic fibrosis. *J. Pediatr.*, **118**, 715–723.

45. European Working Group on CF Genetics (EWGCFG) (1990) Gradient of distribution of the major CF mutation and of its associated haplotype. *Hum. Genet.*, **85**, 436–445.

46. Kerem, E., Corey, M., Kerem, B.-S. *et al.* (1990) The relationship between genotype and phenotype in cystic fibrosis – analysis of the most common mutation (delta-F508). *NEJM*, **323**, 1517–1522.

47. Santis, G., Osborne, L., Knight, R.A. and Hodson, M.E. (1990) Independent genetic determinants of pancreatic and pulmonary status in cystic fibrosis. *Lancet*, **336**, 1081–1084.

48. Johansen, H.K., Nir, M., Høiby, N., Koch, C. and Schwartz, M. (1991) Severity of cystic fibrosis in patients homozygous and heterozygous for ΔF508. *Lancet*, **337**, 631–634.

49. Lanng, S., Schwartz, M., Thorsteinsson, B. and Koch, C. (1991) Endocrine and exocrine pancreatic function and

the delta-F508 mutation in cystic fibrosis. *Clin. Genet.*, **40**, 345–348.

50. Nerup, J., Mandrup-Poulsen, T. and Mølvig, J. (1987) The HLA-IDDM association: implications for etiology and pathogenesis of IDDM. *Diab. Metab. Rev.*, **3**, 779–802.

51. Stutchfield, P.R., O'Halloran, S.M., Smith, C.S. *et al.* (1988) HLA type, islet cell antibodies and glucose intolerance in cystic fibrosis. *Arch. Dis. Child.*, **63**, 1234–1239.

52. Zanelli, P., Neri, T.M., De Fanti, A. *et al.* (1990) *Genetic and immunological markers of preclinical insulin dependent diabetes mellitus (IDDM) in cystic fibrosis (CF)*. Workshop of Cystic Fibrosis, Sestri Uvante, Italy 1990 (abstract).

53. Schwartz, H.P., Bonnard, G.D., Neri, T.M. *et al.* (1984) Histocompatibility antigens in patients with cystic fibrosis and diabetes mellitus. *J. Pediatr.*, **104**, 799–800 (letter).

54. Lanng, S., Thorsteinsson, B., Pociot, F. *et al.* (1993) Diabetes mellitus in cystic fibrosis: genetic and immunological markers. *Acta Paediatr. Scand.*, **82**, 150–154.

55. Carrington, M., Krueger, L.J., Holselaw, D.S. Jr, Iannuzzi, M.C., Dean, M. and Mann, D. (1994) Cystic fibrosis-related diabetes is associated with HLA DQB1 alleles encoding Asp-57 sup(–) molecules. *J. Clin. Immunol.*, **14**, 353–358.

56. Bottazzo, G.F. and Bonifacio, E. (1991) Immune factors in the pathogenesis of insulin-dependent diabetes mellitus, in *Textbook of Diabetes*, (ed. J.C. Pickup and G. Williams), Blackwell Scientific Publications, Oxford pp. 122–140.

57. Garne, S., Petersen, W., Heilmann, C. *et al.* (1985) Beta-cell function in cystic fibrosis. *Pediatr. Res.*, **19**, 629 (abstract).

58. Geffner, M.E., Lippe, B.M., McLaren, N.K. and Riley, W.J. (1988) Role of autoimmunity in insulinopenic and carbohydrate derangements in patients with cystic fibrosis. *J. Pediatr.*, **122**, 419–421.

59. Cucinotta, D., Conti Nibali, S., Arrigo, T. *et al.* (1990) Beta cell function, peripheral sensitivity to insulin and islet cell autoinimunity in cystic fibrosis patients with normal glucose tolerance. *Horm. Res.*, **34**, 33–38.

60. Stahl, M., Girard, J., Rutishauser, M. *et al.* (1974) Endocrine function of the pancreas in cystic fibrosis: evidence for an impaired glucagon and insulin response following arginine infusion. *J. Pediatr.*, **84**, 821–824.

61. Redmond, A.O.B., Buchanan, K.D. and Trimble, E.R. (1977) Insulin and glucagon response to arginine infusion in cystic fibrosis. *Acta Paediatr. Scand.*, **66**, 199–204.

62. Adrian, T.E., McKiernan, J., Johnstone, D.I. *et al.* (1980) Hormonal abnormalities of the pancreas and gut in cystic fibrosis. *Gastroenterology*, **79**, 460–465.

63. Ross, S.A., Morrison, D. and McArthur, R.G. (1981) Hypersecretion of gastric inhibitory polypeptide in nondiabetic children with cystic fibrosis. *Pediatrics*, **67**, 252–254.

64. Allen, J.M., Penketh, A.R.L. and Adrian, T.E. (1983) Adult cystic fibrosis: postprandial response of gut regulatory peptides. *Gastroenterology*, **85**, 1379–1383.

65. Nousia-Arvanitakis, S., Tomita, T., Desai, N. and Kimmel, J.R. (1985) Pancreatic polypeptide in cystic fibrosis. *Arch. Pathol. Lab. Med.*, **109**, 722–726.

66. Lamers, C.B.H.W., Jansen, J.B.M.J., Hafkenscheid, J.C.M. and Jongerius, C.M. (1990) Evaluation of tests of exocrine and endocrine pancreatic function in older patients with cystic fibrosis. *Pancreas*, **5**, 65–69.

67. Hamdi, I., Green, M., Shneerson, J.M., Palmer, C.R. and Hales, C.N. (1993) Proinsulin, proinsulin intermediate and insulin in cystic fibrosis. *Clin. Endocrin.*, **39**, 21–26.

68. Lanng, S., Thorsteinsson, B., Røder, M.E. *et al.* Pancreas and gut hormone reponses to oral glucose and intravenous glucagon in cystic fibrosis patients with normal, impaired, and diabetic glucose tolerance. *Acta Endocrin.*, **128**, 207–214.

69. Meacham, L.R., Caplan, D.B., McKean, L.P., Buchanan, C.N., Parks, J.S. and Culler, F.L. (1993) Preservation of somatostatin secretion in cystic fibrosis patients with diabetes. *Arch. Dis. Child.*, **68**, 123–125.

70. Rakotoambinina, B., Delaisi, B., Laborde, K. *et al.* (1994) Insulin responses to intravenous glucose and the hyperglycemic clamp in cystic fibrosis patients with different degrees of glucose tolerance. *Pediatr. Res.*, **36**, 667–671.

71. Hinds, A., Sheehan, A.G. and Parsons, G. (1995) Tolbutamide causes a modest increase in insulin secretion in cystic fibrosis patients with impaired glucose tolerance. *Metabolism*, **44**, 13–18.

72. Binder, C. (1991) C-peptide and B-cell function in diabetes mellitus, in *Textbook of Diabetes*, (eds J.C. Pickup and G. Williams), Blackwell Scientific Publications, Oxford, pp. 348–354.

73. Sjoberg, R.J. and Kidd, G.S. (1989) Pancreatic diabetes mellitus. *Diabetes Care*, **12**, 715–724.

74. Kendall, D.M., Sutherland, D.E.R., Najarian, J.S. *et al.* Effects of hemipancreatectomy on insulin secretion and glucose tolerance in healthy subjects. *NEJM*, **322**, 898–903.

75. Raskin, P., Aydin, I. and Unger, R.H. (1976) Effect of insulin on the exaggerated glucagon response to arginine stimulation in diabetes mellitus. *Diabetes*, **25**, 227–229.

76. Starke, A., Imamura, T. and Unger, R.H. (1987) Relationship of glucagon suppression by insulin and somatostatin to the ambient glucose concentration. *J. Clin. Invest.*, **79**, 20–24.

77. Adrian, T.E., Bestermann, H.S., Mallinson, C.N. *et al.* (1979) Impaired pancreatic polypeptide release in chronic pancreatitis with steatorrhoea. *Gut*, **20**, 98–101.

78. Larsen, S. (1992) Diabetes mellitus secondary to chronic pancreatitis. *Dan. Med. Bull.*, **40**, 153–162.

79. Kreymann, B. and Bloom, S.R. (1991) Glucagon and the gut hormones in diabetes mellitus, in *Textbook of Diabetes*, (eds J.C. Pickup and G. Williams). Blackwell Scientific Publications, Oxford, pp. 313–324.

80. Davis, T.M.E., Batten, J.C., Rudenski, A.S. and Turner, R.C. (1987) Insulin sensitivity and beta-cell function assessed by C-peptide in young adults with cystic fibrosis. *Eur. J. Clin. Invest.*, **17**, 12–15.

81. Holl, R.W., Wolf, A., Rank, M. and Heinze, E. (1993) Reduced pancreatic insulin release and impaired

peripheral insulin sensitivity contribute to high incidence of diabetes mellitus in young adults with cystic fibrosis. *Diabetes*, **42**, (Suppl. I), 60A.

82. Andersen, O., Garne, S., Heilmann, C. *et al*. (1988) Glucose tolerance and insulin receptor binding to monocytes and erythrocytes in patients with cystic fibrosis. *Acta Paediatr. Scand*., **77**, 67–71.

83. DeFronzo, R.A., Tobin, J.D. and Andres, R. (1979) Glucose clamp technique: a method for quantifying insulin secretion and resistance. *Am. J. Physiol*., **237**, E214–E223.

84. Cucinotta, D., De Luca, F., Gigante, A. *et al*. (1994) No changes of insulin sensitivity in cystic fibrosis patients with different degrees of glucose tolerance: an epidemiological and longitudinal study. *Eur. J. Endocrinol*., **130**, 253–258.

85. Lanng, S., Thorsteinsson, B., Røder, M., Nerup, J. and Koch, C. (1994) Insulin sensitivity and insulin clearance in cystic fibrosis patients with normal and diabetic glucose tolerance. *Clin. Endocrinol*., **41**, 217–223.

86. Ahmad, T., Nelson, R. and Taylor, R. (1994) Insulin sensitivity and metabolic clearance rate of insulin in cystic fibrosis. *Metabolism*, **43**, 163–167.

87. Moran, A., Pyzdrowski, K.L., Weinreb, J. *et al*. (1994) Insulin sensitivity in cystic fibrosis. *Diabetes*, **43**, 1020–1026.

88. Austin, A., Kalhan, S.C., Orenstein, D., Nixon, P. and Arslanian, S. (1994) Roles of insulin resistance and β-cell dysfunction in the pathogenesis of glucose intolerance in cystic fibrosis. *J. Clin. Endocrinol. Metab*., **79**, 80–85.

89. Lippe, B.M., Kaplan, S.A., Neufeld, N.D., Smith, A. and Scott, M. (1980) Insulin receptors in cystic fibrosis: increased receptor number altered affinity. *Pediatrics*, **65**, 1018–1022.

90. Lanng, S., Thorsteinsson, B., Nerup, J. and Koch, C. (1992) Influence of the development of diabetes mellitus on clinical status in patients with cystic fibrosis. *Eur. J. Pediatr*., **151**, 684–687.

91. Lanng, S., Thorsteinsson, B., Nerup, J. and Koch, C. (1994) Diabetes mellitus in cystic fibrosis: effect of insulin therapy on lung function and infections. *Acta Paediatr*., **83**, 849–853.

92. Hodson, M.E. (1992) Diabetes mellitus and cystic fibrosis. *Baillière's Clin. Endocrinol. Metab*., **6**, 797–805.

93. Allen, J.L. (1986) Progressive nephropathy in a patient with cystic fibrosis and diabetes. *NEJM*, **315**, 764.

94. Dolan, T.F. (1986) Microangiopathy in a young adult with cystic fibrosis and diabetes mellitus.*NEJM*, 314, 991–992.

95. Zipf, W.B., Kien, C.L., Horswill, C.A., McCoy, K.S., O'Dorisio, T. and Pinyerd, B.L. (1991) Effect of tolbutamide on growth and body composition of nondiabetic children with cystic fibrosis. *Pediatr. Res*., **30**, 309–314.

96. Culler, F.L., McKean, L.P., Buchanan, C.N., Caplan, D.B. and Meacham, L.R. (1993) Glipizide treatment of patients with cystic fibrosis and impaired glucose tolerance. *J. Pediatr. Gastroenterol. Nutr*., **18**, 375–378.

97. Shwachman, H., Kulczycki, L.L., Mueller, H.L. and Flake,

C.G. (1962) Nasal polyposis in patients with cystic fibrosis. *Pediatrics*, **30**, 389–401.

98. Taylor, B., Evans, J.N.G. and Hope, G.A. (1982) Upper respiratory tract in cystic fibrosis. *Arch. Dis. Child*., **49**, 133–136.

99. Bak-Pedersen, K. and Kildegaard Larsen, P. (1979) Inflammatory middle ear diseases in patients with cystic fibrosis. *Acta Otolaryngol*., **360**, 138–140.

100. Stern, R.C., Boat, T.F., Wood, R.E. *et al*. (1982) Treatment and prognosis of nasal polyps in cystic fibrosis. *Am. J. Dis. Child*., **136**, 1067–1070.

101. Davis, P.B. and di Sant'Agnese, P.A. (1984) Diagnosis and treatment of cystic fibrosis: an update. *Chest*, **85**, 802–809.

102. De Gaudemar, I., Contencin, P., Van den Abbeele, Y. *et al*. (1996) Is nasal polyposis in cystic fibrosis a direct manifestation of genetic mutation or a complication of chronic infection? *Rhinology*, **34**, 194–197.

103. Neely, J., Harrison, G.M., Jerger, J.F. *et al*. (1972) The otolaryngologic aspects of cystic fibrosis. *Am. Acad. Ophthal. Oto. Trans*., **76**, 313–324.

104. Sørensen, H., Mygind, N., Tygstrup, I. and Flensborg, E.W. (1977) Histology of nasal polyps of different etiology. *Rhinology*, **15**, 121–128.

105. Tos, M., Mogensen, C. and Thomsen, J. (1977) Nasal polyps in cystic fibrosis. *J. Laryngol. Otol*., **91**, 827–835.

106. Rowe-Jones, J.M., Shembekar, M., Trendell-Smith, N. and Mackay, I.S. (1997) Polypoidal rhinosinusitis in cystic fibrosis: a clinical and histopathological study. *Clin. Otolaryngol*., **22**, 161–171.

107. Triglia, J.-M. and Nicollas, R. (1997) Nasal and sinus polyposis in children. *Laryngoscope*, **107**, 963–966.

108. Jaffe, B.F., Strome, M., Khaw, K.-T. and Shwachman, H. (1977) Nasal polypectomi and sinus surgery for cystic fibrosis – a 10 year review. *Otol. Clin. North Am*., **10**, 81–90.

109. Cepero, R., Smith, R.J., Catlin, F.I. *et al*. (1987) Cystic fibrosis: an otolaryngologic perspective. *Otolaryngol. Head Neck Surg*., **97**, 356–360.

110. Reilly, J.S., Kenna, M.A., Stool, S.E. and Bluestone, C.D. (1985) Nasal surgery in children with cystic fibrosis: complications and risk management. *Laryngoscope*, **95**, 1491–1493.

111. Crockett, D.M., McGill, T.J., Healy, G.B. *et al*. (1987) Nasal and paranasal sinus surgery in children with cystic fibrosis. *Ann. Otol. Rhinol. Laryngol*., **96**, 367–372.

112. Wang, D., Levasseur-Acker, G.M., Jankowski, R. et al. (1997) HLA class II antigens and T lymphocytes in human nasal epithelial cells. Modulation of the HLA class II gene transcripts by gamma interferon. *Clin. Exper. Allergy*, **27**, 306–314.

113. Gharib, R., Allen, R.P., Joos, H.A. and Bravo, L.R. (1964) Paranasal sinuses in cystic fibrosis. *Am. J. Dis. Child*., **108**, 499–502.

114. Ledesma-Medina, J., Osman, M.Z. and Girdany, B.R. (1980) Abnormal paranasal sinuses in patients with cystic fibrosis of the pancreas. *Pediatr. Radiol*., **9**, 61–64.

115. Møller, N.E. and Thomsen, J. (1978) Mucocele of the paranasal sinuses in cystic fibrosis. *J. Laryngol. Otol.*, **92**, 1025–1027.

116. Kingdom, T.T., Lee, K.C., FitzSimmons, S.C. and Cropp, G.J. (1996) Clinical characteristics and genotype analysis of patients with cystic fibrosis and nasal polyposis requiring surgery. *Arch. Otolaryngol. Head Neck Surg.*, **122**, 1209–1213.

117. Koch, C., McKenzie, S.G., Kaplowitz, H. *et al.* (1997) International practice patterns by age and severity of lung disease in cystic fibrosis: data from the epidemiologic registry of cystic fibrosis (ERCF). *Pediatr. Pulmonol.*, **24**, 147–154.

118. Johnson, S. and Knox, A.J. (1994) Arthropathy in cystic fibrosis. *Respir. Med.*, **88**, 567–570.

119. Taussig, L.M., Landau, L.I. and Marks, M.I. (1984) Respiratory system, in *Cystic Fibrosis*, (ed. L.M. Taussig), Thième-Stratton, New York, pp. 115–174.

120. Lemen, R.J., Gates, A.J., Mathe, A.A. *et al.* (1978) Relationship among digital clubbing, disease severity, and serum prostaglandins $F_2\alpha$ and E concentration in cystic fibrosis patients. *A. Rev. Respir. Dis.*, **117**, 639.

121. Grossmann, H., Denning, C.R. and Baker, D.H. (1964) Hypertrophic osteoarthropathy in cystic fibrosis. *Am. J. Dis. Child.* **129**, 1–6.

122. Athreya, B.H., Borns, P. and Rosenlund, M.L. (1975) Cystic fibrosis and hypertrophic osteoarthropathy in children. *Am. J. Dis. Child.*, **129**, 634–637.

123. Braude, S., Kennedy, A., Hodson, M. *et al.* (1984) Hypertrophic osteoarthropathy in cystic fibrosis. *BMJ*, **288**, 822–823.

124. Nathanson, I. and Riddlesberger, M.M. (1980) Pulmonary hypertrophic osteoarthropathy in cystic fibrosis. *Radiology*, **135**, 649–651.

125. Newman, A.J. and Ansell, B.M. (1979) Episodic arthritis in children with cystic fibrosis. *J. Pediatr.*, **94**, 594–596.

126. Schidlow, D.V., Goldsmith, D.P., Palmer, J. and Huang, N.N. (1984) Arthritis in cystic fibrosis. *Arch. Dis. Child.*, **59**, 377–379.

127. Rush, P.J., Shore, A., Coblentz, C. *et al.* (1986) The musculosceletal manifestations of cystic fibrosis. *Semin. Arthritis Rheum.*, **15**, 213–225.

128. Dixey, J., Redington, A.N., Butler, R.C. *et al.* (1988) The arthropathy of cystic fibrosis. *Ann. Rheum. Dis.*, **47**, 218–223.

129. Pertuiset, E., Menkes, C.J., Lenoir, G. *et al.* (1992) Cystic fibrosis arthritis. A report of five cases. *Br. J. Rheumatol.*, **31**, 535–538.

130. Wulffraat, N.M., de Graeff-Meeder, E.R., Rijkers, G.T. *et al.* (1994) Prevalence of circulating immune complexes in patients with cystic fibrosis and arthritis. *J. Pediatr.*, **125**, 374–378.

131. Benjamin, C.M. and Clague, R.B. (1990) Psoriatic or cystic fibrosis arthropathy? Difficulty with diagnosis and management. *Br. J. Rheumatol.*, **29**, 301–302.

132. Soden, M., Tempany, E. and Bresnihan, B. (1989) Sarcoid arthropathy in cystic fibrosis. *Br. J. Rheumatol.*, **28**, 341–343.

133. Hassan, J., Feighery, C., Bresnihan, B. and Whelan, A. (1992) Prevalence of anti-Fab antibodies in patients with autoimmune and infectious diseases. *Clin. Exp. Immunol.*, **89**, 423–426.

134. Taccetti, G., Campana, S., Marianelli, L. and Turchini, S. (1995) Cystic fibrosis and episodic arthritis. *J. Pediatr.*, **126**, 848–849.

135. de Graeff-Meeder, E.R., Rijkers, G.T., Voorhorst-Ogink, M. *et al.* (1993) Antibodies to human HSP60 in patients with juvenile chronic arthritis, diabetes mellitus, and cystic fibrosis. *Pediatr. Res.*, **34**, 424–428.

136. Zhao, M.H., Jayne, D.R.W., Ardiles, L.G. *et al.* (1996) Autoantibodies against bactericidal/permeability-increasing protein in patients with cystic fibrosis. *Q. J. Med.*, **89**, 259–265.

137. Nielsen, H.E., Lundh, S., Jacobsen, S.V. and Høiby, N. (1978) Hypergammaglobulinemic purpura in cystic fibrosis. *Acta Paediatr. Scand.*, **67**, 443–447.

138. Fradin, M.S., Kalb, R.E. and Grossman, M.E. (1987) Recurrent cutaneous vasculitis in cystic fibrosis. *Pediatr. Dermatol.*, **4**, 108–111.

139. Finnegan, M.J., Hinchcliffe, J., Russell-Jones, D. *et al.* (1989) Vasculitis complicating cystic fibrosis. *Q. J. Med.*, **72**, 609–621.

140. Summers, G.D. and Webley, M. (1986) Episodic arthritis in cystic fibrosis: a case report. *Br. J. Rheumatol.*, **25**, 393–395.

141. Rush, P.J., Gladman, D.D., Shore, A. and Anhorn, K.A.B. (1991) Absence of an association between HLA typing in cystic fibrosis arthritis and hypertrophic osteoarthropathy. *Ann. Rheum. Dis.*, **50**, 763–764.

142. Titò, L., Prez Ayuso, R., Navarro, S. *et al.* (1987) Generalized amyloidosis: a rare complication of cystic fibrosis. *Pancreas*, **2**, 233–236.

143. Bontempini, L., Ghimenton, C., Colombari, R. *et al.* (1987) Secondary amyloidosis and cystic fibrosis. A morphologic and histochemical study of five cases. *Histol. Histopathol.*, **2**, 413–416.

144. Skinner, M., Pinnette, A., Travis W.D. *et al.* (1988) Isolation and sequence analysis of amyloid protein AA from a patient with cystic fibrosis. *J. Lab. Clin. Med.*, **112**, 413–417.

145. Smith, J.W., Colombo, J.L. and McDonald, T.L. (1992) Comparison of serum amyloid A and C-reactive protein as indicators of lung inflammation in corticosteroid treated and non-corticosteroid treated cystic fibrosis patients. *J. Clin. Lab. Anal.*, **6**, 219–224.

146. Samuels, M.H., Thompson, N., Leichty, D. and Ridgway, E.C. (1995) Amyloid goiter in cystic fibrosis. *Thyroid*, **5**, 213–215.

147. Gaffney, K., Gibbons, D., Keogh, B. and FitzGerald, M.X. (1993) Amyloidosis complicating cystic fibrosis. *Thorax*, **48**, 949–950.

148. Alvarez-Sala, R., Prados, C., Sastre Marcos, J.et al. (1994) Amyloid goitre and hypothyroidism secondary to cystic fibrosis. *Postgrad. Med. J.*, **71**, 307–308.

149. Couce, M., O'Brien, T.D., Moran, A. *et al*. (1996) Diabetes mellitus in cystic fibrosis is characterized by islet amyloidosis. *J. Clin. Endocrinol. Metab*., **81**, 1267–1272.

150. Dolan. T.F. and Gibson, L.E. (1971) Complications of iodide therapy in patients with cystic fibrosis. *Pediatr. Pharmacol. Therapeut*., **79**, 684–687.

151. Devuyst, O., Golstein, P.E., Sanches, M.V. *et. al*. (1997) Expression of CFTR in human and bovine thyroid epithelium. *Am. J. Physiol*., **272**, C1299–C1308.

152. Azizi, F., Bentley, D., Vagenakis, K. *et al*. (1974) Abnormal thyroid function and response to iodides in patients with cystic fibrosis. *Trans. Assoc. Am. Physicians*, pp. 111–117.

153. Baran, D., Wolter, R., Bourdoux, P. and Ermans, A.M. (1979) Increased serum TSH response to TRH in cystic fibrosis. *Monogr. Paediat*., **10**, 114–118.

154. Segall-Blank, M., Vagenakis, A.G., Shwachman, H. *et al*. (1981) Thyroid gland function and pituitary TSH reserve in patients with cystic fibrosis. *J. Pediatr*., **98**, 218–222.

155. De Luca, F., Trimarchi, F., Sferlazzas, C. *et al*. (1982) Thyroid function in children with cystic fibrosis. *Eur. J. Pediatr*., **138**, 327–330.

156. Sack. J., Blau, H., Amado, O. and Katznelson, D. (1983) Thyroid function in cystic fibrosis patients compared with healthy Israeli children. *Isr. J. Med. Sci*., **19**, 17–19.

157. Borel, D.M. and Reddy, J.K. (1973) Excessive lipofuscin accumulation in the thyroid gland in mucoviscidosis. *Arch. Pathol*., **96**, 269–271.

158. Rosenlund, M.L., Selekman, J.A., Hong, K.K. and Kritchevsky, D. (1977) Dietary essential fattty acids in cystic fibrosis. *Pediatr*., **59**, 428–432.

159. Kauf, E., Dawczynski, H., Jahreis, G. *et al*. (1994) Sodium selenite therapy and thyroid-hormone status in cystic fibrosis and congenital hypothyroidism. *Biol. Trace Elem. Res*., **40**, 247–253.

160. Al-Awqati, Q. (1995) Regulation of ion channels by ABC transporters that secrete ATP. *Science*, **269**, 805–806.

161. Crawford, I. Maloney, P.C., Zeitlin, P.L. *et al*. (1991) Immunocytochemical localization of the cystic fibrosis gene product. *Proc. Natl Acad. Sci. USA*, **88**, 9262–9266.

162. Morales, M.M. Carroll, T.P., Morita, T. *et al*. (1996) Both the wild type and a functional isoform of CFTR are expressed in kidney. *Am. J. Physiol*., **270**, (*Renal Fluid Electrolyte Physiol*., **39**), F1038–F1048.

163. Stanton, B.A. (1997) Cystic fibrosis transmembrane conductance regulator (CFTR) and renal function. *Wien Klin. Wochenschr*.; **109**, 457–464.

164. Stenvinkel, P., Hjelte, L., Alvan, G. *et al*. (1991) Decreased renal clearance of sodium in cystic fibrosis. *Acta Paediatr. Scand*., **80**, 194–198.

165. Donckerwolcke, R.A.. van-Diemen-Steenwoorde, R.,, van-der-Laag, J. *et al*. (1992) Impaired diluting segment chloride reabsorption in patients with cystic fibrosis. *Child Nephrol. Urol*., **12**, 186-191.

166. Spino, M. (1991) Pharmacokineties of drugs in cystic fibrosis. *Clin. Rev. Allergy*, **9**,169–210.

167. Strandvik, B., Berg, U., Kallner, A. and Kusoffsky, E. (1989) Effect on renal function of essential fatty acid supplementation in cystic fibrosis. *J. Pediatr*., **115**, 242–250.

168. McNicholas, C.M., Guggino, W.B., Schwiedbert, E.M. *et al*. (1996) Sensitivity of a renal K^+ channel (ROMK2) to the inhibitory sulfonylurea compound glibenclamide is enhanced by coexpression with the ATP-binding cassette transporter cystic fibrosis transmembrane regulator. *Proc. Natl Acad. Sci. USA*, **93**, 8083–8088.

169. Hanaoka, K., Devuyst, O., Schwiebert, E.M. *et al*. (1996) A role for CFTR in human autosomal dominant polycystic kidney disease. *Am. J. Physiol*., **270**, (*Cell Physiol*., **39**), C389–C399.

170. Davidow, C.J., Maser, R.L., Rome, L.A. *et al*. (1996) The cystic fibrosis transmembrane conductance regulator mediates transepithelial fluid secretion by human autosomal dominant polycystic kidney disease epithelium *in vitro*. *Kidney Internat*., **50**, 208–218.

171. Brill, S.R., Ross, K.E. and Davidow, C.J. (1996) Immunolocalization of ion transport proteins in human autosomal dominant polycystic kidney epithelial cells. *Proc. Natl Acad. Sci. USA*, **93**, 10206–10211.

172. Katz, S.M., Krueger, L.J. and Falkner, B. (1988) Microscopic nephrocalcinosis in cystic fibrosis. *NEJM*, **319**, 263–266.

173. Bentur, L., Kerem, E., Couper, R. *et al*. (1990) Renal calcium handling in cystic fibrosis: lack of evidence for a primary renal defect. *J. Pediatr*., **116**, 556–560.

174. Strandvik, B. and Hjelte, L. (1993) Nephrolithiasis in cystic fibrosis. *Acta Paediatr*., **82**, 306–307.

175. Chidekel, A.S. and Dolan, T.F. (1996) Cystic fibrosis and calcium oxalate nephrolithiasis. *Yale J. Biol. Med*., **69**, 317–321.

Osteoporosis

176. Consensus Development Conference (1991) Prophylaxis and treatment of osteoporosis. *Osteoporosis International*, **1**, 114–117.

177. Ralston, S.H. (1996) Pathophysiology of osteoporosis, in *Osteoporosis*, (ed. J. Compston), Royal College of Physicians, London, p. 35.

178. Compston, J.E., Cooper, C. and Kanis, J.A. (1995) Bone densitometry in clinical practice. *BMJ*, **310**, 1507–1510.

179. Bhudhikanok, G.S., Lim, J., Marcus, R., Harkins, A., Moss, R.B. and Bachrach, L.K. (1996) Correlates of osteopenia in patients with cystic fibrosis. *Pediatrics*, **97**, 103–111.

180. Gibbens, D.T., Gilsanz, V., Boechat, M.I., Duffer, D., Carlston, M.E. and Wang, C. (1988) Osteoporosis in cystic fibrosis. *J. Pediatr*., **113**, 295–300.

181. Henderson, R.C. and Madsen, C.D. (1996) Bone density in children and adolescents with cystic fibrosis. *J. Pediatr*., **128**, 28–34.

182. Haworth, C.S., Selby, P.L., Webb, A.K. *et al*. (1999) Low bone mineral density in adults with cystic fibrosis. *Thorax*, **54**, 961–967.

183. Aris, R.M., Renner, J., Lester, G., Riggs, D., Neuringer, I.P. and Ontjes, D.A. (1996) Severe osteoporosis, increased

fractures and kyphosis in adults with late stage cystic fibrosis. *Pediatr. Pulmonol.*, (Suppl. 13), 317.

184. Cummings, S.R., Black, D.M., Nevitt, M.C. *et al*. (1993) Bone density at various sites for prediction of hip fractures. *Lancet*, **341**, 72–75.

185. Henderson, R.C. and Specter, B.B. (1994) Kyphosis and fractures in children and young adults with cystic fibrosis. *J. Pediatr.*, **125**, 208–212.

186. Aris, R.M., Renner, J.B., Winders, A.D. *et al*. (1998) Increased rate of fractures and severe kyphosis: sequelae of living into adulthood with cystic fibrosis. *Ann. Intern. Med.*, **128**, 186–193.

187. Elkin, S.L., Compston, J.E. and Hodson, M.E. (1998) Age distribution and rate of fracture in patients with cystic fibrosis. *Current Research in Osteoporosis and Bone Mineral Measurement*, **9**, 102.

188. Ferrari, S.L., Nicod, L.P. and Hamacher, J. (1996) Osteoporosis in patients undergoing lung transplantation. *Eur. Respir. J.*, **9**, 2378–2382.

189. Gallagher, J.C. (1998) Vitamin D treatment in osteoporosis and osteomalacia, in *Osteoporosis*, (ed. J.C. Stevenson and R. Lindsay), Chapman & Hall Medical, London, pp. 243–262.

190. Ott, S.M. and Aitken, M.L. (1998) Osteoporosis in patients with cystic fibrosis. *Clin. Chest Med.*, **19**, (3), 560–562.

191. Elkin, S.L., Fairney, A., Burgess, J. and Hodson, M.E. (1998) Hypovitaminosis D in patients attending a national cystic fibrosis centre. *Thorax*, **53**, (S4), A19.

192. Johnston, C.C., Miller, J.Z., Slemenda, C.W. *et al*. (1992) Calcium supplementation and increases in bone mineral density in children. *NEJM*, **327**, 82–87.

193. National Institutes of Health (1994) Optimal calcium intake: NIH Consensus Statement. *Nutrition*, **12**, 1–31.

194. Aris, R.M., Neuringer, I.P., Weiner, M.A., Egan, T.M. and Ontjes, D.A. (1996) Severe osteoporosis before and after lung transplantation. *Chest*, **109**, 1176–1183.

195. Haworth, C.S., Selby, P.L., Webb, A.K., Mawer, E.B., Adams, J.E. and Freemont, T.J. (1998) Severe bone pain after intravenous pamidronate in adult patients with cystic fibrosis. *Lancet*, **352**, (9142), 1753–1754.

16

Psychological aspects of cystic fibrosis

B. LASK

Introduction	339	Care-givers	344
Children with cystic fibrosis	339	Management	345
Adults with cystic fibrosis	342	Conclusion	346
The family	343	References	346

INTRODUCTION

Do psychosocial assessments and interventions add anything of clinical value to the management of people with cystic fibrosis and their families? The committed mental health worker and many pediatricians and respiratory physicians would say that such a contribution is invaluable. Indeed, in the United Kingdom the demand for such a service far exceeds the supply, yet the skeptic might reasonably argue that there is limited evidence to warrant this attitude.

The vast literature on the psychosocial aspects of CF should guide us towards resolution of this dichotomy. The earlier reports which seemed to indicate that children with CF had a high incidence of psychopathology, particularly anxiety, depression and poor social functioning, are either anecdotal or limited by methodological flaws, including the use of small, biased samples, unstandardized questionnaires, the subjectivity of the psychological assessment, the absence of comparison groups, and the use of inappropriate statistical methods[1]. We need therefore to give more serious consideration to recent research, with its much improved methodology. Emphasis will be placed on findings from controlled studies where possible, as uncontrolled studies give rise to yet more confusion and contradiction. Even so, we have to accept that because different researchers use a wide range of informants, assessment approaches and instruments, and either no or different control groups, age ranges and degrees of severity of CF, it is inevitable that these studies will to some extent produce mixed results. Hopefully, as the prognosis continues to improve so too will psychosocial well-being.

Psychosocial aspects of CF may be considered under five main headings: (1) children with CF; (2) adults with CF; (3) the family; (4) care-givers and (5) management.

CHILDREN WITH CYSTIC FIBROSIS

Psychosocial adaptation

It is very difficult to ascertain the true incidence of satisfactory adaptation to CF. There has been considerable variation in the figures quoted, and this is almost certainly due to the multiple methodological problems in such studies (see above). Findings vary from, at one extreme, the suggestion that children with CF are as well adjusted as their healthy peers[2,3], to the other extreme, that 53 per cent of a sample of 36 children with CF had a psychiatric disorder, compared with 17 per cent of a matched control group[4]. A meta-analysis of relevant studies has suggested that children with CF are as well adjusted as healthy children and children with other chronic diseases[5].

Kashani et al.[3] have suggested that the infrequent finding of psychopathology in CF children results from the fact that they are receiving sufficient care and attention from healthcare professionals, social service groups and/or family, to offset any increases in psychopathology which might be associated with the illness. They propose that the results should be interpreted with caution, and more effort made to control for confounding variables. The variables that may have a mediating effect include age, gender, disease severity, coping mechanisms, intelligence, family circumstances and family functioning.

Age does appear to act as a mediating variable. For example, in the studies reported from the Hospital for Sick Children, Toronto, 41 preschool children showed no significant excess of behavior problems when compared to healthy controls[6]. In contrast, 108 children aged 6–11 years had a 23 per cent prevalence of psychiatric disorder, compared with l5 per cent of their healthy siblings[7]. In 85 adolescents aged 12–15 years, there were higher symptom scores than published standardized norms, but not reaching statistical significance[8]. In addition there is some evidence that adults with CF have a higher incidence of emotional disorder than do adolescents[9]. This is discussed further in the section below on adults with CF.

It is difficult to compare the Toronto findings with others in that there is a far greater overlap in age range in other studies. For example, Kashani et al.[3] compared 30 patients aged 7–17 years with 30 matched controls. Few differences emerged between the two groups. However, age was not found to be a significant predictor of psychopathology among or between children with CF and controls.

When children with CF are compared with other clinical populations, the former show a slight tendency to be psychologically healthier. For instance, Burke et al.[10] found that children with CF had a lower lifetime prevalence of depression than children with inflammatory bowel disease, although there was no difference between the groups in the current prevalence of depression or anxiety, or the lifetime prevalence of anxiety, each of which was comparable to that of the normal population. In a comparison of 65 children with CF (aged 6–18 years) with 239 children with various central nervous system (CNS) disorders, and 360 healthy controls, severe psychiatric impairment was found in 11 per cent of the CF group, 30 per cent of the CNS group and 11 per cent of the control group[11].

Gender also appears to be a significant mediating factor in adaptation. Cowen et al.[9] reported greater emotional disturbance in females at all ages, and the same workers suggested that males enjoy better protection by virtue of more complete integration of their illness into their self-perception[8]. Sawyer et al. found that adolescent girls, but not boys were less well adjusted than their healthy peers[12]. Similar findings have been reported in adults[13] (see below).

Bluebond-Langner[14] has described six periods in the natural history of the disease which correlate with illness severity:

1. the first year following diagnosis;
2. the years up to the first exacerbation;
3. the time between the first exacerbation and increasing hospitalization;
4. the period of increasing complications;
5. the period of increasing deterioration;
6. the terminal phase.

Clearly, illness severity has to be considered as a mediating variable. Some correlation has been found between illness severity and psychosocial adaptation. Steinhauser and Schindler[15] initially found illness severity to be less significant than family variables, but in a later study[4] they found illness severity to be the most important variable in predicting adaptation. The Toronto group[8,9] found no correlation between illness severity and adaptation. This is in accord with the findings of the Great Ormond Street Hospital group[16]. In a study of 51 children awaiting heart–lung transplantation, i.e. those children at the most severe stage of the illness, 25 per cent had a psychiatric disorder and 60 per cent had a degree of impairment of their psychosocial functioning, both figures being higher than are generally reported in CF. In contrast, the Toronto group[8,9] found no correlation between illness severity and adaptation. It may be, however, that illness severity is more relevant in childhood and in adult life, than in adolescence[9].

Denial is frequently quoted as a protective factor in adjustment to CF. This is a difficult process to evaluate, but several authors, for example Simmons et al.[8] and Sawyer et al.[12], have suggested that males tend to use denial with more success. Bluebond-Langner[14] has criticized the term 'denial', recommending instead the use of the concept 'compartmentalization of information'. In developing this theme Christian and D'Auria[17] have noted that adolescents with CF use a variety of protective strategies for reducing their sense of difference from their peers: (1) keeping secrets, (2) hiding visible differences and (3) discovering a new baseline. Good friends were a critical source of support.

Notwithstanding the methodological flaws and differences, numerous studies have suggested that the intelligence quotient of most CF patients falls within the normal range[18,19], although it has been shown that over half the children with CF were delayed in two or more subjects[18], with the conclusion that the child's overall level of anxiety and general response to school were mediating variables. However, no definite relationship has been found between IQ and psychosocial adjustment[20].

Family factors are important variables to take into account when considering the CF patient's adaptation. These include family circumstances such as size, structure, socio-economic status, financial well-being, and parental health, reactions and attitudes to the illness, and communication patterns. Although it is likely that there is a complex and significant interaction between individual and family variables, rarely have family factors been controlled in studies of individual adaptation, thus it is not possible to make definitive statements about their relevance. Family adaptation is discussed in more detail below.

Adherence

Adherence to treatment, including medication, diet and physiotherapy, is clearly essential for satisfactory control of CF. Numerous authors have commented on adherence, but there is little convincing literature documenting the extent of the problem, not least because it is so difficult to define poor adherence in the absence of valid and reliable measures[21]. D'Angelo and Lask have argued that adherence should be conceptualized as a continuum, on which the extremes of either complete or non-adherence are very rare[22]. Most young people are partially adherent and therefore partial adherence should be considered the norm, although not the ideal. Zeltzer et al.[23] considered CF patients to be the most compliant of patients with chronic illness, but this may be due to the fact that they are rarely asymptomatic, and therefore do not suffer the immediate consequence of partial adherence. Most studies attempting to report on adherence rates have focused on young children whose parents are responsible for implementing treatment. Patterson[24] has reported that family expressiveness – open and direct expression of feeling – is positively correlated with treatment adherence.

Czajkowski and Koocher[25] have commented on the problems of defining adherence. In their evaluation of a new assessment tool for measuring adherence, they selected the following objective criteria: cooperation in daily physiotherapy, adherence to diet, taking all medication, cooperating in all routine investigations and recording all daily inputs and outputs. Of 40 patients aged 13–23 years, 14 (35 per cent) were deemed to be 'noncompliant'. Proportionately, more females than males were poor 'compliers' and the oldest age segment was the least 'compliant'. More recent studies have reported a wide variation in rates of adherence, with adults being the least adherent[26–28].

Koocher et al.[29] have described a typology of poor adherence in CF: (1) inadequate knowledge, (2) psychosocial resistance, and (3) educated nonadherence, and they suggest that clinical use of this conceptual framework may enhance diagnostic and treatment efforts. In particular, management will differ from one type to another because the etiology differs[30].

Knowledge

Although it is possible that people with CF resist information about their disease as a way of defending against the threat of a fatal illness, it is also possible that knowledge has a positive effect. However, very few studies have investigated how much CF patients and their relatives know about their disease.

Kulczycki et al[31] found a wide variation in knowledge of their disease in 26 children under 10 years, and Falkman[19] made similar observations in a study of 52 CF patients aged 4–15 years. Nolan et al.[32] assessed knowledge in 28 patients aged 10–21 years and in their parents. Knowledge of disease pathophysiology and treatment was generally comprehensive and detailed, but knowledge of genetics was only fair. Not surprisingly, better results were achieved by children older than 12 compared with those under 12, and by children at a higher education level. Girls knew more than boys, and those children with older parents did better.

The findings regarding parents were similar[32]. Higher parental age and socioeconomic status predicted better knowledge, and mothers knew more than fathers. Finally, Dinwiddie and Ramsay[33] have found no correlation between level of parental knowledge and ability to manage the CF.

Feeding and eating problems

Feeding and eating problems have been reported in a number of studies and particularly in infants[34,35]. This may be due to the fact that the recommended daily intake for children with CF is 130 per cent of normal intake. Stark et al. noted that both preschool children[34] and school-age children with CF[35] consume as much or more than healthy peers, but they are still not achieving the recommended daily intake. Parental anxiety may account for Stark's findings that there appear to be behavioral differences in eating and parental perception of their children's eating. Alternatively, these differences may lead to the inadequate intake. Steinhauser and Schindler[15] reported an eating disorder in 6 out of 36 patients (17 per cent), and Pumariega et al.[36] reported a series of 13 adolescents with CF and an atypical eating disorder. Crist et al.[37] noted excessively long meal-times in 11 out of 21 (55 per cent) young children with CF, delay of eating by talking in 46 per cent, and spitting out food in 41 per cent. Berry et al.[38] attributed nutritional disorders in CF to be secondary to the disease process, but Pumariega et al.[36] argued that psychological factors contribute to poor nutritional intake. This view is strengthened by the observations of distorted body image in those adolescents with eating difficulties[39]. Further, a noteworthy gender difference has been observed[39]. Whereas in females a higher body mass index (BMI) was associated with an elevated drive for thinness and negative effects on meals, in males a higher BMI was associated with better self-image and self-confidence.

Some reports suggest that attention to mother–infant relationships, particularly feeding interactions, can improve nutritional status in babies with CF, thus pointing to important preventive measures[40–42].

Schooling

There are very few reports regarding the relationship between CF and the child's school. In a report of the school experiences of 24 British children with CF, mean age 12 years, as reported by teachers, the majority of the children were making good academic and social progress[43]. Only a minority had sports restrictions. Half the sample had special arrangements at school for medication and physiotherapy, and little time was missed from school. Teachers generally felt ill-informed about CF, but this did not seem to have an adverse effect on the child.

However, it is equally possible that teachers and peers who have little understanding of CF may inhibit the child's ability to participate in normal school activities. In such circumstances school visits may enhance acceptance of children with CF and their needs. Further clarification of the school-based needs of children with CF and their teachers is required, and any such study should take into account the severity of the disease.

ADULTS WITH CYSTIC FIBROSIS

Treating the adult with CF challenges the physician's interpersonal as well as medical resources. Now that well over half of patients with CF will live into adult life, far more information is needed than is available on the psychosocial status and needs of this group[13]. In contrast to the extensive literature on children and adolescents, there is relatively little on adults.

One of the first studies of adults with CF was that of Boyle et al.[44] who noted in 13 patients over the age of 18 that there were four main areas of stress: altered physical appearance, strained interpersonal relationships, social isolation and increased awareness of the future.

More detailed studies have since been reported[9,13,45–54]. Over 700 adult patients have been described in these studies, with a mean age of about 25 years. About one-third were living with their parents and between one-quarter and two-thirds were cohabiting or married. (Perobelli's[48] study is excluded from these data as her findings were so different: 80 per cent of her sample were still living at home, and she believes cultural factors are relevant here.) Between one-third and half of all the patients described were in full-time employment and about a quarter were full-time students.

Many of the findings from these studies are, by and large, similar. Patients generally consider themselves well informed about their illness, although important gaps and misconceptions had been noted. Although patients found CF clinic staff helpful in providing information, immediate family and/or partner were rated as the most valuable in solving general problems of living. The aspects of the illness that bothered some patients most were, in order of frequency: cough. 66 per cent; thinness, 57 per cent; dyspnea or fatigue, 47 per cent, gastrointestinal or bowel symptoms, 38 per cent[13]. Most patients in these reports rated themselves as having mild or moderate disease, and there was a significant difference between patient and physician rating, with the former consistently underrating their severity of illness. A significant minority rarely or never disclosed the fact that they had CF, and between 10 and 20 per cent admitted to poor adherence to treatment.

Some inconsistency between studies emerges in relation to work, social and sexual satisfaction. Strauss and Wellisch[13], for example, reported a high commitment to work, low self-esteem and a poor social life: 71 per cent of the men and 66 per cent of the women dated less than once a month. Boyle et al.[44] and Coffman et al.[49] have noted high levels of sexual dissatisfaction. In contrast, Shepherd et al.[47] found quite the opposite, with high levels of sexual satisfaction, and satisfaction with work and social life. They did, however, note that the unmarried patients had a high level of sexual dissatisfaction, and they postulated that high self-image predisposes both to marriage and sexual satisfaction.

With regard to emotional distress, differences are again reported between studies. Strauss and Wellisch[13] found that 29 per cent felt frustrated by their illness much of the time, and 43 per cent were depressed occasionally or frequently; 20 per cent felt life was not worth living at least once a year; 86 per cent indicated that they were able to express angry feelings only rarely or sometimes. In contrast, others concluded that adults with CF have essentially normal self-concepts and adequate psychosocial adaptation[9,46]. Shepherd et al.[47] found no significant differences in psychosocial adaptation between their patients and a healthy control group.

When considering the correlation between mediating variables, there seems to be a significant relationship between physical and psychological health, disease severity and psychological adjustment, and lung function and coping status. There is some indication that men adjust less well than women, which may in part be due to their inability to procreate.

Although little difference was found in adaptation between those patients still living with their families of origin and those who have left home, other than that the latter group are less adherent[48], autonomy does appear to be a crucial issue. Shepherd et al.[47] found that a subset of adults (43 per cent) enjoy as much autonomy as healthy adults, but that another 30 per cent remained in highly dependent roles, living at home and depending on others for financial support. Surprisingly there was no correlation between degree of autonomy and level of physical health.

Quin[50] has reported that adults with CF find it impossible to get life insurance, loans and mortgages. If they admit to having CF on job application forms, they do not get interviews. Their main aspiration is to own a car and thus reduce their dyspnea and dependence.

In summary, although many adults with CF lead contented and satisfying lives, a substantial proportion are dependent, socially isolated, concerned about their appearance, use minimization and denial as coping measures, and compensate in part for lowered self-esteem and impoverished social life by commitment to their employment. Like their peers, most aspire to good health, satisfying interpersonal relationships and their own transport! An area that has not yet received detailed consideration is that of young adults with CF who become mothers.

THE FAMILY

Information on the family can be categorized under the following headings: (1) the effect of CF on the family; and (2) the effect of family functioning on, and adaptation to, CF and the course of the illness.

Effect on the family

The effect on the family may be considered under a number of different subheadings: effect on the family as a whole, effect on the parents, effect on the marriage, and effect on the well siblings.

CF has a devastating effect on the whole family. It is a major burden: practical, financial and emotional. Bluebond-Langner[14] has noted that the one word she heard parents use repeatedly during the first year following the diagnosis is 'overwhelmed'. Indeed, the disease is so overwhelming that families adopt strategies as a way of containing the intrusions into their lives and preserving as much of their previous normal way of life for as long as possible. These strategies have been considered in relation to the six periods of the disease, as outlined on p. 340.

In period (1), the first year following the diagnosis, families develop a routine for the CF-related tasks and compartmentalize information, i.e. they process and sort out all the new and overwhelming information they receive soon after the diagnosis is made. In period (2), the years between the first annual examination and the first exacerbation, families tend to avoid reminders of CF, redefine what is normal, and reconceptualize the future. Period (3), the time from the first exacerbation to the time of increasing hospitalization, sees an intensification of all these strategies and a reassessment of family priorities. In period (4), the time of increasing complications, it becomes much harder for families to contain the intrusions and their coping strategies are challenged. A new view of the future, a bleaker one, is projected. It is at this time that the siblings come to see CF as a chronic, progressive, incurable disease. In period (5), when there is increasing deterioration, families can no longer use such strategies as avoiding reminders of CF and redefining normal. Their compartmentalization of information is compromised, and their conceptualization of the future and assessment of family priorities change.

Effect on the parents

McCollum and Gibson[51] have also described stages of parental response to CF:

1. The prediagnostic stage is that time between the onset of parental concern for their child's health and the establishment of a diagnosis. It is characterized by repeated fruitless attempts to obtain a diagnosis, accompanied by rising anger and hostility directed at the medical profession.
2. The confrontational stage, distinguished by initial denial, followed by anticipatory mourning, and wanting subsequent pregnancies to replace the patient, but fearing the genetic risk. Anger is common at this stage, directed to the medical profession, the marital partner, and God, but not the child. The parents have difficulty grasping the full meaning and implications of the information given to them.
3. The long-term adaptational stage, the foremost demand of which is the sustaining of a mutually satisfying relationship between the parents and a child who is very likely to die before them.
4. The terminal stage, in which palliative care is implemented.

In considering family reactions to, and coping with, CF we should take account of the stage of the illness, although only rarely is this the case in the literature. The Toronto group[6], however, have reported on the adaptation to CF in the preschool child. They found that parents of healthy preschoolers reported more child-based problems than did parents of children with CF, suggesting that parents who have had to confront the CF diagnosis go on to minimize the normal stresses of this period. Parents in any given family tended to perceive similarly the impact that their child has upon them, a finding also noted by Hymovich and Baker[52].

Fathers of children with CF were more likely than control fathers to rate their family life as positive. Similar findings have been noted by others[4,30]. This may indicate some emotional distancing, a possibility supported by the reports from other studies on fathers' lack of involvement in the management of CF[19,44,53]. In the only published study of father–infant interaction in CF[54], fathers who were more involved in treatment were more positively interactive with their infant. The more highly stressed fathers showed less positive behavior to their infant.

The suggestions above of denial and minimization permeate the literature, and should caution us against taking too rosy a view of family coping. Although some studies have referred to the strengths and adaptability of these families[18,55,56], the intense and long-lasting trauma is bound to take its toll. Turk [57] has pointed out that many families had inadequate time and means for adult activities, and time for self and leisure was not available. There was also a lack of communication between family members, referred to as 'the web of silence', which in turn caused misunderstanding and impaired family functioning. Similar observations have been made by Kulczycki *et al.*[31] and Falkman[19], among others.

In trying to reconcile these opposing views we have to accept that, as is so often the case in CF psychosocial research, many of the studies lack control groups, and objective and normative data, thus casting doubt on their reliability and validity, and limiting their generalizability. Data from self-report measures should be interpreted with particular caution, as should studies that fail to take account of such significant variables as stage or severity of the illness.

The effect of CF on the marital relationship has been explored in a number of studies, although most had important methodological flaws. Allan *et al.*[58], in Australia, found that 33 per cent of marriages were in difficulty. Burton[18], in Britain, noted that 50 per cent of the marriages were severely strained and in 20 per cent the sexual relationship had ceased. A meta-analysis of 14 studies of parents of children with chronic illness has shown that separation and divorce were higher in parents of children with CF than in parents of children with spina bifida and leukaemia, but no higher than the national average[59]. A well-constructed study in Sweden reported lower divorce rates than the national average, but also that 26 per cent of the parents reported deteriorated marriages in reaction to the CF and a majority of parents described an inability to communicate about the CF[19].

De Wet and Cywes[20] have made the very important point that these optimistic findings must be interpreted with care because samples were often biased towards inclusion of stable families, and that absence of divorce cannot be seen to represent marital stability. Nor can it be seen to represent marital satisfaction. Many factors militate against divorce after a marriage has broken down.

Effect on well siblings

The effect of CF on the well siblings has unjustifiably received scant attention. Again, methodological problems impose caution on interpretation of the findings and there are considerable contradictions in the literature for example Breslau *et al.*[60] and Gayton *et al.*[61]. The most useful study to date has been that of Bluebond-Langner[62,63] who studied 175 families containing CF and reported on in-depth observations of 40. She concluded that the well siblings' views and responses are part of a

complex process involving the patient's condition and experience of illness, the sibling's own assessment of this, the parental responses to the patient and the sibling's assessment of these responses. These views and responses are likely to change as the disease progresses. The author did not detect any other mediating variables such as age. She concludes that any help geared to the well sibling must take account of the stage of the disease. The concerns of a child whose brother or sister has had, say, only one exacerbation will clearly differ from those whose brother or sister is at end-stage.

Effect of family functioning on psychosocial adaptation and on the course of the illness

There is increasing evidence that family dysfunction, whether or not this results from the illness, has an adverse effect on the behavior and health status of the child with CF[55,57,64,65]. For example, a correlation has been found between poor family functioning and the number of behavior problems in children with CF[55]. It has been reported that psychopathology in the child correlated first with the severity of the illness and then with two aspects of disturbed family functioning[4]. In the other direction, significant positive correlations have been noted between certain parental coping styles and improvements in the child's physical health[66]. Patterson[24] found that family expressiveness was positively associated with adherence, which in turn was associated with weight/height ratios, a measure of health status. The same team[64] has found that 22 per cent of the variance in 15-month weight and height changes were explained by family stress, family resources and parental coping. Family functioning variables also explained 17 per cent of the variance in 3-month pulmonary functioning changes and 15 per cent of the variance in 3-month weight and height changes.

Wilson *et al.*[65] have reported that children with CF segregated into subgroups of high and low psychological and physical risk, based on specific family attributes. Children in families that were achievement-oriented or that fostered independence were at lower risk for signs of progression of the disease. Angry children from families who encouraged expression of feelings fared better both physically and emotionally than angry children from families who inhibited such expression.

All these findings reinforce the importance of the family in its influence on both the physical and emotional well-being of children with CF.

CARE-GIVERS

There is very little in the literature on the effects of caring for CF on professional staff, nor on what characteristics in such staff make for a better disease course.

Common sense, supported by anecdotal reports, indicates that empathy, warmth and availability are the characteristics most valued by patients and their families. Whereas physicians are valued for their knowledge and expertise, nursing staff are often reported to be more supportive and helpful.

The stress of caring for chronically ill children and young adults with a fatal disease leads to high staff turnover and high levels of burnout, a syndrome consisting of emotional exhaustion and overload, depersonalization and reduced personal accomplishment[67]. Bergman et al.[68] specifically cited aspects of CF care that may lead to burnout. It is a disease with an unpredictable course and a hopeless prognosis; there is long-term contact with the patients and their families and the inevitable development of close relationships; therapy is nonspecific and labor intensive, and in the USA, at least, the healthcare system is unsympathetic to the needs of the chronically sick.

A comparison of CF care-givers with a control group found higher levels of emotional exhaustion, lower levels of depersonalization and equal levels of personal accomplishment[69].

Perhaps the most important study in this area is that of Coady et al.[70]. They studied burnout experienced by social workers employed in CF centers throughout the USA, and reported a significant relationship between team support, supervisory support and low burnout. They conclude that programs can be devised, and institutions structured, to decrease the amount of burnout in staff caring for chronically or terminally ill patients. Of particular value are staff-support groups and supervision.

Burnout is best prevented rather than treated. Preventative and treatment techniques include paying attention to working patterns, such as setting realistic goals, occasionally doing things differently, ensuring adequate breaks from work, with leisure and relaxation, taking things less personally when they go wrong, and ensuring adequate support and supervision from colleagues.

MANAGEMENT

The main objectives of psychosocial management are to enhance adaptation to the disease, improve the quality of life and overcome the associated psychological and social problems that arise from having CF. The models developed for other chronic or life-threatening diseases are likely to be equally applicable to CF. It has been pointed out that studies of several chronic disease interventions, particularly those related to asthma, chronic obstructive pulmonary disease and diabetes, have shown improved aspects of patient functioning, quality of life, healthcare utilization and health status[71].

Techniques that are used in CF include individual approaches, such as teaching self-help skills and promoting knowledge, behavioral approaches for poor adherence to treatment[72], poor nutritional intake[73] and family-oriented approaches, such as parental counseling and education[74,75], parental interpersonal skills training[76] and family therapy. Many centers use group approaches to promote understanding and knowledge and therefore to enhance coping skills for both patient[77] and parents[51,75,77,78]. Summer camps are a popular forum for providing group counseling and education[79,80] and educationally oriented school visits have also been described[41].

There have been some words of caution. For example, De Wet and Cywes[20] have emphasized the need to support and develop family coping mechanisms over the need for individual intervention. Dodge et al.[74] have noted that however well-intentioned the medical adviser may be, many factors militate against effective counseling, including intellectual/educational, psychological and linguistic factors. They suggest that counseling should be a continuing process, and that the same aspects be repeated on more than one occasion so that they may be fully comprehended. Also it is important for medical advisers to be aware of the extent to which adverse psychological reactions may be affecting patients and relatives. For this reason the use of trained counselors should be encouraged and further developed.

It is surprising that, unlike in other diseases, psychosocial interventions in CF have only very rarely been formally evaluated. Schroder et al.[76] have reported a pilot study evaluating a brief educational workshop for improving communication and problem-solving skills of parents of children with CF. Assessments of videotapes of couple interactions by trained raters indicated successful learning of communication skills and improvement in problem-solving skills. Parents scoring low on self-esteem, marital adjustment and family functioning showed significant improvement after treatment.

The effectiveness of a program designed to increase calorie consumption has been evaluated[73]. The intervention involved nutritional education, the establishment of gradually increasing calorie goals, teaching parents contingency management strategies, and a reward program for achieving calorie goals. Although there was no comparison group, calorie intake increased across meals and total calorie intake was 25–43 per cent above baseline, and was maintained at follow-up after 9 months. Significant changes in weight and height were made during treatment and the year following intervention.

McCracken et al.[80] have developed and evaluated a program of self-care intervention for adolescents at summer camp. Compared with controls who received only standard clinic care, the experimental group showed a significant improvement over time on both physical and psychological measures. This is the only controlled evaluation of a psychosocial treatment to be reported and offers a model for further studies.

Future research endeavors should put a high priority on the evaluation of interventions aimed at improving functioning and quality of life of CF patients and their families[71]. Such studies need to be well constructed, with appropriate comparison and control groups, and to avoid the methodological flaws so common in much of the early CF psychosocial research.

CONCLUSION

The overall impact of CF on psychosocial functioning remains unclear, probably because of the different research designs used in different centers. However, there is no doubt that many patients, especially in the mid and later stages of the disease, are in considerable emotional distress. Adherence to treatment is often poor. The effect of CF on the family is profound, but equally the family can have both a positive and negative effect on both adjustment and the course of the illness. Of particular relevance are the mother–child relationship and such family characteristics as achievement orientation, promotion of autonomy and emotional expressiveness. Evidence is beginning to emerge demonstrating the value of psychosocial interventions in improving psychosocial adjustment, family functioning and respiratory function. Further research endeavors should be guided by these findings and, in particular, we should attempt to answer key clinical questions such as:

1. Can we confirm that certain aspects of the mother-child relationship affect the course of the illness?
2. Can we confirm that specific family characteristics affect the course of the illness?
3. What other psychosocial factors affect the course of the illness?
4. How might we anticipate and identify poor adherers?
5. Can we confirm that certain psychosocial interventions do indeed contribute toward an improvement in the course of the illness, as well as toward an enhanced quality of life for both child and family?
6. If so, can we identify the most effective treatments, and those children and families who would most benefit?

Convincing answers to these questions would not only enhance the significance of psychosocial considerations, but also would lead to improved physical and psychological well-being.

REFERENCES

1. Graham, P. (1991) *Child Psychiatry*, (2nd edn), Oxford University Press, Oxford.
2. Drotar, D., Deorstrak, C., Stern, R. *et al*. (1981) Psychological functioning of children with cystic fibrosis. *Pediatrics*, **67**, 338–343.
3. Kashani, J., Barbero, G., Wilfley, D. *et al*. (1988) Psychological concomitants of cystic fibrosis in children and adolescents. *Adolescence*, **23**, 873–880.
4. Steinhauser, H., Schindler, H. and Stephan, H. (1983) Correlation of psychopathology in sick children and an empirical model. *J. Am. Acad. Child Adolesc. Psychiat.*, **22**, 559–564.
5. D'Angelo, S., Fosson, A. and McAninch, C. (1991) The adjustment of children with CF: a meta-analysis of empirical studies. *Pediatr. Pulmonol. Suppl.*, **7**, 287.
6. Cowen, L., Corey, M., Kennan, N. *et al*. (1985) Family adaptation and psychosocial adjustment to cystic fibrosis in the preschool child. *Soc. Sci. Med.*, **20**, 533–560.
7. Simmons, R., Corey, M., Cowen, L. *et al*. (1987) Emotional adjustment of latency age children with cystic fibrosis. *Psychosom. Med.*, **49**, 291–301.
8. Simmons, R., Corey, M., Cowen, L. *et al*. (1985) Emotional adjustment of early adolescents with cystic fibrosis. *Psychosom. Med.*, **47**, 111–19.
9. Cowen, L., Corey, M., Kennan, N. *et al*. (1984) Growing older with cystic fibrosis: psychological adjustment of patients over 16 years old. *Psychosom. Med.*, **46**, 363–369.
10. Burke, P., Meyer, V., Kocoshis, S. *et al*. (1989) Depression and anxiety in paediatric inflammatory bowel disease and cystic fibrosis. *J. Am. Acad. Child Adolesc. Psychiatr.*, **28**, 948–951.
11. Breslau, N. and Marshall, I. (1985) Psychological disturbance in children with physical disabilities. *J. Abnormal Child Psychol.*, **13**, 199–216.
12. Sawyer, S., Rosier, M., Phelan, P. and Bowes, G. (1995) The self image of adolescents with cystic fibrosis. *J. Adolesc. Hlth*, **16**, 204–20.
13. Strauss, G. and Wellisch, D. (1981) Psychosocial adaptation in older cystic fibrosis patients. *J. Chronic Dis.*, **34**, 141–146.
14. Bluebond-Langner, M. (1991) Living with cystic fibrosis: a family affair, in *Young People and Death*, (ed. J. Morgan), Charles Press, Philadelphia.
15. Steinhauser, H. and Schindler, H. (1981) Psychosocial adaptation in children and adolescents with cystic fibrosis. *J. Develop. Behaviour. Pediatr.*, **2**, 74–77.
16. Serrano-Ikkos, E., Lask, B. and Whitehead, B. (1997) Psychosocial morbidity in children, and their families, awaiting heart or a heart-lung transplantation. *J. Psychosom. Res.*, **42**, 253–260.
17. Christian, B. and D'Auria, J. (1997) The child's memories of growing up with cystic fibrosis. *J. Pediatr. Nurs.*, **12**, 3–12.
18. Burton, L. (1975) *The Family Life of Sick Children*, Routledge and Kegan Paul, London.

19. Falkman, C. (1977) Cystic fibrosis: a study of 52 children and adolescents. *Adolescence*, **23**, 873–80.

20. de Wet, B. and Cywes, S. (1984) The psychosocial impact of cystic fibrosis. *South Afr. Med. J.*, **65**, 526–530.

21. Lask, B. (1994) Non adherence in cystic fibrosis: methods, meanings and management. *J. R. Soc. Med. Suppl.*, **21**, 25–27.

22. D'Angelo, S. and Lask, B. (2000) Misuse of adherence, in: *The Illness Mosaic: Psychosocial Issues in Cystic Fibrosis*, (eds M. Bluebond-Langner, D. Angst and B. Lask), Arnold, London.

23. Zeltzer, L., Ellenberger, L. and Rigler, D. (1980) Psychological effects of illness in adolescents. *J. Pediatr.*, **97**, 132–137.

24. Patterson, J. (1985) Critical factors affecting family compliance with home treatment for children with cystic fibrosis. *Fam. Relat.*, **34**, 28–89.

25. Czajkowski, D. and Koocher, G. (1987) Medical compliance and coping with cystic fibrosis. *J. Child Psychol. Psychiatr. Allied Discipl.*, **28**, 311–319.

26. Geiss, S., Hobbs, S., Hammersley-Maerchlein, G. *et al.* (1992) Psychosocial factors related to perceived compliance with cystic fibrosis treatment. *J. Clin. Psychol.*, **48**, 99–103.

27. D'Angelo, S., Kanga, J. and Yates, C. (1992) Compliance with chest physiotherapy in cystic fibrosis. *Pediatr. Pulmonol. Suppl.*, **8**, 320.

28. Schultz, J. and Muser, A. (1992) Barriers to treatment adherence in cystic fibrosis. *Pediatr. Pulmonol. Suppl.*, **8**, 321.

29. Koocher, G., McGrath, M. and Gudens, L. (1990) Typologies of non-adherence in cystic fibrosis. *J. Develop. Behaviour. Pediatr.*, **2**, 353–358.

30. Cramer, J. and Spilker, B. (1991) *Patient Compliance in Medical Practice and Clinical Trials*, Raven Press, New York.

31. Kulczycki, L., Robinson, M. and Berg, C. (1969) Somatic and psychological factors relative to management of patients with cystic fibrosis. *Clin. Proc. Child. Hosp.*, **13**, 217–224.

32. Nolan, T., Demond, K., Herlich, R. and Hardy, S. (1978) Knowledge of cystic fibrosis in patients and their parents. *Pediatrics*, **77**, 229–336.

33. Dinwiddie, R. and Ramsay, S. (1992) Parental knowledge and management of cystic fibrosis. Presented at International Cystic Fibrosis Conference, Dublin.

34. Stark, L., Powers, S., Jelalian, E., Rape, R. and Miller, D. (1994) Modifying problematic mealtime interactions of children with cystic fibrosis and their parents by behavioural parent training. *J. Pediatr. Psychol.*, **19**, 751–768.

35. Stark, L., Mulvihill, M., Jelalian, E. *et al.* (1997) Descriptive analysis of eating behaviour in school age children with cystic fibrosis and healthy controlled children. *Pediatrics*, **99**, 665–671.

36. Pumariega, A., Breiger, D., Pearson, D. *et al.* (1990) Behavioural symptoms in cystic fibrosis v. neurological patients. *Psychosomatics*, **31**, 405–409.

37. Crist, W., McDonnell, P., Beck, M. *et al.* (1992) Behaviour at mealtimes and nutritional intake in the young child with cystic fibrosis. *Pediatr. Pulmonol. Suppl.*, **8**, 321.

38. Berry, H., Kellogg, F., Hunt, K. *et al.* (1975) Dietary supplement and nutrition in children with cystic fibrosis. *Am. J. Dis. Child.*, **129**, 165–171.

39. Smrekar, U., Ellemunter, H., Rothner, G. and Bonch, C. (1992) Eating attitudes and body experience in adolescent and adult CF patients. Paper presented at XIth International Cystic Fibrosis Congress, Ireland.

40. Fischer-Fay, A., Goldberg, S., Simmons, R. and Lewison, H. (1988) Chronic illness and infant–mother attachment: cystic fibrosis. *J. Develop. Behaviour. Pediatr.*, **9**, 266–270.

41. Simmons, R., Goldberg, S., Washington, J., Fispher-Day A., and McKlusky, I. (1995) Infant/mother attachment and nutrition in children with CF. *J. Develop. Behaviour. Pediatr.*, **16**, 183–186.

42. Stein, A. and Fairburn, C. (1994) An infant with cystic fibrosis and a mother with an eating disorder: a difficult combination. *Int. J. Eating Dis.*, **16**, 93–95.

43. Zoritch, B., Eiser, C., Bowyer, D. and Miller, J. (1992) School experience of children with CF: teacher's viewpoint. *Pediatr, Pulmonol. Suppl.*, **8**, 232.

44. Boyle, R., di Sant'Agnese, P. and Sack, L. *et al.* (1976) Emotional adjustment of adolescents and adults with cystic fibrosis. *J. Pediatr.*, **88**, 318–326.

45. di Sant'Agnese, P. and Davis, J. (1979) Cystic fibrosis in adults: 75 cases and review of 232 cases in the literature. *Am. J. Med.*, **66**, 121–131.

46. Moise, J., Drotar, D., Doershuk, C. and Stern, R. (1987) Correlates of psychosocial adjustment among young adults with cystic fibrosis. *J. Develop. Behaviour. Pediatr.*, **8**, 141–148.

47. Shepherd, S., Hovell, M., Harwood, I. *et al.* (1990) A comparative study of the psychosocial assets of adults with cystic fibrosis and their healthy peers. *Chest*, **97**, 1310–1316.

48. Perobelli, S. (1992) The psychosocial situation of independently living adults, in *Cystic Fibrosis, Basic and Clinical Research*, (eds N. Holby and S. Pederson), Excerpta Medica, London.

49. Coffman, C., Levine, S., Althof, S. and Stern, R. (1984) Sexual adaptation among single adults with cystic fibrosis. *Chest*, **86**, 412–418.

50. Quin, S. (1992) Psychosocial needs of adults with cystic fibrosis. Paper presented at XIth International Cystic Fibrosis Congress, Ireland.

51. McCollum, A. and Gibson, L. (1970) Family adaptation to the child with cystic fibrosis. *J. Pediatr.*, **77**, 571–578.

52. Hymovich, D. and Baker, C. (1982) The needs and concerns and coping of parents of children with cystic fibrosis. *Family Relat.*, **34**, 91–97

53. Tavormina, J., Ball, T., Dunn, N. *et al.* (1981) Psychosocial effects on parents of raising a physically handicapped child. *J. Abnorm. Child Psychol.*, **9**, 121–131.

54. Darke, P. and Goldberg, S. (1994) Father infant interaction and parent stress with healthy and medically compromised infants. *Infant Behaviour Develop.*, **17**, 3–14.

55. Lewis, B. and Khan, K. (1982) Family functioning as a mediating variable affecting psychosocial adjustment in children. *J. Pediatr.*, **101**, 636–639.

56. McCubbin, H., McCubbin, M., Patterson, J. *et al.* (1983) CHIP – Coping health inventory for parents: an assessment of parental coping patterns in the care of the chronically ill child. *Marriage Fam.*, **45**, 359–370.

57. Turk, J. (1964) Impact of cystic fibrosis on family functioning. *Pediatrics*, **34**, 67–71.

58. Allan, J., Townley, R. and Phelan, P. (1974) Family response to cystic fibrosis. *Austr. Paediatr. J.*, **10**, 136–146.

59. Begleiter, M., Burry, Y. and Harris, D. (1976) Divorce among parents of children with cystic fibrosis and chronic diseases. *Social Biol.*, **23**, 260–264.

60. Breslau, N., Weitzman, M. and Messenger, K. (1981) Psychological functioning of siblings of disabled children. *Pediatrics*, **67**, 344–353.

61. Gayton, W., Friedman, S., Tavormina, J. and Tucker, F. (1977) Children with cystic fibrosis: psychological test findings of patients, siblings and parents. *Pediatrics*, **58**, 888–894.

62. Bluebond-Langner, M. (1991) Living with cystic fibrosis: the well sibling's perspective. *Med. Anthropol. Quart.*, **5**, 133–152.

63. Bluebond-Langner, M. (1997) *In the Shadow of Illness: Parents and Siblings of the Chronically Ill Child*, Queenstown University Press, New Jersey.

64. Patterson, J., McCubbin, H. and Warwick, W. (1990) The impact of family functioning on health changes in children with cystic fibrosis. *Soc. Sci. Med.*, **31**, 159–164.

65. Wilson, J., Fooson, A., Kangle, J. and D'Angelo, S. (1996) Homeostatic interactions: a longitudinal study of biological, psychosocial and family variables for children with cystic fibrosis. *J. Fam. Ther.*, **2**, 123–140.

66. McCubbin, H. and Patterson, J. (1983) *Systematic Assessment of Family Stress, Resources and Coping*, Department of Family and Social Science, University of Minnesota, St Paul.

67. Maslach, C. and Jackson, E. (1986) *Maslach Burnout Inventors*, (2nd edn), Consulting Psychologists Press, Palo Alto, CA.

68. Bergman, A., West, A. and Lewiston, N. (1979) Social work practice and chronic pediatric illness. *Social Work Hlth Care.*, **4**, 265–274.

69. Lewiston, N., Conley, J. and Blessing-Moore, J. (1981) Measurement of hypothetical burnout in cystic fibrosis. *J. Develop. Behaviour. Pediatr.*, **9**, 266–270.

70. Coady, C., Kent, V. and Davis, P. (1990) Burnout among social workers with patients with cystic fibrosis. *Hlth Social Work*, **15**, 116–124.

71. Eigen, H., Clark, N. and Wolle, J. (1987) Clinical behavioural aspects of cystic fibrosis: directions for future research. *Am. Rev. Resp. Dis.*, **136**, 1509–1513.

72. Stark, L., Miller, S., Phenes, A. and Dradman, R. (1987) Behavioural contracting to increase chest physiotherapy. *Behaviour Modificat.*, **2**, 75–86.

73. Stark, L., Knapp, L., Bowen, A. *et al.* (1993) Increasing calorie consumption in children with cystic fibrosis: replication with 2 year follow-up. *J. Appl. Behaviour Anal.*, **26**, 435–450.

74. Dodge, J., Burton, L., Cull, A. and McCrae, W. (1978) Effectiveness of counselling in cystic fibrosis. *Patient Counselling Hlth Educ.*, First quarter, 8–12.

75. Belmonte, M. and St Germaine, Y. (1973) Psychosocial aspects of the CF family, in *Psychosocial Aspects of Cystic Fibrosis*, (eds P. Patterson, C. Denning and A. Kutshaw), Columbia University Press, New York.

76. Schroder, K., Casodabian, A. and Davis, B. (1988) Interpersonal skills training for parents of children with cystic fibrosis. *Fam. System. Med.*, **6**, 51–68.

77. Madge, S. (1999) Groupwork, in *The Illness Mosaic: Psychosocial Issues in Cystic Fibrosis*, (ed., M. Bluebond-Langner, D. Angst and B. Lask), Chapman & Hall, London.

78. Bryce, M., Rodgers, D. and Rodman, J. (1984) Group intervention techniques with parents of chronically ill children, in *Cystic Fibrosis: Horizons*, (ed. D. Lawson), Wiley, New York.

79. Maxwell, B. and Stone, R. (1992) Learning about CF can be fun. *Pediatr. Pulmonol. Suppl.*, **8**, 322.

80. McCracken, M., Budd, J. and Warwick, W. (1992) A study of self-care intervention for adolescents with cystic fibrosis. *Pediatr. Pulmonol. Suppl.*, **8**, 322.

17

Nontransplant surgery

D. M. GRIFFITHS

Introduction	349	Venous access	355
Meconium ileus	350	Thoracic surgery	356
Meconium peritonitis	351	ENT surgery	357
Abdominal disorders	351	References	357
Nutritional support	354		

INTRODUCTION

Patients with cystic fibrosis (CF) may require surgery for specific CF-related disorders (e.g. meconium ileus) or for conditions that can present difficulty in CF (e.g. intussusception) or for conditions which are identical, but may be missed (e.g. adhesion obstruction). Whatever the operation, there are some general points about operating on patients with CF that need to be noted.

Any patient with CF should have specialist anesthetic input, as even a short general anesthetic produces marked changes in lung function for at least 48 hours after surgery, with the greatest changes in forced expiratory flows, such as FEV_1[1,2].

An experienced anesthetist will be aware of the multisystem problems with CF, and specifically those affecting the lungs (e.g. bronchorrhea; bronchial lability; bullae, with the attendant risk of pneumothorax; and increased oxygen dependency). Unless the general anesthetic is going to being very short, intubation and ventilation are preferable because of the reduced risk of laryngospasm, the control of ventilation in those dependent on their hypoxic drive, the ability to perform endotracheal suction and more rapid awakening[3].

There may be a case for peroperative physiotherapy in sputum-producers, but this has to be balanced against the increased length of the anesthetic.

Moderate cirrhosis may be clinically occult but pro-duce measurable changes in liver function, especially a prolonged prothrombin time. This will require correction with vitamin K prior to surgery.

Any fluid losses in a patient with cystic fibrosis will have a higher than usual sodium content. Thus, in obstruction, fluid will be lost by vomiting and into the bowel lumen and peritoneal cavity. Any pyrexia will produce sweating, which will increase the sodium loss. Despite renal sodium conservation, this sodium loss may become quite marked, and should be consciously looked for and replaced prior to surgery. Pediatricians tend to use 0.18 per cent NaCl saline as their fluid of choice, and this may be inappropriate initially.

Deliberate preoperative starvation, peroperative fluid losses and a variable period of postoperative starvation, possibly together with postoperative vomiting, may produce mild dehydration. Although there may not be a problem in non-CF patients, this combination can make the mucus of CF patients even more viscid than usual. There is therefore a predisposition to postoperative DIOS (distal intestinal obstruction syndrome) and tracheal or bronchial plugging. Deliberate per- and post-operative rehydration, prophylactic antiemetics and the early reintroduction of fluids should minimize these risks.

Following laparotomy for extensive adhesiolysis (especially after previous meconium peritonitis) there may be a prolonged ileus. This author has found rectal domperidone (Motilium®, Sanofi-Winthrop) helpful.

MECONIUM ILEUS

Meconium ileus is the second most common cause of neonatal small intestinal obstruction and the commonest cause of intestinal perforation *in utero*[4]. It is associated with CF in 95 per cent of cases[5], with an incidence of 1 : 15 000–20 000 live births[6]. Thus, about 10–15 per cent of patients with cystic fibrosis present neonatally with meconium ileus. It is a neonatal surgical emergency and the baby needs to be transferred to the regional neonatal surgical unit safely[7].

The abnormally thick intestinal secretions produce a viscid meconium, the stickiness of which is linked to increased albumin[8], decreased carbohydrate[9] and the formation of an insoluble calcium glycoprotein[10]. The meconium sticks firmly to the mucosa, causing obstruction. Classically, the point of obstruction is 10–30 cm above the ileo-cecal valve. Above this point the ileum is dilated, hypertrophied and full of 'inspissated, putty-like, tenacious, thick, sticky, viscid meconium . . . adhering to everything it touches, including the intestinal mucosa and the surgeons gloves'[4] (Fig. 17.1). Below the point of obstruction, the ileum is collapsed and filled with small, hard, pellet-like concretions, which may extend into an unused microcolon.

Clinical features and investigations

There are two types of meconium ileus: simple (or uncomplicated) and complicated. At least a half of all cases of meconium ileus are complicated by volvulus, leading to necrosis, stenosis, atresia, perforation or meconium peritonitis (see below)[11]. A distended, heavy loop of mid- or distal ileum full of meconium tends to volve at the point of obstruction and become ischemic, producing a stenosis, atresia or meconium peritonitis[12]. At delivery there may be 'meconium-stained liquor', which is due to bile-stained vomiting[13]. Postnatally, the baby rapidly develops abdominal distension, fails to pass meconium and continues to vomit green bile. On examination, there may be palpable 'putty filled' loops of bowel, which may be indentable. In complicated meconium ileus the baby may be sicker, with a distended abdomen and a palpable mass due to matted loops of bowel.

Following initial resuscitation with intravenous fluids and the passage of a nasogastric tube, the baby should have a supine abdominal X-ray. This will demonstrate many dilated loops of bowel and may show Neuhauser's sign (Fig. 17.2) – bowel with a ground-glass (soap-bubble) appearance, caused by air within the thick meconium[14]. Complicated meconium ileus may, in addition, show calcification or pneumoperitoneum, but one-third of patients have no additional features[15].

If meconium ileus is suspected, a gastrografin enema should follow. This will demonstrate the microcolon and may reach the pellets in the terminal ileum.

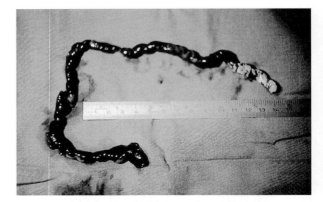

Fig. 17.1 *Inspissated, putty-like, tenacious meconium.*

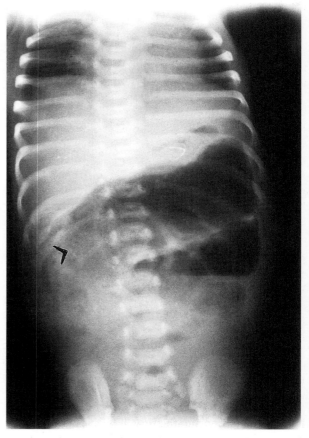

Fig. 17.2 *Neuhauser's sign – the arrowhead demonstrates bowel with a ground-glass (soap-bubble) appearance.*

Treatment

Historically, all babies with meconium ileus came to operation. Now some simple cases can be managed medically, although operation is still necessary for some simple cases and all the complicated ones[4].

Originally, all neonates with meconium ileus had a laparotomy with varying resections, stomata, vented stomata, anastomoses and tubes. The Bishop–Koop vented stoma was very popular[16], but had a significant complication rate. Noblett demonstrated that gastrografin (a mixture of a long-chain benzoic acid compound and Tween 80®, a wetting agent) could be used as a therapeutic as well as a diagnostic enema[17]. In simple meconium ileus, success rates vary from 90 per cent[18] to 50 per cent or less, so that only some neonates with simple meconium ileus avoid surgery.

If the gastrografin enema fails to relieve the obstruction, for whatever reason, or there is a perforation during the enema (up to 25 per cent)[19] or the meconium ileus is complicated, then the neonate requires laparotomy. In simple meconium ileus most surgeons perform an enterotomy well proximal to the point of obstruction and emulsify the meconium with either acetylcysteine (4 per cent, which breaks down sulfur–sulfur bonds) or gastrografin[20,21]. This procedure is time consuming and involves considerable exposure and handling of the ileum and colon. However, it has the major merits of avoiding stomata and tubes, and all the obstructed meconium can be removed at one procedure.

In complicated meconium ileus, the procedure will depend on the pathology, but will usually involve resection of any hypertrophied bowel and an anastomosis. A temporary stoma may be required.

Postoperatively, these babies must be kept well hydrated and oral pancreatic enzymes should be started as soon as possible, to try to prevent reaccumulation of viscid mucus. Pancrex® powder will go down a 6F nasogastric tube, but there is no suitable microsphere preparation yet.

Results

Recent results demonstrate an almost 100 per cent surgical survival rate[22] with good long-term survival, regardless of whether the meconium ileus is simple or complicated[20].

MECONIUM PERITONITIS

Meconium peritonitis is an umbrella description for the changes that can ensue following an *in utero* perforation[4]. It occurs in 1 : 20 000–40 000 live births[23] and may not be due to meconium ileus[4]. The perforation may be due to volvulus of an ileal loop full of meconium or due to pressure necrosis. If the perforation occurs early on, a severe, chemical peritonitis develops, produced by the enzymes in the meconium, causing fibrous adhesions throughout the peritoneal cavity and often sealing the original perforation. Calcification occurs in carnified epithelial cells as early as 12 hours after perforation[24,25]. If the perforation is not sealed, the adhesions fix the bowel loops, enclosing them in a thick-walled cystic cavity that fills with meconium and exudate antenatally, and air and bacteria post-

natally. With a late perforation there is less time for antenatal fibrous fixation, but more generalized peritonitis postnatally.

Clinical features and investigation

These babies have the features of complicated meconium ileus: bile-stained vomiting, abdominal distension and failure to pass meconium are usually present within the first 24 hours. If the perforation is unsealed, bacterial peritonitis and pneumoperitoneum will ensue, causing massive abdominal distension and a tender, red abdominal wall in a sick baby. A meconium cyst may be identifiable antenatally as ascites with surrounding calcification. Plain abdominal X-rays will show extraluminal calcification or the rim of calcification in a cyst with small-bowel obstruction.

Management

Following resuscitation and transfer to a regional neonatal surgical center, a laparotomy is always necessary because of the obstruction. There will be a long operation for the baby to withstand, massive adhesions, and extensive dissection and blood loss. As many of the adhesions as possible are freed, any atresia resected, any perforation, if found, resected and then either a primary anastomosis performed or temporary stoma created. Residual calcium deposits are slowly reabsorbed[4].

All meconium cysts also require difficult surgery. Ideally, the cyst contents should be emptied, the cyst should be removed (decorticated), and the bowel ends found and treated appropriately (anastomosis or stomata)[4].

Six factors improve the prognosis: maturity, early operation, pneumoperitoneum without calcification, generalized peritonitis (implying fewer adhesions), antibiotics for 10 days and total parenteral nutrition (TPN)[23,26].

Results

Postoperatively, all babies with meconium peritonitis will be very unwell and require TPN. Once the bowel is in continuity, attempts should be made to use it, but this may take time. Once the baby and its bowel have recovered from the surgery, they have the same prognosis as that for meconium ileus.

ABDOMINAL DISORDERS

Abdominal pain

All patients can develop abdominal pain, but this does not usually need any surgical input. Some painful abdominal conditions are similar in course and treatment in patients without CF (e.g. urinary calculi). Others can develop in CF and non-CF patients, but there are differences between them (e.g. appendicitis, intussusception, intestinal obstruction). Others only exist in CF (e.g. DIOS) and may cause confusion and delay in diagnosis if they are the only ones considered, or if they are forgotten.

If the pain is severe, then it is sensible to be proactive and involve the surgical team early on. Once any DIOS has been treated adequately, then a contrast enema (gastrografin) may be tried to exclude intussusception, and this may even be therapeutic. Further investigation with ultrasound or CT, followed by oral lavage, may be tried.

However, increasing local tenderness, the presence of a raised white cell count and the patient's overall general condition are of paramount importance in deciding whether to proceed to laparotomy, as it may be impossible to be absolutely accurate preoperatively.

If the patient has had previous abdominal surgery, then although DIOS is more common, the chance of adhesion obstruction or a stricture at the anastomosis must be considered. This applies to 10 per cent of all CF patients, as 60 per cent of those with meconium ileus come to laparotomy, with either a bowel resection and anastomosis, enterotomy or ileostomy (see above). Strictures can cause diarrhea which will not be the usual steatorrhea of cystic fibrosis. If the diarrhea is persistent and resistant to enzyme and dietary manipulation, a stricture needs to be excluded by a suitable radiological investigation.

PAIN WITH A MASS

Cystic fibrosis patients with abdominal pain will often have an abdominal mass. Commonly the pain is periumbilical and colicky, or in the right iliac fossa with a palpable mass. The mass may be inspissated, undigested intestinal contents in the terminal ileum and ascending colon (DIOS), an appendiceal abscess, an intussusception or simply faeces. All of these may progress to partial or complete obstruction.

Distal intestinal obstruction syndrome (DIOS)[27,28]

Although this was originally a surgical problem, there is almost no need for surgery nowadays. The intraluminal, obstructing, undigested food can be flushed out with N-acetylcysteine[29] or gastrografin[30] (either orally, via a gastrostomy or by enema) or by the large-volume flush of a balanced electrolyte solution, e.g. Klean-Prep®[31].

The appendix[32,33]

Appendicitis is less common in CF (1 per cent) than in the normal population (7 per cent)[34], but may present with classical central colicky pain, moving to the right iliac fossa, nausea, vomiting, focal right iliac fossa tenderness and an elevated white cell count. However, because of the frequency of chronic abdominal pain in CF, there is often delay as DIOS is the first diagnosis. Up

to 85 per cent of appendices have perforated at laparotomy[33], although there does not seem to be any special postoperative problem (this compares with a non-CF perforation rate of 10–15 per cent).

Much thought has to gone into trying to find a way to reduce this very high perforation rate. The fundamental delay seems to be simply that appendicitis is not considered early enough. DIOS is not associated with a raised white cell count and marked, localized tenderness, even if a mass is present. Plain abdominal X-ray is unhelpful, although modern ultrasound is becoming more accurate at identifying an inflamed appendix. Contrast enemas, to dislodge the presumed inspissated food, if performed in X-ray, may demonstrate extrinsic compression of the cecum by the appendix abscess, or nonfilling of the appendix[33].

A further 1 per cent of patients with CF may present with an appendix distended with inspissated mucus, with or without histological inflammation[32]. The appendix may be intussuscepting. These patients are cured by appendicectomy.

Intussusception

Intussusception is said to occur in 1 per cent of patients with CF[35], although this was before the introduction of modern pancreatic preparations (1971). The average age of occurrence in CF is much older (9–12 years) than in non-CF children (9 months)[36]. It can mimic DIOS with a nontender mass, central colicky pain, vomiting and rectal bleeding (although this is less common in babies with DIOS than in those with intussusception). Ultrasound is now the normal method of diagnosing intussusception and should show the classical 'doughnut' appearance if the diagnosis is considered (Fig. 17.3)[37], although some authors dispute this[27,38]. A gastrografin, rather than air, enema, may be doubly beneficial, as it will reduce the intussusception and liquefy the intestinal contents. However, the literature suggests that many of these

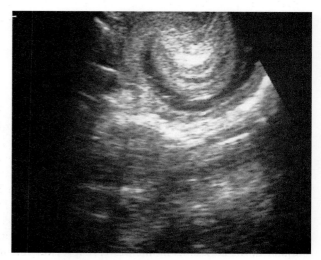

Fig. 17.3 *Ultrasound of intussusception, showing classical ring-doughnut appearance.*

patients are not diagnosed prior to laparotomy or may require surgical reduction. Chronic intussusception may be difficult to diagnose and may be overlooked[39].

Constipation

Some CF patients develop an acquired megacolon with chronic fecal retention and abdominal pain[40]. There is reduced bowel frequency and severe overloading with soiling, which may be confused with diarrhea. Distal colonic obstruction severe enough to require clearance by colonoscopy or even laparotomy has been described[41]. Plain X-ray demonstrates massive colonic faecal masses which need to be removed either medically or under general anesthesia. Subsequently, the pancreatic enzyme supplements need to be increased (so that fat absorption is more than 85 per cent) and the colon stimulated with regular Senokot® until it has shrunk to a normal size and has regained its normal peristaltic activity[33].

Rarer causes of pain with a mass

These include :

- constipation due to opiate use (or abuse); this is frequently seen by surgeons postoperatively, but rarely seen by respiratory physicians;
- Crohn's disease (see Chapter 12);
- ovarian cysts;
- volvulus or adhesion obstruction following previous surgery (commonly for meconium ileus)[42].

ABDOMINAL PAIN WITH NO MASS

Many patients with cystic fibrosis and abdominal pain will have a mass present, but if there is no mass then the nature of the pain may pinpoint the cause.

Symptoms and signs of intestinal obstruction, even after adequate treatment of DIOS

If partial or complete intestinal obstruction persists, then there is a surgical cause which needs to be elucidated[43]. If there has been a previous laparotomy, then adhesions, volvulus and anastomotic stricture are the most common. If not, then consider a colonic stricture[44,45].

Epigastric pain

Gastroesophageal reflux and esophagitis
Heartburn due to regurgitation can occur in up to 26.5 per cent of patients with CF, associated with an increased incidence of regurgitation (20 per cent)[46]. Although relaxation of the lower esophageal sphincter has been identified by one group as the major cause of the reflux[47], this is not always found[46]. Similarly, coughing with raised intra-abdominal pressure could overwhelm the lower esophageal sphincter, leading to gastroesophageal reflux, and physiotherapy has been associated with reflux in cystic fibrosis[48]. However, episodes of reflux can occur unrelated to coughing[46]. Overnight nasogastric feeds via a pump increase the frequency of reflux[46], but do not produce symptoms of esophagitis or aspiration. Esophagitis and severe reflux may present at any age[49].

Treatment should be medical initially, with thickened feeds and solids (in infants), and H_2-receptor blockers, proton-pump inhibitors and prokinetic agents[50]. In addition, vigorous treatment of the chest disease may reduce the amount of coughing, with fewer episodes of vomiting and an improvement in any esophagitis. If medical treatment is unsuccessful and appears to be resulting in a failure to thrive, then a Nissen fundoplication (probably with a gastrostomy for overnight feeds) should be performed.

Gastritis
In some cystic fibrosis patients the basal gastric acid output may be higher than normal and is exacerbated by drugs such as theophylline. Gastric ulcers are very rare unless associated with severe stress[51] or oral steroids. Gastroscopy and biopsy (to exclude *Helicobacter pylori*) are required prior to treatment of any presumed 'gastritis', as esophagitis is much more likely.

Central pain radiating to the back

Pancreatitis can occur at any age and is more common in pancreatic-sufficient patients[52,53]. The pain is typical of pancreatitis, may be relieved by leaning forward and may be associated with vomiting or constipation. The multisystem problems of pancreatitis in non-CF patients have not been found in CF patients. There may be chronic, recurrent abdominal pain or a severe acute attack. Pancreatic serum enzymes, often low in CF, are usually, but not always, raised in patients with pancreatitis. The pancreas may be edematous on ultrasound.

The treatment is primarily medical, with bowel rest initially, analgesia and naso-jejunal feeds. Early refeeding with supplemental pancreatic enzymes may be used when the pain subsides. Chronic, burnt-out pancreatitis may produce severe pain warranting pancreatectomy[54].

Pancreatic cysts are usually very small (up to 1 cm) and asymptomatic. However, they may become enormous, tense and painful, with the pancreas virtually completely replaced by cysts. These cysts are obvious on ultrasound or CT and have been drained both percutaneously by 'skinny needle'[55] and surgically[56]. Pancreatic stones are rarely symptomatic, but chronic abdominal pain associated with stones in the pancreatic duct on ERCP has been treated by lithotripsy[57].

Recurrent abdominal pain with no positive clinical findings

As with any other group of children, some children with CF will have psychosomatic abdominal pain. Prompt exclusion of other causes and firm reassurance is advised, although the literature is full of reports of patients whose abdominal pain was mistreated for years, before their real diagnosis was made[39,42,45]. Very occasionally, Münchhausen by proxy may be suspected.

Extrahepatic biliary duct disease

Although at least 25 per cent of patients with cystic fibrosis have nonfunctioning gallbladders[58], or 'micro gallbladders'[59], at post-mortem and 24 per cent have radiolucent gallstones at post-mortem[60], they are usually asymptomatic.

Biliary colic, cholecystitis and bile duct obstruction are all described in CF and should be managed in the usual way[61]. It is debatable whether laparoscopic cholecystectomy offers any significant advantage over mini-laparotomy in CF patients or non-CF patients[62]. Endoscopic sphincterotomy is the procedure of choice for both common bile duct stones and a distal bile duct stricture due to chronic pancreatitis.

Rectal prolapse

In untreated CF patients, rectal prolapse has been documented in up to 18 per cent[63], with a peak onset at 1–3 years, suggesting that it is related to potty training. The frequency varies with the mode of presentation, from 11 per cent in those with meconium ileus or respiratory problems, to 20 per cent in those with gastrointestinal problems[27]. The prolapse is presumed to occur because of the combination of voluminous, frequent bowel actions, poor nutrition and increased abdominal pressure from coughing.

In some children the tendency to prolapse will disappear prior to any treatment of the CF[63], but the mainstay is adequate pancreatic replacement therapy. This cures at least 75 per cent very rapidly, with most of the rest improving slowly. In some, persistent prolapse ceases to be a problem as they develop muscular tricks to replace it without manual pressure. If the rectal prolapse develops after enzyme treatment has been started, then it is less likely to respond to dietary and enzyme manipulation.

Surgical treatment is therefore reserved for the few who fail medical treatment. Day-case injection with submucosal 5 per cent phenol in almond oil is usually successful[64]. If this fails, then every author says their method is the easiest, fastest, least traumatic or most completely complication-free[63,65]. Major surgery should be avoided[66]. There may still be a few children who present with rectal prolapse as their only symptom of CF, but the vast majority will have other, more obvious manifestations.

Other intestinal diseases

As in any specialty, it is easy to assume that a symptom that is obviously due to the specialty in question, namely CF, is therefore not due to an unrelated disease. Thus, following extensive dietary and enzymatic manipulation, steatorrhea has been found to be due to stagnant loop syndrome, Crohn's disease and even *Giardia lamblia* infection[67,68].

NUTRITIONAL SUPPORT

When the decision to supplement feeding has been made, the choice is between nasogastric[69] and gastrostomy[70] enteral feeds or parenteral nutrition. A jejunostomy[71] is no longer required.

Enteral nutrition (see Chapter 19b)

NASOGASTRIC TUBES

Nasogastric tubes have many advantages. They are cheap, variably comfortable and removable by day, so there is no cosmetic problem. However, re-passing the tube is rarely pleasant, there is a small risk of intra-bronchial placement and there may be nasal irritation or sensitivity to the adhesive. If the tube is left *in situ*, there is a considerable cosmetic problem in an otherwise normal-looking child.

GASTROSTOMY

A gastrostomy is an iatrogenic fistula between the skin and the stomach, and has revolutionized supplemental nutrition in CF. If there are problems with the nasogastric tube or it is anticipated that there will be a long period of nutritional support, then a gastrostomy is much better[70]. Gastrostomies tend to exacerbate any pre-existing gastroesophageal reflux and may cause its development. The risk of gastric varices developing at the gastrostomy is said, by some, to be a contraindication, but if the nutritional need is great enough, the benefits outweigh the risk.

Percutaneous endoscopic gastrostomy (PEG) tubes were used originally, but have been replaced largely by gastrostomy buttons (Fig. 17.4)[72,73], although some patients still prefer a short tube.

The ideal gastrostomy is inserted as a single stage, easily replaceable without a general anesthetic, has a functioning antireflux valve, can neither fall in nor out, and has no dangly bits to be caught by an active child and so accidentally dislodged[74].

Although gastrostomy tubes are excellent for bedridden adults[75], the tube requires a general anesthetic for replacement, has no antireflux valve and is always awkward to disguise under clothes. Gastrostomy buttons can be inserted at open operation (45 minutes), percutaneously (10 minutes), in either a single[74] or two-stage procedure[73]. Some are put in under radiological[76] or laparoscopic control. Feeds can be given by bolus or, more commonly, as a supplement at night using a bedside pump. Although modern gastrostomies fulfil all the

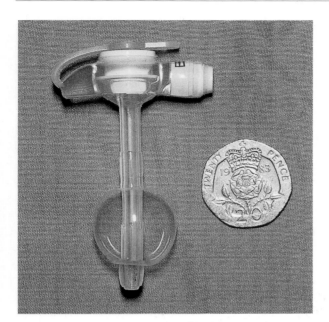

Fig. 17.4 *Mic-Key gastrostomy button.*

requirements of an ideal gastrostomy, there is still considerable room for improvement in both their cost and the durability of the balloon.

COMPLICATIONS

These may be technical, care-related, tube-related or long term.

Technical complications

These include wound dehiscence and infection. More important is separation of the stomach from the back of the anterior abdominal wall, when the stomach will leak its content into the peritoneum, so a formal laparotomy and open reinsertion of gastrostomy is required. Separation may occur either before the stomach is sufficiently fused (soon after PEG or button insertion) or later, following traumatic reinsertion.

Percutaneous damage to a gastro-epiploic artery may cause circulatory collapse requiring a laparotomy. Injury to the liver and pancreas have been reported, with no lasting harm. The colon can be transfixed following both underinflation of the stomach (causing it to remain in the way) or overinflation (rotating the colon up so that the gastrostomy goes into the posterior wall of the stomach). Conservative treatment with antibiotics and removal of the gastrostomy is sufficient and allows subsequent percutaneous reinsertion when all has settled.

Care-related complications

If a tube or button falls out, then, as a gastrostomy is a fistula, it will close remarkably quickly, making reinsertion difficult or impossible without a general anesthetic.

Skin excoriation caused by the leakage of gastric juice is exacerbated by angulation of gastrostomy tubes and is often helped by H_2 antagonists. Persistent leakage should not be treated by inserting a larger-diameter tube or button, as the problem will recur. Instead, the gastrostomy tube or button should be removed and the track allowed to shrink overnight on to a smaller Foley-type catheter, before formal dilatation the following day. The original-sized gastrostomy tube or button can be reinserted as a snug fit. Blockage is prevented by regular flushing of the gastrostomy.

Tube-related

Granulation tissue develops almost universally following insertion of a gastrostomy, irrespective of the type or method of insertion. Eventually it settles down, helped by silver nitrate cautery, Sofradex® ointment or Lyofoam®.

Foley-catheter-type gastrostomy tubes can prolapse through the pylorus and impact in the duodenum. This produces the bizarre symptom complex of pure green bile vomits with perfectly normal feeds through the gastrostomy tube.

Balloon deflation will allow the gastrostomy to fall out. This may be very early, allowing the stomach to separate and requiring a laparotomy, or simply due to the expected corrosion of the balloon, when reinsertion of a new one is all that is required.

Long term

Up to 50 per cent of patients with a gastrostomy may develop gastroesophageal reflux which is sufficient to require medical or even surgical treatment.

VENOUS ACCESS

Short-term lines

There is an increasing trend to treat chest infections requiring intravenous antibiotics using a 'short long line', inserted percutaneously at the elbow or forearm, with the tip in a large central vein. This type of technology developed in neonates and has spread to older children. These can be placed easily and aseptically on the ward under local anesthetic, with sedation if required. They will usually last for the 2–3 weeks required for the course of antibiotics. They are fairly cheap (especially compared to multiple peripheral intravenous cannulas) and much less traumatic for the patient than changing the cannula every 3 or 4 days. Following removal, the vein should have recovered by the next infection, and so can be reused. These lines need as much care and attention as any other central line and are unsuitable for patients requiring more than three or four intravenous courses per year. Any complication other than simple flushable blockage is treated by prompt removal and, if appropriate, another line inserted elsewhere.

TIVAD

A totally implantable venous access device (TIVAD) (Fig. 17.5) consists of a 'port' connected to a central line, both of which are surgically inserted subcutaneously so that there is no external tubing, as in a Hickman or Broviac line[77,78]. This allows unlimited physical activity (including swimming) and the patient's self-image is not affected. TIVAD has become standard treatment for venous access problems and is better than Hickman or Broviac lines, both cosmetically and because, unlike in oncology, it is only used intermittently for short courses of antibiotics. The port is circular, may be made of titanium or plastic, and contains a silicone block. Under the block is a space connected to the central line, which is inserted in the internal jugular vein as far as the right atrial/superior vena caval junction. The port is 'accessed' with a special noncoring needle inserted through the skin, directly into the subsilicone block space. This may be for a monthly flush, or for courses of antibiotics or, rarely, for intravenous feeding.

Indications for TIVAD include established chest infections requiring at least three courses of antibiotics a year, failure to maintain peripheral intravenous access successfully, with four or more intravenous cannulas per week, and a family who can be taught to care for it[77]. Other secondary indications include simple failure to establish intravenous access, and severe needle phobia. Contraindications include superior vena caval obstruction or pulmonary hypertension, both of which may be complications of previous lines, and social reasons, if a family is not going to be able to cope at home.

TIVADs are available in various sizes, but the smaller ones are more difficult to access, may occlude more frequently[79] and are not cosmetically superior. The line may be of silicone or polyurethane, neither with a proven advantage.

TIVADs can be inserted under local anesthetic in adults, but require a 60-minute general anesthetic in children. The optimal position for the port is in the anterior axillary line of the nondominant axilla, so that the patient can help with access. In this position the port is cosmetically invisible and does not prevent arm movement. The central line should be placed in the internal jugular vein by cutdown. The percutaneous subclavian route is contraindicated as pulmonary hyperinflation produces a greater risk of pneumothorax[80].

COMPLICATIONS

TIVADs may get infected, block or become painful. Meticulous care by patients and their carers should ensure that they last at least 2 years. Infection can occur

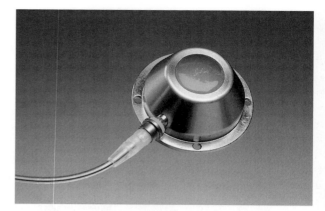

Fig. 17.5 *A totally implantable venous access device (TIVAD).*

in any indwelling line, and the incidence in TIVAD is no greater than with Hickman lines. They may be treated successfully with appropriate antibiotics, without removal (in up to 75 per cent of cases). Blockage may occur due to growth as the line retracts from the superior vena cava. Blood clots in the line are due to inadequate flushing after blood sampling and are less common than in the longer Hickman and Broviac lines. Blockage is very hard to treat as the line cannot be powerfully flushed or 'cleaned' with a guidewire. Urokinase may succeed, but replacement is usually the only option. Pain on injection at the level of the clavicle has been noted, especially in prepubertal girls. This is probably due to endothelial growth over the catheter tip, which results in the infusion being forced back around the catheter within the endothelial sheath, with pain on distension in the neck. Replacement is necessary.

Reservoir protrusion due to cachexia can be treated with repositioning under the pectoralis major. Peri-port infiltration can be avoided altogether by meticulous care when 'accessing' the port and is treated by immediate discontinuation of the infusion. Any infiltration usually settles rapidly with only local measures.

THORACIC SURGERY

Hemoptysis

Hemoptysis is due to bleeding from multiple anastomoses between the bronchial and pulmonary vessels. Although life-threatening hemoptysis is described in association with bronchiectasis in CF, it is very rare. Emergency lobectomy may be required[80].

Pneumothorax

Pneumothorax is rare in children with CF, but increases in frequency with age. This is despite their recurrent lung infections which cause vascular pleural adhesions, which should protect against pneumothorax.

Management is a balance between treating the current symptoms adequately and the difficulties of future transplantation surgery if treatment is too aggressive. If the pneumothorax is asymptomatic, then it may be simply watched. If it is symptomatic, tube drainage may be all that is required, but the recurrence rate is up to 50 per cent[81]. If it persists longer than a week or rapidly reaccumulates or recurs frequently, then more permanent treatment may be required. Video-assisted thoracoscopy is impossible because of the vascular adhesions. Surgical pleurectomy or pleurodesis using talc, if successful, makes future transplantation hazardous[82,83]. A limited, abrasion pleurodesis at thoracotomy using a dry swab may be successful, but recurrent pneumothoraces are difficult and loculated.

Single lobectomy

If there is severe disease (e.g. bronchiectasis) which on extensive investigation using CT and ventilation scans to define the extent of the nonfunctioning lung, is only in one lobe[84], then there is an argument for single lobectomy. This may not effect long-term survival, but will improve quality of life and may help to prevent the spread of bacteria to other lobes[85,86]. Any procedure will need intensive preoperative care with physiotherapy and antibiotics, experienced anesthesia, possible preoperative physiotherapy and sustained pain relief postoperatively with early mobilization.

ENT SURGERY

Despite the importance of other surgical specialities, the most common surgical procedures in cystic fibrosis are for ENT problems[87]. They are not life threatening, but may contribute to considerable distress in an otherwise healthy patient, who may eventually view their medically obvious problem as normal. The CF child is just as likely to have allergic rhinitis, tonsillitis or secretory otitis media as any other child.

The mucus produced in the nose and sinuses may be too viscid for the mucosal cilia to move. This will produce stasis and obstruction with secondary infection and the development of nasal polyps, sinusitis and, rarely, mucoceles and facial deformity[88].

Polyps

These can occur in 10–30 per cent of patients with CF[87] and may be asymptomatic or cause nasal blockage, recurrent rhinitis, rhinorrhea and anosmia. They may be visible on the upper lip (protruding from the nose) or on simple inspection with an otoscope.

Steroid sprays may be effective, unless there is com-plete obstruction, when drops can be tried. Surgical polypectomy will relieve the symptoms and improve the airway, in the knowledge that the polyps will almost certainly recur[89] unless prevented by regular topical steroids.

Sinusitis

The maxillary and ethmoidal sinuses are affected in 90 per cent of patients with cystic fibrosis[90], ranging from mucosal thickening, through opacification, to mucocele formation[91]. Endoscopic sinus surgery has opened up the possibility of more proactive treatment of nasal disease in CF, as marked sinus disease can now be treated better and more easily[92]. Severe polyposis, medialization of the lateral nasal wall, or widening of the nasal bridge require CT scanning with a view to endoscopic sinus surgery.

All patients should have regular assessment of their upper respiratory tract, with inspection of the nasal passages at an annual review. This allows the patient to voice his or her concerns about this 'minor' area.

REFERENCES

1. Lamberty, J.M. and Rubin, B.K. (1985) The management of anaesthesia for patients with cystic fibrosis. *Anaesthesia*, **40**, 448–459.
2. Richardson, V.F., Robertson, C.F., Mowat, A.P. *et al.* (1994) Deterioration in lung function after general anaesthesia in patients with cystic fibrosis. *Acta Paediatr. Scand.*, **73**, 75–79.
3. Wood, K. (1998) Anaesthesia in cystic fibrosis, in *Practical Guidelines for Cystic Fibrosis Care*, (ed.C.M. Hill), Churchill Livingstone, Edinburgh.
4. Ein, S. (1994) Meconium ileus, in *Surgery of the newborn*, (ed. N.V. Freeman *et al.*), Churchill Livingstone, London, pp.139–157.
5. Santulli, T.V. (1980) Meconium ileus, in *Pediatric surgery*. (eds T.M. Holder and K.W. Ashcroft), Saunders, Philadephia, pp. 356–373.
6. Dickson, J.A.S. and Mearns, M.B. (1975) Meconium ileus, in *Recent Advances in Pediatric Surgery*, (ed. A.W. Wilkinson), Churchill Livingstone, Edinburgh, pp.143–155.
7. Bourchier, D. (1994) The transport of surgical neonates, in *Surgery of the Newborn*, (ed. N.V. Freeman), Churchill Livingstone, London, pp. 9–13.
8. Rule, A.H., Baran, D.T. and Shwachman, H. (1990) Quantitative determination of water-soluble protein in meconium. *Pediatrics*, **45**, 847–850.
9. Buchanan, D.J. and Rapoport, S. (1952) Chemical composition of normal meconium and meconium from a patient with meconium ileus. *Pediatrics*, **9**, 304–310.
10. Roelfs, R.E., Gibbs, G.E. and Griffin, G.D. (1967) The

composition of rectal mucus in cystic fibrosis. *Am. J. Dis. Child.*, **113**, 419–421.

11. Lloyd, D.A. (1986) Meconium ileus, in *Pediatric Surgery*, (4th edn), (eds K.J. Welch, J.G. Randolph, M.M. Ravitch, *et al.*), Year Book Medical, Chicago, pp. 849–858.

12. Blanck, C., Oxmian, L. and Robbe, H. (1965) Mucoviscidosis and ileal atresia: a study of 4 cases in the same family. *Acta Pediatr. Scand.*, **55**, 557–565.

13. Griffiths, D.M. and Burge, D.M. (1988) When is meconium-stained liquor actually bile-stained vomiting? *Arch. Dis. Child.*, **63**, 201–202.

14. Neuhauser, E.B.D. (1946) Roentgen changes associated with pancreatic insufficiency in early life. *Radiology*, **46**, 319–328.

15. Leonidas, J.C., Berdon, W.E., Baker, D.H. *et al.* (1970) Meconium ileus and its complication : a re-appraisal of plain film roentgen diagnostic criteria. *Am. J. Roent.*, **108**, 598–609.

16. Bishop, H.C. and Koop, C.E. (1957) Management of meconium ileus: resection, roux-en-y anastamosis and ileostomy irrigation with pancreatic enzymes. *Ann. Surg.*, **145**, 410–414.

17. Noblett, H. (1969) Treatment of uncomplicated meconium ileus by gastrografin enema: a preliminary report. *J. Pediatr. Surg.*, **4**, 190–197.

18. Frech, R.S., McAlister, W.H., Ternberg, J. *et al.* (1970) Meconium ileus relieved by 40% water-soluble contrast enema. *Radiology*, **94**, 341–342.

19. Ein, S.H., Shandling, B., Reiley, B.J. *et al.* (1987) Bowel perforation with non-operative treatment of meconium ileus. *J. Pediatr. Surg.*, **22**, 146–147.

20. Nguyen, L.T., Youssep, S., Guttman, F.M. *et al.* (1986) Meconium ileus: is a stoma necessary? *J. Pediatr. Surg.*, **21**, 766–768.

21. Schiller, M., Grosfeld, J.L. and Morse, T.S. (1971) Non-operative treatment of meconium ileus: an experimental study in rats. *Am. J. Surg.*, **122**, 22–26.

22. Chappell, J.S. (1977) Management of meconium ileus by resection and end-to-end anastamosis. *South Afr. Med. J.*, **52**, 1093–1094.

23. Tibboel, D. and Molenaar, J.C. (1984) Meconium peritonitis – a retrospective, prognostic analysis. *Zeit. Kinderchirurg.*, **39**, 25–28.

24. Heetderks, D.R. Jr and Verbrugge, G.P. (1969) Healed meconium peritonitis presenting as a scrotal mass in an infant. *J. Pediatr. Surg.*, **4**, 363–365.

25. Bendel, W.L. Jr and Michel, M.L. Jr (1953) Meconium peritonitis: review of the literature and report of a case with survival after surgery. *Surgery*, **34**, 321–333.

26. Caresky, J.M., Grosfeld, J.L., Weber, T.R. *et al.* (1982) Giant cystic meconium peritonitis (gcmp): improved management based on clinical and laboratory observations. *J. Pediatr. Surg.*, **17**, 482–489.

27. Littlewood, J.M. (1992) Gastro-intestinal complications in cystic fibrosis. *J. R. Soc. Med.*, **85**, (Suppl. 18), 13–19.

28. Park, R.W. and Grand, R.J. (1981) Gastro-intestinal manifestations of cystic fibrosis : a review. *Gastroenterol.*, **81**, 1143–1161.

29. Hodson, M.E., Mearns, M. and Batten, J. (1976) Meconium ileus equivalent in adults with cystic fibrosis of the pancreas: a report of 6 cases. *BMJ*, **2**, 790–791.

30. O'Halloran, S.M., Gilbert, J., McKendrick, D.M. and Carty, H.M.L. (1986) Gastrografin in acute meconium ileus equivalent. *Arch. Dis. Child.*, **61**, 1128–1130.

31. Cleghorn, G.J., Forstner, C.G., Stringer, D.A. *et al.* (1986) Treatment of distal intestinal obstruction syndrome in cystic fibrosis with a balanced intestinal lavage solution. *Lancet*, **i**, 8–11.

32. Coughlin, J.P., Gauderer, M.W.L., Stern, R.C. *et al.* (1990) The spectrum of appendiceal disease in cystic fibrosis. *J. Pediatr. Surg.*, **25**, 835–839.

33. Shields, M.D., Levison, H., Reisman, J.J. *et al.* (1990) Appendicitis in cystic fibrosis. *Arch. Dis. Child.*, **65**, 307–310.

34. McCarthy, V.P., Mischler, E.H., Hubbard, V.S. *et al.* (1984) Appendiceal abscess in cystic fibrosis: a diagnostic challenge. *Gastroenterology*, **86**, 564–568.

35. Holsclaw, D.H., Rockmans, C. and Shwachman, H. (1971) Intussusception in patients with cystic fibrosis. *Pediatrics*, **48**, 51–58.

36. Turner, D., Rickwood, A.M.K. and Brereton, R.J. (1980) Intussusception in older children. *Arch. Dis. Child.*, **55**, 544–546.

37. Mulvihill, D.M. (1988) Ultrasound findings of chronic intussusception in a patient with cystic fibrosis. *J. Ultrasound. Med.*, **7**, 353–355.

38. Holmes, M., Murphy, V., Taylor, M. and Denham, B. (1991) Intussusception in cystic fibrosis. *Arch. Dis. Child.*, **66**, 726–727.

39. Webb, A.K. and Khan, A. (1989) Chronic intussusception in a young adult with cystic fibrosis. *J. R. Soc. Med.*, **82**, (Suppl. 16), 47–48.

40. Rubinstein, S., Moss, R. and Lewiston, N. (1986) Constipation and meconium ileus equivalent in patients with cystic fibrosis. *Pediatrics*, **78**, 473–479.

41. Apelgren, K.N. and Yuen, J.C. (1989) Distal colonic impaction requiring laparotomy in an adult with cystic fibrosis. *J. Clin. Gastroenterol.*, **11**, 687–690.

42. Dalzell, A.M., Heaf, D.P. and Carty, H.M.L. (1990) Pathology mimicing distal intestinal obstruction syndrome in cystic fibrosis. *Arch. Dis. Child.*, **65**, 540–541.

43. Janik, J.S., Ein, S., Filler, R.M. *et al.* (1981) An assessment of the surgical treatment of adhesive small bowel obstruction in infants and children. *J. Pediatr. Surg.*, **16**, 225–229.

44. Smyth, R.L., van Velzen, D., Smyth, A.R. *et al.* (1994) Stricture of ascending colon in cystic fibrosis and high strength pancreatic enzymes. *Lancet*, **343**, 85–86.

45. Littlewood, J.M. and Hind, C.R.K. (1996) Fibrosing colonopathy in children with cystic fibrosis. *Postgrad. Med. J.*, **72**, (Suppl. 12), S1–S64.

46. Scott, R.B., O'Loughlin, E.V. and Gall, D.G. (1985) Gastro-

oesophageal reflux in patients with cystic fibrosis. *J. Pediatr.*, **106**, 223–227.

47. Cucchiara, S., Santamaria, F., Andreotti, M.R. *et al.* (1991) Mechanism of gastro-oesophageal reflux in cystic fibrosis. *Arch. Dis. Child.*, **66**, 617–622.

48. Foster, A.C., Voyles, J.B., Murray, B.L. *et al.* (1983) 24 hour pH monitoring in children with cystic fibrosis: association of chest physiotherapy to gastro-oesophageal reflux. *Pediatr. Res.*, **17**, 118A(Abs609).

49. Feigelson, J., Girault, F. and Pecau, Y. (1987) Gastro-oesophageal reflux and oesophagitis in cystic fibrosis. *Acta Pediatr. Scand.*, **76**, 989–990.

50. Dab, I. and Malfoot, A. (1988) Gastro-oesophageal reflux: a primary defect in cystic fibrosis. *Scand. J. Gastroenterol. Suppl.*, **143**, 125–131.

51. Oppenheimer, E.H. and Esterley, J.R. (1975) Pathology of cystic fibrosis. review of the literature and comparison with 146 autopsy cases. *Perspect. Pediatr. Pathol.*, **2**, 241–278.

52. Shwachman, H., Lebenthal, E., and Khaw, P.-T. (1995) Recurrent acute pancreatitis in patients with cystic fibrosis with normal pancreatic enzymes. *Pediatrics*, **55**, 86–94.

53. Atlas, A.B., Orenstein, S.R. and Orenstein, D.M. (1992) Pancreatitis in young children with cystic fibrosis. *J. Pediatr.*, **120**, 756–759.

54. Ade-Ajayi, N., Law, C., Burge, D.M. *et al.* (1997) Surgery for pancreatic cystosis with pancreatitis in cystic fibrosis. *Br. J. Surg.*, **84**, 312.

55. Davidson, A.G. (1995) Gastro-intestinal and pancreatic disease in cystic fibrosis, in Cystic Fibrosis, (1st edn), (eds D.M. Geddes and M.E. Hodson), Chapman & Hall London, p. 267.

56. Toth, I.R. and Lang, J.N. (1986) Giant pancreatic retention cyst in cystic fibrosis, a case report. *Pediatr. Pathol.*, **6**, 103–110.

57. Weiss, A.A., Grieg, J.M. and Fache, S. (1991) Lithotripsy of pancreatic stones in a patient with cystic fibrosis: successful treatment of abdominal pain. *Can. J. Gastroenterol.*, **6**, 25–28.

58. L'Heureux, P., Isenberg, J., Sharp, H. *et al.* (1977) Gallbladder disease in cystic fibrosis. *Am. J. Roentgenol.*, **128**, 953–956.

59. Anagnostopoulos, D., Tsagari, N. and Noussia-Arvanitaki, S. (1993) Gallbladder disease in patients with cystic fibrosis. *Eur. J. Pediatr. Surg.*, **3**, 348–351.

60. Vawter, G.F. and Shwachman, H. (1979) Cystic fibrosis in adults: an autopsy study. *Pathol. Ann.*, **14**, 357–382.

61. Roy, C.C., Weber, A.M., McRin, C.C. *et al.* (1982) Hepatobiliary disease in cystic fibrosis: a survey of current issues and concepts. *J. Pediatr. Gastroenterol. Nutr.*, **1**, 469–478.

62. McGinn, F.P., Miles, A.J., Uglow, M. *et al.* (1995) Randomised trial of laparoscopic cholecystectomy and mini-cholecystectomy. *Br. J. Surg.*, **82**, 1374–1377.

63. Stern, R.C., Izant, R.J., Boat, T.F. *et al.* (1982) Treatment and prognosis of rectal prolapse in cystic fibrosis. *Gastroenterol.*, **82**, 707–710.

64. Wyllie, G.G. (1979) The injection treatment of rectal prolapse. *J. Pediatr. Surg.*, **14**, 62–64.

65. Schepens, M.A. and Verhelst, A.A. (1993) Re-appraisal of Ekehorn's rectopexy in the management of rectal prolapse in children. *J. Pediatr. Surg.*, **28**, 1494–1497.

66. Ashcraft, K.W., Amoury, R.A. and Holder, T.M. (1977) Levator repair and posterior suspension for rectal prolapse. *J. Pediatr. Surg.*, **12**, 241–245.

67. Baxter, P.S., Dickson, J.A.S. and Variend, S. *et al.* (1988) Intestinal disease in cystic fibrosis. *Arch. Dis. Child.*, **63**, 1496–1497.

68. Lloyd-Still, J.D. (1994) Crohn's disease and cystic fibrosis. *Dig. Dis. Sci.*, **39**, 880–885.

69. Moore, M.C., Greene, H.L., Donald, W.D. *et al.* (1986) Enteral tube feeding as adjunct therapy in malnourished patients with cystic fibrosis: a clinical study and literature review. *Am. J. Clin. Nutr.*, **44**, 33–41.

70. Moran, B.J., Taylor, M.B. and Johnson, C.D. (1990) Percutaneous endoscopic gastrostomy. *Br. J. Surg.*, **77**, 858–862.

71. Boland, M.P., Patrick, J., Stoski, D.S. *et al.* (1987) Permanent enteral feeding in cystic fibrosis: advantages of a replaceable jejunostomy tube. *J. Pediatr. Surg.*, **22**, 843–847.

72. Gauderer, M.W.L., Ponsky, J.L. and Izant, R.J. (1980) Gastrostomy without laparotomy : a percutaneous endoscopic technique for feeding gastrostomy. *J. Pediatr. Surg.*, **15**, 872–875.

73. Gauderer, M.W.L. (1991) Percutaneous endoscopic gastrostomy: a 10 year experience with 220 children. *J. Pediatr. Surg.*, **26**, 288–294.

74. Griffiths, D.M. (1996) The single stage percutaneous insertion of gastrostomy button insertion: a leap forward. *JPEN*, **20**, 237–239.

75. Norton, B., Homer-Ward, M., Donelly, M.T. *et al.* (1996) A randomised prospective comparison of percutaneous endoscopic gastrostomy and nasogastric tube feeding after acute dysphasic stroke. *Br. Med. J.*, **312**, 13–16.

76. Malden, E.S., Hicks, M.E., Picus, D. *et al.*, (1992) Fluoroscopically guided percutaneous gastrostomy in children. *J. Vasc. Int. Radiol.*, **3**, 673–677.

77. Cassey, J., Ford, W.D.A., O'Brien, L. *et al.* (1988) Totally implantable system for venous access in children with cystic fibrosis. *Clin. Pediatr.*, **27**, 91–95.

78. Wesenberg, F., Flaatten, H., Janssen, C.W. Jr (1993) Central venous catheters with subcutaneous injection port (Port-A-Cath): 8 years clinical follow up with children. *Pediatr. Hematol. Oncol.*, **10**, 233–239.

79. de Backer, A., Vanhulle, A., Otten, J. *et al.* (1993) Totally implantable central venous access devices in paediatric oncology – our experience in 46 patients. *Eur. J. Pediatr. Surg.*, **3**, 101–106.

80. Wood, R.E. (1992) Haemoptysis in cystic fibrosis. *Pediatr. Pulmonol. Suppl.*, **8**, 82–84.

81. Luck, S.R., Raffensperger, J.G., Sullivan, H.J. *et al.* (1977) Management of pneumothorax in children with chronic

pulmonary disease. *J. Thorac. Cardiovasc. Surg.*, **74**, 834–836.

82. Penketh, A.R., Knight, R.K., Hodson, M.E. *et al.* (1982) Management of pneumothorax in adults. *Thorax*, **37**, 850–853.

83. Egon, T.M. (1992) Treatment of pneumothorax in the context of lung transplantation. *Pediatr. Pulmonol. Suppl.*, **8**, 80–81.

84. Stern, R.C., Boat, T.F. and Orenstein, D.M. (1978) Treatment and prognosis of lobar and segmental atelectasis in cystic fibrosis. *Am. Rev. Resp. Dis.*, **118**, 821–826.

85. Lucas, J., Connett, G.J., Lea, R. *et al.* (1996) Lung resection in cystic fibrosis patients with localised pulmonary disease. *Arch. Dis. Child.*, **74**, 449–451.

86. Mearns, M.B., Hodson, C.J., Jackson, A.D.M. *et al.* (1972) Pulmonary resection in cystic fibrosis. *Arch. Dis. Child.*, **47**, 499–508.

87. Stern, A.C., Boat, T.F., Wood, R.E. *et al.* (1982) Treatment and prognosis of nasal polyps in cystic fibrosis. *Am. J. Dis. Child.*, **136**, 1067–1070.

88. Berman, J. and Coleman, B.H. (1977) Nasal aspects of cystic fibrosis in children. *J. Laryngol. Otol.*, **91**, 133–139.

89. Jaffe, B.H., Strome, M., Khaw, K.-T. *et al.* (1977) Nasal polypectomy and sinus surgery for cystic fibrosis – a 10 year review. *Otol. Clin. North Am.*, **10**, 81–90.

90. Gharib, R., Allen, R.P., Joos, H.A. *et al.* (1964) Paranasal sinuses in cystic fibrosis. *Am. J. Dis. Child.*, **108**, 499–502.

91. Møller, N.E. and Thomsen, J. (1978) Mucocele of the paranasal sinuses in cystic fibrosis. *J. Laryngol. Otol.*, **92**, 1025–1027.

92. Cuyler, J.P. (1992) Follow up of endoscopic sinus surgery in children with cystic fibrosis. *Arch. Otolaryngol.*, **118**, 505–506.

18

Lung transplantation

B. P. MADDEN

Introduction	361	Postoperative care	366
Indications and contraindications for transplantation	361	Specific CF-related problems	370
Pretransplant assessment	363	Program of long-term care	371
Patient preparation	364	Results	371
Donor selection and organ procurement	364	Recurrence of disease	372
Donor and recipient matching	365	Quality of life	372
Operative technique	365	Challenges	372
Immunosuppression	366	References	373

INTRODUCTION

Despite improved survival rates, cystic fibrosis (CF) is associated with significant morbidity and mortality. The major cause of death among adult patients is end-stage respiratory failure. It was against this background that the possibility of lung transplantation became a promising therapeutic option for the CF patient. Initially there was much concern about operating on patients with CF on account of the multisystem nature of their disease, together with persisting infection in the upper and lower respiratory tract.

There are, however, advantages in transplanting patients with CF compared to other patients requiring transplantation for end-stage lung disease. CF patients are usually young and extremely well motivated; they are used to taking regular medication, attending outpatient clinics and generally taking an active role in their management. Their parents and family are good at providing support, a factor particularly important while waiting for transplantation and in the early postoperative period. With the identification of the CF gene[1] it would appear that the CF defect is located in the cells and not serum of the affected patient and therefore should not affect transplanted lungs.

The first successful heart–lung transplants for CF were performed in the United Kingdom in 1985[2,3]. Intermediate-term results (5.5 years' experience) of heart–lung transplantation for CF is encouraging but the shortage of donor organs and the complication of obliterative bronchiolitis remain the two major obstacles to be overcome[4]. Single lung transplantation is not usually suitable for CF patients, as the remaining native lung would be a source of infection. En-bloc double-lung transplantation without tracheal revascularization has been associated with poor results, largely due to tracheal anastomotic dehiscence[5]. Bilateral sequential single lung transplantation has become the predominant operative approach to end-stage CF lung disease[6] with comparable outcome to heart–lung transplantation.

INDICATIONS AND CONTRAINDICATIONS FOR TRANSPLANTATION

The selection criteria for heart–lung and bilateral sequential lung transplantation are outlined in Table 18.1. Patients should only be accepted onto the transplant waiting list if they have deteriorating chronic respiratory failure with a severely impaired quality of life in spite of the best available medical treatment. In practice, the forced expiratory volume in one second (FEV_1) is usually less than 30 per cent of the predicted value. Many patients who are referred for assessment will improve significantly if conventional treatment is optimized and therefore will not be considered for transplantation. The patients themselves must positively want a transplant and there should be no intractable psychological instability which may interfere with their capacity to cope with the operation, strict postoperative follow-up and compliance with drug treatments. Contraindications to lung transplantation include active aspergillus or mycobacterial infection, noncompliance with treatment, prednisolone therapy in excess of 10 mg/day or other end-organ failure (unless this is also treatable at the time of transplantation, e.g. by performing combined heart–lung and liver transplantation in patients with coexisting severe liver disease). Gross malnutrition precludes transplantation, as does malignancy unless the patient has been successfully treated and free of recurrence for 5 years prior to transplantation. Significant osteoporosis may contraindicate transplantation as the process can be exacerbated by postoperative steroid therapy. This can lead to vertebral collapse with neurological sequelae in some patients. Serology for hepatitis B must be interpreted with caution as postoperative infection in the presence of immunosuppression can be fatal[6a]. Patients positive for hepatitis C or human immunodeficiency viruses 1 and 2 are contraindicated for transplantation. Other likely risk factors include preoperative ventilation, previous thoracic surgery, pleurectomy, chemical pleurodesis and severe liver disease requiring heart–lung–liver transplantation[4].

It is now a policy in many centers not to ventilate conventionally patients with CF in end-stage respiratory failure. In selected patients it is possible to use nasal intermittent positive pressure ventilation as a bridge to transplantation[7]. This avoids invasion of the airways with an endotracheal tube and thus minimizes the risk of pseudomonal toxemia. Furthermore, patients can be managed on the ward or even at home and do not require nursing in the intensive care unit. The patients are able to adjust the ventilatory support provided by the machine and therefore feel to some degree in control of the situation.

Although previous thoracotomy for pleurodesis or lung resection are not absolute contraindications to transplantation, the procedure carries an increased risk of perioperative bleeding. Techniques to control bleeding (e.g. the use of aprotinin and the argon coagulator) make it possible to operate successfully on many patients who have had previous thoracic surgery. Patients who have had a previous pleurectomy can present considerable difficulties on account of adhesions.

Patients with aspergilloma at the time of assessment are not selected for surgery because of the risk of pleural contamination, which may become a potential source of opportunistic infection in an immunocompromised patient following transplantation. However, patients with a past history of successfully treated aspergilloma have been transplanted. All patients who are being considered for transplantation and produce sputum are carefully screened for *Aspergillus fumigatus*. If the organism is present before transplantation, a course of oral itraconazole together with amphotericin B by nebulizer is recommended, in an attempt to clear the sputum. Patients with a persistently high count ($\geq 10^3$ cfu/mL) are not accepted onto the transplant waiting list. If a patient

Table 18.1 *The selection criteria for heart—lung and bilateral lung transplantation*

Indications
1. Severe respiratory failure in spite of optimal medical therapy
2. Severely impaired quality of life
3. Patient positively wants a transplant

Strong contraindications
1. Active aspergillosis or mycobacterial infection
2. Noncompliance with treatment
3. Prednisolone therapy, >10 mg/day
4. Other end-organ failure
5. Gross malnutrition
6. Malignancy within 5 years
7. Human immunodeficiency viruses 1 and 2
8. Hepatitis B surface antigen and hepatitis C seropositivity
9. *Pseudomonas* or *Burkholderia* species in sputum with no *in vitro* antibiotic sensitivities
10. Significant osteoporosis

Risk factors[a]
1. Preoperative ventilation
2. Previous thoracic surgery (pleurectomy, abrasion pleurodesis)
3. Chemical pleurodesis
4. Severe liver disease necessitating combined heart–lung and liver transplantation

[a]Some centers may not accept these patients.

has a low positive sputum count at the time of lung transplantation, oral itraconazole and amphotericin B by nebulizer are prescribed for the first postoperative month[8]. Active mycobacterial infection is a contraindication to transplantation as, in the presence of immunosuppression, fatal postoperative infection may occur. It is therefore essential that such infection be completely eradicated before surgery. Methicillin-resistant *Staphylococcus aureus* in sputum or mucosal sites does not preclude transplantation. Patients with a pseudomonal species in their sputum to which there is no *in vitro* antibiotic sensitivities would theoretically contraindicate transplantation, but the presence of *Burkholderia cepacia* in sputum does not usually preclude transplantation as the organism is frequently sensitive to antibiotics such as temocillin.

Patients who are noncompliant with treatment or clinic attendance should not be selected for the transplant program. Long-term treatment with high-dose steroid therapy is also a contraindication, although lung transplantation has been performed in patients taking 10 mg/day of prednisolone preoperatively with no added complications. Patients with cushingoid features are excluded until these changes subside with reduction in steroid therapy, as long-term steroid therapy may adversely affect tissue healing (and particularly healing of the tracheal anastomosis) after transplantation. Insulin-dependent diabetes mellitus, which is not associated with microvascular complications, is not considered a contraindication to transplantation. In successfully transplanted patients diabetic control usually becomes easier as exercise capacity improves and the number of episodes of respiratory infection are significantly reduced. Severe liver dysfunction may impair the patient's ability to metabolize immunosuppressive drugs after surgery and in patients with portal hypertension a combined heart–lung and liver transplant may be an option[4]. Patients with gross malnutrition must have this addressed with aggressive preoperative nutritional management which may necessitate overnight gastrostomy feeding. Significant osteoporosis, particularly in patients who are at risk of crush fractures, may contraindicate transplantation.

PRETRANSPLANT ASSESSMENT

Patients are admitted to hospital for a period of about 1 week, which enables them to get to know the staff, visit the surgical center and meet some patients who have already been transplanted. While in hospital, a full history and physical examination (which includes height, weight and chest measurements) is performed and assessment of the patient's quality of life and psychosocial suitability is undertaken. There will be a detailed dental and ear, nose and throat examination as chroni-

cally infected sinuses or teeth may become potential sources of postoperative infection[9]. Measurements of lung function include FEV_1, forced vital capacity (FVC) and blood gas analysis at rest and on exertion. Typically, when patients are accepted onto the transplant waiting list, their FEV_1 and FVC are about 30 per cent predicted and oxygen saturation at rest is between 80 and 90 per cent, with marked desaturation on exertion. In addition to chest radiography, a CT scan of the thorax is undertaken to assess the state of the patient's pleura as CF patients often have extensive pleural thickening and adhesions which are essential to document prior to surgery.

Together with clinical evaluation, cardiac assessment involves performing an ECG, two-dimensional echocardiogram and 24-hour Holter monitor. After careful counseling, permission is sought from the CF patient to become a cardiac donor for the domino procedure[2]. When a heart–lung transplant is performed for CF the patient's heart can be transplanted into another patient requiring cardiac transplantation alone. In order for a heart to be considered suitable for domino transplantation, valves and left ventricular function must be normal. Mild to moderate tricuspid regurgitation and right ventricular dysfunction are, however, acceptable.

Blood group and routine hematological and biochemical parameters are measured and abnormalities in hepatic and renal function addressed. With regard to lung transplantation, liver disease may be associated with coagulation disorders and hence perioperative bleeding, or may be a contraindication to postoperative administration of azathioprine. Preoperative assessment of hepatic function includes coagulation screen, serum albumin, bilirubin, alkaline phosphatase, liver enzymes and hepatic ultrasound. If any of these investigations are abnormal, a liver biopsy may be indicated. If the alkaline phosphatase is below 1000 IU/1iter with a normal bilirubin, major problems are unlikely. The outcome of 28 patients who had abnormalities in liver function at the time of transplantation has been fully documented[10].

Serological investigations for infection include those for cytomegalovirus, Epstein–Barr virus, Australia antigen, toxoplasmosis, human immunodeficiency virus and herpes simplex. Microbiological examination of the sputum is undertaken for pathogens, acid-fast bacilli and fungi. It is of paramount importance to know which antipseudomonal antibiotics to prescribe to the patient following transplantation. The majority of patients grow *Pseudomonas aeruginosa* in their sputum preoperatively, although patients with *Burkholderia cepacia* or methicillin-resistant *Staphylococcus aureus* have been successfully transplanted[4]. Some centers have advocated the exclusion of patients with *B. cepacia* in their sputum on account of the high mortality and morbidity associated with this organism[11].

Table 18.2 *Donor selection*

1. No significant cardiac or pulmonary injury
2. <50 years old
3. Nonsmoker
4. No past history of pulmonary, cardiac or malignant disease
5. Clear lung fields on chest radiograph
6. Normal gas exchange
7. No systemic infection
8. Normal ECG

PATIENT PREPARATION

It is essential that patients and their families are fully prepared for the events that may ensue following acceptance onto the transplant waiting list. It should be stressed that unfortunately there are more patients requiring transplantation than available donor organs, and being accepted onto the list does not guarantee that a suitable donor organ will be found for the patient. The patients should also be advised of the risks of transplantation and what to expect in the intensive care unit and during the early postoperative period. They should also understand that following transplantation they will need to take lifelong daily immunosuppressive therapy and will require careful postoperative supervision. It should also be made clear that transplantation is not a cure for CF and that the patient will exchange CF lungs for the discipline of living with transplanted organs. It is also important to point out that obliterative bronchiolitis is a potential long-term complication following successful transplantation. The majority of patients and their families realize that without transplantation the chance of survival is minimal. However, with transplantation there is a good chance that they may obtain a substantial improvement in their quality of life. Thus, even when fully informed, most patients wish to go ahead and be placed on the transplant waiting list.

Once on the waiting list, patients face an uncertain time. It is essential that they can be found at all times and some patients benefit from have an aircall bleep or a portable telephone. During this time, transplant support groups are particularly helpful. These groups are usually organized by transplant nurses, social workers or psychologists and involve patients on the waiting list meeting at regular intervals to discuss progress and problems. Ideally the groups are attended on a monthly basis by a doctor on the transplant team, to answer any questions and keep the group up to date on progress and new developments in the area of transplantation. Patients who have been successfully transplanted regularly attend the groups and give encouragement and advice to those patients awaiting transplantation. During the waiting period, patients who are malnourished have their nutrition improved and, of course, should patients' clinical condition deteriorate they are immediately admitted to hospital for intensive treatment.

DONOR SELECTION AND ORGAN PROCUREMENT

Good donor cardiac and respiratory function are essential to optimize success of cardiac and pulmonary transplantation. The most common cause of brain death in donors is trauma with brain injury. Some guidelines used to determine organ suitability are outlined in Table 18.2. It is appreciated that with increasing demand and scarcity of suitable organs, these criteria are changing. The potential donor should have no significant cardiac or pulmonary injury and be ideally a nonsmoker under the age of 50 years. There should be no past history of pulmonary, cardiac or malignant disease. Chest radiography should reveal clear lung fields and gas exchange should be normal (PaO$_2$ > 15 kPa with an FiO$_2$ of 35 per cent). The donor should be free from systemic infection and ideally not have infected bronchial secretions. Donors may be accepted who have contaminated tracheobronchial secretions or treatable infection, excluding multiresistant *Staphylococcus aureus*. If in doubt, flexible bronchoscopy should be performed to document absence of mucous membrane inflammation or ulceration. Prolonged mechanical ventilation is undesirable, as the incidence of infections and atelectasis is increased.

The donor ECG should be normal. If an arrhythmia or ST segment abnormality is present, echocardiography and perhaps coronary angiography may be needed to exclude organic disease. It is essential that the donor condition is stabilized while organ procurement teams are in transit. This is particularly important in cases of multiorgan donation where several surgical teams are involved.

The distant organ procurement technique involves taking a portable cardiopulmonary bypass machine by the retrieval team to the donor hospital. The donor is cooled on bypass to a core temperature of 8–10°C, the heart is preserved with cold blood potassium cardioplegia solution, and the organs are transported in cold donor blood and packed in ice. Good donor preservation is essential for safe transportation of the donor organs over a long distance and to ensure return of normal cardiac and pulmonary function following transplantation. Ideally, the organ ischemic time (which starts from discontinuation of donor ventilatory support and ends with reperfusion of the transplanted organs) should be kept to under 5 hours. Research is ongoing to improve preservation and this has allowed for successful transplantation of organs with longer ischemic times. This enables successful procurement of donor organs from further afield and therefore increases the size of the available donor pool. An alternative method of preserving the donor lungs by first giving intravenous prostacycline followed by a single cold-flush technique into the pulmonary artery has been described[12]. The pulmonary preservation fluid contains several additives, including mannitol and prostacycline.

DONOR AND RECIPIENT MATCHING

Matching criteria are based on ABO blood group compatibility, size of thoracic cage and cytomegalovirus (CMV) antibody status. Potential recipients are also screened for preformed antibodies against a panel of HLA antigens.

Ideally the donor lungs should be slightly smaller than the recipient chest cavity, as organs that are too big may predispose to atelectasis and uneven ventilation due to compression. On the other hand, lungs that are too small may fail to obliterate the pleural space, with the potential risks of air leak, pleural effusion or empyema formation. CMV infection is a major cause of morbidity and mortality following lung transplantation[13]. The organism can be transmitted by donor organs or blood products. CMV-negative recipients should therefore receive CMV-negative donor organs and blood products wherever possible, in an attempt to minimize postoperative infection, as CMV-negative antibody recipients of CMV-positive donor organs have a higher incidence of primary CMV pneumonitis.

OPERATIVE TECHNIQUE

The technique of heart–lung transplantation consists of tracheal, aortic and right-atrial anastomoses. If the recipient's heart is subsequently used as part of a domino transplant, bicaval anastomoses replace the right-atrial anastomoses[15]. Donor and recipient operations must be well coordinated to keep organ ischemic time to a minimum. Following extraction of the recipient's organs, hemostasis must be achieved in the posterior mediastinum and the phrenic, vagal and recurrent laryngeal nerves must be protected. Recipient peritracheal tissue and long length of trachea are left intact to maximize healing of the tracheal anastomosis. The low incidence of tracheal dehiscence associated with heart–lung transplantation, together with the low incidence of accelerated coronary atherosclerosis among CF heart–lung transplant recipients[4], has become a strong argument for the application of heart and lung transplantation in patients with CF.

The heart from a CF patient who undergoes heart–lung transplantation is now routinely donated for cardiac transplantation to a patient with end-stage cardiac disease associated with a moderate reversible elevation in pulmonary vascular resistance[2]. As the donor heart has already been conditioned to cope with elevated pulmonary artery pressure secondary to the pre-existing CF pulmonary disease, the 'primed' right ventricle is better able to cope with the recipient's pulmonary vascular resistance during the perioperative period. In a series of 103 domino procedures reported, 58 were from patients with CF[15].

With increasing numbers of centers performing cardiac transplantation, the number of heart–lung donor blocs is declining significantly. This has resulted in a worldwide decline in the number of heart–lung transplants performed. Today the predominant operative approach to end-stage CF lung disease is bilateral sequential single lung transplantation. However, healing of the tracheal anastomosis following en-bloc double-lung transplantation or of the bronchial anastomoses following bilateral sequential lung transplantation is still a problem. Ischemia to the anastomosis as a result of interruption of the coronary bronchial collaterals can lead to dehiscence or granulation tissue formation. The latter can promote sputum retention and therefore facilitate the development of pulmonary infection, which in itself can be a stimulus for further granulation tissue formation. Should granulation tissue form at the level of the airway anastomosis it can often be successfully treated using Nd:YAG laser therapy[15a]. Studies to improve vascularity of the bronchial anastomosis with an abdominal omental wrap were encouraging[16], although the need for this procedure has been challenged in a prospective randomized trial comparing different types of wrap versus no wrap for the bronchial anastomosis after isolated lung transplantation[17]. Early results of direct revascularization of the bronchial arteries using the internal mammary artery are encouraging in en-bloc double-lung transplantation[17] and may reduce the high incidence of tracheal anastomotic dehiscence observed after this procedure[18].

Single-lung transplantation would be inappropriate for CF due to the risk of the transplanted lung becoming infected by sputum overspill from the remaining CF native lung. En-bloc double-lung transplantation with direct revascularization of the bronchial arteries is, however, a logical option, as is bilateral single-lung transplantation[19]. This latter procedure is done via a transverse thoracosternotomy and involves sequential replacement of the two lungs. Advantages include separate bronchial anastomoses to reduce ischemic airway complications and improved exposure to permit better visualization of bleeding points and thus reduce intraoperative hemorrhage. In some cases the procedure can be performed without the need for full cardiopulmonary bypass. Intermediate and long-term results of bilateral lung transplantation for CF are comparable to those observed with heart–lung transplantation.

Living lobar donor lung transplantation for CF is associated with short and intermediate-term results which are comparable to cadaveric lung transplantation with respect to survival, function and incidence of complications[20]. Following bilateral pneumonectomy, the recipient receives a bilateral sequential transplant of a lower lobe from each of two living donors[21]. There must be detailed independent clinical and psychosocial assessments to ensure that the donors and recipients are fully aware of the risks attendant on lobectomy and on transplantation. It is essential that undue pressure is not being brought to bear on the donors or on healthy siblings of the CF patient to become donors. It should also be remembered that CF can run in families and therefore more than one child can be affected. As parents can theoretically only donate one lobe each, they should not be put in a position of having to choose between children. Recent work with cadaveric lobar transplantation, whereby an adult cadaveric single lung is divided into two lobes, for a smaller bilateral lung recipient, suggests that this may be an encouraging option for selected pediatric candidates[22].

IMMUNOSUPPRESSION

Patients are routinely immunosuppressed with azathioprine and cyclosporin-A after transplantation. Episodes of acute graft rejection are treated with intravenous methylprednisolone, occasionally supplemented by antithymocyte globulin. Since its introduction into clinical transplantation in 1978[23] cyclosporin-A has become the immunosuppressive agent of choice[24]. It inhibits the synthesis of interleukin-2 thereby preventing the clonal expansion of helper T cells. It is given with pre-med in a dose of 6–10 mg/kg (depending on the patient's renal function) and thereafter the dose is adjusted to maintain levels of 500 ng/mL (whole blood monoclonal antibody assay) in the first postoperative month and 250–350 ng/mL thereafter, renal function permitting. If patients become oliguric or serum creatinine rises in excess of 200 µmol/L cyclosporin-A is stopped and patients are immunosuppressed with prednisolone instead. In addition to nephrotoxicity, cyclosporin-A is hepatotoxic and has a side-effect profile that includes hypertension, hyperkalaemia, convulsions, gum hypertrophy, hirsutism and susceptibility to lymphoproliferative disorders.

Azathioprine is an antimetabolite that was first used in renal transplantation in 1961[25]. It affects cellular proliferation, including both B and T cells. The drug is administered orally at a dose of 0–2 mg/kg/day and is discontinued in the presence of leukopenia (white blood cell count below 4.0×10^9/liter in peripheral blood) or thrombocytopenia. The drug can occasionally cause cholestatic liver disease and its dose may have to be monitored in CF patients with coexisting liver disease. Pancreatitis is uncommonly encountered.

Methylprednisolone is given for episodes of acute pulmonary rejection. The dose is 10 mg/kg/day intravenously on three consecutive days for children and 1 g daily intravenously on three consecutive days for adults. If patients develop a severe acute rejection episode, the intravenous treatment is followed by a reducing dose of oral prednisolone, commencing with 1 mg/kg/day. Prednisolone is also prescribed for those patients who are intolerant of cyclosporin-A on account of renal impairment or those who experience more than three acute rejection episodes in the first 3 postoperative months (when a maintenance dose of 0.2 mg/kg/day is employed in addition to azathioprine and cyclosporin-A). Episodes of acute rejection not responding to steroid therapy may be treated in addition by antithymocyte globulin of rabbit or horse origin. Other immunosuppressive agents available include tacrolimus rapamycin and mycophenolate mofetil, although the precise role of these agents for lung transplant recipients requires clarification from prospective clinical trials (which are currently in progress).

POSTOPERATIVE CARE

Following lung transplantation, patients with CF may experience medical problems common to all lung transplant recipients (Table 18.3) in addition to specific problems relating to their primary disease (Table 18.4)[26, 27].

Infection

For the first 10 postoperative days patients are prescribed antipseudomonal antibiotics intravenously. The choice of drug is based on the immediate preoperative sputum culture and sensitivity result. Sputum specimens are sent on a daily basis postoperatively and antibiotics are adjusted as appropriate. In practice, aminoglycosides are

Table 18.3 *Common medical problems after lung transplantation*

1. Infection
2. Acute rejection
3. Grand mal seizures
4. Lymphoproliferative disorders
5. Obliterative bronchiolitis
6. Complications of immunosuppression

Table 18.4 *Specific CF-related problems*

1. Malnutrition
2. Upper respiratory tract infection
3. Malabsorption of cyclosporin-A
4. Diabetes mellitus
5. Salt loss
6. Bowel obstruction
7. Liver disease

avoided because of the synergism with cyclosporin-A in promoting nephrotoxicity. Flucloxacillin is prescribed while central lines and chest drains are *in situ*. All positive sputum cultures are treated during the first 2 postoperative months and thereafter only clinical respiratory tract infections are treated. Patients are prescribed aciclovir for the first 3 postoperative months and lifelong colistin sulfate inhalation (1 megaunit twice daily during the first 3 postoperative months and thereafter 1 megaunit daily) via a face mask. It is believed that this latter treatment is responsible for the low incidence of pseudomonal respiratory infections observed after the second postoperative month[4]. Patients also receive lifelong prophylactic co-trimoxazole against *Pneumocystis carinii*, taken every third day. In those patients intolerant of co-trimoxazole, pentamidine isethionate by inhalation is prescribed every second week.

Common pathogenic organisms causing pulmonary infection after lung transplantation are listed in Table 18.5. Presenting symptoms are variable and include cough (which may be productive of purulent sputum), dyspnea, pyrexia or reduction in lung function. Chest radiograph may be normal or demonstrate interstitial shadowing and arterial blood hypoxemia may be present. It is frequently impossible to diagnose pulmonary infection reliably on the basis of clinical findings and chest radiograph and to differentiate it from acute pulmonary rejection. It is most important, therefore, that should patients develop cough, pyrexia, reduction in exercise capacity or lung function tests, or have an abnormality on chest radiograph, fibreoptic bronchoscopy be performed as a matter of urgency. During this procedure:

1. the appearance of the airway anastomosis is observed;
2. sputum and bronchoalveolar lavage fluid specimens are sent for bacterial culture and sensitivity and opportunistic pathogen screen (culture for *Aspergillus fumigatus*, *Candida albicans*, *Mycobacterium tuberculosis*, *Legionella pneumophila*, *Pneumocystis carinii*; monoclonal immunofluorescence test and detection of early antigen fluorescent foci (DEAFF) for CMV); and
3. three transbronchial lung biopsies are taken from the lower lobe if there is a diffuse abnormality on chest radiograph or from the appropriate lobe for localized shadowing, using a cupped forceps[28].

Table 18.5 *Common pulmonary pathogens after lung transplantation*

Bacterial:	*Pseudomonas aeruginosa*, *Staphylococcus aureus*, *Haemophilus influenzae*, *Streptococcus pneumoniae*
Viral:	CMV
Fungi:	*Aspergillus fumigatus*, *Candida albicans*
Protozoa:	*Toxoplasma gondii*, *Pneumocystis carinii*

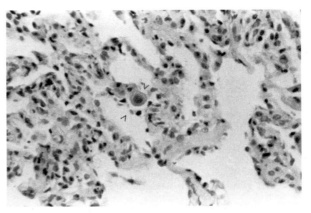

Fig. 18.1 *Transbronchial biopsy from a patient with CMV pneumonitis demonstrating a CMV inclusion body (arrowhead). Hematoxylin and eosin, medium power.*

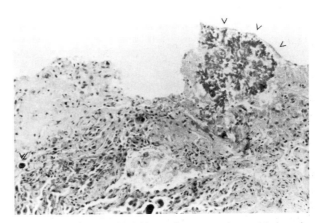

Fig. 18.2 *Transbronchial biopsy from a patient with invasive aspergillosis. The fungal hyphae are clearly seen (arrowheads). CMV inclusion bodies are also present (V/). Hematoxylin and eosin, medium power.*

Fluoroscopy may or may not be employed while taking transbronchial biopsies.

Pathogenic bacterial organisms, if present, are usually isolated from bronchoalveolar lavage fluid specimens. They are treated with appropriate antibiotics. CMV pneumonitis, fungal and protozoal respiratory infections can be diagnosed reliably on transbronchial lung biopsy specimens[28] (Figs 18.1 and 18.2). The former is treated with ganciclovir and, if necessary, hyperimmune globulin to CMV or occasionally foscarnet. *Aspergillus fumigatus* can be treated with itraconazole or liposomal amphotericin B and *Candida albicans* with fluconazole or amphotericin B. *Toxoplasma gondii* is treated with sulfadiazine and pyrimethamine and *Pneumocystis carinii* with co-trimoxazole.

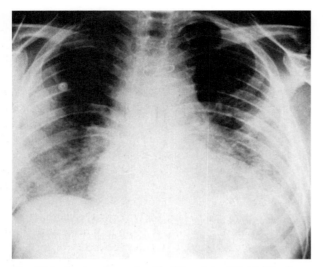

Fig. 18.3 *Chest radiograph with diffuse interstitial infiltration – acute rejection.*

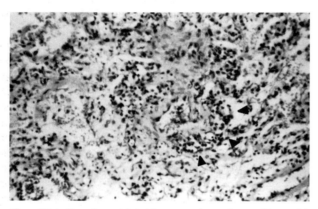

Fig. 18.4 *Transbronchial biopsy perivascular cuffing with mononuclear cells (arrowheads) – acute rejection. Hematoxylin and eosin, medium power.*

Acute rejection

Acute rejection is common and most frequently encountered during the first 3 postoperative months[4]. Typically, the first episodes occur between the tenth and fourteenth postoperative days. Features of acute rejection include pyrexia, cough and reduction in lung function. During the first postoperative month, the chest radiograph may be abnormal, demonstrating interstitial shadowing, pleural effusions or septal lines (Fig. 18.3). The diagnosis is confirmed by transbronchial biopsy, which may demonstrate perivascular cuffing with mononuclear cells[29] (Fig. 18.4). Treatment consists of intravenous methylprednisolone, which may be supplemented by oral prednisolone as outlined above or by antithymocyte globulin.

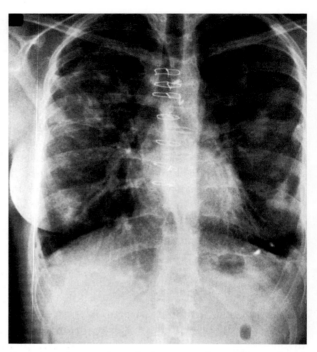

Fig. 18.5 *Chest radiograph from a patient with B-cell pulmonary lymphoproliferative disorder.*

Grand mal seizures

These are frequently of metabolic origin and are particularly common among patients on intravenous cyclosporin-A. Possible causes include elevated cyclosporin-A levels, hypomagnesemia, hypokalemia, hyponatremia and hypoglycemia. If there is no obvious metabolic cause, then CT or MRI brain scan is indicated to exclude intracranial hemorrhage, infarction or infection. A lumbar puncture may be necessary to exclude infection.

Lymphoproliferative disorders

These disorders may be of B- or T-cell type and their clinical presentation can be very variable. Patients may present with pyrexia, a history of weight loss, malaise or anorexia, rash, change in bowel habit or a noticeable mass. Sometimes they are asymptomatic and a mass is noted on routine chest radiograph (Fig. 18.5). Physical examination may be normal or a rash, tonsillar enlargement, lymphadenopathy or palpable mass may be noted.

It is essential that masses are biopsied. In the chest this may be facilitated by CT scanning. The B-cell disorders are usually associated with Epstein–Barr virus, and patients' serum may demonstrate monoclonal or polyclonal antibody activation to this agent. There is a wide variety of histopathological appearances; thus, accurate diagnosis depends on identifying Epstein–Barr virus in biopsy material by immunohistochemical staining or *in situ* hybridization. Initial treatment is conservative irrespective of the histopathologial appearances and clonality. It comprises reduction in immunosuppression and treatment with high-dose aciclovir for B-cell disorders. The T-cell disorders are not usually associated with an intercurrent viral infection, and treatment is aimed at reducing immunosuppression alone. Up to 60 per cent of patients respond to conservative measures. Conventional lymphoma therapy is required in clinically aggressive cases, which typically occur late after transplantation; these disorders have a poor prognosis.

Obliterative bronchiolitis

This remains the most serious late complication following lung transplantation, affecting up to 40 per cent of adult patients[4,15]. It is a clinical diagnosis of progressive airflow obstruction often in the presence of infection. The patient usually presents with cough, reduced exercise capacity and deterioration in lung function. The chest radiograph is typically normal or may show hyperexpanded lung fields. Although the diagnosis may be confirmed histologically (Fig. 18.6) transbronchial biopsies are usually normal, as the affected bronchioles are peripheral and randomly distributed in the lung and therefore not usually sampled at biopsy. CF patients have a similar incidence of obliterative bronchiolitis when compared with non-CF heart–lung transplant recipients[4]. When patients are diagnosed as having obliterative bronchiolitis, their immunosuppression is augmented

with the addition of oral prednisolone, 1 mg/kg/day for a period of 2–4 weeks. Thereafter the dose of prednisolone is reduced over a period of time to a maintenance dose of 0.2 mg/kg/day, in addition to their cyclosporin-A and azathioprine. Other potential therapeutic options include substituting tacrolimus and mycophenolate mofetil for cyclosporin A and azathioprine respectively, or the use of total lymphoid irradiation. Unfortunately only a minority of patients will demonstrate an improvement in lung function on this regime. The majority will either stabilize or their respiratory function will progressively decline to the extent that respiratory failure ensures. At this stage the only remaining treatment option available is retransplantation[15,30]. The results of repeat heart–lung transplantation for patients with obliterative bronchiolitis have not been good, although results of single-lung transplantation for this condition are more encouraging[15], with 1 year actuarial survival of approximately 30 per cent. Some centers have a policy not to retransplant patients with obliterative bronchiolitis on account of limited donor organ availability in conjunction with the poor results of retransplantation.

The etiology of obliterative bronchiolitis remains unclear. A relationship between acute persistent episodes of lung rejection and subsequent development of obliterative bronchiolitis has been suggested[31] and an association between viral infection and obliterative bronchiolitis has been reported[32]. Viral infection may facilitate enhanced MHC class II expression on epithelium and endothelial cells in the graft and a host immunological response may be directed against these targets. Furthermore, it is suggested that the condition is more commonly encountered among younger lung transplant recipients[33]. It may well be that obliterative bronchiolitis represents a final common pathway to pulmonary injury. Further studies may implicate several etiological factors, including acute rejection, viral infection, bacterial infection and chronic pulmonary allograft rejection. Bacterial infection may be an important factor. As the lungs are denervated, ciliary beat frequency is discordinate and therefore an important aspect of local host defense is lost[34]. Persistent bacterial infection at the level of the small airways may facilitate the development of obliterative bronchiolitis. It is essential therefore that rapid and reliable early diagnosis of acute rejection and pulmonary infection is made in an attempt to reduce the incidence of obliterative bronchiolitis.

Studies are needed urgently to determine the etiology of this condition so that effective measures can be made to prevent its occurrence. At the present time retransplantation is the only effective management if augmentation of immunosuppression fails. Further experience with tacrolimus, total lymphoid irradiation, mycophenolate mofetil and rapamycin in the management of this condition is awaited.

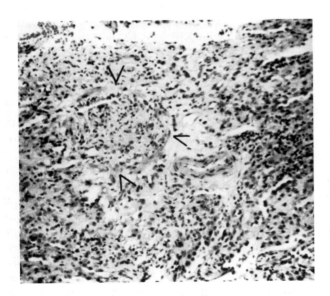

Fig. 18.6 *Transbronchial biopsy of obliterative bronchiolitis. The lumen of the small bronchiole is obstructed by fibrous tissue (arrowheads). Note also lymphocytic infiltration in the surrounding parenchyma. Hematoxylin and eosin, medium power.*

Complications of immunosuppression

Cyclosporin-A has been associated with a variety of side-effects, including renal impairment, hirsutism, gum hypertrophy, hypertension and increased susceptibility to lymphoproliferative disorders and grand mal seizures. Similar side-effects can occur with tacrolimus, and this agent can also lead to diabetes mellitus. Azathioprine can cause bone-marrow suppression, cholestatic jaundice and pancreatitis. Mycophenolate is less likely to cause bone marrow suppression.

It should be remembered that a variety of drugs can interact with immunosuppressive therapy. Thus erythromycin, itraconazole, ketoconazole and fluconazole may increase plasma cyclosporin-A or tacrolimus levels, whereas anticonvulsants or antituberculous drugs may reduce plasma levels as a consequence of liver enzyme induction. It is essential therefore that, when agents known to interfere with immunosuppressive therapy are prescribed, the dose of the immunosuppressive agent is adjusted approximately and blood concentrations are monitored frequently to avoid the risks of toxicity or of rejection caused by subtherapeutic concentrations. Amphotericin, aminoglycosides, lincosamides and nonsteroidal anti-inflammatory agents can potentiate renal impairment when prescribed in conjunction with cyclosporin-A or tacrolimus. Co-trimoxazole and ganciclovir can cause bone-marrow suppression. This may necessitate stopping or reducing the dose of azathioprine. The dose of azathioprine must be reduced by 75 per cent if patients are also prescribed allopurinol.

SPECIFIC CF-RELATED PROBLEMS

Malnutrition

It is essential to commence oral feeding early in the postoperative period as soon as bowel sounds have returned. Patients are routinely prescribed elemental diet supplemented with medium-chain triglycerides and carbohydrates via a nasogastric tube or a gastrostomy or jejenostomy feeding tube. If patients are unable to tolerate nasogastric feeding, on account of gastric atony secondary to vagal nerve injury, total parenteral nutrition is prescribed. The usual protein, lipid and sugar solutions are used with vitamin and mineral supplementation. Close attention is paid to serum hematological and biochemical parameters and, because of the potential risk of infection with this form of feeding in immunocompromised patients, conversion to the nasogastric or oral routes is made as soon as possible.

Upper respiratory tract infection

Following lung transplantation CF changes persist in the mucosa above the anastomosis and patients are typically colonized with *Pseudomonas aeruginosa* in the upper respiratory tract. It is most important to prevent infection in this area from contaminating the transplant lungs. Indeed, this was originally a concern against performing lung transplantation in CF. Colistin sulfate inhalation via a face mask is prescribed lifelong for CF patients after lung transplantation, and this is believed to be an important factor in minimizing the incidence of lower respiratory tract infection with *Pseudomonas aeruginosa* after surgery[4,10,26]. Although not routinely performed, some CF patients may benefit from maxillary sinus antrostomy and repeated sinus lavage after surgery[9]. Those who develop local obstruction secondary to polyp formation are referred to an ENT surgeon. Patients are also advised to perform daily postural drainage even when there is minimal sputum production, as impaired ciliary motility in the denervated transplanted lung may promote sputum retention[34].

Malabsorption of cyclosporin-A

Cyclosporin-A is lipophilic and its poor absorption explains the higher oral requirement in CF patients compared to non-CF patients after transplantation[35]. On account of this, the drug is usually administered intravenously in the early postoperative period. The oral dose prescribed is commonly in the range of 10–30 mg/kg body weight in two divided doses, and the dose is adjusted in the light of trough whole-blood levels. Pancreatic enzyme supplements are taken with cyclosporin-A to aid absorption. For those patients with gross malabsorption, it may be necessary to take cyclosporin-A three or four times per day or to take calcium antagonist drugs in addition to elevate blood levels.

Diabetes mellitus

This condition may be exacerbated in the early postoperative period on account of stress, steroid therapy or total parenteral nutrition. Blood sugar levels are controlled with insulin as appropriate. After the early postoperative period, diabetes mellitus is not usually a significant problem as patients' exercise capacity improves significantly and the incidence of respiratory infections is substantially reduced.

Salt loss

During the early postoperative period, patients are maintained in a warm intensive care unit and are often on dopamine (<5 µg/kg/min) and diuretics, both of which enhance urinary sodium excretion. On account of their disease, CF patients are prone to salt loss and thus sodium depletion may occur. It is most important to monitor electrolyte balance closely and sodium supplementation is prescribed as appropriate. Hyponatremia can sometimes be a cause of grand mal seizures following transplantation.

Bowel obstruction

Patients who develop meconium ileus equivalent are treated with oral (and if necessary enemas) of N-acetylcysteine. Any factors that may exacerbate this situation (e.g. analgesic agents containing codeine) should be stopped. The majority of patients will settle on this form of treatment and laparotomy with intestinal resection is very rarely necessary.

Liver disease

Patients with CF associated with end-stage respiratory failure and severe liver disease with portal hypertension require combined bilateral lung and liver transplantation. Those patients with impaired hepatic function in the absence of portal hypertension may experience a further deterioration in hepatic function after surgery, secondary to a combination of factors, including the effects of cardiopulmonary bypass, hypotension, multiple blood transfusions or hypoxia. It may be necessary to modulate the doses of potentially hepatotoxic drugs (such as azathioprine and cyclosporin-A) in the early postoperative period. The effect of lung transplantation on liver disease in a large series of CF patients has been reported[10].

PROGRAM OF LONG-TERM CARE

Following discharge from hospital, patients are managed by the transplant unit in collaboration with the referring CF center. Each patient receives a home microspirometer on discharge and measures FEV_1 and FVC on a daily basis. Should they experience a greater than 15 per cent reduction in lung function on home testing, or develop a cough, pyrexia in excess of 37.5°C or reduction in exercise tolerance, they are advised to contact the transplant center. Patients are initially required to attend outpatient clinics on a weekly basis during the first month after hospital discharge but thereafter the frequency of outpatient appointments becomes less and eventually the majority of patients attend the transplant center for review every 6 months. In between, they attend their local hospital for routine hematological and biochemical investigations together with cyclosporin-A level (at least monthly for stable patients with malabsorption) and lung function

testing. The results are faxed to the transplant center and any changes in immunosuppression are made as appropriate.

The referring center is encouraged to play an active role in the management of the CF patient following lung transplantation and, indeed, should patients develop problems, the majority will present to their local center. In such situations early communication and, if necessary, prompt referral to the transplant center is essential.

RESULTS

The largest experience in heart–lung transplantation for CF has been obtained in the UK[2–4]. A series of 79 CF patients who underwent heart–lung transplantation[4] (three of whom underwent combined heart–lung and liver transplantation) was reported with actuarial patient survival for the whole group of 69 per cent at 1 year and 52 per cent at 2 years. Twenty-three patients had one or more possible high-risk factors, and survival of these patients was 64 per cent at 1 year and 57 per cent at 2 years, compared with 71 per cent and 49 per cent, respectively, in the low-risk group ($n = 56$; Fig. 18.7). The difference between both groups was significant to 3 months ($P < 0.05$) but thereafter there was no statistically significant difference between the groups. Presumably this finding reflects bleeding, infection and multiorgan failure, which were more common in the high-risk group during the early postoperative period[4]. Lung function improved quickly during the first 3 postoperative months, with a substantial improvement over pretransplant values. The mean values of FEV_1 and FVC before surgery were 20–30 per cent of their predicted values and the mean FEV_1 at 1, 2 and 3 years after surgery was 67 per cent, 70 per cent and 60 per cent predicted, respectively, with corresponding values for FVC of 71 per cent, 70 per cent and 66 per cent predicted, respectively.

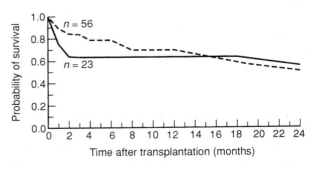

Fig. 18.7 *Survival of high-risk (——) versus low-risk (----) patients in heart–lung transplantation for cystic fibrosis. High-risk group = preoperative ventilation, thoracic surgery, heart–lung–liver transplantation, pleurodesis. (Reproduced with permission from the* Lancet.*)*

Most patients were well enough to return to their normal activities (e.g. school, work, higher education) between 6 and 12 months after transplantation. Obliterative bronchiolitis was the most serious late complication and cause of late death.

Bilateral sequential lung transplantation is the most commonly performed transplant procedure worldwide for CF patients[6]. En-bloc double-lung transplantation is now rarely performed due to the high hospital mortality in this patient group. The 1996 St Louis International Registry reported 1-, 2- and 3-year actuarial survival of 70 per cent, 62 per cent and 53 per cent, respectively, for bilateral lung transplantation for CF[6]. Interestingly, a comparison of CF patients to other transplant diagnoses of emphysema, primary pulmonary hypertension and pulmonary fibrosis shows that CF patients had the highest rate of survival of all groups. The incidence of obliterative bronchiolitis is similar to that of heart and lung transplant recipients.

One-year actuarial survival following living-related lobar transplantation for CF is 70 per cent[20]. Mean FEV_1 and FVC are approximately 70 per cent of predicted values by the end of the first postoperative year and pulmonary hemodynamics are normal. Interestingly, acute rejection is often unilateral and the incidence of obliterative bronchiolitis is comparable to that of bilateral lung and to heart and lung transplant recipients[6,20].

RECURRENCE OF DISEASE

In CF there is an abnormally high (more negative) potential difference across the respiratory epithelium[36]. Following the advent of successful lung transplantation for CF, the question was raised as to whether the donor lungs would regain the elevated potential difference found in the CF host airways. *In vivo* measurements of airway potential difference after heart–lung transplantation have suggested that the CF membrane defect has not occurred in the donor lungs after up to 2 years' follow-up[37]. Above the tracheal anastomosis the upper airways still retain the CF epithelial defect and may remain colonized with *P. aeruginosa*, as previously mentioned.

QUALITY OF LIFE

There is no doubt that the quality of life after successful transplantation is better than before. Many patients have returned to school, work or higher education after surgery. Some have married and others have gone on overseas holidays. Lung transplant recipients have been shown to enjoy improved levels of social and emotional well-being[38].

CHALLENGES

Shortage of suitable donor organs remains a serious issue and continued efforts must be made to ensure that the subject of organ donation is raised in a caring and compassionate way with relatives of potential donors fulfilling the brainstem death criteria. Lung transplantation for CF is a costly procedure because large doses of cyclosporin-A are needed on account of malabsorption. However, it is less expensive than caring for a chronically sick patient with CF who requires frequent hospital admissions and intravenous antibiotics. Furthermore, the quality of life is much better for the successfully transplanted patient[38].

The timing of surgery is vital: it must not be too early as approximately 30 per cent of patients die during the first postoperative year; nor must it be too late as suitable donor organs may not be found in time or the patient may be too ill to be successfully transplanted. It is of paramount importance that only those patients who have had maximum medical treatment be considered for transplant surgery.

Obliterative bronchiolitis remains a serious problem which needs to be addressed. It is hoped that the development of newer immunosuppressive agents and modalities (tacrolimus, mycophenolate mofetil, rapamycin, total lymphoid irradiation), together with improved diagnosis and treatment of rejection and pulmonary infection, will reduce the incidence of this condition.

It is important that we give psychosocial support not only to the patients and their relatives while they are on the transplant waiting list but also to the relatives whose loved ones died and to the patients who do well. This latter group may require support in adjusting to a more normal lifestyle after many years of ill health.

The majority of lung transplants for CF have been performed on patients in their twenties and thirties. There is a definite impression that younger patients do not do as well and that there is a higher incidence of obliterative bronchiolitis in lung transplant recipients under the age of 10 years[33]. It would therefore seem appropriate that great care is taken to avoid putting young patients on the transplant waiting list who would still respond to conventional medical treatment.

The shortage of donor organs remains the major limiting factor to lung transplantation. There are more patients on the transplant waiting list than available donor organs and thus many patients die awaiting surgery. In an attempt to overcome this problem, transplant centers are investigating the use of animal organs for human transplantation (xenografting). Ideally, suitable animals should have organs of comparable size and anatomy to humans and be easy to breed. Pigs fulfill these criteria and extensive research into porcine xenografting is being carried out.

Hyperacute rejection leading to early graft failure following xenografting is the most serious complication. It is believed to reflect the effects of preformed cross-reacting antibodies and local complement activation. Platelet activating factor and thromboxane B_2 may also play an important role[39,40]. Discordant xenotransplants (e.g. pig to human) result in hyperacute rejection (HAR) because of the presence of high levels of antidonor species in the recipient. The most important factor in determining whether HAR will occur is the specific pattern of glycosylation of proteins and lipids on the vascular endothelium of the two species. Humans express ABO histo-blood group oligosaccharides whereas pigs express α-galactosyl (αGAL) epitopes instead. Higher primates have anti-GAL antibodies, which are developed soon after birth as a response to colonization of the bowel by α-GAL-expressing microorganisms. Consequently, a transplanted organ from a pig will be hyperacutely rejected by antibody-mediated complement activation. Efforts are being made to 'humanize' the pig myocytes by genetic manipulation (i.e. transgenic induction of expression of a human decay accelerating factor for complement on their surface), thus avoiding (or reducing the severity of) the host immunological response. Prolonged xenograft survival in animal models has been demonstrated with 15-deoxyspergualin used in combination with total lymphoid irradiation[41], plasma exchange or absorption of antibodies by porcine kidney profusion[42], monoclonal antibody against CD4[43] and splenectomy[44]. It was hoped that the application of these and other techniques would enable xenografting to become a future option for transplanting CF patients. However, there remains the serious concern of possible transmission of infection from pigs to humans (zoonosis). As a consequence, many countries have abandoned research into xenotransplantation and therefore its future role in human lung transplantation remains uncertain at this time.

REFERENCES

1. Rommens, J.M., Ianuzzi, M.C., Kerrem, B. *et al*. (1989) Identification of the cystic fibrosis gene: chromosome walking and jumping. *Science*, **245**, 1059–1065.
2. Yacoub, M.H., Banner, N.R., Khaghani, A. *et al*. (1990) Heart–lung transplantation for cystic fibrosis and subsequent domino heart transplantation. *J. Heart Transplant.*, **9**, 459–467.
3. Scott, J., Higenbottam, T., Hutter, J. *et al*. (1988) Heart–lung transplantation for cystic fibrosis. *Lancet*, **ii**, 192–194.
4. Madden, B.P., Hodson, M.E., Tsang, V. *et al*. (1992) Intermediate-term results of heart–lung transplantation for cystic fibrosis. *Lancet*, **339**, 1583–1587.
5. Patterson, G.A. (1989) Double lung transplantation. *Pediatr. Pulmonol.*, **4**, 56–57.
6. Yankaskas, J., Mallory, G and the Consensus Committee. (1996) Lung transplantation in cystic fibrosis: Consensus conference statement. *Concepts in Care*, CF Foundation, Vol. 7, Section 2, pp. 1–19.
6a. Stemenkovic, S.A., Alphonso, N. Rice, P. and Madden, B.P. (1999) Recurrence of hepatitis B after single lung transplantation. *J. Heart Lung Transplant.*, **18**, 1246–1250.
7. Hodson, M.E., Madden, B.P., Steven, M.H. *et al*. (1991) Non-invasive mechanical ventilation for cystic fibrosis patients: a bridge to transplantation. *Eur. Respir. J.*, **4**, 524–527.
8. Madden, B.P., Chan, C.M., Kamalvand, K., Siddiqi, A.J., Vuddamalay, P. and Hodson, M.E. (1993) *Aspergillus* infection in patients with cystic fibrosis following lung transplantation, in *Clinical Ecology of Cystic Fibrosis*, (eds H. Escobar, F. Baquero and L. Suarez), Excerpta Medica, International Congress Series 1034, Elsevier Science, Amsterdam, pp. 189–194.
9. Lewiston, N., King, V., Umetsu, D. *et al*. (1991) Cystic fibrosis patients who have undergone heart–lung transplantation benefit from maxillary sinus antrostomy and repeated sinus lavage. *Transplant Proc.*, **23**, 1207–1208.
10. Madden, B.P., Kamalvand, K., Chan, C.M. *et al*. (1993) The medical management of patients with cystic fibrosis following heart-lung transplantation. *Eur. Respir. J.*, **6**, 965–970.
11. Snell, G.I., de Hoyos, A., Krajden, M., Winton, T. and Maurer, J. (1993) *Pseudomonas cepacia* in lung transplant recipients with cystic fibrosis. *Chest*, **103**, 466–471.
12. Wallwork, J., Jones, K., Cavarocchi, N. *et al*. (1987) Distant procurement of organs for clinical heart–lung transplants using a single flush technique. *Transplantation*, **44**, 654–658.
13. Hutter, J.A., Wreghitt, T., Scott, J.P. *et al*. (1989) The importance of cytomegalovirus in heart lung transplant recipients. *Chest*, **95**, 627–631.
14. Yacoub, M.H., Khaghani, A., Aravot, D. *et al*. (1988) Cardiac transplantation from live donors. *J. Am. Coll. Cardiol.*, **11**, 102A.
15. Madden, B., Radley-Smith, R., Hodson, M. *et al*. Medium term results of heart and lung transplantation. *J. Heart Lung Transplant.*, **11**, s241–s243.
15a. Madden, B.P., Kumar, P., Sayer, R. and Murday, A.J. (1997) Successful resection of obstructing airway granulation tissue following lung transplantation using endobronchial laser (Nd:YAG) therapy. *Eur. J. Cardiothorac. Surg.*, **12**, 480–485.
16. Lima, O., Goldberg, M., Peters, W.J. *et al*. (1982) Bronchial omentopexy in canine lung transplantation. *J. Thorac. Cardiovasc. Surg.*, **83**, 418–421.
17. Khaghani, A., Tadjkarimi, S., Daly, R. *et al*. (1994) The influence of different types of wraps versus no wrap in single lung transplantation. A prospective randomised trial. *J. Heart Lung Transplant.*, **13**, 767–773.
18. Patterson, G.A., Todd, T.R., Cooper, J.D. *et al*. (1990) Airway complications after double lung transplantation. *J. Thorac. Cardiovasc. Surg.*, **99**, 14–21.

19. Pasque, M.K., Cooper, J.D., Kaiser, L.R. *et al.* (1990) Improved technique for bilateral lung transplantation: rationale and initial clinical experience. *Ann. Thorac. Surg.*, **49**, 785–791.

20. Starnes, V.A., Barr, M., Cohen, R. *et al.* (1996) Living donor lobar lung transplantation experience: Intermediate results. *J. Thorac. Cardiovasc. Surg.*, **112**, 1284–1291.

21. Starnes, V.A., Barr, M.L., Cohen, R.G. *et al.* (1994) Lobar transplantation. Indications, technique and outcome. *J. Thorac. Cardiovasc. Surg.*, **108**, 403–411.

22. Couetil, J.P., Grousset, A., Benaim, D. *et al.* (1994–95) Experimental model of pulmonary bipartition with bilateral lobe transplantation in dogs and application to clinical medicine. *Chirurgie*, **120**, 512–517.

23. Calne, R.Y., White, D.J.G., Thiru, S. *et al.* (1978) Cyclosporin A in patients receiving renal allografts from cadaver donors. *Lancet*, **ii**, 1323–1327.

24. Kahan, BD. (1989) Cyclosporin. *NEJM*, **321**, 1725–1738.

25. Calne, R. (1961) Inhibition of the rejection of renal homografts in dogs by purine analogues. *Transplant. Bull.*, **28**, 65–81.

26. Madden, B.P. (1991) Post operative care and follow-up after heart–lung transplantation. *Paediatr. Pulmonol. Suppl.*, **6**, 132–133.

27. Madden, B.P., Hodson, M.E. and Yacoub, M. (1992) Heart–lung transplantation for cystic fibrosis. *BMJ*, **304**, 835–836.

28. Pomerance, A., Madden, B.P., Burke, M. and Yacoub, M. (1995) Transbronchial biopsy in heart and lung transplantation: Clinicopathologic correlations. *J. Heart Lung Transplant.*, **14**, 761–773.

29. Higenbottam, T., Stewart, S., Penketh, A. and Wallwork, J. (1988) Transbronchial lung biopsy for the diagnosis of rejection in heart–lung transplant patients. *Transplantation*, **46**, 532–539.

30. Madden, B.P., Khaghani, A. and Yacoub, M. (1991) Successful retransplantation of the heart and lungs in an adult with cystic fibrosis. *J. R. Soc. Med.*, **84**, 561.

31. Scott, J.P., Sharples, L., Mullins, P. *et al.* (1991) Further studies on the natural history of obliterative bronchiolitis following heart–lung transplantation. *Transplant. Proc.*, **23**, 1201–1202.

32. Griffith, B.P., Paradis, I.L., Zeevi, A. *et al.* (1988) Immunology mediated disease of the airways after pulmonary transplantation. *Ann. Surg.*, **208**, 371–379.

33. Whitehead, B., Helms, P., Goodwin, M. *et al.* (1991) Heart–lung transplantation for cystic fibrosis. Outcome. *Arch. Dis. Child.*, **66**, 1022–1026.

34. Shankar, S., Fulsham, L., Read, R. *et al.* (1991) Mucociliary function after lung transplantation. *Transplant. Proc.*, **23**, (1), 1222–1223.

35. Cooney, G.F., Fiel, S.B., Shaw, L.M. and Cavarocchi, N.C. (1990) Cyclosporin bioavailability in heart–lung transplant candidates with cystic fibrosis. *Transplantation*, **49**, 821–823.

36. Knowles, M.D., Gatzy, J. and Boucher, R. (1981) Increased bioelectric potential difference across respiratory epithelia in cystic fibrosis. *NEJM*, **305**, 1489–1495.

37. Alton, E.W.F.W., Khaghani, A., Taylor, R.F.H. *et al.* (1991) Effect of heart–lung transplantation on airway potential difference in patients with and without cystic fibrosis. *Eur. Respir. J.*, **4**, 5–9.

38. Squier, H.C., Ries, A.L., Kaplan, R.M. *et al.* (1995) Quality of well-being predicts survival in transplantation candidates. *Am. J. Respir. Crit. Care Med.*, **152**, 2032–2036.

39. Makowka, L., Chapman, F.A., Cramer, D.V. *et al.* (1990) Platelet-activating factor and hyperacute rejection. The effect of a platelet-activating factor antagonist, SRI 63-441, on rejection of xenografts and allografts in sensitised hosts. *Transplantation*, **50**, 359–365.

40. Hammer, C., Schutz, A., Pratschke, J. *et al.* (1992) Bridging to transplant: allogeneic heart transplantation after xenografting. *J. Heart Lung Transplant.*, **11**, S182–S188.

41. Marchman, W., Araneda, D., De Masi, R. *et al.* (1992) Prolongation of xenograft survival after combination therapy with 15-deoxyspergualin and total-lymphoid irradiation in the hamster-to-rat cardiac xenograft model. *Transplantation*, **53**, 30–34.

42. Fischel, R.J., Matas, A.J., Platt, J.L. *et al.* (1992) Cardiac xenografting in the pig-to-rhesus monkey model: manipulation of antiendothelial antibody prolongs survival. *J. Heart Lung Transplant.*, **11**, 965–973.

43. Kemp, E., Dieperink, H., Jensenius, J.C. *et al.* (1990) Hope for successful xenografting by immunosuppression with monoclonal antibody against CD4, total lymphoid irradiation and cyclosporine. Six months' survival of hamster heart transplanted into rat. *Scand. J. Urol. Nephrol.*, **24**, 79–80.

44. Monden, M., Valdivia, L.A., Gotoh, M. *et al.* (1989) A crucial effect of splenectomy on prolonging cardiac xenograft survival in combination with cyclosporin. *Surgery*, **105**, 535–542.

19

Paramedical issues

19a Physiotherapy *J. A. Pryor and B. A. Webber*	376
Introduction	376
Excess bronchial secretions	376
Breathlessness	381
Chest wall stiffness	382
Exercise tolerance	382
Physiotherapy for complications	382
Conclusion	383
19b Dietary treatment of cystic fibrosis *S. Poole, A. McAlweenie and F. Ashworth*	384
Introduction	384
Causes of malnutrition	384
Nutritional requirements	386
Dietary management	388
Nutritional intervention	388
Specific dietary complications	393
Conclusion	395
19c Nursing *F. Duncan-Skingle and F. Foster*	396
Introduction	396
Impact of CF on the family following diagnosis	396
Coping with treatment	397
School	397
Adolescence	397
Transition to the adult setting	398
Late diagnosis	398
Outpatient care	399
Inpatient care	399
Home care	401
Relationships	402
Fertility and pregnancy	402
Disease progression	402
Deteriorating health	402
Transplantation	404
Terminal phase	404
Bereavement counseling	405
How does the nurse cope with the stress of caring for CF patients?	405
19d Cystic fibrosis home care *F. Duncan-Skingle and E. Bramwell*	406
Introduction	406
The advantages of home care	407
The disadvantages of home care	407
The organization of home care	407
Conducting a home-care visit	408
Specific aspects of home-care nursing of CF patients	409
Contracts for home care	411
Summary	412
19e Social work *N. Cloutman*	413
Introduction	413
Children and young families	413
Growing up with cystic fibrosis	414
Employment	414
Housing	415
Relationships and marriage	415
Making adjustment to deteriorating health	416
The social worker's role in transplant assessment	416
Bereavement	417
Conclusion	417
19f Occupational therapy *V. Otley Groom*	419
Introduction	419
Assessment	419
Interventions	419
Oxygen provision and equipment	422
References	424

Physiotherapy

J. A. PRYOR AND B. A. WEBBER

INTRODUCTION

Physiotherapy is recognized as an integral part of the management of patients with cystic fibrosis and is one of the aspects of treatment that contributes to improvement in quality of life. It has been suggested that knowledge of the condition and understanding of treatment have an impact on adherence[1]. Adherence with physiotherapy is also improved if the physiotherapist understands the patients' views and beliefs and is increased in patients who perceive physical benefits from physiotherapy[2].

Assessment and reassessment of patients are essential for effective management. The individual's needs will change as she or he progresses from infancy, through school, college, university and work, but it is important to encourage as normal a lifestyle as possible while making time to include regular physiotherapy.

Physiotherapy can assist in the treatment of excess bronchial secretions, breathlessness, chest wall stiffness and pain of musculoskeletal origin, and reduced exercise tolerance.

EXCESS BRONCHIAL SECRETIONS

Many pediatricians acknowledge early evidence of inflammation and infection in the lungs[3,4] and, in an attempt to delay the destructive process of infection, recommend introducing physiotherapy at the time of diagnosis even if the infant or child is asymptomatic. If physiotherapy becomes an accepted part of life, adherence will probably be better than if it is introduced at a later stage.

A close bonding usually develops between the parents and the child, and it is important that both parents are involved. The siblings should also be included in the care of the affected child and should be given sufficient atten-

tion so that they feel that they are involved in the family activities.

For the infant and small child, physiotherapy is passive and internationally, apart from some variations, the techniques to encourage the clearance of secretions commonly include gravity-assisted positions and chest clapping to stimulate coughing. Appropriate positions for drainage may be indicated on assessment, but the apical segments of the upper lobes (Fig. 19.1) should be included until the child begins to walk. If no specific

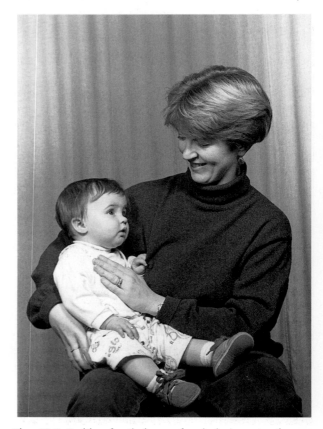

Fig. 19.1 *Position for drainage of apical segments of upper lobes. (Reproduced with the parents' permission.)*

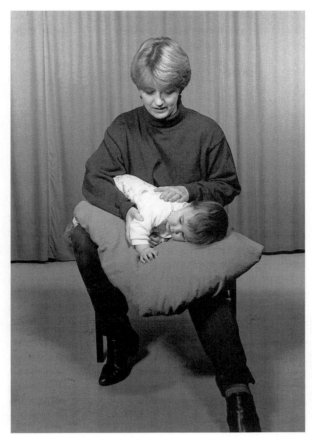

Fig. 19.2 *One of the gravity-assisted positions for drainage of the right lower lobe. (Reproduced with the parents' permission.)*

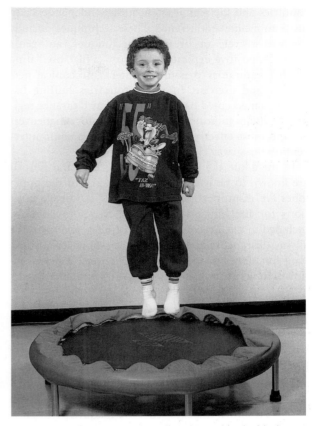

Fig. 19.4 *Bouncing on a trampoline. (Reproduced with the parents' permission.)*

areas of the lungs are affected, the recommendations from clinical practice are to use the gravity-assisted positions of sitting and side lying. When the infant is tilted downwards on his or her parent's knee he or she can be angled to drain the middle lobe, lingula and each lower lobe (Fig. 19.2). Bouncing games on the parent's knees can be introduced at an early stage to make physiotherapy enjoyable.

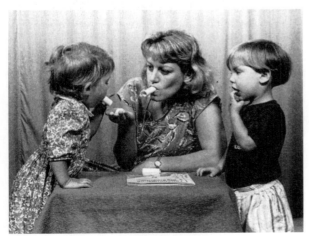

Fig. 19.3 *Huffing games. (Reproduced with the parents' permission.)*

Infants with CF have a higher than normal incidence of gastroesophageal reflux, but there is conflicting evidence as to whether this is exacerbated by the head-down position[5–7]. When an increase is suspected, the effect of positioning must be assessed. Gastroesophageal reflux may be exacerbated by the vigorous techniques used in some parts of the world, rather than the head-down tipped position.

Treatment sessions should be given before feeds, for 5–10 minutes, and usually twice a day. During episodes of infection the frequency and duration of these sessions will need to be increased.

Cough swabs may assist in the identification of pathogenic organisms. Nasopharyngeal suction should only be used when a sputum specimen is essential or an infant is distressed by excess secretions.

When the child is about 2 years of age he or she can begin to participate in breathing exercises. Huffing games (Fig. 19.3) can be used to introduce huffing. A foam-rubber wedge or cushions will probably be more comfortable for the child than continuing positioning on the parent's knees. To make physiotherapy sessions fun, activities such as bouncing on a trampoline (Fig. 19.4), 'wheelbarrows' or skipping can be included.

For the child, adolescent and adult, different airway clearance techniques have been developed in different countries and the regimens encourage independence in order to facilitate adherence. These techniques[8] include the active cycle of breathing techniques, autogenic drainage, positive expiratory pressure (PEP), oscillating positive expiratory pressure (Flutter), mechanical percussion and exercise. In many countries huffing has become an accepted part of these airway clearance regimens. Studies indicate that forced expiratory maneuvers are the most effective part of physiotherapeutic intervention for airway clearance[9].

In the adult, the areas of bronchiectasis and fibrosis are known to be irregularly distributed, but the upper lobes are disproportionately involved[10]. Drainage positions for the upper lobes should therefore often be included in the airway clearance regimen. Several of the airway clearance techniques have been shown to improve lung function, and a relationship between a deterioration in lung function and mortality has been identified[11].

Active cycle of breathing techniques

When a child can huff effectively, the active cycle of breathing techniques (ACBT) can be introduced in appropriate gravity-assisted positions.

The more passive techniques of postural drainage have been shown to be less effective than ACBT in gravity-assisted positions[12] and, using these techniques, many people are able to carry out their own treatment independent of assistance[13].

The active cycle of breathing techniques is a cycle of breathing control, thoracic expansion exercises and the forced expiration technique. Breathing control is normal breathing, at tidal volume, using the lower chest with the upper chest and shoulders as relaxed as possible. It is used in the rest periods between the more active parts of the cycle.

Thoracic expansion exercises are deep-breathing exercises emphasizing inspiration. Expiration is passive and relaxed. An increase in lung volume reduces the resistance within the collateral ventilatory system[14] and allows air to flow behind secretions to assist in mobilizing them. Interdependence, the expanding forces exerted between adjacent alveoli, also aids lung re-expansion[15]. This effect is greater at high lung volumes.

The forced expiration technique is one or two huffs or forced expirations combined with periods of breathing control. Huffing to a low lung volume is necessary to loosen and clear secretions from the more peripheral airways. When secretions have reached the upper airways, a huff or cough from a high lung volume can be used to clear them. The dynamic collapse and compression of the airways downstream of the equal pressure point[16] is an important part of the clearance mechanism of a forced expiratory maneuver, huff or cough. The length of the huff and the force of contraction of the muscles of expiration should be adapted for each individual to max-

imize air flow and minimize airway collapse. The huff should never be a violent maneuver. When forced expirations are combined with breathing control there is no increase in airflow obstruction[12,17].

The ACBT is carried out in positions as indicated on assessment. An example of the cycle is:

1. breathing control;
2. 3–4 thoracic expansion exercises with or without chest clapping or chest shaking;
3. breathing control;
4. 1–2 huffs with or without chest compression;
5. breathing control.

The cycle is adapted to suit the individual and it may be preferable to repeat the thoracic expansion exercises and the pause for breathing control before going on to the huffs. The length of the pauses will vary. In a patient with bronchospasm or unstable airways, or in one who is debilitated and fatigues easily, longer pauses are more appropriate. Paroxysmal coughing is exhausting and ineffective and can be minimized by adapting the length of the huff and using breathing control.

The cycle is continued until the huff or cough has remained dry-sounding and nonproductive during two consecutive cycles. A treatment session usually includes drainage of only two or three positions as it is likely that a minimum of 10 minutes will be necessary for each productive position.

Many patients benefit from the use of gravity-assisted positions[18] but the ACBT is also effective in the sitting position. When secretions are minimal, or when it is more convenient, for example at college, work (Fig. 19.5) or on holiday, the sitting position can be used and may improve adherence. When the head-down tipped position is recommended, a postural drainage frame which supports the whole body may be of value in the home (Fig. 19.6).

The length of time for treatment, the number of treatments in a day and the positions for treatment will vary and will be determined on assessment. It is recommended that patients are reassessed at least every 6 months by a physiotherapist to check and update techniques.

From the age of 8 or 9 years children can begin to do some of the treatment themselves and gradually learn to be independent of their parents. Adolescents often prefer to take full responsibility for their treatment and this can often continue throughout adult life. Many patients will benefit from assistance with treatment during periods of an exacerbation of a bronchopulmonary infection (Fig. 19.7) and some frail patients will always need assistance.

A physiotherapy treatment regimen needs to be effective, efficient, comfortable and easy to use. The active cycle of breathing techniques fulfills these criteria. It has also been shown to improve lung function[19]. Studies of postural drainage, chest clapping and forced expirations have shown a fall in skin oxygen tension or oxygen satu-

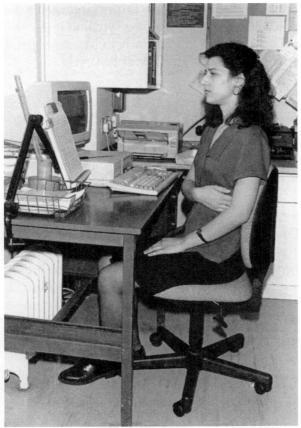

Fig. 19.5 *Active cycle of breathing techniques in sitting. (Reproduced with permission of the patient.)*

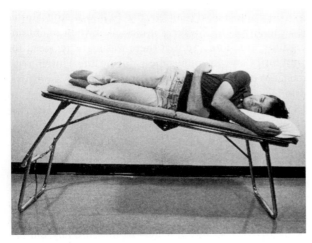

Fig. 19.6 *Frame for postural drainage at home. (Reproduced with permission of the patient.)*

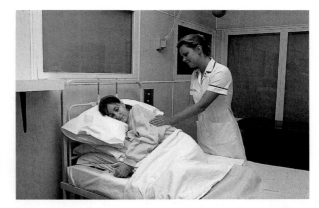

Fig. 19.7 *Active cycle of breathing techniques with assistance. (Reproduced with permission of the patient.)*

Autogenic drainage

Autogenic drainage (AD) aims to maximize air flow within the airways to aid mucus clearance. Controlled breathing at differing lung volumes is used to reach the highest possible air flow in different generations of bronchi[23]. The Belgian method[8] recognizes three phases:

1. 'Unstick' – this phase is carried out at a low lung volume and helps to loosen the peripherally situated secretions.
2. 'Collect' – breathing around mid lung volume facilitates collection of secretions in the upper airways.
3. 'Evacuate' – breathing at high lung volume facilitates clearance of secretions from the upper airways.

Patients soon learn to feel the level at which secretions are situated. Breathing in should be slow, with a hold of about 3 seconds encouraged at the end of each inspiration. This facilitates filling of lung segments.

When AD was compared with postural drainage and percussion, sputum production was significantly increased with AD[24] and AD does not cause oxygen desaturation[25]. It requires considerable patient cooperation and may be most feasible for adolescents over 12 years of age and for adults[26].

The Germans have modified the technique of autogenic drainage, as breathing to a very low lung volume in the 'unstick' phase can be uncomfortable for the breathless patient. In modified autogenic drainage (MAD)[8] the patient breathes around tidal volume while breath holding for 2–3 seconds at the end of each inspiration. Coughing is used to clear secretions as soon as they reach the larynx.

Positive expiratory pressure

The positive expiratory pressure (PEP) mask incorporates a one-way valve, expiratory orifice resistor and manometer (Fig. 19.8). The positive expiratory pressure

ration[20,21]. In contrast, a study of ACBT showed no fall in oxygen saturation, the differences being the inclusion of thoracic expansion exercises during chest clapping, and periods of breathing control following huffing[22].

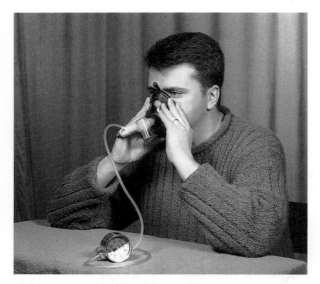

Fig. 19.8 *Positive expiratory pressure (PEP). (Reproduced with permission of the patient.)*

generated helps to keep the airways open and allows air to track behind secretions to assist in mobilizing them[27]. In the sitting position, the patient leans forward with his or her elbows supported on a table. He or she holds the mask firmly over the nose and mouth and breathes at tidal volume with a slightly active expiration for about 6–10 breaths. The expiratory pressure should be between 10 and 20cmH₂O during mid-expiration[27]. The lung volume should be kept up by avoiding complete expiration.

After a period of PEP, huffing or coughing is used to clear secretions from the upper airways. The duration and frequency of each treatment is adapted to the individual patient. About 10–15 minutes twice a day is often recommended[8].

PEP has been shown to increase sputum yield and improve transcutaneous oxygen tension when compared with postural drainage, percussion and breathing exercises[20]. Lung function has been shown to improve with PEP in a long-term study when compared with postural drainage and percussion[28]. A study[18] comparing an unassisted treatment using PEP with an unassisted treatment using ACBT did not show any advantage in the use of PEP. A further study demonstrated a temporary increase in lung volume with PEP, but there was no increase in mucus transport[29].

High-pressure PEP is a modified form of PEP mask treatment utilizing forced expiratory maneuvers through the expiratory resistor[8,30]. By using high pressure, 40–100cmH₂O, secretions may be mobilized more easily in patients with unstable airways. This technique is only recommended where lung-function equipment is available for regular reassessment of the appropriate expiratory resistance.

Oscillating positive expiratory pressure (Flutter)

The Flutter is a pipe-shaped device which provides both positive expiratory pressure and an oscillation of the air within the airways as the patient breathes out (Fig. 19.9).

A slow deep breath in with a breath hold of 3–5 seconds is followed by a breath out through the Flutter at a faster rate than normal. The angle of the device is adjusted to obtain maximal oscillation. After 4–8 breaths many patients use huffing, either through the Flutter or without the Flutter, to clear secretions.

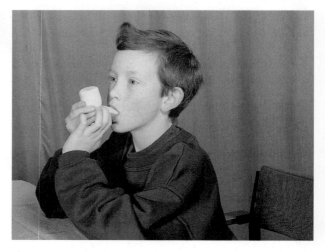

Fig. 19.9 *Oscillating positive expiratory pressure (Flutter). (Reproduced with the parents' permission.)*

A long-term study comparing PEP with the Flutter indicated that the Flutter is not as effective in maintaining lung function, and that there was a greater need for antibiotics and hospitalization during the Flutter regimen[31]. When the Flutter was compared with a postural drainage regimen including up to 10 positions in 15 minutes, more sputum was expectorated with the Flutter[32].

Mechanical percussion and vibration

Mechanical percussors have been shown to increase intrathoracic pressure[33], but other workers could not demonstrate any clinical benefit as measured by sputum clearance or lung function[34]. Vibratory jackets, for example ThAIRapy, utilize the principle of mechanical percussion, and the Hayek Oscillator can be used to deliver high-frequency external oscillations with intermittent chest compressions.

A review of mechanical percussion, vibration, high-frequency oscillation and chest wall compression has been undertaken[35]. Mechanical vibration may increase mucociliary clearance and high-frequency chest wall compression may be more effective than oral high-frequency oscillation, but further work needs to be undertaken on the frequency of the vibration, and the optimal frequency may vary from patient to patient.

In countries where patients are already using independent airway clearance techniques, the more expensive and cumbersome alternative of mechanical percussion is unlikely to be cost effective or improve quality of life.

Exercise

The mucociliary clearance effect of exercise has been compared with that of the active cycle of breathing techniques[36]. This study concluded that exercise should be used in addition to the regimen of ACBT but not as a substitute. Bilton et al.[37] could find no objective difference in sputum expectoration when exercise either preceded or followed physiotherapy.

Summary

Patients should be encouraged to use the regimen which is most effective and efficient for them. In a survey of patients' views on physiotherapy, their reasons for using airway clearance techniques included: 'Makes my breathing easier', 'It stops me from coughing at other times' and 'I feel better afterwards'. Their reasons for not using airway clearance techniques included: 'Not enough time', 'Feel very well' and 'Too tired'[2].

Clinical benefit for the use of airway clearance devices (e.g. PEP, Flutter) or an increase in adherence to treatment, should be identified before a device is recommended in preference to one of the regimens that do not incur additional equipment costs (e.g. ACBT, AD).

Inhalation of drugs

Bronchodilator drugs may be prescribed and these should be inhaled before treatment to clear secretions. Nebulized bronchodilators should be used only if there is additional clinical benefit to inhalation with a simpler device (e.g. metered dose or dry-powder inhaler).

Normal saline (0.9 per cent) or hypertonic saline (3–7 per cent) inhaled before physiotherapy may assist in the clearance of secretions[38–41]. Mucolytic agents, for example N-acetylcysteine (Parvolex®), should be used with caution. A reduction in sputum viscosity does not necessarily increase sputum clearance and bronchospasm may be induced. If hypertonic saline or mucolytic agents are to be inhaled, a test dose is necessary with recordings of peak expiratory flow rate or FEV_1 before and after the first inhalation to identify any increase in airflow obstruction.

Inhaled antibiotics should be taken after treatment to clear secretions. Spirometry should be recorded before and after the first dose to detect an increase in airflow obstruction[42]. If this effect should occur, it can usually be minimized by the inhalation of a bronchodilator. Exhalation of antibiotics should be via a one-way valve and effective filter, or vented out of the window via wide-bore tubing (Fig. 19.10). This is to prevent dispersion of the antibiotic into the air which may result in environmental organisms becoming resistant to the antibiotic or other people in the vicinity receiving a subtherapeutic dose[43,44].

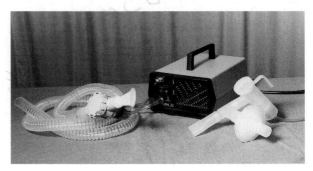

Fig. 19.10 *Equipment for nebulized antibiotics (acknowledgements to Medic-Aid Ltd and PariMedical Ltd).*

The optimal time for inhalation of dornase alfa (Pulmozyme® – DNase) in relation to physiotherapy has not yet been identified and needs to be assessed for each individual, if it is prescribed. Some patients benefit most by inhaling the drug about 30 minutes before physiotherapy, while others find that it takes several hours to reach a maximal effect. The latter, who take it after one physiotherapy session, find that the next session is more productive. Pulmozyme® requires isotonic conditions and a neutral pH for maximal activity. It should therefore be nebulized on its own and a period of at least 30 minutes should elapse between Pulmozyme® and the administration of other drugs, e.g. antibiotics, which may be either acidic or alkaline.

Nebulizers must be cleaned and dried thoroughly after each treatment to reduce the possibility of bacterial infection[45]. Air compressors should be serviced regularly[46].

BREATHLESSNESS

Breathing control can be used to minimize breathlessness and should be encouraged when breathlessness on exertion becomes noticeable, for example when walking up stairs and hills. Breathlessness at rest can be helped by the use of positions that optimize the length tension status of the diaphragm[47,48]. In the high side lying position (Fig. 19.11) the curvature of the dependent part of the diaphragm is probably increased by the position of the abdominal contents, and this effect, combined with

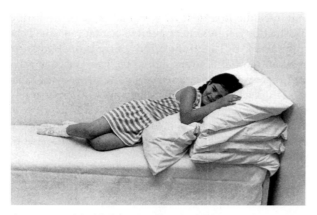

Fig. 19.11 *High side lying to relieve breathlessness. (Reproduced with the parents' permission.)*

relaxation of the head, neck and shoulders, facilitates breathing control. Other useful positions include sitting or standing leaning forward.

CHEST WALL STIFFNESS

Posture and thoracic mobility exercises will help to maintain normal function of the thoracic cage, but with increasing chest disease and hyperinflation of the chest, passive mobilization techniques, active assisted and active exercises may improve posture and lung function, and reduce chest wall pain[49].

EXERCISE TOLERANCE

Exercise is important to improve general physical fitness. It has been shown to increase exercise tolerance and cardiorespiratory fitness, to reduce breathlessness and may improve self-esteem (Chapter 20). Children should take part in normal school games when possible and adults should be encouraged to take some form of exercise regularly. Some patients prefer to exercise after using airway clearance techniques, either because they are too breathless to exercise until they have cleared their secretions or they find it more socially acceptable to be coughing less while participating in sports. Other patients prefer to exercise before treatment. A sport that the family can all enjoy is an easy way in which to include exercise in daily life.

PHYSIOTHERAPY FOR COMPLICATIONS

Acute exacerbation of a bronchopulmonary infection

Airway clearance techniques will be adapted as indicated on assessment. If oxygen therapy is prescribed, it should be continued throughout treatment. When secretions are very tenacious, heated high humidification should be considered, either continuously with oxygen therapy or for 10–15 minutes before physiotherapy.

Intermittent positive pressure breathing (IPPB) may be used to reduce the work of breathing or to assist in the clearance of secretions, but would be contraindicated if the patient has a history of pneumothoraces.

Noninvasive ventilation (NIV)[50] may be used to improve ventilation, particularly overnight, and the physiotherapist may be involved when the patient is initially set up on the ventilator.

Transmission of infection

Thorough hand washing by health professionals between patients is essential to minimize the possibility of transmission of infection. This has been demonstrated in patients with *Burkholderia cepacia*[51].

It has been shown that segregation of patients colonized with *B. cepacia* limits the spread of this organism[52]. Patients should be cared for in single rooms and their physiotherapy undertaken away from other patients. They should also be encouraged not to congregate with other patients and should be seen in a separate area in outpatient clinics. Care must also be taken when considering group exercise activities for patients with different pathogenic organisms.

Hemoptysis

Blood streaking of sputum is a frequent occurrence in patients with CF but is not usually a reason to alter the physiotherapy regimen. In cases of frank hemoptysis it is appropriate to discontinue physiotherapy temporarily until the bleeding begins to settle. Positioning may need to be modified and chest clapping withheld, but it is important to restart treatment as soon as possible to avoid the accumulation of old blood in the airways and retention of sputum. If embolization is necessary, physiotherapy can be restarted soon after the procedure.

Pneumothorax

A small pneumothorax is not a contraindication to chest physiotherapy, but when a large pneumothorax requires intercostal drainage, physiotherapy should be withheld until the drain has been inserted.

If surgical intervention is undertaken, physiotherapy should be restarted as soon as possible postoperatively. High humidification, probably combined with oxygen therapy, will assist the clearance of secretions. Effective analgesia is essential.

Pregnancy

In the later stages of pregnancy the respiratory system is compromised and lung function reduced. Modified gravity-assisted positions will probably be more appropriate for use during airway clearance. After the birth, intensive physiotherapy should be continued as the reduction in lung function persists for some time.

Transplantation

The physiotherapist should be involved both before and after heart–lung and lung transplantation. Cardiopulmonary rehabilitation programs have demonstrated improvements in exercise ability and quality of life in patients awaiting transplantation surgery[53].

Postoperatively, rehabilitation is essential to gain maximum benefit from surgery and to improve quality of life. Due to denervation of the lungs below the tracheal anastomosis the normal awareness of excess bronchial secretions is lost and cilial function is less effective. Early recognition of signs of a chest infection is particularly important to prevent pooling of secretions in the transplanted lung, which may lead to bronchiectasis. Patients should be encouraged to continue a short, daily session of breathing exercises and this should be increased as necessary during periods of chest infection.

Terminal care

The physiotherapist plays an important part in the life of patients with CF, and even when physiotherapy may no longer be effective it is important that support in the terminal stages is not withdrawn.

Appropriate positioning can help the breathless patient (Fig. 19.11) and a modified airway clearance technique can be used to clear secretions from the upper airways. Occasionally, adjuncts such as intermittent positive pressure breathing may also be of value. Nasotracheal suction is not indicated as it would cause distress and serve no useful purpose at this stage.

CONCLUSION

Physiotherapy must be adapted to suit the changing needs of the patient. Many patients will be under the care of more than one hospital and medical team and it is important that good communication exists both between teams and within teams to avoid confusion for the patient and the family. A regular review by a physiotherapist should identify any problems related to physiotherapy and provide an opportunity for remotivation, encouragement and changes in treatment plans as appropriate. Physiotherapy is an essential part of the management of CF, but programs must be discussed and agreed with parents and/or patients and should be realistic to optimize adherence and obtain a balance between sufficient treatment and quality of life.

Continued research in physiotherapy should lead to more effective management in the future.

Dietary treatment of cystic fibrosis

S. POOLE, A. McALWEENIE AND F. ASHWORTH

INTRODUCTION

Dietary assessment and nutritional advice are an important aspect of treatment for patients with cystic fibrosis (CF). Potential nutritional problems are multifactorial, and include maldigestion with subsequent malabsorption, increased requirements and poor dietary intake resulting in malnutrition. There is strong indication that improvement in nutritional status leads to an improvement in the prognosis for these patients[54–56]. However, dietary advice must be practical and adapted to suit the patient's lifestyle, particularly for adolescents and young adults. It should not be seen as another pressure and just one more treatment by patients who already spend a lot of their time carrying out other therapies.

The role of nutrition in the treatment of CF achieved prominence in the late 1970s. At this time, Toronto followed an aggressive nutritional policy advocating a high energy, high fat diet. They compared two CF populations and found a marked difference in mean age of survival: 21 years in Boston and 30 years in Toronto[57]. In Toronto males and females were taller and males were heavier than in Boston. The main difference in the management of these patients was the different nutritional approach.

The aim of dietary treatment should be to obtain normal growth and development from the time of diagnosis and to maintain this through to adult life. However, this becomes difficult in patients with severe lung disease, as a close relationship has been found between nutritional status and the degree of respiratory impairment. In adults weight loss most often reflects poor control of bronchopulmonary infection[58]. A multidisciplinary approach to optimizing nutrition intervention is essential[58a].

CAUSES OF MALNUTRITION

Malabsorption/maldigestion

Energy losses within the stool accounts for some of the increased dietary requirements in CF. In approximately 85 per cent of patients, significant intestinal malabsorption is present from infancy, and eventually 95 per cent of CF patients are affected[59]. Treatment with pancreatin preparations usually reduces steatorrhea[60]. However, in some patients with supposedly good symptomatic control, stool energy losses have been shown to be three times greater in CF patients compared with controls who have similar energy intakes: 10.6 per cent of gross energy intake was lost in the stools of CF patients compared with a normal loss of 3.5 per cent in controls[61].

Although faecal fat excretion is the most common measure of malabsorption in CF, Murphy et al. reported that stool lipid accounted for around 41 per cent of faecal energy in CF patients who were on their habitual pancreatic replacement treatment. A further 30 per cent of energy within the stool is derived from colonic bacteria. This is similar in both CF patients and healthy controls[61].

Appropriate use of pancreatic enzyme supplements is essential to minimize energy losses. Educating the patients on how to adjust the dosage and timing of the pancreatic supplements according to individual dietary intake is essential for the effective control of steathorrhea[62,63]. Providing an understanding of the constituent nutrients within foods, including main meals, snacks and milk, will enable the patients to take the appropriate supplementation for their diet. This is an important role for the dietitian as patients are often unaware that enzymes are necessary for digesting protein and carbohydrate as well as fat. Enzyme requirements will vary significantly between patients; in addition, each patient will have daily variations in their diet and consequently their own daily enzyme use will fluctuate. Regular dietary assessment, review of enzyme dose and education by the dietitian should be emphasized.

Pancreatin in the form of enteric coated microspheres is recommended for almost all pancreatic insufficient (PI) patients. For infants and young children who are unable to swallow the capsules, the microspheres can be mixed with an acid food (such as fruit purée or other food of suitable consistency) and given on a spoon. If mixed with an alkaline food (above pH 5), there is some deterioration in the enteric coating and leakage of enzymes can occur within 10 minutes. Therefore yoghurt and fruit, which have an acid pH 4 or less, are probably most appropriate as a medium[64]. It is important to note that the microspheres should be mixed with food and not chewed as this will destroy the enteric coating. As enzyme doses vary widely and many patients have a high requirement, the dose should be spread throughout the meal if feasible. However, taking capsules several times during a meal may prove difficult for children to administer, and may decrease compliance. Pancreatin powder or scoops of microspheres can be used for some babies and young children[65]. Care should be taken to ensure that the powder is not taken without first being mixed with a small amount of food.

There is little evidence to suggest that very high intakes of pancreatic enzyme are necessary even in the many patients with poorly controlled malabsorption[66]. Most clinicians rely on a history of abdominal symptoms, such as frequent, offensive, bulky stools and changes in body weight to regulate the enzyme dose. However, abdominal symptoms in CF may not be entirely due to insufficient pancreatic enzyme replacement[67,68]. It is very important to determine whether symptoms are due to fat malabsorption (confirmed by faecal fat assessment), before advising an increase to an inappropriately high dose of pancreatic enzymes[69]. In 1993 fibrosing colonopathy was described as a rare complication in children[70] with CF and there appears to be a dose-related association between pancreatic enzyme replacements, particularly the high-strength preparations, and its development[71]. Colonic strictures have occurred in patients who took doses of more than 6000 IU lipase/kg/meal. The 1995 UK Committee on Safety of Medicine (CSM)[72] recommended that 'it would be prudent for patients with CF not to exceed a daily dose of enzymes equivalent of 10 000 IU lipase per kg body weight per day'. Also in 1995 the US Cystic Fibrosis Foundation and Food and Drug Administration conference recommended the following guidelines on the use of enzymes[73]:

- Infants: 2000–4000 IU lipase/120 mL feed or 450–900 IU lipase/ gram of fat.
- Children: 500–4000 IU lipase/gram of fat/day or a mean of 1800 IU lipase/gram fat /day.

In the UK the high-strength enzymes are now rarely used in children under the age of 15. Adult patients who have high enzyme requirements may find it advantageous and help aid compliance if they can take a lower number of high-strength capsules. All patients taking any enzyme preparation should be monitored closely to ensure that the dosage is not allowed to gradually increase to an inadvisably high level. Care must always be taken when changing to another enzyme supplement. The final dosage should be achieved on the basis of stool characteristics due to variations in individual requirements. In those patients who still have uncontrolled malabsorption and who may be receiving the maximum dose of pancreatic enzymes, it may be appropriate to use a H_2 blocker or proton pump inhibitor as an adjunctive therapy.

Energy requirements in CF

Energy requirements in CF will vary depending on nutritional state, age and lung function[74,75,75a]. It appears that deteriorating lung function is the major factor associated with increased resting energy expenditure (REE)[76]. Little, if any, increase in REE is seen in healthy, normally nourished CF males with good lung function[77]. It is interesting to note that patients with moderate lung disease adapt to an increased REE by reducing their activity levels and thereby maintaining their total energy expenditure (TEE). In subjects with pancreatic insufficiency, there will be variable losses of both fat and nitrogen in the stools, as well as the influence of deteriorating lung function affecting energy requirements. In an assessment of dietary energy requirements, both these factors should considered. Some workers[78] have reported that there may be a basic defect in CF influencing energy requirements but others have recently shown this may not be the case[79]. It has also been suggested that there is a genetic component relating to increased energy requirements. Those patients who are homozygous for ΔF_{508} may have an increased REE, but this has also now been disputed[77,80]. During periods of rapid growth (such as the first 2 years of life and during puberty), there is an increased energy demand, which should also be accounted for when assessing energy requirements.

Dietary intake

Anorexia is common in CF and can become more of a problem especially during recurrent chest infections. This may lead to a chronically poor appetite. Subjects with CF may have voracious appetites before diagnosis and this is usually the result of long-standing steatorrhea[81]; when this is corrected the appetite tends to subside. Inadequate energy intake has been shown to be one of the major factors contributing to malnutrition in CF[82,83,83a]. Improving energy intake is therefore the area to be targeted. Studies have shown that some patients do meet their energy requirements, particularly if they receive dietetic contact[84,85]. Actual energy intakes in healthy patients with CF have not been well documented.

There are many factors contributing to a poor dietary intake in CF. Such problems include foul-tasting sputum, coughing with possible subsequent vomiting, abdominal symptoms and gastroesophageal reflux (GOR).

Regular dietary assessment and counseling from a dietitian has been shown to lead to an improvement in energy intake. In one UK pediatric clinic, patients who had had no regular contact with a dietitian were reported to have had mean energy intakes of 97 per cent of that recommended for age. Those who had seen a dietitian at least twice within the previous year had a mean energy intake of 119 per cent of that recommended for age[85]. In 1994 the average energy intake of 50 patients in a clinic, age range 0.75–25 years, was found to be 97 per cent (57–169 per cent) of the respective recommended for age[86]. Intakes can also be improved with behavioral nutrition education[86a].

Other factors contributing to a poor dietary intake include dietary dislikes, emotional and psychological problems and social pressures. For dietary advice to be effective, long-term education and support of the individual is essential. The advice will often conflict with current information on 'healthy eating' for the family, and reassurances are needed by parents or spouses that a diet which does not restrict fat, sugar or salt is really being recommended! Parents and adults may also worry that a high saturated fat intake may lead to future cardiac problems. A high-fat diet in CF patients with pancreatic insufficiency has not been found to raise serum lipid levels, however, patients with normal pancreatic function should be monitored[86b].

The financial cost of a high energy diet may also be a factor leading to suboptimal intakes. Practical advice from a dietitian on economical ways to achieve dietary requirements can be helpful.

NUTRITIONAL REQUIREMENTS

Energy

When calculating energy requirements, all the factors, such as faecal energy losses, increased basal metabolic rate (BMR), catch-up growth and frequency of infection, need to be taken into consideration. It has been demonstrated that normal rates of weight gain are achieved once absorbed energy intakes reach 100–110 per cent of requirements[87]. For patients with normal growth and good control of fat malabsorption, total daily energy requirements should be equivalent to the normal dietary reference values (DRV) for age and sex[81]. In those patients who are failing to grow adequately and who may also have deteriorating lung function, energy require-

ments can be calculated using formulae based on their BMR, level of activity and coefficients of fat absorption[81].

For ease in clinical practice, some workers have suggested using a simple formula for calculating energy requirements in patients who are failing to thrive[87]. This involves calculating 120–150 per cent of the normal energy requirements for age and sex[88,89]. As many patients will have differing levels of fat malabsorption and degree of lung disease, it would seem more prudent to use a method of assessment which accurately reflects the individual. Indirect calorimetry gives an accurate assessment of basal energy requirements but is costly and time consuming in everyday clinical practice.

In practice, dietitians calculate patients' energy requirements based on a knowledge of the dietary history and an estimation of 120–150 per cent of that recommended for age and sex.

It should be noted that some medical treatments are known to affect energy requirements. Intravenous antibiotic therapy can reduce energy expenditure in CF[90,90a], and use of inhaled bronchodilators can result in increased REE of about 10 per cent over a 3-hour period[91].

An assessment of current dietary energy intake should be made by the dietitian on diagnosis or at referral. Appropriate advice should be given to achieve an increased intake if the patient is below 90 per cent predicted weight for height or if there has been recent weight loss. The main indicators of an adequate energy intake are weight gain and growth in children and the maintenance of at least 90 per cent weight for height in adults[81].

The dietary energy goal should be practical and achievable for each patient. This is more important than an accurate calculation of individual needs, which is often impossible due to the many variable factors[92]. Realistically, if weight gain or growth is poor for an individual patient then a 20–30 per cent increase in their own usual energy intake should be aimed for initially and then reviewed regularly to monitor improvement in nutritional status[93].

Protein

There are no definitive recommendations for dietary protein requirements. However, total body protein synthesis and metabolism in CF has been investigated[94]. This study showed protein synthesis to be markedly decreased in those with acute infection while protein catabolism was increased in those with chronic but stable pulmonary infection. There are also losses of malabsorbed protein in the stool in CF. A diet that is high in protein as well as energy is therefore appropriate[95]. It has been suggested that protein intakes should be as high as 200 per cent of the requirement[96]. In practice the majority of the patients with CF have little difficulty in achieving this level of intake, therefore specific advice and supplementation are not required.

Fat

Historically, a low-fat diet was recommended up until the late 1970s to help alleviate the amount of steatorrhea in CF stools. However, in 1979 results from the Toronto clinic[57] showed near normal growth on a normal fat diet, and in 1983 Pencharz stated that there was no evidence to support the continued use of low-fat diets in CF[97]. Following this, fat was actively encouraged with the aim of achieving at least 35 per cent of dietary energy derived from fat[85]. This radical change in diet therapy has been a major contributor to the improved nutritional status of CF patients today.

It has taken many years for some patients, especially the older ones, to adapt to a higher fat diet. This is due to both food preferences and to anxiety about tolerating higher fat intakes without abdominal discomfort. Compliance with pancreatic enzyme therapy and appropriate adjustment of dosage is important in order to tolerate the increased fat intakes. The increased efficacy of the enteric coated microspheres has greatly improved tolerance of long-chain tryglyceride (LCT) within the diet. Therefore the use of medium-chain triglyceride (MCT) as an additional source of energy is no longer necessary. However, it may still be used as a source of fat in supplementary enteral feeds.

Low plasma levels of essential fatty acids (EFAs) have been reported in CF patients[98] who have pancreatic insufficiency. This could be due to EFA being lost as unabsorbed fat or related to a specific defect in fatty acid metabolism. Although oral or intravenous supplements of EFAs will correct the low plasma and cell membrane levels, there is little evidence of clinical benefit, therefore supplementation is not currently routine practice[85,96,99,100,100a,100b].

Vitamins and minerals

Most centers in the UK advise that pancreatic insufficient (PI) patients take routine fat-soluble vitamin supplementation, as clinical deficiencies have been seen in these patients[100]. Absorption of water-soluble vitamins is thought to be normal in CF and clinical deficiencies of vitamin B complex, vitamin C and folate have not been recorded. However as the CF diet can often be suboptimal, some centers advise a multivitamin preparation as a source of both fat- and water-soluble vitamins. Vitamin B$_{12}$ supplementation may be necessary, however, in those patients who have undergone ileal resection and show biochemical evidence of pernicious anemia[101].

Due to fat malabsorption, low serum levels of vitamins E, A and D are more common in PI patients[102], but deficiency of vitamins A and E have been found to be independent of pancreatic function[102a]. Some centers

therefore screen both PI and pancreatic sufficient (PS) patients. Clinical vitamin E deficiency, including neurological abnormalities, has been recorded. Most patients with PI are prescribed oral supplementation daily, (e.g. 25–250 mg vitamin E for children and adolescents and 100–400 mg for adult patients), although some centers monitor serum vitamin E levels and titrate the dosage of supplements accordingly[81]. However, there is some question as to whether serum levels of the fat-soluble vitamins are a true indicator of vitamin status. Further studies are needed to assess the vitamin status and requirements of patients both with and without symptomatic steatorrhea.

Vitamins A and D are given either daily within a multivitamin BPC preparation or as vitamin A and D capsules at twice the normal recommended dosage for age. However, we must be aware of the risk of hypervitaminosis[103,104]. This has been reported in an infant following excessive supplementation and also in an adult supplemented with 10 000 IU retinol palmitate[93]. Therefore there is a need for further investigation of vitamin A requirements and consequently supplementation in CF. A large intake of vitamin A is of particular concern during pregnancy in a CF patient as it is with the normal population, due to the risk of birth defects from vitamin toxicity. Serum vitamin D levels and bone densities have been found to be low in CF patients, putting them at risk of osteoporosis. Due to malabsorption, poor dietary vitamin D intake and little sun exposure in some countries, there is some suggestion that vitamin D supplements should be increased[104a].

If vitamin K supplementation is required, as judged by a prolonged prothrombin time and a tendency toward excessive bleeding[105], this can be given either orally, preferably in the water-miscible form (10 mg/day for adults), or by injection. There is also evidence of subclinical deficiencies of vitamin K[106]. To aid compliance, vitamin supplementation should be available in an easy-to-take form.

Trace element status is usually well maintained in CF[102]. Mineral supplements are not usually necessary; however, iron, zinc and selenium deficiencies have been described and iron supplements may occasionally be required[107,108]. Little research on dietary intake of these nutrients has been carried out.

Dietary fiber

The recommended energy-dense diet in CF is, by definition, low in dietary fiber. As fiber is an important factor in the etiology of constipation, it is plausible that some of the abdominal discomfort experienced by CF patients is due to faecal loading rather than malabsorption *per se*. Further research is needed to evaluate this. However, it seems prudent to ensure that patients should include dietary fiber and have an adequate fluid intake in their daily diet, while still achieving a high energy intake. In those patients who are unwell and find it difficult to meet their increased energy requirements, the inclusion of dietary fiber would not be a priority. Some workers have shown that children with CF had lower than average intakes of dietary fiber compared to non-CF age-matched controls[109]. They also compared the mean dietary fiber intakes in children with CF who were troubled with moderate or severe abdominal pain with those who had occasional but mild abdominal symptoms. This was shown to be significantly lower in these children with the more frequent and severe pain.

DIETARY MANAGEMENT

Feeding and behavioral problems

Dietary intervention in CF should not be considered by patients or their families to be a special diet and should not be in any way restrictive. Good eating patterns should be established during childhood and parents reassured that food refusal and dietary manipulation are normal toddler and childhood behavior. Although it is important to maintain an adequate nutritional intake, if this is overemphasized in early childhood, it may cause behavioral problems related to food intake later on in life. As with other chronic diseases, food fads, fussy eating and food manipulation can become a problem, children can refuse to take pancreatic enzymes and may spend hours at the table consuming very little food. This may result in the child consuming a very limited diet and 'filling up' on milk or juice. Mealtimes may then become very difficult. It may be appropriate in this situation to enlist the help of a clinical psychologist who can work with the dietitian and help the parents cope with and eventually overcome these problems.

General practical advice

Establishing a regular daily eating and enzyme pattern is important. Ideally, the overall increased energy and protein requirements should be taken as ordinary food, rather than relying on special dietary supplements. Many children and adults who are well nourished and have few chest infections can easily achieve their requirements with 'normal foods' when given some practical dietetic advice. Patients and carers should be given information on how to increase the energy density of meals and which high-calorie snacks and drinks (milkshakes, nuts, crisps, full-fat yoghurts) they should select in order to transform a normal diet into a high-energy one.

All dietary advice should be practical, achievable, economical and suited to the individual's lifestyle. Adolescent and young adult patients, who are learning to be independent and may be living away from home for the first time, are at risk of potential nutritional problems. They are often living alone, existing on a student loan or low income and find the increased quantities of food required costly. In addition, they lack the facilities or the time to prepare and eat full meals and snacks. It is important that this group of patients receives practical advice on maintaining weight.

Infant feeding

Breast feeding for infants with CF is encouraged as long as they are thriving well. Breast milk has several advantages over modified formula milks, particularly for infants with CF. It is better absorbed then formula milk due to the relatively small size of fat particles, it provides protection against infection, both bacterial and viral, and also contains some lipase to aid digestion[106,110]. Both breast-feeding or feeding with a modified milk require pancreatic enzyme supplements to be given with each feed. If the mother is breast-feeding it is important to ensure that the infant does not retain any enzymes in his or her mouth during feeding, as these enzymes may cause soreness of the nipples or to the infant's mouth and gums. Determination of the exact dose is difficult. It is usually appropriate to begin with a quarter of a capsule or scoop given with fruit purée or 2000–4000 units of lipase/feed and to monitor stools, abdominal symptoms and weight gain. It is important to have regular contact with parents at this time to monitor the child's progress and provide reassurance.

If the baby is receiving a modified milk or is breast-feeding and is failing to thrive, the modified formula or expressed breast milk can be fortified either with a glucose polymer or a combined fat and carbohydrate supplement. It may also be appropriate to concentrate infant formula by adding an extra scoop of powder to improve the energy and protein content of the milk. If the fat content of the milk is increased by using a fat and glucose powder, then pancreatic enzyme supplements need to be increased correspondingly. This needs to be done under dietetic supervision. Weaning should be encouraged as for a normal child but with the possible addition of fat in the solid food if this is necessary.

NUTRITIONAL INTERVENTION

Dietary supplements

If optimal weight gain and growth in children, or maintenance of weight in adults, is not achieved with normal food and snacks and adequate pancreatic enzyme replacement, supplementation of the diet should be considered. This may be reserved for times of acute chest infection. Oral dietary supplements taken regularly may be recommended and should be given between or after meals so that appetite and normal dietary intake are not impaired. It is important that they supplement the diet and do not become a substitute for meals, as no nutritional benefit would then be gained. There have been few studies into the long-term effectiveness of nutritional supplements; however, one small study failed to show significant benefit of supplements to justify their routine use for extended periods[111]. In one study using a high-energy supplement, significant weight gain was achieved under dietetic supervision[111a]. Therefore care should be taken to use them only when absolutely necessary. It is worth noting that some patients may rely on nutritional supplements too heavily and consequently neglect 'normal' foods. The supplements often contain added vitamin and minerals, it is therefore necessary to monitor patients' intake of these drinks in order to check that they are not receiving an undesirable amount of these micronutrients from combined nutritional and vitamin supplements.

The use of dietary supplements varies widely between centers. There are a large number of commercial food supplements (Table 19.1); however, home-made milkshake-type drinks are often the first choice, if practicable. They are based on products that are readily available at home, may be cheaper and may also be higher in energy than many commercially available feeds, for example:

1. 1 pint (560 mL) full-cream milk
   2 oz (50 g) milk powder
   2 oz (50 g) glucose/glucose polymer
   Flavoring
   Contains: 851 kcal/3557 kJ

2. [quarter] pint (180 mL) full-cream milk
   2 oz (50 g) ice-cream
   1 oz (25 g) milk powder
   1 oz (25 g) glucose polymer/glucose
   Flavoring
   Contains: 522 kcal/2181 kJ

Further practical dietary advice and recipe ideas are available in booklets appropriate for both pediatric and adult patients from the UK Cystic Fibrosis Trust[112].

Some whole-protein milk-based sip feeds are available as powders to be reconstituted with milk up to a recommended maximum of 2 kcal(8.36kJ)/mL. The liquid ready-to-drink supplements contain between 1 kcal(4.18kJ)/mL and 1.5 kcal(6.27kJ)/mL, with the more energy-dense products being preferred. These are very convenient and palatable for some (but not all) patients to take to school or work. However, they are comparatively expensive and have a limited range of fla-

Table 19.1 *Oral dietary supplements*

Supplement	Examples	Energy content	Uses
Glucose polymer powders (100% carbohydrate)	Polycose, Polycal, Maxijul S.S, Caloreen	3.8 kcal(15.8kJ) per 10g	May be added to food and drinks to increase energy content
Liquid carbohydrate (various flavors)	Maxijul, Polycal, Hycal, Calsip	2.5 kcal(10.4kJ)/mL	Used less frequently, may be useful while patient is on clear fluids following MIE/DIOS
Milk-based drinks containing whole protein (various flavors)	Fresubin, Ensure plus, Fortisip, Entera, Fortifresh Clinutren 1.5	1 kcal(4.18kJ)/mL or 1.5 kcal(6.27kJ)/mL	Palatable, flavored drinks useful as a regular supplement to the diet. Aim to use at least 1.5 kcal/mL so that a smaller volume is required
Milk-based powder containing whole protein (various flavors)	Scandishake	2 kcal(8.36kJ)/mL reconstituted with full-fat milk	Palatable, high-energy milkshakes can be used to fortify food.
Fat emulsions (MCT and LCT based)	Liquigen, Calogen	4 kcal(16.7kJ)/mL 4.5 kcal(18.8kJ)/mL	50% fat : water Emulsions may be added to milk-based foods, drinks and enteral feeds
Fruit-juice-based drinks containing whole protein (various flavors) + fat free	Provide Extra, Fortijuice, Enlive	1.25 kcal(5.2kJ)/mL	Used for variety and for those who cannot take a milk-based supplement
Combined fat and glucose powder/liquids	Duocal, MCT Duocal,	4.9 kcal(20.5kJ)/mL	May be added to infant milk

These products were ACBS listed for the UK Jan. 2000

vors, which become monotonous if the same drink is taken every day for many years! More recently, fruit-juice-based nutritional supplements containing 1.25 kcal(5.2kJ)/mL have been used more in these patients and some have found them to be more palatable than the milk-based drinks.

Artificial methods of nutritional support

More invasive methods of nutritional intervention have been practiced successfully by many centers during the past decade. These more aggressive methods of intervention are appropriate for patients who are unable to maintain adequate nutritional status in spite of intensive dietary counseling, optimal pancreatic enzyme replacement therapy and oral dietary supplementation. Various routes have been evaluated, including nasogastric, gastrostomy, jejunostomy and intravenous (Fig. 19.12).

PARENTERAL FEEDING

Several studies have shown a clinical improvement in nutritional status with supplementary parental feeding[113,114,115]. Shepherd *et al.* administered parenteral nutrition to CF patients, providing 90–100 per cent of the recommended allowance and permitted oral food intake *ad libitum*, so that patients received a total nutritional intake of over 130 per cent of their recommended for a period of 3 weeks. Improvements in weight gain and respiratory function were demonstrated after 6 months. Patient numbers were small in this study and similar results have not been demonstrated in other studies.

The cost, risk of metabolic complications and technical complexity of administering parenteral nutrition, especially at home, mean that this is not a routine therapy for CF patients. However, there may be incidences when parenteral nutrition may be the only option. For example, in the acute hospitalized situation, when enteral feeding is inappropriate or physically difficult, parenteral feeding can be effective in the short term (e.g. acute nasally ventilated patients, hyperemesis in preg-

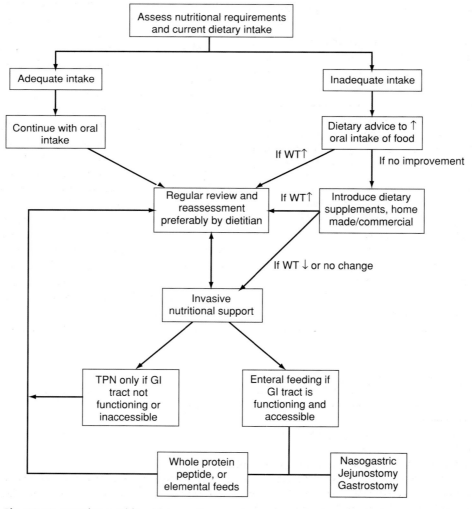

Fig. 19.12 *Assessing nutritional intervention.*

nancy, abdominal ileus). This method of supplementary feeding must be monitored carefully by trained staff to prevent metabolic complications.

ENTERAL FEEDING

Enteral feeding is generally the method of choice for supplementary feeding. It has been associated with improvements in body fat, height, lean body mass, increase in total body nitrogen and improved muscle strength[116]. Some workers have reported improvements in lung function[117]. Most enteral regimes usually involve administering feeds nocturnally over 8–10 hours to allow the patients to eat and drink normally during the day. Several studies have shown weight gain and an improvement in nutritional status with nasogastric[118,119], gastrostomy[117] and jejunostomy[120,121] feeding. The nasogastric or gastrostomy route is used most commonly in the UK.

When considering patients for enteral feeding, ideally they should already have received maximal dietary advice, and be making every effort to take an adequate intake orally. Patients should consent to supplementary feeding prior to introducing it. In our experience those patients who are motivated and eat fairly well but are not achieving their requirements are more likely to benefit from enteral feeding. The advantages and disadvantages of both the nasogastric and gastrostomy feeding should be discussed well in advance. The most appropriate route can then be chosen for the inidividual. Both these routes have been used successfully throughout the UK. Gastroesophageal reflux (GOR) and abdominal bloating are problems experienced by patients during enteral feeding. It is therefore important to be aware of these problems and treat if appropriate, with metoclopramide and cisapride.

Nasogastric

A fine-bore nasogastric tube is generally used in the UK, as these are made of soft, flexible material and narrow enough not to cause nasal irritation (e.g. 6 FR in children or 8 FR in adults). Patients are taught to pass the tube themselves each night and remove it in the morning before their first session of physiotherapy, to prevent it being dislodged by coughing. Prior to commencing the feed, the tube's position should always be checked. The effectiveness of nasogastric feeding is variable between CF centers and also between individual CF patients. It has been found to be particularly successful for short-term feeding during an acute illness or following recent weight loss, although some patients have used this successfully long term at home. However, some individual patients, often in the adult population, have found that they are unable to tolerate the nasogastric tube. This can be due to the presence of nasal polyps or to interruptions to feeding by frequent dislodgement of the tube following bouts of coughing. Patients receiving regular NIPPV have also found this difficult to tolerate, due to the nasogastric tube breaking the seal of the ventilator mask, therefore making ventilation ineffective.

Gastrostomy

Percutaneous endoscopic gastrostomy (PEG) is increasingly the route of choice in many centers. It is the preferred route as it does not require nightly insertion and is not at risk of being dislodged during coughing, and is an acceptable method of long-term feeding, even in patients with severe lung disease. However, some patients feel that for cosmetic and psychological reasons they do not want a permanent feeding tube *in situ*. These factors must be considered when assessing patients for supplementary feeding.

Following PEG insertion, (usually under local anaesthetic with appropriate sedation for adult patients and general anesthetic for the children) feeding can be commenced within 12 hours, depending on local policy (Table 19.2). Feeding regimes should be adapted to suit individual requirements and tolerance. Keeping the rate of feed administration down to 50–75 mL/hour will help prevent abdominal distension. Low rates may be advisable for the week following insertion until any abdominal discomfort has settled. Gastric motility stimulants may help if distension persists.

Once the feeding regime has been established, this regime can generally be followed during episodes of acute infection and may even be increased if oral intake diminishes during these times. It may also be appropriate to administer bolus daytime feeds and medication via the PEG, especially if other treatments interfere with the normal regime.

Following the insertion of a gastrostomy tube, the

Table 19.2 *Example of feeding regime following insertion of PEG*

1. 2 hours rest, i.e. nil by mouth and nothing administered via gastrostomy
2. 6 hours sterile water, 50mL/hour
3. Commence feed of 0.5 kcal(2.09kJ)/mL until 8.00a.m.
4. Flush tube with 20mL sterile water
5. Recommence nocturnal feed at 50mL/hour, 1 kcal(4.18kJ)/mL
6. If tolerated, increase volume and strength of feed, alternate nights until final volume and strength are achieved
7. The gastrostomy tube should be flushed before and after every feed with 20mL water, using a 50mL syringe (a 50mL syringe is required to prevent excess pressure at the distal end of the tube)

patients will require intensive follow-up when they are first discharged home in order to discuss any practical or physical problems that may occur. This helps them gain confidence in managing the tube. The time spent educating patients on self-management prior to discharge will ensure that supplementary feeding is successful.

What type of feed?

Many commercial feeds are now available for enteral feeding (Table 19.3) The most appropriate feed for each patient should be chosen on an individual basis.

Whole-protein feeds

These have the advantage of being convenient as they are 'ready to feed'. A 1.5 kcal(6.27kJ)/mL preparation is preferred as this is more energy dense and will provide 1500 kcal(6270 kJ) in a liter. The administration of the feed may be complicated by the difficulty of achieving optimal pancreatic enzyme replacement therapy (PERT), particularly by adult patients, and for those requiring high doses with their food, as the overall daily intake needs to be considered to prevent exceeding the maximum recommendation. Enzyme capsules should ideally be spread throughout the feed but this is obviously not practical with a nocturnal feed. They therefore tend to be given in two doses, one at the beginning and one at the end of the feed. Many patients tolerate this extremely well, although it may lead to some malabsorption of the feed. It may be that those patients with less severe pancreatic and lung disease do better with whole-protein feeds than very sick patients with added complications. Further studies are needed to assess the absorption of the different feeds with pancreatic enzymes.

Peptide-based feeds

These are available as either liquid or powder preparations. Some contain a high proportion of fat as medium-chain triglycerides (MCT). They have a lower osmolality than elemental feeds and may require fewer pancreatic enzyme supplements than whole-protein feeds.

However, the dosage of pancreatic enzymes will vary depending on the percentage of MCT and LCT fat within the feed. Patients' requirements for enzymes with these feeds should be assessed and monitored.

Elemental feeds

These are usually available as nutritionally complete powdered feeds based on amino acids, glucose and a high proportion of MCT fat. Previously perceived as being low in fat, the newer elemental formulations have as comparable a fat content as standard, whole-protein feeds, but the disadvantage is that these have to be reconstituted. The powder is mixed with sterile water (cooled, boiled water for patients at home) and the concentration is increased according to patient tolerance. Despite the high osmolality, some patients can tolerate concentrations of up to 2 kcal(8.36kJ)/mL (providing 2000 kcal (8360 kJ) in 1 liter). Due to the high osmolality of this feed, the strength should be increased gradually over 1–2 weeks and the patients should be monitored regularly. Concentrations of 2.2–2.5 kcal(9.2–10.5kJ)/mL have been achieved and well tolerated. With the advantage of providing a high-energy feed of low volume, these are ideal for patients with advanced disease, abdominal bloating, GOR or short bowel syndrome[121a].

Although some studies have shown that pancreatic enzyme supplements are still required for MCT-containing and elemental feeds[65,122], in practice we have found that the majority of patients can improve their nutritional status using supplements of an elemental feed (with 83 per cent of fat as MCT) without the use of enzymes. The early studies assessing the absorption of elemental feeds suggest that the absorption of MCT is improved with pancreatic enzymes. Care must be taken in interpreting these results as the elemental feeds differ in their composition, particularly in the concentration of MCT, and it has yet to be shown that the absorption of those with more than 80 per cent of fat as MCT is improved with concurrent use of pancreatic enzyme therapy. In one study the absorption of fat from a semi-

Table 19.3 *Commercial feeds widely used for nocturnal feeding in the UK*

Feed type	Example	Form	Pancreatic enzyme requirement
Whole-protein feed	Nutrison Energy Nutrison Paediatric Energy Plus, Ensure Plus, Entera, Clinifeed 1.5	Liquid feeds (ready to feed) 1.5 kcal(6.27kJ)/mL	Require pancreatic enzymes
Semi-elemental (peptide-based feed)	Perative, Nutrison Pepti, Survimed OPD, MCT Pepdite 2+, Peptamen, Pepdite 2+ Nutrison MCT	Liquid or powdered preparations	May require a smaller dose of enzymes than whole-protein feed
Elemental feed (amino acid based); some high in MCT fat	Emsogen, Elemental 028, Elemental 028 Extra	Powdered modular feeds	Symptomatically do not appear to require enzymes but no evidence to support this
Pediatric whole protein	Paediasure, Nutrini, Nutrini extra	Liquid feeds 1–1.5 kcal(4.18–6.27kJ)/mL	

elemental feed without using enzymes and a standard feed with enzymes, was compared. There was little difference in the coefficient of fat absorption between the two feeds and malabsorption of MCT fat in the semi-elemental feed contributed minimally to fat malabsorption[122a]. Whether the feed used is elemental or semi-elemental is also likely to be an important factor in deciding whether or not patients require pancreatic enzymes. Until research can demonstrate a feed that is effectively absorbed in patients with CF, without the use of enzymes, CF centers will continue to use a feed that is most acceptable to the individual patient.

The use of high fat feeds in CF has also created some debate. Kane et al.[123] compared the effects of low-, medium- and high-carbohydrate formula feeds in CF patients and found that an increased respiratory quotient was produced with high-carbohydrate feeds. They also examined whether the increase in V_{CO_2} and ventilatory demands by high-carbohydrate feeds could be detrimental to patients with moderate to severe lung disease. They concluded that despite the highest increase in V_{CO_2} after a high-carbohydrate formula the patients, who were clinically stable, were able to increase their minute volume sufficiently to prevent worse hypoxia or CO_2 retention. Despite this, there yet remains insufficient evidence to justify the use of high-fat feeds as it may be difficult to ascertain true alterations in V_{CO_2} when these feeds are used as a supplement to a mixed diet. Further research is needed in this area.

SPECIFIC DIETARY COMPLICATIONS

CF-related diabetes mellitus (CFRD)

The incidence of diabetes mellitus in CF is thought to be between 8 and 15 per cent, depending on the diagnostic criteria used and the age of groups studied. As patients live longer, more of the older CF population will develop diabetes. The occurrence of CF-related diabetes mellitus (CFRD) has been associated with deterioration in clinical and nutritional status prior to diagnosis[124] and has been shown to occur in children above 10 years of age. There may be impaired glucose tolerance in as many as 40 per cent of patients[125]; an increasing problem with adolescent and adult patients. A survey of a clinic in Copenhagen indicated that as many as 5 per cent of the patients over the age of 15 years develop impaired glucose tolerance or CFRD each year. A survey of the adult clinic population at Royal Brompton Hospital showed a prevalence of 14.5 per cent in March 1996. The patients presented at a median age of 21 years by a variety of diagnostic methods (B. Yung et al., personal communication). Members of the CF team should be aware of those patients who may be at risk of developing CFRD; this is important for the prompt and effective control of this increasing complication.

The dietary management of CFRD varies from that of non-CF-related diabetes[125,126,126a]. It involves achieving a high energy intake without compromising diabetic control: the emphasis being on maintaining or improving the patient's nutritional status.

The British Diabetic Associations 1991 guidelines[127] on the management of diabetes mellitus recommended a low-fat diet (<30 per cent total energy) and one high in unrefined carbohydrates. This low-energy diet could be highly detrimental to someone with CFRD (Table 19.4)[128]. Instead, the dietary intake of a patient with CFRD should be assessed and modifications made to the timing and distribution of carbohydrate eaten throughout the day. Fat in the diet is actively encouraged in order to maintain a high-energy intake (aim for 40 per cent energy from fat). As CF patients tend to have high intakes of refined sugars, so advice is given to moderate these and it is suggested that these are taken in conjunction with other foods or after meals and to avoid binges that could cause rapid surges in blood glucose levels.

Table 19.4 *Comparison of dietary guidelines in diabetes mellitus, cystic fibrosis and CFRD*

	DM	CF	CFRD
Energy	100% normal if not overweight aim BMI 19–24 kg/m²	120–150% of normal requirement for age and sex	120–150% normal requirement for sex and age
Fat	<30% Energy	30–40% energy	At least 35% energy
Sugar	Restriction to <25 g/day	Allowed FREELY to increase energy	Allow in conjunction with meals, e.g. puddings, milkshakes with a meal
Salt	Low intake	Increased intake	Increased intake
Fiber/starchy carbohydrate	High-fiber intake recommended, regular complex carbohydrate	No recommendation currently	Carbohydrate advised at each meal and between meals; no specific advice on fiber
Snacks	Scheduled meal plan	Snacks encouraged, both sweet and savory in order to achieve high energy intake	Regular savory snacks encouraged, e.g. cheese sandwiches, crisps, milk, nuts, fruit

Some dietary supplements taken regularly by the patients may need to be changed to those with a lower sugar concentration.

Dietary advice is very much individualized, and diabetic control gained by making adjustments to the insulin dosage or other medication rather than restrictions made to the diet. Achieving diabetic control using dietary means alone is not recommended and may compromise the patient's nutritional status.

For the successful management of CFRD, a flexible yet simplified approach to the use of oral hypoglycemic agents and insulin should be adopted, in conjunction with the expertise of a dietitian specializing in cystic fibrosis(Table 19.5). All members of the CF team should be aware of how important the treatment of diabetes is, and that the dietary advice is unique to the patient with CFRD. Prompt management following diagnosis is emphasized. Patients are taught to monitor blood sugar levels as necessary. They should be aware of how to manage hypoglycemic episodes and to maintain blood sugar levels during exercise and illness.

Pregnancy and lactation

For women with CF who are considering pregnancy, optimizing their nutritional status is extremely important, as maternal nutritional status is a major factor influencing the success of a pregnancy. A low preconceptual weight is a risk factor for poor pregnancy outcome[128a]. Due to the increase in tissue mass and in metabolic activity during pregnancy, dietary energy requirements are raised. Although the increase in estimated average requirement (EAR) for pregnancy in the UK is given as 0.8 MJ/day (200 kcal/day) during the last trimester, this is raised in women who are underweight at the beginning of pregnancy[129]. The combination of the increased energy needs of a moderately well CF woman (of perhaps 110–120 per cent of normal) and the increased requirements for pregnancy in the third trimester, can often create a nutritional problem[129]. Achieving nutritional requirements can be even more challenging if the patient is suffering with nausea and deteriorating lung function. Education to improve nutritional intake during the first and second trimesters is important as during the third trimester these patients may also be more breathless. At this time, the use of energy-dense foods, snacks and supplements can be useful.

General nutritional advice must also be given to women with CF who are considering pregnancy. Folic acid supplementation (400 mg/day) is routinely recommended for all women, both preconceptually and for the first 12 weeks of pregnancy[130]. Information on safe foods and the avoidance of listeriosis, salmonellosis and toxoplasmosis is also appropriate.

Further research is needed concerning supplementation with vitamin A in CF pregnant women. For pregnant women in the general population it is recommended that vitamin A supplements and foods containing high levels of vitamin A should be avoided[131]. Most CF centers currently continue to use vitamin A supplements for women with CF; however, dietary intake and vitamin status should be monitored regularly throughout pregnancy.

Initial reports suggested that the breast milk of a mother with CF was high in sodium and therefore breast feeding was contraindicated[132]. However, more recent studies have concluded that there was no evidence of raised sodium concentrations within breast milk, and that the other constituents were also within the normal range[133,134]. If mothers with CF do wish to breast feed, it is important to ensure that their nutritional status is carefully monitored and support given to help them maintain an adequate dietary intake during this period of high nutritional requirements.

Celiac disease

The incidence of celiac disease in CF is thought to be 1 : 220[135], which is above that expected in the general population. However, there is no conclusive evidence for an abnormal link between CF and celiac disease. For the small group of CF patients with celiac disease, practical advice, combining a gluten-free and high-energy diet is recommended. Gluten-free bread, biscuits and cakes for snacks should be consumed.

Distal intestinal obstruction syndrome (DIOS)/Meconium ileus equivalent (MIE)

Following an episode of distal intestinal obstruction syndrome (DIOS)/meconium ileus equivalent (MIE), the patient's dietary intake and PERT should be reviewed.

Table 19.5 *General dietary advice in CFRD*

- Eat regularly 3 meals and 3 snacks each day
- Sugar should be taken in moderate amounts spread out during the day, generally as part of or immediately after a meal
- Avoid glucose polymers and drinks containing high levels of glucose
- Try to maintain a high fat dietary intake
- Continue with usual nutritional supplements – unless they are causing sharp rises in blood glucose
- Adjust timing and dosage of insulin or oral hypoglycemic agent rather than impose dietary restrictions to achieve good control of blood sugars

This is generally done by the dietitian asking the patient to complete a 3-day diet and enzyme diary. This is then used to assess whether he or she is taking an appropriate distribution of enzymes, particularly with snacks and milk-based drinks, and to assess whether the diet includes an adequate fiber and fluid intake.

CONCLUSION

The dietary management of CF patients is often more complex than might be supposed. Regular contact with a dietitian who can offer simple, practical dietary advice will help to prevent a decline in nutritional status and may have the added advantage of improving quality of life and possibly prognosis for some patients. However, overemphasis of the importance of nutrition to the younger patients and their parents should be avoided. In addition, supervised nutritional support, either oral, enteral or parenteral, should be actively offered to patients with severe lung disease who are struggling to achieve their individual dietary requirements.

Nursing

F. DUNCAN-SKINGLE AND F. FOSTER

INTRODUCTION

The important nursing issues that will be discussed in this chapter include supporting the family and patient from diagnosis to the terminal stage of the disease; the counseling and educational needs of the family, child and adult; examining the implications of the patient's nursing needs during admissions to hospital, outpatient visits and in the community. The problems of late diagnosis, relationships, fertility and pregnancy will also be addressed, together with issues of deteriorating health, the implications of a possible transplantation, terminal care, and bereavement care. The effects of all this on the nurse who provides care will be examined.

Caring for the patient with CF can be challenging and gratifying for the nurse. As part of the healthcare team nurses can do a considerable amount to help parents and patients to overcome their many problems. It is often the alert health visitor or practice nurse who may lead the way to diagnosis. As the course of the disease may be protracted and uncertain, it is often the nurses who provide the mainstay of support, education and counseling over the years. This should help the patient and relatives to live life to the full within any limitations they may have.

It is especially useful for the nurse to make early contact with each family member who is going to play a caring role and to make it clear that she is available to answer questions and listen to their fears and problems[136]. By helping families cope with life stress, the health of the child maybe indirectly improved [137].

The diagnosis may be made at birth following meconium ileus (10 per cent), or by routine neonatal screening. This is only available in some regions at present. Diagnosis may be delayed for months or years due to the insidious progress of the disorder. If there has been long-term anxiety about their child's health due to delayed diagnosis, the parents often experience a degree of relief to have a diagnosis and plan for treatment[136]. They may also feel gratification that their instincts had been correct and not imagined.

After the initial diagnosis has been made it is important that parents are given the basic facts about the disease, and nursing care must be aimed at establishing the confidence and trust of parents. The families will have many questions and they will need time to appraise the situation and mobilize coping resources. It is important that good rapport with the healthcare team is established in order to ensure that the parents learn adequately how to treat their children and to help minimize the problems they will face in the long term. It should be remembered that children with chronic conditions such as CF and their parents require lifelong ongoing education and support[138].

IMPACT OF CF ON THE FAMILY FOLLOWING DIAGNOSIS

The diagnosis of CF may have a devastating impact on all family members. Potentially there can be many difficulties for the family. The parents often feel bereaved, with changing expectations for their family unit. They will grieve for their child's future, experience guilt, denial and anger, but hopefully they will move on to acceptance, although this may never be achieved. The hope for further children will be a cause for concern. Future pregnancies should be discussed, ensuring that the couple understand the risks of having another child with CF and also ensuring that they are aware of improved life expectancy and improved treatment regimes. However, it should be remembered that to tell parents 'your child could live until 30 years of age' is not such a good deal. Genetic counseling should always be available.

The parents may become depressed and feel overburdened with responsibility. They may come to terms with the situation at different stages. This places further burden on the parent who has come to terms with the situation, who may feel that he or she has two sick children to cope with: their partner and their child[136]. Where parents are not traveling together through adaptation, the family unit may be severely disrupted.

The diagnosis of CF has reverberations throughout the extended family. Grandparents may feel guilty and there may be recriminations from both sides of the family with the familiar cry of 'it's never been in our family'. Parents and siblings will require counseling regarding the effects that a diagnosis of CF may have on them. Are they carriers? Should other family members be tested?

Healthy siblings of the affected child will have their own worries and fears. They will, if old enough, be sympathetic with their parents and brother/sister, but at the same time may feel confused or angry and resent any loss of attention they feel they ought to receive. Siblings should be included in decision making if appropriate, especially if there is a CF brother or sister who is reaching the final stage of the disease. They also need support and information as they may feel guilty over past behavior and feelings toward their CF brother/sister. It is important for the nurse to realize and try to understand the family dynamics so that he/she can help promote, maintain and restore family health. Interactions between the family members and society should be as normal as possible.

COPING WITH TREATMENT

The investment of time and energy in keeping a child with CF as well as possible is considerable. Children are often not cooperative, they get bored and, when very young, will not understand the need for treatment regimes, they may feel they are being punished and isolated. The nurse can be helpful in offering advice and suggesting techniques on how to deal with this situation, e.g. physiotherapy can be done while listening to music. Sometimes there is maternal denial of the seriousness of the diagnosis and this may mean that home physiotherapy may be sparse. In contrast, other mothers may enforce strict treatment regimes rigidly, which can lead to poor compliance in older children. The need for flexibility within treatment regimes is imperative. Parents need to be reassured that missing one treatment is not going to harm their child. If possible, treatment should be fun and only a part of life, and it should be kept in perspective. There is also potential for conflict between partners about tasks; fathers may lose interest in their families and become marginalized, resulting in the mother becoming even more burdened, and this may lead to marital breakdown[139].

It should be part of the nurse's role to help the fam-

ily recognize the problems that may arise. Parents should be encouraged to share the load and have other family members (e.g. aunts, uncles, grandparents, siblings) conversant with treatment, especially physiotherapy, so there will be willing helpers to allow time to be allocated for each individual's needs and wishes. The needs of the CF child should not necessarily supersede the needs of the other family members. However, it may be hard for the family to recognize this and adjust accordingly. It may be easy to place the CF child in a privileged position, thus creating tensions and jealousy among family members.

SCHOOL

It is essential that going to school is encouraged and that schools and teachers are aware and knowledgeable about the child's health. However, it may be during adolescence that going to school becomes more difficult, at a time when school attendance is very important. Frequent hospital attendance may mean that ground is lost and adolescents will be reluctant to join a more junior year, opting out rather than attending school. Nurses can encourage people on both sides of the educational fence to find the best solution to the problem. The nurse should also be able to support the staff at the school, provide education about CF and help to find solutions to problems (e.g. an area to perform physiotherapy, administration of intravenous antibiotics and allowing pupils to carry pancreatic enzymes).

Encouraging achievement at school is essential, for with good care someone with CF should be able to pursue further education and compete in the job market with everyone else. Financial independence is just as important for someone with CF as it is for any other teenager.

ADOLESCENCE

The normal process of adolescence involves achieving more mature relationships with peers of both sexes, coming to terms with their sexuality, gaining emotional independence from their parents, accepting a changing physique, preparing for a career and hopefully financial independence. Illness and physical disability are not a part of normal adolescent life. It can also be an extremely taxing time for any family, but may become more so for a family where there is a child with CF. Having a chronic disease heightens the difference between peer groups at a time when being one of the herd is of paramount importance.

This is often the time when young people with CF exert their independence and rebel against treatment; they may become noncompliant and may well use their disease as the ultimate weapon against their parents. Some adolescents will seek more information about their disease so that they can rationally build up coping methods which may involve, to a greater or lesser degree, denial of their disease. Others wish to have no further information and totally deny the existence of CF, not even mentioning it to friends[140].

Obviously, every family will have different experiences during this time, some parents will find it extremely difficult to allow sick children the freedom they need to grow and mature. Parents often feel that they have 'control' over the disease during childhood, but once the child begins to exert authority the parents, and especially the mother, may feel left out and fearful that all their good work in keeping the child well will be to no avail. It is essential during this difficult time that the nurse reassures the families that all will be well and encourages the parents to let go and tells them that this sort of behavior is normal for teenagers. Indeed, it may at times be difficult for some families to discern between normal adolescent behavior and problems that have arisen purely from CF. It should be remembered that adolescents with CF will have their fair share of the normal adolescent fears and prejudices.

Responsibility for care should be beginning to be transferred from the parent to the child, as soon as the adolescent is seen to be capable of taking care of him- or herself, and has the maturity to understand what is expected of him or her. A few adolescents will not wish to fulfil this role and will indeed never gain full independence from their parents; although this is not necessarily a healthy attitude, it may have to be accepted as the norm for that family. Every family tackles these situations at a different pace.

Sometimes the fact that the adolescent sees that someone other than their parents trusts them is enough to encourage them to take responsibility for themselves. During this time continuing support, education and reassurance are essential. The nurse's role is as an adviser, being nonjudgemental and empathetic to all the family's needs.

The teenage years may coincidentally be a time when CF becomes a larger issue in the patient's life. Increasing age may mean increasing symptoms and hospital admissions. During admissions patients may notice that there are people who are better or worse than they are. As the patient progresses through adulthood, complications of CF may arise and at times difficult issues may have to be faced.

TRANSITION TO THE ADULT SETTING

There will come a time when a transition has to be made between the pediatric services and the adult facilities. Ideally this should happen at approximately 16 years, but

may occur earlier if the child feels mature enough to cope with the move, but should not be left any later than 18 years or regression may occur. The transition should always be a planned process. It will always be a difficult time, not least for the family but also for the pediatrician. Patients and family are keenly aware of the ultimate nature of the disease and may feel depressed by the thought of moving to an adult clinic as it may bring the concept of death closer.

Parents and their child with CF tend to feel secure with the pediatrician whom they have known for many years. However, if transition is viewed as a natural progression, prepared for adequately and seen as a continuation of care rather than a break, it should be regarded as a positive milestone towards maturity and independence for the patient.

In the pediatric setting the nurse should encourage the older patient to have a private consultation with their doctor, before inviting the parents to come in, so positively encouraging independence and promoting responsibility.

Parents need to be reassured that they will not be thrust out into the wilderness of the waiting room when their son or daughter visits the adult physician and made to feel superfluous. They will still have an active supporting role to play but may have to stand back and allow their child to take control of his or her own life, develop maturity and accept managing the treatment of his or her disease.

LATE DIAGNOSIS

It should be remembered that although the majority of people with CF are diagnosed in childhood, some will be diagnosed in adult life. They may have suffered minor symptoms that have been dismissed or not seen as a whole. They may have been referred via ENT consultations for sinus disease or nasal polyps and, in some cases, following infertility investigations. Before the diagnosis of CF is accepted, all clinical features and investigations should be considered carefully[141].

Confirmation of a diagnosis of CF in the older patient can be as devastating to them as it is to a parent of a child. It changes their perception of themselves, it may distort their body image, and diminish their feelings of self-worth. Diagnosis may make them fearful for the future and bring a sudden confrontation with their own mortality.

For men infertility can undermine their masculinity and heighten sexual anxiety. Careful counseling, empathy and understanding by the nurse involved is very important. Reassurance should be given that sexual peformance is unaffected, and intercourse can take place as normal.

OUTPATIENT CARE

Regular visits to the outpatient department become an important part of the life of the family with a CF child. It has been shown that children with CF should be seen at a regional center for some of their care, so the nurses and medical staff can adopt an objective view of their progress[142]. At the clinic the family will come into contact with a specialist nurse. The clinical nurse specialist (CNS) offers continuity of care, provides a key person for the family to relate to, should have a high level of interpersonal skill and be able to offer advice, provide a shoulder to cry on and a listening ear[143]. She or he will also be able to liaise with other paramedical staff while being an advocate for the family's needs. The CNS will be able to continue assessing the family's and child's knowledge of the disease, while helping them adapt to any clinical or treatment changes. The outpatient department should be a center for multifocused care involving all disciplines, so that close monitoring of the patient is maintained. If the child is well, a 2–3 monthly outpatient appointment may be the only contact the family has with the hospital, so it is important that the nurse in clinic ensures that maximum benefit is derived from the visit and that knowledge levels are monitored and maintained. It is essential that nurses remember that CF involves all the family and it is good practice to ask about the health and behavior of unaffected siblings and to offer advice as necessary and to encourage and congratulate parents on the care they are giving.

INPATIENT CARE

Hopefully with vigilant outpatient care and follow-up at a CF center, pediatric inpatient care should be kept to a minimum. However, there are inevitably times when admission is necessary. The first admission to hospital for treatment of a chest infection is always traumatic for all concerned. It intensifies normal parental anxiety and is always accompanied by fear that it is a serious problem. The family need much reassurance and knowledge at this time, so that they understand the reasons for and are happy with the need for admission.

Nurses need to remember the pressures that are brought to bear on the family when a child is admitted to hospital[144]. There may be other children at home to be looked after. Home may be some distance from the hospital. Both parents may have to work to contribute to the family purse. They may also feel guilty that they have failed their child in some way and thereby precipitated the admission.

It is important to ensure that the parents' investment of time and energy in their child is recognized and reassurance is given that they had done all they could and the admission was inevitable. From child's point of view, a pediatric ward is an alien, terrifying environment on a first admission. It is important that all aspects of their care are explained to them so as to gain their confidence. They will be fearful of pain and discomfort; the use of topical anesthetic creams (e.g. Emla®)[145] is useful to help dispel the fear of venepuncture. Obviously with small children venous access can be very difficult. The child may feel discomfort if he is kept still for long periods of time. Parents also feel guilty and upset about the distress their child is suffering. The child may feel restricted in lifestyle and mobility, so it is vital that a play therapist is introduced as early as possible in order to minimize trauma and aid the child's adjustment to the strange new environment.

The nurse's involvement plays a large part in helping families cope with this crisis in their lives. Some parents are willing to perform many of the nursing tasks in hospital and although they should be encouraged, the nurse should make sure that, first, she does not feel threatened by such actions and, second, that she is able to discern between what the parents are capable of and what they are not, and be able to take over when they no longer feel able to care for their child. Some families will abdicate from care while their child is in hospital and see it as a time when the burden of responsibility can be placed elsewhere. They may become immobilized by the whole situation and feel incapable of doing anything for their child except simple basic tasks. Nurses must not judge people's actions at this time; coping mechanisms are different for all individuals and we must bear in mind that most families cope with their children more than adequately for months and years on end with no problems at all. While in hospital it is an ideal time to reinforce education, and to check up and follow through any problems that may have arisen since the last visit.

Young adults being admitted to hospital for the first time will have all the fears that children have. Ideally they should be in a designated young people's area, preferably in single rooms to prevent cross-infection. There should be adequate recreation facilities, and nurses skilled in coping with the needs of young people. Many may be very afraid and aware of their mortality due to their knowledge of the disease, and some will have lost friends with CF.

While on the ward they will be given some responsibility for their own treatment, as more patients are now being taught how to cope with treatment methods that in the past would have been the nurses' responsibility (e.g. intravenous therapy). The CNS should be available for counseling, consultation and support. She will also participate in clinical procedures, especially in promoting new methods of management. She will be a familiar face both in the ward and outpatient clinic.

Some of the basic nursing care required by the CF patient and how it should be delivered is shown in Table 19.6.

Table 19.6 *Some of the basic nursing care required by the CF patient and its delivery*

Problems	Aims/actions	Outcome/action
Treatment of chest infections; ineffective airway clearance due to increased pulmonary secretions	Reduce symptoms caused by an infective exacerbation and help the patient to maintain a clear airway	• Encourage physiotherapy • Bronchodilators are given before physiotherapy if prescribed • Monitor mobility and breathlessness. If breathless, assist in positioning patient comfortably and encourage mobilization when able • Report changes in the amount, quality and color of sputum • Provide mouthwash if sputum is foul tasting, after nebulized antibiotics, after steroid inhalers • Encourage good posture and exercise if appropriate • Give prescribed nebulized therapy in the form of bronchodilators and/or nebulized antibiotics and/or DNase (see p. 381 for order of medication delivery) • Give oxygen therapy as prescribed by the doctor • Frequently assess the respiratory status, i.e. respiratory rate, pulmonary function tests, Sao_2
Effective and safe handling of intravenous therapy	Minimize the problems associated with intravenous therapy	• Administer antibiotics as prescribed. In young children and adolescents Emla® cream placed on proposed venepuncture site 1 hour prior to insertion of cannulae is advisable • Ensure cannulae or Huber needle, if implantable port used, is secure[146] • Check site regularly for signs of phlebitis • Follow correct procedure for i.v. drug administration • Check aminoglycoside levels and ensure correct dose is given, getting the prescribed dose changed if necessary • Observe for side-effects and report if any occur and/or stop infusion
	Promote self-administration of intravenous drugs	• Teach the patient how to reconstitute i.v. drugs and method of delivery • Teach safety aspects of care of line or port for handling and administering drugs and clean techniques for reducing infection risk • Understand action of drugs and what to observe for in possible side-effects • Assess competency of either patient and/or relative according to standards. All should be reassessed for each course of intravenous antibiotics • Advise on disposal of sharps • Provide with emergency contact telephone numbers • Provide details of home care services
Malabsorption of food and poor dietary intake	Ensure patients' calorie intake is sufficient for their energy expenditure and steatorrhea is adequately controlled	• Refer to dietitian • Monitor weekly weight • Monitor dietary input • Report any weight loss • Encourage high calorie snacks

Table 19.6 *contd.* *Some of the basic nursing care required by the CF patient and its delivery*

Problems	Aims/actions	Outcome/action
	Maintain a reasonable weight with methods that are acceptable to the patient	• Ensure pancreatic enzymes are taken with all meals and snacks (small babies may require a medium such as fruit purée to take their enzymes) • Monitor bowel actions to ensure that steatorrhea is well controlled • Ideally encourage the patient to eat little and often if very breathless • Ensure that referral to a dietician has been made • Weigh at regular intervals but not so regularly that it becomes an anxiety to the patient • Ensure patient is able to eat meal, e.g. positioned properly in bed or chair. May need assistance if very breathless • Encourage use of supplements if recommended by dietician
	Provide care if alternative feeding methods used	**Nasogastric feeding:** • Ensure tube is correctly positioned • Teach patient to repass own tube if appropriate • Check that feed is correct for patient • Monitor flow rates of feed so that the correct amount is delivered over the prescribed time, e.g. l liter over 12 h **Percutaneous endoscopic gastrostomy feeding tubes[147]:** • Observe site, redress daily with clean, dry dressing when newly formed stoma, until dry. After 2 weeks patient will be able to bathe fully and to swim. Attention should be paid to drying the stoma carefully otherwise soreness will occur • Teach patient how to care for stoma site • Observe patient for discomfort and bloating during and after administration of feed • Give prescribed antiemetic as necessary • Ensure correct amount is given over the period of time • Feeds should always be administered and controlled with a feeding pump **Total parenteral nutrition (TPN):** • Ensure scrupulous attention to intravenous site • Careful monitoring of vital signs in order to detect infection or reactions to TPN • Check intravenous drugs against the prescribed regimen

HOME CARE

In some areas, support for the patient and family at home may be available. This may be a special home-care nurse or team, or a specialist nurse from the hospital coming out into the community. These nurses can offer support and advice in the home setting, away from the often threatening atmosphere of the hospital. They can carry on the educative process begun in hospital, especially of families of newly diagnosed children, and provide support for families dealing with new equipment or treatment regimes, such as home intravenous therapy. They may be trained to take blood or change cannulae, lines or port needles and extend their role to care for patients with a gastrostomy or using home NIPPV. The nurse also provides a liaison with the family doctor, health visitors, schools, colleges or places of work in order to promote as normal a lifestyle as possible. It should be recognized that families are expected to provide full nursing care at home and much pressure is brought to bear on families to assume and absorb these extra burdens. Support at home is very important, but there may be times when hospital admission is preferable, and advisable for all concerned as it allows the family to have some pressure removed and gives the patient permission to be sick. The need for admission to hospital is not a failure on the relatives' part and should not be judged as such. Instead, we should positively praise them for the part their care has played in keeping the patient at home for so long.

RELATIONSHIPS

As with any young people, starting relationships with members of the opposite sex becomes increasingly more important as time progresses; this is no different for people with CF. However, many factors may influence whether a permanent lasting relationship may be achieved. Many patients yearn for someone who will care for them as a person and not as someone who has CF. Some experience rejection and pain along the way, and will often counter this by a reluctance to admit to having CF until a firm relationship is built. Some lack confidence and feel unattractive, pointing out their lack of stature, thinness and cough with sputum production as particularly unattractive features. Boys, in particular, may feel less than masculine, especially in view of their almost certain infertility. The nurse should have an awareness of the problems they are facing, be able to offer advice and time, on a one to one basis, to discuss these problems and possible solutions and give encouragement[148]. It has been found that there is no predictable relationship between sexual adaptation and severity of disease. With good support, sexual adaptation is normal[149]. However, there is some indication that a minority of adolescents and adults with CF will have fewer social relationships and form fewer intimate relationships outside the home than their peers[150].

Fear of involving others in their illness may deter some people with CF from trying to form relationships. Young people with CF may feel it is unfair to become involved with someone if they are going to die young and may also shy away from the emotional investment that such a relationship may involve. It is important that they are afforded the opportunity to bring their partner along for counseling, education and advice, so that informed discussion is opened up by both sides of the relationship. If a permanent relationship is formed, it is essential that issues such as pregnancy, infertility and early mortality are discussed.

FERTILITY AND PREGNANCY

It is vital that all males are aware that infertility occurs in about 96 per cent of men with CF. Ideally, they should be informed at an early age in a nonthreatening environment so that they grow up with the knowledge and awareness that not all men, even those without CF, can father children. If the subject is not discussed and the patient is suddenly confronted with this fact, it can be devastating. Some men may grieve acutely for the children they may never have. They may feel that there will be nothing left to mark their passing if they die young. Reassurance and understanding from nursing staff can help the patient come to terms with this situation. Advice about possible methods of 'fathering' children should be given (e.g. artificial insemination by donor sperm, fostering, adoption and techniques for harvesting sperm from the testes)[151].

Obviously, contraceptive advice should be available to both sexes, for although the male is unlikely to impregnate anyone, he should be aware of the concepts of safe sex. For the female, the best method of contraception is the pill, but other forms should be discussed[152].

If a couple wish to start a pregnancy, good counseling is essential so that they understand the risks involved. The unaffected partner should be offered carrier screening to ensure that accurate information regarding the risk to the child of inheriting CF can be assessed. The health of the girl with CF should be assessed and her capability of looking after a toddler. Also she should be informed of the risk to her own health. It is possible that an irreversible decline in lung function may occur[153]. The couple should be aware that the CF mother may not live long enough to see her child grow up. However, if the couple wish to proceed with pregnancy, the nurse should be nonjudgemental whatever her personal beliefs are, and the patient should be aware that support will be available whatever her decision. Opportunity should be afforded to discuss prenatal screening if desired or necessary.

DISEASE PROGRESSION

As the person with CF gets older, the likelihood of the occurrence of complications and medical intervention increases. The nursing activities required for specific complications are shown in Table 19.7.

DETERIORATING HEALTH

It is easy for nurses not to recognize deterioration in the health of a patient who they may see regularly and who always responds positively when asked how they are. It is vitally important that nurses observe beyond the initial

Table 19.7 *Nursing activities required for specific complications*

Problems	Aims	Actions
Poor venous access	Make venepuncture as untraumatic as possible and reduce damage to venous system	• Ensure that antibiotics are sufficiently diluted to reduce irritation in vein • Promptly remove cannulae if problems occur, to reduce risk of damage to vein • Advise patient of other methods of venous access, e.g. long intravenous line, Hickman line, totally implantable venous access system • Educate patient on how to use various venous access systems and their individual flushing regimes • Use of aids to extend the life of cannulae, e.g. GTN patches and steroids[154,155]
Hemoptysis	Help allay fears. Promote cessation of bleeding	• Reassurance • Encourage physiotherapy with supervision • Observe amount and type of hemoptysis • Report increase and frequency • If embolization of bronchial artery is necessary, frequent temperature, pulse, respiration, blood pressure, pedal pulses and leg color will need to be observed, as well as leg movements. Pressure maintained on access site and necessary analgesia given
Pneumothorax	Relieve breathlessness and promote healing of air leak	• Report sudden onset of breathlessness or chest pain. Be aware of implications • Care of patient with chest drain, observe drainage from chest drain. Report any change in drainage activity • Teach patient about chest drainage safety • Give necessary analgesia • Promote mobility if possible • If suction is required, ensure correct settings are maintained
Diabetes[156]	Control and monitor hyperglycemia	• Record blood glucose levels at regular intervals (maybe 2 hourly in the newly diagnosed diabetic) • Give insulin or oral hypoglycemic as per regime • Monitor symptoms of hyperglycemia, e.g. weight and weight loss, polyuria and polydipsia • Educate patient about diabetes, hypo- and hyperglycemic episodes and self-administration of insulin • Educate patient how to monitor blood glucose levels and record same • Educate on care of the skin and nails • Remember that steroid use may precipitate a diabetic state. Ensure that patient is monitored for potential development of diabetes when taking steroids • Annual assessment to prevent and control retinopathy[157]
Meconium ileus equivalent (MIE) or distal ileus obstructive syndrome (DIOS)[158]	Promote return to previous bowel habits	• Give prescribed laxatives and enemas • Monitor bowel movements, frequency and type • Observe for dehydration and abdominal distension • Administer prescribed intravenous fluids if nil by mouth • Give appropriate analgesia and antiemetic if required
Possible need for ventilatory assistance via nasal route (i.e. NIPPV)[159]	Reduce anxiety of patient and relative, and promote good compliance with equipment	• Ensure that patient understands what is happening and is happy with this course of action • Reassure and remain with the patient while NIPPV being introduced. Give anxiolytics if prescribed • Educate patient about safety issues, e.g. no drinking and eating while being ventilated due to increased risk of inhalation • Ensure that the patient and relatives know how to disconnect from the machine if necessary • Advise on the meaning of the alarms and significance of the different ones • Observe and record length of time on and off NIPPV • Promote good skin care around mask area. Keep clean and dry. Ensure bridge of nose is relieved of pressure as much as possible. Agents such as Granuflex® or Spencoderm® may be employed as aids in relieving pressure
Coping with the terminal stages of cystic fibrosis	Relieve symptoms	• Encourage patients, relatives and staff to communicate with each other • Allow patients and relatives time and space to be alone • Help them to listen to each other's need • Be prepared to answer questions honestly • Help patients to maintain independence for as long as possible • Alleviate feelings of isolation, anxiety and fear • Control symptoms of breathlessness, pain and any other symptoms that may occur, to ensure that a comfortable, dignified death is achieved. The use of opiates may be helpful • Provide support for family and friends prior to and following death[160] • Bereavement follow-up support

assessment and realize that maybe John is more breathless than on a previous admission, and may need more help or may not be able to be as independent and self-caring as he had been in the past. Obviously it is also difficult for the patient to admit the need for more help and most will struggle to maintain physical independence for as long as possible. This independence may have been hard fought for, and to see it slipping away can leave the patient with a feeling of loss of control and it is important that nurses encourage patients to maintain as much control as possible over their lives.

Deteriorating health often starts insidiously and results in the introduction of new treatment regimes and progresses to incorporating new items of equipment or invasive techniques, such as implantable ports to aid venous access or gastrostomies to improve nutritional status. This passes finally into the terminal phase of illness, when issues such as lung transplantation may have to be considered[161]. Throughout, it is imperative that nurses recognize how needy patients are at this time. What may be only a nebulizer to us is another reminder to them that they have a disease that will eventually kill them. Patients with CF suffer many bereavements throughout their lives, and this is not just the loss of CF friends and relatives but will include the smaller losses, such as having extra treatments, inability to catch the bus to work any more, needing oxygen at home, or loss of friends due to social isolation. This may culminate in loss of independence and the need to return to the family home for care and support, where they may feel that they are a burden in spite of having devoted parents. This will cause inevitable strain on both sides and may include financial, physical and emotional hardship.

TRANSPLANTATION

The subject of possible lung transplantation may be raised by either the patient or the doctor. Some patients may not wish to address this issue or even recognize how sick they are, and so they may be shocked when transplantation is discussed. In many ways they are being asked to address their own mortality; although recognizing it in their peers with CF, they may not see themselves in the same position. Many patients and relatives are confident that they will be the ones to beat the disease.

Transplantation may not be an option for all patients. Some will be unsuitable on medical grounds, others may not wish to be considered for moral, ethical or religious reasons.

If transplantation is an option, patients will face a battery of tests and will need to be aware of the reasons for them. They will also need reassurance, support and education during this period so that they know what they will face before and after transplantation. They need to know that the waiting time may be very long but that

there is always someone at the end of the phone if they need a shoulder to lean on. Many people will die waiting for donor organs. The high mortality rate (50 per cent) of people awaiting donor organs has caused some families and transplant teams to pursue the concept of live-lobe donation. This technique is still in its early days and is not an option for all. There are many ethical, medical and moral issues to be considered from both the donor's and the recipient's point of view. Families need help with the adjustments that have to be made pre- and post-transplantation, both physically and psychologically.

TERMINAL PHASE

Many patients will die on the transplant waiting list, others may not wish to be considered or may be unsuitable for this treatment. It is the nurse's role to help prepare the patient for death without destroying all hope. The possibility of dying may be difficult for the patient to address. He will not wish to fail his parents or even the doctors and nurses who are caring for him, but there may come a point when death is inevitable. It should be remembered that caring for the dying patient may be the most significant thing we do for him; sometimes all we can do is hold his hand and be there for him. It is important that everyone is aware of what is happening to the patient, and good lines of communication are kept open between family, patient and staff. Saying 'goodbye' is difficult for all concerned and we need to encourage an open environment so that the patient does not feel isolated by people trying to avoid what is happening. However, hard it may be for the nurse, it can never be as difficult as it is for the family and the person dying. We must reassure the patient and families that adequate medication will be given to control symptoms and that there will be plenty of support for them.

Good terminal care is essential. Honesty is always the best policy. Patients are very knowledgeable about their disease and usually know when they are going to die. They will share their fears with the person they feel confident with.

> I know you feel insecure, don't know what to say, don't know what to do. But please believe me, if you care, you can't go wrong. Just admit you care. That is really for what we search. We may ask for whys and wherefores, but we don't really expect answers. Don't run away . . . Wait . . . All I want to know is that there will be someone to hold my hand when I need it. I am afraid. Death may get to be a routine with you, but it is new to me. You may not see me as unique, but I've never died before. To me it is pretty unique.
>
> You whisper about my youth, but when one is dying is he really so young any more? I have lots I wish we would talk about. It really would not take much of your time because you are in here quite a bit anyway. If only

we could be honest, both admit our fears, touch one another. If you really care, would you lose so much of your valuable professionalism if you even cried with me? Just person to person? Then it might not be so hard to die . . . in a hospital . . . with friends close by.'[162]

Relatives and nurses are often surprised by how well prepared some CF patients are about their impending death. Many will have written wills and discussed funeral arrangements or left letters discussing disposal of possessions. It is often difficult for relatives to hear or see these things, but it is important for the dying person to say or do them.

BEREAVEMENT COUNSELING

Relatives should be able to return to the ward following the death of a patient and bereavement counseling should be available. Some families will wish to cut ties completely, viewing hospitals as too difficult to return to, others will wish to continue returning because they feel their loved one is still around. Nurses should remember that care of these families does not cease with death, but carries on in a supportive role.

For the nurse having to sit with a newly grieving family it is often very difficult. It will remind us of our own mortality and vulnerability, and we are rarely left without some feelings of a sense of failure and helplessness. Families will ask many questions, often over and over again, needing reassurance. Sometimes we have to accept that some problems have no solutions and that all we can give is ourselves.

HOW DOES THE NURSE COPE WITH THE STRESS OF CARING FOR CF PATIENTS?

It has been recognized that nurses caring for patients with CF may suffer from stress 'burnout'. Bergman *et al.*[163] identified aspects of care of CF patients that may precipitate burnout.

People with CF have a mean life expectancy of 31.5 years in the UK, males slightly more than females, but the clinical course is unpredictable[164]. Nurses working with CF patients over a long period of time may develop close relationships with the patient and family. It can be very difficult for a young nurse (or any team member) to cope with the death of a patient who may be their own age and could be a peer. It is essential that time, space and support is given to all the team, otherwise one could lose a potentially valuable resource for the future. If a patient dies on the unit, it should be remembered that the team will grieve as well. This is a healthy outcome and time for multidisciplinary team support should not be overlooked.

If the CF unit has been very busy with many very sick or dying patients members of staff may exhibit symptoms or signs of burnout. This may include clock watching, taking extended breaks, avoiding patients and their relatives, failure to concentrate on what patients are saying and displaying a cynical or judgemental attitude towards them. All these have a direct negative consequence for the patient[165]. The team member may also be suffering from emotional exhaustion, have low personal esteem and may experience feelings of depersonalization. With good team support these signs should be recognized and acted upon. Some nurses may feel that working with chronic illness is not for them, but those that do this work will find it a rewarding experience.

CF units could be potentially gloomy, but the reverse is usually true, with much fun and laughter and patients encouraging and supporting each other. It has often been said to us 'Don't you find your job depressing?'. Our reply is 'It is a privilege to work with these young people and it is a positive, challenging and rewarding role'. If you allow CF patients the opportunity and listen to what they say about their lives and their philosophy for living, they will teach us a great deal. The majority of patients yearn for life and try to fill that life with all the experiences and challenges it can give them. It is our responsibility to encourage and support them in all their endeavors. We should all remember this: 'I have cystic fibrosis, I am not cystic fibrosis' (quote from CF patient aged 26 years).

Cystic fibrosis home care

F. DUNCAN-SKINGLE AND E. BRAMWELL

INTRODUCTION

Home care is not a new concept in the management of cystic fibrosis (CF). Patients and their families have for many years focused their energies on daily treatment in a bid to control and reduce the impact of this progressive, life-threatening disease (e.g. twice-daily physiotherapy, adherence to drug regimes such as enzymes and antibiotics). Over the past decade there has been an increasing trend to move care from the hospital to the home, including high-technology healthcare (HTHC). In North America this is defined as 'the provision of equipment, drugs and services to the patient at home for the purpose of restoring and maintaining his or her maximal level of comfort, function and health'[166]. A number of schemes and services have been developed to enable patients to be nursed and cared for at home, including renal and peritoneal dialysis, intravenous antibiotics or cytotoxic therapy, enteral and parenteral nutrition, respiratory support, and the use of ventilators and oxygen therapy.

Economic forces and NHS reforms in the UK are partially behind the movement of care from hospital to the home[167]. Other factors in the trend towards home care have been improvements in the socio-economics of the population and thereby the home environment. The rapid development in medical technology has made equipment more portable and user-friendly (e.g. disposable devices for the administration of intravenous antibiotics). Not least in the drive towards home care is the patient's choice in wishing for the provision of treatment at home[168]. Research indicates that being at home may be more conducive to a speedy recovery and reduces the risks of hospital acquired infection[169]. For many patients the preference for home treatment also ensures a greater sense of control over their treatment and therefore over their disease[170]. Hospital teams need to be able to evaluate not only how patients and families cope with these treatments, but also the emotional demands of managing high-technology equipment for treatment at home.

For patients with CF, their first introduction to home HTHC would probably be intravenous antibiotics. The purpose of all the services developed is to enable an earlier discharge from hospital and reduce the need for frequent hospital admissions. By providing a high level of nursing support at home and identical treatment to that provided in hospital, it also ensures that there is optimal use of scarce resources and improves patient care. The health professions need to work in partnership with the patient and family. The patient and family will need appropriate education if they are to manage their treatment at home effectively with a minimum of risk and complications[171]. The hospital nurse specialist should provide the appropriate education, with the home-care team supporting the patient on his or her return home.

The role of the specialist home-care nurse is to provide education and support, clinical assessment and advice in the home setting. The home-care service may be appropriate for visiting the patient and family of the newly diagnosed, those with sibling problems, or those needing education with regard to managing their illness. Visits to schools, to those on intravenous antibiotics (IVAB) or on recently introduced treatments, also to patients awaiting transplantation, may be beneficial. The home-care nurse must ensure that good liaison is maintained with the family doctor and the hospital. The role and scope of the specialist home-care nurse will include all aspects of the patient's treatment management from diagnosis to the terminal stage of their disease.

It is important that the patient's and family's needs are understood and addressed. Home care can impose considerable strain on carers and patients. Any additional treatment needs to be negotiated between the patient and the hospital specialist team, with a realistic understanding of the demands and pressures put on the patient and the family. Although the patients and carers become experts in their knowledge and treatment of the disease, professional help is beneficial in supporting patients with lifelong illnesses[172].

Over the past 10 years hospitals in the UK, Europe and further afield have provided services to young people with cystic fibrosis at home by developing support networks for the patient and family. These services are supported by government legislation[173]. This legislation has set out strategies to enable patients to have a greater say in their treatment management and to maximize their independence within the constraints of their disease.

Some of the advantages and disadvantages of home care are set out below, and should be taken into consideration before the patient is discharged.

THE ADVANTAGES OF HOME CARE

These include reduced hospital admissions or patient's length of stay. Many aspects of treatment, for example intravenous antibiotics, can be administered at home as effectively as in hospital, although there is some evidence to show that patients suffer less fatigue in hospital, possibly because they have to do more for themselves at home[174]. Other advantages are:

- The risk of hospital acquired infection to the patient is greatly reduced out of a hospital setting[175].
- Patients can tailor their treatment program to their day.
- Being admitted into hospital can be disruptive, and reducing the need for admission can improve quality of life without compromising the efficacy or safety of treatment[176].
- The ability to attend school, college and work avoids disruption to normal daily activities.
- There are many benefits of a specialist nurse visiting a sick child at home. It is now recognized that hospitalization can contribute to subsequent behavioral problems[177].
- Technological developments have produced disposable, safe delivery systems for intravenous antibiotics, which have given the patient more flexibility, autonomy and confidence in administering intravenous antibiotics at home[178].

THE DISADVANTAGES OF HOME CARE

- Escalating demands on the patient and family.
- Additional treatment may increase the stress the family is under and the home becomes more like hospital.
- Carers may have to change their lifestyle/working pattern.
- The carer may have to give up or take time off from work, causing financial problems.
- The patient may feel overwhelmed and isolated. The

hospital may provide a safe haven and remove the stress of having to care for oneself.
- The responsibility for time-consuming and difficult therapies can be all consuming and result in nonadherence[179].
- Professional advice and assistance will not be as readily available.
- Pressure on hospital beds may encourage physicians to discharge the patient early or presume that home care is a satisfactory alternative.

THE ORGANIZATION OF HOME CARE

Nurses undertaking home care are part of a hospital-based multidisciplinary specialist team. They should have excellent clinical skills and an in-depth knowledge of CF. They should be good communicators, with the ability to teach both patients and staff, while undertaking an active interest in research and evidence-based practice. A diploma in counseling is an advantage. Vehicles will be necessary to enable the home nurses to travel to patients' homes and to carry the equipment required to ensure satisfactory clinical visits. The vehicles used by the home-care team should be equipped with a spirometer, pulse oximeter, weighing scales, sphygmomanometer, syringes, needles, dressing packs, sharps bins, a cool box for specimens, nebulizer spare parts, etc. On occasions the nurses may need to carry oxygen, nasal inspiratory positive pressure ventilator (NIPPV), tipping bed and nebulizer compressors.

The nurse should also carry a telephone to enable her to communicate with patients and the hospital. Clinical advice, as well as laboratory results, can be sought from the specialist team. Many practical problems are dealt with early by using the telephone. The nurse will also need patient records and information leaflets, and a laptop computer is useful for data collection.

General practitioner liaison

The key to successful care in the community is effective communication and liaison between all involved with the patient[180]. As more treatment is taking place in the home, community nurses are being encouraged to be flexible in their roles (UKCC Scope of professional practice 1992). Other pediatric or adult home-care teams may be involved with the patients, so it is imperative that all agencies are aware of their roles to coordinate not duplicate the care.

The aim of the specialist home-care team is to complement the primary healthcare teams. Good liaison between the hospital CF specialist team and the primary healthcare team (PHCT) is essential. Much of the medical and nursing needs of the person with CF are complex, and many PHCTs will feel out of their depth without this close liaison[181]. This may also be an opportunity to share the latest information on research and new treatments available.

Providing education and advice for community nurses ensures that the response to the patient's acute care needs is achieved more promptly and more health professionals are available to that person. It was thought that the growth of community specialist nurses would threaten and fragment care and undermine the role of the district nurse. This is not our experience. It has been a positive development for the primary healthcare teams, the hospital team and the patient.

Hospital liaison

Effective communication with the multidisciplinary team is important to ensure optimum care. Liaison by mobile phone and regular contact with the team can be a challenge but weekly multidisciplinary team meetings where the patients are discussed can be a useful forum for sharing information about the patients at home or in hospital. This meeting can also provide peer support for the home-care nurse, who may otherwise be professionally isolated.

Referral to a specialist home-care nurse can be either via the specialist hospital team of which she is a member, the primary healthcare team or by direct referral from a patient already known to the team.

Discharge planning

Careful discharge planning is essential. The patient's physical and psychological fitness for discharge should be assessed. The drug regimen and the length of treatment that is to be managed at home, the suitability of the home situation and the impact on the rest of family life must be considered[182].

- Patient and carer have to have confidence in the hospital team planning their discharge and need to be reassured that safe care is possible at home.
- They must understand the drug regimen and length of treatment, side-effects and adverse reactions[183].
- They should have had appropriate education and have shown the skills and confidence to administer the treatment.
- They must understand the use and management of the patient's venous access, if appropriate (i.e. short or long cannulae or implantable venous access port).
- Patient and carer must be confident that their GP has knowledge of their treatment regime.
- They must know the name and telephone number of their specialist team and be assured that advice is available 24 hours a day.
- They must know the name, telephone number and delivery times of drugs from the commercial home-care company, if appropriate.
- Patient and carer must understand the safe disposal of drugs, clinical waste and sharps. This is often undertaken by the commercial home-care company. Otherwise waste must be returned to the hospital for safe disposal.
- They should know the date and time that the home-care nurse is going to visit and that the nurse will notify them if she is going to be more than 30 minutes late.
- They should also feel confident that lung function, oxygen saturation and weight are monitored the same as in hospital and should know the appointment date and time of their next hospital outpatient visit.
- Domiciliary physiotherapy services are sometimes available. There is some evidence of improved compliance to physiotherapy if it is demonstrated in the home[184].

CONDUCTING A HOME-CARE VISIT

People with CF, as with most people, have daily commitments, but in addition they have a time-consuming

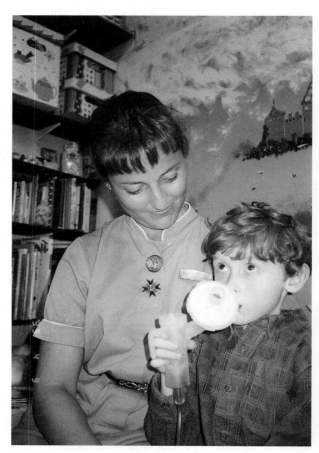

Fig. 19.13 *Conducting a home-care visit. (Reproduced with the parents' permission.)*

treatment regime. It is important that a home visit is anticipated favorably and is not viewed as a burden that produces more anxiety. A time to visit should be arranged, if possible, to fit in with the patient's commitments.

The nurse should be able to monitor weight, lung function and oxygen saturation (Fig. 19.13). She should be able to educate, counsel and advise the patient/carer on every aspect of their disease or know where to seek advice.

It is important to document each visit. Any clinical intervention or instruction, who was present at the visit, and when is the next hospital/home appointment. It is useful to document the time spent on the visit and how long it took the nurse to travel to the patient and travel time between patients. This information may help with the future development of the service.

SPECIFIC ASPECTS OF HOME-CARE NURSING OF CF PATIENTS

The newly diagnosed patient

Diagnosis of CF has a devastating impact on the family. In addition to having come to terms with their child having a potentially life-threatening disease, parents will be expected to meet the treatment needs arising from the child's illness. Patient/carer education is vital in the care of individuals with chronic conditions such as CF, and should be ongoing and constantly under review. Frequent visits to the family home, especially in the first few weeks may be necessary. As time progresses this can be adapted to the needs of the patient and family. It has been noticed that specialist nurses, skilled in their specific field, can improve the knowledge of patients and carers and ensure better health outcomes with appropriate care and support[185].

Parents of children with CF face substantial demands on their time and emotions. They sometimes feel overwhelmed by the responsibility for administering treatment, providing twice-daily chest physiotherapy, in addition to monitoring the child's respiratory and nutritional status. There may be an economic burden created, due to loss of income, when undertaking medical care, as well as the daily physical and emotional strain of rearing a child with a chronic illness. There is also the long-term psychological impact of a disorder that is both inherited and lethal.

The home-care nurse can provide education on all aspects of treatment and management of the disease. This may include genetic counseling and advice on screening before future pregnancies; this may extend to other family members who may be concerned about their carrier status. There is often a psychosocial transition, by which the family moves from seeing themselves as a healthy family to accepting the reality of a long-term health problem. The home-care team can help in this process by enabling the family, and encouraging them to provide a flexible framework to exist within. They should also be reassured that their feelings and behavior are entirely normal during this process.

Family and siblings

A child or adult with a chronic illness seriously affects the entire family[186]. Mothers usually shoulder the burden of the child's care and treatment[187] and often suffer significantly more psychological distress than mothers of healthy children.

Many adjustments are necessary to enable the family to care for a child with CF, support in the community is received from friends, family, work colleagues and the professional care-givers. By providing home care and support, it reduces the emotional trauma to the whole family, by minimizing the separation of the child from family and home. The benefit to the siblings of the sick child is to ensure that the family unit is preserved, therefore reducing their stress[188]. Parents are less anxious, have a greater sense of being in control, and an increased capacity for learning new care skills; they prefer home care[189].

School visits

If a child is unwell, the family will have concerns for his or her education and how he or she will cope at school. Explanation of treatment management and the care necessary for these children while they are at school can be given to the school with the parents' consent. This will reduce the anxiety for both the mother and the teachers. Routine visits to the school can be arranged with follow-up as necessary. Some children may need additional assistance at school. This may mean that the school will require additional resources.

Home intravenous antibiotics (IVAB)

Lung infections may require intravenous antibiotic therapy. This is frequently undertaken at home. Being admitted to hospital leads to disruption in the patient's personal life. So remaining at home enables patients to tailor their treatment programs to their own timetables, maintaining both self-sufficiency and optimum treatment. Home intravenous therapy requires careful discharge planning from hospital to ensure that treatment is appropriate and manageable. It is important that the patient is closely monitored and followed up on discharge. Accessible support, such as a home-care nurse should be involved, where possible[175]. Before deciding whether home IVABs are appropriate, certain aspects should be considered[190]. Occasionally it may be inadvisable to send a patient home on IVABs. Exclusion criteria may include:

- poor manual dexterity;
- poor comprehension of instructions, even after adequate and sometimes lengthy education;
- insufficient carer or social support[191];
- poor standards of hygiene and no telephone facility;
- inability to undertake the additional treatment associated with an exacerbation, e.g. physiotherapy[192];
- noncompliance with physiotherapy during an exacerbation[193];
- noncompliance with IVAB therapy[194];
- emotional instability[191];
- poor visual acuity.

Patients requiring intravenous antibiotics at home will have their venous access established and first dose administered in hospital with supervision. They will wait for at least 1 hour prior to discharge home. This reduces the risks of anaphylaxis and inspires confidence in both patient and carer. It is advisable to have a protocol for teaching and assessing the patient's ability to administer IVABs at home.

SUGGESTED PROTOCOL FOR TEACHING PATIENTS/CARERS PRIOR TO DISCHARGE ON HOME IVABS

The patient/carer must actively wish to do IVABs at home. When discharged from hospital the patient/carer will need to know:

- the principles of home IVABs;
- how to manage an infusion pump (e.g. Intermate);
- how to set up, reconstitute and draw up IVABs, also saline flush and/or Hepsal®;
- order of administration;
- principles of asepsis;
- how to prevent, recognize and be aware of and respond to complications, including catheter-related sepsis, occlusion and reaction to drugs (i.e. sensitivity);
- how to store and check drugs, diluents and syringes at home;
- how to store other equipment, and how it is delivered by the company (if appropriate);
- safe disposal of sharps and removal from home;
- name and telephone number of the healthcare professionals who will be available to provide advice 24 hours a day;
- date, time and arrangements for aminoglycoside blood levels, if appropriate;
- date of follow-up clinic or home visit.

The protocol should be used with a standard audit tool. There must be an appropriate protocol for monitoring aminoglycoside levels, monitoring the patient's clinical condition and removal of the venous access on completion of the antibiotic course. Attention should be paid to psychosocial issues that may need addressing.

If progress has not been maintained, then an early referral back to hospital may be necessary. The option to complete IVAB in hospital should always be explored with the patient at each episode.

DEVICES FOR INTRAVENOUS DELIVERY

Over the past few years there has been a proliferation of new devices and pumps available to aid the administration of intravenous drugs. These include elastomeric infusion systems that may be prefilled and delivered to the home. It is vital that patients are educated in their use and are familiar with the device that may be supplied to them[195].

Awaiting transplantation

Lung transplantation has become an option for patients with end-stage respiratory failure secondary to CF[196]. Many of these patients will wait at home for donor lungs for considerable lengths of time. Regular clinical assessment, support and reassurance during this period is essential, in conjunction with hospital follow-up visits.

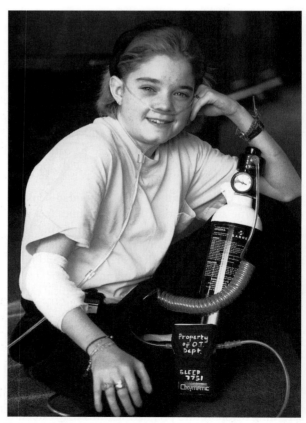

Fig. 19.14 *CF patient on oxygen awaiting lung transplantation. Oxygen delivered via an oxilite and nasal cannulae. (Reproduced with the parents' permission.)*

These visits to hospital are often exhausting for the very sick patient, taking them 2–3 days to recover from an outpatient visit.

It is often necessary for the family to provide 24-hour care. This has a major impact on family life. It is important not to underestimate this burden on the family[197]. Due to the limited availability of cadavaric organs and the natural history of the disease, many of these patients will die awaiting transplantation[198]. It is therefore necessary to support both the patient and family in preparing them for the possibility of death, while not totally destroying hope.

Continuous assessment of these patients is essential for effective management of the disease. Many may have complex treatment regimes to cope with, including overnight entral or gastrostomy feeds and IVAB, continuous oxygen, and for some nasal inspiratory positive pressure ventilation (NIPPV)[199]. The family needs support to develop the skills to carry out these complicated treatments, which also require a great deal of personal stamina. They should be given the opportunity to opt out, without feeling that they are letting their loved one down. The home-care nurse needs to be aware and sensitive to these issues. Good liaison between the hospital and community teams is important to ensure that re-referral back to hospital is achieved quickly and efficiently should it be necessary.

Introducing new treatments

The information that CF patients require becomes important as survival into adult life continues to improve. It has been shown that the clinical nurse specialist undertaking education and support is both necessary and beneficial and can help smooth the introduction of new treatment regimes[200]. Examples of such treatment regimes are: after insertion of a gastrostomy, insertion of an implantable venous access port, nebulized antibiotic therapy and IVAB treatment, and introduction to and monitoring of oxygen therapy or NIPPV, which is sometimes used for ventilatory support for the seriously ill patient while waiting for transplantation[201].

After a gastrostomy tube is inserted the patient is followed-up by the home-care team to reinforce correct care of the stoma and to monitor the site. If there are problems with the feed, then referral to the dietetic service can be made. Any new drugs and nebulizers can be monitored in the same way, giving the patient reassurance and confidence in their use.

Oxygen therapy may be introduced in the hospital but will require installation of an oxygen concentrator at home, for nightly or more continuous use. In the past, oxygen has been initiated when the patient is in the terminal stage and therefore patients and families may perceive its use as a poor prognostic sign. The psychosocial impact of beginning oxygen therapy cannot be underestimated. Families may need to be reassured of the benefits of oxygen therapy at home in addition to the safety aspects that need to be considered. Monitoring by the home-care team and observing for overuse with its potentially serious side-effects is crucial.

Family calendars and noticeboards become full of telephone numbers of the hospital, home-care company, oxygen delivery services, as well as dates for frequent visits from the home-care nurse and clinic outpatient appointments.

Terminal care and bereavement

Even with the best clinical treatment and advancements in research many young patients die; some may wish to die at home. Good terminal care is essential. The home-care team can provide the care and support that is necessary, liaising with other community teams and the hospital to enable the patient to die with dignity at home.

Caring for a loved one who is dying has an enormous impact on the family. There are many emotions involved as they try to come to terms with their impending loss. The support required at this time should never be underestimated, it should reflect the family's wishes while ensuring that other patients' needs are not overlooked.

Follow-up for the newly bereaved family should be provided, helping them to come to terms with their loss[202,203]. The extent of the follow-up depends on the family's needs and wishes. It may be necessary to see the parents and the siblings separately as their grief may be at different stages.

CONTRACTS FOR HOME CARE

These must ensure cost-saving options, but no cost compromising in terms of patient safety, comfort or clinical outcome. However, it is recognized that patients who receive these services from a commercial company have few complaints and that the use of delivery system devices saves patients/carers considerable time in the reconstitution of drugs and are very convenient for patients[204]. Purchasing from a commercial home-care company must be monitored by the specialist team to ensure expertise and the correct infrastructure to provide the requirements of their patients. Purchasers are also keen to have more research-based evidence concerning the use of HTHC at home to justify the use of their resources[205].

SUMMARY

Political forces and financial resources and restraints often determine the future of developments, such as specialist home care. Many people have tried to estimate the financial savings to hospitals by providing HTHC at home[206,207]. The present UK government is trying to change the professional power base of healthcare from hospital dominance to community-based care. There is, however, some recognition of the importance of the overlap between primary and secondary care[208].

CF home care has many advantages for selected patients. In the interests of patients we must ensure that this flexibility for treatment is maintained and that change in healthcare is not just cost driven. Home care is here to stay on the grounds of patient preference and convenience. It should be of a high quality and there should be equity of access to this type of service for all patients with CF.

'Being at home allows me to be with my family and lead a more normal life' (quote from a CF patient, 1998).

Social work

N. CLOUTMAN

INTRODUCTION

This section outlines the contribution of the hospital-based social worker to patient care within a specialist cystic fibrosis unit. The social work brief will inevitably be dictated by prevailing social attitudes, social and economic policy and the legislative framework that governs health and social care.

In most developed countries today ideas that support empowerment, independence and personal choice are having a potent influence on the design of services for people with chronic illnesses and disability. Supporting people and their carers to live independently in the community makes economic sense and usually provides better opportunities for people to lead more fulfilling lives[209]. The social worker, therefore, seeks to consider the individual and his carers in order to support their choices, and to act as an advocate for them. Within a specialized clinical framework the social worker is in a unique position to develop an understanding of the needs of people with cystic fibrosis (CF) and to convey these to social services departments and other resource providers in the community.

Specialist knowledge of cystic fibrosis can also have a bearing on the quality of service the social worker is able to provide directly to those affected and to their families. A survey carried out by Barnardo's in 1987 demonstrated that many families had negative experiences of social workers and of other helping professionals, due to the latter's limited knowledge of cystic fibrosis. The conclusion was that a real understanding of the condition was necessary in order to enhance services, and to generate confidence in those receiving them[210].

Within the multidisciplinary team, therefore, the social worker brings a particular perspective in which she attempts to address the experience and needs of the whole person in relation to his illness, and in the context of his family and the community.

The tasks of the hospital social worker can be summarized as follows:

1. Assessment of psychosocial care needs, including discharge planning and risk assessment.
2. Planning care in the community.
3. Assisting and supporting partners or informal carers and, in the case of children and young people, parent carers.
4. Counseling for personal or family difficulties encountered as a result of illness and, associated with this, changing ability and needs.
5. Bereavement counseling.
6. Practical assistance and advice on welfare rights, employment, care of dependants, etc.

It is important to acknowledge that there are some areas of overlap between the social worker's role and that of other professionals such as psychologists and clinical nurse specialists. There is thus potential for duplication, competition or exclusion. Close contact, clear communication and good professional accountability are important if this is to be prevented.

In the following pages the various emotional and practical difficulties that can be experienced by those living with CF are discussed in relation to the role of the social worker.

CHILDREN AND YOUNG FAMILIES

The level of concern experienced by young families with children who have CF is very high. Inevitably the arrival of an affected child will have a considerable impact on the family. There may, as a result, be significant changes to family life, and in the roles and relationships within it. It is not unusual for parents to experience anxiety and depression, and there may be added feelings of guilt and anger resulting from the genetic nature of CF[211]. Any pre-existing marital conflicts may be heightened, whereas a more stable marital relationship can be strengthened by the arrival of a child with CF[212]. Parental concern for the affected child, together with the very real demands of his treatment requirements, may lead to siblings feeling neglected and resentful[213].

The Barnado's survey on the experiences and needs of families showed that parents had difficulties in accepting the diagnosis of CF and in getting the information and education they required. A sense of isolation was commonly experienced. Parents were often unable to obtain either the practical and financial help or the emotional support they needed[210]. Appropriate support in the early stages of the child's life is essential if major stress is to be prevented. Clear information at the time of diagnosis followed by ongoing support can have a major bearing on the family's capacity to face up to and live with CF[214].

A family's ability to cope influences the young person's developing adjustment to his condition[215,216]. Many young adults who live a full life, yet accept the limitations CF imposes upon them, report that they have been supported and encouraged during childhood by parents who were open about their condition, but who did not 'fuss'. Others who have perceived their families as anxious or protective may lack confidence in their own ability to lead a full and active life. Conversely, they may respond by not giving sufficient attention to their treatment needs. For yet others who have grown up in an environment where their CF was denied, the later progress of the disease may be particularly difficult to manage and accept.

GROWING UP WITH CYSTIC FIBROSIS

During recent years advances in medicine have greatly increased the life expectancy of people with CF. This very positive development brings with it new practical and emotional issues for those affected and for their families[216].

Adolesence is a stage of crucial transition. Conflicts between dependency and independence, and the struggles of both parent and child in letting go, can lead to stormy interactions. This may be intensified for the young person with CF who has throughout childhood required a great deal of care and attention from his parents. It may be further complicated in that the nature of CF gives the adolescent the means to rebel in ways that can endanger him and deeply concern those close to him[217]. When conflicts do arise, outsiders, including helping professionals, can fall into the trap of siding with one party or other, viewing a 'noncompliant' child or 'overprotective' parent as the cause of the difficulty.

It is important, however, that both parent and child can have their own views and experiences validated and understood before there can be any possibility of their beginning to listen to and understand one another. This kind of help can be offered through joint or individual work by a social worker.

Most young people with CF move into adulthood normally and without undue difficulty. However, if relationships have been very intense and enmeshed, difficulties about letting go and breaking away can continue into adulthood.

EMPLOYMENT

The transition into adulthood brings with it many practical issues. When seeking employment the young person is faced with the question of what is realistic, both in terms of his current and his future health. There is also the very difficult question of whether or not to tell prospective employers[218]. Although many employers are accepting and sympathetic, others are very ready to reject applicants on the grounds of any possibility of ill health. In this situation the social worker's task is not so much to advise but to help the young person explore and consider what action feels most appropriate for him. Often people decide that truth is the best policy on entering employment. Others omit to inform employers about their CF at this stage, but then do so later, once secure that their qualities as an employee are recognized and valued.

A recent survey of 866 CF adults in the UK showed that 54 per cent were in paid employment compared with 69 per cent of the general population over 16 years[219]. Men were more likely to be employed than women. Of the unemployed, 30 per cent were students and the remainder were unable to work because they were too sick or unable to find work. Of employed adults, 56 per cent had had less than 2 weeks' sick leave in the previous year and only 6.7 per cent had more than 12 weeks' sick leave.

Vulnerability to recurrent infections often necessitates periodic interruptions to employment. The increasing frequency of such interruptions, or the progress of CF, can confront the individual with the question of stopping work altogether. This brings with it not only the prospect of financial hardship, but can result in considerable emotional turbulence. An individual's status, sense of purpose, identity and self-esteem are often invested in the work he does, and can thus be deeply shaken by the loss of employment. The opportunity to talk through both the practical and emotional implications of giving up work is often a very crucial part of the process in which this decision is made. In this context the social worker can offer the necessary emotional support, as well as helping the individual to seek alternative resources in terms of finance and possibly occupation.

Interruptions and loss of work necessitate claims for welfare benefits. Benefits systems (in many countries) can be difficult to negotiate. Information is not always easy for the claimant to obtain, and claims may be subject to considerable delays. Enquiries about benefits constitute a high proportion of social work referrals in the

Cystic Fibrosis Department. Much social work time is spent in advising clients about benefits, and in negotiating and advocating on their behalf.

HOUSING

For the young adult establishing independence, the acquisition of housing is often very important but can be difficult for somebody with CF. Public-sector housing is limited, and increasingly a young person wishes to buy a home. Some people with CF have done this successfully. However, many others are excluded either by limitations on their working and earning capacity, or by difficulty in obtaining necessary insurances. In this situation the only possibility of independent living lies in obtaining special needs accommodation For an applicant to be considered, social work support as well as medical back-up is usually required.

A UK survey of adults with CF carried out in 1990 showed that 56 per cent of men and 48 per cent of women with CF still lived with their parents[219].

RELATIONSHIPS AND MARRIAGE

Many people with cystic fibrosis enter satisfactory and secure partnerships. However, this difficult developmental milestone can hold some additional complications for them. There may be realistic anxieties about how much the partner understands about the condition and might cope in the future. The very nature of CF and sometimes the absence of outward signs may mean that the partner has little insight into what might lie ahead. This might be compounded when the partner with CF, still relatively well, uses denial as a means of maintaining a positive attitude[220].

> *Example*: Jennifer, a 19-year-old girl with CF, had been fit and active. She worked full-time, led a full social life and had become engaged to be married. When her condition deteriorated significantly her fiancé was clearly shocked and withdrew. After Jennifer had stabilized sufficiently, their engagement was broken by mutual agreement. Subsequently Jennifer's functioning and mobility were much more limited and she needed a great deal of care from her parents. Although distressed about the breakdown of her engagement, she also felt relieved that the crises had occurred before rather than after the marriage.

This example highlights the importance of the availability for new couples of counseling by social workers, nurses or others who have a good knowledge and understanding of CF. It is important to stress that the difficulties described in this example do not always occur. Most partners remain devoted and loving through critical and terminal illness.

In any situation the establishment of new partnerships can give rise to parental opposition. Although this is not always the case when somebody has CF, such opposition can become focused on the disease. The parents of the partner without CF may have difficulty in understanding the condition and may be very frightened by it. They may feel anxious or disappointed that their offspring has become involved with somebody with an illness or disability. The parents of the young adult with CF may feel protective and have difficulty in letting go. Those facing this situation can experience intense conflict and feel torn between parent and partner. He or she may require a great deal of help in working out his or her own needs or wishes in the face of such family pressures. The social worker with a good understanding of family systems and dynamics could usefully work with the family as a whole.

For young women contemplating a long-term partnership, there generally arises the question of having children. Clearly, a medical or nursing consultation regarding the advisability, the outlook and risks involved is of prime importance[212]. Such a consultation can be complemented by the opportunity to talk the issues through with a social worker whose nonmedical role enables her to offer some objectivity and neutrality.

In recent years there has been a significant rise in the occurrence of pregnancy and childbirth in young women with CF. The increased possibility of motherhood is clearly a positive step in terms of fulfilment in the affected person's life, and many young women with CF are now bringing up their children very happily and successfully. However, difficulties can arise. Where the mother's health is compromised, the demands of caring for young children may become problematic. When this is the case, the social worker may play a part in helping the mother and father to identify resources within their own families and in negotiating support from parents and siblings. In other cases support from outside the family may be required, and the hospital social worker may need to liaise with local authorities to mobilize services such as home care, and day nursery places. In situations where the health and life expectancy of a mother is poor, she and her partner will need to think about the emotional impact on their child or children, and about how to communicate with them about what is happening. This can be very difficult at a time when the parents themselves are having to cope with emotions arising from change, loss and the possibility of impending death. In such circumstances the help of an outside professional such as a social worker or a psychologist can be particularly valuable.

Young men with CF often find it more difficult than women to establish partnerships[218]. The 1990 adult survey carried out in the UK showed that 34 per cent of CF adults were married or cohabiting, compared with 61 per cent in the general population. Women were significantly more likely to be married or cohabiting than men, with 44 per cent of women to 26 per cent of men in such relationships. In this area, many CF-affected men experience a lack of confidence, which is closely associated with poor body image. Many talk of fearing that they would be 'Too much of a responsibility for a partner to take on'. Despite the fact that the caring role is traditionally ascribed to women, it does seem that the 'sick role' greatly conflicts with what society expects of young men, i.e. strength, control, competence, etc.

The likelihood of infertility in CF affected men, with its implications for sexual confidence, is undoubtedly pertinent to their difficulties in establishing partnerships. While the recent development of epididymal sperm aspiration greatly improves their chances of reproducing, it is too early yet to gauge how this will impact upon relationship patterns.

In the meantime, the difficulties experienced by some young men in this area can give rise to a great deal of frustration and depression. The social worker may offer support and the opportunity to talk through such feelings, which can bring relief. It may also be appropriate for her to refer the person on for more specialized long-term therapeutic help that could bring about emotional changes.

MAKING ADJUSTMENT TO DETERIORATING HEALTH

Struggles about moving into independent adulthood are compounded by the likelihood of progressive deterioration, and thus the possibility of reverting to increased dependency. For the young adult this may mean again becoming reliant upon a parent from whom independence has been achieved. Adjustments involved for both parent and child can be difficult[221]. The parent may hold back, fearing that to do otherwise might be clumsy or intrusive. The patient may feel angry and frustrated by renewed dependency.

The progression of cystic fibrosis can require major adjustments for couples. The partner with CF is likely to become more dependent and to make greater demands. The other partner may have to give up work or withdraw from other commitments in order to become a carer. The losses involved can cause stresses for both parties, and in turn may create strains on the relationship. It may be that both partners need close support by a social worker and by other professionals in order that they can understand, accept and tolerate what is happening.

The hospital team always attempts to enable the deteriorating CF patient to remain at home for as long and as much as possible. At the Royal Brompton Hospital the establishment of a home-care service by clinical nurse specialists has done much to facilitate this. The social worker's role in liaising with local services, and in mobilizing resources, such as adequate home care and appro-

priate welfare benefits, is also an important part of discharge planning.

A significant deterioration in health is perhaps particularly difficult for the isolated adult living alone. In this situation hospital or nursing home care may be the only realistic alternative. However, the combination of a good family doctor and a home-care team may allow for a better quality of life if these resources can be mobilized.

THE SOCIAL WORKER'S ROLE IN TRANSPLANT ASSESSMENT

A social work report is always completed as part of the assessment program for lung transplant surgery. The purpose of this report is not to make recommendations regarding the suitability of the person for transplant surgery, but to identify his coping strategies, family supports, emotional, practical and financial needs. It also gives the patient and his family the opportunity to talk through the experience of being confronted with the possibility of transplant surgery.

Transplant surgery is clearly a huge life event, which for many people is understandably difficult to accept and come to terms with. At the same time it is not uncommon for people to fear expressing reservations which they feel could adversely affect their chances of being placed on the waiting list. It is important for the social worker to help the patient talk through these complex feelings and, if appropriate, to enable him to ask for more time before making a decision to go on the list.

When making a social work assessment for transplant surgery, it is always important to consider the interactions and dynamics between the patient and his family, and to consider 'who is the transplant for?'. From time to time, particularly with children and adolescents, it may be that the patient's own needs and wishes become unclear in the light of the parents' anxiety for him to go forward for transplant surgery.

Example: N, a 16-year-old boy with CF, had grown up in the sole care of his father, a caring but anxious man whose emotional dependency upon his son was great. N had been placed on the waiting list for heart–lung transplant surgery 2 years before. When donor organs became available N became highly distressed and refused surgery. Subsequently it emerged that at the time of the assessment (done elsewhere), N had had little opportunity to explore and talk through his feelings, and that he had gone onto the list because he felt his father wanted him to. Sadly, N's refusal of the transplant led to great conflict between father and son during the period shortly before N's death.

This case highlights how important it is that there should be good information and preparation at the assessment stage.

Having been placed on the transplant waiting list, the patient and his family are faced with a very difficult and uncertain waiting period[222]. Loss of function and of mobility will have necessitated role adjustments within couples and families. Some families will have had to uproot themselves from their home, community or even country, in order to be within reasonable proximity to the appropriate transplant center. In such circumstances the family is likely to be very isolated, and it is important that the social worker not only maintains a close contact but helps the family to establish contact with appropriate community supports.

In this situation additional living expenses are likely to be incurred, and may not be met by welfare benefits. When this is the case, the social worker may need to help the family raise money from voluntary organizations.

Perhaps the greatest difficulty about the waiting period is the uncertainty about if and when donor organs will become available. The patient and his family must struggle to find a balance between the hope which is necessary to maintain a positive attitude, and a sense of reality regarding the possibility of there being no transplant, or of surgery not working out. This balance will vary from one individual to another and it is important for the social worker and others supporting the family to respect that denial is a necessary and valid defence at times. At the same time, the patient and family must be given the opportunity to air fears and concerns when they need to.

The recent development of lobe transplantation from live donors presents a means by which uncertainties associated with conventional transplant surgery can be overcome. However, this procedure also gives rise to moral and ethical issues that need to be addressed carefully and debated by the multidisciplinary team. The interests of organ donors as well as recipients need to be considered, and the motivation of donors requires careful exploration and understanding. In this context it is important to ensure that decisions have not resulted from factors such as family pressures or any unresolved feelings the potential donor has towards the patient. Siblings may be particularly vulnerable if they have experienced feelings of jealousy, rivalry and guilt arising from this. In the course of her contribution to the assessment, the social worker could play an important role in exploring these issues with the patient and the family.

BEREAVEMENT

When death occurs, those left behind have often spent long periods supporting and caring for a sick partner or child. Bereavement research has shown that the grieving process can be more complex for those who have been carers. Having lost the person he or she has loved, the carer is faced with the additional loss of his or her own role, and of the sense of purpose associated with this[223].

Grief needs to be fully expressed in order that it can be worked through and resolved[224]. This requires that the bereaved person is fully supported through this process. For some people it may be possible to gain such support from family or friends. For others it is not, especially if potential supporters are also grieving. Thus there may be a place for outside professional support. In some cases this can be offered by the hospital social worker. However, there are times when this is not possible, either because of geographical distance or due to emotional pain associated with returning to hospital. Referral by the social worker to an outside agency may then be appropriate. Families living with CF often derive a great deal of support from each other, particularly if, as the disease has progressed, long periods have been spent in hospital, where others are in the same position. It is understandable therefore that people who have lost a child, sibling or partner through CF sometimes want to continue sharing their experiences with other such families. Support groups run within CF centers for bereaved relatives can sometimes be an appropriate way of meeting this need. Many bereaved relatives like to maintain an interest and involvement with activities concerning CF. It is not uncommon for those recently bereaved to channel energy into fund raising for the benefit of those with the disease. Such activity can be a healthy way of finding meaning in the loss and of mitigating the pain of grief. However, problems can arise if such activities are too frantic and are used to 'take flight' from the reality of the loss.

With the increase of women and potentially of men with CF, having children, there is also the possibility of children experiencing the early loss of a parent. Children grieve very differently to adults and their needs can often be overlooked or misunderstood. That the child is allowed to grieve is of paramount importance for his future emotional development. However, where adults in the family are also grieving, they may have difficulty in providing the necessary support to the child. Prior to and following the death of a parent, the social worker can help families to find ways of communicating with children. She can also help to facilitate a referral for ongoing psychological help where required[225].

Research has shown that there is a close correlation between suppressed grief and mental health problems[224]. It is therefore important for social workers, clinical nurse specialists or others supporting the bereaved adult or children to address situations where grief is being denied.

CONCLUSION

Advances in medical treatment have greatly increased the life expectancy and potential opportunities available for people with CF. This, together with the psychosocial impact of developments such as transplant surgery, home nasal ventilators, etc., results in constant changes in needs.

In order to ensure that quality as well as longevity of life is optimized, medical advances must be accompanied by social work and support services which are sensitive and responsive to such changing needs. These services need to be based both in the CF unit and also in the community. The correct balance needs to be struck between such professionals and self-help groups run by local CF organizations.

Finally, it should be stressed that empowerment is always an important objective for any effective social work or support service. The efforts of professionals and of organizations need therefore to be made with rather than for people with CF[218]. There are considerable strengths and resources within this group who have first-hand knowledge of the condition, needs and the problems encountered. The thoughts and ideas of those with CF, and of their families must therefore play an important part in shaping the development of services available to them.

Occupational therapy

V. OTLEY GROOM

INTRODUCTION

Patients with cystic fibrosis (CF) lead active and independent lives until the natural history of the disease becomes unpredictable and medical complications increase, which in turn begin to restrict and control their lifestyle[226]. Occupational therapists assess 'the physical, psychological and social functions of the individual, identify areas of dysfunction and involve the individual in a structured programme of activity to overcome disability'[227]. They always follow a process starting with a screening assessment, leading to selected interventions, evaluation, further intervention if required and then discharge with follow-up if needed.

As Bluebond-Langer describes in *Natural History of Cystic Fibrosis*[228] a person with CF has several stages to his or her disease:

1. First year following the diagnosis of CF.
2. Months and years following a diagnosis of the disease when a child is relatively healthy, up to the first major exacerbation which requires hospitalization.
3. The time between the first exacerbation when the CF patient is relatively stable up to increased hospitalization.
4. Increasing complications, for example, diabetes, shortness of breath, intermittent use of oxygen during hospitalization.
5. Increasing deterioration, e.g. regular use of oxygen, activity restricted by the disease.
6. Terminal phase of the illness.

Although issues can arise at each stage of the disease, the occupational therapist's unique and specialist skills are best employed as a person with CF begins to experience limitations to their ordinary life (i.e. occupational dysfunction) and increasing medical complications occur (stage 4 onwards).

With any intervention, a person with CF should be given responsibility for solving his or her own problems and maximizing their own independence according to their own individually defined needs[229]. This is the central philosophy to an effective contract between therapist and patient.

ASSESSMENT

The quality and effect of the occupational therapist's treatment is dependent on the accuracy and relevance of his or her assessments. This enables the therapist to establish a baseline that reviews previous functional status, combined with client-selected desired activities of daily living. The occupational therapist and person with CF then jointly set treatment goals, and the therapist, guided by this, will select an appropriate frame of reference. The assessment should be informal with a discrete structure and good therapeutic rapport. From the interview, patients are asked to identify particular occupational component areas that they find difficult (Table 19.8), how they perceive their current performance and their satisfaction with performing them.

It is important to remember that an initial assessment does not need to be completed in one interview, but can be the result of several contacts, and a comprehensive assessment of need is built up over time.

INTERVENTIONS

Given that CF is a disease that reduces the life span of individuals, it is important to optimize quality of life wherever possible, as with all respiratory disease[230]. The following occupational therapy interventions should be considered if indicated:

- functional assessment;
- stress management;
- energy conservation;

Table 19.8 *Assessment for occupational therapy*

Occupational component areas	Areas to be assessed
Motor	Strength and endurance
	Shortness of breath on exertion
	Range of motion
	Posture
	Mobility and transfers (bath, bed, chair, car, stairs)
	Pressure relief
	Pain
Body functioning	Motivation
	Volition
	Anxiety
	Stress
	Affect
Socio-cultural	Behavior
	Beliefs
	Values
Spiritual	Self-concepts
	Coping mechanisms
	Emotional status and effect
Self-care	Meal preparation
	Housework
	Personal self-care
	Personal activities of daily living
Leisure	Hobbies
	Sports activities
	Play
Productivity	Work
	Home management
	Volunteering/caring for others
Environment	Physical
	Social
	Cultural

- independence equipment provision;
- pressure relief;
- wheelchair provision;
- discharge planning;
- informal counseling and problem solving.

Functional assessments

In establishing a patient's current level of functional ability, the occupational therapist needs to assess the patient by using familiar activities that are relevant to the individual. Use of functional assessment aids identification of problems experienced by the patient and is appropriate to use as a therapeutic medium to restore his or her independence[231]. This will, in turn, improve the patient's satisfaction and performance of occupational roles[232]. A variety of functional treatments can then be used, including transfers, functional mobilizing, personal activities of daily living and domestic activities of daily living (e.g. managing in the kitchen).

Stress management and relaxation

The aim of stress management is to teach individuals to be aware of how stress affects their day-to-day living, by identifying the causes of stress and understanding the effects of stress, physically, psychologically and behaviorally, and how this impacts on health. Next, establishment of a balance of healthy and unhealthy stress within their lifestyles should be identified. Finally, control and alleviation of stress is required, by teaching one of a range of techniques.

When there is a deterioration in an indiviual's physical or psychological condition, stress responses and anxiety can become excessive or prolonged, indicating the need for stress management education. Stress management has been shown to reduce the patient's perception of anxiety[233] and to increase feelings of well-being[234] and the patient's ability to cope with the disease process[235].

Stress management can be offered on an individual or group basis, depending on the individual patient's need and on the resources available. Some patients prefer two introductory sessions with home practice and audio tapes, whereas many benefit from a more formal structured program, encompassing cognitive behavioral techniques, individually or as a group with other cystic fibrosis or respiratory patients.

Relaxation has been shown in several studies to improve quality of life significantly and to reduce feelings of anxiety[236]. It does not always improve basal spirometry; however, it is shown to improve mood, an area which must always be addressed as it affects symptom reporting and patient's perception of ability to cope with the disease process[235]. Relaxation techniques offered should be tailored to the individual's preferred style, but should include one of the following techniques.

PROGRESSIVE MUSCLE RELAXATION

This is a method involving tensing and relaxing each part of the body in turn and the aim is to learn the difference between a tense and relaxed muscle group[237].

AUTOGENIC RELAXATION

This is a cognitive approach, teaching the patients how to feel and experience tension in different body areas. This technique focuses on breathing tension out of the body and encouraging the patient to think about sensations and feelings of warmth, heaviness, loose limbs and of sinking into their base of support[238].

GUIDED IMAGERY

This technique often involves the therapist taking the patient on an imaginary mental journey, enabling them to use their cognitive processes to achieve a feeling of well-being and relaxation. This is often a more advanced approach which can be used once a therapeutic relationship has been established[239].

BIOFEEDBACK

This technique can also be used but requires close monitoring and a minimum of six sessions to effectively utilise the techniques[240].

Energy conservation

Low energy is a factor associated with all chronic illness. Patients with CF will often experience low energy, frequent hospitalization and inability to carry out normal tasks, and they are no longer able to make the most of their body's available energy. Energy conservation strategies provide coping mechanisms for the individual to deal with loss of energy[241] and to reduce energy expenditure during college, work or activities of daily living[242].

Work simplification can be employed, enabling the activity undertaken to be broken into simpler, manageable parts (Table 19.9).

Pacing principles should be used with all activities and

Table 19.9 *Work simplification – parts principle*

P	Preplan and prioritize all activities of daily living
A	Avoid unnecessary activities and repetition
R	Rest often and frequently to maintain an achievable healthy balance
T	Time, particularly when ensuring there is enough time to complete a desired activity
S	Slow, rhythmical movements should always be utilized

the importance of avoiding overactivity emphasized. Overactivity, when many activities are undertaken in one day, results in the patient being unable to carry out ordinary, simply achieved tasks in subsequent days. This leads to anxiety and increased effort in breathing, decreased self-esteem and a resultant loss of independence and self-control over the patient's own life.

Carried out correctly, energy conservation maximizes functional ability and helps the patient with CF to increase performance and independence in their desired activities of daily living[243].

Independence equipment provision and pressure relief

The provision of assistive equipment within home or hospital environment maintains the patient's functional independence[244], retains the patient's perception of privacy and dignity with self-care[245]. Using the information gained from the functional assessment, appropriate equipment should be selected and tried. If equipment is not available within the hospital, contact should be made with community services to ensure that home assessment and provision of appropriate independence equipment is coordinated and provided as quickly as possible.

Housing adaptations should also be considered. This may include bath rails, stair rails, stair lifts, ramps and extensions to housing. Provision of independence equipment is an adjunct to energy conservation and also helps simplify a routine task for both patient and, where appropriate, carer[246].

PRESSURE RELIEF

Pressure relief reduces the risk of pressure sore development[247] and assists in the comfort and positioning of an individual, particularly as they reach palliative stage. It is important that patients who are potentially at risk of developing pressure sores are identified through standardized assessment, e.g. the Waterlow score. This is to establish a level of pressure relief risk in order to maintain and improve tissue status and prevent further breakdown of skin. It is important for an occupational therapist to loan and advise and educate on different pressure-relieving devices, including chair and wheelchair cushions, special mattresses, elbow pads and bed booties.

Wheelchair provision

Dyspnea, fatigue and reduced exercise tolerance are often symptoms experienced by patients with CF. These all impact on mobility. The provision of a wheelchair when the patient is experiencing shortness of breath and low energy gives a patient independence with internal and external mobility[248]. It also allows the patient to participate in social activities and events, both in hospital and when at home in their own community. Any patient requiring a wheelchair should be assessed by an accredited wheelchair assessor in order to prescribe a chair which best suits their individual needs. Factors that need to be considered when assessing are:

- patient's physical size (height, weight measurements);
- purpose the chair will be used for (internal/external mobility);
- environmental considerations (home layout, access, transportation);
- patient's oxygen requirements;
- needs of the carers;
- psychological adjustment to 'disability' label.

Discharge planning

As part of a multidisciplinary team, occupational therapists have an important role in discharge planning for a patient with CF. Where indicated, predischarge visits are found to be comprehensive and helpful to patients and carers when planning a safe discharge[249]. Otherwise, close liaison with community occupational therapists for postdischarge home visits should be arranged if required. In conjunction with the social worker, occupational therapists should liaise with community services in order to provide any necessary care and assistance identified during hospitalization. The occupational therapist's assessment will need to be given to a social worker to ensure that they have the objective assessment of a patient's functional needs and will enable the social worker to request services to meet these needs.

Advice to patients and their carers regarding home layout, suitability of housing, assistance with rehousing and adaptations can also be given. These roles depend on the individual hospital's approach to discharge planning, but it is essential that they are considered when patients reach the terminal stage of their disease.

Informal counseling, problem solving and advice

As a member of the multidisciplinary team and as trained informal counselors and problem-solvers, occupational therapists, along with psychologists and social workers, can assist with informal counseling.

OXYGEN PROVISION AND EQUIPMENT

There is enormous variability in prescription and adherence to present guidelines regarding provision of short-burst oxygen therapy, ambulatory oxygen and long-term oxygen therapy. When assessing whether a patient requires oxygen, the following should be considered:

- arterial blood gas tensions should have been measured;
- optimum medical management should have been carried out;
- depending on whether prescription is for ambulatory or long-term oxygen, establishment of oxygen desaturation on exercise and improvement in exercise capacity should be demonstrated with the use of ambulatory oxygen.

It is also important to consider the psychological factors prior to prescribing oxygen, to consider whether the patient will be able to use the oxygen equipment or device at home and be able to refill or coordinate changeover of cylinders.

Prescription of oxygen

Long-term oxygen may be prescribed in patients with CF when the Pao_2 is less than 8 kPa in the presence of nocturnal hypoxemia, secondary polycythemia, pulmonary hypertension or peripheral edema. Patients with CF develop exercise desaturation, and studies have shown that supplemental oxygen may improve exercise capacity in these patients[250].

The medical practitioner should always prescribe oxygen as a result of standardized tests. The following information must always be obtained when organizing domiciliary oxygen equipment:

- oxygen saturations at rest and on activity;
- liters of oxygen per minute;
- hours per day;
- method of oxygen delivery;
- mask or cannulae.

Education of the patient

Following prescription of oxygen, demonstration and education should be provided to patients to ensure they understand how to use the equipment, the benefits and contraindications. It is important when educating patients that they become completely familiar and confident with the oxygen equipment that they are required to use. Competence is required with refilling. Information on health and safety precautions, using oxygen in the home and travel advice are all essential.

Domiciliary oxygen equipment

- cylinders
- concentrators
- ambulatory or portable oxygen
- conservers (Oxymatic system)
- liquid oxygen.

OXYGEN CYLINDERS

These contain compressed oxygen and deliver the gas through a regulator valve. Flow rate can be variable or fixed, depending on the specification of the regulator. Cylinders can vary in size and provide oxygen under high pressure. The advantage of cylinders is that the oxygen is cool and dry. Disadvantages are the storage of bulky cylinders in the patient's home and the frequent collection and delivery of cylinders if a patient requires a high flow rate. They are not a suitable arrangement for patients prescribed oxygen for more than 12 hours/day.

OXYGEN CONCENTRATOR

These are mains-powered devices that concentrate oxygen from the atmosphere. The device concentrates room air and passes it under pressure through a cylindrical bed of xeolite which removes the nitrogen and concentrates the oxygen. The device has two chambers and ensures a continuous flow of oxygen as long as it is connected to electricity. These can be installed in the patient's home and are low-flow devices, unlike hospital oxygen which is delivered under pressure.

The flow rate of concentrators is adjustable between 0 and 5 liters/minute and, if additional oxygen is required, two concentrators can be used in tandem. As the flow rate increases, however, oxygen concentration can decrease. This is an important consideration when high flow rates are prescribed. Although not easily portable, the concentrators can be moved and taken away on holiday or when staying with friends.

The main advantages are that they never run out, the oxygen is delivered at room temperature and there are no delivery or storage problems. The disadvantages are a lower, limited maximal flow rate (8 liters per minute when used in tandem) and that they not only concentrate room air but also any smells and odors within the room.

AMBULATORY OXYGEN (PORTABLE)

Assessments should include a walking test, which can be performed by an occupational therapist, physiotherapist or nurse. Prior to carrying out the test, practice walks should be performed and the test should be carried out both on air and supplemental oxygen. Ambulatory oxygen should therefore be prescribed on exercise with an improvement of more than 10 per cent above baseline in walking distance or breathlessness scores with supplemental oxygen compared to air in a cylinder. In the prescription of oxygen, measurement of walking distance as well as pulse oximetry and dyspnea scores should be included.

Ambulatory oxygen is provided via small cylinders, which should always be supplied with a carry case. It is important when providing this equipment to ensure that patients can carry it, and if they are unable, that a partner can carry it or that a suitable lightweight trolley is provided.

In the UK, portables are PD11 (cannot be refilled and repeat prescription is required by a pharmacist) or portable 230 liters/minute cylinders (refillable by using a larger pressurized cylinder). These can be carried round by the patients while carrying out normal activities of daily living. On a flow rate of 2 liters/min they last up to 1 hour 50 minutes.

Advantages are that, if patients can carry the cylinders, ambulatory oxygen can allow them to leave a fixed source of continuous oxygen at home and go out, either walking or in a wheelchair. Disadvantages to patients are that the cylinders are heavy, complex to refill, and there are potential health and safety hazards if not used correctly. They are really only suitable for short periods of time and, although designed as portable, are often too heavy and difficult for patients to carry when they have low energy and breathlessness.

CONSERVER DEVICES

These are also suitable for ambulatory oxygen provision and are portable. They are inspiratory-activated devices which conserve the amount of oxygen used and allow portable cylinders to last for longer periods of time. Oxygen is conserved by providing short bursts at specific times during the inspiratory part of the respiratory cycle. This then enables the device to last for a longer period of time (up to 14 hours on 1 liter/min), dependent on the flow rate of the individual patient, but it is important to remember that they can only be used with cannulae, so if a specific percentage of oxygen is required, they are not a suitable device. They are not routinely available within the UK, and are more frequently found in Ireland and the USA.

Advantages are that these devices are lightweight, portable and last considerably longer than ordinary portable cylinders (up to six times as long). The disadvantages are that these devices can only be used with a cannulae. If the patient has severe exercise desaturation, they may not be appropriate. They are ideal only for patients on a flow rate of up to 2–3 liters/min.

LIQUID OXYGEN

Liquid oxygen is provided in insulated tanks at a temperature of −240°F with a vaporizer that converts the liquid oxygen into gaseous oxygen when the system is used. These can be used to provide long-term oxygen therapy and contain larger volumes than the gas systems. They can also deliver higher flow rates, up to 8 liters/min. However, the cylinders require refilling with liquid oxygen, delivered by lorry usually at least once a week.

This is limited within the UK and not available on ordinary prescription. It is more widely available in the USA and some European countries and is often used as the main method of providing oxygen. Liquid oxygen is stored in a large tank in the patient's home, from which it can be decanted into an additional portable device and used by the patient.

Advantages are that the ambulatory unit is more lightweight than the metal portable cylinders, and is easy to use and to refill. The disadvantages are that liquid oxygen is expensive, requires a weekly delivery and is not readily available within the UK without a private prescription.

Important considerations when a patient is being discharged home on oxygen

When prescribing or arranging domiciliary oxygen, it is essential that the patient's lifestyle is considered. Does the patient require it for school or for work? Does the patient require oxygen to be arranged not only in one home but maybe in a college flat? Does he or she intend to travel on holiday or visit friends or family at weekends?

The requirement for long-term domiciliary oxygen can be complicated and difficult for patients who want to lead independent and active lives. It is important to problem solve with them, considering the individual situations they may find themselves in when requiring to utilize additional or alternative oxygen delivery methods. Special arrangements may be necessary for patients who travel, particularly by air (see Chapter 10).

REFERENCES

Physiotherapy

1. Conway, S. P., Pond, M. N., Watson, A. and Hamnett, T. (1996) Knowledge of adult patients with cystic fibrosis about their illness. *Thorax*, **51**, 34–38.
2. Carr, L., Smith, R.E., Pryor, J.A. and Partridge, C. (1996) Cystic fibrosis patients' views and beliefs about chest clearance and exercise – a pilot study. *Physiotherapy*, **82**, 621–627.
3. Birrer, P., McElvaney, N.G., Rüdeberg, A. *et al.* (1994) Protease–antiprotease imbalance in the lungs of children with cystic fibrosis. *Am. J. Respir. Crit. Care Med.*, **150**, 207–213.
4. Khan, T. Z., Wagener, J. S., Bost, T. *et al.* (1995) Early pulmonary inflammation in infants with cystic fibrosis. *Am. J. Respir. Crit. Care Med.*, **151**, 1075–1082.
5. Phillips, G.E., Pike, S.E., Rosenthal, M. and Bush, A. (1998) Holding the baby: head downwards positioning for physiotherapy does not cause gastro-oesophageal reflux. *Eur. Respir. J.*, **12**, 954–957.
6. Button, B.M., Heine, R.G., Catto-Smith, A.G. *et al.* (1997) Postural drainage and gastro-oesophageal reflux in infants with cystic fibrosis. *Arch. Dis. Child.*, **76**, 148–150.
7. Taylor, C.J. and Threlfall, D. (1997) Postural drainage techniques and gastro-oesophageal reflux in cystic fibrosis. *Lancet*, **349**, 1567–1568.
8. International Physiotherapy Group for Cystic Fibrosis (IPG/CF) (1995) *Physiotherapy in the treatment of cystic fibrosis (CF)*, (2nd edn), IPG/CF.
9. van der Schans, C.P. and Rubin, B.K. (1997) Chest physical therapy and therapeutic devices for mucus clearance. Are they useful? *Pediatr. Pulmonol. Suppl.*, **14**, 120–121.
10. Tomashefski, J.F., Bruce, M., Goldberg, H.I. and Dearborn, D.G. (1986) Regional distribution of macroscopic lung disease in cystic fibrosis. *Am. Rev. Respir. Dis.*, **133**, 535–540.
11. Kerem, E., Reisman, J., Corey, M. *et al.* (1992) Prediction of mortality in patients with cystic fibrosis. *NEJM*, **326**, 1187–1191.
12. Pryor, J.A., Webber, B.A., Hodson, M.E. and Batten, J.C. (1979) Evaluation of the forced expiration technique as an adjunct to postural drainage in treatment of cystic fibrosis. *BMJ*, **2**, 417–418.
13. Pryor, J.A. and Webber, B.A. (1979) An evaluation of the forced expiration technique as an adjunct to postural drainage. *Physiotherapy*, **65**, 304–307.
14. Menkes, H.A. and Traystman, R.J. (1977) Collateral ventilation. *Am. Rev. Respir. Dis.*, **116**, 287–309.
15. Mead, J., Takishima, T. and Leith, D. (1970) Stress distribution in lungs: a model of pulmonary elasticity. *J. Appl. Physiol.*, **28**, 596–608.
16. West, J.B. (1992) *Pulmonary pathophysiology*, (4th edn), Williams and Wilkins, Baltimore.
17. Pryor, J.A., Webber, B.A., Hodson, M.E. and Warner, J.O. (1994) The Flutter VRP1 as an adjunct to chest physiotherapy in cystic fibrosis. *Resp. Med.*, **88**, 677–681.
18. Hofmeyr, J.L., Webber, B.A. and Hodson, M.E. (1986) Evaluation of positive expiratory pressure as an adjunct to chest physiotherapy in the treatment of cystic fibrosis. *Thorax*, **41**, 951–954.
19. Webber, B.A., Hofmeyr, J.L., Morgan, M.D.L. and Hodson, M.E. (1986) Effects of postural drainage, incorporating the forced expiration technique, on pulmonary function in cystic fibrosis. *Brit. J. Dis. Chest.*, **80**, 353–359.
20. Falk, M., Kelstrup, M., Andersen, J.B. *et al.* (1984) Improving the ketchup bottle method with positive

expiratory pressure, PEP, in cystic fibrosis. *Eur. J. Resp. Dis.*, **65**, 423–432.

21. McDonnell, T., McNicholas, W.T. and FitzGerald, M.X. (1986) Hypoxaemia during chest physiotherapy in patients with cystic fibrosis. *Irish J. Med. Sci.*, **155**, 345–348.

22. Pryor, J.A., Webber, B.A. and Hodson, M.E. (1990) Effect of chest physiotherapy on oxygen saturation in patients with cystic fibrosis. *Thorax*, **45**, 77.

23. Schöni, M.H. (1989) Autogenic drainage: a modern approach to physiotherapy in cystic fibrosis. *J. Royal Soc. Med.*, **82**, (Suppl. 16), 32–37.

24. Davidson, A.G.F., McIlwaine, P.M., Wong, L.T.K. *et al.* (1988) Physiotherapy in cystic fibrosis: a comparative trial of positive expiratory pressure, autogenic drainage and conventional percussion and drainage techniques. *Pediatr. Pulmonol. Suppl.*, **2**, 132.

25. McIlwaine, M., Davidson, A.G.F., Wong, L.T.K. and Pirie, G. (1991) The effect of chest physiotherapy by postural drainage and autogenic drainage on oxygen saturation in cystic fibrosis. *Pediatr. Pulmonol. Suppl.*, **6**, 291.

26. Davidson, A.G.F. and McIlwaine, M. (1995) Airway clearance techniques in cystic fibrosis. *New Insights into Cystic Fibrosis*, **3**, (1), 6–11.

27. Falk, M. and Andersen, J.B. (1991) Positive expiratory pressure (PEP) mask, in *Respiratory Care*, (ed. J.A. Pryor), Churchill Livingstone, Edinburgh, pp. 51–63.

28. McIlwaine, P.M., Wong, L.T., Peacock, D. and Davidson, A.G.F. (1997) Long-term comparative trial of conventional postural drainage and percussion versus positive expiratory pressure physiotherapy in the treatment of cystic fibrosis. *J. Pediatr.*, **131**, 570–574.

29. van der Schans, C.P., van der Mark, Th.W., de Vries, G. *et al.* (1991) Effect of positive expiratory pressure breathing in patients with cystic fibrosis. *Thorax*, **46**, 252–256.

30. Oberwaldner, B., Evans, J.C. and Zach, M.S. (1986) Forced expirations against a variable resistance: a new chest physiotherapy method in cystic fibrosis. *Pediatr. Pulmonol.*, **2**, 358–367.

31. McIlwaine, P.M., Wong, L.T.K., Peacock, D. and Davidson, A.G.F. (1997) 'Flutter versus PEP': a long-term comparative trial of positive expiratory pressure (PEP) versus oscillating positive expiratory pressure (Flutter) physiotherapy techniques. *Pediatr. Pulmonol. Suppl.*, **14**, 299.

32. Konstan, M.H., Stern, R.C. and Doershuk, C.F. (1994) Efficacy of the Flutter device for airway mucus clearance in patients with cystic fibrosis. *J. Pediatr.*, **124**, 689–693.

33. Flower, K.A., Eden, R.I., Lomax, L. *et al.* (1979) New mechanical aid to physiotherapy in cystic fibrosis. *BMJ*, **2**, 630–631.

34. Pryor, J.A., Parker, R.A. and Webber, B.A. (1981) A comparison of mechanical and manual percussion as adjuncts to postural drainage in the treatment of cystic fibrosis in adolescents and adults. *Physiotherapy*, **67**, 140–141.

35. Goodwin, M.J. (1994) Mechanical chest stimulation as a physiotherapy aid. *Med. Engin. Physics*, **16**, 267–272.

36. Salh, W., Bilton, D., Dodd, M. and Webb, A.K. (1989) Effect of exercise and physiotherapy in aiding sputum expectoration in adults with cystic fibrosis. *Thorax*, **44**, 1006–1008.

37. Bilton, D., Dodd, M.E., Abbot, J.V. and Webb, A.K. (1992) The benefits of exercise combined with physiotherapy in the treatment of adults with cystic fibrosis. *Resp. Med.*, **86**, 507–511.

38. Pavia, D., Thomson, M.L. and Clarke, S.W. (1978) Enhanced clearance of secretions from the human lung after the administration of hypertonic saline aerosol. *Am. Rev. Respir. Dis.*, **117**, 199–203.

39. Sutton, P.P., Gemmell, H.G., Innes, N. *et al.* (1988) Use of nebulised saline and nebulised terbutaline as an adjunct to chest physiotherapy. *Thorax*, **43**, 57–60.

40. Eng, P.A., Morton, J., Douglass, J.A. *et al.* (1996) Short-term efficacy of ultrasonically nebulized hypertonic saline in cystic fibrosis. *Pediatr. Pulmonol.*, **21**, 77–83.

41. Robinson, M., Hemming, A.L., Regnis J.A. *et al.* (1997) Effect of increasing doses of hypertonic saline on mucociliary clearance in patients with cystic fibrosis. *Thorax*, **52**, 900–903.

42. Webb, A.K. and Dodd, M.E. (1997) Nebulised antibiotics for adults with cystic fibrosis. *Thorax*, **52**, (Suppl. 2), S69–S71.

43. Sanderson, P.J. (1984) Common bacterial pathogens and resistance to antibiotics. *BMJ*, **289**, 638–639.

44. Smaldone, G.C., Vinciguerra, C. and Marchese, J. (1991) Detection of inhaled pentamidine in health care workers. *NEJM*, **325**, 891–892.

45. Hutchinson, G.R., Parker, S., Pryor, J.A. *et al.* (1996) Home-use nebulizers: a potential primary source of *Burkholderia cepacia* and other colistin-resistant, gram-negative bacteria in patients with cystic fibrosis. *J. Clin. Microbiol.*, **34**, 584–587.

46. Dodd, M.E., Hanley, S.P., Johnson, S.C. and Webb, A.K. (1995) District nebuliser compressor service: reliability and costs. *Thorax*, **50**, 82–84.

47. Sharp, J.T., Drutz, W.S., Moisan, T. *et al.* (1980) Postural relief of dyspnea in severe chronic obstructive pulmonary disease. *Am. Rev. Respir. Dis.*, **122**, 201–211.

48. Dean, E. (1985) Effect of body position on pulmonary function. *Phys. Ther.*, **65**, 613–618.

49. Potter, H.M. (1998) Musculoskeletal dysfunction, in *Physiotherapy for Respiratory and Cardiac Problems*, (eds J.A. Pryor and B.A. Webber), (2nd edn), Churchill Livingstone, Edinburgh, pp. 192–200.

50. Piper, A.J. and Ellis, E.R. (1998) Non-invasive ventilation, in *Physiotherapy for Respiratory and Cardiac Problems*, (eds J.A. Pryor and B.A. Webber), (2nd edn), Churchill Livingstone, Edinburgh, pp. 101–120.

51. LiPuma, J.J., Dasen, S.E., Nielson, D.W. *et al.* (1990) Person-to-person transmission of *Pseudomonas cepacia* between patients with cystic fibrosis. *Lancet*, **336**, 1094–1096.

52. Muhdi, K., Edenborough, F.P., Gumery, L. *et al*. (1996) Outcome for patients colonised with *Burkholderia cepacia* in a Birmingham adult cystic fibrosis clinic and the end of an epidemic. *Thorax*, **51**, 374–377.

53. Bray, C.E. (1998) Cardiopulmonary transplantation, in *Physiotherapy for Respiratory and Cardiac Problems*, (eds J.A. Pryor and B.A. Webber), (2nd edn), Churchill Livingstone, Edinburgh, pp. 413–427.

Dietary treatment of cystic fibrosis

54. Kraemar, R., Rudeberg, A., Hadorn, B. and Rossi E. (1976) Relative underweight in cystic fibrosis and its prognostic value. *Acta Paediatr. Scand*., **67**, 33–37.

55. Shale, D.J. (1997) Predicting survival in cystic fibrosis. *Thorax*, **52**, 309.

56. Hayllar, K.M., Williams, S.G., Wise, A.E. *et al*. (1997) A prognostic model for the prediction of survival in cystic fibrosis. *Thorax*, **52**, 313–317.

57. Corey, M.., McLaughlin, F.J., Williams, M., and Levison, H. (1988) A comparison of survival, growth, and pulmonary function in patients with cystic fibrosis in Boston and Toronto. *J. Clin. Epidemiol*., **41**, 588–591.

58. Koch, C. and Høiby, N. (1991) Cystic fibrosis: management of CF in different countries. Cystic fibrosis in Copenhagen. *Thorax*, **46**, (5), 383–386.

58a. Creveling, S., Light, M., Gardner, P. *et al*. (1997) Cystic fibrosis, nutrition, and the healthcare team. *J. Am. Diet. Assoc.*, **97** (10 Suppl. 2), S186–191.

59. Shwachman, H. (1975) Gastrointestinal manifestations of cystic fibrosis. *Pediatr. Clin. North Am*., **22**, 787.

60. Zentler Munro, P.L. (1983) In *Cystic Fibrosis*, (eds M.E. Hodson, A.P. Norman and J.C. Batten), Ballière Tindall, London, pp. 144–163.

61. Murphy, J.L., Wootton, S.A., Bond, S.A. and Jackson, A.A.(1991) Energy content of stools in normal healthy controls and patients with cystic fibrosis. *Arch. Dis. Child*., **66**, 495–500.

62. Morrison, G., Morrison, J., Redmond, A., Byers, C., McCracken, K. and Dodge, J.A. (1991) Pancreatic enzyme supplements in cystic fibrosis [letter]. *Lancet*, **338**, (8782–8783), 1596–1597.

63. Owen, G., Peters, T.J., Dawson, S. and Goodchild, M.C. (1991) Pancreatic enzyme supplement dosage in cystic fibrosis [letter]. *Lancet*, **338**, (8775), 1153.

64. Winnie, G.B., Standler, N.A., Fulton, J.A., McCoy, A. and Virji, M.A.(1996) pH acceptable foods vehicles for oral pancreatic enzyme supplements. *Paediatr. Pulmonol. Suppl*., **13**, 322 (abstract 408).

65. Brennan, J., Ellis, L., Kalnins, D. *et al*. (1991) Do infants with cystic fibrosis and pancreatic insufficiency require a predigested formula? *Paediatr. Pulmonol. Suppl*., **6**, 296 (abstract 264)..

66. Phelan, P.D. and Bowes, G. (1991) Cystic Fibrosis.7. Management of cystic fibrosis in different countries. Cystic fibrosis in Melbourne. *Thorax*, **46**, (5), 383–384.

67. Brady, M.S., Rickard, K., Yu, P.L. and Eigen, H. (1991) Effectiveness and safety of small vs large doses of enteric coated pancreatic enzymes in reducing steatorrhoea in children with cystic fibrosis: A prospective randomised study. *Paediatr. Pulmonol*., **10**, 79–85.

68. Baxter, P.S., Dickson, J.A.S., Variend, S. and Taylor, C.J. (1988) Intestinal disease in cystic fibrosis. *Arch. Dis. Child*., **63**, 1496–1497.

69. Robinson, P.J. and Sly, P.D. (1990) High dose pancreatic enzymes in cystic fibrosis. *Arch. Dis. Child*., **65**, 311–315

70. Smyth, R.L., van Velzen, D.K., Smyth, A.R., Lloyd, D.A. and Heaf, D.P.(1994) Strictures of ascending colon in cystic fibrosis and high strength pancreatic enzymes. *Lancet*, **343**, 85–86.

71. Smyth, R.L., Ashby, D., O'Hea, U. *et al*. (1995) Fibrosing colonopathy in cystic fibrosis; results of a case control study. *Lancet*, **346**, 1247–1251.

72. Littlewood, J.M. and Hind, C.R.K. (eds) (1996) Fibrosing colonopathy in children with cystic fibrosis. *Postgrad. Med. J*., **72** (845), 129–130.

73. Borowitz, D.S., Grand, R.J., Durie, P.R., and the Consensus Committee (1995) Use of pancreatic enzyme supplements for patients with cystic fibrosis in the context of fibrosing colonopathy. *J. Paediatr*., **127**, 681–684.

74. Booth, I.W. (1991) The nutritional consequences of gastrointestinal disease in adolescence. *Acta Paediatr. Scand. Suppl*., **37**, (3), 91–102.

75. Vaisman, N., Pencharz, P.B., Corey, M., Canny, G.J. and Hahn, E. (1987) Energy expenditure of patients with cystic fibrosis. *J. Pediatr*., **111**, 496–500.

75a. Dodge, J.A. and O'Rawe, A.M. (1996) Nutritional aspects of cystic fibrosis (Review). *Euro. J. Gastroenterol. Hepat.*, **8**, (8), 739–743.

76. O'Rawe, A., McIntosh, I., Dodge, J.A. *et al*. (1992) Increased energy expenditure in cystic fibrosis is associated with specific mutations. *Clin. Sci*., **82**, 71–76.

77. Fried, M.D., Durie, P.R., Tsui, L.C., Corey, M., Levison, H. and Pencharz, P.B., (1991) The cystic fibrosis gene and resting energy expenditure. *J. Paediatr*., **119**, 913–916.

78. Buchdahl, R.M., Cox, M., Fulleylove, C. *et al*. (1988) Increased resting energy expenditure in cystic fibrosis. *J. Appl. Physiol*., **64**, (5), 1810–1816.

79. Wainwright, C., Dean, B., McCowan, J., Grear, R., Shepherd, R. and Francis, P. (1996) Resting energy expenditure is abnormal early in CF infants and is unrelated to lung function. *Paediatr. Pulmonol*., **13**, 315 (abstract 383).

80. O'Rawe, A., Dodge, J.A., Redmond, A.O.B., McIntosh, I. and Brock, D.J.H. (1990) Gene/energy interaction in cystic fibrosis. *Lancet*, **ii**, 552–553.

81. Ramsey, B.W., Farrell, P.M., Pencharz, P., and the Consensus Committee. (1992) Nutritional assessment and management in cystic fibrosis: a consensus report. *Am. J. Clin. Nutr*., **55**, 108–116.

82. Daniels, L.A. (1984) Collection of dietary data from children with cystic fibrosis: some problems and practicalities. *Hum. Nutr. Appl. Nutr.*, **38A**, 110–118.

83. Bell, L., Durie, P. and Forstner, G.G. (1984) What do children with cystic fibrosis eat? *J. Pediatr. Gastrenterol. Nutr.*, **3**, (Suppl. 1), s137–s146.

83a. Kawchak, D.A., Zhao, H., Scanlin, T.F. *et al.* (1996) Longitudinal, prospective analysis of dietary intake in children with cystic fibrosis. *J. Pediatr.*, **129**, (1), 119–129.

84. Bell, L., Linton, W., Carey, M.L., Durie, P. and Forstner, G.G. (1981) Nutrient intakes of adolescents with cystic fibrosis. *J. Can. Dietetic Assoc.*, **42**, (1), 62–71.

85. Littlewood, J.M. and MacDonald, A. (1987) Rationale of modern dietary recommendations in cystic fibrosis. *J. R. Soc. Med.*, (Suppl. 15), **80**, 16–23.

86. Morrison, J.M., O'Rawe, A., McCracken, K.J., Redmond, A.O.B. and Dodge, J.A. (1994) Energy intake and losses in CF. *J. Hum. Nut. Diet.*, **7**, 39–46.

86a. Stark, L.J., Bowen, A.M., Tyc, V.L. *et al.* (1990) A behavioral approach to increasing calorie consumption in children with cystic fibrosis. *J. Pediatr. Psych.*, **15**, (3), 309–326.

86b. Slesinski, M.J., Gloninger, M.F., Constantino, J.P. *et al.* (1994) Lipid levels in adults with cystic fibrosis. *J. Am. Diet Assoc.*, **94**, 402–408.

87. Parsons, H.G., Beandry, P., Dumas, A. and Pencharz, P.B. (1983) Energy needs and growth in children with cystic fibrosis. *J. Pediatr. Gastroenterol. Nutr.*, **2**, 44–49.

88. Roy, C.C., Darling, P. and Weber, A.M. (1994) A rational approach to meeting macro and micro nutrient needs in cystic fibrosis. *J. Paediatr. Gastroenterol. Nutr.*, **S**, (Suppl. 1), 54–162.

89. Haymans, H.A.S. (1989) Gastrointestinal dysfunction and its effect on nutrition in cystic fibrosis. *Acta Paediatr. Scand. Suppl.*, **363**, 74–77.

90. Elborn, J.S. and Bell, S.C. (1996) Airway inflammation and nutritional status in adults with cystic fibrosis. *Paediatr. Pulmonol. Suppl.*, **13**, 163, S11.4.

90a. Vic, P., Ategbo, S., Gottrand, F. *et al.* (1997) Nutritional impact of antipseudomonas intravenous antibiotic courses in cystic fibrosis. *Arch. Dis. Child.*, **76**, (5), 437–440.

91. Spicher, V., Roulet, M., and Schutz, Y. (1991) Assessment of total energy expenditure in free living patients with cystic fibrosis. *J. Paediatr.*, **118**, 865–872.

92. Dodge, J.A. (1988) Nutritional requirements in cystic fibrosis: A review. *J. Pediatr. Gastroenterol. Nutr.*, **7**, (Suppl. 1), S8–S11.

93. MacDonald, A .(1996) Nutritional management of cystic fibrosis. *Arch. Dis. Child.*, **74**, (1), 81–87.

94. Holt, T.L., Ward, L.C., Francis, P.J., Isles, A., Cooksley, W.G. and Shepherd, R.W. (1985) Whole body protein turnover in malnourished cystic fibrosis patients and its relationship to pulmonary disease. *Am. J. Clin. Nutr.*, **41**, 1061–1066.

95. Dodge, J.A. (1985) The nutritional state and nutrition. *Acta Paediatr. Scand. Suppl.*, **317**, 31–37.

96. Goodchild, M.C. (1986) Practical management of nutrition and gastrointestinal tract in cystic fibrosis. *J. R. Soc. Med.*, **79**, (Suppl. 12), 32–35.

97. Pencharz, P.B. (1983) Energy intakes and low-fat diets in children with cystic fibrosis. *J. Paediatr. Gastroenterol. Nutr.*, **2**, 400–402.

98. Kusoffsky, E., Strandvik, B. and Troell, S. (1983) Prospective study of fatty acid supplementation over 3 years in patients with cystic fibrosis. *J. Paediatr. Gastroenterol. Nutr.*, **2**, 434–438.

99. Chase, H.P., Cotton, E.K. and Elliott, R.B. (1979) Intravenous linoleic acid supplementation in children with cystic fibrosis. *Pediatrics*, **64**, 207–213.

100. Pencharz, P.B. and Durie, P.R. (1993) Nutritional management of cystic fibrosis. *Ann. Rev. Nutr.*, **13**, 111–136.

100a. Roulet, M., Frascardo, P., Rappaz, I. and Pilet, M. (1997) Essential fatty acid deficiency in well nourished young cystic fibrosis patients. *Euro. J. Pediatr.*, **156**, (12), 952–956.

100b. Henderson, W.R., Astley, S.J., McCready, M.M. *et al.* (1994) Oral absorption of omega-3 fatty acids in patients with cystic fibrosis who have pancreatic insufficiency and in healthy control subjects. *J. Pediatr.*, **124**, 400–408.

101. Congden, P.J., Bruce, G., Rothburn, M.M. *et al.* (1981) Vitamin status in treated patients with cystic fibrosis. *Arch. Dis. Child.*, **56**, 708–714.

102. Kelleher, J. (1987) Laboratory measurement of nutrition in cystic fibrosis. *J. R. Soc. Med.*, **80**, (Suppl. 15), 28–29.

102a. Lancellotti, L., D'Orazio, C., Mastella, G. *et al.* (1996) Deficiency of vitamins A and E in cystic fibrosis is independent of pancreatic function and current enzyme and vitamin supplementation. *Euro. J. Pediatr.*, **155**, (4), 281–285.

103. Eid, N.S., Shoemaker, L.R. and Samies, T.D. (1990) Vitamin A in cystic fibrosis; case report and review of the literature. *J. Pediatr.Gastroenterol. Nutr.*, **10**, 265–269.

104. James, D.R., Owen, G., Campbell, I.A. and Goodchild, M.C. (1992) Vitamin A absorption in cystic fibrosis, risk of hypervitaminosis A. *Gut*, **33**, 707–710.

104a. Henderson, R.C. and Madsen, C.D. (1996) Bone density in children and adolescents with cystic fibrosis. *J. Pediatr.*, **128**, (1), 28–34.

105. Goodchild, M. and Dodge, J.A. (1985) *Cystic fibrosis, manual of diagnosis and management*, (2nd edn), Ballière Tindall.

106. Rashid, M., Durie, P., Kalnins, D. *et al.* (1996) Prevelance of Vitamin K deficiency in children with cystic fibrosis. *Pediatr. Pulmonol. Suppl.*, **13**, 313 (abstract 377).

107. Kelleher, J., Goode, H.F., Field, H.P., Walker, B.E., Miller, M.G. and Littlewood, J.M. (1986) Essential element nutritional status in cystic fibrosis. *Hum. Nutr. Appl. Nutr.*, **40A**, 79–84.

108. Stead, R.J., Redington, A.N., Hinks, L.J., Clayton, B.E.,

Hodson, M.E. and Batten, J.C. (1985) Selenium deficiency and possible increased risk of carcinoma in adults with cystic fibrosis. *Lancet*, **ii**, 862–863.

109. Gavin, J., Ellis, J., Dewar, A.L., Rolles, C.J. and Connett, C.J. (1997) Dietary fibre and the occurance of gut symptoms in cystic fibrosis. *Arch. Dis. Child.*, **76**, 35–37.

110. Thomas, B. (ed.) (1994) *Manual of Dietetic Practice*, (2nd edn), Blackwell Scientific Publications. Oxford.

111. Kalnins, D., Durie, P.B., Corey, M., Ellis, L., Pencharz, P. and Tullis, E. (1996) Are oral supplements effective in the nutritional management of adolescents and adults with cystic fibrosis? *Pediatr. Pulmonol. Suppl.*, **13**, 314 (abstract 381).

111a. Skypala, I., Ashworth, F.A., Hodson, M.E. *et al.* (1998) Oral nutritional supplements promote significant weight gain in cystic fibrosis patients. *J. Hum. Nutr. Diet.* **11**, 95–104.

112. MacDonald, A. (1992) Nutritional management of cystic fibrosis. Cystic Fibrosis Research Trust, 5 Blyth Road, Bromley, Kent, BR1 3RS.

113. Lester, L.A., Rothberg, R.M., Dawson, G., Lopez, A.L. and Corpuz, Z. (1986) Supplemental parenteral nutrition in cystic fibrosis. *J Parent. Ent. Nutr.*, **10**, (3), 289–295.

114. Shepherd, R., Cooksley, W.G.E. and Cooke, W.D.D. (1980) Improved growth and clinical, nutritional and respiratory changes in response to nutritional therapy in cystic fibrosis. *J. Pediatr.*, **97**, (3), 351–357.

115. Skeie, B., Askanazi, J., Rothkopf, M.M., Rosenbaum, S.H., Kvetan, V. and Ross, E. (1987) Improved exercise tolerance with long term parenteral nutrition in cystic fibrosis. *Crit. Care Med.*, **15**, (10), 960–962.

116. Moore, M.C., Greene, H.L., Donald, W.D. and Dunn, G.D. (1986) Enteral tube feeding as adjunct therapy in malnourished patients with cystic fibrosis: a clinical study and literature review. *Am. J. Clin. Nutr.*, **44**, 33–41.

117. Steinkamp, G. and Von der Hardt, H. (1994) Improvement of nutritional status and lung function after long-term nocturnal gastrostomy feedings in cystic fibrosis. *J. Paediatr.*, **124**, (2), 244–249.

118. Smith, D.L., Clark, J.M. and Stableforth, D.E. (1994) A nocturnal nasogastric feeding programme in cystic fibrosis adults. *J. Hum. Nutr. Dietet.*, **7**, (4), 257–262.

119. Levy, L.D., Durie, P.R., Pencharz, P.B. and Corey, M.L. (1985) Effects of long term nutritional rehabilitation on body composition and clinical status in malnourished children and adolescents with cystic fibrosis. *J. Pediatr.*, **107**, 225–230.

120. Boland, M.P., Patrick, J., Stoski, D.S. and Soucy, P. (1987) Permanent enteral feeding in cystic fibrosis: advantages of a replaceable jejunostomy tube. *J. Pediatr. Surg.*, **22**, (9), 843–847.

121. Boland, M.P., MacDonald, N.E., Stoski, D.S., Soucy, P. and Patrick, J. (1986) Chronic jejunostomy feeding with a non-elemental formula in undernourished patients with cystic fibrosis. *Lancet*, **i**, 232–234.

121a. Williams, S.G., Ashworth, F.A., McAlweenie, A. *et al.*

(1999) Percutaneous endoscopic gastrostomy feeding in children and adults with cystic fibrosis. *GUT*, **44**, (1), 87–90.

122. Durie, P.R., Newth, C.J., Forstner, G.G. and Gall, D.G. (1980) Malabsorption of medium chain triglycerides in infants with cystic fibrosis: correction with pancreatic enzyme supplements. *J. Pediatr.*, **96**, 862.

122a. Erskine, J.M., Lingard, C.D., Sontag, M.K. *et al.* (1998) Enteral nutrition for patients with cystic fibrosis: comparison of a semi-elemental and non-elemental formula. *J. Pediatr.*, **132**, (2), 265–269.

123. Kane, R.E., Hobbs, P.J. and Black, P.G. (1990) Comparison of low, medium and high carbohydrate formulas for night time enteral feedings in cystic fibrosis patients. *J. Parent. Ent. Nutr.*, **14**, (1), 47–52.

124. Finkelstein, S.M., Wielinski, C.L., Elliott, G.R. *et al.* (1988) Diabetes mellitus associated with cystic fibrosis. *J. Pediatr.*, **112**, 373–377.

125. Lanng, S., Thorsteinsson, B., Nerup, J. and Koch, C. (1992) Influence of the development of diabetes mellitus on clinical status in patients with cystic fibrosis. *Eur. J. Paediatr.*, **151**, 684–687.

126. Cystic Fibrosis Foundation (1990) *Cystic Fibrosis Foundation concensus conferences on Diabetes*, Cystic Fibrosis Foundation, USA, Vol. 1, section IV, pp.1–8.

126a. Ashworth, F.A., Bramwell, E.C., Yung, B. *et al.* (1999) The management of Cystic Fibrosis related diabetes. *Brit. J. Homecare*, **1**, (4), 136–140.

127. British Diabetic Association (1991) Dietary recommendations for people with diabetes: an update for the 1990's. *J. Hum. Nutr. Dietet.*, **4**, 393–412.

128. Mueller, D. (1990) Nutrition for CF patients with diabetes mellitus. *Pediatr. Pulmonol. Suppl.*, **5**, 109, S 7.2.

128a. Kotloff, R.M., FitzSimmons, S.C. and Fiel, S.B. (1992) Fertility and pregnancy in patients with cystic fibrosis. *Clin. Chest. Med.*, **13**, 623–635.

129. HMSO (1991) *Dietary reference values for food, energy and nutrients for the United Kingdom*, HMSO Report on Health and Social Subjects, 41, HMSO, London.

130. Department of Health (1992) *Folic acid and the prevention of neural tube defects*. Report from an expert advisory panel., HMSO, London.

131. Chief Medical Officer (1990) *Women cautioned: watch your vitamin intake*, Department of Health press release no. 90/507, London.

132. Whitelaw, A. and Butterfield, A. (1977) High breast milk sodium in CF. *Lancet*, **ii**, 1288.

133. Alpert, S.E. and Cormier, A.D. (1983) Normal electrolyte and protein content in milk from mothers with CF: an explanation for the initial report of elevated milk sodium concentration. *J. Pediatr.*, **102**, 77–80.

134. Stead, R.J., Brueton, M.J., Hodson, M.E. and Batten, J.C. (1987) Should mothers with CF breast feed? (letter) *Arch. Dis. Child.*, **62**, (4), 433.

135. Valletta, E.A. and Mastella, G. (1988) Incidence of coeliac disease in a cystic fibrosis population. *Acta Paediatr. Scand.*, **78**, 784–785.

Nursing

136. Whyte, D.A. (1992) A family nursing approach to the care of a child with a chronic illness. *J. Adv. Nurs.*, **17**, 317–327.

137. Van Os, D.K., Clark, C.G., Turner, C.W. and Herbst, J.J. (1985) Life stress and cystic fibrosis. *West. J. Nurs. Res.*, **7**, 301–315.

138. Cooper, M. (1992) Playing the game. *Nurs. Stand.*, **6**, (21), 22–23.

139. Aspin, A.J. (1991) Psychological consequences of cystic fibrosis in adults. *Br. J. Hosp. Med.*, **45**, 368–371.

140. Gode, R.O. and Smith, M.S. (1983) Development: self, family, friends and school, in *Effects of Chronic Disorders on Adolescents*, (ed. M.S. Scott), John Wright, Bristol, pp. 31–44.

141. Goodchild, M.C. and Dodge, J.A. (1985) *Cystic fibrosis Manual of Diagnosis and Management*, Ballière Tindall, London, pp. 43–44.

142. Phelan, P. and Key, E. (1984) Cystic fibrosis mortality in England and Wales and in Victoria, Australia 1976–80. *Arch. Dis. Child.*, **59**, 71–73.

143. Stewart, A. (1984) The primary care team's role. *Nurs. Times*, 23 May, 34–35.

144. Bowlby, J. (1953) *Child Care and the Growth of Love*, Penguin, Harmondsworth.

145. Morton, N.S. (1993) Balanced analgesia for children. *Nurs. Stand. Suppl.*, **7**, (21), 8–10.

146. Stead, R.J., Davidson, T.I., Duncan, F.R. *et al.* (1987) Use of a totally implantable system for venous access in cystic fibrosis. *Thorax*, **42**, 149–150.

147. Fellow, I.W. and Mansell, P.I. (1980) Percutaneous endoscopic gastrostomy. *Intensive Ther. Clin. Monitor.*, June/July, 179–180.

148. Mackenzie, H. (1988) Teenagers in hospital. *Nurs. Times*, **84**, 58–61.

149. Coffman, C.B., Levine, S.B., Althof, S.E. and Stern, R.C. (1984) Sexual adaptation among single young adults with cystic fibrosis. *Chest*, **86**, 412–418.

150. Dibble, S.L. and Savedra, M.C. (1988) Cystic fibrosis in adolescence: a new challenge. *Paediatr. Nurs.*, **14**, 299–303.

151. Silber, S.J., Ord, T., Balmaceda, J. *et al.* (1990) Congenital absence of the vas deferens. The fertilizing capacity of human epididymal sperm. *NEJM.*, **323**, 1788–1792.

152. Stead, R.J., Grimmer, S.F., Rogers, S.M. *et al.* (1987) Pharmacokinetics of contraceptive steroids in patients with CF. *Thorax*, **42**, 59–64.

153. Canney, G.J., Corey, M., Livingstone, R.A. *et al.* (1991) Pregnancy and cystic fibrosis. *Obstet. Gynecol.*, **77**, 850–853.

154. Khawaja, H.T., Campbell, M.J. and Weaver, P.C. (1988) Effect of transdermal glyceryl trinitrate on the survival of peripheral intravenous infusions: a double-blind prospective clinical study. *Br. J. Surg.*, **75**, 1212–1215.

155. Hecker, J.F. (1992) Review. Potential for extending survival of peripheral intravenous infusions. *BMJ*, **304**, 619–624.

156. Hodson, M.E. (1992) Diabetes mellitus and cystic fibrosis. *Baillières Clin. Endocrinol. Metab.*, **6**, 797–805.

157. Yung, B., Landers, A., Mathalone, B., Gyi, K.M. and Hodson, M.E. (1998) Diabetic retinopathy in adult patients with CF related diabetes. *Resp. Med.*, **92**, 871–872.

158. Davidson, A.C., Harrison, K., Steinfort, C.L. and Geddes, D.M. (1987) Distal intestinal obstruction syndrome in cystic fibrosis treated by oral intestinal lavage and a case of recurrent obstruction despite normal pancreatic function. *Thorax*, **42**, 518–541.

159. Hodson, M.E., Madden, B.P., Steven, M.H. *et al.* (1991) Non-invasive mechanical ventilation for cystic fibrosis patients – a potential bridge to transplantation. *Eur. Respir. J.*, **4**, 524–527.

160. Charnock, A. (1983) Care of the dying. *Nurs. Times*, 21 Sept., 64.

161. Geddes, D.M. and Hodson, M.E. (1989) The role of heart and lung transplantation in the treatment of cystic fibrosis. *J. R. Soc. Med.*, **82**, (Suppl. 16), 49–53.

162. Anon. (1983) Death in the first person. *Nurs. Times*, 21 Sept., 64.

163. Bergman, A., West, A. and Leviston, N. (1979) Social work practice and chronic paediatric illness. *Soc. Work Hlth Care*, **4**, 265–274.

164. Dodge, J.A., Morison, S., Lewis, P.A. *et al.* (the U.K. Cystic Fibrosis Survey Management Committee) (1997) 1968–1995: incidence, population and survival. *Arch. Dis. Child.*, **77**, (6), 493–496.

165. Coady, C.A., Kent, V.D. and Davis, P.A. (1990) Burnout amongst social workers working with CF. *Hlth Soc. Work*, May, 116–124.

Cystic fibrosis home care

166. Council on Scientific Affairs (1990) Home care in the 1990s. *J. Am. Med. Assoc.*, **263**, 1241–1244.

167. NHS Management Executive (1995) *Purchasing high-tech health care for patients at home*, EL95(5), NHSME, Leeds.

168. Leen, G. (1992) *An assessment of stress experienced by parents in administering home intravenous treatment to their child with cystic fibrosis*. XIth Inter, CF Congress Dublin.

169. Brooks, R. (1996) Your place or mine. *Hlth Services J.*, April, 35.

170. Fay, L. and Evans, M. (1997) Direct line to home. *Nursing Times*, **93**, (37), 29–30.

171. Van Aalderen, W.M.C., Mannes, G.P.M., Bosma, E.S., Roorda, R.J. and Heymans, H.A.S. (1995) Home care in cystic fibrosis patients. *Eur. Respir. J.*, **8**, 172–175.

172. Kiettke, U., Magdorf, K., Staab, D., Paul, K. and Wahn, U. (1998) Can home therapy replace hospital intravenous antibiotic therapy in patients with cystic fibrosis in Germany? Department of Paediatric Pneumology and

Immunology, Virchow Clinic of Humboldt University, Heckeshorn Chest Hospital, Berlin, Germany.

173.   Secretary of State for Health (1997) *The New NHS: Modern Dependable*, HMSO, London.

174.   Wolter, J.M., Bowler, S.D., Nolan, J.G. and McCotteck, JG. (1997) Home intravenous therapy in cystic fibrosis: a prospective randomised trial examining clinical, quality of life and cost aspects. *Eur. Resp. J.*, **10**, 896–900.

175.   Kayley, J., Berendt, A.R., Snelling, M.J.M. *et al.* (1996) *Safe intravenous antibiotic therapy at home: experience of an UK based programme*, The British Society for Antimicrobial Chemotherapy, pp. 1023–1029.

176.   Pilling, M. and Walley, T. (1997) Effective high tech homecare services. *Hlth Soci Care Commun.*, **5**, (2), 134–146.

177.   Hughes, S. (1993) Meeting a need. *Nursing Times*, **89**, (39), 36–37.

178.   Duncan-Skingle, F. and Bramwell, E. (1992) Home help. *Nursing Times*, **88**, (31), 34–35.

179.   Aspin, A.J. (1991) Psychological consequences of cystic fibrosis in adults. *Br. J. Hosp. Med.*, **45**, 368–371.

180.   Worth, A., Tierney, A. and Lockerbie, L. (1994) Community nurses and discharge planning. *Nursing Standard*, **8**, (21), 25–30.

181.   Gnanapragasam, S., Hanchet, S., Mills, J. and Hill, M. (1995) Paediatric homecare team. *Nursing Times*, **91**, (9), 28–30.

182.   Cohen, P. (1997) Intravenous therapy at home. *Nursing Times*, **93**, (15), 42.

183.   Kei-Cheung Chuk, P. (1997) Clinical nurse specialists and quality patient care. *J. Adv. Nursing*, **26**, 501–506.

184.   Rogers, D., and Goodchild M.C. (1996) Role of a domiciliary physiotherapist in the treatment of children with cystic fibrosis. *Physiotherapy*, **82**, 396–402.

185.   Oldham, D. (1997) Nurse-led asthma clinic in an Asian community. *Nursing Times*, **93**, (13), 58–59.

186.   Sawyer, E. (1992) Family functioning when children have cystic fibrosis. *J. Paediatr. Nursing*, **7**, (5), 304–310.

187.   Nagy, S. and Unger, J.A. (1990) The adaptation of mothers and fathers to children with cystic fibrosis: a comparison. *CHC*, **19**, (3), 147–153.

188.   Bradley, S. (1997) Better late than never? An evaluation of community nursing services for children in the UK. *J. Clin. Nursing*, **6**, 411–418.

189.   While, A. (1991) An evaluation of pediatric home care schemes. *J. Adv. Nursing*, **16**, 1413–1421.

190.   Conway, A. (1996) Home intravenous therapy for bronchiectasis patients *Nursing Times*, **92**, (45), 34–35.

191.   Plumer, A.L. (1987) *Principles and practices of intravenous therapy*, (4th edn), Little, Brown and Co., Boston.

192.   Pryor, J.A. and Webber, B.A. (1998) *Physiotherapy for respiratory and cardiac problems*, (2nd edn), Churchill Livingstone, Edinburgh, chapter 20, p. 469.

193.   Carr, L., Pryor, J.A. and Hodson, M.E. (1995) Self chest clapping. *Physiotherapy*, **81**, (12), 753–757.

194.   Stephenson, K. (1989) Giving antibiotics at home. *Nursing Standard*, **3**, (40), 24–25.

195.   Bramwell, E.C., Halpin, D.M.G., Duncan-Skingle, F., Hodson, M.E. and Geddes, G.M. (1995) Home treatment of patients with cystic fibrosis using the 'Intermate': the first year's experience. *J. Adv. Nursing*, **22**, 1063–1067.

196.   Elborn, J.S,. Shale. D.J. and Britton, J.R. (1994) Heart–lung transplantation in cystic fibrosis: predictions for the next decade in England and Wales. *Resp. Med.*, **88**, (2), 135–138 (abstract).

197.   Duncan-Skingle, F. and Foster, F. (1991) Heart–lung transplantation – the other part of the story. *ACFA*, Dec., 6.

198.   Sharples, L., Hathaway, T., Dennis, C., Caine, N., Higenbottam, T. and Wailwork, J. (1993) Prognosis of patients with cystic fibrosis awaiting heart and lung transplantation. *J. Heart Lung Transplant.*, **12**, (4), 669–673.

199.   Sexton, B. (1998) Assisted ventilation in cystic fibrosis: Nursing Care. *Nursing Standard*, **12**, (52), 52–54.

200.   Dyer, J. (1997) Cystic fibrosis nurse specialist: a key role. *J. R. Soc. Med.*, **90**, (Suppl. 31), 21–25.

201.   Hodson, M.E., Madden, M., Steven, M.H., Tsang, V.T. and Yaeoub, M.H. (1991) Non-invasive mechanical ventilation for cystic fibrosis. Patients, a potential bridge to transplantation. *Eur. Resp. J.*, **4**, 524–527.

202.   Bluebond Langner, M. (1996) *In the Shadow of Illness*, Princetown University Press, chapter 11, pp. 135–196.

203.   While, A., Citrone, C. and Cornish, J. (1995) A study of the needs and provisions for families caring for children with life-limited incurable disorders. Executive Summary, Department of Nursing Studies King's College London.

204.   Pilling, M. and Walley, T. (1997) Parentral antibiotics at home in cystic fibrosis: experiences and attitudes of recipients. *Hlth Soc. Care Commun.*, **5**, (3), 209–212.

205.   Pilling, M. and Walley, T. (1996) Contracting for high-tech health care for patients at home: a survey of purchaser responses. *J. Managt. Med.*, **10**, (6), 17–23.

206.   Nathwani, D. and Davey, P. (1996) Intravenous antimicrobial therapy in the community underused, inadequately resources, or irrelevant to healthcare in Britain? *BMJ*, **313**, 1541–1543.

207.   Community Health Services (1996) UK Domiciliary Care Market Report, pp. 38–45.

208.   Vettner, N. (1995) *The Hospital From Centre of Excellence to Community Support*, Chapman & Hall, London, chapter 10, pp. 182–197.

Social work

209.   Griffiths, R. (1989) *Community Care: An Agenda for Action*. HMSO, London.

210.   Neale, T. (1987) Future service development, in *Cystic Fibrosis Project: A survey of the Needs of Families in the Midlands Area*, Barnardos, Midlands, pp. 47–48.

211. Homrighausen Zander, J. (1989) The family, in *Cystic Fibrosis. A Guide for Patient and Family*, (ed. D.N. Orenstein), Raven Press, New York, 121–128.

212. Norman, A.P. and Hodson, M.E. (1983) Emotional and social aspects of treatment, in *Cystic Fibrosis*, (eds M.E. Hodson, A. Norman and J.C. Batten), Baillière Tindall, London, pp. 242–258.

213. Bluebond-Langer, M. (1990) Living with cystic fibrosis. The well siblings' perspective. *Pediatr. Pulmonol.*, **5**, 177–178.

214. Warwick, W.J. (1989) Faith, hope and control as factors in cystic fibrosis. *Pediatr. Pulmonol.*, **4**, 77–79.

215. Lask, B. (1990) Depression, denial, and reality. *Pediatr. Pulmonol.*, **5**, 179.

216. Pinkerton, P., Trauer, T., Duncan, F. *et al.* (1985) Cystic fibrosis in adult life – a study of coping patterns. *Lancet*, **i**, 761–763.

217. Orenstein, D.M. and Rogers, D.R. (1989) Daily life, in *Cystic Fibrosis. A Guide for Patient and Family*, (ed. D.M. Orenstein), Raven Press, New York, 95–99.

218. Harris, A. and Super, M. (1991) *Cystic Fibrosis, The Facts*, Oxford University Press, Oxford.

219. Walters, S., Britton, J. and Hodson, M.E. (1993) Demographic and social characteristics of adults with cystic fibrosis in the United Kingdom. *BMJ*, **306**, 549–552.

220. Perobelli, S. (1992) The psychosocial situation of CF adults living independently, in *Cystic Fibrosis, Basic and Clinical Research*, (eds N. Høiby and S.S. Pedersen), Elsevier Science Publishers, Amsterdam, pp. 193–200.

221. Charmaz, K. (1992) The effects of intrusive illness on self-concept: adult patients' perspectives. *Pediatr. Pulmonol.*, **8**, 230–231.

222. Duncan Skingle, F. (1992) Quality of life after heart lung transplantation (HLT), in *Cystic Fibrosis, Basic and Clinical Research*, (eds N. Høiby and S.S. Pedersen), Elsevier Science Publishers, Amsterdam, pp. 201–203.

223. Pincus, L. (1976) *Death and the Family*, Faber and Faber, London.

224. Parkes, C.M. (1972) *Bereavement: Studies of Grief in Adult Life*. Tavistock, London.

225. Smith S.C. and Pennells M, (1995) Interventions with Bereaved Children. Jessica Kingsley Publishers, London.

Occupational therapy

226. Bluebond-Langer, M. (1991) Living with cystic fibrosis: a family affair, in *Young People and Death*, (ed. J. Morgan), Charles Press, Philadelphia.

227. Hagerdorn, R. (1997) *Foundations for Practice in Occupational Therapy*, Churchill Livingstone, Edinburgh, p.5

228. Bluebond-Langer, M. (1991) *Natural History of Cystic Fibrosis*. Philadelphia.

229. LIACE, (1991) *Occupational Therapy Guidelines for Client-Centred Practice*, CAOT, Toronto, Canada.

230. McSweeney, A. J., Grant, I., Heaton, R.K., Adams, K.M. and Timmins, R.M. (1982) Life quality of patients with chronic obstructive pulmonary disease. *Arch. Intern. Med.*, **142**, 473–478.

231. Eakin, P. (1991) Outcome of therapy in stroke rehabilitation 'Do we know what we are doing?' *Br. J. Occupat. Ther.*, **54**, (8), 305–307.

232. Law, M., Baptiste, S. *et al.* (1994) *Canadian Occupational Performance Measure*, (2nd edn) CAOT, Ontario, Canada.

233. Shriver, A.C., Dekker, F.N. *et al.* (1990) Quality of life in elderly patients with chronic nonspecific lung disease in family practice. *Chest*, **98**, 894–899.

234. Sachs, G., Haber, P., Speiss, K. and Moser, G. (1993) Effectiveness of relaxation groups in patients with chronic respiratory tract diseases. *Wien. Klin. Hochensch.*, **105**, **21**, 603–610.

235. Wijkestra, PJ., Van Atterna, R., Kraau, J. *et al.* (1994) Quality of life in patients with chronic obstructive pulmonary disease improves after rehabilitation at home. *Eur. Resp. J.*, **7**, 269–273.

236. Shriver, A.C., Dekker, F.N. *et al.* (1990) Quality of life in elderly patients with chronic nonspecific lung disease in family practice. *Chest*, **98**, 894–899.

237. Salt, V.L. and Kerr, K.M. (1997) Mitchell's simple physiological relaxation and Jacobson's progressive relaxation techniques: a comparison. *Physiotherapy*, **83**, (4), 200–207.

238. Renfroe, K.L. (1988) Effect of progressive relaxation on dyspnea and state anxiety in patients with chronic obstructive pulmonary disease. *Heart and Lung: J. Crit. Care*, **17**, (4), 408–413.

239. Royle, J.A., Blythe, J., Ingram, C., DiCenso, A., Bhatnager, N. and Potvin, C. (1996) The research utilisation process: the use of guided imagery to reduce anxiety. *Can. Oncol. Nursing J.*, **6**, (1), 20–25.

240. Delk, K.K., Gevirtz, R., Hicks, D.A., Carden, F. and Rucker, R. (1994) The effects of biofeedback assisted breathing retraining on lung functions in patients with cystic fibrosis. *Chest: Cardiopulmon. J.*, **105**, (1), 23–28.

241. Dewees, J.A. (19XX) Ten simple solutions in the workplace. *Am. J. Occupat. Ther.*, **14**, (3), 4–5

242. Gilbert, D.W. (1965) Energy expenditures for the disabled homemaker. *Am. J. Occupat. Ther.*, **19**, (6), 321–328.

243. Parent, L.H. (1986) Energy: the illusive factor in daily activity. *Occupat. Ther. Hlth Care*, **3**, (1), 5–15.

244. Helm, M. (1987) *Occupational Therapy with the Elderly*, Churchill Livingstone, London.

245. Mandiestam, M. (1992) *How to get Equipment for Disability*. Jessica Kinglsey Publishers, London.

246. Judge, F. and McClusky, J. (1996) Bathing and toileting equipment for the elderly. *Br. J. Ther. Rehabil.*, **3**, (3), 128–134.

247. Hoffman, A., Geelkeren, R.H. *et al.* (1994) Pressure sores and pressure relieving mattresses, controlled clinical trial. *Lancet*, **343**, 560–571.

248. Kavanagh, J. and Cornwell, M. (1996) The role of the

wheelchair in the mobility chain. *Br. J. Ther. Rehabil.*, **3**, (2), 69–74.

249.   Bore, J. (1994) Occupational therapy home visits: a satisfactory service? *Br. J. Occupat. Ther.*, **57**, (3), 85–88.

250.   Nixon, P.A., Orenstein, D.M., Curtis, S.E. *et al*. (1990) Oxygen supplementation during exercise in cystic fibrosis. *Am. Rev. Respir. Dis.,* **142**, 807–811.

20

Exercise and training for adults with cystic fibrosis

A. K. WEBB AND M. E. DODD

Introduction	433	Exercise training programs	439
Exercise responses and training in health	433	Conclusion	443
Exercise limitations in cystic fibrosis	434	References	444
Studies of exercise testing and training programs in cystic fibrosis	437		

INTRODUCTION

Exercise training programs for patients with cystic fibrosis (CF) are increasingly seen to have a therapeutic role[1-6]. Exercise can be a pleasurable addition to the domiciliary discipline of complex self-care which includes chest clearance, optimal nutrition, multiple oral and inhaled medications, and sometimes intravenous antibiotics. In general, the benefits of exercise have been viewed as enhancing sputum clearance[6], reducing breathlessness[5] and improving patient mobility. As a consequence, CF patients can mix more easily with their peers and enjoy a better quality of life with a better exercise capacity[7]. As CF patients now have a mean survival into the fourth decade of life[8] the factors that improve survival are being evaluated. Nutrition and pulmonary function are the best prognostic indices of survival[9-10]. They correlate strongly with each other and best values are achieved when care is delivered by a multidisciplinary team from a CF center[11]. Additionally, components of fitness such as peak work capacity and peak oxygen consumption are associated with a better prognosis for CF patients, as has been suggested by some retrospective studies[12-13], but there are no long-term prospective published studies to confirm this work.

During their educational years CF patients with mild to moderate disease can usually participate both socially and competitively in sporting activities at the same level as their healthy peers. Sporting activities are often compulsory at school and facilities for exercise are readily available. However, when the CF child becomes an adult and commences employment, exercise often ceases. In addition, there is increasing concern relating to the decreased levels of fitness and habitual activity for the population as a whole. At the same time, respiratory disease, the main cause of death in CF, is progressing[14]. A more sedentary lifestyle is adopted, with a reduction in cardiorespiratory reserve and decreased exercise efficiency. Quality of life declines and the patient becomes more disabled and demoralized, with a consequent impact upon quality of life. The prescription of individualized exercise programs may remedy this decline. The majority of unfit CF patients with mild to moderate disease have the capacity to exercise and increase fitness in a manner similar to their peers[15-16]. Patients who because of advanced disease have very limited exercise capacity should not be excluded from training programs and may have most to gain from an increase in function. Patient mobility can be maintained for patients with the severest disease awaiting organ transplantation. It is therefore important to measure the exercise limits of CF patients with all grades of disease severity and, using this information, recommend individualized, safe and effective training programs.

EXERCISE RESPONSES AND TRAINING IN HEALTH

In health, exercise capacity is constrained by circulatory rather than ventilatory limits. Muscles fatigue and exercise ceases once the limits of stroke volume, cardiac frequency and oxygen delivery have been reached.

The most commonly used physiological measurements of exercise capacity are oxygen consumption ($\dot{V}O_2$) and peak work capacity (PWC). The oxygen consumption reflects the supply of oxygen by the cardiorespiratory system and its uptake by working muscles.

The maximum oxygen uptake ($\dot{V}O_2$max) represents the efficiency of the cardiorespiratory system to deliver oxygen to working muscles and the ability of these muscles to endure sustained use and can usefully be defined as follows:

$$\dot{V}O_2\text{max} = \text{stroke volume} \times \text{heart rate} \times \text{arteriovenous oxygen difference.}$$

From the above equation it can be seen that several physiological adaptations following training will influence the $\dot{V}O_2$max.

During exercise, ventilation rises in a linear fashion until oxygen consumption reaches a level of 60–70 per cent of $\dot{V}O_2$max[17]. At this point, oxygen supply becomes inadequate to meet demand, anaerobic metabolism begins and lactic acid accumulates. The consequent increased CO_2 production due to buffering by bicarbonate and then acidosis leads to increasing ventilatory drive and there is an upward inflexion of ventilation. This point is referred to as the anaerobic threshold and occurs early in untrained subjects. During exercise, ventilation can increase from 5 liters/min at rest to 180 liters/min in the trained athelete. This is achieved by changes in tidal volume (V_T) and breathing frequency (bf) and adjustments in the duty cycle of breathing (T_I/T_{tot}) which is defined as the ratio of inspiratory time (T_I) to total breath duration T_{tot}, resulting in alterations to inspiratory ($V_T \backslash T_I$) and expiratory flow rates. Tidal volume (V_T) increases with exercise until it reaches a maximum value of 60 per cent of vital capacity and then ventilation continues to rise due to increased breathing frequency. Inspiratory and expiratory times are balanced to increase V_T and allow the lungs to empty to maintain functional residual capacity. Consequently, flow is maintained to preserve alveolar ventilation. Breathing patterns are adapted in health and disease to minimize the sense of effort arising in the respiratory muscles. There is more even matching of ventilation and perfusion with increasing exercise which reduces the physiological dead space. Exercise becomes limited finally when the symptoms of breathlessness or muscular fatigue exceed that which the person is prepared to tolerate. The sense of muscle fatigue becomes most acute when muscle metabolism enters the anaerobic phase and lactic acid accumulates due to inadequate oxygen supply.

Before training, the cardiac limits to exercise are cardiac frequency and the size of the stroke volume. Following training, stroke volume increases due to cardiac hypertrophy with an increase in wall thickness and chamber size; cardiac output is higher at maximal exer-

cise and more oxygen will be delivered to muscles at a lower heart rate for a given level of activity.

In trained skeletal muscle, structural and biochemical changes take place. There is an increase in muscle capillary and fiber size. At a cellular level, the mitochondria and mitochondrial enzymes increase. A greater supply of oxygen is delivered by the cardiorespiratory system and more efficiently extracted by skeletal muscle, which accounts for the widening of the arteriovenous oxygen difference following training. These changes permit exercise to continue aerobically for a longer period of time. Training delays the onset of lactic acid accumulation, improves lactic acid tolerance and increases the time allowed for comfortable aerobic exercise[18]. The purpose of a training program should be to increase endurance rather than increase the level of maximum exercise. Training will increase the $\dot{V}O_2$max in both health and disease and the degree of improvement is inversely related to initial fitness.

The purpose of training in both health and disease is to promote those physiological adaptations which will increase fitness and improve exercise performance. Fitness can be defined broadly as the capacity to endure more exercise without discomfort following training.

EXERCISE LIMITATIONS IN CYSTIC FIBROSIS

The exercise capacity of CF patients is limited by the impaired mechanics of diseased lungs and compromised gas exchange[19–21]. Lower levels of activity in CF children have also been related to poor nutritional status[22] and diminished exercise capacity in both CF children and adults may be correlated with both the quality and quantity of muscle (see below). Although pulmonary function and nutrition are the most important correlates of peak oxygen consumption[19–21], $\dot{V}O_2$ peak is also influenced by age, gender, height, hemoglobin concentration, motivation, conditioning and muscle mass. At higher levels of pulmonary function, neither the forced expiratory volume in one second (FEV_1) nor body mass index (BMI: weight in kilogram divided by (height in meters)^2) as a measure of nutritional status is a good predictor of peak performance in an individual[23].

Ventilatory mechanics during exercise

One of the earliest observed abnormalities of pulmonary function in CF is an increase in the physiological dead space which increases with disease severity[19]. In health and in patients with mild CF the resting ratio of physiological dead space to tidal volume (V_D/V_T) is 25–35 per cent and decreases with exercise due to the increase in tidal volume. In patients with severe disease, this resting ratio is high and increases with exercise due to a limited tidal volume and severe mismatching of ventilation and perfusion. Ventilation is higher for a given workload.

In health, tidal volume increases to 60 per cent of vital capacity during exercise[24]. CF patients with mild to moderate disease (FEV_1 60 per cent predicted) can exercise to almost the same degree as their normal peers but those patients with severe disease (FEV_1 less than 40 per cent predicted) have little capacity to increase their tidal volume during exercise. Breathing frequency must increase in order to maintain alveolar ventilation. This compensatory mechanism aggravates dynamic hyperinflation of the lungs. The increased breathing frequency also creates excessive work for the respiratory muscles and exercise ceases.

During exercise, minute ventilation is maintained by balancing inspiratory and expiratory flow rates. Regnis *et al.* have studied the changes in lung volume and breathing patterns that take place during exercise in CF patients with severe lung disease[25]. These patients (mean FEV_1 29 per cent predicted) increased their end-expiratory lung volume during exercise, which minimized expiratory flow limitation but resulted in hyperinflation, limited work capacity and an inability to increase tidal volume. These patients were only able to triple their inspiratory and expiratory flow rates at maximal exercise. In the same study, patients with moderately severe disease (FEV_1 as low as 50 per cent predicted) were able to increase expiratory flow rates eightfold and normalize end-expiratory lung volume.

HYPERCAPNIA DURING EXERCISE

Concern has been expressed about the development of hypercapnia during progressive exercise in CF patients with advanced disease. Coates *et al.* have studied the effect of severe airflow limitation, physiological dead space and the timing components of ventilation upon gas exchange with increasing exercise[26]. All patients had advanced lung disease but the group that retained carbon dioxide (CO_2) were characterized by lower values for FEV_1, a greater arterial oxygen desaturation and a rise in end-tidal CO_2; there was a significantly smaller maximal exercise ventilation. T_I/T_{tot} (the ratio of time spent in inspiration to total respiratory time) was reduced. It is suggested that hypercapnia was associated in this group with a cutoff in inspiration causing a reduction in tidal volume and ventilation. In this study, although CO_2 retention occurred during the initial stages of exercise, the rise ceased half way through exercise and did not imply the onset of respiratory failure. Hypercapnia can be considered an economical response to the excessive work of breathing whereby the effort of ventilation and dyspnea is minimized.

Rochester[27] has suggested that the adoption of a similar breathing pattern and associated hypercapnia in patients with chronic obstructive airways disease (COAD) may forestall inspiratory muscle fatigue.

However, not all CF patients with severe disease retain CO_2 during exercise. The pattern of respiratory mechanical response may be constitutionally determined by the inherent CO_2 sensitivity which may show wide variation in CF[28]. In contrast, studies in CF children have demonstrated a normal neural drive to breathing as expressed by the $P_{0.1}$ (pressure generated at the mouth in the first 100 ms of inspiration through an occluded mouthpiece). Ventilatory response was diminished with worsening lung disease and characterized by an increase in breathing frequency and no increase in tidal volume[29]. A recent study has shown impaired carbon dioxide excretion during maximal exercise testing of CF patients with mild lung disease[30]. Arterialized blood samples rather than end-tidal CO_2 were used for gas analysis. The authors attributed their findings primarily to the increased physiological dead space ventilation consequent upon ventilation perfusion mismatch, although an alternative explanation might be an 'adaptive' blunting of the ventilatory response to acidosis.

HYPOXIA DURING EXERCISE

The majority of CF patients are able to preserve their arterial oxygen pressure during exercise but significant desaturation occurs with severe disease. Studies have reported the following predictors for exercise-induced arterial oxygen desaturation: an FEV_1 of less than 50 per cent of vital capacity[31]; an FEV_1 less than or equal to 60 per cent predicted[20]; and if the diffusing capacity (DLCO) of the lungs was greater than 80 per cent predicted then no desaturation during exercise occurred, but all patients desaturated during exercise if the DLCO was less than 65 per cent predicted[32].

Resting oxygen saturation is a less predictable factor for oxygen desaturation during exercise[31]. Hypoxic patients on the steep slope of the oxygen dissociation curve will have large drops in SaO_2 compared with relatively small drops in PaO_2. Inability to correct the exercise hypoxia in severe disease may be due to a failure to maximize cardiac adaptations with training or alter fixed ventilation perfusion mismatch.

It is important to try and predict hypoxia in CF patients in order to advise what precautions they should take for recreational activities of daily living, for travel and during exercise. CF patients are ambitious in their exercise activities and partake in parachuting, bunji-jumping and skiing. Skiing can provide the hazardous combination of extreme exercise and high altitude in potentially very hypoxemic patients, with sometimes disastrous consequences[33]. Hypoxic challenge studies using 15 per cent oxygen have been performed in the laboratory to simulate the degree of oxygen desaturation that may occur during commercial flight or skiing at altitude[34]. These studies offer useful information for advising patients who may need supplementary oxygen during air travel or who should be advised against vigorous holidays at altitude. Although many studies have evaluated the predictors of oxygen desaturation, apart from hypoxic patients exercising at altitude there are no other reports of adverse outcomes associated with desaturation.

Muscle strength and fatigue during exercise

Respiratory muscle strength, as measured by maximal static inspiratory and expiratory pressures, may be marginally reduced or supranormal in stable CF patients with moderate disease[35,36]. However, another study reported a marked reduction in maximal expiratory and inspiratory pressures in poorly nourished, hyperinflated CF adult males[37]. Although severe lung disease may compromise the efficiency of the respiratory muscles, a study of diaphragm power in CF has shown that weakness was most strongly correlated with malnutrition[38]. Clearly there is a strong interrelationship between nutrition and muscle function. If muscle bulk is reduced, CF patients will not be able to maintain the same level and duration of exercise as their peers. Lands et al. found that peak sprint work performed by CF patients during a Wingate test (a measure of maximal leg muscle performance) was reduced[21]. However, sprint work achieved was normal when corrected for lean body mass, suggesting that the problem was one of reduced muscle quantity. A larger study of adolescent CF males using the Wingate protocol found that peak and absolute peak power outputs were reduced compared to healthy controls even when corrected for lean body mass; the greatest power reduction occurred in those patients with the worst nutritional status (BMI <17.5)[39]. Both the quantity and quality of CF muscle may thus contribute to exercise capacity. The few direct studies of CF skeletal muscle do show abnormalities of function. Szeinberg et al. found a leftward shift in the force–frequency response in CF malnourished patients, consistent with selective atrophy of type 2 (fast twitch) muscle fibers[37]; this finding would be consistent with the described reduction in anaerobic/sprint capacity of CF patients[39,40]. At a cellular level, oxidative enzyme dynamics, particularily with regard to adenosine triphosphate (ATP) formation in the mitochondria of skeletal muscle, are impaired[41–43]. Although muscle quality may be abnormal, the most likely contributory factors to diminished exercise capacity are decreased muscle bulk associated with poor nutritional status and deconditioning due to inactivity and ill health.

Keens et al. reported that CF patients had 36 per cent higher ventilatory muscle endurance compared to controls before commencing a training program[44]. It was suggested this was due to the chronic training stress of breathing against an increased inspiratory load. More recent work has confirmed that inspiratory muscle strength and fatigue is similar for CF patients and controls, and also independent of lean body mass and leg strength[45]. This independence of inspiratory muscle strength in CF represents a selective training effect due to chronic lung disease, complementing the work by Keens et al.[44].

CF patients have a well-documented pubertal delay[46]. Boas et al. showed that although nutritional factors were the major factor accounting for anaerobic output, a small but significant component was accounted for by testosterone, emphasizing the importance of sexual maturity in improving exercise capacity[39]. Testosterone probably influences muscle quality as well as improving muscle quantity.

As discussed, muscle quantity plays an important role in defining the limits of exercise capacity, but it is not clear as to what degree muscular fatigue limits exercise compared with ventilatory factors. A study of exercise in CF adults found that overall muscle effort scores were greater than breathlessness scores for both CF patients and controls, implying that peripheral muscle fatigue was a greater limiting factor than breathlessness for the CF patients[47]. However, for levels of FEV_1 less than 40 per cent predicted, breathlessness and muscular effort scores were similar, confirming that ventilation was becoming the limiting factor.

CF patients also perceived muscular fatigue as similar for both arm and leg ergometry[48]. Although measured infrequently, lactate levels for CF patients are a true reflection of peripheral muscle effort except when respiratory function is so severe that exercise is primarily ventilatory limited[30,48].

In all patients with chronic airflow limitation and hyperinflation the oxygen cost of breathing is increased and then exaggerated during exercise. During maximal exercise the oxygen consumption of the respiratory muscles can reach 35–40 per cent (normal value 10–15 per cent) of whole-body $\dot{V}O_2$[49]. Respiratory and nonrespiratory muscles will compete with each other for oxygen, muscles fatigue and exercise ceases.

It has been recognized for many years that the resting energy expenditure (REE) of CF patients is elevated[50]. This elevation has been attributed to the basic genetic defect, chronic pulmonary infection and the work of breathing associated with altered lung mechanics. Resting energy expenditure correlates negatively with lung function and nutritional status for CF patients[51] and of the limited studies undertaken during exercise, no differences were found in energy expenditure during 30 and 50 watts walking[52].

Nutrition and exercise tolerance

Although pulmonary disease correlates with exercise tolerance, especially in those CF patients with an FEV_1 less than 50 per cent predicted, nutritional status – an independent contributory factor[20,53] – may be of greater importance. Different measurement techniques have shown that CF patients have a decrease in both fat mass and lean muscle mass[54]. Early studies have shown that better nutrition improves prognosis[10] and supplemental nutrition results in positive changes in body composition and growth velocity with no decline in pulmonary function[55].

Recent studies have shown that nutritional status may play a more important role than respiratory function for maintaining anaerobic and aerobic exercise over both the short and long term[39,53]. The study by Moorcroft et al. showed that despite a significant decrease in FEV_1 (63 mL/annum) over 6 years there was a significant increase in BMI (19 to >20.9) with no change in $\dot{V}O_2$ max. It can be speculated that an improved BMI may have contributed to the maintenance of exercise capacity.

The appreciation that lean tissue wasting with consequent decreased muscle mass can impair exercise performance[56] has led to the adoption of a policy of nutritional supplementation in order to improve exercise tolerance. Some studies have found an improvement in peak work capacity and respiratory and skeletal muscle strength following nutritional supplementation[57,58] but other studies have not been so encouraging and found no change for either variable[59]. It is intriguing to speculate whether, if CF patients can gain weight with supplemental feeding, an accompanying exercise program will convert the additional weight into useful functional lean muscle mass. Although there are brief reports of such benefit[60-63], no prospective controlled trial has currently been undertaken to answer this important question.

Cardiac limitations to exercise

Pulmonary hypertension and abnormal right ventricular function were demonstrated in early cardiac catheterization studies of patients with severe CF[64,65]. Predominant right heart disease has distracted attention from anatomical and functional abnormalities of the left ventricle, which may have important implications for exercise[66,67]. Two-dimensional echocardiography has shown ventricular interdependence in severe CF where the enlarged right ventricle compresses the left ventricle[68]. This will result in decreased left ventricular filling and a diminished stroke volume at rest and during exercise. A decreased stroke volume has also been recorded in CF patients with good respiratory function and has been attributed to hyperinflation causing impairment of right ventricular function[69].

Perrault et al. studied changes in cardiac output during exercise in the upright and supine positions in CF patients with a range of disease severity. Cardiac output increased to the same degree with both exercising positions in controls and patients with mild to moderate disease, but was reduced in severe disease[70]. However, there was a reduction in stroke index with the change from erect to supine position at rest for all CF patients compared to controls, suggesting a limitation in diastolic reserve when ventricular preload is increased.

Overall, the cardiovascular responses in CF are relatively normal for a given workload[19,71]. For patients with mild to moderate disease, an almost normal maximal heart rate is achieved with exercise, but with a rapid rise in the heart rate[53].

The greatest reduction in stroke volume occurs in patients with severe disease[72] and with poor nutrition[20]. Stroke volume will also be reduced in patients who are inactive due to ill health.

STUDIES OF EXERCISE TESTING AND TRAINING PROGRAMS IN CYSTIC FIBROSIS

Over the past two decades considerable research has been undertaken evaluating the benefits of exercise for CF patients. Exercise programs have studied different aspects of training, which are discussed below. Slowly, as the results of these studies have been published, there has been increased perception of the multiple advantages by which patients may benefit from undertaking regular exercise. Equally, it is important to include all patients from the fittest to the sickest in exercise training. Healthy patients who maintain fitness may lead a better quality of life[7] and potentially improve their prognosis[12,13]. Patients with severe disease, awaiting a transplant, can remain mobile with a good morale while undertaking carefully monitored and specifically tailored exercise programs[73].

Although prescriptive exercise training monitored tightly in the hospital setting is valid evidence of the benefits of training, it is even more important to encourage the patient to continue exercise at home. It is an important component of self-care which the patient enjoys[74,75].

General exercise testing and training programs

Early studies considered the cardiorespiratory adjustments and adaptations that occur during maximal exercise in CF patients with a range of disease severity[15,71]. Patients with mild to moderate disease achieved peak minute ventilation, work rate and heart rate similar to normal controls. However, patients with severe disease had a reduced work capacity, significant exercise-induced arterial oxygen desaturation and increased end-tidal CO_2 despite a high minute ventilation. The authors cautioned, although there is currently no evidence base, that exercise should not be prescribed which would result in an arterial oxygen desaturation of greater than 5 per cent or a decrease below an absolute value of 80 per cent.

Subsequent to these preliminary studies of exercise

limits, supervised studies of general exercise training (usually cycling or running) have confirmed that CF patients with a range of disease severity can improve their exercise tolerance[3–5,16,61,76]. Specific patient benefits from these studies included an increase in respiratory muscle endurance[16], a reduction in residual volume[4,5], improvement in overall endurance[76], an increase in sputum expectoration associated with a training effect[3], and maintenance of pulmonary function[61]. In the home environment following a 3-month of cycle training there was a reduction in the degree of limitation measured by an activities of living questionnaire[77].

The only long-term study (3 years) of a general training program showed a significantly lower rate of decline in vital capacity and an improved sense of well being[78]. Currently no studies have examined the effects of a change in lifestyle.

Training specific muscle groups

Preliminary studies having shown that CF patients with mild to moderate disease can improve their exercise tolerance with general fitness programs, attention then turned to the training of specific muscles groups; namely the upper and lower body muscles and the respiratory muscles. However, it is self-evident that a general exercise program of sufficient intensity will involve and train these specific muscle groups to some degree.

UPPER AND LOWER BODY MUSCLE TRAINING

The upper body and arms are used for many functions of daily living. Patients with airflow limitation can develop severe breathlessness when they use their upper limbs but can perform more exercise when they use only their lower limbs[79]. It is probable that arm work overloads already hard working accessory muscles, resulting in premature dyspnea. Furthermore, the excessive ventilatory demands of arm exercise leads to dyssynchronous movements of abdomen and chest wall.

Lake et al. studied the benefits resulting from exercise training of upper and lower limbs separately and a combination of both programs in 28 patients with chronic air-flow limitation[80]. There was an improvement in performance which was specific to those muscles being trained. Thus upper-limb performance improved with arm ergometry. There was no crossover benefit for the separate training of arms and legs.

Strauss et al. studied the benefits of variable weight training in CF patients, which included both an aerobic and anaerobic component[81]. In the first part of the study, patients used light weights with a high number of repetitions (aerobic and anaerobic) and during the final month heavier weights with fewer repetitions (anaerobic) were used. Significant increases in body weight, muscle size and strength were recorded. No measurements were made of exercise tolerance or respiratory

muscle endurance. Residual volume decreased: a finding reported in previous exercise studies[4,5]. These pulmonary changes were attributed to bigger and stronger upper-body muscles providing greater mobility to the chest wall.

Only two studies have evaluated the physiological responses to arm exercise in CF patients[48,82]. In the study by Alison et al., both controls and CF patients performed less arm than leg exercise and ventilation was higher for both groups with arm work. Arm work was only less than controls in those CF patients with severe lung disease (FEV$_1$ <40 per cent predicted). The study concluded that arm work capacity in CF patients was well preserved until severe lung disease developed. In the study by Moorcroft et al. arm work was less than leg work for the whole CF group. The ratio of arm to leg work was closer at lower values of FEV$_1$ per cent predicted where pulmonary function is the limiting factor, whereas at higher lung volumes peripheral muscle mass and conditioning are the determining factors, as in the normal population. In agreement with Alison et al., ventilation was higher for arm work with an alteration in breathing patterns, but Moorcroft showed muscular fatigue was the limiting factor to exercise, not breathlessness.

RESPIRATORY MUSCLE TRAINING

Interest has increasingly focused on the pathophysiology of the respiratory muscles in pulmonary disease[83]. Research has centered on the question as to whether inspiratory muscle training will increase strength and/or endurance and delay fatigue[84].

Keens et al. specifically studied respiratory muscle endurance in CF patients[44]. In this study patients with CF had an initial 36 per cent higher ventilatory muscle endurance than controls when performing 15 minutes of normocapnic hyperpnea. Some of the patients then participated in a specific ventilatory muscle endurance training program, performing 25 minutes of daily maximal hyperpnea 5 days a week for 4 weeks. They increased their endurance by 51.6 per cent when compared to controls, who improved by only 22.1 per cent. A further group took part in daily intensive swimming and canoeing (upper body exercise) for 4 weeks and were able to increase their ventilatory muscle endurance by 56.7 per cent. The authors commented that specific respiratory muscle training is tedious but demonstrated the same objectives could be achieved with upper body endurance exercise. It is doubtful that the majority of patients would have the time to exercise daily at this intensity.

Asher et al. evaluated the effect of inspiratory muscle training on the development of strength, endurance and exercise performance[85]. The patients (mean FEV$_1$ 35 per cent predicted) breathed through an inspiratory resistance for 15 minutes twice daily for 4 weeks and acted as their own controls. Although there was an improvement in respiratory muscle strength and endurance, there was no improvement in exercise performance with progressive and submaximal exercise testing. The results evaluating muscle fatigue in Asher's study were inconclusive, although inspiratory muscle training in COPD patients showed a delay in the development of muscle fatigue[86].

A study of inspiratory muscle training in young children resulted in improvements in inspiratory muscle strength, pulmonary function and exercise tolerance[87], but a recent physiological study of respiratory muscles in CF children found that the strength and fatigue of respiratory muscles was well preserved, probably as a selective training effect due to chronic lung disease[45]. On this basis, the authors question the utility of imposing inspiratory muscle training on a patient group who have problems complying with the excessive requirements of self-care.

THE ABDOMINAL MUSCLES

In health, the abdominal expiratory muscles do not participate in quiet breathing but are recruited during exercise, when lung volume is elevated and they then act against a greater resistive load. During exercise, the force of contraction increases with a higher minute ventilation and the end-expiratory lung volume is reduced. The abdominal muscles also enhance diaphragmatic action during inspiration by increasing diaphragmatic length at the beginning of inspiration and so augmenting greater inspiratory pressure. However, CF patients have a higher tonic abdominal activity than controls during quiet breathing, probably as a response to pulmonary hyperinflation[88].

A group of patients with severe COAD who received 3 weeks' abdominal physiotherapy training increased their abdominal muscle strength and exercise tolerance[89]. No studies of abdominal muscle training or their function during exercise have been undertaken in CF.

EXERCISE TRAINING PROGRAMS

Greater understanding of both the physiological limitations of the lung during exercise and previous exercise studies provide a suitable basis for the prescription of safe and effective training programs. The patient and physician have a common interest in exercise. Patients have an awareness of being unfit and are keen to exercise because it increases social mixing, reduces breathlessness, improves morale and improves overall quality of life. The physician wants to improve cardiorespiratory fitness, stabilize lung function and as a consequence influence survival.

Training programs in CF have established the factors limiting exercise and provided protocols for the provision of safe exercise. As the result of an individual exercise test, each patient can then be prescribed a level of exercise from which an appropriate training effect will

result. It is then crucial for the patient to continue and maintain an effective level of exercise in the community.

Assessing exercise capacity

Maximal exercise capacity ($\dot{V}_{O_2}$max) will differ for the individual CF adult according to disease severity and level of fitness. The association of FEV_1 and $\dot{V}_{O_2}$ peak is closest at low lung volumes (below 50 per cent predicted) where ventilatory mechanics determine exercise capacity. At higher lung volumes, where a ventilatory limit is unlikely to be reached, other factors such as habitual activity, muscle mass, motivation and conditioning are of importance. A progressive exercise test will define the limits set by the severity of the lung disease and the level of fitness (Table 20.1). Knowledge of these limits allows exercise to be set at acceptable levels which can be performed regularly.

When assessing exercise capacity in CF patients it is important to have some awareness of their usual activities of daily living. Limits defined by a maximal exercise test may be far removed from the ability to pursue everyday activities. Also CF patients with mild to moderate disease have a considerable variation in their maximal oxygen consumption, which cannot be predicted from resting pulmonary function. A questionnaire measure of self-reported habitual activity levels[90] found similar scores for CF adults and controls except for those patients with an FEV_1 of less than 50 per cent predicted, where there was some reduction[91]. The measurements and equipment required for exercise testing are outined in Table 20.2. The choice of protocol depends on the equipment available, the disease severity and levels of fitness of the patient. An electronic bicycle ergometer is used for assessing exercise limits in our patients[92]. The starting workload and increments (8–25 watt) are selected according to the patient's weight, fitness and disease severity. The increments are increased at one-minute intervals and the measurements are recorded at rest, towards the end of each minute and one minute after the cessation of exercise.

The shuttle walk, an externally-paced incremental test, correlates with $\dot{V}_{O_2}$ in COPD[93]. This test has been modified and validated to measure peak exercise performance in adults with CF[94].

Exhaustion, either due to muscular fatigue or breathlessness, should occur within 5–10 minutes. It is important to record symptoms limiting exercise in CF. The two main limiting symptoms are breathlessness and muscular fatigue. Borg or visual analog scale (VAS) scores are useful for comparing and evaluating these symptoms. Lactate levels are a useful measurement of effort limitation related to muscular fatigue, but are not routinely used except in the research setting.

As with chronic obstructive pulmonary disease, dyspnea scores in CF are poorly correlated with resting

Table 20.1 *Patient (a) who trains regularly and achieves a higher $\dot{V}o_2$max, heart rate and ventilation at maximum exercise than patient (b), who is untrained but of similar disease severity*

Patient	FEV$_1$ (L)	(% pred)	Weight (kg)	$\dot{V}o_2$max (mL/kg/min)	$\dot{V}o_2$ (liters/min)	$\dot{V}$E (liters/min)	HR (beats/min)	Load (watts)	Sat (%)
a	2.5	(78%)	51	29.2	1.49	46.0	182	150	93
b	2.4	(80%)	47	20.6	0.97	32.0	144	87	94

Table 20.2 *Measurements and equipment required for assessing exercise capacity*

Measurements	Equipment
Peak work capacity	Bicycle – resistance
	Treadmill – speed and incline
	Walking – speed and distance
Peak heart rate	Cardiac monitor
	Pulse meter
	Fingers
Oxygen saturation	Pulse oximeter
Spirometry pre- and post exercise	Spirometer
Perceived breathlessness and muscular fatigue	Borg or VAS scores
Respiratory rate	Count or 'on-line'
Ventilation (VE,V_T, Ti$_{TOT}$, RR)	On-line system
Oxygen uptake	
CO_2 output	
End-tidal CO_2	
Blood lactate	Lactate analyzer or blood to laboratory
Pao$_2$ and Paco$_2$	Arterial line

back.

pulmonary function[95]. Most CF patients score muscular fatigue higher than breathlessness at peak exercise, except in those patients with severe pulmonary disease where breathlessness scores are similar or may be higher[96].

Safety precautions during testing should include personnel trained in resuscitation; oxygen and appropriate drugs used for resuscitation should be immediately available in the exercise department.

Provision of training programs

Before providing home exercise programs the following factors should be taken into consideration: disease severity, initial fitness and the need both to make exercise enjoyable and integrate the program with social and work commitments in order to optimize compliance. The prescription of exercise must be carefully tailored for the individual patient. A training effect is lost within 2–3 weeks after ceasing exercise[97] and benevolent supervision is required to maintain motivation.

WHAT SORT OF EXERCISE?

Most young adults with CF with mild to moderate disease can participate in exercise of their choice and interest to the level of their peers. This can include rugby, running, swimming, tennis, bicycling and weight training. The comparative benefits of these individual activities have not been compared. Initially exercise should be provided to improve cardiorespiratory fitness. The perceived benefits for the patient will be a reduction in breathlessness and muscle fatigue. Aerobic endurance exercises involving large muscle groups will achieve this objective.

Many patients would like to improve their body image. A combination of anaerobic and aerobic weight training will increase muscle bulk, chest wall flexibility and strength and is popular with the patients. Two suggested programs for weight training are the Pyramid method and that of De Lorms and Watkins. One study of weight training has reported an increase in body weight[81]. Strength training for children is not necessarily contraindicated but should be approached with extreme care. Growing bones are sensitive to stress, especially repetitive loading and the epiphysial plate is susceptible to injury before full growth is complete. It is important to provide a varied program and ensure joints are not subjected to repetitive loading.

Specific inspiratory muscle training has been extensively studied and shown no advantage over upper-body exercises. Patients find it tedious to perform and it should not be recommended for recreational activity.

It is preferable for patients to participate in an exercise activity of their own choice which they will enjoy. Some adults do not have the time or inclination. For these patients we provide standardized exercise routines. The 5BX and XBX physical fitness programs for men and women are ideal for this group[98]. Suitable equipment to use at home can include ergometer cycles, dumb-bells, small trampolines and rowing machines. The increase of health/gym clubs in the community has provided a ready outlet for CF patients to continue recreational or prescribed exercise at home. Some clubs can be expensive but reduced rates can often be negotiated with a sympathetic manager.

Exercise programs initiated in the hospital setting can be continued successfully at home with an improvement in maximal work capacity and an increase in the activities of daily living[77].

INTENSITY OF EXERCISE

In order to achieve a training effect the exercise must make reasonable demands on the physical capacity and must be progressive. The limits of the patient's ability to exercise maximally will have already been established.

From this information work can be initiated at a level of 50–60 per cent of $\dot{V}O_2$max or 50 per cent of PWC[20,99]. In mildly affected patients, the recommendation for achieving 70–85 per cent of measured maximum heart rate can be used to attain fitness[16]. Exercise should be set at a level which will cause breathlessness without distress[100]. Measurement of blood lactate levels at the anaerobic threshold have provided a useful additional measurement of the intensity of exercise required for training and can be reduced with training in patients with moderately severe COAD[101].

FREQUENCY AND DURATION OF EXERCISE

Patients with lung disease take longer to reach a steady state than healthy subjects[102]. A minimum of 15 minutes exercise (additional to a warm up and cool down period) three times a week are required. Ideally 30 minutes of exercise 5–6 days a week are recommended. Patients with severe disease are unable to tolerate this level initially and the exercise session should begin at 5 minutes' duration and increase slowly. Five to ten weeks of a progressive exercise program are needed to achieve substantial gains in a training effect[103].

ASSESSING EXERCISE TRAINING

It is important to evaluate continuously the benefits of patient exercise; this also acts as an encouragement to the patient. The testing modality used should be similar to the training modality and involve the same muscle groups as those being trained. Submaximal rather than repeated maximal tests can be used and the lactate or ventilatory threshold used as a marker of changing aerobic fitness. Submaximal tests are patient acceptable and reproducible. Reviewed diary cards are used to monitor exercise sessions and to provide encouragement and motivation. Activity questionnaires, activity monitors, reduced respiratory exacerbations, hospitalization and time off work/school are all outcome measures of training programs.

Exercising the patient with advanced lung disease

A maximal exercise test defines the limits of exercise of those patients with severe lung disease. There is no evidence that carefully tailored training programs are harmful for these patients and they should not be excluded from exercise. Indeed with careful supervision they can, over a period of months, increase their work capacity (Fig. 20.1). Interval training may be appropriate for these patients. Exercise-induced desaturation and breathlessness are minimized, permitting increased exercise tolerance. It is important to encourage patients who are listed for heart–lung transplantation to maintain mobility and morale. Patients who are dependent on oxygen and nasal intermittent positive pressure ventilation (NIPPV) can safely be mobilized on a treadmill using their ventilator and their oxygen requirements matched to inspiratory flow (Fig. 20.2).

Another mechanism for relieving the respiratory work of breathing during exercise for patients with severe lung disease is the application of continuous positive airway pressure (CPAP)[104]. The beneficial results of CPAP were reduced oxygen consumption, dyspnea and transdiaphragmatic pressure and an increased exercise tolerance.

OXYGEN SUPPLEMENTATION

The role of supplemental oxygen with the purpose of improving exercise performance has been evaluated and the evidence is conflicting[105,106] (Table 20.3). It is accepted that oxygen desaturation is minimized. Patients may ventilate less for a given level of exercise and the work of breathing is reduced. End-tidal carbon dioxide may rise.

The provision of oxygen during exercise prevents the transient rise in pulmonary artery pressure[64], although there is no evidence that brief reductions in exercise saturation lead to any permanent change in pulmonary artery pressure. Although concern is expressed about

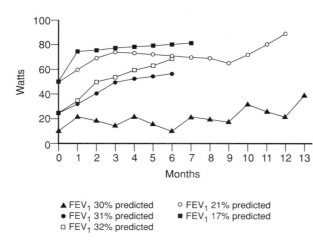

Fig. 20.1 *Slow improvement in work capacity in patients with severe lung disease, performing steady-state exercise. Patients exercise frequently on a cycle ergometer at a work rate limited by breathlessness.*

oxygen desaturation during exercise, it occurs to a greater extent during sleep in patients with both severe and moderate disease[107]. Oxygen supplementation during training may permit a higher work rate and increased duration for lower levels of breathlessness and exercise tolerance will improve. For patients with severe disease and awaiting transplantation, maintenance of mobility is

Table 20.3 *The debated benefits of oxygen supplementation at peak exercise in patients with severe disease*

Peak exercise	Nixon *et al.*[106]	Marcus *et al.*[105]
$\downarrow Sa_{O_2}$	Minimized	Minimized
HR	$\downarrow$	$\leftrightarrow$
VE	$\downarrow$	$\leftrightarrow$
PE_{CO_2}	$\uparrow$	$\uparrow$
PWC	$\leftrightarrow$	$\uparrow$
V_{O_2}	$\leftrightarrow$	$\uparrow$

crucial. Out of the hospital setting, the prescription of liquid oxygen for continuous usage has considerably improved patient mobility and quality of life[108] (Fig. 20.3).

Compliance with exercise

It is essential to maintain interest and compliance with exercise because fitness is readily lost when training is discontinued[97,109]. Compliance with home exercise is variable[77,110].

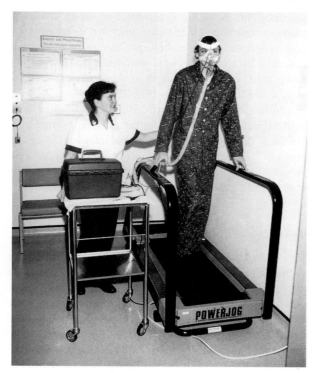

Fig. 20.2 *A hypoxic CF adult patient awaiting transplantation, exercising comfortably on a treadmill. (Reproduced with permission from ref. 73.)*

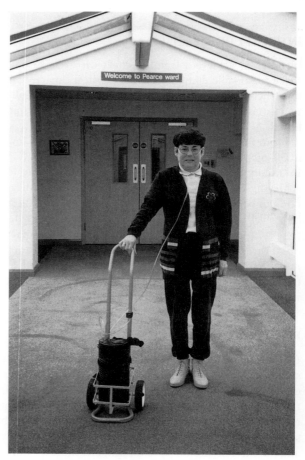

Fig. 20.3 *A hypoxic patient awaiting transplantation, pushing liquid oxygen and improving mobility and some quality of life. (Reproduced with permission of the patient.)*

Regular review of the level of exercise and patient contact encourages motivation and compliance. The timetabling for regular exercise should be integrated with daily lifestyle. The majority of patients feel they do not do enough exercise and would like to do more (Fig. 20.4a,b). A positive and encouraging approach to exercise should be adopted by the medical team to achieve that aim (Table 20.4).

It is important that compliance with chest clearance continues and should not be replaced by exercise[6,111]. Both modalities have complementary benefits which the patients prefer[3,6] (see chapter 19, Physiotherapy). Exercise is seen in a different light from other forms of self-therapy[75]. We should consider our patients' preferences, their beliefs and health perceptions when discussing a program of self-care. For some it may not be easy to maintain exercise over a 12-month period, but patients enjoy the extra exercise and feel satisfied with the level of exercise achieved (Fig. 20.5a,b,c).

Precautions and exercise

Exercise should temporarily cease for the following medical problems: pneumothorax, infective exacerbations associated with fever, persistent hemoptysis, transient arthralgia and arthritis. If patients are undertaking regular exercise in a hot climate they should be advised to take salt tablets and fluid to avoid dehydration. Exercise-induced bronchoconstriction is rare in CF. This can be monitored with pre- and postexercise spirometry and controlled with pre-exercise bronchodilators, if a problem. Exercise for the diabetic patient should be encouraged with the precaution of taking extra carbohydrate prior to exercise.

The transmissibility of microorganisms between patients necessitates special precautions. Currently, patients with *Burkholderia cepacia* should not use the same rebreathing exercise equipment as other patients, nor should they communally exercise with CF patients who are not colonized with *Burkholderia cepacia*.

It is salutary that despite the well-recognized benefits of exercise for CF patients a minority of CF patients are offered well-defined exercise programs as part of home care. Although 98 per cent of specialist centers in the USA and UK recommended exercise as therapy, only 22 per cent organized exercise programs[112,113].

Some sporting activities may carry a medical risk[114]. Contact sports, bungee jumping and parachute jumping are not advised for patients with portal hypertension and signifcant enlargement of the spleen and liver. Those patients with air trapping and sinus disease should avoid scuba diving. Skiing, fierce aerobic exercise at altitude for the hypoxic patient, and contact sports for those with confirmed osteoporosis are also contraindicated.

Table 20.4 *Essential aspects of an exercise program*

Enquire about and encourage exercise
Assess exercise capacity with formal testing
Provide individual exercise advice based on preference, fitness
  and disease severity
Supply equipment and training
Use outside agencies, e.g. gyms and Sports Development
  Officers
Monitor progress
Incorporate exercise into inpatient treatment

CONCLUSION

Over the past 5 years continuing exercise research and training in CF patients has provided a much clearer focus as to the short- and long-term benefits of exercise. Most importantly there is a clearer realization that aerobic fitness is correlated with a better prognosis in healthy populations and CF patients[12,13,115].

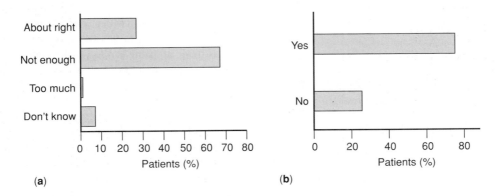

Fig. 20.4 **(a)** *Patients'* (n = 129) *awareness of their level of exercise, and* **(b)** *their wish to do more exercise.*

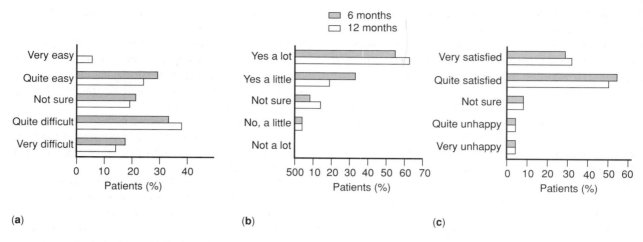

Fig. 20.5 *Patients' awareness of* (**a**) *the ease of maintaining an exercise program;* (**b**) *the enjoyment of an exercise program; and* (**c**) *their satisfaction with their training over 6 months and 12 months* (n = 24).

In many ways the objectives of exercise for CF patients are much more ambitious than those for COPD patients, where emphasis is mainly based upon achieving a better QOL by decreasing limitations imposed by breathlessness. With CF patients the main aims are to maintain lung function, improve body mass index and consequently increase survival. Recent exercise studies would suggest these objectives are possible, but equally the exercise programs require patient cooperation and practice in the home setting. Mean survival of CF patients is only into the fourth decade of life and improving quality of life (morbidity) may be an equally important reality for the patient. Care must be taken not to make the burden of already overloaded self-care increasingly onerous for the patient.

Although knowledge of the benefits of exercise has increased considerably over the past 10 years, many unanswered questions are worthy of further research (Table 20.5).

Table 20.5   *Future questions and exercise in cystic fibrosis*

Can CF patients comply beneficially with long-term exercise at home?

What are the relative merits of respiratory function and nutrition in maintaining and improving exercise performance?

Can supplemental nutrition combined with exercise result in increased muscle mass?

Do the components of ventilation change with training?

Should breathing patterns be changed with exercise?

Is there sufficient evidence to show that regular exercise for CF patients improves mortality?

REFERENCES

1. Zach, M., Oberwaldner, B. and Hausler, F. (1981) Effect of swimming on forced expiration and sputum clearance in cystic fibrosis. *Lancet*, **11**, 1201–1203.
2. Stanghelle, J.K., Michalsen, H. and Skyberg, D. (1988) Five year follow up of pulmonary function and peak oxygen uptake in 16-year-old boys with special regard to the influence of regular physical exercise. *Int. J. Sports Med.*, **9**,19–24.
3. Salh, W., Bilton, D., Dodd, M. *et al*. (1989) Effect of exercise and physiotherapy in aiding sputum expectoration in adults with cystic fibrosis. *Thorax*, **44**,1006–1008.
4. Andreasson, B., Jonson, B., Kornfalt, R. *et al*. (1987) Long-term effects of physical exercise on working capacity and pulmonary function in cystic fibrosis. *Acta Paediatr. Scand.*, **76**, 70–75.
5. O'Neill, P.A., Dodd, M.E., Phillips, B. *et al*. (1987) Regular exercise and reduction of breathlessness in cystic fibrosis.*Br. J. Dis. Chest*, **81**, 62–69.
6. Bilton, D., Dodd, M., Abbott, J. *et al*. (1992) The benefits of exercise combined with physiotherapy in the treatment of adults with cystic fibrosis. *Respir. Med.*, **86**, 507–512.
7. De Jong, W., Kaptein, A.A., van der Schans, C.P. *et al*. (1997) Quality of life in patients with cystic fibrosis. *Pediatr. Pulmonol.*, **23**, 95–100.
8. Dodge, J.A., Morison, S., Lewis, P.A. *et al*. (1997) Incidence, population and survival of cystic fibrosis in the UK, 1968–95. *Arch. Dis. Child.*, **77**, 493–496.
9. Kraemer, R., Rudeberg, A., Hadorn, B. *et al*. (1978) E. Relative underweight in cystic fibrosis and its prognostic value. *Acta Paediatr. Scand.*, **67**, 33–37.
10. Corey, M., McLaughlin, F.J., Williams, M. *et al*. (1988) A comparison of survival, growth and pulmonary function

in patients with cystic fibrosis in Boston and Toronto. *J. Clin. Epidemiol.*, **41**, 583–591.

11. Mahadeva, R., Webb, A.K.,Westerbeek, R.C. *et al*. (1998) Clinical outcome in relation to care in centres specializing in cystic fibrosis: a cross sectional study. *BMJ*, **316**, 1771–1775.

12. Nixon, P.A.,Orenstein, D.M., Kelsey, S.F. *et al*. (1992) The prognostic value of exercise testing in patients with cystic fibrosis. *NEJM*, **237**, 1785–1788.

13. Moorcroft, A.J., Dodd, M.E. and Webb, A.K. (1997) Exercise testing and prognosis in cystic fibrosis. *Thorax*, **52**, 291–293.

14. Kerem, E., Reisman, J., Corey, M. *et al*. (1992) Predictions of mortality in patients with cystic fibrosis. *NEJM*, **326**, 1187–1191.

15. Cerny, F.J., Pullano, T.P. and Cropp, G.J.A. (1982) Cardiorespiratory adaptations to exercise in cystic fibrosis. *Am. Rev. Resp. Dis.*, **126**, 217–220.

16. Orenstein, D.M., Franklin, B.A., Doershuk, C.F. *et al*. (1981) Exercise conditioning and cardiopulmonary fitness in cystic fibrosis. *Chest*, **80**, 392–398.

17. Spiro, S. (1977) Exercise testing in clinical medicine. *Br. J. Dis. Chest*, **71**, 145–172.

18. Mayes, R., Hardman, A.E. and Williams, C. (1987) The influence of training on endurance and blood lactate concentration during submaximal exercise. *Br. J. Sports Med.*, **21**, 119–124.

19. Godfrey, S. and Mearns, M. (1971) Pulmonary function and response to exercise in cystic fibrosis. *Arch. Dis. Child.*, **46**, 144–151.

20. Marcotte, J.E., Grisdale, R.K., Levison, H. *et al*. (1986) Multiple factors limit exercise capacity in cystic fibrosis. *Pediatr. Pulmonol.*, **2**, 274–281.

21. Lands, L.C., Heigenhauser, J.F. and Jones, N.L. (1992) Analysis of factors limiting maximal exercise performance in cystic fibrosis. *Clin. Sci.*, **83**, 391–397.

22. Boucher, G.P., Lands, L.C., Hay, J.A. *et al*. (1997) Activity levels and the relationship to lung function and nutritional status in children with cystic fibrosis. *Am. J. Phys. Med. Rehabil.*, **76**, 311–315.

23. Orenstein, D.M. and Noyes, B.E. (1993) Cystic fibrosis in *Principles and practice of pulmonary rehabilitation*, (eds R. Cassaburi and T.L. Petty), W.B. Saunders, Philadelphia, pp. 439–458.

24. Cotes, J.E. (1979) *Lung Function, Assessment and Application in Medicine*, (4th edn), Blackwell Scientific, Oxford.

25. Regnis, J.A., Alison, J.A., Henke, K.G. *et al*. (1991) Changes in end-expiratory lung volume during exercise in cystic fibrosis relate to severity of lung disease. *Am. Rev. Respir. Dis.*, **144**, 507–512.

26. Coates, A.L., Canny, G., Zinman, R. *et al*. (1988) The effects of chronic airflow limitation, increased dead space and the pattern of ventilation on gas exchange during maximal exercise in advanced cystic fibrosis. *Am. Rev. Respir. Dis.*, **138**, 1524–1531.

27. Rochester, D.F. (1991) Editorial.Respiratory muscle weakness, pattern of breathing, and CO_2 retention in chronic obstructive pulmonary disease. *Am. Rev. Respir. Dis.*, **143**, 901–903.

28. Coates, A.L., Desmond, K., Milic Emili, J. *et al*. (1981) Ventilation, respiratory centre output and contribution of the rib cage and abdominal components to ventilation during CO_2 breathing in children with cystic fibrosis. *Am. Rev. Respir. Dis.*, **124**, 526–530.

29. Bureau, M.A., Lupien, L. and Begin, R. (1981) Neural drive and ventilatory strategy of breathing in normal children and in patients with cystic fibrosis and asthma. *Pediatrics*, **68**, 187–194.

30. McLoughlin, P., McKeogh, D., Byrne, P. *et al*. (1997) Assessment of fitness in patients with cystic fibrosis and mild lung disease. *Thorax*, **52**, 425–430.

31. Henke, K.G. and Orenstein, D.M. (1984) Oxygen saturation during exercise in cystic fibrosis. *Am. Rev. Respir. Dis.*, **129**, 708–711.

32. Lebecque, P., Lapierre, J.G., Lamarre, A. *et al*. (1987) Diffusion capacity and oxygen desaturation effects on exercise in patients with cystic fibrosis. *Chest*, **91**, 693–697.

33. Speechly-Dick, M.E., Rimmer, S.J. and Hodson, M.E. (1992) Exacerbations of cystic fibrosis after holidays at high altitude – a cautionary tale. *Resp. Med.*, **86**, 55–56.

34. Oades, J., Buchdahl, R. and Bush, A. (1994) Prediction of hypoxaemia at high altitude in children with cystic fibrosis. *BMJ*, **308**, 15–18.

35. Mier, A., Redington, A., Brophy, C. *et al*. (1990) Respiratory muscle function in cystic fibrosis. *Thorax*, **45**, 750–752.

36. O'Neill, S., Leahy, F., Pasterkamp, H. *et al*. (1983) The effects of chronic hyperinflation, nutritional status and posture on respiratory muscle strength in cystic fibrosis. *Am. Rev. Respir. Dis.*, **128**, 1051–1054.

37. Szeinberg, A., England, S., Mindorff, C. *et al*. (1985) Inspiratory and expiratory pressures are reduced in hyperinflated, malnourished young adult male patients with cystic fibrosis. *Am. Rev. Respir. Dis.*, **132**, 766–769.

38. Pradhal, U., Polese, G., Braggion, C. *et al*. (1994) Determinants of maximal transdiaphragmatic pressure in adults with cystic fibrosis. *Am. J. Resp. Care Med.*, **150**, 167–173.

39. Boas, S.R., Joswiak, M.L., Nixon, P.A. *et al*. (1996) Factors limiting anaerobic performance in adolescent males with cystic fibrosis. *Med. Sci. Sports Exercise*, **28**, 291–298.

40. Cabrera, M.E., Lough, M.D., Doershuk, C.F. *et al*. (1993) Anaerobic performance assessed by the Wingate test in patients with cystic fibrosis. *Pediatr. Exercise Sci.*, **5**, 78–87.

41. DeMeer, K., Jeneson, J.A.L., Gulmans, V.A.M. *et al*. (1995) Efficiency of oxidative work performance of skeletal muscle in patients with cystic fibrosis. *Thorax*, **50**, 980–983.

42. Shapiro, B.I. (1989) Evidence for a mitochondrial lesion in cystic fibrosis. *Life Sci.*, **44**, 1327–1334.

43. Dechecchi, M.C., Cirella, E., Cabrini, G. *et al*. (1988) The K_m of NADH dehydrogenase is decreased in mitochondria of cystic fibrosis cells. *Enzyme*, **40**, 45–50.

44. Keens, T.G., Krastins, I.R.B., Wannamaker, E.M. *et al*.

(1977) Ventilatory muscle endurance training in normal subjects and patients with cystic fibrosis. *Am. Rev. Respir. Dis.*, **116**, 853–860.

45. Lands, L.C., Heigenhauser, J.F. and Jones, N.L. (1993) Respiratory and peripheral muscle function in cystic fibrosis. *Am. Rev. Respir. Dis.*, **147**, 865–869.

46. Reiter, E.O., Stern, R.C. and Root, A.W. (1981) The reproductive endocrine system in CF. Basal gonadotrophins and sex steroid levels. *Am. J. Dis. Child.*, **135**, 422–426.

47. Moorcroft, A.J., Dodd, M.E., Haworth, C. *et al.* (1997) Exercise limitation and symptoms at peak cycle ergometry in adults with cystic fibrosis. *Thorax*, **52**, S6 A5.

48. Moorcroft, A.J., Dodd, M.E. and Webb, A.K. (1997) Exercise capacity, ventilation, and symptoms at peak arm versus peak leg ergometry in cystic fibrosis. *Pediatr. Pulmonol.*, **S14**, 300–301.

49. Levison, H. and Cherniack, R.M. (1968) Ventilatory cost of exercise in chronic obstructive pulmonary disease. *J. Appl. Physiol.*, **25**, 21–27.

50. Bell, S.C., Saunders, M.J., Elborn, J.S. *et al.* (1996) Resting energy expenditure and oxygen cost of breathing in patients with cystic fibrosis. *Thorax*, **51**, 126–131.

51. Vaisman, N., Pencharz, P.B., Corey, M. *et al.* (1987) Energy expenditure of patients with cystic fibrosis. *J. Pediatr.*, **111**, 496–500.

52. Grunow, J.E., Azcue, M.P., Berall, G. *et al.* (1993) Energy expenditure in cystic fibrosis during ctivities of daily living. *J. Pediatr.*, **122**, 243–246.

53. Moorcroft, J.A., Dodd, M.E. and Webb, A.K. (1997) Long-term change in exercise capacity, body mass and pulmonary function in adults with cystic fibrosis. *Chest*, **111**, 338–343.

54. Newby, M.J., Keim, N.L. and Brown, D.L. (1990) Body composition of adult cystic fibrosis patients and control subjects as determined by densitometry, bioelectrical impedance, total-body electrical conductivity, skinfold measurements, and deuterium oxide dilution. *Am. J. Clin. Nutrit.*, **52**, 209–213.

55. Levy, D.L., Durie, P.R., Pencharz, P.B. *et al.* (1985) Effect of long-term nutritional rehabilitation of body composition and clinical status in malnourished children and adolescents with cystic fibrosis. *J. Pediatr.*, **107**, 225–230.

56. Coates, A.L., Boyce, P., Muller, D. *et al.* (1980) The role of nutritional status, airways obstruction, hypoxia, and abnormalities in serum lipid composition in limiting exercise tolerance in children with cystic fibrosis. *Acta Pediatr. Scand.*, **69**, 353–358.

57. Coates, A.L., Charge, T.D., Drury, D. *et al.* (1991) Nutritional rehabilitation and changes in respiratory strength, function and maximal exercise capacity in cystic fibrosis. *Pediatr. Pulmonol.*, **S6**, 286.

58. Hanning, R.M., Blimkie, C.J.R., Bar-Or, O. *et al.* (1993) Relationships among nutritional status and skeletal and respiratory muscle function in cystic fibrosis: does early dietary supplementation make a difference. *Am. J. Clin. Nutr.*, **57**, 580–587.

59. Kirvela, O., Stern, R.C., Askanazi, J. *et al.* (1993) Long term parenteral nutrition in cystic fibrosis. *Nutrition*, **9**, 119–126.

60. Bakker, W. (1992) Nutritional state and lung disease in cystic fibrosis. *Neth. J. Med.*, **41**, 130–136.

61. Heijerman, H.G.M., Bakker, W., Sterk, P.J. *et al.* (1992) Long-term effects of exercise training and hyperalimentation in adult cystic fibrosis patients with severe pulmonary dysfunction. *Int. J. Rehabil. Res.*, **16**, 22–27.

62. Heijerman, H.G. (1993) Chronic obstructive lung disease and respiratory muscle function: the role of nutrition and exercise training in cystic fibrosis. *Respir. Med.*, **SB**, 49–51.

63. Skeie, B., Askanazi, J., Rothkopf, M.M. *et al.* (1987) Improved exercise tolerance with long-term parenteral nutrition in cystic fibrosis. *Crit. Care Med.*, **15**, 960–962.

64. Goldring, R.M., Fishman, A.P., Turino, G.M. *et al.* (1964) Pulmonary hypertension and cor pulmonale in cystic fibrosis of the pancreas. *J. Pediatr.*, **65**, 501–524.

65. Siassi, B., Moss, A.J. and Dooley, R.R. (1971) Clinical recognition of cor pulmonale in cystic fibrosis. *J. Pediatr.*, **78**, 794–805.

66. Oppenheimer, E.H. and Esterly, J.R. (1973) Myocardial lesions in patients with cystic fibrosis of the pancreas. *Johns Hopkins Med. J.*, **133**, 252–261.

67. de Wolf, D., Franken, P., Piepsz, A. *et al.* (1998) Left ventricular perfusion deficit in patients with cystic fibrosis. *Pediatr. Pulmonol.*, **25**, (2), 93–98.

68. Jacobstein, M.D., Hirschfeld, S.S., Winnie, G. *et al.* (1981) Ventricular interdependence in severe cystic fibrosis. *Chest*, **80**, 399–404.

69. Pianosi, P. and Pelech, J. (1996) Stroke volume during exercise in cystic fibrosis. *Am. J. Respir. Care Med.*, **153**, 1105–1109.

70. Perrault, H., Coughlan, M., Marcotte, J.E. *et al.* (1992) Comparison of cardiac output determinants in response to upright and supine exercise in patients with cystic fibrosis. *Chest*, **101**, 42–51.

71. Cropp, G.J., Pullano, T.P., Cerny, F.J. *et al.* (1982) Exercise tolerance and cardiorespiratory adjustments at peak work capacity in cystic fibrosis. *Am. Rev. Respir. Dis.*, **126**, 211–216.

72. Hortop, J., Desmond, K.J. and Coates, A.L. (1988) The mechanical effects of expiratory flow limitation on cardiac performance in cystic fibrosis. *Am. Rev. Respir. Dis.*, **137**, 132–137.

73. Webb, A.K., Egan, J. and Dodd, M.E. (1996) Clinical management of cystic fibrosis patients awaiting immediately following lung transplantation, in *Cystic Fibrosis: Current Topics*, Vol. 3 (eds J.A. Dodge, D.J.H. Brock and J.H. Widdicombe), Wiley and Sons, Chichester.

74. Abbott, J., Dodd, M., Bilton, D. *et al.* (1994) Treatment compliance in adults with cystic fibrosis. *Thorax*, **49**, 115–120.

75. Abbott, J., Dodd, M.E. and Webb, A.K. (1996) Health perceptions and treatment adherence in adults with cystic fibrosis. *Thorax*, **51**, 1233–1238.

76. Freeman, W., Stableforth, D.E., Cayton, R. *et al.* (1993) Endurance exercise capacity in adults with cystic fibrosis. *Respir. Med.*, **87**, 252–257.

77. De Jong, W., Grevink, R.G., Roorda, R.J. *et al.* (1994) Effect of a home exercise training program in patients with cystic fibrosis. *Chest*, **105**, 463–468.

78. Reisman, J.J.J., Schneiderman-Walker, M., Corey, D. *et al.* (1995) The role of an organised exercise program in cystic fibrosis – a three year study. *Paediatr. Pulmonol. Suppl.*, **12**, 261.

79. Celli, B.R., Rassulo, J. and Make, B.J. (1986) Dyssynchronous breathing during arm but not leg exercise in patients with chronic airflow obstruction. *NEJM*, **314**, 1485–1490.

80. Lake, F.R., Henderson, K., Briffa, T. *et al.* (1990) Upper-limb and lower-limb exercise training in patients with chronic airflow obstruction. *Chest*, **97**, 1077–1082.

81. Strauss, G.D., Osher, A., Wang, C. *et al.* (1987) Variable weight training in cystic fibrosis. *Chest*, **92**, 273–276.

82. Alison, J.A., Regnis, J.A., Donnelly, P.M. *et al.* (1997) Evaluation of supported upper limb exercise capacity in patients with cystic fibrosis. *Am. J. Respir. Crit. Care Med.*, **156**, 1541–1548.

83. Roussos, C. and Macklem, P. (1982) The respiratory muscles. *NEJM*, **13**, 786–797.

84. Flenley, D.C. (1985) Short review: inspiratory muscle training. *Eur. J. Respir. Dis.*, **67**, 153–158.

85. Asher, M.I., Pardy, R.L. and Coates, A.L. (1982) The effects of inspiratory muscle training in patients with cystic fibrosis. *Am. Rev. Respir. Dis.*, **126**, 855–859.

86. Pardy, R.L., Rivington, R.N., Despas, P.J. *et al.* (1981) The effects of inspiratory muscle training on exercise performance in chronic airflow limitation. *Am. Rev. Resp. Dis.*, **123**, 426–433.

87. Sawyer, E.H. and Clanton, T.L. (1993) Improved pulmonary function and exercise tolerance with inspiratory muscle conditioning in children with cystic fibrosis. *Chest*, **104**, 1490–1497.

88. Cerny, F., Armitage, L. and Hirsch, J.A. (1992) Respiratory and abdominal muscle responses to expiratory threshold loading in cystic fibrosis. *J. Appl. Physiol.*, **72**, 842–850.

89. Vergeret, J., Kays, C., Choukroun, M.L. *et al.* (1987) Expiratory muscles and exercise limitation in patients with chronic obstructive pulmonary disease. *Respiration*, **52**, 181–188.

90. Baeke, J.A.H., Burema, J. and Frijters, E.R. (1982) A short questionnaire for measurement of habitual physical activity in epidemiological studies. *Am. J. Clin. Nutrit.*, **36**, 936–942.

91. Moorcroft, A.J., Abbott, J., Dodd, M.E. *et al.* (1996) Assessment of habitual levels of physical activity in cystic fibrosis. *Pediatr. Pulmonol.*, **S13**.

92. Jones, N.L. (1988) *Clinical Exercise Testing*, (3rd edn), WB Saunders, Philadelphia, USA, pp. 306–307.

93. Singh, S.J., Morgan, M.D.L. and Scott, S. (1992) Development of a shuttle walking test of disability in patients with chronic airways obstruction. *Thorax*, **47**, 1019–1024.

94. Bradley, J.M., Howard, J.L., Wallace, E.S. *et al.* (1999) The validity of a modified shuttle test in adult cystic fibrosis. *Thorax*, **54**, 437–439.

95. de Jong, W., van der Schans, G.P.M., Mannes, W.M.C. *et al.* (1997) Relationship between dyspnoea, pulmonary function function and exercise capacity in patients with cystic fibrosis. *Respir. Med.*, **1**, 41–46.

96. Moorcroft, A.J., Dodd, M.E. and Webb, A.K. (1996) Muscular fatigue, ventilation and perception of limitation at peak exercise in adults with cystic fibrosis. *Pediatr. Pulmonol.*, **S13**, 306.

97. Coyle, E.F., Martin, W.H., Sinacore, D.R. *et al.* (1984) Time course of loss of adaptions after stopping prolonged intense endurance training. *J. Appl. Physiol.*, **57**, 1857–1864.

98. Royal Canadian Airforce (1983) *Physical fitness. 5BX; the 11 minute exercise plan for men XBX; the 12 minute exercise plan for women*. Penguin, Harmondsworth, Middlesex.

99. Astrand, P.O. and Rodahl, K. (1977) *Textbook of Work Physiology*, McGraw-Hill, London.

100. Dodd, M.E. (1991) Exercise in cystic fibrosis adults, in *International Perspectives in Physical Therapy – 7 Respiratory Care*, (ed. J.A. Pryor), Churchill Livingstone, Edinburgh, pp. 27–50.

101. Casaburi, R., Patessio, A., Ioli, F. *et al.* (1991) Reductions in exercise lactic acidosis and ventilation as a result of exercise training in patients with obstructive lung disease. *Am. Rev. Respir. Dis.*, **143**, 9–18.

102. Spiro, S., Hahn, H.L., Edwards, R.H. *et al.* (1974) Cardiorespiratory adaptations at the start of exercise in normal subjects and in patients with chronic obstructive bronchitis. *Clin. Sci. Molec. Med.*, **47**, 165–170.

103. Casaburi, R. (1992) Principles of exercise training. *Chest*, **101**, 263–267.

104. Henke, K., Regnis, J.A. and Bye, P.T. (1993) Benefits of continuous positive airway pressure during exercise in cystic fibrosis and relationship to disease severity. *Am. Rev. Respir. Dis.*, **148**, 1272–1276.

105. Marcus, C.L., Bader, D., Stabile, M. *et al.* (1992) Supplemental oxygen and exercise performance in patients with cystic fibrosis with severe pulmonary disease. *Chest*, **105**, 52–57.

106. Nixon, P.A., Orenstein, D.M., Curtis, S.E. *et al.* (1990) Oxygen supplementation during exercise in cystic fibrosis. *Am. Rev. Respir. Dis.*, **142**, 807–811.

107. Coffey, M.J., Fitzgerald, M.X. and McNicholas, W.T. (1991) Comparison of oxygen desaturation during sleep and exercise in patients with cystic fibrosis. *Chest*, **100**, 659–662.

108. Dodd, M.E., Haworth, C.S. and Webb, A.K. (1998) A practical approach to oxygen therapy in cystic fibrosis. *J. R. Soc. Med.*, **91**, (Suppl. 34), 30–39.

109. Coyle, E.F., Martin, W.H., Bloomfield, S.A. *et al.* (1985)

Effects of detraining on responses to submaximal exercise. *J. Appl. Physiol.*, **59**, 853–859.

110. Holzer, F.R., Schnall, R. and Landau, L.I. (1982) The effect of a home exercise programme in children with cystic fibrosis and asthma. *Aus. Paediatr. J.*, **20**, 297–302.
111. Zach, M.S., Oberwaldener, B. and Hausler, F. (1982) Cystic fibrosis: physical exercise versus chest physiotherapy. *Arch. Dis. Child.*, **57**, 587–589.
112. Kaplan, T.A., ZeBranek, J.D. and McKey, R. (1991) Use of exercise in the management of cystic fibrosis: short communication about a survey of cystic fibrosis referral centres. *Pediatr. Pulmonol.*, **10**, 205–207.
113. Samuels, S., Samuels, M., Dinwiddie, R. *et al.* (1995) A survey of physiotherapy techniques used in specialist clinics for cystic fibrosis in the UK. *Physiotherapy*, **81**, 279–283.
114. Webb, A.K. and Dodd, M.E. (1999) Exercise and sport in cystic fibrosis: benefits and risks. *B. J. Sports. Med.*, **33**, 77–78.
115. Blair, S.N., Kohl, H.W., Paffenbarger, R.S. *et al.* (1989) Physical fitness and all-cause mortality: a prospective study of healthy men and women. *JAMA*, **262**, 2395–2401.

21

Future prospects

M. STERN AND D. M. GEDDES

Introduction	449	Antimicrobial approaches	457
Gene and protein therapy	449	Ethical considerations	457
Ion-transport therapy	454	References	458
Anti-inflammatory approaches	455		

INTRODUCTION

The cornerstones of CF medical treatment remain nutrition, antibiotics and physiotherapy. There are, however, a number of promising new approaches which may add considerably to these traditional treatments. The most fundamental of these is gene therapy; less visionary but potentially as important is drug therapy aimed at correction of the abnormality in airway epithelial cell ion transport. Both of these two approaches are probably best suited to patients with early or even presymptomatic disease. In contrast, a third group of new treatments may prove useful in patients with established lung damage; these include a variety of anti-inflammatory and antimicrobial approaches. This chapter will discuss each of these new treatments, as well as exploring the difficult issue of assessing new treatments in presymptomatic disease.

GENE AND PROTEIN THERAPY

The identification and cloning of the cystic fibrosis (CF) gene with subsequent characterization of its protein (CFTR)[1-3] has opened the way for gene and protein therapy. The simple idea is to administer the normal CF gene or protein as if it were a drug. In theory, this should result in restoration of normal cellular function and so prevent or treat the disease. Early results were encouraging when insertion of either protein or gene restored ion transport towards normal in a variety of cell systems. Subsequent progress has been slower as it has proved much more diffi-

cult to do this *in vivo*. It is likely that the technical problems will be overcome but few agree on how long it will take.

Protein therapy

Normal human CFTR can be made by recombinant protein technology, albeit at high cost and low yield. This normal protein can correct ion transport in CF cells and there is some evidence of similar correction *in vivo* in the CF transgenic mouse[4]. However, turnover of CFTR is rapid and so the half-life of any topically delivered protein is likely to be very short. Topical delivery is inefficient and only a small fraction of the protein is incorporated into the cell membrane. Unless and until these problems of cost, inefficiency and transience are solved, protein therapy is unlikely to reach clinical trials.

Gene therapy

THEORY

Three challenges need to be met for safe and successful gene therapy in CF: optimization of the therapeutic gene, efficient gene transfer *in vivo* and targeting of the correct cells. In spite of an enormous international effort, none of these problems has yet been solved.

THE GENE

The ideal would be to insert the normal version of the CF gene, complete with all its associated promoters and regulatory elements, into the correct site in chromosome 7, where it would continue to work normally until the death of the cell. Existing therapeutic genes fall far short of this ideal. The usual compromise is to use the coding region of the gene driven by a viral promoter; the therapeutic gene is thus much smaller and easier to use but is not subject to physiological regulation and tends to be transcribed only transiently due to either 'promoter shutdown', plasmid degradation and/or cell death. Much work is currently going into the development of CFTR 'mini-genes'[5]. In addition to the CFTR-coding region, these will contain all the necessary regulatory elements. However, the latter have not yet been fully identified and are thus not ready for clinical use. Another intriguing way round some of these problems is to use small-fragment homologous recombination[6]. Wild-type oligonucleotide sequences spanning the mutated region of the gene are administered and incorporated through homologous recombination. This should subsequently, in theory, correct the defect.

Other problems with existing therapeutic genes stem from their production in bacteria. They contain antibiotic-resistance genes, which are incorporated to allow selection of the bacteria in culture. Furthermore, bacterial DNA can cause inflammation in humans.

EFFICIENT GENE TRANSFER

Two main classes of gene delivery systems are currently in use: viral and nonviral. The former include retrovirus, adenovirus, adeno-associated virus and a few others, while the latter include liposomes with or without DNA condensation agents or attached chemicals intended to bind to receptors or to assist escape from endosomes. Each system has advantages and disadvantages. For example, on the one hand viral coat proteins assist gene transfer but, on the other, are proinflammatory or immunogenic. As a result, viruses are efficient *in vitro* but less so *in vivo*. Current viral research aims to retain the efficiency advantages and delete the proinflammatory and immunogenic disadvantages. In contrast, lipids lack both the efficiency advantages and toxicity disadvantages of viruses. Current lipid research thus aims to modify liposomes chemically to incorporate advantageous viral features. The two strands of work may meet half way.

VIRAL VECTORS

Retroviral vectors are in use for *ex vivo* gene transfer in a variety of diseases. They were used in early *in vitro* experiments to correct the CFTR defect[7] but have not been developed for clinical use in CF for a number of reasons. First, most retroviral vectors transfect only dividing cells and are therefore not suited for the transfection of fully differentiated lung epithelial cells. Second, while, potentially, integration of the vector into the host genome allows permanent correction, there are also potential safety problems associated with integration of viral DNA into the genome. These problems still need to be resolved.

Adenoviral vectors

These are particularly well suited to airway gene therapy since they can transfect nondividing cells and are tropic for the airway epithelium. The virus has a relatively large genome which can accomodate *CFTR* cDNA (Fig. 21.1)[8]. Disadvantages include acute inflammation and immunogenicity which may impair or block gene transfer, especially on repeat administration. Thus, in common with many vectors, adenoviral gene transfer is at least 100-fold less efficient *in vivo* than *in vitro*. Although wild-type adenovirus can cause serious human disease, there is reassuring experience with the use of modified adenovirus in vaccination programs. Similarly, the possibility of recombination between the viral vector and wild-type virus has not been a problem in practice.

Adeno-associated virus

This is a single-stranded DNA parvovirus. It does not cause human disease and requires a helper virus for replication. It can only carry a small therapeutic gene (≤4.7 kb)[9] but may cause less inflammation or immungenicity than adenovirus. Integration of the transferred gene into chromosome 19 has been

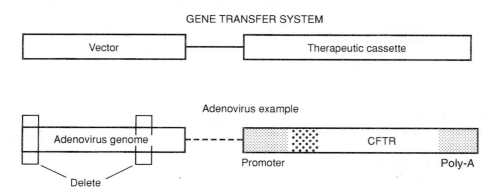

GENE TRANSFER SYSTEM

Fig. 21.1 *Adenovirus-based gene-transfer system.*

reported[10]. One advantage of such integration is prolongation of protein expression; a disadvantage would be the alteration of the host genome, resulting in unpredictable side-effects. However, transgene integration was not found in a recent CF volunteer trial[11].

NONVIRAL VECTORS

Plasmid DNA can combine with a variety of synthetic chemicals which have the dual role of condensing the large molecule and of facilitating entry into the cell. Cationic lipids, usually in the form of cationic liposomes[12–13], associate with DNA and the resulting complex enters the cell either by receptor-mediated endocytosis or possibly by direct entry into the cytoplasm following fusion with the cell membrane (Fig. 21.2). The surface charge on the lipid may not be essential, and neutral and even anionic lipids are being evaluated.

A large number of lipids have been assessed as gene-transfer agents. Structure–function relationships are being worked out and a variety of additional modifications are being tested (e.g. antibodies to cell-surface antigens, poly-L-lysine, viral entry proteins). Nonviral gene transfer by receptor-mediated endocytosis is also being explored using nonlipid systems[14–15]. These use polycations such as poly-L-lysine or protamine to condense the DNA together with receptor-binding chemicals, such as transferrin, or antibodies, e.g. to the polymeric IgA receptor.

Both viral and nonviral systems work much better *in vitro* than *in vivo*. This inefficiency is probably due to a variety of cell-surface defenses which limit access to the cell membrane, such as respiratory mucus, the cilia and the glycocalyx. To date, systematic comparison between viral and nonviral systems has not been made.

CELL TARGETS

Gene therapy for CF pulmonary disease is at present being directed at the airway epithelium for three main reasons: first, CFTR is present in the apical membrane of epithelial cells[16]; second, a number of defects of epithelial cell function have been linked with disease – in particular ion transport and antibacterial defenses; and third, because the epithelium is accessible for topical delivery. Nevertheless, the airway submucosal glands also express CFTR[16] and these glands produce the majority of the airway mucus. It is therefore possible that efficient gene transfer to the epithelium will not be enough for clinical benefit, in which case alternative gene delivery will need to be developed to target the submucosal glands.

Other sites in the body, for example bile duct, pancreas and gut, might also be treated by either topical or systemic gene therapy. At present these sites are not a major focus of research because access is more difficult and because the lung is the main site of clinical disease. Systemic, or conceivably fetal, gene therapy may one day be developed in an attempt to provide whole-body correction.

PROGRESS TO DATE

Advances have been rapid in the laboratory but difficult to translate into clinical practice. *In vivo* gene transfer is more difficult and low levels of correction reported so far in clinical trials show that there is still a long way to go.

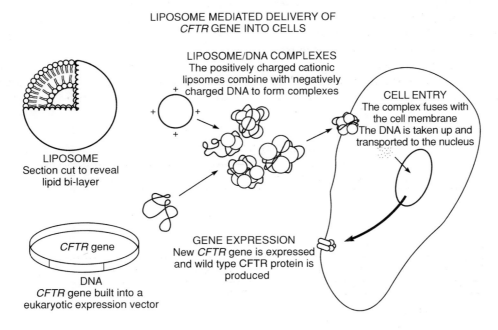

Fig. 21.2 *Liposome-based gene-transfer system.*

Table 21.1 *Clinical trials of CFTR gene transfer*

Country	Center	Gene delivery system	Target organ(s)	Subjects	Reference/under way (u/w)
USA	University of Iowa College of Medicine, Iowa	Adenovirus	Nose	3	26
USA	The New York Hospital–Cornell Medical Center, New York	Adenovirus	Nose and lungs	4	27
USA	University of North Carolina at Chapel Hill, Chapel Hill	Adenovirus	Nose	12	28
USA	University of Iowa College of Medicine, Iowa	Adenovirus	Nose	8	29
France	Hospice Civils, Lyon and Trangene, Strasbourg	Adenovirus	Nose and lungs	6	30
USA	University of Cincinatti	Adenovirus	Nose and lungs		*
USA	Washington/Seattle/Massachussetts	Adenovirus	Lungs		*
USA	The New York Hospital–Cornell Medical Center, New York	Adenovirus	Lungs	14	31
USA	University of Pennsylvania, Pittsburgh	Adenovirus	Lungs	11	32
Switzerland	Hopital Cantonal, Geneva	Adenovirus	Nose		*
France	Lyon	Adenovirus	Nose (repeat dose)		33
USA	Stanford University Medical Center, Stanford, California	Adeno-associated virus (AAV) Phase I	Maxillary sinus	10	11
USA	Stanford University Medical Center, Stanford, California	(AAV) Phase II	Maxillary sinus	23	34
UK	Royal Brompton Hospital, National Heart and Lung Institute, London	Cationic liposomes	Nose	15	35
UK	University of Oxford/University of Cambridge	Cationic liposomes	Nose	12	36
UK	MRC Human Genetics Unit, Western General Hospital, Royal Infirmary, University of Edinburgh	Cationic liposomes	Nose	16	37
USA	University of Iowa College of Medicine, Iowa	Cationic liposomes	Nose	12	38
UK	Royal Brompton Hospital, National Heart and Lung Institute, London	Cationic liposomes	Nose and lungs	16	39
UK	University of Oxford/University of Cambridge	Cationic liposomes	Nose (repeat dose)		*
USA	University of Alabama, Birmingham	Cationic liposomes	Lungs		*
USA	University of North Carolina at Chapel Hill, Chapel Hill	Liposomes	Nose		*

* Underway or completed, but not yet reported

Laboratory studies

The ion-transport properties of CFTR can be demonstrated following gene transfer into individual cells and CF cell lines can be corrected using a wide range of viral and nonviral vectors in association with the expression of CFTR mRNA and protein[17-20].

In vivo the results are very variable. Adenoviral vectors can transfer a variety of genes into the lungs of a cotton rat[21-22] – a species particularly susceptible to adenoviral infection. Both adenovirus[23] and adeno-associated virus[9] show variable transfer of marker genes into other small animals and monkeys, often associated with inflammation. This may be a reaction to the transgene protein product or to viral proteins. Liposomes can transfer marker genes *in vivo* in mice, rats and monkeys with relatively less inflammation. In transgenic CF mice, *CFTR* gene transfer using liposome vectors has corrected the chloride-transport defect[24-25]. Transgene expression *in vivo* is transient – approximately 1 week, regardless of vector. However, with the development of new gene-delivery systems, many of these problems are being overcome.

Clinical studies

A number of trials using adenoviral vectors to transfer *CFTR* cDNA to CF adult volunteers have been undertaken and many reported[26-33] (Table 21.1). Some early studies reported acute inflammation probably related to local instillation of a high viral load. There has been some evidence of gene transfer as determined by detection of mRNA or CFTR protein but this was inconsistent and failed to identify which cells were transfected. Electrophysiological correction has been claimed in some studies but the methodology has not been validated. Only one study was double blind and this showed limited evidence of gene transfer at the highest dose but no evidence of functional correction.

Two clinical trials using adeno-associated virus have been reported[11,34]. No significant side-effects have been observed and some evidence of correction of the chloride-transport defect has been suggested.

Liposome–plasmid complexes have been tested in eight clinical trials at least[35-39]. Of these, five were conducted in the UK and were all double-blind studies. Three trials with similar design showed partial correction of the chloride-transport defect in the nose[35-37]. In a further trial using lipid 67 (Genzyme) the complex was delivered to both nose and lungs by nebulization[39]. Partial, but significant, correction of chloride transport was seen at both sites. Administration of the gene–lipid complexes to the lungs in this trial was associated with a transient febrile reaction which did not occur in the control group, who received the lipid on its own. This side effect may be attributable to the bacterial origin of the DNA[40]. None of these studies showed any correction of the sodium-transport defect and vector-specific mRNA was only found inconsistently.

FUTURE DIRECTIONS

While most research effort has so far been directed towards techniques of gene transfer and correction of the chloride-channel defect *in vitro*, this is only the beginning. A number of key questions are now being addressed.

How much gene transfer is needed?

A number of observations point to the possibility that only low levels of transfection may be needed for clinical benefit. First, expression of CFTR in normal lungs is relatively low compared to that found, for example, in the kidneys[16]. Second, the fact that carriers of a mutant gene (i.e. heterozygotes) are entirely healthy implies that CFTR levels of 50 per cent are adequate. Further, *in vitro* studies in which CF and normal cells were mixed[41], show that 6–10 per cent of wild-type cells are sufficient for normal chloride transport. In contrast, however, more than 50 per cent of wild-type cells are needed for normal sodium transport[42]. So far, clinical studies have shown only partial correction of chloride transport, in line with transfection of less than 5 per cent of cells. If chloride-transport correction alone is needed, then success may be in sight, but if sodium transport must also be normalized, there is still a long way to go.

How often?

The duration of correction following gene transfer and its relation to vector and dose needs to be defined. Unless permanent correction of stem cells is achieved, treatment will need to be repeated at weekly or monthly intervals (the turnover time of the airway epithelium is measured in months). Although there are limited data showing prolonged presence of transferred cDNA following gene transfer, mRNA and function appear to fade after a week or so.

Control of expression

mRNA levels for CFTR are very low (1–2 copies/cell) in the airway epithelium. This suggests that only low levels of expression are required for normal function, which may make adequate gene transfer easier to achieve. Conversely, it raises the possibility of risk from overexpression and, ideally, control elements will be needed as well as simply a copy of the normal gene.

Host defenses

Repeated administration of viral vectors induces a host immune response. This may cause inflammation and impair gene transfer on repeat dosing. Preliminary data suggest that host immunity may be less of a problem when very low viral doses are given, but efforts to block host immunity continue to be researched and have focused on three strategies. The first has been to delete viral genes encoding potentially immunogenic proteins[43]. The second has been to suppress the host's ability to react to viral proteins, by using immunosuppressive agents such as cyclosporin. Finally, a further approach has been to selectively inhibit the immune response with the use of anti-T-cell monoclonal antibodies[44].

Theoretically, similar considerations regarding host response may apply to the expression of normal CFTR, which might be treated as a foreign protein by the immune system. Fortunately, clinical experience from protein replacement in other monogenic diseases, such as hemophilia, suggests that this seldom limits treatment.

CONCLUSIONS

Progress in gene therapy research has been most encouraging and the pace will accelerate. Many difficulties remain unresolved, however, and issues of safety become more and more important as the outlook for CF continues to improve. These issues will need to be addressed before phase III trials can begin.

ION-TRANSPORT THERAPY

Introduction

Pharmacological agents that target and modulate the ion-transport defects associated with CF are being tested both *in vitro* and *in vivo*. Ion-transport pharmacotherapy remains a promising area of research, with some advantages over gene therapy. First, a number of drugs with well-characterized ion-transport pharmacology also have well-characterized safety and toxicity profiles. Second, drug therapy does not have to be targeted at specific cells; a systemically active drug could, in theory, correct the chloride-channel defect at all sites. Finally, protocols for the regulation and testing of new drugs, or new applications of existing drugs, are well established and pose no new or special ethical or safety considerations.

Theory (Fig. 21.3)

The agents under investigation may be divided according to three different strategies. The first is to improve the function of mutant CFTR. The second is to enhance chloride transport by activating alternative chloride channels. The third is to reduce the increased airway sodium transport.

IMPROVING MUTANT CFTR

The most common CFTR mutation, ΔF_{508}-CFTR, results in a protein that is retained in the cells' endoplasmic reticulum, where it is degraded. One strategy to correct the defect is to use a known transcriptional regulator, sodium-4-phenylbutyrate (4-PBA), which upregulates gene expression. This enables a greater fraction of ΔF_{508}-CFTR to avoid degradation and traffic through the Golgi

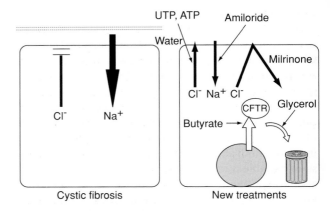

Fig. 21.3 *Ion-transport-modifying drug approaches.*

apparatus and then appear at the cell surface. Proof of this principle has been demonstrated in CF cells *in vitro*, and more recently, 4-PBA has been the subject of a placebo-controlled clinical trial[45]. Eighteen CF patients were randomized to receive 19 g/day or placebo for 1 week. Small but statistically significant improvements in epithelial CFTR chloride-channel function were demonstrable, and there were no important side-effects due to the therapy.

An alternative strategy to improve the function of mutant CFTR is to use glycerol, which corrects its processing (folding) defect. This reduces the amount of mutant CFTR which is degraded in the endoplasmic reticulum and so increases trafficking to the membrane. No clinical trial data are yet available, although *in vitro* studies have demonstrated restoration of CFTR channel function following treatment with glycerol. Yet a further alternative strategy is to increase the chloride-transport function of any mutant CFTR which reaches the membrane by using agents such as the phophodiesterase inhibitors IBMX or milrinone. Although there are some supportive *in vitro* data, these agents seem to have little, if any, effect *in vivo* in CF mice or CF volunteers.

A number of xanthines have recently been identified which act directly on CFTR and enhance chloride-channel activity. These include 8-cyclopentyl-1,3-dipropyl-xanthine (CPX) and 1,3-diallyl-8-cyclohexylxanthine (DAX) which, in addition, act preferentially on CF cells because of increased affinity of mutant CFTR for binding. A phase I multicenter clinical study of CPX has been undertaken and the report is awaited.

STIMULATION OF ALTERNATIVE CHLORIDE CHANNELS

Chloride secretion mediated through the protein kinase A and C pathways is defective in CF. However, that produced by elevation of intracellular calcium appears to function normally. Several agents are known to act through this pathway, with bradykinin and the triphosphate nucleotides ATP and UTP being perhaps the most clinically relevant. Using cultured airway epithelial cells, Manson et al.[46] have shown that both nucleotides can produce an increase in chloride secretion (and intracellular calcium) in CF cells. Using in vivo measurements of nasal PD as a marker of chloride secretion, a subsequent study[47] has demonstrated an increase in response to both ATP and UTP in CF patients. Interestingly, the PD rose to similar levels in non-CF and CF subjects, suggesting the restitution of previously absent chloride transport in CF airways. The PD response was maintained during perfusion of the drugs into the nasal cavity, although data regarding the time course of action following cessation of topical drug application have not been published.

UTP has subsequently been both further characterized and also evaluated for clinical use. It is now known to stimulate chloride secretion across airway epithelia via extracellular P2Y2 receptors, and is also thought to inhibit sodium transport[48]. It stimulates ciliary beat frequency and goblet cell degranulation, useful adjuncts to its effects on chloride secretion, with respect to treatment of CF. Initial studies have demonstrated that aerosolized UTP is safe after short-term and long-term use in animals and after short-term dosing of normal and CF human subjects[49]. More recently, a double-blind placebo-controlled rising-dose study of aerosolized UTP in CF patients has been undertaken[50]. No safety problems were noted and efficacy data are awaited.

SODIUM ABSORPTION

The diuretic amiloride has been shown both in vivo and in vitro to inhibit sodium transport across normal epithelial cells as well as the hyperabsorption of sodium characteristic of CF[51]. These observations underlie the hypothesis that inhalation of aerosolized amiloride in vivo might inhibit excessive sodium and water absorption in CF airway epithelia and thus improve the rheology and clearance of airway secretions. Initial in vivo studies in sheep confirmed that it was possible to deliver sufficient quantities of aerosolized amiloride directly to the airways to inhibit sodium and water absorption, and the earliest human clinical studies of inhaled amiloride confirmed safety[52]. Further studies demonstrated improved pulmonary mucociliary clearance following administration of inhaled amiloride, both acutely and over a 3-week period[53]. A 24-week double-blind crossover study of nebulized amiloride in a small number of CF patients followed[54]. The data that emerged suggested that amiloride improved the rheological and clearance properties of the sputum and lessened the decline in lung function seen when CF patients were taken off all other treatments. However, these encouraging results were not sustained in a number of further clinical trials, which were unable to document additional beneficial effects of amiloride when added to standard current therapy[55–57]. Clinical trial data on the use of amiloride in pediatric patients with CF remains limited, although safety has been confirmed in two reported studies[58–59]. A Glaxo Pharmaceuticals-sponsored multicenter, placebo-controlled clinical study of the safety and efficiency of amiloride in CF patients down to the age of 10 years has been undertaken, but no positive results have been reported.

There are many derivatives of amiloride with different durations of action and minor differences in pharmacological profiles. One example is benzamil, which has been tested topically in the nasal epithelium of CF patients in two separate studies[60–61]. Both studies concluded that this agent has a similar maximal effect on nasal potential difference as amiloride, but a more prolonged duration of action suggesting that it might be more useful clinically then amiloride. This hypothesis has however not been tested in the lungs of CF patients.

Conclusion

There have been a number of promising preliminary studies of ion-transport drugs in CF, but none can yet be recommended for routine use. At present, the best prospects are for a combined approach with a sodium-channel-blocking drug and a stimulator of chloride secretion. So far only topical administration has been explored and the ideal of a systemically active drug which specifically corrects the CF ion-transport abnormality remains only speculative.

ANTI-INFLAMMATORY APPROACHES

Theory

There is overwhelming evidence that the inflammatory processes directed against the colonizing organisms in the lungs not only fail to eradicate these organisms but also produce a cycle of immune hyperresponsiveness as well as neutrophil- and cytokine-mediated tissue damage. The failure to eradicate the organisms is, in part, due to the fact that local conditions appear to favor colonization and growth; in part, due to various defenses employed by the bacteria (e.g. alginate production and microcolony formation); and, in part, due to the products of inflammation themselves. In particular, the proteolytic enzymes released by inflammatory cells may break down other immune products and so actually render these immune processes ineffective. For example, neutrophil elastase[62] cleaves chemotactic factors, breaks down some complement components and inactivates immunoglobulins. In this way an inflammatory response can be considered as excessive in that it actually inhibits its own antimicrobial actions. At the same time, many inflammatory mediators, once released, may damage local host tissues and set up a cycle of chronic inflammatory damage and scarring. This damage then favors further bacterial growth, as local mechanisms of bacterial inhibition and clearance are themselves impaired or destroyed. While many mediators are released during airway inflammation, recent attention has focused on neutrophil elastase and free radicals.

Several ways of countering this inflammatory damage have been proposed. These range from relatively specific therapy directed at proteolytic enzymes, such as α_1-antitrypsin[63], to more general anti-inflammatory drugs, both steroidal (e.g. prednisolone) and nonsteroidal (e.g. ibuprofen). The current evidence favors ibuprofen but not systemic steroids. Other anti-inflammatory agents such as the antioxidant gluthathione, and immunosuppressive drugs such as methotrexate, azathioprine or cyclosporin-A, have also been proposed. These latter agents have not yet been evaluated in CF. For all of these anti-inflammatory and anti-immune approaches there are theoretical risks of uncontrolled infection.

Corticosteroids

Prednisolone has been used for many years with benefit in CF patients with associated allergic bronchopulmonary aspergillosis, immune-mediated arthritis and resistant bronchospasm. It has not, however, been used routinely in the management of CF. One trial has suggested that at a dose of 2 mg/kg, given on alternate days, prednisolone produced a reduction in respiratory problems and improved lung function[64]. A follow-up study, however, has demonstrated that side-effects of this treatment outweigh benefits[65]. However, as the potent anti-inflammatory action of corticosteroids remains a good rationale for therapy, and as the inhaled route is likely to cause fewer side-effects, the benefits of using inhaled steroids on a long-term basis have been investigated. Randomized placebo-controlled trials of inhaled fluticasone and budesonide have been undertaken in London and Copenhagen respectively. While the results of the former study are pending, the latter study[66] demonstrated short-term benefit in patients with CF and chronic *P. aeruginosa* infection who also had hyperreactive airways. Prolonged studies in larger numbers of patients will be necessary to determine long-term benefit of this treatment.

Ibuprofen

Ibuprofen in high doses has been shown to inhibit migration, adherence and aggregation of neutrophils, as well as the release of lysosomal enzymes. Furthermore, in a rat model that mimics CF, high-dose ibuprofen significantly reduced lung inflammation without increasing the burden of *P. aeruginosa*[67].

The first double-blind human clinical trial of ibuprofen for CF has been reported[68]. Eighty-five CF patients with mild lung disease ($FEV_1 > 60$ per cent predicted) were randomized to receive high-dose ibuprofen or placebo orally twice daily for 4 years. FEV_1 was selected as the primary outcome measure, although percentage of ideal body weight, a chest X-ray score and the frequency of hospital admissions were also assessed. The data suggested that ibuprofen, taken consistently for 4 years, was safe and that it significantly slowed progression of lung disease in CF patients over 5 years of age in whom disease was mild from the outset. Of note, however, was that this effect was particularly evident in patients who completed the treatment and who were initially less than 13 years old, and not demonstrable in older patients. This younger group consisted of a very small sample of only 36 patients. Thus, although the results are encouraging, further studies are required to confirm the benefits of this agent.

α_1-Antitrypsin (AAT)

This is the most important of a number of antiproteases which protect the lungs from proteolytic enzymes. While its deficiency was originally associated with lung disease in the form of emphysema, it is now clear that low circulating levels of AAT also predispose to bronchiectasis. Furthermore, in chronic pulmonary inflammation the amount of AAT, although normal, appears to be inadequate to balance the amount of proteolytic enzyme released. Since replacement AAT therapy may be valuable in the deficiency state, considerable progress has already been made in investigating this form of therapy. Human AAT can be prepared from donor blood and both infusions and aerosol delivery have been shown to provide normal levels of AAT in the lung epithelial lining fluid (ELF) in AAT-deficient subjects.

In CF, preliminary studies[54] have shown normal levels of AAT in ELF, but high levels of neutrophil elastase in ELF which swamp the AAT activity. Further, it has been demonstrated that aerosol AAT elevates the levels in ELF three- to sixfold and that the levels remain approximately twice normal up to 12 hours after administration. Neutrophil killing of *P. aeruginosa* is inhibited by ELF from CF patients (presumably because of the excess neutrophil elastase) but returns to normal following aerosol treatment with AAT.

Both the theory and these preliminary studies suggest a possible role for AAT in modifying the airway inflammation and enhancing bacterial killing in CF. There are not, however, as yet any supporting clinical data. Furthermore, *Pseudomonas* colonization occurs in CF before there is gross inflammation and this treatment might only be appropriate for the more severely affected patients, in whom many other factors are contributing to their deterioration. A transgenic sheep has recently been bred with the ability to secrete human AAT in its milk[69] and the derived human protein is currently being investigated for its effect in CF patients with moderately severe lung disease.

An alternative antiprotease is the secretory leukoprotease inhibitor (SLP1). This is probably a less important system than α_1-antitrypsin but is also subject to much current investigation. More recently, a new antielastase agent, DMP-777 (DuPont Merck)[70] has been tested in a multicenter phase I clinical trial designed to evaluate its safety and most effective dose required.

Finally, a single clinical study has shown promising results using oral pentoxyphylline[71]. This compound inhibits tumor necrosis factor-α (TNFα) transcription and also has stimulatory effects on neutrophils. In a small placebo-controlled study lasting 6 months, pentoxyphylline significantly reduced sputum levels of elastase and this was associated with beneficial changes in lung-function decline and infective exacerbations which just failed to reach 5 per cent significance.

ANTIMICROBIAL APPROACHES

Effective prevention of *P. aeruginosa* infection could greatly reduce the decline in pulmonary function which is part of the natural history of CF, and which progresses more quickly after colonization. Strategies that have been considered include antipseudomonas immunization, inhibition of bacterial adherence and improvement of airway surface antimicrobial properties. To accelerate the development of new antipseudomonal therapies, a Pseudomonas Genome Project has been established in the USA. The project, a collaborative effort between the Cystic Fibrosis Foundation, the University of Washington Genome Center and industry, has determined the complete sequence of *P. aeruginosa* strain PAO1, the isolate that has been most widely used for genetic and biochemical studies of this organism. The estimated size of the genome is 5.94 million base pairs, including more than 5000 genes, and a 2-year period has been needed to complete the task of sequencing.

Immunization

This concept seems somewhat illogical since humoral immunity is not impaired in CF and high immunoglobulin levels are the rule. However, IgG levels correlate negatively with lung function and, interestingly, CF patients with hypogammaglobulinemia have significantly better lung function than most CF patients. Clinical trials of immunization have been disappointing to date, and a study of passive immunization with MEP-rich intravenous immunoglobulin has shown no benefit on respiratory status when compared with standard intravenous immunoglobulin. It may be, however, that benefit would ensue if immunization were to precede rather than follow colonization.

Inhibition of bacterial adherence

P. aeruginosa adheres to airway epithelium by interaction between pili and cell-surface asialoganglioside receptors[72]. Theoretically, inhibition of adherence by blocking these receptors could be beneficial. However, studies have demonstrated inflammatory mediator release on binding of either pilin or antibody to this receptor on CF cells, highlighting a potential problem. Neuraminidase inhibitors have been studied for other diseases, such as influenza, and might find application in CF. Similarly, oligosaccharides are being developed as competitive inhibitors of adherence for use in other infective diseases. In particular, high molecular weight dextrans and diphosphatidylglycerol liposomes have nonspecific antiadhesive properties. Aerosolized dextran has been shown to prevent pulmonary infection in a mouse model of *P. aeruginosa* pneumonia[73] and clinical trials of dextran in CF patients are planned.

Airway surface liquid defenses

Defensins, lysozyme and lactoferrin are all normal antimicrobial defenses found in airway surface liquid. The effect of these may be reduced in CF due to the altered ionic environment[74]. A considerable effort is therefore going into the modification, or amplification of endogenous levels or, alternatively, the production of synthetic agents to augment their action.

ETHICAL CONSIDERATIONS

The more fundamental treatments such as gene and ion-transport therapy will take many years to develop and their assessment will raise new ethical issues. They will, at least in theory, be most likely to benefit the patient if they are given very early, and ideally should be started before the lungs become colonized by bacteria and before vicious cycles of inflammatory damage begin. Indeed, it may well be that these treatments will prove relatively ineffective once the lungs are damaged, since in this situation persistent bacterial growth is a consequence of this damage and its secondary effect on lung clearance mechanisms, rather than due to the genetic defect itself. These arguments are particularly worrying as there is a natural preference to try out new treatments on those with the most severe disease who are most in need of new drugs and who may therefore be ready to accept the attendant risks.

Thus, if it is accepted that presymptomatic patients are the most likely to benefit, then difficult ethical issues must be addressed. Will it be justified to give new treatments to children for many years in order to see whether lung disease is delayed or prevented? In the past, when

CF was almost fatal in early life, this approach would have been more easily accepted than today, when 80 per cent of patients with CF survive to the age of 20 and many are virtually free of symptoms. If the prognosis continues to improve, then these issues will become even more difficult, particularly with entirely new treatments such as gene therapy. In this situation a short-term safety record would not be particularly reassuring and a long-term safety record could only be obtained by long-term studies in humans.

Nevertheless, in spite of the formidable difficulties, both scientific and ethical, the future has never looked brighter for people with CF. Not only are a number of entirely new treatments, which may prevent lung damage, being very actively researched, but progress in transplantation is giving new hope to those with end-stage disease. For patients with moderate disease, conventional treatment is leading to an ever better outlook.

REFERENCES

1. Rommens, J.M., Iannuzzi, M.C., Kerem, B-S. *et al.* (1989) Identification of the cystic fibrosis gene: Chromosome walking and jumping. *Science*, **245**, 1059–1065.
2. Riordan, J.R., Rommens, J.M., Kerem, B.S. *et al.* (1989) Identification of the cystic fibrosis gene: Cloning and characterization of complementary DNA. *Science*, **245**, 1066–1073.
3. Kerem, B.S., Rommens, J.M., Buchanan, J.A. *et al.* (1989) Identification of the cystic fibrosis gene: Genetic analysis *Science*, **245**, 1073–1080.
4. Ramjeesingh, M., Huan, L-J., Li, C. *et al.* (1998). Assessment of the efficacy of *in vivo* CFTR protein replacement therapy in CF mice. *Hum. Gene Ther.*, **19**, (4), 521–528.
5. Burke, D.T., Carle, G.F. and Olson, M.V. (1987) Cloning of large segments of exogenous DNA into yeast by means of artificial chromosome vectors. *Science*, **236**, 806–812.
6. Goncz, K.K., Kunzelmann, K., Zu, Z. and Gruenert, D.C. (1998) Targeted replacement of normal and mutant CFTR sequences in human airway epithelial cells using DNA fragments. *Hum. Mol. Genet.*, **7**, (12), 1913–1919.
7. Rich, D.P., Anderson, M.P., Gregory, R.J. *et al.* (1990). Expression of cystic fibrosis transmembrane conductance regulator corrects defective chloride regulation in cystic fibrosis airway epithelial cells. *Nature*, **347**, 358–363.
8. Haj-Ahmad, Y. and Graham, F.L. (1986) Development of a helper-independent human adenovirus vector and its use in the transfer of the herpes simplex virus thymidine kinase gene. *J. Virol.*, **57**, (1), 267–274.
9. Flotte, T., Solow, R., Owens, R.A., Afione, S., Zietlin, P. and Carter, B.J. (1992) Adeno-associated virus vectors and complementation of cystic fibrosis. *Am. J. Resp. Cell Mol. Biol.*, **7**, (3), 349–356.
10. Duan, D., Fisher, K.J., Burda, J.F. and Engelhardt, J.F. (1997) Structural and functional heterogeneity of integrated recombinant AAV genomes. *Virus Res.*, **48**, (1), 41–56.
11. Wagner, J.A., Reynolds, T., Moran, M.L. *et al.* (1998) Efficient and persistent transfer of AAV-CFTR in maxillary sinus. *Lancet*, **351**, (9117), 1702–1703.
12. Felgner, PL, Gadek, T.R., Holm, M. *et al.* (1987). Lipofection: A highly efficient lipid-mediated DNA-transfection procedure. *Proc. Natl Acad. Sci. USA*, **84**, 7413–7417.
13. Gao, X. and Huang, L. (1991) A novel cationic liposome for efficient transfection of mammalian cells. *Biochem. Biophys. Res. Comm.*, **179**, 280–285.
14. Wagner, E., Zenke, M., Cotten, M., Beug, H, and Birnstiel, M.L. (1990) Transferrin–polycation conjugates as carriers for DNA uptake into cells. *Proc. Natl Acad. Sci. USA*, **87**, 3410–3414.
15. Cotton, M., Langle-Rouault, R., Kirlappos, H. *et al.* (1990) Transferrin-polycation-mediated introduction of DNA into human leukemic cells: Stimulation by agents that affect the survival of transfected DNA or modulate transferrin receptor levels. *Proc. Natl Acad. Sci. USA*, **87**, 4033–4037.
16. Englehardt, J.F., Zepeda, M., Cohn, J.A. *et al.* (1994) Expression of the cystic fibrosis gene in adult human lung. *J. Clin. Invest.*, **93**, 737–749.
17. Drumm, M.L., Popoe, H.A., Cliff, W.H. *et al.* (1990) Correction of the cystic fibrosis defect in vitro by retrovirus-mediated gene transfer. *Cell*, **62**, 1227–1233.
18. Rich, D.P., Anderson, M.P., Gregory, R.J. *et al.* (1990) Expression of cystic fibrosis transmembrane conductance regulator corrects defective chloride regulation in cystic fibrosis. *Nature*, **347**, 358–363.
19. Olsen, J.C., Johnson, L.G., Stutts, M.J. *et al.* (1992) Correction of the apical membrane chloride permeability defect in polarized cystic fibrosis airway epithelia following retroviral-mediated gene transfer. *Hum. Gene Ther.*, **3**, (3), 253–266.
20. Anderson, M.P., Rich, P., Gregory, R.J. *et al.* (1991) Generation of cAMP-activated chloride currents by expression of CFTR. *Science*, **251**, 679–682.
21. Rosenfeld, M.A., Siegfried, W., Yoshimura, K. *et al.* (1991) Adenovirus-mediated transfer of a recombinant alpha I antitrypsin gene to the lung epithelium *in vivo*. *Science*, **252**, 431–434.
22. Rosenfeld, M.A., Yoshimura, K., Trapnell, B.C. *et al.* (1992) *In vivo* transfer of the human cystic fibrosis transmembrane conductance regulator gene in the airway epithelium. *Cell*, **68**, 143–155.
23. Canonico, A.E., Conary, J.T., Meyrick, B.O. and Brigham, K.L. (1994) Aerosol and intravenous administration of human α1-antitrypsin gene to the lungs of rabbits. *Am. J. Resp. Cell Mol. Biol.*, **10**, 24–29.
24. Alton, E.W.F.W., Middleton, P.G., Caplen, N.J. *et al.* (1993) Non-invasive liposome-mediated gene delivery can correct the ion transport defect in cystic fibrosis mutant mice. *Nature Genetics*, **5**, 135–142.

25. Hyde, S.C., Gill, D.R., Higgens, C.F. *et al.* (1993) Correction of the ion transport defect in CF transgenic mice by gene therapy. *Nature*, **362**, 250–255.

26. Zabner, J., Couture, L.A., Gregory, R.J., Graham, S.M., Smith, A.E. and Welsh, M.J. (1993) Adenovirus-mediated gene transfer transiently corrects the choride transport defect in nasal epithelia of patients with CF. *Cell*, **75**, 207–216.

27. Crystal, R.G., McElvaney, N.G., Rosenfeld, M.A. *et al.* (1994) Adminsistration of an adenovirus containing the human CFTR cDNA to the respiratory tract of individuals with cystic fibrosis. *Nature Genetics*, **8**, 42–51.

28. Knowles, M.R., Hohneker, K.W., Zhou, Z. *et al.* (1995) A controlled study of adenoviral-vector-mediated gene transfer in the nasal epithelium of patients with cystic fibrosis. *NEJM*, **333**, 823–831.

29. Zabner, J., Ramsay, B.W., Meeker, D.P. *et al.* (1996) Repeat administration of an adenovirus vector encoding cystic fibrosis transmemebrane conductance regulator to the nasal epithelium of patients with cystic fibrosis. *J. Clin. Invest.*, **97**, (6), 1504–1511.

30. Bellon, G, Michel-Calemard, L., Thouvenot, D. *et al.* (1997) Aerosol adminstration of a recombinant adenovirus expressing CFTR to cystic fibrosis patients: a phase I clinical trial. *Hum. Gene Ther.*, **8**, (1), 15–25.

31. Harvey, B.G., Leopold, P.L., Hackett, N.R. *et al.* (1999) Airway epithelial CFTR mRNA expression in cystic fibrosis patients after repetitive administration of a recombinant adenovirus. *J. Clin. Invest.* **104**, (9), 1245–1255.

32. Zuckerman, J.B., Robinson, C.B., McCoy, K.S. *et al.* (1999) A phase I study of adenovirus-mediated transfer of the human cystic fibrosis transmembrane conductance regulator gene to a lung segment of individuals with cystic fibrosis. *Hum. Gene Ther.* **10**, (18), 2973–2985.

33. Bellon, G., Fau, C., Michel, L. *et al.* (1999) CFTR gene transfer by repeated administration of recombinant adenovirus to the nasal mucosa of cystic fibrosis patients. *Pediatr. Pulmonol. Suppl.*, **19**, 210.

34. Wagner, J.A., Mesner, A.H., Moran, M.L. *et al.* (1999) A phase II double-blind randomised controlled clinical trial of tgAVCF using maxillary sinus delivery in CF patients with antrostomies. *Paediatr. Pulmonol. Suppl.*, **19**, 209.

35. Caplen, N.J., Alton, E.W.F.W., Middleton, P. *et al.* (1995) Liposome mediated CFTR gene transfer to the nasal epithelium of patients with cytic fibrosis. *Nature Med.*, **1**, 39–46.

36. Gill D.R., Southern, K.W., Mofford, K.A. *et al.* (1997) A placebo controlled study of liposome-mediated gene transfer to the nasal epithelium of patients with cystic fibrosis. *Gene Ther.*, **4**, (3), 199–209.

37. Porteus, D.J., Dorin, J.R., McLachlan, G. *et al.* (1997) Evidence for safety and efficacy of DOTAP cationic liposome-mediated CFTR gene transfer to the nasal epithelium of patients with cystic fibrosis. *Gene Ther.*, **4**, (3), 210–218.

38. Zabner, J., Cheng, S., Meeker, D. *et al.* (1997) Comparison of DNA–lipid complexes and DNA alone for gene transfer to cystic fibrosis airway epithelium *in vivo*. *J. Clin. Invest.*, **100**, (6), 1529–1537.

39. Alton, E.W.F.W., Stern, M., Farley, R. *et al.* (1999) Cationic lipid-mediated CFTR gene transfer to the lungs and nose of patients with cystic fibrosis: a double-blind placebo-controlled trial. *Lancet*, **353**, 947–954.

40. Schwartz, D.A., Quinn, T.J., Thorne, P.S. *et al.* (1997) CpG motifs in bacterial DNA cause inflammation in the lower respiratory tract. *J. Clin. Invest.*, **100**, 68–73.

41. Johnson, L.G., Olsen, J.C., Sarkadi, B., Morre, K.I., Swanstrom, R. and Boucher, R.C. (1992) Efficiency of gene transfer for restoration of normal airway epithelial function in cystic fibrosis. *Nature Genetics*, **2**, 21–25.

42. Johnson, L.G., Boyles, S.E., Wilson, J.M. and Boucher, R.C. (1995) Normalisation of raised sodium absorption and raised calcium mediated chloride secretion by adenovirus mediated expression of cystic fibrosis transmembrane conductance regulator in primary human cystic fibrosis airway epithelial cells. *J. Clin. Invest.*, **95**, (3), 1377–1382.

43. Engelhardt, J.F., Ye, X., Dorantz, B. and Wilson, J.M. (1994) Ablation of E2A in recombinant adenoviruses improves transgene persistence and decreases inflammatory responses in mouse liver. *Proc. Natl Acad. Sci. USA*, **91**, 6196–6200.

44. Zsengeller, Z.K., Boivin, G.P., Sawchuck, S.S., Trapnell, B.C., Whitsett, J.A. and Hirsh, R. (1997) Anti-T cell receptor antibody prolongs transgene expression and reduces lung inflammation after adenovirus-mediated gene transfer. *Hum. Gene Ther.*, **8**, 935–941.

45. Rubenstein, R.C. and Zeitlin, P.L. (1998) A pilot clinical trial of sodium-4-phenylbtyrate (Buphenyl) in delta F508 homozygous cystic fibrosis patients: partial restoration of nasal epithelial CFTR function. *Am. J. Respir. Crit. Care Med.*, **157**, (2), 484–490.

46. Manson, S.J., Paradiso, A.M. and Boucher, R.C. (1991) Regulation of transepithelial ion transport and intracellular calcium by extracellular ATP in human normal and cystic fibrosis airway epithelium. *Br. J. Pharmacol.*, **103**, 1649–1656.

47. Knowles, M.R., Clarke, L.L. and Boucher, R.C. (1991) Activation by extracellular nucleotides of chloride secretion in the airway epithelia of patients with cystic fibrosis. *NEJM*, **325**, 533–538.

48. Devor, D.C. and Pilewski, J.M. (1997) UTP inhibits Na^+ absorption in normal and CF human airway epithelia. *Pediatr. Pulmonol. Suppl.*, **14**, 242.

49. Bennet, W.D., Olivier, K.N., Zemen, K.L. *et al.* (1996) Effect of uridine-5-triphophotate plus amiloride on mucociliary clearance in adult cystic fibrosis. *Am. J. Respir. Crit. Care Med.*, **153**, (2), 1796–1801.

50. Noone, P.G., Hohneker, K.W., Winders J.M., Retch-Bogart, G.Z., Boucher, P.R.C. and Knowles, M.R. (1997) Efficacy and safety of repeated doses of aerosolized uridine-5-triphosphate in patients with mild to moderate cystic fibrosis. *Pediatr. Pulmonol. Suppl.*, **14**, 274.

51. Knowles, M.R., Gatzy, J. and Boucher, R.C. (1981)

Increased bioelectric potential difference across respiratory epithelia in cystic fibrosis. *NEJM*, **305**, 1489–1495

52. Knowles, M.R., Church, N.L., Waller, W.E., Gatzy, J.T. and Boucher, R.C. (1992) Amiloride in cystic fibrosis: safety, pharmacokinetics, and efficacy in the treatment of pulmonary disease, in *Amiloride and its analogues: unique cation transport inhibitors*, (eds E.T. Cragoe, T.R. Kleyman and J. Simichowitz), VCH Publishers, New York, pp. 301–306.

53. App, E.M., King, M., Helfesrieder, R., Kohler, D. and Matthys, H. (1990) Acute and long-term amiloride inhalation in cystic fibrosis lung disease. *Am. Rev. Resp. Dis.*, **141**, 605–612.

54. Knowles, M.R., Church, N.L., Waltner, W.E. *et al.* (1990) A pilot study of aerosolised amiloride for the treatment of cystic fibrosis lung disease. *NEJM*, **332**, 1189–1194.

55. Graham, A., Hasani, A., Alton, E.W.F.W. *et al.* (1993) No added benefit from nebulised amiloride in patients with cystic fibrosis. *Eur. Resp. J.*, **6**, 1243–1248.

56. Robinson, M., Donnelly, P.M., Donnelly, J., Torzillo, P. and Bye, P.T.P. (1995) Effect of long-term inhalation of amiloride on lung function and exercise capacity in adults with cystic fibrosis. *Am. Rev. Resp. Dis. Suppl.*, **12**, A20.

57. Bowler, J.M., Kelman, E., Worthington, D. *et al.* (1995) Nebulised amiloride in respiratory exacerbations of cystic fibrosis: a randomised controlled trial. *Arch. Dis. Child.*, **73**, (5), 427–430.

58. Anderson, W.R., Church, N.L., Wisniewski, M.E. and Hsyu, P.H. (1995) Effects of aerosolised amiloride on pulmonary function in children with cystic fibrosis. *Resp. Crit. Care Med.*, **151**, (4), A19.

59. Church, N.L., Hsyu, P.H., Wisniewski, M.E. and Anderson, W.H. (1995) Safety trial of nebulised amiloride in children with cystic fibrosis. *Resp. Crit. Care Med.*, **151**, (4), A19.

60. Hoffman, T., Stutts, M.J., Ziersch, A. *et al.* (1998) Effects of topically delivered benzamil and amiloride on nasal potential difference in cystic fibrosis. *Am. J. Crit. Care Med.*, **157**, (6 Pt 1), 1844–1849.

61. Rodgers, H.C. and Knox, A.J. (1999). The effect of topical benzamil and amiloride on nasal potential difference in cystic fibrosis. *Eur. Resp. J.*, **14**, (3), 693–696.

62. Berger, M. (1991) Inflammation in the lung in cystic fibrosis. *Clin. Rev. Allergy*, **9**, 119–142.

63. McElvaney, N.G., Hubbard, R.C., Birrer, P. *et al.* (1991) Aerosol alpha I antitrypsin treatment for cystic fibrosis. *Lancet*, **337**, 392–394.

64. Auerbach, H.S., Williams, M. and Kilpatrick, J.A. (1985) Alternate day prednisolone reduces morbidity and improves pulmonary function in cystic fibrosis. *Lancet*, **2**, (8457), 686–688.

65. Rosenstein, B.J. and Eigen, H. (1991) Risks of alternate day prednisolone in patients with CF. *Pediatrics*, **87**, 245–246.

66. Bisgaard, H., Pederson, S.S., Nielsoen, K.G. *et al.* (1997) Controlled trial of inhaled budesonide in patients with cystic fibrosis and chronic bronchopulmonary *Pseudomonas aeruginosa* infection. *Am. J. Respir. Crit. Care Med.*, **156**, (4 Pt 1), 1190–1196.

67. Konstan, M.W., Vargo, K.M. and Davis, P.B. (1991) Ibuprofen attenuates the inflammatory response to *Pseudomonas aeruginosa* in a rat model of chronic pulmonary infection: implications for antiinflammatory therapy in cystic fibrosis. *Am. Rev. Respir. Dis.*, **141**, 186–192.

68. Konstan, M.W., Byard, P.J., Hoppel, C.L. and Davis, P.B. (1995) Effect of high dose ibuprofen in patients with cystic fibrosis. *NEJM*, **332**, (13), 848–854.

69. Carver, A., Wright, G., Cottom, D. *et al.* (1992) Expression of human alpha 1 antitrypsin in transgenic sheep. *Cytotechnology*, **9**, (1–3), 77–84.

70. Raghaven, K.S., Gray, D.B., Scholtz, T.H., Nemeth, G.A. and Hussain, M.A. (1997) Degradation kinetics of DMP-77, an elastase inhibitor. *Pharm. Res.*, **13**, (12), 1815–1820.

71. Aronoff, S.C., Quinn, F.J., Carpenter, L.S. and Novick, W.J. (1994) Effects of pentoxyphylline on sputum neutrophil elastase and pulmonary function in patients with cystic fibrosis: preliminary observations. *J. Paediatr.*, **125**, (6, Part 1), 992–997.

72. Saiman, L. and Prince, A. (1993) *Pseudomonas aeruginosa* pilli bind to asialo-GM1 which is increased on the surface of cystic fibrosis epithelial cells. *J. Clin. Invest.*, **92**, 1875–1880.

73. Bryan, R., Feldman, M., Jawetz, S.C. *et al.* (1999) The effects of aerosolised dextran in a mouse model of *Pseudomonas aeruginosa* pulmonary infection. *J. Infect. Dis.*, **179**, 1449–1458.

74. Smith, J.J., Travis, J.M., Greenberg, E.P. and Welsh, M.J. (1996) Cystic fibrosis airway epithelia fail to kill bacteria because of abnormal airway surface fluid. *Cell*, **85**, 229–236.

Index

Note: page numbers in *italics* refer to tables, those in **bold** refer to figures.

3849 mutation 52–3, 191
A455E mutation 38, 39
  dominant mild allele 191
  genotype–phenotype correlation 50
  sweat gland function *51*, 52
abdominal disorders, surgery 351–4
abdominal pain 351–3
  with mass 352–3
  with no mass 353
abortion, spontaneous 306
abscess, endobronchial 145
N-acetylcysteine 212–13, 269, 277, 282, 352
  bowel obstruction post-lung
    transplantation 371
  inhaled 381
aciclovir 367, 369
acrodermatitis enteropathica 151
active cycle of breathing techniques 212,
  378–9
adeno-associated virus vectors for gene
  therapy 450, *452*, 453
adenovirus 85
  gene therapy vectors 450, *452*, 453
adherence to treatment *see* compliance
adhesiolysis, laparotomy 349
adolescence
  conflicts 414
  disease complications 398
  nursing support 397–8
  responsibility for care 398
adoption 304
adrenal gland hyperplasia 151
adulthood
  health deterioration 416
  transition to 414–15
African–American population 22
age
  at diagnosis 2, **3**
  emotional disorders 340
  lung function 4
  lung transplantation 372
  microbial colonization 5, **6**
  prognosis 10
air travel 170, 231, 435, 436
airway
  clearance
    enhancement 212–14
    techniques 212
  compliance measurement 210
  epithelial lining fluid 456

NaCl concentration 112–13
  extrathoracic 163
  inflammation
    dornase alfa 226
    preceding bacterial infection 110–11
  obstruction 209
    index 165
  resistance measurement 210
  secretions
    neutrophil serine proteinases 119–20
    viscoelasticity 212
airway disease 160–5
  atopic 121
  bronchial hyperreactivity 163–4
  extrathoracic airways 163
  intrapulmonary airways 160–3
  lung volumes 164–5
  see also bronchiectasis; bronchiolitis;
    bronchitis; lung disease
airway epithelium
  CFTR on apical membrane 65
  CFTR protein 34–5
  chloride channel 65
  chloride transport 65–6
  gene therapy target 451
  membrane composition 111–12
  sodium ion absorption 64
airway submucosal glands, CFTR protein 35
airway surface liquid
  abnormal composition 204
  defenses 457
airway wall compliance 161–2
alanine 271
albumin serum levels 263
albuterol, inhaled 213
Alcaligenes xylosoxidans 211
alginate
  mucoid 92
  P. aeruginosa 114
alginate–toxin A vaccine 125
alkaline phosphatase 178, 292
allelic heterogeneity 194
allergic bronchopulmonary aspergillosis 7,
  55, 121–2
  adults 219
  chest pain 220
  chest physiotherapy 228
  corticosteroid therapy 126, 225, 228
  diagnosis 228
  incidence 94, 121, 227

lower respiratory tract 142
  testing 86
α-cell function 318
altitude 170–1, 231
  exercise 435, 436, 443
  hypoxia 170
aluminium hydroxide 267
alveolar macrophages
  IGF-1 production 123
  IgG blocking effect on *P. aeruginosa*
    phagocytosis 116
alveolar type II cells 34
amantidine 225
amenorrhea, secondary 305
amikacin 217, 223, *224*
amiloride 226, 455
  inhalation 84
aminoglycosides 215, *216*, 217, 223
  hepatic encephalopathy 297
  inhaled 217
  renal clearance 328
amniocentesis 179
amniotic fluid
  analysis 178–9
  cultured cells 178
  direct mutation analysis of cells 179
amoxycillin 222
amphotericin B 363, 367
ampicillin 222
amylase
  pancreatitis 270
  salivary 272
amyloid A fibril protein 325
amyloid goiter 163
amyloidosis 325–6
anesthesia, surgical 349
anger 343
angiography 227
animal models 76
anorexia 385
  nervosa 183
anovulatory cycles 305
antacids 267
anti-inflammatory therapy 126–7
  strategies 455–7
anti-T-cell monoclonal antibodies 454
antibacterial therapy, microbial colonization
  85
antibiotics 215, *216*, 217
  delivery devices 410

antibiotics – *contd.*
  GI motility 272
  inhaled 217, 381
  intravenous 406, 409–10
  lung infections *89*
  renal clearance 328
  resistance 90, 92, 215, 222, 223
  safety in pregnancy *308*
  therapy monitoring 217
antibody
  production 115–16
  response 93
antidepressants in terminal care 230
antielastase agents 457
antiendomysial antibody test 281
antigen presentation 109
antimicrobial chemotherapy *87, 88*, 222–5,
  457
antinuclear antibodies 324
antioxidants 248
  deficiency 283
antiprotease agents 214, 226
antireticulin antibody test 281
antithymocyte globulin 366, 368
α_1-antitrypsin 214, 226, 456–7
antiviral agents 225
AP-1 and AP-2 binding sites 31
apocrine glands 151
apoptosis
  intracellular acidification 76
  neutrophils 117
appendicitis 277–8, 352
appetite 385
arachidonic acid, calcium-linked generation
  67
arm exercise 438
arterial oxygen saturation 210–11
arthritis 324–5
arthropathy 7, 324–5
  episodic 151
artificial insemination 304
ascites 296–7
asialoganglioside 1 111
asialoganglioside receptors 457
asialoglycoproteins 204
aspergilloma 362
Aspergillus 5, **6**, 94
  adult infections 218, **219**
  invasion in lung transplantation 228
  lower respiratory tract infection 142–3
  see also allergic bronchopulmonary
    aspergillosis
Aspergillus fumigatus 86, 121–2
  adult infections 219, 227–8
  infant colonization 211
  lower respiratory tract infection 142
  lung transplantation 367
    contraindication 362
assisted reproductive technology 304–5
at-risk couple identification *see* carrier
  status; carrier testing
atelectasis
  lobar 211, 212, 226, **227**
  patchy 212
ATP 455
  hydrolysis 73, 75
  transport 73, 75
atrial natriuretic peptide 167

auto-PEEP 167, 168
autoantibodies 324–5
autogenic drainage 212, 378, 379
autogenic relaxation 421
autonomy 342
  principle 194
autosomal dominant polycystic kidney
  disease 327
axonemes, multiple 142
azathioprine 366, 370, 371, 456
azithromycin 222
azlocillin 217, 223, 224
azoospermia 53, 303, 304
  obstructive 187, 305
aztreonam 217, 223

B cells
  disorders 368–9
  S. aureus 123
β-lactam antibiotics 215, 223
  renal clearance 328
bacterial adherence inhibition 457
bacterial colonization, prognostic factor
  10–11
bacterial infections 85–94
  antibiotic sensitivity testing 86
  CFTR mutations 112
  cultures 85–6
  evaluation 85
  lower respiratory tract 142
  monitoring 86, 87
  phage typing 86
  predictive value 85
  secondary 143
  typing methods 86
  see also bronchiolitis; bronchitis;
    individual bacteria; lung infections
bacterial phenotype 114
bactericidal/permeability-increasing protein
  324, 325
bacteriological diagnosis 85
balloon tamponade 296
band ligation 296
Barrett's esophagus 148, 273, 274, **275**, 283
basal metabolic rate 54–5
  energy requirements 386
beclomethasone dipropionate 214
bed, tipping 407
behavioral problems 388
benzamil 455
bereavement 411
  counseling 405
  social worker role 417
beta cells
  function 317–18
  islet amyloid polypeptide 326
bi-level positive airway pressure 168
bicarbonate 67
  CFTR mediation of secretion 69
  decreased secretion 264
  ORDIC channel 69
bile acids 290, 294
bile duct 149–50
  atresia 297
  collagen deposition 290
  destruction 290
  extrahepatic disease 297–8, 354
  intrahepatic 290

  epithelial cells 289
  obstruction 296, 298, 354
  stenosis 150, 297
  see also common bile duct obstruction
bile salts
  loss 297–8
  pancreatic enzyme therapy 267–8
biliary cirrhosis 289
  clinical features 291
  liver transplantation 295
  ultrasound scoring system 293
  ursodeoxycholic acid therapy 294
biliary colic 298, 354
biliary epithelial cells, intrahepatic 289
biliary fibrosis, focal 150
biliary plugs 289
biliary stones 149
biliary tract, gene therapy 295
bioelectrical impedance analysis 250
biofeedback 421
birth prevalence reduction 193
birthweight 248
Bishop–Koop vented stoma 351
bisphosphonate 332
blood 69–70
blood gas analysis 163, 172
body composition measurement 250
body image 440
body mass, bone mineral density 331
body mass index 245
  decline 249
  gender difference 341
  insulin therapy in diabetes mellitus 320,
    321
bone
  age 302
  body mass 250, 331
  density measurement 329–30
  disease management 332
  fractures 151
  loss 329
  pathology 151
  physiology 329
  remodeling 329
bone mineral density 246
  body mass 331
  fracture risk 330
  measurement 329, 330
  nutritional support 331
  soap bubble appearance 269
  steroids 331
bowel
  ground-glass (soap-bubble) appearance
    269, 350
  obstruction 371
  rest 270
bowel loops 350
  distended 269
bradykinin 455
brainstem auditory potentials, impaired 151
Brasfield scoring system 207, 232
breast, lobar atrophy 151
breast milk 388
  analysis 309
  composition 394
breast-feeding 263, 309, 388
  lactose intolerance 279
  pancreatic enzyme preparations 265–6

breath sounds 206
breathing
  exercises 377
  mechanics 166
  oxygen cost 436
  patterns 434
breathlessness 440
  physiotherapy 381–2
  see also dyspnea
Brisket disease 170
bronchi 143–5
  evolution of changes 146
  plugging 144
bronchial artery
  ligation 227
  occlusion 227, **228**
  rupture 146–7
  surgical resection 227
bronchial cells, sodium resorption 113
bronchial hyperreactivity 121–2, 163–4
bronchial hyperresponsiveness 221
bronchial secretions, excess 376–8
bronchial wall thickening 187
bronchiectasis 144, 204
  CT imaging 220
  disseminated 55
  D$_L$CO 165
  evolution 146
  hemoptysis 220
bronchioles 143–5
  plugging 144, 204
bronchiolitis 144, 145, 204
  infants 211–12
  obliterative 145, 147, 364, 369, 372
bronchitis
  acute 144
  chronic 55
  ulcerative 144
bronchoconstriction, hypoxia 170
bronchodilators/bronchodilator therapy
    213–14
  adults 225
  beneficial response determination 161
  inhaled 381
  lung function deterioration 161, 162
  respiratory failure 229
  safety in pregnancy *308*
  terminal care 230
bronchopulmonary infection, acute
    exacerbation 382
bronchopulmonary sepsis 157
budesonide 226, 456
  inhaled 214
Burkholderia, culture 85, 86
Burkholderia cepacia 5, 89–90
  antibiotics 224
    resistance 90, 224
  chest radiography **225**
  clinical patterns of infection 90
  colonization 10
  cross-infection 219
  culture media 85, 86
  diagnostic evaluation 187
  epidemic 89–90
  genovars 89
  incidence 87, 218
  infant colonization 211
  infection transmission 382

lower respiratory tract infection 142
lung transplantation contraindication 363
microbiology 222
mucin binding 112
prevalence 89, 218
rebreathing exercise equipment 443
survival determination 10–11
transmission risk 90
virulence factors 115
burnout 345, 405

C-peptide concentration 317
C-reactive protein 325–6
C3bi receptors 113
CAAT sequence 31
calcium
  bone mass 331
  dietary 331, 332
  glucocorticoid therapy 331
  kidney metabolism 327–8
calcium ions
  chloride channel activity 66
  heterozygotes 75
  intracellular in fibroblasts 70–1
  red blood cells 69
  sodium ion transport regulation 66
  white blood cells 70
calcium oxalate crystaluria 328
calcium-binding proteins, CF antigen 70
calmodulin 72
calmodulin kinase 66
calnexin 38, 74
calorie intake increase 345
cAMP defective pathway 62, 65
cancer *see* malignant disease
Candida 211
  lower respiratory tract infection 143
  lung transplantation 367
  vaginitis 83
capsular polysaccharides of *S. aureus*
    114–15
carbenicillin 223, 224
carbon dioxide
  end tidal 437
  impaired excretion 169
  retention with exercise 435
carbon monoxide transfer 165, 170
cardiac limitations with exercise 437
cardiac output 434
  exercise 169, 437
cardiopulmonary physiology 157
  measurements 157–8
  see also heart
care system
  arrangements 231
  see also home care; self-care
carers 344–5
  needs 406–7
  protocol for home intravenous antibiotics
    410
carnitine deficiency 291
β-carotene 248
carotid bodies 151
carrier screening 179, 193, 194
  couples 40, 195–6
  pregnancy 307
  school-age 194

take-up rates 195
trials 195
carrier status 39, 193
  apparent 192
  idiopathic pancreatitis 270
  males 53
carrier testing
  cascade 196–7
  parental 179
  population-based 40
cascade testing 196–7
catalase 120, 121
cathepsin G 117, 119–20
Caucasian population 15–16
  CFTR gene frequency 21
CD11b 113
CD18 119
cDNA libraries 29
cefsuladin 223
ceftazidime *216*, 217, 223, 224
cefulodin 217
celiac disease 148, 280–1
  dietary requirements 394
celiac syndrome 280
cell culture 76
cell-mediated immunity, defects 142
central nervous system, pathology 151
cephalosporins *216*, 217, 222
cervical mucus 150, 305
cervicitis 150
cervix
  erosions 150
  mucous gland hyperplasia 150
CF antigen 70
CF cell lines, immortalized 76
CF pancreatic cell line 33
CF phenotype 13–14
  carrier frequency 15
  definition 14–15
  incidence 14, 15–17
  life-span analysis 17–20
  non-Caucasian groups 16
  racial groups 15–17
  seasonal effects 17
  sex ratio 17
  survival 20–1
CF transmembrane conductance regulator
  see CFTR
CF-causing mutations 183–4
CFTR 29, 61, 72–5
  abnormalities 13
  absent 38
  airway submucosal glands 35
  alleles 190–1
    analyzable 194
    dominant mild 191, 192
    single mutant 191–2
  apical membrane of airway epithelium 65
  ATP transport 73, 75
  bicarbonate secretion mediation 69
  cellular localization 33–5
  chloride channel 32, 33, 49, 65, 73–4
    activity 63
    bidirectional 34
    epithelium 37
    function 33, 75
    kidney 70
  chloride ion conductance 72

CFTR – *contd.*
　chloride transport function increase 454
　dephosphorylation by membrane-
　　associated phosphatases 32
　endocytosis 75
　endosomes 72
　exocytosis 75
　expression 204
　　fetal tissue 34
　　kidney 327
　　thyroid 327
　folding 39
　　defect 454
　function 56, 72–3
　　organ system involvement 56–7
　genotype
　　bacterial colonization 51
　　lung disease 50–1, 55
　　male infertility 53–4
　　pancreatic disease 51
　　phenotypic features 54–5
　　sweat gland disease 52–3
　heterozygotes 75
　in vivo expression 31
　intracellular acidification 76
　intracellular transport promotion 38
　ion-transport properties 453
　localization 73–4
　mini-genes 450
　mistrafficking 76
　mRNA 33, 192, 453
　　airway surface epithelium localization
　　　34–5
　　cellular localization 33–5
　　expression in kidney 327
　　expression pattern 34
　　in vivo expression 31
　　pancreatic ductal cells 34
　　uterus 35
　mutations 4, 112
　　analysis sensitivity 39
　　bacterial infections 112
　　classes 74
　　detection rate 38
　　function improvement 454
　　T cells 122
　pancreatic abnormality 261
　Pseudomonas receptor 76
　R domain 73
　regulation 72–3
　　other ion channels 74
　renal cyst genesis 70
　seminiferous tubules 35
　single-channel characteristics 72–3
　sodium channel regulation 33
　structure **30**, 72
　sweat gland localization 34
　therapeutic delivery 449
　transcripts 33
　truncated 38
CFTR gene 13
　animal models 41–2
　3 bp deletion 35
　cDNA transfer 453
　cloning 35
　coding region sequence 29, 30
　cross-species analysis of DNA sequence
　　30–1

　defective 15
　　distribution 21–2
　epidemiology 21–2
　exon 10 disruption 41
　expression 31, 73
　　fetal tissue 34
　frequency 21
　heterogeneity 190
　heterozygote advantage 37
　intron 8 polymorphism 192
　microsatellites 37
　mutations 13, 21, 35–7, 49, 183
　　CBAVD 53
　　CFTR chloride channel function
　　　disruption 37–8
　　distribution **35**
　　exons 36
　　frequency 36
　　intron–exon boundaries 36
　　male carriers 53
　　missense 36, 50
　　origin 37
　　pancreatic function association 51
　　promoter region 36
　　selective advantage 37
　　splice 36
　promoter 30–2, 73
　sequence analysis 36–7
　spermatogenesis 150
　structure 30–2
　5T allele 184, 192
　Tn locus 192
　transcription initiation start sites 32
　see also gene therapy
CFTR-associated disease spectrum
　305
chaperones, CFTR class II mutations 74
Charcot–Leyden crystals 142
chest clapping 378, 379
chest compression *see* high-frequency chest
　compression
chest imaging 187, 207, **208**
chest infection 244, *400*
　see also bronchiolitis; bronchitis; lung
　　infections
chest pain 220
chest physiotherapy 206, 212
　ABPA 228
　chest pain 220
　gastroesophageal reflux 273–4
　respiratory failure 229
chest radiography
　adults 220, **221**
　B. cepacia **225**
　infants 159
Chlamydia 224
chlamydial infection of lower respiratory
　tract 142
chloramphenicol 224
chloride channel
　airway epithelium 65
　CFTR 63, 65, 75
　heart 71
　pancreas 69
　stimulation of alternative 454–5
chloride ion
　conductance 29, 65, 72
　defect

　cAMP-mediated in submucosal glands 67
　pancreas 69
　efflux from fibroblasts 71
　nasal PD measurement 186
　resorption 61
　secretion
　　bicarbonate-dependent 67
　　calcium-regulated 41
　　defect 31
　　gastrointestinal tract 68
　　inhibitors 226
　　mediation 454
　sweat 4, 49, 52
　sweat gland impermeability 62, 63
　sweat test analysis 180–2
　transport 61
　　abnormalities 218
　　airway epithelium 65–6
　　altered pathways 63
　　defect site 62–3
　　gastrointestinal tract 68
　　kidney 70
　　respiratory tract 64–6
　　skin 70, 71
　　sweat glands 62–3
cholangiography 293
cholecystitis 149, 298, 354
cholecystokinin 272
　stimulation test 264
choledocholithiasis 296, 298
cholera resistance 37
cholesterol clefts 145
chorionic villus sampling 178, 179, 307
chromosome 7 28
chromosome walking 28
chymase, mast cell 120
chyme composition 275–6
Chymex test 264
chymotrypsin assay 263
cilia abnormalities 141–2
　see also mucociliary clearance;
　　mucociliary transport
cimetidine 274
ciprofloxacin 223, 224
circulatory mismatch 165–6
cirrhosis 150
　portal hypertension 148
cisapride 274
clarithromycin 222
clavulanic acid 217, 222
clindamycin 222
clines 22
clinical epidemiology 2
　diagnosis 2–4
　lung function 4–5
　medical care provision 11, **12**
　presentation 3–4
　prognosis 9–11
　sociodemographic features 7–9
　treatment 12
clinical presentation 205–7
clinical spectrum 178
Clostridium difficile colitis 83, 281
clubbing 151, 207, 220, 324
co-trimoxazole 222, 367
Cochrane Collaboration 12
cohort survival 18, **19**
cold air challenge 164

Cole's growth assessment slide rule 245, 246
colistin sulfate 217
    inhalation 367
colistinethate 217
colitis 83
    Clostridium difficile 281
colomycin 224
colonic obstruction, clearance 353
colonic strictures 148
colonopathy, fibrosing 146, 264, 265, 282–3
common bile duct obstruction 290
    stricture 296
community nurses 407, 408
compartmentalization of information 340, 343
complement, neutrophil elastase 118
complement C3 325
compliance
    children 341
    exercise 442–3
    lung transplantation 363
    physiotherapy 376
    studies 166
    treatment 341
complications 6–7
    adult respiratory disease 226–9
    childhood respiratory disease 211–12
computed tomography
    chest imaging 187, 220
    paranasal sinuses 187
    see also high-resolution computed tomography; quantitative computed tomography
conductivity
    sweat test 181, **182**
    see also total body electrical conductivity
congenital bilateral absence of the vas deferens 4, 53
    CFTR gene mutations 187
    deltaF$_{508}$ heterozygosity 150
    diagnosis 187–8
    mutations 53
        associated 184
    R117H splicing variants 53
    sweat electrolytes 187
constipation 277
    surgery 353
continuous positive airway pressure 168, 229
    exercise 442
contraception/contraceptive advice 303, 306, 402
Cooperman score 232
copper–zinc superoxide dismutase 69
cor pulmonale 147, 167, 218
    desaturation during sleep 168
    D$_L$CO 165
    end-stage respiratory disease 228
corticosteroids 225–6
    ABPA 126, 225, 228
    anti-inflammatory use 456
    inhaled 456
    respiratory failure 229
    see also glucocorticosteroids; steroids
cost–benefit analysis, screening 40
cough 205
    chest pain 220
    stress incontinence 306

terminal care 230
    vomiting 386
counseling
    bereavement 405
    continuing process 345
    dietary 386
    family 397
    informal by occupational therapist 422
    pregnancy 307, 402
    relationships 415
    social workers 415
    see also genetic counseling
couples screening *see* carrier screening
cows' milk enteropathy 279–80
cows' milk intolerance 279–80
craniofacial morphology 151
Creon 252
Crispin scoring system 207, 232
Crohn's disease 148, 280, 283
cromolyn sodium 214
cross-infection, adults 219
Cullen's sign 270
cushingoid features 363
cyanosis 207, 220
cyclosporin-A 366, 368, 370, 371
    anti-inflammatory activity 456
    host suppression in gene therapy 453
    malabsorption 370
cysteine proteinases 120
cytogenetic studies 27–8
cytokines 123–4
    immunomodulatory 93
    proinflammatory 93, 123
cytomegalovirus
    antibody status 365
    infection 150
    lung transplantation 367

deltaF$_{508}$ mutation 3, 29
    with A455E 50
    age 37
    animal models 76
    Caucasian populations 190
    DNA testing of allele 191
    evolution 37
    frequency 35, 36, 190
    heterozygosity 50
        CBAVD 150
    homozygosity 9, 50
        pubertal delay 246
    lung disease 55
    meconium ileus 54, 268
    occurrence 21
    pancreatic function 51
    pancreatic insufficiency 316
    pancreatic status 262
    prevalence 183, *184*
    processing defect 38
    R117H splicing variants 53
    relative frequency 22
    selective advantage 37
    sweat gland function 52
deltaF$_{508}$-CFTR 38
deltaF$_{508}$/5T compound heterozygotes 192
deltaF$_{508}$/R117H compound heterozygote 9–10
death
    impending 404–5
    see also bereavement; terminal care

deep-throat culture 85
β-defensin-1 83
defensins 457
defining CF 15
delayed gastric emptying 274, 276
delayed intestinal transit time 283
demographic features 8
dendritic cells 109
denial 340, 343
    adolescents 398
15-deoxyspergualin 373
dependence 342, 343
desaturation
    exercise 169, 422
    oxygen therapy 171
    sleep 168
desmosines 118
dextran, high-molecular weight 457
diabetes mellitus 6–7
    α-cell function 318
    beta-cell function 317–18
    C-peptide concentration 317
    CF clinical status in prediabetes 320
    clinical features 319–21
    diagnosis 315–16
    dietary requirements 393–4
    dietary supplements 394
    entero-insular axis 319
    etiology 316–17
    HLA-DR type 317
    incidence 314–15
    insulin dependent 315, 318, 319
    insulin sensitivity 319
    insulin therapy 320, 322–3
    late complications 321
    lung transplantation 363, 370
    medical therapy 322–3
    microvascular complications 321
    non-insulin dependent 315, 318, 319
    nursing *403*
    nutritional management 321–2
    nutritional status 251, 393
    pathogenesis 316–17
    pathophysiology 317–19
    prevalence 314–15
    survival 320–1
    treatment 321–3
    women 306
diagnosis 178
    age at 2, **3**
    clinical features 178, *179*
    criteria 49, *50*, 178–88
    errors 186
    family impact 396–7
    home care 409
    late 398
    misclassification 191
    mutation analysis 183–4
    neonatal screening 189–93
    nursing 396
    parental response 343
    post-mortem 188
    postnatal 179–88
    preimplantation 179
    prenatal 39, 178–9
diagnostic strategies 14–15
diaphragm 439
    hypertrophy 166

dietary complications 393–5
dietary fiber 387–8
dietary intake 385–6
dietary management 388
dietary supplements 388–90
dietary treatment 384
diphosphatidylglycerol liposomes 457
disaccharidases 178
  intestinal 271
discharge planning 408, 422
disease locus, chromosomal location 28
disease progression, nursing 402, *403*
distal intestinal obstruction syndrome 6, **7**,
    148, 271, 276–7
  abdominal pain 352
  clinical presentation 277
  diagnosis 277
  dietary complications 394–5
  laboratory investigations 277
  nursing *403*
  pathophysiology 276–7
  postoperative 349
  surgery 352
  therapy 277
diuretics 296, 455
D$_L$CO *see* whole lung carbon monoxide
    transfer
DMP-777 457
DNA fragments 28
DNase
  hypersensitive sites 32
  see also recombinant human DNase
docosahexaenoic acid 247
domperidone 349
dornase alfa 213, 226, 381
  respiratory failure 229
doughnut appearance, intussusception 352
drug therapy, aggressive 141
dual energy X-ray absorptiometry 246, 250,
    329–30
dyspareunia 306
dyspnea 220
  scores 440
  terminal care 230
  see also breathlessness

eating problems 341, 388
eccrine glands 151
education 8
eicosapentaenoic acid 247
ejaculate, small volume 304
elastase 117, 118
  measurement 263
  pancreatic 187
  see also neutrophil elastase
elastic recoil 166
elastin-split products 118
electrolytes, analysis 180–1
elemental feeds 392–3
embolization **228**
  indications 227
emesis 205
emotional disorders 340
emotional distress, adults 342
emotional investment 402
emphysema 146
  detection 171

employment 8–9, 414–15
empyema 229
ENaC sodium channel 74
encephalopathy 297
end-stage respiratory failure 410
endocervix 71
endocrine system
  abnormalities 251
  pathology 151
endocytosis, CFTR 75
endoplasmic reticulum 38
endosomes
  acidification 111
  CFTR 72
energy
  conservation 421
  expenditure 252
  intake 251
  nutritional requirements 385, 386
  oral supplements 246
ENT surgery 357
enteral feeding 354–5, 391–3
  commercial feeds 392
  overnight 411
enteric infections 281–3
Enterobacteriaceae 86–7
enterokinase 271
enteropathy
  cows' milk 279–80
  gluten-induced 280
environmental deprivation 183
eosinophils
  ABPA 142
  recruitment markers 121
epidemiological method 14
epidemiology 13–15
  CFTR gene 21–2
  complexity 22
  healthcare effectiveness 20–1
epididymal sperm aspiration 416
epididymis 71
  abnormalities 150
  absence 303
epigastric pain 353
epithelial cells
  biliary intrahepatic 289
  host defense mechanism 76
  potential difference 61–2
  Pseudomonas ingestion 76
  see also airway epithelium; kidney, tubule
    epithelial cells; nasal polyps, epithelial
    cells; thyroid gland, epithelial cells
epithelium
  asialoglycoproteins 204
  CFTR chloride channel function 37
Epstein–Barr virus 147, 368–9
equipment provision for independence 421,
    422
erythema nodosum 324
erythromycin 222
Escherichia coli 94
esophageal pH probe monitoring 212
esophagitis 274
  surgery 353
esophagus
  potential difference 68, 69
  varices 148, 150
essential fatty acids 247

GI tract 271
  motility 272
  plasma levels 387
estradiol 303
  CFTR function inhibition 69
estrogen, delayed puberty 303, 331
ethambutol 225
ethics 457–8
ethinyl estradiol 303
ethmoiditis, chronic 206
ethnic background 179
ethnic intermarriage 22
etiology of CF 13–14
evidence-based medicine 12
exercise 168–70, 378
  altitude 435, 436, 444
  benefits 433
  bronchial hyperreactivity measurement
    164
  capacity 422, 433–4
    assessment 439–40
  carbon dioxide retention 435
  cardiac limitations 437
  cardiac output 169, 437
  compliance 443
  CPAP 442
  desaturation 169, 422
  diagnostic studies 169–70
  duration 441
  fatigue 436
  FEV$_1$ 435
  frequency 441
  heart rate 437
  hypercapnia 435
  hypoxia 435–6
  intensity 441
  intolerance 121
  limitations 434–7
  lower body training 438
  mucociliary clearance 381
  muscle strength 436
  NIPPV 441
  oxygen supplementation 441–2
  peak performance 439
  performance 10, 434
  precautions 443
  prognostic studies 170
  quality of life 433, 437
  rebreathing equipment 443
  testing 172, 437–9
  therapeutic studies 170
  tolerance 10, 170, 438
    adults 220
    nutrition 436–7
    physiotherapy 382
  training 170, 437, 438
    assessment 441
    programs 433, 439–43
  transplant waiting list 437, 441
  treadmill 441, **442**
  types 440–1
  upper body training 438
  ventilation limitation 170
  ventilatory mechanics 434–6
  weight-bearing 331, 332
exhaustion 439
exocytosis, CFTR 75
exoenzyme S 113

exons, nucleotide sequence 30
exotoxin A 113, 124
expectoration 205
expiratory flow rate 434
extracellular protein toxins 113
extrathoracic airways 163
ezrin 75

failure to thrive 3, **4**
fallopian tubes 71
family
    communication 344
    coping 343–4
        ability 414
        mechanisms 345
        with treatment 397
    factors 340–1
    functioning 344
    home care of child 409
    impact of diagnosis 396–7
    involvement in care 376
    needs 406–7, 414
    oxygen therapy at home 411
    psychosocial factors 343–4
    relationship with nurses 405
    social worker support 413–14
    strategies 343
    support networks 407
fat
    digestion 263
    fecal analysis 187
    fecal excretion 263, 264
    globules in stools 263
    high-fat feeds 393
    malabsorption 263, 387
        oxalate load 328
    nutritional requirements 387
fat body mass 250
fat-free mass estimation 246
fatigue, exercise 436
fatty acids *see* essential fatty acids; ω-3 fatty
    acids
fecal fat analysis 187
feeding
    infant 252, 254
    problems 341
feeding problems 388
$FEF_{25-75\%}$ (decline in flow at midpoint of vital
    capacity) 209
fertility 402, 415
    see also infertility
fetal mutation analysis 179
fever, low-grade 205
fibroblasts
    chloride efflux 71
    heterozygotes 75
    intracellular calcium 70–1
fibrosing colonopathy 146, 264, 265, 282–3
fish oil preparations 126
fitness 434
flow volume curves, partial 159
flucloxacillin 222, 367
fluconazole 367
fluticasone 456
Flutter 212, 378, 380
folate 247
Foley catheter 355
forced expiration technique 378

forced expiratory maneuvers 378
forced expiratory volume 4, **5**
    adults 221
    bronchodilator therapy response
        determination 161
    decrease 209
    exercise 435
    insulin therapy 320
    lung function measurement 50
    lung transplantation indications 361–2
    measurement 210
        post-lung transplantation 371
    pregnant women 306
    pretransplant assessment 363
    prognostic factor 10
    risk factors for decline 209
forced vital capacity 4, 161, 162
    adults 221
    decline 209
    measurement post-lung transplantation
        371
    pretransplant assessment 363
    prognostic factor 10
formula feeds 388
    predigested 252
foscarnet 367
frame-shift mutations 38
fruit-juice based nutritional supplements
    390
functional residual capacity 210
functional status 11
fundoplication procedures 274
fungal infections
    lower respiratory tract 142–3
    see also Aspergillus; Candida

G85E mutation 52
G542X mutation 36
    evolution 37
    incidence 190
    meconium ileus 54, 268
G551D mutation 36, 190
    animal models 76
    lung disease 76
    meconium ileus 54
    mouse models 42
    nasal polyposis 54
G551S mutation, sweat gland function 52
gallbladder 297
    cancer 298
    nonfunctioning 354
    pathology 149
gallstones 297, 298
gamma globulin therapy 226
    P. aeruginosa 126
ganciclovir 367
gas dilution techniques 210
gas exchange 165–6
gas trapping marker 10
gastric acid secretion 271, 353
gastric emptying 274–6
    delayed 274, 276
gastric inhibitory polypeptide 317, 319
gastrin 272
gastritis 278, 353
gastroesophageal reflux 212, 272–4
    chest physiotherapy 273–4
    clinical presentation *273*, 274

diagnosis 274
dietary intake 386
etiology 272–3
gastrostomy 355
pathogenesis 272–3
physiotherapy 377
pregnancy 307
pulmonary disease 273–4
surgery 353
therapy 274
gastroesophagography 212
gastrografin 269, 277
    enema 350, 351, 352
gastrointestinal dysmotility 264, 272–8
    syndrome 272
gastrointestinal tract 271–83
    chloride transport 68, 271
    ion transport 271
    malignancies 283, 298
        carcinoma 7, 148
    mucosal abnormalities 271
    pathology 147–8
    perforation 278
        meconium peritonitis 351
    sodium transport 68, 271
    see also intestinal obstruction; small
        bowel
gastrostomy 354–5
    buttons 354, 355
    complications 355
gastrostomy feeding 391–2
    overnight 411
gene
    cloning 76
    identification 27–9
    isolation in genetic diseases 27
gene therapy 84–5, 171, 226, 449–51, *452,*
    453–4
    anti-T-cell monoclonal antibodies 454
    cell targets 451
    clinical studies *452,* 453
    cyclosporin for host suppression 453
    efficient transfer 450
    ethical issues 457
    expression control 453
    gene 449–50
        transfer 450–1, 453
    host defenses 453–4
    laboratory studies 453
    mini-genes 450
    vectors 450–1, 453
    viral gene deletion 453
    viral vectors 450–1, 453
gene transplantation, replacement vector 42
general practitioner liaison 407–8
genetic counseling 39, 178, 307, 396
    cascade testing 197
genetic screening
    high school age 194
    uptake 40
genetic testing 14, 39
    general public 40
    male 150–1
    National Institutes of Health concensus 40–1
genetics, positional/reverse 28
genitourinary tract
    evaluation 187–8
    pathology 150–1

genomic DNA, cloned 29
genotype 13–14
  chest infection severity 252
  homozygote 21
  organ disease relationship 50–5
  P. aeruginosa 5
  pancreatic phenotype correlation 262
  rare 21
genotype–phenotype relationship 56
gentamicin 217, 223, 224
giardiasis 281–2
Gibson–Cooke sweat test method 180, **181**
glibenclamide 322
glipizide 322
globlet cells, bronchiolitis 145
glucagon 272, 317
glucagon-like peptide-1 317, 319
glucocorticoid therapy 331
glucocorticosteroids 123
  see also corticosteroids; steroids
glucose
  active transport-mediated absorption in GI
    tract 271
  fasting plasma level 315, 316
  intolerance 319
    nutritional state 251
    pubertal delay 246
  tolerance
    insulin sensitivity 319
    normal 314–15
  see also impaired glucose tolerance; oral
    glucose tolerance test
gamma-glutamyl transpeptidase 178, 292
glutathione 456
  supplementation 248
gluten-free diet 281
gluten-induced enteropathy 280
glycerol
  CFTR folding defect correction 454
  deltaF$_{508}$ processing defect 38
glycine 267
glycosuria 315, 316
Glypressin 296
goblet cell abnormalities 271
goiter 326
  amyloid 163
Golgi, CFTR glycosylation 38
Golgi apparatus, intestinal mucosa 271
Golytely 277
grand mal seizures 368
  hyponatremia 371
Gray–Turner's sign 270
grieving 417
growth 6, **7**, 243, 248–50, **253**, 254
  adolescence 301–3
  assessment 207
  catch-up **253**, 254
  children 248–9
  evaluation 244
  factors influencing 250–2
  infant 248, 252, 254
  measurement 244–8
  pulmonary function 301, 302
  rate of gain 246–7
  spurt 301
    delay 250
  UK patients 249, **250**
growth hormone 123

grunting 210
guided imagery 421

H$_2$-receptor blockers 270, 353
Haemophilus influenzae 5, **6**, 84, 85
  adult infections 218, 219
  antibiotics 217, 222
  β-lactamase producing 88
  culture media 85–6
  diagnostic evaluation 187
  incidence 87
  infant colonization 211
  intermittent infection 218
  lower respiratory tract infection 142
  lung pathology progression 86
  mucin binding 112
  strains 88
  treatment 88–9
  vaccine 125
Hardy–Weinburg equilibrium 190
Harrison's sulci 220
Hayek Oscillator 380
HbA$_{1c}$ 319
  values 315–16
health deterioration 402, 404
  adjustment to 416
healthcare
  effectiveness 20–1
  high-technology 406, 411, 412
heart 167–8
  chloride ion channel 71
  failure 228
  monitoring for pretransplant assessment
    363
  rate with exercise 170, 437
  see also cardiac output; cardiopulmonary
    physiology
heart–lung transplantation 21, 147, 361
  clubbing regression 324
  donor availability 365
  heart donation 365
  liver disease 297
  operative technique 365–6
  physiotherapy 383
heart–lung–liver transplantation 295
heat shock proteins see Hsp
height 6, **7**, 243
  assessment 245
Helicobacter infection 278
Helicobacter pylori 283
helium dilution
  lung volumes 159, 160
  technique 164, 210
helium total lung capacity 165
helper T cells see T-helper cells
hemoglobin, capillary blood 207
hemoptysis **7**, 220, 227
  bronchial artery rupture 146–7
  nursing 403
  physiotherapy 382
  surgery 356
  terminal 147
hepatic encephalopathy 297
hepatitis
  giant-cell 150
  see also liver disease
hepatitis B 362
hepatitis C 362

hepatocytes, injury 290
hepatomegaly, chronic liver disease marker
  291–2
Hering–Breuer reflex 210
heterozygote screening 193–7
  allelic heterogeneity 194
  before pregnancy 194–5
  cascade testing 196–7
  during pregnancy 195–6, 197
  neonatal 190, 191–2
  school-age 194
heterozygotes 75
  compound 9–10, 191, 192
  detection 39–40
  incorrect scoring 191
  parental 193
high-frequency chest compression 212
high-resolution computed tomography 207
high-technology healthcare 406, 411, 412
hip replacement 151
histamine challenge 172
histiocytes, lipid-filled 145
HIV infection 362
HLA class II antigens 323
HLA DBQ locus 291
HLA-DR type, diabetes mellitus 317
home care 406–12
  advantages 407
  clinical nurse specialists 416
  contracts 411
  disadvantages 407
  discharge planning 408
  equipment 407
  general practitioner liaison 407–8
  hospital liaison 408
  medical technology 406
  newly diagnosed patient 409
  nurse 406
  nursing 401–2
  organization 407
  treatment 229–30
  visit 408–9
home intravenous antibiotics 409–10, 411
  delivery devices 410
home intravenous therapy programs 217,
  229–30
hospital liaison 408
host defense
  defects 142
  gene therapy 453–4
host factors
  bacterial airway colonization 110–13
  pathological processes in respiratory tract
    126
host inflammatory response modulation
  212
host proteinase release 110
host response 93
housing 415
  adaptations 421, 422
  special needs 415
HpaII restriction enzyme 29
Hsp60 324–5
Hsp70 38, 74
Hsp90 74
huffing 378, 379
  games 377
humoral immune response 115–16

hydrogen peroxide scavengers 120
p-hydroxyphenylacetic acid 282
hypercapnia 169, 210
    exercise 435
    sleep 168
hypergammaglobulinaemia 123
hyperglycemia 319
hyperimmune globulin preparations 125–6,
    367
hyperinflation
    assessment 206
    diaphragam hypertrophy 166
    progressive 209
hyperoxia 171
hypersplenism 297
hypertonic saline, expectoration aid 164
hypertrophic pulmonary osteoarthropathy
    151, 220, 324
hypogammaglobulinemia 142
hypoglycemia 323
hypogonadism 331
hyponatremia, grand mal seizures 371
hypothyroidism 151, 326
hypoxemia 210
    sleep 168
hypoxia 170–1
    altitude 170
    bronchoconstriction 170
    exercise 435–6
    nocturnal 229
    pulmonary artery pressure 171
hypoxic challenge 172

ibuprofen 126, 214, 226, 456
    anti-inflammatory therapy 456
IgA antigliadin antibody test 280–1
IgA polymeric receptor 451
IgG antibodies 324
    reponse 93
    subclasses 116
IgM antibodies 324
ileal brake phenomenon 272
ileal loop, volvulus 351
ileus, postoperative 349
imaging
    adult respiratory disease 220–1
    chest 187, 207, **208**
    lung function deterioration detection 171
    techniques for lung function in infants
        158–9
    ventilation scans 158–9
        isotope 159, 220
    see also chest radiography; computed
        tomography; high-resolution computed
        tomography; magnetic resonance
        cholangio-pancreatography; magnetic
        resonance imaging; quantitative
        computed tomography
iminodiacetic acid 293
imipenem 223
immune complexes 115–16
immune hyperresponsiveness 455
immunization 457
    measles 222
    travel 231
    see also vaccination
immunoglobulins *see* Ig; intravenous
    immunoglobulin

immunological hyperresponsiveness 225–6
immunological therapeutic strategies 124,
    125–7
immunology 109–10
immunoprophylaxis 124–5
immunoreactive trypsin screening 189–90
    DNA combination 190–1, **192**
    heterozygotes 192
immunoreactive trypsinogen 262
    pancreatitis 270
immunosuppression
    advanced pulmonary disease 122
    complications 370
    drug interactions 370
    lung transplantation 366, 372
immunotherapy 125–6
impaired glucose tolerance 7, 314
in vitro fertilization 39
incidence of CF 14–17
    variation 15
incretins 319
independence, equipment provision 421, 422
index case relatives 197
indomethacin, intestinal damage 282
inducible nitric oxide synthase 124
infant mortality rate 16, 20
infants
    feeding 252, 254, 388
    growth 252, 254
    lung-function studies 158–60
    malnourished 266
    pancreatic enzyme preparation dosage
        266
    see also breast-feeding
infections
    transmission 382
    vulnerability 414
    see also bacterial infections; fungal
        infections
infertility 309
    female 150, 305
    late diagnosis 398
    male 49, 303–4, 402, 416
        CFTR genotype 53–4
inflammation
    chronic 109
    preceding bacterial lung infection 110–11
    T cells in impaired control 122
    type shift 126
inflammatory bowel disease 280, 283
inflammatory defense mechanisms 84, 85
inflammatory mediators 455–6
inflammatory products 110
inflammatory response
    chronic 110
    modulation 214–15
inflammatory system activation, cytokines
    123
influenza
    resistance 37
    vaccination 125, 222
influenza A 85, 225
    CF patient deterioration 125
injection sclerotherapy 296
inpatient care, nursing 399, *400–1*
inspiratory flow rate 434
inspiratory muscle
    strength 436

    training 438–9, 441
insulin 317, 394
    clearance rate 319
    deficiency 251
    resistance 319
    response **318**
    secretion stimulation 322
    sensitivity 319
    therapy 322–3
        clinical status in diabetes 320, 321
insulin-like growth factor 1 123, 251
insulinopenia 316, 318
interferon-gamma 124
    recombinant 126
interleukin-1 93, 123
interleukin-2 123
    NO inhibition 124
interleukin-3 122
interleukin-4 122
interleukin-5 122
interleukin-6 93, 123
interleukin-8 93, 123
    infant lung 110, **111**
interleukin-10 76, 93, 122
interleukin-12 123
intermittent positive pressure breathing 382
intermittent positive pressure ventilation 168
    nasal 362
    see also nasal inspiratory positive pressure
        ventilation
intestinal lavage solution 277
intestinal modifiers, human disease 56
intestinal obstruction 4, 350
    animal models 76
    fetal 179
    in utero 179
    neonatal 49, 54
    null mutant mice 41
    surgery 353
intestinal permeability 282, 283
intestinal transit time, delayed 283
intracellular acidification, CFTR 76
intracellular defects 72
intracellular organelles, defective
    acidification 83
intracytoplasmic sperm injection **304**, 305
intrapulmonary airways
    large airways 160–3
    small airways 160, **161**
intrauterine insemination 305
intravenous immunoglobulin 214–15, 226
intravenous therapy *400*
intussusception 148, 278
    surgery 352–3
ion transport, intestinal 271
ion-transport therapy 454–5
    ethical issues 457
ipratropium bromide 214
islet cells 316
    amyloidosis 326
    function 149, 316, 317–18
islet-cell cytoplasmic antibodies 317
isoniazid 225
isoproterenol, GI motility 272
itraconazole 228, 363, 367

jaundice 296
joint pathology 151

kidney 327–8
    CFTR chloride channel 70
    chloride transport 70
    pathology 150
    renal cyst 70
    sodium transport 70
    tubule epithelial cells 327
    see also renal calcinosis
Klebsiella 94
    bronchiolitis 212
    infant colonization 211
knowledge of disease 341
    promotion 345
kyphosis 151
    spinal 206, 220

L206W mutation and sweat gland function 52
lactase, activity loss 279
lactation
    dietary complications 394
    see also breast-feeding
lactic acid
    blood level measurement 441
    muscle 436
        fatigue 439
        training 434
lactic acidosis 169
lactitol 297
lactoferrin 457
lactose intolerance 279, 280
lactulose 277, 297
laparotomy, meconium ileus 350–1
laryngeal braking 210
Lautropia mirabilis 94
lean body mass 250
left ventricular perfusion defects 168
Legionella pneumophila 94
leptins 251
leucine aminopeptidase 178
leukocyte integrins 119
life expectancy 414
life span, international differences 20–1
linkage analysis 28
lipase
    dosage level 265
    duodenal 263
    gastric 271
    human milk 263
    lingual 272
    pancreatitis 270
lipids
    gene transfer 451
    stool 384
lipopolysaccharide
    P. aeruginosa 92–3
    vaccine 124
liposomes 451, 452, 453, 457
liver
    enzymes 7
    fatty infiltration 291
    function tests 247
    pathology 149–50
    transplantation 150, 251, 294–5
        pulmonary contraindications 295
liver disease 54, 289
    bile acid therapy 294
    clinical features 291

complications 295–7
familial concordance 291
gene therapy 295
heart–lung transplantation 297
histological assessment 294
immune mechanisms 291
investigations 292–3
lung transplantation 297, 371
    contraindication 363
management 294–5
nutritional state 251
pathogenesis 289–91
prognostic value 291–2
ultrasound scoring system 292–3
variceal hemorrhage 291, 295, 296
    see also hepatitis; portal hypertension
lobectomy 366
    single 357
long-chain triglycerides 387, 392
lower esophageal sphincter pressure 272
lower respiratory tract 142–7
    bacterial infection 142
    bronchi/bronchioles 143–5, 146
    fungal infection 142–3
    lung parenchyma 145–6
    pulmonary vasculature 146–7
    viral infections 143
lung
    auscultation 206
    cysts 146
    diffusing capacity 435
    drainage
        lobes 376–7
        postural 212, 378, 379
    fetal
        CFTR expression 34
        mucin accumulation 143
    hyperinflation 159, 165
    normal development 158
    parenchyma 145–6
    rejection 147
    volume measurement 164–5
    see also pulmonary entries
lung disease
    advanced 441–2
    CFTR genotype 50–1, 55
    deltaF$_{508}$ 50, 55
    development effects 158
    exercise 441–2
    G551D mutation 76
    gastroesophageal reflux 273–4
    nasal polyp relationship 324
    severity with deltaF$_{508}$ and A455E
        mutations 50
    variability 49
    work capacity 441, 442
lung function 4–5
    centiles 158
    growth velocity 301, 302
    imaging for deterioration detection 171
    measurement 50, 157–8,
        209–10
    microbial colonization 5
    MPO correlation 121
    nutritional status 5
    prognostic factor 10
    resting energy expenditure 54–5
    studies in infants 158–60

testing 208–10
    in clinical practice 171–2
lung infections
    antibiotics 89
    energy expenditure 252
    insulin therapy in diabetes mellitus 320,
        321
    lung transplantation 147, 366–7
    nursing 400
    physiotherapy 377
    prediabetes 320
    repeat 144
    treatment 215, 216, 217
    weight gain 244
lung transplantation 141, 361
    ABPA complication 121
    acute rejection 368
    age 372
    Aspergillus invasion 228
    assessment for 229
    bilateral sequential single 361, 365, 366
    bowel obstruction 371
    cadaveric 366
    complications 147
    contraindications 362–3
    diabetes mellitus 363, 370
    disease recurrence 372
    donor selection 364–5
    donor–recipient matching 365
    grand mal seizures 368, 371
    immunosuppression 366
        complications 370
    indications 361–3
    infections 366–7
        opportunist 147
    liver disease 297, 363, 371
    living lobar donor 365–6, 404, 417
    long-term care 371
    lymphoproliferative disorders 368–9
    malnutrition 370
    nursing 404
    obliterative bronchiolitis 369, 372
    operative technique 365–6
    organ availability 372
    organ procurement 364–5
    patient preparation 364
    physiotherapy 383
    postoperative care 366–70
    pretransplant assessment 363
    pulmonary infections 367
    quality of life 364, 372
    rejection 373
    results 371–2
    salt loss 370–1
    social worker role in assessment 416–17
    support groups 364
    survival 372
    timing of surgery 372
    transbronchial biopsy 367, 368
    upper respiratory tract infection 370
    waiting for 410–11, 437, 442
    waiting list 417
        death on 404
    xenografting 372, 373
lung–liver transplantation 295
lymphocytes
    cytotoxic response activated with
        allogenic cells 122

function 122–3
  IGF-1 production 123
  neutrophil elastase-mediated receptor
    cleavage 119
lymphoid irradiation 372
lymphoproliferative disorders 368–9
  post-transplant 147
lysozyme 457

Macroduct sweat test method 180, **181**
macrophages 109
  Fc gamma receptors 116
  vitamin E deficiency 148
  see also alveolar macrophages
magnetic resonance cholangio-
  pancreatography 293
magnetic resonance imaging 220
  liver disease 293
magnetometers 166
malabsorption 384–5
  acrodermatitis enteropathica 151
  fat 263, 387
  nursing *400–1*
  nutritional state 251
  osteoporosis risk factor 330–1
  pancreatic secretory capacity loss 263
  pancreatic tissue loss 149
  selenium deficiency 148
  steatorrhoea 150
maldigestion 384–5
male carriers of mutations 53
male infertility 49, 303–4, 402, 416
  CFTR genotype 53–4
malignant disease 148, 283, 298
  susceptibility 7
malnutrition 3, **4**, 249
  causes 384–5
  infants 266
  lung function 171
  lung transplantation 370
    contraindication 363
  stroke volume 171
manganese ions 69
marital relationships 344
marriage 415–16
mast cell chymase 120
maximum expiratory flow–volume loop 221
measles immunization 222
mechanical percussion 378, 380–1
meconium
  cyst 351
  peritonitis 179, 278, 351
  viscid 350
meconium ileus 4, 49, 54, 148, 268–9
  clinical presentation 269, 350
  complicated 350
  deltaF$_{508}$ mutation 54
  demonstration in fetus 261
  diagnosis 269
  equivalent 148, 276–7, 371
    dietary complications 394–5
    nursing *403*
  G542X mutation 54
  G551D mutation 54
  investigations 350
  laparotomy 350–1
  medical management 350, 351
  mortality 17

mouse models 42
  mutations 268
  pathophysiology 268–9
  surgery 350–1
  therapy 269
  treatment 350–1
meconium plug
  fetal gastrointestinal tract 147–8
  syndrome 148, 269
medical care provision 11, **12**
medium-chain triglycerides 268
  enteral feeds 392–3
  infant formula 252
megacolon 353
membrane-bound protein toxins 113
menarche 150
  age at 246, 302
  delay 250
menopause, bone loss 329
meropenem 223
MET flanking marker for CF gene 28
metabolic rate 54–5
metaproterenol *213*
methacholine, bronchial hyperreactivity
  measurement 163–4
methicillin-resistant *Staphylococcus aureus*
  see MRSA
methotrexate 456
methylprednisolone 366, 368
metronidazole 281, 282
mezlocillin 217, 223
microbial colonization, lung function *5*
microbiology
  adult respiratory disease 221–2
  pretransplant assessment 363
microscopic epididymal sperm aspiration
  304–5, 309
microvillar intestinal enzymes 178, 179
mid upper-arm circumference 246
milk shakes 389
milk-based sip feeds, whole-protein 389
minerals 247
minute ventilation 437
missense mutations 36, 50
mitochondria
  abnormalities 72
  intestinal mucosa 271
mixing index 159, 164
mobility maintenance 442
model systems 76
molecular pathology 37–9
Moraxella catarrhalis 94
mortality, age-specific 17–18
mother–infant relationships 341
motilin 272
mouse models 41, 42, 55–6
MRSA 88, 219
  lung transplantation 363
*Msp*I restriction enzyme 29
MUC5B gene 67
MUC7 gene 67
mucin 271–2
  fetal lungs 143
  genes 67
  intestinal 271
  respiratory 112
  submandibular glands 71
mucocele 323–4

mucociliary clearance 212
  amiloride 455
  defective 112
  exercise 381
  hypertonic saline 164
  impaired 112, 212
  mechanical vibration 380–1
  viral infections 143
mucociliary transport, mouse models 41
mucoid exopolysaccharide 116
mucolytic agents 212–13, 225, 381
mucosal surfaces, microbial entry 110
mucous cysts, nasal polyps 141
mucous glands
  hyperplasia in cervix 150
  hyperplastic 141
mucous plugging, submucosal glands 204, **205**
mucus
  airways 144
  hypersecretion 119–20
    in bronchioles 145
    from bronchial epithelium 143
  plugs 142
mucus glycoproteins, sulfation 67, 83
multi-drug-resistant transporter 271
multiple inert gas technique 169–70
Münchausen syndrome by proxy 183, 353
muscle
  abdominal 439
  expiratory 439
  fatigue 436, 439
  lean tissue wasting 437
  lower body training 438
  pathology 151
  progressive relaxation 421
  strength
    exercise 436
    nutritional supplementation 437
  testosterone effects 436
  trained 434
  training specific groups 438–9
  upper body training 438
  see also inspiratory muscle; respiratory
    muscle
mutation analysis 183–4
  sensitivity 184
mycetomas 228
mycobacteria
  atypical 219, 225
  culture 86
  incidence 87
  infant colonization 211
  lung transplantation contraindication 363
Mycobacterium tuberculosis 219, 225
  sputum culture 222
mycophenolate mofetil 366, 369, 370, 372
Mycoplasma pneumoniae 224
myeloperoxidase 120–1
myeloperoxidase-induced oxidation 127
myocardial fibrosis 168
myocardium, exercise 169

N1303K mutation 36
  evolution 37
Na$^+$/2Cl$^-$/K$^+$ cotransporter 63, 64
Na$^+$,K$^+$-ATPase 61
  airway epithelial cell sodium ion
    absorption 64

Na+,K+-ATPase – contd.
  epithelial cell potential difference 61–2
  sodium ion absorption 66
nasal epithelium, potential difference 64,
  65, 185
  measurement 184–6
nasal inspiratory positive pressure
  ventilation 362, 407, 411
  exercise 441
nasal mucosa, cilia abnormalities 141–2
nasal obstruction, polyps 141
nasal polyposis, G551D 54
nasal polyps **7**, 54, 141, 323–4
  epithelial cells 323
  lung disease relationship 324
  nasal PD measurement 186
  presentation 206
  surgery 357
nasogastric feeding 391
  tubes 354, 391
nasopharynx, inspection 206
National Institutes of Health concensus on
  genetic testing 40–1
nebulizers 381, 407
neomycin 297
neonatal screening 2–3, 189–93
  IRT 189–90
    combined with DNA 190–1
  justification 193
nephrocalcinosis 150
nepthrolithiasis 328
netilmicin 217, 223
neuraminidase inhibitors 457
neutrophil elastase 117–18, 118–20, 214
  excess production 218
  inflammatory response 455, 456
  inhibitors 126
neutrophil gelatinase 120
neutrophils
  activation 110, 117–21
  airway influx 110–11
  apoptosis 117
  chemoattractants 117
  enzymatic activities 118
  impaired function 113
  infant lung 110, **111**
  reactive oxygen species 114
  serine proteases 117
  stimulation at low neutrophil elastase
    levels 119
  T-helper cells 122
Nissen fundoplication 274, 353
nitric oxide 124
nitric oxide synthase 124
nitrogen washout gas dilution techniques
  210
non-Caucasian populations 16–17
  CFTR-defective gene incidence 22
non-steroidal anti-inflammatory drugs 126,
  214, *308*
Norman–Chrispin score 193
Northern score 232
nuclear factor-κB
  activation inhibition 126
  transcription factor pathway 75, 76
nucleotide-binding domains 30, 73
null mutant mice 41
nurses, clinical specialists 416

nursing 396
  disease progression 402, *403*
  education 397
  family relationship 405
  family support 397
  home care 401–2, 406
    visits 408–9
  inpatient care 399, *400–1*
  outpatient care 399
  primary healthcare teams 407–8
  stress 405
  transition to adult services 398
nutrition 248–50
  children 248–9
  exercise tolerance 436–7
  UK patients 249, **250**
nutritional intervention/support 388–93
  artificial methods 390–3
  bone mineral density 331, 332
  dietary supplements 388–90
  enteral nutrition 354–5
  muscle strength 437
  nursing *400–1*
  peak work capacity 437
nutritional requirements 386–8
  pregnancy 394
nutritional status 6, 11, 302
  assessment 207
  evaluation 244
  factors influencing 250–2
  genetic backgoround 56
  laboratory investigations 247–8
  lung function *5*
  measurement 244–8
  pregnancy 252, 307
  prognosis 243–4

occupational therapy 419
  assessment 419, *420*
  discharge planning 422
  energy conservation 421
  functional assessment 420
  independence equipment provision 420,
    421, 422
  informal counseling 422
  interventions 419–22
  oxygen provision and equipment 422–4
  problem solving 422
  relaxation 420–1
  stress management 420–1
25-OH vitamin D 331
ω-3 fatty acids 126, 247
omeprazole 274
opsonophagocytosis 118–19
oral contraceptives 306
oral glucose tolerance test 314, 315, 316
oral hypoglycemic agents 394
ORCC channel 39, 74
ORDIC channel 65–6
  bicarbonate 69
  CFTR channel comparison 72–3
  skin 70
  white blood cells 70
organ procurement 364–5
organ transplantation
  liver disease 297
  lung–liver 295
  support groups 364

see also heart–lung transplantation;
    heart–lung–liver transplantation; liver,
    transplantation
oropharynx 271–2
  inspection 206
oscillating Flutter device 212, 378, 380
oscillation, high-frequency 380
osmolality, sweat test 181
osteoarthropathy, hypertrophic pulmonary
  151, 220, 324
osteomyelitis 323
osteoporosis 151, 247, 329–32
  lung transplantation contraindication
    362, 363
  risk factors 330–1
  sport contraindications 443
outpatient care 399
outpatient visits, lung transplantation
  waiting list 410–11
outwardly rectifying chloride channel *see*
  ORCC channel
ovaries, follicular cysts 150
overaeration 187
oxalate, urinary excretion 150
oxandrolone 302
oxygen
  alveolar–arterial difference measurement
    221
  ambulatory 423
  arterial desaturation 437
  arterial saturation 210–11
  concentrators 423
  conserver devices 423
  consumption 434
  cost in breathing 436
  cylinders 423
  discharge to home 424
  domiciliary equipment 423–4
  liquid 423–4, **442**, 442
  long-term therapy 424
  maximum uptake 434
  partial pressure 231
  patient education 422
  peak consumption 434
  peak uptake 10
  prescription 422
  provision and equipment 422–4
  radicals 120–2
  supplementation 309, 407, 441–2
    air flight 170
  therapy 171, 411
    desaturation 171
    right-sided heart failure 228
  transcutaneous 163
    tension 172, 378–9, 380

P2Y2 receptors 455
P67L mutation, dominant mild allele 191
P547H mutation 38
pain, central 353
palliative care 343
pancreas 261
  adenocarcinoma 149
  chloride ion defect 69
  cysts 353
    giant 270
  enzyme concentration 261
  exocrine function assessment 186–7

function
  decline 186
  deltaF$_{508}$ mutation 51
  fat absorption 243
  R117H 51
interstitial fibrosis 149
laboratory assessment of function 263–4
microcysts 270
multiple cystosis 270
pathology 148–9, 261–2
pathophysiology 261–2
phenotype correlation with CF genotype 262
secretions 261
  heterozygotes 192
stones 271
see also islet cells
pancreatic disease 49
  CFTR genotype 51
  G85E 52
  mouse models 42
  sweat chloride association 52
  see also pancreatitis
pancreatic duct obstruction 51
pancreatic elastase 187
pancreatic enzyme preparations/replacement
  therapy 251, 264
  acid-resistant 243
  adjustment 274–7
  adjuvants 267–8
  bile salts 267–8
  constipation 277
  with cyclosporin-A 370
  DIOS 277
  dosage 264, 265, 266, 283, 385
  energy loss minimizations 384–5
  enteric-coated 265
  fat intake 387
  gastric emptying 276
  high strength 282, 385
    colonic strictures 148
  inadequate therapeutic response 267
  infants 252, 388
  initiation 274–7
  potency 264
  rectal prolapse 354
  safety in pregnancy 308
pancreatic insufficiency 3, 262–8
  clinical presentation 263
  gastric emptying 276
  sweat test 263
  therapy 264
pancreatic polypeptide cells 317, 318–19
pancreatic sufficiency 261, 262–8
  function abnormalities 263
pancreatic-associated protein 262
pancreatic-sufficient patients 243–4
pancreatic-sufficient phenotype 10, 262
pancreatin preparations 385
  steatorrhea 384
pancreatitis 269–70, 353
  carrier state 270
  clinical presentation 270
  diagnosis 270
  pain 353
  recurrent 149
  therapy 270
  see also pancreatic disease

pancreolauryl test 264
pantoprazole 274
paracentesis 297
parainfluenza viruses 85
paranasal sinus evaluation 187
parenteral nutrition 171, 351, 390–1
parenthood 304, 309–10
  support 415
parents
  heterozygosity 193
  inpatient care 399
  knowledge of disease 321
  newly diagnosed patient 409
  nurse contact 396
  perception of eating 341
  psychosocial effects 343–4
patient
  evaluation 205
  needs 406–7
  protocol for home intravenous antibiotics 410
  support networks 407
PDZ motifs 75
peak expiratory flow rate 161
peak minute ventilation 437
peak work capacity 434, 437
  nutritional supplementation 437
pectus carinatum see sternum bowing
penicillins 216, 217
  allergic reactions 217
pentamidine isethionate 367
pentoxyfylline 126, 214, 226, 457
peptic ulcer disease 278
peptide-based feeds 392
percussion 212
percutaneous endoscopic gastrostomy 391
  tubes 354
pertussis immunization 222
phage typing 86
phagocytosis, neutrophil-mediated 118
phenacin 113
phenotype 13
  atypical 52, 186–8
  bacterial 114
  genetic background 56
  pancreatic-sufficient 10
  sweat gland function 51
  variability 49–50, 51
  see also CF phenotype
phenotype–genotype relationship 14, 49
phenotypic features 178, 179
physical activity 331
physical examination of children 205–6
physical health 342
physical signs, adults 220
physiotherapy 222, 376
  breathlessness 381–2
  for complications 382–3
  excess bronchial secretions 376–81
  exercise tolerance 382
  family help 397
  see also chest physiotherapy
pilin 457
pilocarpine iontophoresis 180, **181**
piperacillin 217, 223
piroxicam 126
Pitressin 227
pJ3.11 flanking marker for CF gene 28

plasmid DNA 451
platelet dysfunction, drug-induced 227
plethysmography 159, 165
  whole-body 210
pleural adhesions, vascular 357
pleurectomy, surgical 357
pleurisy, chest pain 220
pleurodesis, surgical 357
pneumatosis intestinalis 283
Pneumocystis carinii 367
pneumonectomy, bilateral 366
pneumonia
  endogenous lipoid 145
  parenchymal changes 146
  staphylococcal 212
pneumothorax 147, 218, **221**, 226–7
  CT imaging 220
  nursing 403
  physiotherapy 382
  surgery 356–7
poly-L-lysine 451
polycystic kidney disease, adult 70
polyhydramnios 269
polymorphonuclear leukocytes 84, 109
  airway damage 214
polymorphonuclear neutrophils 120–1
polymyxin B 217
polypectomy 357
population, epidemiological method 14
population-based screening 39, 40
portal hypertension 148, 150, 295
  complications 297
  lung transplantation contraindication 363
  sport contraindications 444
positional genetics 28
positive airway pressure, bi-level 168
positive end-expiratory pressure 167
positive expiratory pressure 378, 379–80
  high-pressure 380
  mask 212, 380
  oscillating 378, 380
post-mortem diagnosis 188
postnatal diagnosis 179–88
postural drainage 212, 378, **379**
potassium, total body 250
potassium ions
  efflux from salivary glands 71
  transport 67
predictive index for survival 292
prednisolone 366, 368, 369
  anti-inflammatory therapy 126, 456
prednisone 214, 225
Pregestimil 252
pregnancy 306–7, 308, 309, 402
  counseling 307, 402
  dietary complications 394
  drug use 307, 308, 309
  heterozygote testing 193
  nutritional requirements 394
  nutritional status 252, 307
  physiotherapy 383
  planned 307
  respiratory status 306–7
  screening
    before 194–5
    during 195–6, 197
    tests 194

pregnancy – contd.
  testing 40
  vitamin A 394
preimplantation diagnosis 179
prenatal carrier status 178
prenatal diagnosis 39, 178–9
prenatal screening programs 179
pressure relief 421
primary healthcare teams 407–8
problem solving 422
progesterone
  CFTR function inhibition 69
  cyclical 303
prognosis 9–11, 83
  alginate production 92
  neonatal screening 193
  new therapies 458
  nutritional state 243–4
prognostic exercise studies 170
prolactin, sweat formation 63
proline residues of transport proteins 39
promoter mutations 36
prostaglandin E 207
prostaglandin F$_{2\alpha}$ 207
prostaglandins, GI motility 272
protamine 451
proteases 214
protein
  dietary restriction 297
  digestion 263
  nutritional requirements 386–7
  therapy 449
protein A 115
protein kinase A 30, 31, 32, 33, 454
  chloride ion channel regulation 65, 66
protein kinase C 32, 33, 62, 454
  sodium ion transport regulation 66
protein in vitamin K absence 263
proteinase 3 117
proteinase
  inhibitors 117–18
  pathogenesis hypothesis 126
α$_1$-proteinase inhibitor 117–18
  aerosolized 127
proteoglycans 289
Proteus 94
prothrombin time, pancreatic insufficiency 263
proton-pump inhibitors 270, 274, 353
protriptyline 221
pseudo-Bartter's syndrome 247
Pseudomonas aeruginosa
  adherence inhibition 457
  age at first colonization 10
  alginate production 114
  alkaline phosphatase 113
  antibiotics 217, 223–4
    aerosol 224
    resistance 92, 223
  antimicrobial therapy 457
  β-lactamase production 92
  biofilms 92
  bronchiolitis 212
  CFTR binding sites 75, 76
  colonization 2, 5, 91–2
    chronic 86
    rate 51
    secondary 85

complement deposition 92
cross-infection 91
culture 85–6
defective CFTR-mediated uptake 83
diagnostic evaluation 187
elastase 113
empyema 229
flagella vaccine 125
gamma globulin therapy 126
hyperimmune globulin preparations 125–6
identification 211
IgG subclasses of antibodies 116
immune complexes 116
immunoprophylaxis 124–5
incidence 87
infection 85
  chronic 92–3
  propensity 204
  risk 90–1
lipopolysaccharide 92–3, 113
lower respiratory tract infection 142
lung pathology progression 86
lung transplantation 147, 370
  contraindication 363
morbidity/mortality 83, 84
mucin binding 112
oropharyngeal cultures 211
parasitic traits 118
patient segregation 91
phenotype 114, 125
  switch 114
polyagglutinability 92–3
prevalence 5, 93, 94, 211, 218
proteinases 113
RSV association 90
serine proteases 114
survival determination 10
T cells 122
toxins 92
treatment 93
virulence 118
  determinants 113
  factors 92
Pseudomonas cepacia see Burkholderia cepacia
Pseudomonas Genome Project 457
Pseudomonas ingestion, epithelial cells 76
psoriasis 324
psychological health
  adults 342
  children 340
psychopathology, children 339–40
psychosocial adaptation
  adults 342–3
  care-givers 345
  children 339–41
  families 343–4
psychosocial management 345–6
pubertal status 246
puberty
  delayed 243, 246, 250, 302–3, 332, 436
    bone loss 331
  induction 302
pulmonary amyloidosis 147
pulmonary arterial branches, intimal fibrosis 146
pulmonary artery pressure 167
  hypoxia 171

pulmonary circulation 167
pulmonary hemorrhage 218
pulmonary hypertension 146, 147, 218
  incidence 147
pulmonary regurgitation 167
pulmonary vascular resistance 167
pulmonary vasculature 146–7
  see also lung
Pulmozyme 213, 381
pulse oximetry 172, 210–11
pyoverdin 113
pyrazinamide 225
pyrexia, microbiology 222
pyrimethamine 367

Q1291H mutation 36
quality of life
  exercise 433, 437
  heart–lung transplantation 21
  liquid oxygen **442**, 442
  lung transplantation 364, 372
quantitative computed tomography 329, 330
quinolones, renal clearance 328

R117-1G mutation 190–1
R117H mutation
  CBAVD 53
  diagnosis 184
  dominant mild allele 191
  genotype–phenotype correlation 50
  incidence 190
  lung function 51
  mild pancreatic disease association 50–1
  pancreatic function 51
  splicing variants 5T and 7T 53
  sweat gland function 52
R334W mutation, sweat gland function 52
racial background 179
racial groups 15–17
radionuclide gastroesophagography 212
radionuclide imaging of liver 293–4
ranitidine 274
rapamycin 366, 369, 372
rapid thoracic compression technique 210
reactive oxygen species, neutrophils 114
rebreathing exercise equipment 443
recombinant human DNase 85, 213
  aerosolized 213
  inhalation 85
recreational activities 435
rectal mucosa 68
rectal prolapse 282, 354
  mucosal 148
red blood cells 69
relationships 415–16
  counseling 415
  sexual 309, 402
relatives of index cases 197
relaxation 420–1
renal calcinosis 328
  see also kidney
renal cyst genesis 70
reproductive health 301
  female 305–7, 308, 309
  male 303–5
residual volume to total lung capacity
  ratio 210

respiration, observation 206
respiratory disease
    adults 218
    microbiology in adults 218–19
    progression and exercise 433
    treatment in children 212–15, *216*, 217
    see also bronchiectasis; bronchiolitis;
        bronchitis; lung disease
respiratory epithelial cells 110
respiratory failure
    adult 229
    end-stage 362
respiratory infection *see* bronchiectasis;
    bronchiolitis; bronchitis; lung infections
respiratory mechanics 166–7
    compliance studies 166
respiratory muscles 222
    diagnostic studies 166
    endurance 438
    fatigue 439
    length–tension curve 166
    oxygen consumption 166
    strength 439
        determinants 166
    training 166–7, 438–9
respiratory pathogen identification 211
respiratory status 302
    pregnancy 306–7
respiratory symptoms 205
    age of onset 219–20
respiratory syncytial virus 85, 211
    P. aeruginosa predisposition 90, 125
respiratory system, adult 218
    care systems 231
    complications 226–9
    home treatment 229–30
    investigations 220–2
    microbiology 218–19
    physical signs 220
    scoring systems 231–2
    symptoms 219–20
    terminal care 230–1
    travel 231
    treatment 222–6
respiratory system, pediatrics 204
    clinical presentation 205–7
    complications 211–12
    laboratory assessment 208–11
    radiographic assessment 207, **208**
    treatment of disease 212–15, *216*, 217
respiratory tract
    chloride transport 64–6
    microbiology 187
    normal physiology 64
    pathology 141–7
    see also lower respiratory tract; upper
        respiratory tract
respiratory virus infections *see* viral
    infections
resting energy expenditure 250, 252, 385
    elevation 436
restriction fragment length polymorphisms
    27, 28, **29**
retinol 271
retroviral vectors for gene therapy 450–1
reverse genetics 28
rhamnolipids 113
rheumatoid factor 324

rhinovirus 85
ribavirin 211
rifampicin 225
right ventricle 167
right ventricular ejection fraction 167
right-sided heart failure 228
RNA hybridization 29
ROMK2 potassium channel 74–5
RV/TLC 10

safe sex 402
salbutamol *213*
    airway wall compliance 161
    exercise tolerance 170
    GI motility 272
salivary glands 271–2
    potassium efflux 71
salmeterol 225
Salmonella typhi 281
salt depletion 247
    lung transplantation 370–1
sarcoid arthropathy 324
Schamroth's sign 207
school-age screening 194
schooling 342, 397, 409
    sport 433
sclerosing cholangitis 150
    liver transplantation 295
scoring systems 231–2
screening
    cost–benefit analysis 40
    couple 40, 195–6
    heterozygote 193–7
    neonatal 189–93
    prenatal programs 179, 195–6, *197*
    school-age 194
    two-step (sequential) 40, 195–6
    see also heterozygote screening; neonatal
        screening
secretin 272
secretin–cholecystokinin stimulation test
    264
secretin–pancreozymin stimulation test 264
secretory leukocyte proteinase inhibitor 118
    antiprotease activity 457
    recombinant 127, 226
selective advantage of CF gene mutations 37
selenium 248
    deficiency 148, 283
    supplementation 248
self-care 421
    accepting responsibility 398
    intervention program 345–6, 443
self-esteem 342, 343
    late diagnosis 398
self-help skills 345
semen analysis 304
seminal vesicles
    abnormalities 150
    absence 303
seminiferous tubules, CFTR protein 35
serine proteases, *P. aeruginosa* 114
serine protein elastase 117
serological investigations, pretransplant
    assessment 363
Sertoli cells 71

serum amyloid A protein 325
severity of illness 340
    correlation between organs 49
    exercise 437
    family functioning 344
    patient rating 342
sex
    age-secific mortality 17–18
    body mass index 341
    emotional disorders 340
    prognostic factor 10
    ratio 17
sex steroids, delayed puberty 302, 303
sexual characteristics, secondary 150
sexual function 309, 402
    late diagnosis 398
sexual health 301
    female 305–7, *308*, 309
sexual satisfaction 342
shunt fraction measurement 165–6
shuttle walk 439
Shwachman score 165, 167, 193, 231–2
siblings
    healthy 397
    home care of child 409
    well 344
sibship concordance 49–50
sinus disease 54
sinusitis 323–4
    nasal polyposis 206
    surgery 357
skeletal age estimation 246
skeletal maturity delay 250
skiing 435, 443
skin
    chloride ion transport 70, 71
    ORDIC channels 70
    pathology 151
skinfold measurements 246
sleep 168
small airway obstruction 209
small bowel
    bacterial overgrowth syndrome 282
    biopsy 281
    brush border 271
    delayed transit 276
    obstruction with meconium ileus 350
small left colon syndrome 269
smoking 222
social life 342, 343
social workers 345, 413
    bereavement support 417
    counseling 415
    family support 415
    hospital 413
    transplant assessment 416–17
    welfare benefits 415
socio-economic indicators 11
sociodemographic features 7–9
sodium
    absorption 455
    absorption inhibitiors 226
    dietary restriction 296
    excretion in lung transplantation 371
    replacement prior to surgery 349
    resorption into bronchial cells 113
    sweat test analysis 180–2
sodium bicarbonate 267

sodium chloride concentration, airway
  epithelial lining fluids 112–13
sodium cromoglycate see cromolyn sodium
sodium ion–glucose cotransporter 68
sodium ions
  absorption and Na⁺,K⁺-ATPase 66
  airway epithelial cell absorption 64
  resorption 61
  transport 61, 63, 66
    abnormalities 218
    gastrointestinal tract 68
    kidney 70
sodium selenite therapy 326
sodium-4-phenylbutyrate 454
specialist centers
  care 11, 83
  survival 20, 21, 83
spermatogenesis
  CFTR gene 150
  defective 303
spermatozoa, abnormal 35
sphincterotomy, endoscopic 354
spinal cord degeneration 151
spinal kyphosis 206, 220
spirometry 166, 171–2, 207
splenomegaly 297
splice mutations 36
sports
  medical risk 443
  schooling 433
sputum 386
  expectoration 438
  retention and terminal care 230
  viscosity 85
squeeze partial flow volume curves 161
squeeze technique 159
stagnant-loop syndrome 269, 282
Staphylococcus aureus 83, 84, 87
  adult colonization 218, 219
  antibiotics 217
  antimicrobial therapy 222
  B cells 123
  bronchiolitis 212
  bronchitis 144
  capsular polysaccharides 114–15
  culture media 85
  diagnostic evaluation 187
  eradication 88
  incidence 87
  infant colonization 211
  lower respiratory tract infection 142
  lung 85
    pathology progression 86
  mucin binding 112
  pneumonia 212
  prophylaxis 87–8
  respiratory tract damage 87–8
  superantigens 115
  T cells 122–3
  vaccine 125
  see also MRSA
starvation, preoperative 349
steatorrhea 4, 186, 387
  causes 354
  control 264
  malabsorption 150
  pancreatic insufficiency 263
  pancreatin preparations 384

Stenotrophomonas maltophilia 211, 218, 219
step test 163
sternum bowing 206, 220
steroids
  bone effects 331
  inhaled 214
  lung transplantation contraindication 363
  terminal care 230
  weight gain 246–7
  see also corticosteroids;
    glucocorticosteroids
stool
  chymotrypsin assay 263
  elastase 263
  fat globules 263
  lipid 384
  softener 277
stop-codon mutations 38
strength training 440
Streptococcus pneumoniae 85, 93–4
  incidence 87
stress
  carers 345
  management 420–1
  nursing 405
stress incontinence 306
stroke volume 169, 434, 437
  index 168
  malnutrition 171
submandibular glands, mucin 71
submaxillary gland enlargement 272
submucosal glands 66–7
  cAMP-mediated chloride ion defect 67
  hypertrophy 143
  mucous plugging 204, 205
sulfadiazine 367
sulfate ions, sweat gland perfusion 62
sulfonylureas 322
superantigens, S. aureus 115
superoxide anion radical 120–1
support networks 407
surgery 349
  abdominal disorders 351–4
  ENT 357
  gastrostomy 354–5
  meconium ileus 350–1
  meconium peritonitis 351
  nasal polyps 357
  sinusitis 357
  thoracic 356–7
    previous to lung transplantation 362
  venous access 355–6
survival
  CFP 20–1
  cohort 18, 19
  current 17–18
  diabetes mellitus 320–1
  historical improvement 17
  lung transplantation 372
  patterns 18, 19
  predictive index 292
sweat
  electrolytes in CABVD 187
  production 62
sweat chloride 2, 4, 49, 52
  pancreatic disease association 52
sweat duct
  apical membrane 38

potential difference 62
sweat gland
  disease and CFTR genotype 52–3
  dysfunction 49
  eccrine 151
  normal physiology 61–2
  reabsorptive duct 62–3
  secretory coil 61, 62
  VIP-ergic innervation 63
sweat gland function
  A455E 51, 52
  deltaF₅₀₈ mutation 52
  G85E 52
  G551S 52
  L206W 52
  phenotype 51
  R117H 52
  R334W 52
sweat test 2, 61, 179–83
  conductivity 181, 182
  diagnostic criteria 182
  efficiency 191
  error sources 182–3
  inconsistent results 183
  indications 180
  methodology 180
  osmolality 181
  pancreatic insufficiency 263
  postnatal 178
  quality assurance 182–3
  recall rate 191
  repeat 182, 183
  reporting 181–2
  sample analysis 180–2
  sample collection 180, 181
  sodium absorption 63
sympathomimetic agents 214
synovitis with progressive erosive disease
  324
syntaxin 75
systematic reviews 12

T cells
  CFTR mutations 122
  disorders 368–9
  impaired control of inflammation 122
  neutrophil elastase 119
  P. aeruginosa 122
  S. aureus 122–3
  suppressor activity 122
T-helper 1 subset 122
  NO inhibition of proliferation 124
T-helper 2 subset 122
T-helper cells 109, 122
5T mutation
  allele 192
  diagnosis 184
tacrolimus 366, 369, 370, 372
taurine 267
  supplementation 294
taurine chloramine 121
teichoic acid 115
teicoplanin 222
temocillin 224
terbutaline 213
terminal care 230–1, 411
  nursing 403, 404–5
  physiotherapy 383

terminal illness 343
testicular function 303
testis, retroversion 304
testosterone
   delayed puberty 202, 302
   muscle effects 436
   replacement 331, 332
tetracycline 222
theophylline 214, 221, 225
   exercise tolerance 170
   GI motility 272
therapeutic exercise studies 170
therapy vest 212
thoracic expansion exercises 378
thoracic gas volume 159
thoracic index 206
thoracic surgery 356–7
   previous to lung transplantation 362
thoracoscopy, video-assisted 357
thrombocytopenia 227
thyroglobulin, hyposialylation 327
thyroid gland 151, 326–7
   epithelial cells 327
thyroid stimulating hormone 326
thyrotropin-releasing hormone 326
thyroxine (T_4) 326, 327
ticarcillin 217, 223, 224
tidal volume 169, 434, 435
tight junctions 271
tissue trans-glutaminase test 281
tobramycin 217, 223, 224
   for inhalation (TOBI™) 217, 224
tolbutamide 322
toloxapol 126
total body electrical conductivity 250
total body potassium 250
total energy expenditure 385
total lymphoid irradiation 372
total parenteral nutrition 351
totally implantable venous access device
   356
Toxoplasma gondii, lung transplantation 367
trace elements 247, 387
trachea
   anatomy 161
   mucociliary transport in mouse models
      41
   stenosis 147
tracheal compliance 161
training 434
   programs 437–8
      provision 440–1
   see also exercise, training
trampolining 377
transcutaneous oxygen 163
   tension 172, 378–9, 380
transexamic acid 227
transferrin 451
transjugular intrahepatic portal systemic
   shunt 296
travel, respiratory disease 231
treadmill exercise 441, **442**
tri-iodothyronine (T_3) 326, 327
tricuspid regurgitation 167
trimethoprim–sulfamethoxazole 224

trypsin
   mucolytic use 212
   see also immunoreactive trypsin screening
tube feeding 266
   nasogastric 354, 391
tuberculosis resistance 37
tumor necrosis factor α 93, 123
   inhibition 457
typhoid resistance 37

ubiquitin-proteosome system 38, 74
ulcerative colitis 280
ultrasonography, prenatal 179
upper respiratory tract
   infection in lung transplantation 370
   pathology 141–2
uridine triphosphate 226, 455
urogenital system
   evaluation 187–8
   pathology 150–1
urolithiasis 150
ursodeoxycholic acid 268, 294
   therapy 251, 296, 298
uterus, CFTR mRNA 35

vaccination
   P. aeruginosa 124–5
   prophylactic 85
   see also immunization
vaginal yeast infections 306
vaginitis 83, 150
vancomycin 222, 281
variceal hemorrhage 291, 295, 296
vas deferens 71
   absence 150, 303
   bilateral absence 49
   see also congenital bilateral absence of the
      vas deferens
vasculitis 325
vasoactive intestinal peptide (VIP)-ergic
   innervation of sweat glands 63
vasoconstrictor drugs 296
vasopressin 296
venous access 355–6, *403*
ventilation:perfusion matching 169–70
ventilation
   exercise 434–5, 437
      limitation 170
   inequalities 165
   noninvasive 382
   nursing assistance *403*
   perfusion imbalance 218
   total 169
ventilation scans
   infants 158–9
   isotope 159, 220
   lung function prediction 159
ventilatory muscle endurance 436, 438
ventricular filling 437
vibration, mechanical 380–1
viral infections
   adults 219
   lower respiratory tract 143, 145
   respiratory 85
   vaccines 125

viral vectors for gene therapy 450–1
virilization 302–3
vital capacity 438
   decline in flow at midpoint ($FEF_{25-75\%}$) 209
vitamin A
   deficiency 247, 263, 330, 387
   fecal loss 271
   pregnancy 394
   supplementation 295, 387
vitamin B_{12} 247
   supplementation 387
vitamin C 247, 248
vitamin D
   deficiency 247, 263, 330–1, 387
      osteoporosis 331, 332, 387
   glucocorticoid therapy 331
   supplementation 387
vitamin E 248
   deficiency 148, 151, 247, 263, 283, 330,
      387
   supplementation 387
vitamin K
   administration prior to surgery 349
   deficiency 151, 227, 247, 330
   supplementation 387
vitamins
   fat-soluble supplementation 387
   safety in pregnancy *308*
vocal cord dysfunction 163
voltage-sensitive organic osmolyte/anion
   channel 66
volvulus 278–9

W1282X mutation 36
walk test 163
water movement 67–8
weaning 388
weight (body) 6, **7**, 243, **253**, 254
   assessment 245
   chest infection 244
   rate of gain 246–7
weight training 441
weighted spirometer technique 166
welfare benefits 415
   transplantation waiting list 417
wheelchair provision 422
wheezing 121
   frequency 205
white blood cells 70
whole lung carbon monoxide transfer (D_LCO)
   165
whole-body plethysmography 210
whole-protein feeds 392
Wisconsin scoring system 207, 232
work capacity, lung disease 441, **442**

xanthines 454
xenografting 372, 373

zinc ions 69